AJN

1987 NURSING BOARDS REVIEW

FOR THE NCLEX-RN EXAMINATION

Coordinators for this Edition

Janis P. Bellack, RN, MN. *Associate Professor, Parent-Child Nursing Graduate Program, University of Kentucky College of Nursing, Lexington, KY*

Phyllis Gorney Cooper, RN, MN. *Educator and Consultant, Los Angeles, CA*

Patricia E. Downing, RN, MN. *Formerly with School of Nursing, University of California, San Francisco, CA*

Edwina A. McConnell, RN, MS. *Independent Nurse Consultant; Part-time staff nurse, Madison General Hospital, Madison, WI*

Marybeth Young, RN, MSN. *Assistant Professor, Maternal-Child Nursing, Niehoff School of Nursing, Loyola University, Chicago, IL*

Contributing Authors

Ida M. Androwich, RN, MS. *ANA Certified Family Nurse Practitioner; Assistant Professor, Niehoff School of Nursing, Loyola University, Chicago, IL*

Cecily Lynn Betz, RN, PhD. *Assistant Clinical Professor, UCLA School of Nursing, Los Angeles, CA*

Carolyn V. Billings, RN, MSN. *ANA Certified Specialist in Psychiatric and Mental Health Nursing; Nurse Psychotherapist, Independent Practice; Nursing Consultant, Raleigh, NC*

Suzette Cardin, RN, MS, CCRN. *Head Nurse, Coronary Care Unit, Coronary Observation Unit, UCLA Medical Center, Los Angeles, CA*

Virginia L. Cassmeyer, RN, MSN. *Associate Professor, University of Kansas School of Nursing, Kansas City, KS*

Olivian De Souza, RN, MSN. *Instructor, Henry Ford Community College, Dearborn, MI*

Gita Dhillon, RN, MEd. *Associate Professor, The American University, Washington, DC*

Cynthia Dunsmore, RN, MSN. *Lecturer, Department of Maternal-Child Nursing, University of Illinois College of Nursing, Chicago, IL*

Carolyn Vas Fore, RN, MSN. *Assistant Professor, University of Kentucky, College of Nursing, Lexington, KY*

Elizabeth Anne Gomez, RN, MSN. *Clinical Nurse Specialist in Neonatology, Instructor in Pediatric Nursing, University Hospitals of Cleveland, Case Western Reserve University, Cleveland, OH*

E. Ingvarda Hanson, RN, MSN. *Associate Professor, Wayne State University, Detroit, MI*

Alene Harrison, RN, MS. *Associate Professor, Assistant Chairperson, Department of Nursing, Wilkes College, Wilkes Barre, PA*

Anne C. Holland, RN, MSN. *Assistant Coordinator, Memorial Hospital, Worcester, MA*

Ann L. Jessop, RN, MSN. *Instructor, McLennan Community College, Waco, TX*

Michele M. Kamradt, RN, EdD. *Assistant Professor, Elmhurst College, Elmhurst, IL*

Alma Joel Labunski, RN, MSN. *Director, Division of Nursing and Natural Sciences; Associate Professor of Nursing, Kendall College, Evanston, IL*

Judith K. Leavitt, RN, MEd. *Professor of Nursing, Tompkins Cortland Community College, Dryden, NY*

Mariann C. Lovell, RN, MS. *Assistant Professor, Senior Level Coordinator, Wright State University, Dayton, OH*

Michele A. Michael, RN, PhD. *Assistant Professor, George Mason University, Fairfax, VA*

Jerry R. Myhan, RN, MSN. *Assistant Professor of Nursing, Harding University School of Nursing, Searcy, AR*

B. Patricia Nix, RN, MSN. *Instructor of Nursing, Henry Ford Community College, Dearborn, MI*

Paulette D. Rollant, RN, MSN, CCRN. *Assistant Professor, Critical Care Graduate Faculty, Emory University School of Nursing, Atlanta, GA*

Judith K. Sands, RN, EdD. *Assistant Professor, University of Virginia, Charlottesville, VA*

Mary Charles Santopietro, RN, MS, EdM, EdD, CS. *Clinical Director, Suburban Hospital, Bethesda, MD; Clinical Lecturer, George Mason University, Fairfax, VA*

Victoria Schoolcraft, RN, MSN. *Associate Professor, Assistant Director, Baccalaureate Program, University of Oklahoma College of Nursing, Oklahoma City, OK*

Diane S. Smith, RN, MSN, CS. *Certified Clinical Specialist, Psychiatric Nursing, Psychiatric Center of Michigan, Detroit, MI*

Karen Stefaniak, RN, MSN. *Assistant Professor Maternal-Child Nursing, Eastern Kentucky University, Richmond, KY*

Diane Morrison Taylor, RN, MSN. *Assistant Professor, School of Nursing, University of Texas at Arlington, Arlington, TX*

Quilla D. B. Turner, RN, PhD. *Assistant Professor, University of Pittsburgh School of Nursing, Pittsburgh, PA*

Deborah L. Ulrich, RN, MA. *Assistant Professor Maternal-Child Nursing, Wright State University, Dayton, OH*

Francene Weatherby, RNC, MSN. *Assistant Professor of Nursing, University of Oklahoma College of Nursing, Oklahoma City, OK*

Gail D. Wegner, RN, MS. *Associate Professor of Nursing, Purdue University, Calumet, Hammond, IN*

Contributors Previous Editions

Kay Bensing, RN, MA. *Formerly with Pierce College, Woodland Hills, CA*

Carol W. Kennedy, RN, PhD. *Assistant Professor, Ohio State University School of Nursing, Columbus, OH*

Deborah Koniak, RN, EdD. *Assistant Dean, Continuing Education; Assistant Professor, Maternal-Child Health Nursing, University of California, Los Angeles, CA*

Beverly Kopala, RN, MS. *Assistant Professor, Maternal-Child Health Nursing, Niehoff School of Nursing, Loyola University, Chicago, IL*

Karen Krejci, RN, MSN. *Instructor, Mount St. Mary's College, Los Angeles, CA*

Esther Matassarin-Jacobs, RN, MEd, MSN. *Assistant Professor, Medical-Surgical Nursing, Loyola University, Chicago, IL*

Joan Reighley, RN, MN. *Certified ANA Specialist of Psychiatric and Mental Health Nursing; Psychotherapist, private practice; Assistant Professor, West Los Angeles College, Los Angeles, CA*

Constance M. Ritzman, RN, MSN. *Assistant Professor, Loyola University, Chicago, IL*

Ann M. Schofield, RN, MS. *Lecturer, California State University, Los Angeles, CA*

THE AMERICAN JOURNAL OF NURSING COMPANY

AJN

1987 NURSING BOARDS REVIEW

FOR THE NCLEX-RN EXAMINATION

A NURSECO BOOK

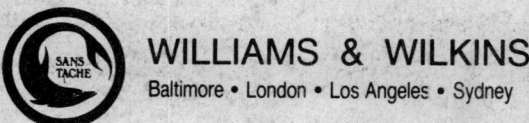

WILLIAMS & WILKINS
Baltimore • London • Los Angeles • Sydney

Editors: Rose Mary Carroll-Johnson, RN, MN
Margo C. Neal, RN, MN

Copyright © 1986 by the American Journal of Nursing Company

A NURSECO BOOK
Published by Williams & Wilkins, 428 East Preston Street, Baltimore, MD 21202, U.S.A.

All rights reserved. No part of this book may be reproduced in any form or by any electronic or mechanical means, including information storage and retrieval systems, without permission in writing from the publisher except by a reviewer who may quote brief passages in a review.

First Edition 1983.
Second Edition 1983.
Third Edition 1984.
Fourth Edition 1985.
Fifth Edition 1986.

Printed in the United States of America

ISBN: 0-683-09503-X

Contents

Section 1: Preparing for the NCLEX 1
PREPARING FOR SUCCESS ON THE NCLEX-RN 3
STRESS-REDUCTION TECHNIQUES 7

Section 2: Nursing Care of the Client with Psychosocial Problems 11

INTRODUCTION 13
Overview 13
Scope of the Profession 13
Interpersonal Relationships 14
Roles Assumed by the Nurse 14
Locations of Practice 15
Psychosocial Characteristics of the Healthy Client 15

THERAPEUTIC USE OF SELF 19
Theoretical Knowledge Base 19
Nurse-Client Relationship 23
Nursing Process 25
Treatment Modalities 26

LOSS, DEATH AND DYING 28
General Concepts 28
  Overview 28
  Application of the Nursing Process to the Client Experiencing a Loss 29
Selected Health Problems 29
  A. Loss 29
  B. Death and Dying 30

LEGAL ASPECTS OF PSYCHIATRIC NURSING 34
Civil Procedures 34
Criminal Procedures 35
Territories 35
Judicial Precedents 35
Role of the Nurse 35

ANXIOUS BEHAVIOR 36
General Concepts 36
  Overview 36
  Application of the Nursing Process to the Client Exhibiting Anxious Behavior 36
Selected Health Problems 37
  A. Anxiety 37
  B. Phobias 40
  C. Dissociative Reactions 41
  D. Obsessive-Compulsive Disorders 41
  E. Anorexia Nervosa 42
  F. Psychosomatic Disorders 43
  G. Conversion Disorders 45
  H. Post-Traumatic Stress Disorders 46

CONFUSED BEHAVIOR 48
General Concepts 48
  Overview 48
  Application of the Nursing Process to the Client Exhibiting Confused Behavior 48

Selected Health Problems 48
  Chronic Confusion 48

ELATED-DEPRESSIVE BEHAVIOR 50
General Concepts 50
  Overview 50
  Application of the Nursing Process to the Client with an Affective Disorder 50
Selected Health Problems 52
  A. Depression 52
  B. Elation and Hyperactive Behavior 58

SOCIALLY MALADAPTIVE/ACTING OUT BEHAVIOR 60
General Concepts 60
  Overview 60
  Application of the Nursing Process to the Client Exhibiting Maladaptive Behavior 60
Selected Health Problems 61
  A. Violence in the Family 61
  B. Hostile, Aggressive, and Assaultive Behavior 64
  C. Acting Out 67
  D. Sexual Acting Out 68
  E. Antisocial Behavior 72

SUSPICIOUS BEHAVIOR 75
General Concepts 75
  Overview 75
  Application of the Nursing Process to the Client Exhibiting Suspicious Behavior 75
Selected Health Problem 75
  Paranoia 75

WITHDRAWN BEHAVIOR 77
General Concepts 77
  Overview 77
  Application of the Nursing Process to the Client Exhibiting Withdrawn Behavior 82
Selected Health Problems 86
  A. Paranoid Schizophrenia 86
  B. Catatonic Schizophrenia 86
  C. Undifferentiated Schizophrenia 87
  D. Childhood Schizophrenia 87
  E. Psychotic Disorders not Elsewhere Classified 87

SUBSTANCE USE DISORDERS 89
General Concepts 89
  Overview 89
  Application of the Nursing Process to the Client with a Substance Use Disorder 90
Selected Health Problems 91
  A. Alcohol 91
  B. Drugs Other than Alcohol 96

GLOSSARY 98

REPRINTS 105
Hardiman, M. "Interviewing? Or Social Chit-Chat?" 107
Neal, M. et al. "Assessment of Mental Status." 110
———. "Stress Management." 112

DiMotto, J. "Relaxation." *114*
Neal, M. Et al. "Behavior Modification." *119*
Westercamp, T. "Suicide." *121*
Harris, E. "Sedative-Hypnotic Drugs." *124*
DeGennaro, M. et al. "Antidepressant Drug Therapy." *130*
Harris, E. "Lithium." *136*
———. "Antipsychotic Medications." *142*
———. "Extrapyramidal Side Effects of Antipsychotic Medications." *150*

Section 3: Nursing Care of the Adult 157

THE HEALTHY ADULT 159

SURGERY 164
Overview 164
Perioperative Period 164
Discharge 167

OXYGENATION 170
General Concepts 170
  Overview 170
  Application of the Nursing Process to the Client with Oxygenation Problems 172
Selected Health Problems 176
  A. Cardiopulmonary Arrest 176
  B. Shock 178
  C. Angina Pectoris 179
  D. Myocardial Infarction 181
  E. Dysrhythmias 185
  F. Congestive Heart Failure 188
  G. Hypertension 191
  H. Peripheral Vascular Disease 193
  I. Chronic Obstructive Pulmonary Disease (COPD) or Chronic Obstructive Lung Disease (COLD) 196
  J. Pneumonia 199
  K. Tuberculosis 201
  L. Chest Tubes and Chest Surgery 203
  M. Cancer of the Lung 205

NUTRITION AND METABOLISM 208

PART ONE: THE DIGESTIVE TRACT 208
General Concepts 208
  Overview 208
  Application of the Nursing Process to the Client with Digestive Tract Problems 210
Selected Health Problems 217
  A. Hiatus Hernia 217
  B. Gastritis 217
  C. Peptic Ulcer Disease 218
  D. Diverticulosis/Diverticulitis 224
  E. Appendicitis 225
  F. Cholecystitis with Cholelithiasis 225
  G. Pancreatitis 226
  H. Hepatitis 227
  I. Cirrhosis 229
  J. Complications of Liver Disease: Esophageal Varices, Ascites, Hepatic Encephalopathy 231

PART TWO: THE ENDOCRINE SYSTEM 233
General Concepts 233
  Overview 233
  Application of the Nursing Process to the Client with Endocrine System Problems 235
Selected Health Problems 236
  A. Hyperpituitarism 236
  B. Hypopituitarism 236
  C. Hyperthyroidism 237
  D. Hypothyroidism 238
  E. Hyperparathyroidism 239
  F. Hypoparathyroidism 240
  G. Hyperfunction of the Adrenal Glands 240
  H. Hyposecretion of the Adrenal Glands 241
  I. Hypofunction of the Pancreas: Diabetes Mellitus 243

ELIMINATION 250

PART ONE: THE KIDNEYS 250
General Concepts 250
  Overview 250
  Application of the Nursing Process to the Client with Kidney Problems 252
Selected Health Problems 257
  A. Cystitis/Pyelonephritis 257
  B. Urinary Calculi 258
  C. Cancer of the Bladder 259
  D. Acute Renal Failure 260
  E. Chronic Renal Failure 262
  F. Dialysis 264
  G. Kidney Transplantation 270
  H. Benign Prostatic Hypertrophy 271
  I. Cancer of the Prostate 273

PART TWO: THE LARGE BOWEL 274
General Concepts 274
  Overview 274
  Application of the Nursing Process to the Client with Large Bowel Problems 274
Selected Health Problems 276
  A. Alteration in Normal Bowel Evacuation 276
  B. Inflammatory Bowel Disease (Regional Enteritis, Crohn's Disease, Ulcerative Colitis) 277
  C. Total Colectomy with Ileostomy 280
  D. Mechanical Obstruction of the Colon 281
  E. Cancer of the Colon 282
  F. Hemorrhoids or Anal Fissure 282

SAFETY AND SECURITY 285
General Concepts 285
  Overview 285
  Application of the Nursing Process to the Client with Safety and Security Problems 288
Selected Health Problems of the Nervous System 293
  A. Acute Head Injury 293
  B. Intracranial Surgery 294
  C. Cerebrovascular Accident 295
  D. Meningitis 296
  E. Spinal Cord Injuries 297
  F. Parkinson's Disease (Parkinsonism) 299
  G. Multiple Sclerosis 300
  H. Epilepsy 302
  I. Myasthenia Gravis 304
Selected Health Problems of the Sensory System 306
  A. Cataracts 306
  B. Retinal Detachment 307
  C. Glaucoma 308
  D. Nasal Problems Requiring Surgery 309
  E. Epistaxis 309
  F. Cancer of the Larynx 310

ACTIVITY AND REST 313
General Concepts 313
  Overview 313
  Application of the Nursing Process to the Client with Activity and Rest Problems 314
Selected Health Problems 315
  A. Fractures 315
  B. Fractured Hip (Proximal End of Femur) 317
  C. Amputation 318
  D. Arthritis 319
  E. Collagen Disease 322
  F. Herniated Nucleus Pulposus 323

CELLULAR ABERRATION 326
General Concepts 326
  Overview 326
  Application of the Nursing Process to the Client with Cancer 327
Selected Health Problems 332
  A. Cancer of the Lung 332
  B. Cancer of the Bladder 332

C. Cancer of the Prostate 332
D. Cancer of the Colon 332
E. Cancer of the Larynx 332
F. Cancer of the Cervix 332
G. Cancer of the Breast 333

REPRINTS 337
Heidrich, G. et al. "Helping the Patient in Pain." 339
Long, M. et al. "Hypertension: What Patients Need to Know." 345
Neal, M. et al. "Hyperalimentation." 351
Chambers, J. "Bowel Management in Dialysis Patients." 352
"The Person with a Spinal Cord Injury." 354

Section 4: Nursing Care of the Childbearing Family 373

FEMALE REPRODUCTIVE ANATOMY AND PHYSIOLOGY 375

ANTEPARTAL CARE 381
General Concepts 381
   Normal Childbearing 381
   Overview of Management 385
   Application of the Nursing Process to Normal Childbearing, Antepartal Care 386
   High-Risk Childbearing 389
   Application of the Nursing Process to High-Risk Childbearing 394
Selected Health Problems 394
   A. Abortion 394
   B. Incompetent Cervical Os 395
   C. Ectopic Pregnancy 395
   D. Hydatidiform Mole 396
   E. Placenta Previa 397
   F. Abruptio Placentae 398
   G. Pregnancy-Induced Hypertension 399
   H. Diabetes 401
   I. Cardiac Disorders 402
   J. Anemia 404
   K. Infections 404
   L. Multiple Gestation 405
   M. Adolescent Pregnancy 407

INTRAPARTAL CARE 408
General Concepts 408
   Normal Childbearing 408
   Ongoing Management and Nursing Care 411
   Application of the Nursing Process to Normal Childbearing, Intrapartal Care 416
Selected Health Problems 420
   A. Dystocia 421
   B. Premature Labor 423
   C. Emergency Birth 425
   D. Induction 425
   E. Episiotomy 426
   F. Forceps 427
   G. Vacuum Extraction 428
   H. Cesarean Birth 428
   I. Rupture of the Uterus 430
   J. Amniotic Fluid Embolism 430

POSTPARTAL CARE 432
General Concepts 432
   Normal Childbearing 432
   Application of the Nursing Process to Normal Childbearing, Postpartal Care 434
Selected Health Problems 437
   A. Postpartum Hemorrhage 437
   B. Hematoma 438
   C. Puerperal Infection 439
   D. Mastitis 440
   E. Postpartum Cystitis 441
   F. Uterine Prolapse With or Without Cystocele or Rectocele 441
   G. Uterine Fibroids 442
   H. Pulmonary Embolus 443
   I. Psychologic Maladaptations 443

THE NORMAL NEONATE 444
Definition 444
General Characteristics 444
Specific Body Parts 445
Systems Adaptations 448
Gestational Age Variations 450
Application of the Nursing Process to the Normal Neonate 452

THE HIGH-RISK NEONATE 457
General Concepts 457
   Definition 457
   Antepartum Risk Factors 457
Selected Health Problems 457
   A. Hypothermia 457
   B. Neonatal Jaundice 457
   C. Respiratory Distress 459
   D. Hypoglycemia 461
   E. Neonatal Infection 462
   F. Neonatal Narcotic Drug Addiction 463
   G. Fetal Alcohol Syndrome 463
   H. Intracranial Hemorrhage 464
   I. Brain Injuries 464
   J. Neonatal Necrotizing Enterocolitis 465
   K. Congenital Anomalies 465
   L. Parental Reaction to a Sick, Disabled, or Malformed Infant 466

REPRINTS 469
Neal, M. "Birth Control: Permanent Methods." 471
_____. "Birth Control: Temporary Methods." 473
_____. "Drugs: Birth Control Pills." 476
Floyd, C. "Pregnancy after Reproductive Failure." 478
Hoffmaster, J. "Detecting and Treating Pregnancy-Induced Hypertension: A Review." 482
Perley, N. et al. "Herpes Genitalis and the Childbearing Cycle." 490
Grad, R. et al. "Obstetrical Analgesics and Anesthesia: Methods of Relief for the Patient in Labor." 495
Blackburn, S. "The Neonatal ICU: A High Risk Environment." 499
Pearson, L. "Climacteric." 504

Section 5: Nursing Care of the Child 511

THE HEALTHY CHILD 513

THE ILL AND HOSPITALIZED CHILD 525

OXYGENATION 532
General Concepts 532
   Overview 532
   Application of the Nursing Process to the Child with Respiratory Problems 532
Selected Health Problems Resulting in an Interference with Respiration 533
   A. Sudden Infant Death Syndrome or "Crib Death" 533
   B. Acute Spasmodic Laryngitis (Spasmodic Croup) 534
   C. Acute Epiglottitis 534
   D. Laryngotracheobronchitis 535
   E. Bronchiolitis 536
   F. Bronchial Asthma 536
   Application of the Nursing Process to the Child with Cardiac Problems 538
Selected Health Problems Resulting in an Interference with Cardiac Functioning 540
   Congenital Cardiac Disorders 540
   Rheumatic Fever 545

Application of the Nursing Process to the Child with Hematologic Problems 546
Selected Health Problems Resulting in an Interference with Formed Elements of the Blood
   A. *Iron-Deficiency Anemia* 547
   B. *Sickle Cell Anemia* 548
   C. *Hemophilia* 550

NUTRITION AND METABOLISM 552
General Concepts 552
   Overview 552
   Application of Nursing Process to the Child with Problems of Nutrition and Metabolism 552
Selected Health Problems 553
   A. *Failure to Thrive Syndrome* 553
   B. *Vomiting and Diarrhea* 554
   C. *Pyloric Stenosis* 556
   D. *Cleft Lip and Palate* 556
   E. *Cystic Fibrosis* 558
   F. *Insulin-Dependent Diabetes Mellitus* 560

ELIMINATION 562
General Concepts 562
   Overview 562
   Application of the Nursing Process to the Child with Elimination Problems 562
Selected Health Problems 563
   A. *Hypospadias* 563
   B. *Urinary Tract Infection* 564
   C. *Nephrosis and Nephritis* 564
   D. *Lower GI Obstruction* 566

SAFETY AND SECURITY 568
General Concepts 568
   Overview 568
   Application of the Nursing Process to the Child with Neurologic or Sensory Problems 568
Selected Health Problems: Neurologic and Sensory Deficits 570
   A. *Mental Retardation* 570
   B. *Down's Syndrome (Mongolism)* 571
   C. *Cerebral Palsy* 572
   D. *Hydrocephalus* 573
   E. *Spina Bifida* 574
   F. *Seizure Disorders* 575
   G. *Bacterial Meningitis* 577
   H. *Otitis Media* 578
   I. *Tonsillitis, Tonsillectomy and Adenoidectomy* 579
Application of the Nursing Process to the Child with a Communicable Disease 580
Selected Health Problems: Communicable Diseases, Skin Infections, Infestations 580
   A. *Communicable Diseases* 580
   B. *Sexually Transmitted Diseases* 582
   C. *Common Skin Infections and Infestations* 584
   D. *Pinworms* 584

Application of the Nursing Process to the Child with an Interference with Safety 584
Selected Health Problems: Interference with Safety 584
   A. *Poisonous Ingestions* 584
   B. *Burns* 589

ACTIVITY AND REST 595
General Concepts 595
   Overview 595
   Application of the Nursing Process to the Child with Interferences with Activity and Rest 595
Selected Health Problems 599
   A. *Congenital Club Foot* 599
   B. *Congenital Hip Dysplasia* 599
   C. *Scoliosis* 600
   D. *Osteomyelitis* 601

CELLULAR ABERRATION (CHILDHOOD CANCER) 602
General Concepts 602
   Overview 602
   Application of the Nursing Process to the Child with Cancer 602
Selected Health Problems 606
   A. *Leukemia* 606
   B. *Hodgkin's Disease* 608
   C. *Brain Tumors* 609
   D. *Neuroblastoma* 611
   E. *Wilm's Tumor (Nephroblastoma)* 611

REPRINTS 615
Sheredy, C. "Factors to Consider when Assessing Responses to Pain." 617
Sacksteder, S. "Congenital Cardiac Defects: Embryology and Fetal Circulation." 620
Ruble, I. "Childhood Nocturnal Enuresis." 624
Meier, E. "Evaluating Head Trauma in Infants and Children." 630
Coughlin, M. "Teaching Children about their Seizures and Medications." 634
Jackson, P. "Ventriculo-peritoneal Shunts." 636
Seleckman, J. "Immunization: What's It All About?" 642

Section 6: Questions and Answers 649

BOOK ONE QUESTIONS 651
BOOK ONE ANSWERS 662
BOOK TWO QUESTIONS 667
BOOK TWO ANSWERS 677
BOOK THREE QUESTIONS 682
BOOK THREE ANSWERS 693
BOOK FOUR QUESTIONS 698
BOOK FOUR ANSWERS 710

Tables and Figures

Section 2: Nursing Care of the Client with Psychosocial Problems

TABLES
2.1 Theoretical Models 20
2.2 Social Determinants of Mental Health and Illness 21
2.3 Life-Cycle Stages 22
2.4 Communication Skills in the Nurse-Client Relationship 24
2.5 Manifestations of Anxiety 37
2.6 Minor Tranquilizers 39
2.7 Antidepressants 51
2.8 Suicide Methods 55
2.9 Major Tranquilizers 80
2.10 Side Effects of Major Tranquilizers 81
2.11 Selected Problem Behaviors and Interventions 83

Section 3: Nursing Care of the Adult

TABLES
3.1 General Anesthesia 166
3.2 Regional Anesthesia 166
3.3 Stages of General Anesthesia 166
3.4 Calculating IV Rates 167
3.5 Analgesics 168
3.6 Emergency Drugs 177
3.7 Coronary Vasodilators 181
3.8 Adrenergic Blockers 181
3.9 Blood Tests For Myocardial Infarction 183
3.10 Anticoagulants 184
3.11 Anticoagulant Antagonists 184
3.12 Approximate Sodium Content in Selected Food Items 185
3.13 Cholesterol and Saturated Fat Content in Selected Food Items 186
3.14 Congestive Heart Failure 188
3.15 Cardiac Glycosides 189
3.16 Antihypertensives 191
3.17 Foods High in Potassium 192
3.18 Adrenergics 195
3.19 Bronchodilators (Xanthine Derivatives) 197
3.20 Expectorants 198
3.21 Mucolytics 198
3.22 Antibiotics 200
3.23 Antituberculous Drugs 202
3.24 Gastrointestinal Hormones 208
3.25 Digestive Enzymes 209
3.26 Acid-Base Imbalance 212
3.27 Fluid Imbalance 213
3.28 Electrolyte Imbalances 214
3.29 Drug Therapy for Peptic Ulcer Disease 220
3.30 Dietary Worksheet 221
3.31 Sample Therapeutic Diets 222
3.32 Hormones 234
3.33 Steroids 242
3.34 Hypoglycemics 244
3.35 Diabetic Meal Planning with Exchange Lists 245
3.36 Differentiating Hypoglycemia from Ketoacidosis 247
3.37 Laboratory Tests Used to Evaluate Renal Function 253
3.38 Urinary Antiseptics 257
3.39 Sulfonamides 257
3.40 Diuretics 262
3.41 Modifications of Food, Fluid, and Electrolyte Intake in Renal Failure 264
3.42 Low Protein Diet Sample Menu 265
3.43 Prostatectomies 272
3.44 Laxatives 276
3.45 Antidiarrheals 277
3.46 Comparison of Crohn's Disease and Ulcerative Colitis 278
3.47 Foods to be *Avoided* on Low Residue Diets 279
3.48 Cranial Nerves 286
3.49 Parasympathetic and Sympathetic Effects 287
3.50 Spinal Cord 297
3.51 Antiparkinsonian Drugs 300
3.52 Anticonvulsants 303
3.53 Cholinergics 304
3.54 Anticholinergics 305
3.55 Anti-Inflammatory Drugs 321
3.56 Chemotherapeutic Agents 329
3.57 Antiemetics 332

FIGURES
3.1 The Normal Heart 171
3.2 Pressures in the Vascular System 172
3.3 Areas of Auscultation of Heart Valves 173
3.4 Pulmonary Volumes and Capacities of an Adult 175
3.5 Distribution of Typical Anginal Pain 180
3.6 Coronary Blood Supply 182
3.7 Myocardial Infarction 182
3.8 Typical Enzyme Patterns After an Acute Myocardial Infarction 183
3.9 Pattern for Rotating Tourniquets 190
3.10 Common Manifestations of Chronic Arterial and Venous Peripheral Vascular Disease 194
3.11 Water-Seal Chest Drainage 204
3.12 Pleur-evac System 205
3.13 Components of the Kidney 251
3.14 Components and Functions of the Nephron 251
3.15 Schematic Representation of Dialysis 266
3.16 Normal Male Anatomy 271
3.17 The Eye (Horizontal Section) 287
3.18 Decorticate Posturing 290
3.19 Decerebrate Posturing 291
3.20 Areas of the Brain that Control Certain Motor and Sensory Functions 296

Section 4: Nursing Care of the Childbearing Family

TABLES
4.1 Assessment of Fertility/Infertility 379
4.2 Signs and Symptoms of Pregnancy 384

x TABLES AND FIGURES

4.3 Naegele's Rule 386
4.4 McDonald's Rule 386
4.5 Recommended Dietary Allowances for Females Aged 11-50 389
4.6 Pregnant Woman's Daily Food Intake 390
4.7 Laboratory Studies of Fetal Well-being 391
4.8 Classification of Eclampsia 399
4.9 Magnesium Sulfate 401
4.10 Baseline FHR—No Contractions 411
4.11 Decelerations in FHR During Contractions 413
4.12 Stages and Phases of Labor 415
4.13 Uterine Dysfunction in Labor 420
4.14 Ritodrine Hydrochloride 424
4.15 Bishop's Scale 426
4.16 Oxytocin 427
4.17 Lochia Changes 432
4.18 Maternal Psychologic Adaptation 434
4.19 Nutritional Comparison of Human and Cow's Milk 450
4.20 High-Risk Conditions for Neonates by Gestational Age and Growth Classification 451
4.21 Apgar Scoring Chart 453

FIGURES
4.1 Female Pelvis 375
4.2 Female External Reproductive Organs 377
4.3 Female Internal Organs 377
4.4 Basal Body Temperature (28-Day Cycle) 378
4.5 Common Site of Ectopic Pregnancy 395
4.6 Hydaditiform Mole 396
4.7 Placenta Previa 397
4.8 Abruptio Placentae 398
4.9 Six Possible Fetal Positions with Cephalic Presentation 409
4.10 Tracing of Normal Fetal Heart Rate 410
4.11 Types of Decelerations in Fetal Heart Rate 412
4.12 Tracing of Acceleration of Fetal Heart Rate in Response to Uterine Activity 413
4.13 Assessment of Uterine Contractions 414
4.14 Friedman Curve 422
4.15 Types of Episiotomies 427
4.16 Types of Cesarian Incisions 429
4.17 Bones, Fontanels, and Sutures of Newborn's Skull 446

4.18 Newborn Maturity Rating and Classification 454
4.19 Rh Sensitization 458
4.20 Silverman-Andersen Scale 460

Section 5: Nursing Care of the Child

TABLES
5.1 Erikson's First Five Stages of Psychosocial Development 514
5.2 Vital Sign Ranges in Children 515
5.3 Average Daily Caloric Needs of Infants and Children 515
5.4 American Academy of Pediatrics Recommended Immunization Schedule 516
5.5 Contraindications for Immunization 517
5.6 Commonly Used Pediatric Restraints 526
5.7 Medication and Temperature Guide 529
5.8 Medication Administration for Young Children 530
5.9 Medications Used to Treat Bronchial Asthma 537
5.10 Cardiac Catheterization in Children: Nursing Considerations 539
5.11 Normal Blood Cells 547
5.12 Insulin-Dependent Diabetes in the Child 560
5.13 Comparison of Nephrosis and Nephritis 565
5.14 Levels of Mental Retardation 571
5.15 Signs of Increased Intracranial Pressure in Infants and Older Children 574
5.16 Sexually Transmitted Diseases 582
5.17 Common Skin Infections and Infestations 585
5.18 Commonly Ingested Poisonous Substances 586
5.19 Systemic Responses to Burn Injury 589
5.20 Types of Traction 596
5.21 Commonly Used Chemotherapeutic Drugs 603
5.22 Staging of Hodgkin's Disease 608

FIGURES
5.1 Normal and Abnormal Hearts 541
5.2 Common Modes of Genetic Transmission 549
5.3 Estimation of Burn Surface Area 590
5.4 Types of Traction 597
5.5 Petalled Cast Edges 599

Foreword

Taking a test is not an activity that most of us cherish. It is stressful regardless of how well prepared we are. Each of you has spent a large portion of your education learning concepts, principles, and theories that pertain to nursing. You have learned about a myriad of nursing responses to health disruptions. The culmination of your learning and experiences comes in the taking of the NCLEX—the registered nurse licensure examination.

You have been taught to assess, plan, implement, and evaluate. You will once again use the same set of problem-solving steps as you approach the test. The *AJN 1987 Nursing Boards Review* is a tool for assessing your current knowledge and calming your fears about the examination.

Two major factors likely to influence your success on the NCLEX are your level of nursing knowledge, your ability to apply that knowledge, and your level of test anxiety. Some degree of anxiety is beneficial for successful test taking; excessive anxiety impairs the ability to think clearly and critically. By systematically studying this review, you can determine your level of readiness for the examination and plan ways to improve in any areas where you feel deficient.

By using this book, you can become less anxious about test taking through a review of your nursing knowledge, and sample NCLEX-type questions that reinforce the knowledge.

Best wishes for success with NCLEX and throughout your nursing career.

Jeanette Lancaster, RN, PhD
Dean and Professor
Wright State University
Miami Valley School of Nursing
Dayton, Ohio

Preface

Taking an examination is always a stressful procedure. The level of anxiety in any classroom during finals week is so high one can feel the energy it generates. And when the examinations you are facing are the basis for your licensure as a member of your chosen profession, no wonder the thought of those upcoming State Boards has you in a state.

Churn no more!

This book has been designed to make you comfortable and confident in taking and passing the NCLEX (National Council Licensure Examination). In addition to its clinical excellence and its focus on the elements of the nursing process and of decision making, it concentrates on your test-taking abilities and teaches you how to use them to your best advantage. An important aspect of this is stress reduction and so the first section of the book presents relaxation techniques. As you know, the test is multiple-choice and a calm attitude helps you use your best judgment.

The clinical aspects of the book have been developed by expert curriculum committees whose members are all top nurses, masters or doctorally prepared, and experienced in teaching in the AJN Nursing Boards Review courses. All of us at the AJN Company and Williams & Wilkins are most grateful to these talented, knowledgeable, conscientious faculty members. They have spent many hours tailoring the subject matter in the best way possible to trigger your thinking and buttress your learning.

Finally, a word about the AJN Nursing Boards Review course. If you want a still greater sense of security about your exam, please do call us for information about the AJN Nursing Boards Review, or fill out the coupon you'll find at the back of this book. Our toll-free number is 800/223-2282; in New York State, call 212/582-8820 collect.

One thing more—our very best wishes to you for success in the exam and throughout your nursing career.

Thelma M. Schorr, RN
President and Publisher
American Journal of Nursing Company

Introduction

Whether you are graduating from a two-year, three-year, or baccalaureate nursing program, you face one important step on the way to establishing yourself as a registered nurse. That step, as we all know, is passing the state board examination, or the NCLEX, as it is now called (NCLEX stands for National Council Licensure Examination.)

Although your education has prepared you well for this series of tests, every RN preparing to take the NCLEX feels the need for a comprehensive review of her or his nursing studies prior to the big day. The *AJN 1987 Nursing Boards Review* provides a comprehensive review of nursing knowledge to prepare you, the graduate nurse, to successfully complete the NCLEX.

To use this book most effectively, read the first section on preparing for the examination and stress-reduction techniques. A firm grasp and application of the knowledge in this section will go a long way toward helping you review content and answer the test questions in a relaxed, calm manner. And review this section frequently; it will reinforce the principles that will have you in top form by examination day.

Review one clinical area at a time. Stay with that area until you feel comfortable with your knowledge mastery of it. Do the sections in any order you wish or as they are ordered in the book. If you run across subject matter with which you are unfamiliar, take time to look it up in your textbooks.

Keep in mind that NCLEX emphasizes nursing role and nursing process in caring for the healthy, as well as the ill, client. This emphasis matches the basic concept of the newly revised exam to test "application of the principles of nursing rather than recall of facts." (Dvorak, E. et al. *The National Council Licensure Examination for Registered Nurses*. Chicago: Chicago Review Press, 1982.)

NCLEX has two focuses. The first is on the steps of the nursing process: assessment, planning and implementation (including setting and establishing priorities for client goals), and evaluation. Second, the focus is on the locus of control in decision making. Is a given decision made by the client? The nurse? Or is it a shared decision? The entire exam consists of four different test parts, each part containing a series of questions regarding nursing care of the adult, child, childbearing family, and emotionally troubled client.

The entire test will be graded as a whole, rather than in separate sections as in the years before 1982. Consider each question carefully. Don't leave questions blank; make a reasonable guess. You will not be penalized for guessing. Of course, your chances of being correct are greater if you can narrow down the four choices to two.

Judicious use of this book, either alone or in conjunction with a review class, will prepare you for successful completion of the licensure exam. It is important to keep in mind, however, not to rely on a review book to teach you new knowledge, but rather to recap and serve as a key to the nursing knowledge you already have. Many students have found marking content with a highlighting pen helpful for quick second-time-through checks.

A particularly valuable feature of this review book is the inclusion of a fine collection of articles from the *American Journal of Nursing* itself. They have been included to enhance the review material. Be sure to read them.

Another feature of this book is its reflection of the women's movement. Aware that language has played a role in reinforcing inequality between the sexes—to the loss of men as well as women—we have attempted to use language in a way that reinforces equality. The most vexing problem in avoiding sexist language is what to do about the "he-she" pronoun. No unisex substitute exists.

We have attempted to avoid stereotyping the nurse as "she" and the client as "he" by alternating the use of the masculine and feminine pronouns. In some sections, the client is referred to as she and, in others, as he.

We have attempted to deal with one or two

parents similarly. Often, there may be only one parent alone, or with a "significant other" who is not the child's parent. This term, too, has been included, sometimes alternately with "partner." Significant other, of course, has a wider scope, referring to anyone—grandparent, brother, sister, roommate, housekeeper—who is significant and personally close in the life of a client of any age.

Whether you see either of these terms, "parent, significant other," in the singular or plural, the point to remember in writing the NCLEX and in the practice of your profession is that your responsibility to your client includes considering the client's relationship with all of his or her significant others.

Finally, over 375 sample questions, written in the style of the examination, are provided. They have been purposefully mixed and not included at the end of each section in order to more closely simulate the actual test situation.

How do you know if you have enough knowledge to pass NCLEX or not? This is difficult to answer; however, the persons who write the NCLEX advise their readers that 75 percent correct answers is a good cutoff point. In other words, if you are wrong more than 25 percent of the time, you need to spend more time reviewing.

Those of us from the American Journal of Nursing Company and Williams & Wilkins who have worked on the production of this book wish you the very best of luck with your review efforts, the examinations, and ultimately, with your nursing career.

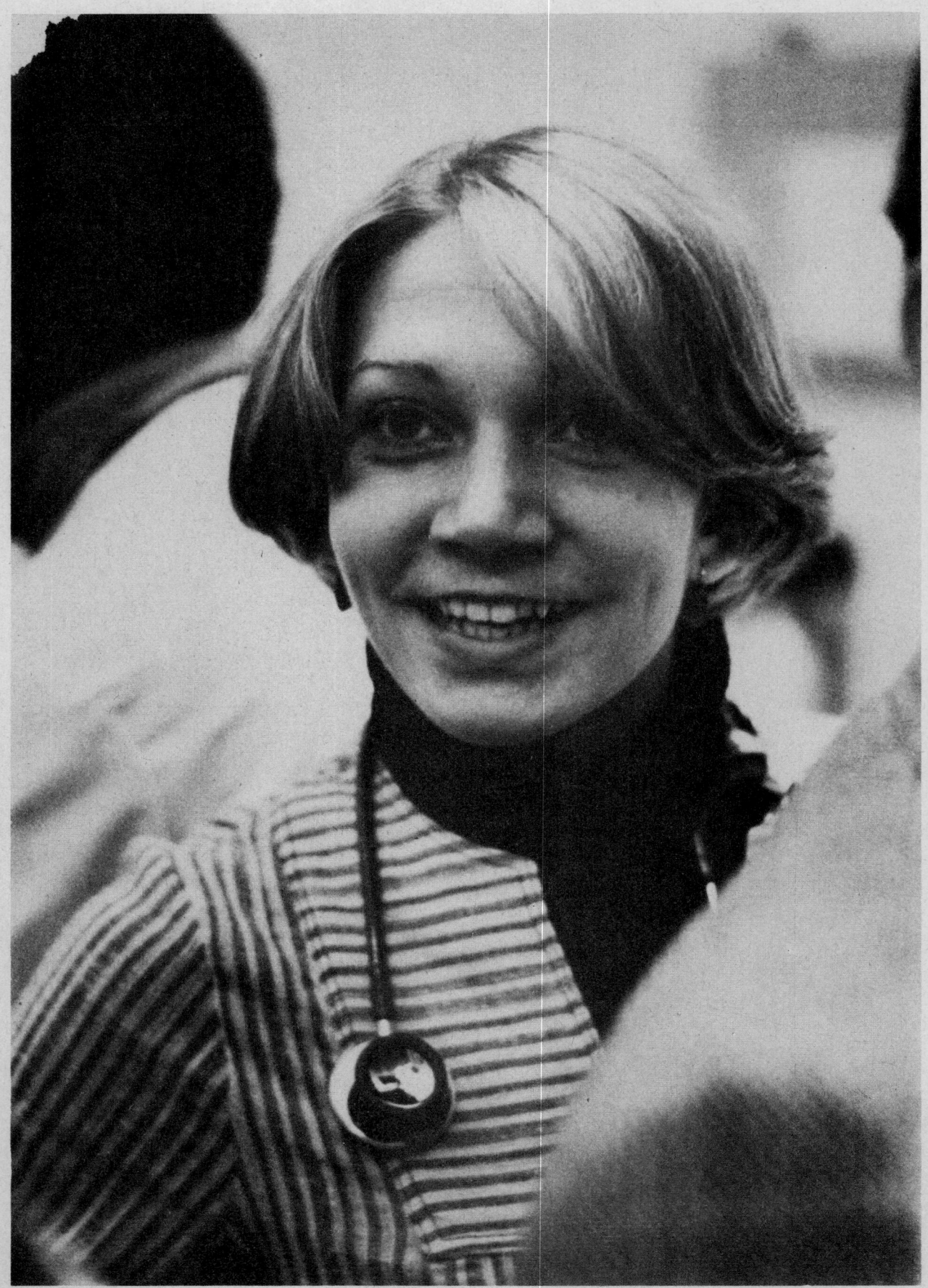

Section 1
Preparing for the NCLEX

Joan Reighley, RN, MN
Marybeth Young, RN, MSN

Section 1: Preparing for the NCLEX

PREPARING FOR SUCCESS ON THE NCLEX-RN 3
STRESS-REDUCTION TECHNIQUES 7

Preparing for Success on the NCLEX-RN

Marybeth Young, RN, MSN

As you prepare to take the National Council Licensure Examination, or NCLEX-RN, you may feel somewhat overwhelmed with insecurity and excitement. Most graduate nurses feel that way. But planned preparation for the test can increase your confidence.

The examination that you will take serves as an entry into professional nursing practice. You want to succeed! To do well you must be able to demonstrate your nursing knowledge on a multiple-choice test. Because many factors influence the outcome, begin your preparation with an evaluation of personal strengths and limitations in knowledge and experience. Then plan a review schedule to meet your individual needs.

In the process of completing a nursing program, you have acquired knowledge and skills enabling you to give safe care to clients with varied health problems. You have learned the practical value of problem solving through written daily care plans. These cognitive abilities will transfer to the testing situation. And they can help you to establish that you are a safe beginning practitioner of nursing.

The New Test: Nursing Process and Locus of Control

It is necessary to understand the testing process well in advance of the testing date. The National Council of State Boards of Nursing has developed a test plan focusing on the measurement of safe nursing behaviors. There is no distinct separation of clinical specialties. You will take an integrated exam with situations describing a variety of client problems. One situation and set of test items may deal with the needs of the hospitalized child and family; the next may focus on the care of the chronically ill adult.

In each of the four test sections, there will be a mix of test questions describing individuals at all developmental levels. Emphasis will be placed on common health problems. From a pool of items developed by experts in clinical practice and education, a totally different test is compiled for each testing date.

Keep in mind that the examination will test nursing behaviors that affect client well-being. These nursing actions are relevant, as they are based on studies of actual nurse–client situations (Jacobs et al. 1978). To help yourself clearly understand the behaviors expected of the safe practitioner of nursing, reflect on past clinical evaluations. The expectations for practice are based on the Standards of Practice developed by the American Nurses' Association. As an example, the nurse is expected to properly position a client to prevent complications of immobility. A test item may ask you how to implement a plan for positioning a client following a cerebrovascular accident.

The framework for the integrated test is the nursing process. You have used this approach in problem solving for many clients. Each phase of the process will be tested equally in the examination.

The five-step process is

1. Assessing by gathering data, observing, and listening to what is reported by the client and family
2. Analyzing data to identify problems, establish a nursing diagnosis, and set goals
3. Planning nursing interventions with client/family to meet specific needs
4. Implementing the plan of care
5. Evaluating the client's response in terms of goal achievement.

Test items based on the nursing process will be based on real-life situations. But instead of creatively setting goals and developing a plan of care, you will be presented with a case study and a set of multiple-choice items related to it. You will apply your nursing knowledge and judgment to determine the ONE best response to each question.

Examples of how the nursing process may be used to provide a framework for examination items follow.

1. Items that focus on assessment may require that you suggest additional observations. If more data are needed as a basis for care, you will need to understand the rationale. You may be asked to select appropriate subjective or objective assessments pertinent to a particular client. You will be expected to be familiar with commonly used diagnostic tests.
2. Some test items will ask you to interpret data given. You will be required to identify specific problems based on information gathered and assessments made. You will be asked to differentiate between normal and abnormal test results. Short- and long-range goals will be set to meet the specific needs that have been identified.
3. Planning of care may involve the nurse and health care team in some situations. In others, the family and client take an active part in such planning. You will need to understand the rationale for the plan.
4. Implementation of care may be tested in a variety of ways. You will be asked about proper preparation and administration of medications and intravenous fluids. Safety measures are an important aspect of therapy. Ongoing surveillance is expected during treatment.
5. Evaluation of care may be tested by asking you to look at the outcomes of medication or other therapy. You may be asked to determine the effectiveness of preoperative or discharge teaching. Refer back to the goals identified for a specific client. Evaluation should reflect the outcome of these goals.

This review text and the test items included use the nursing process as a framework. You will see that the problem-solving approach is logical and relevant for the safe beginning practice of the nurse.

The second focus of the NCLEX examination is locus of control, or systems of health care decision making. As a professional nurse, you take part in the client's decisions about health care. At times, the client is quite independent and uses the nurse for guidance or teaching. For example, a couple may seek information from the nurse in a family planning clinic. They are in control of their situation, and may or may not learn. They make decisions for themselves.

Other clients may be totally dependent on the nurse for decisions and care. For example, in the immediate postoperative period, the nurse assumes responsibility for direct care.

Most frequently, the nurse and client SHARE decision making and participation in care. For example, the young adult with sensory disturbance following an eye injury may be partially dependent on the nurse for some aspects of care. However some degree of control and decision making are possible. Expect to find that the majority of test situations in the NCLEX exam involve shared decision making. In actual clinical practice, this is most often the case.

The test plan identifies additional areas of knowledge basic to safe nursing practice. These include an understanding of normal physiologic functioning, basic human needs, pharmacology, nutrition and fluid/electrolyte balance. The nurse who practices safely considers developmental needs when planning care. Psycho/social/cultural influences on health are important aspects of nursing knowledge. These were all a part of your curriculum, in support courses or in integrated content. They provide a basis for holistic nursing.

In summary, the test plan has a clearly defined framework based on the nursing process, systems of decision making, and the characteristics of safe nursing practice. Knowledge of this plan will enable you to prepare thoughtfully for the examination.

Totaling the Score

Format and scoring of the examination are of concern to you as a candidate for licensure. One minute is allotted for each of the 93–94 items in each test section. Your score will be based on the demonstration and application of knowledge for the entire 375 questions. The raw score, or total of correct responses, is placed on a conversion table of statistically treated scores on a range of about 800 to 3,200. The passing score, 1,600, reflects minimal competency, based on a set standard or criterion. At this time, successful passing of the examination permits licensure by endorsement in every state.

Guessing on this examination may benefit you, as it is scored on the basis of the total number of correct responses. Items not answered do not count for or against you. Neither incorrect answers nor guesses are subtracted from the raw score.

Personal Preparation

Now that you have a general idea of the focus of NCLEX, set some personal goals for preparation and review.

As you read content outlines and test items, you may find you have good recall of prior knowledge. Take credit for a good education! Have confidence in your ability to apply that knowledge. When you uncover a deficit, remedy it through reading and use of this review text.

Consider your intellectual readiness for the test itself. Strategies to deal with multiple-choice items can be learned, practiced in advance, and used during the test.

Be aware that emotions may interfere with memory and performance during a lengthy examination. Anticipate that you may become confused by or even angry at some items. You may even feel that you could have written better options! Emotions can interfere with concentration and lead to frustration and loss of time and energy. Whatever the emotional response, realize that you have the power to manage feelings. Use the relaxation techniques and imagery suggested in this review text. You will find that stress management improves mental abilities during an examination.

Anxiety about the licensure examination can be diminished if you anticipate the testing situation. Just as expectant parents are urged to take a test drive to the birthing center before labor begins, consider a trip to the test site. Plan for your personal needs during the days of testing: headache remedies, hard candies, a bag lunch, a sweater. Whatever you do to promote your physical comfort may also reduce anxiety.

Choosing the Answers

There are many proven strategies that can affect your intellectual performance of the test. First, and most important, get into the habit of reading carefully. Do not skim over the situation hurriedly. Read the question. Pause a moment and try to think of the appropriate assessment or nursing action. Be alert for key words such as FIRST, ALWAYS, and NEVER. Then read *all* the options. Select the one closest to what you would do in such a situation. If no option seems obviously the best, narrow the options to two possible responses by eliminating the least correct. Then reread those options carefully, focusing on specific differences. An educated guess may be indicated if you are uncertain about the decision. Practice this approach to test items. You will build confidence in your ability to think critically.

In some cases, each of the options will seem equally correct. Or, you may read four unfamiliar responses and find a decision impossible. Do not waste precious time studying that question. Omit it for the present. Mark the item number in the space provided for "notes" and proceed with other items. When you have completed the test, return to those difficult items. Ultimately, you may find a random guess is necessary. Remember, there is no penalty for guessing.

This approach will also help with those situations that are totally unfamiliar to you. Even content you had previously known thoroughly may be difficult to recall during the test. Go on to other items and return later to the challenges. Given time, memory may serve you well.

Try to visualize the nurse–client interactions occurring in ideal health settings. And avoid reading into an item something not specified by the test writers. For example, assume that nourishing liquids are available on all shifts. Do not imagine that the client has food preferences similar to yours!

Avoid changing answers indiscriminately. If you complete the test early and decide to review your responses, you may be tempted to change some. Occasionally, inspiration leads to a better response. But an overused eraser can destroy confidence in your problem-solving abilities.

Practice taking multiple-choice tests to improve your skills. Use the questions included in this book. Simulate the time limit of one minute for each item. Try to respond to each item, even if it is not familiar to you. Realize that as a graduate nurse you can apply principles to related problems. For example, your knowledge of perineal care following an episiotomy can be applied to comfort measures suggested after a hemorrhoidectomy.

Approach priority questions thoughtfully. Many times, all options are appropriate, but the situation calls for a FIRST nursing action. One way to approach such an item is to treat each statement as a TRUE/FALSE option. For example if you are asked to identify a priority nursing intervention in delivery room care of the neonate, would you first

1. establish a patent airway
2. promote maternal bonding
3. prevent heat loss
4. record the Apgar score?

Two choices appear most correct: the first and third options. But if the infant's airway is obstructed, heat conservation is a secondary concern. One- and five-minute assessments of the Apgar score are important. Recording of that data is not a priority here.

When planning actual client care, it is relatively easy to identify a priority problem and several appropriate interventions. But you are seldom asked to select one most important nursing action. If you have difficulty making such a choice, ask yourself, "Will my client be endangered if I do NOT carry out this intervention first?"

Communications items should be approached carefully. As you read the situation and questions, clarify whether you are asked to communicate therapeutically, provide teaching, or give information. For example, the client who asks about the length of a recovery room stay may be asking for a time interval, or indicating a need to express feelings about fears related to surgery. Careful reading of the items should provide you with cues.

Perhaps, as you read the options, you will have the feeling that none reflects the way you would really respond to a client. Try to be objective. Look for a statement that reflects effective communication and meets the specific needs at the moment.

A key strategy in test taking is to answer each test item to the best of your ability, then mentally and emotionally move on to the next test item. Dwelling on a previous question can reduce concentration on the next. If a decision troubles you, note the number and reexamine it later.

A careful approach to math calculations may save time and prevent errors. Label all parts of the work: minims, milliliters per hour, drops per minute. Just as such identification promotes client safety in a real situation, it may lead you to the correct test response as well.

Contrary to rumors, there are no hidden tricks in the NCLEX test. Nor is there a pattern of correct responses, such as "When in doubt, select the second response." That is not true! Remember that the questions are carefully edited. Computer selection ensures that answers are randomly sequenced.

Be skeptical about all test rumors. A friend who tells you that the scoring was just changed, or that one health problem is NEVER on the test may mean well but be misinformed. One myth often repeated is that partial credit is given for a "second best" response. That is not true! There is one single best response. And remember, your score depends on the total number of correct responses! So a primary goal during the two testing days is to proceed carefully but quickly. Do watch the time, and complete each test section

In Conclusion

As the date of testing approaches, continue to practice test-taking strategies and stress-reduction techniques. Expect that some items will be very difficult, but be confident in your abilities to apply nursing knowledge.

You can do well on the NCLEX examination with thoughtful preparation and review. This is your opportunity to prove to yourself and your peers that you are a SAFE practitioner of nursing.

References

Jacobs, A. et al. *Critical Requirements for Safe Effective Nursing Practice.* Kansas City, MO: American Nurses' Association, 1978.

Test Plan for the Registered Nurse State Board Test Pool Examination. Chicago: National Council of State Boards of Nursing, 1980.

Young, M. "Preparation for State Boards." *Imprint.* April 1980:50–51, 94–95, 100.

Young, M. and Kopala, B. "Plan for Success: Preparing for the 1982 State Boards." *Imprint.* December 1981:50–51, 70–71, 85.

Stress-Reduction Techniques

Joan Reighley, RN, MN

As you begin your planned review for the NCLEX, consider including stress-management techniques in your study plan. Why? Because stress management can lower anxiety and improve concentration during your study time and during the examination. Successful test taking and stress management are learned skills and must be practiced consistently.

To begin, assess your own stress level by reading "Stress Management" in the reprint section following *The Client with Psychosocial Problems*.

Next, identify your test-taking strengths and stressors. Examples of strengths may include previous successful test taking, experience with multiple-choice questions and timed tests, reading and vocabulary skills, knowledge of nursing process and nursing interventions, problem-solving skills, and health habits such as a daily exercise and relaxation program and adequate nutrition.

Examples of stressors may include pressure from a timed test, difficulty in discriminating the best response, generalized test-taking anxiety, lack of a consistent study and stress-management program, and emotions such as fear of failure, anger at being tested, feelings of powerlessness, and others.

Your strengths can be put to use to help decrease your stress level. Take time now to write down a list of your strengths; then make a list of your stressors. Making a written list helps you to identify them. If you have difficulty identifying your strengths, ask a friend, teacher, or counselor to assist you. Asking for help is strength in itself.

Develop a written plan for stress management to use during your study time and during the examination time. Again, writing out the plan will help to make it more concrete. The following techniques will help you to cope with studying and test taking.

Imagery

Imagination is energy that can be used to move toward a desired goal. Instead of using your imagination to scare yourself, imagine yourself taking the test successfully and with ease. The positive image will then pull you toward what you want. See yourself as you would like to be during the test taking. Imagine yourself as alert, confident, calm, effective, prepared, relaxed—whatever you would like to be. Be aware of your negative thoughts or images that tend to creep in. Replace them with positive thoughts and images.

Use your imagination to remember positive experiences and positive self-images instead of scaring yourself. Most of us have great skill at scaring ourselves: "What if...", "I can't do it," "I'll fail the exam." Let yourself be open to the idea that the better you are at scaring yourself, the better you will be at using your imagination to learn and be successful at test taking.

Positive Affirmations

Create positive, active, new statements about yourself as you would like to be: "I am relaxed." "I am preparing for the exam." "I am confident and excited." "I am able to pass multiple-choice tests." "I know how to take timed tests." "I am able to choose the correct answer."

Write out the statements and place them on your mirror, steering wheel, refrigerator, desk, or any place where they will catch your eye. Repeat the statements to yourself several times daily. Be specific! Be positive! Be brief!

Doubts and negative thoughts and images are some of the ways we stop ourselves from being effective and relaxed. Become aware of how you scare yourself, and you can begin to program yourself for success.

Mental Exercises

Learn mental exercises. They will help you to create a sense of peace and tranquility and to relax muscles. Examples:

- **Progressive Relaxation**: concentrate on relaxing successive sets of muscles from the tips of your toes to the top of your head. This may include tightening one set of muscles and then letting go of the muscles to a count of six. "I'm holding tight the muscles in my hand and arm . . . one, two, three, four, five, six. I'm letting go of the muscles in my arm . . . one, two, three, four, five, six." The holding lasts 15 to 30 seconds and the letting go lasts an equal amount of time. An alternative way to do progressive relaxation is to focus by saying, "My feet are becoming relaxed and warm. My ankles are becoming relaxed and warm." Then progressively focus on successive parts of the body.

- **Autogenic-Training Exercises**: repeat verbal formulas with passive concentration and a relaxed posture. "My body is becoming warm and relaxed. I am beginning to feel quiet and relaxed. My right arm is warm and relaxed. My heart beat is calm and regular. My lungs breathe for me. My forehead is cool. My jaw is relaxed and easy."

Integrate the progressive relaxation and autogenic training exercises with your study and work schedule. Plan to do them for 5 to 10 minutes three or four times daily at a regular time, such as before or after meals, before classes or study times, lunch hour, as an alternative to coffee breaks.

Physical Exercise

Daily physical exercise will help you stay alert and relaxed as well as decrease your anxiety level. Include exercise that is fun for you. Walk, run, dance, swim, garden! Do exercises or yoga! Jump rope! Do stretching breaks! Give yourself 10 minutes of activity for each hour of studying.

Rehearsal

Let yourself rehearse taking the NCLEX by studying in the following way:

1. Set aside 30 minutes each day to answer 30 test questions, timing yourself with a kitchen timer or alarm clock. If you are unable to finish 30 questions in 30 minutes, give yourself 10 minutes longer and then gradually decrease time each day, until you are able to successfully answer 30 questions in 30 minutes.
2. Utilize strategies for multiple-choice questions as suggested earlier in, "Test-Taking Strategies."
3. Check your answers for accuracy and utilize this review book to clarify information on questions you get wrong. Do not time yourself when checking answers or reviewing.
4. Set aside 45 minutes each day to answer 45 questions; follow the same procedure as above. Gradually increase the time and number of questions until you can answer 95 questions in 90 minutes. Let your practice be as much like the testing situation as possible.

Set realistic goals for yourself in studying and stress management. Remember to utilize your strengths to help you cope with your stressors. Daily use of imagery, positive affirmations, relaxation exercises, short exercise breaks, and role rehearsal will allow you to study for the NCLEX effectively and to reach your goal of a passing score and the privilege to put RN after your name.

Copyright © Nurseco, 1983. Used with permission.

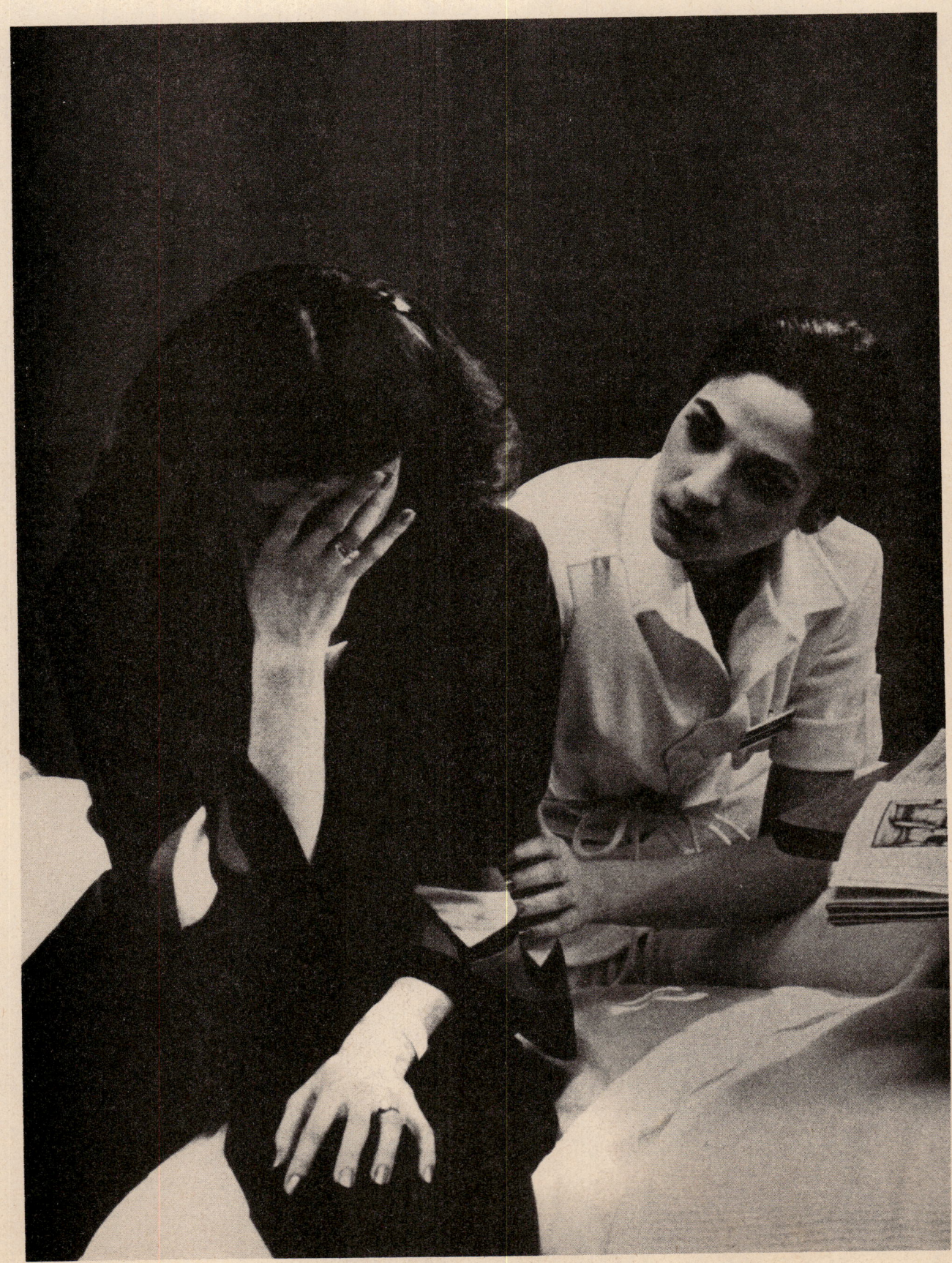

Section 2
Nursing Care of the Client with Psychosocial Problems

Phyllis Cooper, RN, MN, Coordinator

Carolyn V. Billings, RN, MSN
E. Ingvarda Hanson, RN, MSN
Alene Harrison, RN, MS
Ann L. Jessop, RN, MSN
Carol W. Kennedy, RN, PhD
Joan Reighley, RN, MN
Constance M. Ritzman, RN, MSN
Mary Charles Santopietro, RN, MS, EdM, EdD, CS
Victoria Schoolcraft, RN, MSN
Diane S. Smith, RN, MSN, CS
Diane Morrison Taylor, RN, MSN
Gail D. Wegner, RN, MS

Section 2: Nursing Care of the Client with Psychosocial Problems

INTRODUCTION 13
Overview 13
Scope of the Profession 13
Interpersonal Relationships 14
Roles Assumed by the Nurse 14
Locations of Practice 15
Psychosocial Characteristics of the Healthy Client 15

THERAPEUTIC USE OF SELF 19
Theoretical Knowledge Base 19
Nurse-Client Relationship 23
Nursing Process 25
Treatment Modalities 26

LOSS, DEATH AND DYING 28
General Concepts 28
  Overview 28
  Application of the Nursing Process to the Client Experiencing a Loss 29
Selected Health Problems 29
  A. Loss 29
  B. Death and Dying 30

LEGAL ASPECTS OF PSYCHIATRIC NURSING 34
Civil Procedures 34
Criminal Procedures 35
Territories 35
Judicial Precedents 35
Role of the Nurse 35

ANXIOUS BEHAVIOR 36
General Concepts 36
  Overview 36
  Application of the Nursing Process to the Client Exhibiting Anxious Behavior 36
Selected Health Problems 37
  A. Anxiety 37
  B. Phobias 40
  C. Dissociative Reactions 41
  D. Obsessive-Compulsive Disorders 41
  E. Anorexia Nervosa 42
  F. Psychosomatic Disorders 43
  G. Conversion Disorders 45
  H. Post-Traumatic Stress Disorders 46

CONFUSED BEHAVIOR 48
General Concepts 48
  Overview 48
  Application of the Nursing Process to the Client Exhibiting Confused Behavior 48
Selected Health Problems 48
  Chronic Confusion 48

ELATED-DEPRESSIVE BEHAVIOR 50
General Concepts 50
  Overview 50
  Application of the Nursing Process to the Client with an Affective Disorder 50
Selected Health Problems 52
  A. Depression 52
  B. Elation and Hyperactive Behavior 58

SOCIALLY MALADAPTIVE/ACTING OUT BEHAVIOR 60
General Concepts 60
  Overview 60
  Application of the Nursing Process to the Client Exhibiting Maladaptive Behavior 60
Selected Health Problems 61
  A. Violence in the Family 61
  B. Hostile, Aggressive, and Assaultive Behavior 64
  C. Acting Out 67
  D. Sexual Acting Out 68
  E. Antisocial Behavior 72

SUSPICIOUS BEHAVIOR 75
General Concepts 75
  Overview 75
  Application of the Nursing Process to the Client Exhibiting Suspicious Behavior 75
Selected Health Problem 75
  Paranoia 75

WITHDRAWN BEHAVIOR 77
General Concepts 77
  Overview 77
  Application of the Nursing Process to the Client Exhibiting Withdrawn Behavior 82
Selected Health Problems 86
  A. Paranoid Schizophrenia 86
  B. Catatonic Schizophrenia 86
  C. Undifferentiated Schizophrenia 87
  D. Childhood Schizophrenia 87
  E. Psychotic Disorders not Elsewhere Classified 87

SUBSTANCE USE DISORDERS 89
General Concepts 89
  Overview 89
  Application of the Nursing Process to the Client with a Substance Use Disorder 90
Selected Health Problems 91
  A. Alcohol 91
  B. Drugs Other than Alcohol 96

GLOSSARY 98
REPRINTS 105

Introduction

A. **Overview**
1. Psychiatric Nursing: a specialized area of nursing that operates on two levels. The *scientific* aspect focuses on understanding theories of human behavior, while the *art* of psychiatric nursing focuses on the purposeful use of self. Both concepts are directed toward preventing and alleviating mental illness and are concerned with the promotion of optimal mental health for individuals, families, and society.

    Today's nurse faces the task of using a holistic and biopsychosocial approach to safe care in all areas of nursing practice. In order to do this, the nurse needs knowledge of the human lifespan and developmental theories; also essential is verbal and nonverbal therapeutic communication, which is used from infancy through senescence. He or she must also consider the great diversity of sociocultural values and practices. A holistic approach enhances the quality and quantity of nursing care.

    Psychiatric nursing practice focuses on two broad areas. The *dependent* area involves the implementation and coordination of physicians' orders. The *independent* area is the assessment of the client's nursing needs and the development and implementation of individual nursing care plans. These plans are based on the nursing process. They include the initiation, development, and termination of therapeutic relationships between nurses and clients in all settings of nursing practice.

    The psychiatric nurse works in collaboration and coordination with a variety of other health care professionals, all working for the benefit of the client. Thus a high degree of interdependence with colleagues from other professions is inherent and essential.

    This section reviews content that is general to all nursing—that is, communicating with clients and the nurse-client relationship—as well as content that is specific to psychiatric nursing. The NCLEX-RN examination will test your knowledge of communication and interpersonal relationships in *all* sections of the examination.

2. *DSM-III*: the sections in this book are organized in the format of client problem behaviors and the *Diagnostic and Statistical Manual of Mental Disorders*, 3rd Ed. (American Psychiatric Association: 1980). The *DSM-III* categorizes and codes psychiatric diagnoses. These categories and codes are used by physicians and other health care providers to make diagnoses, to compile statistics, to apply for grants, and to report for third-party payment (insurance). Each diagnosis includes a description of diagnostic criteria. NCLEX will not ask you to diagnose the client's disorder.

B. **Scope of the Profession**
1. Scientific Focus: on human behavior
    a. To understand biopsychosocial principles underlying emotional problems
    b. To be aware of safe and effective treatment measures such as psychotherapy, medications, ECT
2. Purposeful Use of Self
    a. To apply principles of the nurse-client relationship to all interactions
    b. To be aware of one's self as a principal in the relationship and countertransference issues
    c. To recognize and use one's own feelings and reactions as a guide to increasing

empathy and trust, and understanding the client
    d. To act as an appropriate behavioral/social role-model
3. **Dependent Practice:** implementation and coordination of physician's orders
    a. Know important aspects of each client problem in order to assess and report findings accurately
    b. Apply knowledge and use skills therapeutically in assessment and treatment
    c. Work collaboratively, sharing information about the client's progress
4. **Independent Practice:** utilization of the nursing process and development of individualized nursing care plans
    a. Assess client's nursing needs
        1) interview the client in order to determine strengths and weaknesses
        2) observe verbal and nonverbal behaviors including dress, mannerisms, gestures, affect, thought processes, orientation, defense mechanisms, judgment, and insight
    b. Analyze and identify client health needs and goals
        1) analyze assessment data to make nursing diagnoses
        2) specify a short-term goal/expected outcome for each nursing diagnosis
        3) set a long-term goal/expected outcome
    c. Plan and implement interventions
        1) specify nursing interventions that will meet each short-term goal; establish a suitable environment for implementation (i.e., a therapeutic milieu)
        2) elicit the *client's* participation in his care
        3) include nursing actions such as setting limits on unacceptable behavior without rejecting the client as a person, increasing or decreasing environmental stimuli, and providing individually appropriate activities
    d. Evaluate client response to nursing interventions
        1) based on the effect of the intervention on the client's behavior, client's concerns, and achievement of short-term goals
        2) done by the individual nurse as well as by the total staff involved in the care
        3) revise nursing care plan as necessary

C. **Interpersonal Relationships**
  1. Therapeutic Relationships
      a. Between nurse and individual client include
          1) the initiation, development, and termination of a therapeutic relationship (objective, professional, empathetic interactions)
          2) the nurse's role modeling appropriate behavior
          3) the nurse's treating the client as a unique individual worthy of respect, and not focusing solely on the client's symptoms
          4) the nurse's being consistent and reliable in increasing the client's trust and security, and decreasing defensive acting-out behavior
      b. In a group include
          1) working with clients concerning the here-and-now living problems they confront
          2) providing information and role modeling
          3) clients getting feedback from other group members
  2. Collaboration with Other Professionals
      a. Coordinating and planning holistic health care
      b. Sharing implementation of the care plan according to skills needed, e.g., physical therapist, occupational therapist, rehabilitation counselor
      c. Working interdependently with other health professionals

D. **Roles Assumed by the Nurse:** nurses are involved directly in the care of the client and may assume many different, overlapping roles
  1. Therapist
      a. Therapy focusing on problems of daily living may be done
          1) on a one-to-one basis (nurse-client communication); focus is on problem solving
          2) in groups such as assertiveness groups, grooming groups, adolescent groups; focus is on dealing with specific problems, providing emotional support and reality

orientation, and increasing social skills and social acceptance
- b. Individual Psychotherapy
  1) therapist and client meet regularly; the client learns to identify own problems and practices new ways of handling them
  2) the client has the opportunity to develop a close relationship with another person (the therapist), to grow from that experience, and to generalize new insights and behavior to other areas of his life
- c. Group Psychotherapy: nurse may be group leader or coleader
- d. Family Therapy
  1) the therapist meets with the client and the family in various combinations
  2) family dynamics are stressed and scapegoating of the "identified patient" is decreased
- e. Sociotherapy: within the community mental health movement, psychiatric nurses provide services aimed at prevention of mental illness and reinforcement of healthy adaptation; specifically, this is done by teaching, by developing therapeutic relationships, and by recognizing early indications of problems and intervening appropriately
2. Surrogate Parent: the nurse is perceived in the role of nurturer, authority figure, parent as part of therapy with adults and children
3. Teacher: the nurse educates the client regarding biopsychosocial health needs, medications, nutrition, and productive ways of interacting and coping with stress
4. Social Agent: the nurse
   a. Assists the client to utilize community agencies and social networks
   b. Helps people learn about mental health, mental illness, and the prevention of mental illness
5. Coordinator of client care
6. Patient Advocate
7. Researcher
8. Administrator
9. Supervisor
10. Expanded and advanced roles as nurse clinical specialists

E. **Locations of Practice:** the role of the nurse is often dictated by the type of mental health facility
1. In Hospitals: the type of involvement the nurse has in client care varies with the theoretical model in use at the individual facility; the nurse may
   a. Work under direction of psychiatrists
   b. Formulate care plans
   c. Observe, support, and listen to clients
   d. Assist clients in developing new behaviors
   e. Provide clients with an environment to try new behaviors
   f. Administer medicines and physical nursing care
2. In Community Mental Health Centers:
   a. The nurse may
      1) provide out-client care using a variety of therapies
      2) do primary prevention in the community through
         a) classes designed to fulfill community needs
         b) crisis intervention
   b. There is a blurring of roles
      1) psychiatrists, psychologists, social workers, psychiatric nurses, and community mental health care workers work together in counseling, home visits, record keeping
      2) psychiatrists prescribe drugs; nurses administer medications; both may do physical exams

F. **Psychosocial Characteristics of the Healthy Client**
1. Young Adult Years (20–40)
   a. Cognitive Development
      1) thinking and learning are problem-centered
      2) thinks at an abstract level and compares ideas mentally or verbally with previous memories, knowledge, and experience
      3) learns formally and informally by emphasizing principles and concepts
      4) objective, realistic
   b. Emotional Development
      1) sexuality is a powerful determinant
      2) expected to be responsible, have good impulse control
      3) Erikson's task: intimacy vs self-isolation or self-absorption

- c. Moral/Religious Development
  1) challenges values, principles defined by parents and identifies those to be retained or modified
  2) values become individualized, integrated, and provide basis for future ethical decision making
- d. Body-Image Development
  1) body image is flexible, subject to constant revision, may not reflect actual body structure
  2) a social creation
  3) close interdependence between body image and personality, self-concept, and identity; may be altered by illness, injury, disability
- e. Life-Style Options
  1) separates from parents in 20s and develops peer relationships
  2) makes decisions regarding types of relationships to form (marriage, child rearing, communal, homosexual)
  3) settles into career
  4) establishes leisure activities
- f. Developmental Tasks
  1) accepts self: stabilizing self-concept and body image
  2) establishes independence
  3) establishes a vocation to make worthwhile contributions
  4) learns to appraise and express love responsibly
  5) establishes intimate bond with another
  6) establishes and manages residence
  7) finds congenial social group
  8) decides on option of a family
  9) formulates philosophy of life
  10) establishes role in community

2. Middle Adult Years (40–65)
   a. Cognitive Development
      1) goal-oriented
      2) enhanced by experiences, motivation
      3) decreased memory functioning
      4) less retained from oral information
      5) continued learning emphasized
      6) emphasis on realistic thinking
      7) problem-centered thinking
      8) attitudes may be less flexible
   b. Emotional Development
      1) transitional, self-assessment period
      2) channels emotional drives without losing initiative and vigor
      3) masters environment
      4) controls emotional responses
      5) values age and life experiences
      6) Erikson's task: generativity vs self-absorption and stagnation
   c. Moral/Religious Development
      1) integrates new concepts from wider sources
      2) beliefs are less dogmatic
      3) personal philosophy offers comfort, happiness
   d. Body-Image Development
      1) adapts to climacteric; changes accepted as part of maturity
      2) reinforces positive self-concept
      3) prefers experiences, insights, values of current age
   e. Life-Style Options
      1) reflects work ethic
      2) increasing leisure time
      3) differentiates compulsive work and play from healthy work and play
      4) recognizes self-creativity
      5) increases preparation for retirement
   f. Developmental Tasks
      1) develops new satisfaction as a mate; supportive to mate; develops sense of unity with mate
      2) assists offspring to become happy, responsible adults
      3) takes pride in accomplishments of self and spouse
      4) balances work with other roles
      5) assists aging parents
      6) achieves social and civic responsibility
      7) maintains active organizational membership
      8) accepts physical changes of middle age
      9) makes an art of friendship
      10) balances leisure with service pursuits
      11) develops more depth of personal philosophy by reevaluating values and examining assets

3. Elderly (Over 65)
   a. Cognitive Development
      1) may decrease as a result of physiologic deterioration
      2) environmental events may affect cognition
         a) loss of self-esteem
         b) isolation
      3) must deal with a will, financial status, and property

- **b.** Emotional Development
  - 1) reflects on meaningfulness of life, puts success and failure into perspective
  - 2) sense of wisdom, knowledge, and self-reliance, of being able to cope with whatever comes along
  - 3) Erikson's task: integrity vs despair
- **c.** Moral/Religious Development
  - 1) may become more spiritually oriented
  - 2) value system changes from a material orientation to a more value-oriented outlook
- **d.** Body-Image Development
  - 1) must integrate continued physiologic changes
  - 2) may see body as less dependable, therefore less desirable
- **e.** Life-Style Options
  - 1) may depend on finances, family situation, state of health
  - 2) increased leisure time upon retirement
  - 3) adjusting to fixed income
  - 4) developing new hobbies and friends
- **f.** Developmental Tasks
  - 1) continued self-development (recognizing positive experience of aging)
  - 2) adapting to family responsibilities
  - 3) maintaining self-worth, pride, and usefulness
  - 4) dealing with loss of spouse, friends, upcoming end to life

I. Sexuality and Cultural Components Related to the Healthy Client
- **a.** Sexuality
  - 1) sexuality: an intrinsic part of each human
    - a) biologic, sociocultural, psychologic, and ethical components
    - b) significant part of Maslow's higher-order needs
    - c) integral part of Erikson's task for early adulthood: intimacy vs isolation
  - 2) definitions
    - a) *gender:* internal sense of masculinity or femininity
    - b) *sexual role behavior:* all we do to disclose ourselves as male or female to others
    - c) *self-concept/self-esteem:* the perceptions each individual has of self
    - d) *body image:* a person's opinion of the appearance, function, and separateness of his body; a component of self-concept
  - 3) sexual role dissatisfaction can occur with a wide variety of problems/disease states
    - a) common physical problems
      - spinal cord injuries, neuromuscular disease
      - cancer of reproductive organs, genitals
      - diabetes mellitus
      - hypertensive drug regimens
      - cardiac problems (fear)
      - advancing age, menopause
      - colostomy
      - obesity
      - venereal diseases
      - infertility
      - endocrine disorders
      - chronic illness
      - rectal, prostate carcinoma
    - b) common bio/psycho/social problems
      - disturbances in body image, self-concept
      - homosexuality, lesbianism
      - transvestitism, transexualism
      - orgasmic dysfunction, impotency
      - post-traumatic stress disorder
    - c) drugs that adversely affect sexuality
      - alcohol
      - antipsychotic tranquilizers, antidepressants, MAO inhibitors
      - antihypertensives
      - chemotherapeutic agents
      - hormones and hormone antagonists
  - 4) sexual functioning is multidimensional and influenced by a large number of variables; "normal" functioning is relative to each individual, the individual's life-style, culture, and values.
  - 5) a critical part of nursing care of the client with respect to sexual role function is that the nurse understand his/her own thoughts, feelings,

beliefs, and misconceptions about this sensitive area.
6) psychosocial support/counseling with client and significant others includes
   a) realizing that surgery in most instances will not change ability to have sexual intercourse
   b) verbalizing feelings/concerns/fears
   c) encouraging client to maximize unaltered sexual characteristics
   d) realizing and verbalizing other characteristics that are part of client's individuality

b. Cultural Variables
1) definition: culture is the organized system of behavior or way of life for an identified social group. It includes knowledge, art, beliefs, morals, laws, customs, and values that are transmitted from one generation to another.
2) psychosocial support for client and significant others includes
   a) awareness of the components of a cultural orientation
      • social institutions: family, religion, education, economics, politics
      • communication systems
   b) identifying client's specific, culturally related nursing care needs
   c) tailoring interventions to be consistent with cultural practices of client

Therapeutic Use of Self

A. Theoretical Knowledge Base
Nursing interventions in the realm of human behavior are based on a variety of theories. Table 2.1 provides an overview of the most prominent ones. Table 2.3 compares the stages of the life cycle as proposed by three theorists. The components of these constructs most applicable to nursing practice are:
1. Stages of Psychosexual Development (Freud): each stage must be negotiated successfully to avoid arrest at any one stage and mental illness.
   a. Oral Stage (0-18 months)
      1) sexual gratification and sustenance derived through the mouth; expression of dependent drives
      2) pleasure of biting; aggressive drives develop (8-18 months)
      3) infant learns to differentiate between self and mother; body image develops
   b. Anal Stage (18 months-3 years)
      1) anal and excretory satisfaction
      2) excretory control learned; associated concepts of cleanliness, punctuality, self-control, personal independence learned
      3) shame and disgust learned
   c. Phallic or Oedipal Stage (3-6 years)
      1) pleasure-giving zone centers on the genitals
      2) child forms deep attachment to parent of opposite sex
      3) child experiences intense competition with parent of same sex
      4) conflict is resolved by identifying with parent of same sex
      5) development of sexual identity; establishment of male and female roles
      6) development of guilt
   d. Latency Stage (6-12 years)
      1) limited sexual image
      2) major socialization outside the home
      3) intellectual and social growth involving school, establishment of friendships
      4) inner control over aggressive-destructive impulses is attained
   e. Genital Stage (12-20 years)
      1) sexuality again focuses on genital organs
      2) learns to become independent from parents and responsible for self
      3) learns to establish identity
      4) learns to become intimate with someone of opposite sex
2. Stages of Psychosocial Development (Erikson): focus on psychosocial crises and developmental tasks. Each crisis must be successfully resolved so the individual will be able to meet subsequent crises.
   a. Trust vs Mistrust (0-18 months): exchanges with parents lay basis for trust or mistrust of others in later life
   b. Autonomy vs Shame and Doubt (18 months-3 years): self-control, personal independence, and self-worth develop through successful management of this crisis
   c. Initiative vs Guilt (3-6 years): successful resolution of this crisis teaches the ability to share, to compete, and to be self-motivated; child learns to control jealousy, rage, envy, guilt
   d. Industry vs Inferiority (6-12 years): child develops capacity to master skills, to work and play in groups, and to grow intellectually; failure results in sense of inferiority
   e. Identity vs Role Diffusion (12-20 years): sense of self and identity apart from

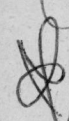

Table 2.1 Theoretical Models

Models/Proponents	Assumptions	Treatment
Medical-Biologic	Emotional disturbance is an illness or defect. Illness is located in body or is biochemical. Disease entities can be diagnosed, classified, and labeled.	Physical/somatic: surgery, ECT, chemotherapy. Therapists: physicians, others treating under MD's orders
Psychoanalytic (Freud, Erikson)	Emotional disturbance stems from emotionally painful experiences. Feelings are repressed. Unresolved, unconscious conflicts remain in the mind. Symptoms and defense mechanisms develop.	Therapy uncovers roots of conflicts through interviews within long-term therapy. Therapists: psychoanalysts, usually MDs
Social-Interpersonal (Sullivan, Peplau)	Emotional disturbance results from problematic interpersonal interaction. Client is seen as a subsystem of larger systems (e.g., family and community).	Client is approached in a holistic way. Intervention includes health promotion/illness prevention and alteration of harmful environments. Constructive interpersonal relationship is developed with therapist. Therapists: physician or nurse
Behavioral (Pavlov, Skinner, Wolpe)	Behavior can be modified by operant conditioning. • behavior that is reinforced tends to be repeated. • behavior that is ignored tends to be eliminated. Knowing the cause of the behavior is not helpful in treating deviant behavior.	Treatment aims at eliminating unwanted behavior by ignoring it and reinforcing wanted behavior. Response to behavior by therapists must be consistent. Therapists: physicians, nurses, psychologists, trained assistants
Community Mental Health	When stresses and supports are in balance, the individual is socially competent. Emotional disturbance results from imbalance between stresses and supports (see table 2.2). • too much stress and not enough support leads to social disorientation and disintegration. • too much support and too little stress leads to social dependence, immobility, regression.	Treatment is aimed at maintaining or restoring balance between stresses and supports. Levels of prevention of mental illness • *primary:* promotion of mental health and disease prevention (anticipatory guidance, education, community organization, crisis prevention). • *secondary:* early treatment to prevent long-term illness (screening, early diagnosis, case finding, brief hospitalization, crisis intervention). • *tertiary:* treatment of chronic, long-term problems (halfway houses, partial hospitalization, day hospitals). Therapists: physicians, nurses, social workers, psychologists, other trained mental health workers

THERAPEUTIC USE OF SELF 21

Table 2.2 Social Determinants of Mental Health and Illness

Stress	Individual	Support
Social • poverty • poor housing • unemployment • crowding • high rate of mobility	Genetic information Constitutional traits Developmental traits • coping mechanisms • ego strength	Social • churches and synagogues • schools • social welfare agencies

Personal
• maturational
  –adolescence
  –aging
• role changes
• situational
  –loss
  –divorce
  –separation
  –illness
		Personal
		• family network
		• friends
		• clergy
		• bartender
		• hairdresser

parents; failure results in unclear sense of self and role

f. Intimacy vs Isolation (20–40 years): individual learns to establish relationship with partner and gratifying social relationships; failure results in isolation from intimates and social peers

g. Generativity vs Stagnation (40–60 years): adult achieves productivity at home, at work, and in the community; this includes the rearing of children

h. Integrity vs Despair (60–death): individual views past and remaining life as a satisfying whole; failure leads to despair and increasing dependence

3. Defense Mechanisms (Freud)
   a. Psychologic techniques the personality develops to manage anxiety, aggressive impulses, hostilities, resentments, frustrations, and conflicts between the id (pleasure-seeking impulses) and the superego (inhibiting)
   b. Used by both mentally healthy and mentally ill persons
   c. Measure of mental health is determined by the degree that defense mechanisms
      1) distort the personality
      2) dominate behavior
      3) disturb adjustment with others
   d. Specific Defense Mechanisms
      1) *suppression**: the conscious, deliberate forgetting of unacceptable or painful thoughts, impulses, feelings, or acts
      2) *repression**: unconscious, involuntary forgetting of unacceptable or painful thoughts, impulses, feelings, or acts
      3) *isolation:* separating thought and affect, allowing only the former to come to consciousness; it is a compromise mechanism
      4) *dissociation:* walling off certain areas of the personality from consciousness
      5) *denial**: treating obvious reality factors as though they do not exist, because they are consciously intolerable
      6) *rationalization:* attempting to justify feelings, behavior, and motives that would otherwise be intolerable, by offering a socially acceptable, intellectual, and apparently logical explanation for an act or decision
      7) *symbolization:* using an object or idea as a substitute or to represent some other object or idea
      8) *idealization:* conscious or unconscious overestimation of another's attributes, e.g., hero worship
      9) *identification:* attaching to one's self certain qualities associated with others; it operates unconsciously and is a significant mechanism in superego development

*Most commonly referred to in psychiatric conditions.

Table 2.3 Life-Cycle Stages

Stage	Age	Common Name	Freud	Erikson	Sullivan	Tasks
I.	Birth–18 mo.	Infancy	Oral	Trust vs mistrust	Development of a self-system. Others gratify needs and satisfy wishes.	Dependent drives. Aggressive drive. Differentiation from mother.
II.	18 mo.–3 yr.	Toddler	Anal	Autonomy vs shame and doubt	Acculturation. Delay gratification.	Shame, disgust. Control, cleanliness. Punctuality. Independence. Self-worth.
III.	3–6 yr.	Play age	Phallic or Oedipal	Initiative vs guilt	Playmates: forms satisfactory relationships with peers.	Guilt, values. Establishment of masculine or feminine role. Sharing, competing. Self-motivation.
IV.	6–12 yr.	School age	Latency	Industry vs inferiority	Chums: relates to a friend of the same sex.	Intellectual and social growth. Mastery of skills. Establishment of friendships. Work and play in groups. Control over aggressive-destructive impulses.
V.	12–20 yr.	Adolescence	Genital	Identity vs identity/role diffusion	Early: satisfactory relationships with members of the opposite sex. Late: intimate relationship with a member of the opposite sex.	Independence from parents. Responsibility for self. Establish independent identity. Acceptance of sexual and peer relationships.
VI.	20–40 yr.	Young adult		Intimacy vs isolation		Establish intimate relationship with a partner. Gratifying social relationships. Work adjustment.
VII.	40–60 yr.	Middle age		Generativity vs. absorption or stagnation		Productivity at home, work, community. Can include reproductivity and child rearing.
VIII.	60 yr.–death	Older adult		Integrity vs despair		Fulfillment. Increased dependence. Death of friends, spouse, self.

10) *introjection:* incorporating the traits of others, internalizing feelings toward others
11) *conversion:* the unconscious expression of mental conflict by means of a physical symptom
12) *compensation*:* putting forth extra effort to achieve in one area to offset real or imagined deficiencies in another area
13) *substitution:* unconsciously replacing an unobtainable or unacceptable goal with a goal that is more acceptable or obtainable; the process is more direct and less subtle than sublimation
14) *sublimation*:* directing energy from unacceptable drives into socially acceptable behavior
15) *reaction formation*:* expressing unacceptable wishes or behavior by opposite overt behavior
16) *undoing*:* thinking or doing one thing for the purpose of neutralizing something objectionable that was thought or done before
17) *displacement*:* transferring unacceptable feelings aroused by one object or situation to a more acceptable substitute
18) *projection*:* unconsciously attributing one's own unacceptable qualities and emotions to others
19) *ideas of reference:* believing that one is the object of special and ill-disposed attention by others
20) *fantasy:* satisfying needs by daydreaming
21) *regression*:* going back to an earlier level of emotional development and organization
22) *fixation:* never advancing the level of emotional development beyond that in which one feels comfortable
23) *withdrawal:* separating oneself from interpersonal relationships in order to avoid emotional expression or responsiveness

B. Nurse-Client Relationship
1. Purpose: to provide counseling, crisis intervention, or individual therapy
2. Characteristics
   a. Mutually defined relationship
   b. Mutually collaborative
   c. Goal-directed
   d. Interpersonal techniques facilitate communication
   e. Development of therapeutic relationship fostered
   f. Relationship differs from friendship
      1) specific boundaries established
      2) purpose, time, and place of interaction are specific
      3) professional demeanor and objectivity maintained
   g. Nurse assists client with problem resolution
   h. Successful relationship leads to mutual growth for client and nurse
3. Facts to remember
   a. It is not a friendship
   b. Its main benefit is to the client
   c. It presents an opportunity to the client to deal with the problems that brought him to treatment
   d. The nurse's approach to the relationship is crucial to the client's being able to express his feelings
   e. Increased experience and education allow the nurse to have more discretion in relating to clients, but new practitioners should "go by the book"
4. Therapeutic Communication: review table 2.4, "Communication Skills in the Nurse-Client Relationship"
   a. Interpersonal techniques that facilitate communication are the principal tools for the nurse and many NCLEX-RN items relate to these.
   b. Techniques listed as "blocks" may *sometimes* be used effectively by experienced practitioners; however, new graduates should avoid selecting such techniques.
   c. The NCLEX-RN will test for the ability to identify the *best* technique in a situation, as well as to distinguish therapeutic from nontherapeutic communication.
5. Phases of the Nurse-Client Relationship
   a. *Initiating or Orientating Phase:* establishes boundaries
      1) when, how long, how often nurse will meet with client
      2) focus of relationship spelled out to client
      3) usually time of anxiety for client and nurse
         a) client may come late to meetings or miss them

Table 2.4 Communication Skills in the Nurse-Client Relationship

Therapeutic Interpersonal Techniques

Using silence	
Accepting	Yes, uh hmm, I follow what you said (nodding).
Giving recognition	Good morning, Mr. S. You've tooled a leather wallet. I notice that you've combed your hair.
Offering self	I'll sit with you a while. I'll stay here with you. I'm interested in your comfort.
Broad opening statement	Is there something you'd like to talk about? What are you thinking about? Where would you like to begin?
Using general leads	Go on. And then? Tell me about it.
Placing the event in time or in sequence	What seemed to lead up to. . .? Was this before or after. . .? When did this happen?
Sharing observations	You appear tense. Are you uncomfortable when you. . .? I notice that you're biting your lips. It makes me uncomfortable when you. . . .
Encouraging description of perceptions	Was it something like. . .? Have you had similar experiences?
Reflecting	*Client:* I can't sleep. I stay awake all night. *Nurse:* You have difficulty sleeping.
Focusing	This point seems worth looking at more closely.
Exploring	Tell me more about that. Would you describe it more fully? What kind of work?
Giving information	My name is. . . Visiting hours are. . . My purpose in being here is. . . I'm taking you to the . . . .
Presenting reality	I see no one else in the room. That sound was a car backfiring. Your mother is not here; I'm a nurse.
Voicing doubt	Isn't that unusual? Really?
Clarifying	Tell me whether my understanding of it agrees with yours. Are you using this word to convey the idea? I'm not sure that I understand what you're saying.
Verbalizing inferred thoughts and feelings	*Client:* I can't talk to you or to anyone. It's a waste of time. *Nurse:* Is it your feeling that no one understands? *Client:* My wife pushes me around just like my mother and sister did. *Nurse:* Is it your impression that women are domineering?
Encouraging	What are your feelings in regard to. . .? Does this contribute to your discomfort?
Suggesting collaboration	Perhaps you and I can discover what produces your anxiety.
Summarizing	Have I got this straight? You've said that. . . During the past hour, you and I have discussed. . . .
Encouraging formulation of a plan of action	Next time this comes up, what might you do to handle it?

    b) client may exhibit nervous mannerisms
    c) client may sit silently, hallucinate, or exhibit delusions
    d) nurse may be more likely to use responses that block communication, because of own anxiety
    e) neither nurse nor client view each other as unique human beings

    4) preparation for termination begins at this stage
    5) client will test boundaries set by the nurse
 b. *Working Phase:* exhibits reduction of anxiety in both client and nurse
    1) client accepts boundaries of relationship
    2) nurse uses interpersonal skills that foster communication

Table 2.4 Continued

Blocks to Therapeutic Communication

False reassurance	Everything will be all right. You don't need to worry. You're doing fine.
Giving advice	What you should do is... Why don't you...?
Giving approval	That's the right attitude. That's the thing to do.
Requesting an explanation	Why are you upset? Why did you do that?
Agreeing with the client	I agree with you. You must be right.
Expressing disapproval	You should stop worrying like this. You shouldn't do that.
Belittling the client's feelings	I know just how you feel. Everyone gets depressed at times.
Disagreeing with the client	You're wrong. That's not true. No, it isn't.
Defending	Your doctor is quite capable. This hospital is well equipped. She's a very good nurse.

     3) client confronts problems and feelings
     4) client develops insights, learns methods of coping and problem solving
         a) begins to come to meetings on time
         b) uses the time with nurse as a "working" time
     5) nurse and client see each other as unique people
  c. *Terminating Phase:* begins when work of relationship is over and builds on preparation made during orientation phase
     1) client and nurse summarize and evaluate work of relationship
     2) both express thoughts and feelings about termination
     3) client may have high anxiety in this stage, exhibited as
         a) hostility
         b) disparagement of relationship
         c) hallucinations, delusions
         d) regressive behaviors
         e) recall of other separation experiences
     4) initial boundaries of relationship should be maintained during termination
     5) termination can be difficult for both client and nurse

C. Nursing Process
1. Assessment: observing, interviewing, and examining the client to determine problem areas and strengths
   a. Note the "ABCs"
      1) *A*ppearance: dress, grooming, affect
      2) *B*ehavior: gestures, mannerisms, activity level
      3) *C*ommunication: appropriateness, clarity, disorder, expression of feelings
   b. Gather information on thought processes, orientation, judgment, insight, work and/or school history, drug and alcohol history
   c. Complete appropriate components of mental-status examination
   d. Complete a review of systems to uncover any outstanding physiological disturbances that affect emotional status
2. Analysis: evaluating information gathered during assessment and making nursing diagnosis
3. Goals (Expected Outcomes) and Interventions: developing client goals and nursing interventions to meet them; these plans will reflect the health team's plan for treatment, will be guides for psychiatric aides and other personnel who give care
4. Implementation: carrying out the nursing care plan; provide suitable environment for client based on behavior, i.e., setting

limits, increasing or decreasing stimuli, providing activities
5. Evaluation: appraising client's response to nursing interventions and modifying the plan as necessary

D. Treatment Modalities
1. Psychotherapy
   a. Definition: goal-oriented, corrective emotional experience with a therapist in order to effect behavioral change, which may include
      1) increased well-being
      2) improved psychologic performance
      3) improved social performance
   b. Length of Treatment
      1) may be long term, to allow client to gain insight and slowly take on new coping mechanisms
      2) may be short term, such as crisis intervention
2. Crisis Intervention
   a. Definition: a time-limited (approximately 6 weeks), directive approach to help a client cope with a crisis
      1) person is in crisis when traditional methods of coping are not effective
      2) crises tend to resolve after several weeks, however, if the present one is ineffectively resolved, the person may have lost some ability to cope with future crises
   b. Therapy
      1) includes helping an individual or family cope with an immediate problem
      2) does not go into cause
      3) does not require insight as does traditional therapy
      4) deals directly and briefly with the situation the individual is in
         a) clarifies situation and identifies problem
         b) teaches client new coping skills
         c) identifies and mobilizes external and internal resources
      5) attempts to return client to at least the previous level of coping
      6) helps persons in crisis become amenable to change because the crisis is intolerable (this is the motivation-of-crisis work)
      7) helps the client learn to problem solve and thus client may grow because of the intervention
      8) is the kind of intervention that may prevent maladaptation into more serious psychiatric symptoms
   c. The process of therapy includes
      1) establishing a nurse-client relationship
      2) being as active and directive as necessary to help client deal with crisis
      3) helping the client to establish therapeutic goals
      4) reinforcing that the relationship is time-limited and therefore it is necessary to establish a termination date
      5) actively encouraging the client to express feelings and emotions regarding the crisis situation
      6) assisting the client to develop new and more effective coping mechanisms
      7) the client taking more responsibility in subsequent sessions (if there is more than one)
      8) a time-limited span: may take from one to several sessions, but is not a long-term process
3. Milieu Therapy: stresses the development of interpersonal and personal skills in a conducive environment
   a. Activities: include client government, occupational and recreational therapy
   b. Requirements: close collaboration between staff and clients toward mutually defined goals
   c. Heavy emphasis on maintaining independence of clients
   d. Clients are responsible for their own behavior
4. Therapeutic Groups: more closely resemble real-life situations than one-to-one therapy
   a. Leading these groups requires training beyond basic nursing education
   b. Beginning nurse may colead a group
   c. Group members provide feedback for each other
   d. Variety of responses and reactions available for behavior displayed in group setting
   e. Three stages of development
      1) group orientation and development of identity
      2) group interaction and observation of dynamics
      3) resolution of dynamics and production of insights

- **f.** Members may examine patterns of relating to each other and authority figures in supportive atmosphere
- **g.** Group therapy more economical than one-to-one therapy; there are usually two therapists and 7-10 clients
- **h.** The goals and purposes are essentially the same as in one-to-one therapy
5. Family Therapy: focuses on the family rather than on the individual
    - **a.** Major Problem: intolerance of differences
        1) healthy family can tolerate differences
        2) maladjusted family experiences differences as threats to individual identity and family unity; conflicts lead to splits, coalitions, scapegoating
    - **b.** Major Objective: to reestablish rational communication between family members
        1) family can reassess and recognize alliances
        2) family can resolve to accept differences between members
    - **c.** Important difference between family therapy and group therapy
        1) in family therapy, the participants enter therapy with a long-standing system of roles and interactions, which the nurse-therapist must learn
        2) in group therapy, the relationship between participants begins with the 1st session; they have no history of a relationship
6. Self-Help Groups: use persons who have themselves surmounted problems. Nurses may serve as consultants/resource persons.
    - **a.** Recovery, Inc.
        1) a consumer-funded group consisting of former mental clients and persons with nervous disorders
        2) focus is on the use of will power in avoiding deviant behavior
    - **b.** Other Self-Help Groups
        1) Parents without Partners
        2) groups for colostomy clients
        3) parents whose children have terminal diseases
        4) Overeaters Anonymous
        5) Reach for Recovery
        6) Alcoholics Anonymous (see page 93)
        7) Narcotics Anonymous (see page 98)

Loss, Death and Dying

General Concepts
A. Overview
1. Every human being experiences several losses during a lifetime, e.g., loss of a relationship or health, loss of a loved one, change in life-style. People deal with loss by grieving and integrating the subsequent changes into their life.
   a. Responses to loss vary greatly depending upon the individual's personality, previous experience with losses, and value of the person or thing lost.
   b. Behavior during normal grieving is similar to that seen in a depressed person, e.g., crying, fatigue, feelings of emptiness. Unlike grief, depression is a chronic state characterized by low self-esteem.
2. Definitions
   a. *Loss:* the anticipated or actual removal of something or someone of value to a person
   b. *Grief:* the normal emotional responses to a loss, which subside after a reasonable time
   c. *Unresolved grief:* failure to complete the grieving process and cope successfully with the loss because of social and psychologic factors
      1) socially unspeakable loss, e.g., suicide
      2) uncertainty over loss, e.g., person missing in action
      3) need to be strong and in control
      4) ambivalence over lost object or person
      5) overwhelmed by multiple losses
      6) reawakens an old, unresolved loss
   d. *Mourning:* the expression of sorrow with outward signs of grief as a result of a perceived or threatened loss
   e. *Grief and Mourning Process:* the process a person goes through in adapting to a loss; this process is triggered by an *actual* or a *threatened* loss
3.
4. The grief and mourning process, according to Engel
   a. Three Stages *Grief*
      1) *shock and disbelief:* usually lasts 1–7 days
      2) *developing awareness* of the loss: lasts several weeks to months
      3) *restitution:* takes a year or more
   b. Adaptive responses to a loss are
      1) first stage: crying, screaming, denial
      2) second stage: blaming self or bargaining; alternating between first-stage behaviors and asking questions about living with the loss
      3) third stage: making plans for the future, speaking comfortably about loss
   c. Maladaptive responses to a loss are
      1) first stage: absence of crying or verbal expression of loss
      2) second stage: persistent guilt and low self-esteem
      3) third stage: isolation of self, lack of interest in living
      4) any time: any kind of destructive behavior
5. According to Kubler-Ross (the theorist most often associated with death and dying), there are five stages in the grief and mourning process of the dying person (these stages can be applied in evaluating other losses).
   a. *Denial:* may last from a few minutes at one extreme to the remainder of the time the person lives; it allows the person to mobilize defenses to cope with the terminal process

Never challenge denial or a delusion

b. *Anger:* is expressed when the person begins to realize what is happening and that it can no longer be denied
c. *Bargaining:* is usually done with God (e.g., an effort to get more time in exchange for church participation)
d. *Depression:* results from loss of function and also the anticipated loss of everything and everyone of value
e. *Acceptance:* is almost devoid of feelings about the loss; the dying person has found some peace and often wishes to be left alone or to associate with only one or two persons

6. A child's understanding and responses to death depend on
   a. Age
      1) preschooler can't differentiate between death and absence
      2) from 5-6 years old, they see death as something others experience, begin to accept death as a fact, believe death is reversible
      3) from 6-9 years old, children associate death with injury; personify death (someone bad carries them away)
      4) from 9-10 years old, they recognize everyone must die
      5) early adolescents understand permanency of death; difficult to see self dying before having a chance to live; may experience resentment, withdrawal, see self as different from others; also concerned about possible different reaction of others (e.g., withdrawal of friends)
   b. Previous experience with death: relatives, friends, pets, family responses to death
   c. Knowledge of what is happening
   d. Other influences
      1) whether child is hospitalized; staff behavior
      2) parents' anxieties
      3) reaction of other family members, siblings

7. Children will convey their feelings and level of understanding of their impending death through symbols (drawings, stories, play with toys and other children) and behaviors such as anger, fear, hostility, withdrawal.

B. **Application of the Nursing Process to the Client Experiencing a Loss**
   1. Assessment
      a. Current Behavior
         1) stage of grief and mourning
         2) adaptive or maladaptive
      b. Previous Losses
      c. Support System
   2. Goal, Plan/Implementation, and Evaluation

   Goal: Client will receive reinforcement for adaptive behaviors; will move through the grief and mourning process within an acceptable time frame.

   Plan/Implementation
   - allow the client to utilize own method of coping as long as he is not physically destructive
   - reinforce adaptive behavior; remember that suicidal ideation is not adaptive in any stage
   - tell client that it is normal and expected to grieve over a loss
   - help client to express feelings ("You look sad. What are you feeling right now?"); listen attentively and with empathy
   - be alert to indications that client is moving into next stage of grieving

   Evaluation: Client responds adaptively to the loss (e.g., talks about the specific loss; asks questions about the future).

Selected Health Problems

A. Loss (Other than Death and Dying)

1. **General Information: types of loss**
   a. Physical losses include loss of
      1) a body part, e.g., a breast
      2) usual function of a body part, e.g., paralysis of a limb
      3) a valued object, e.g., a house
      4) economic changes
      5) loss of youth, beauty, health
      6) a significant other, either through loss of a relationship or through death
   b. Psychologic losses include loss of
      1) meaning in life, beliefs, or values
      2) status, recognition, prestige
      3) meaningful work, creative abilities
      4) self-esteem and self-worth
      5) nurturance and sense of belonging
      6) loss of expected outcome, e.g., stillborn infant
      7) changes in role identity, self-concept

30 SECTION 2: NURSING CARE OF THE CLIENT WITH PSYCHOSOCIAL PROBLEMS

2. **Nursing Process**
   a. **Assessment** (refer to page 29)
      1) specific loss
      2) meaning of loss to client
   b. **Goals, Plans/Implementation, and Evaluation**

   Goal 1: Client will respond adaptively to the loss.
   Plan/Implementation
   - allow client to cry, express anger, or exhibit other adaptive responses to the loss
   - provide support for adaptive behavior (e.g., "It must be very difficult for you right now.")
   - help client to express feelings (e.g., "Other clients in your situation often feel sad or angry. How do you feel?")

   Evaluation: Client exhibits adaptive behaviors (e.g., cries, feels sad).

   Goal 2: Client begins to move to second stage of the grief and mourning process.
   Plan/Implementation
   - continue to help client to express feelings
   - when client asks questions about living with loss, tell him only what he wants to know at this time (in-depth teaching can be done later when client is ready)
   - reinforce all adaptive behaviors
   - expect that client will alternate between behaviors of the first and second stages

   Evaluation: Client asks questions about adapting to the loss; cries less frequently.

B. **Death and Dying**
   1. **General Information**
      a. Responses to the dying process are highly individualized and may be greatly influenced by the client's physical status as well as his own personality. The interaction of client and family will have a strong bearing on the client's healthy progression through the process.
      b. Nurse's Responses
         1) in order to be effective in helping the dying person, the nurse must focus on her own beliefs, feelings, and behaviors in regard to death
         2) unless the nurse becomes aware of her own feelings, fears, and beliefs about death, she may unwittingly inhibit her client's expression of feelings; her own feelings will become more powerful than her desire to help
         3) as the nurse understands her own feelings, she increases her ability to be empathetic to others' feelings
         4) by looking at her beliefs about death and how people should respond to death, she can be aware when she is expecting others to respond in accordance with her belief system
      c. Establishing Priorities
         1) priorities may be determined by the client's psychologic and physical status
            a) at some point, pain or fatigue may demand more attention than the psychologic factors
            b) a client who cannot keep any food down or cannot feel relief from pain needs the nurse to respond to those factors immediately
         2) the next most important action is to assist the client to deal with the manifestations of whatever stage he is in
         3) assist the family to interact in healthy ways with client by healthy role modeling, discussing illness and death with the client

   2. **Nursing Process**
      a. **Assessment**
         1) physical condition and relationship to psychologic stimulus
         2) knowledge of and response to diagnosis; people respond to dying similarly to the way they have responded to other major crises
         3) stage in dying process: the stage can fluctuate, or client/family may be in more than one stage at a given time
            a) current behavior
            b) current affect and feelings expressed
         4) support from significant others
         5) expectations and resources
         6) feelings about being in hospital or elsewhere
         7) family assessment
            a) perception of diagnosis and prognosis; stage of loss
            b) feelings and their influence on client
            c) communication patterns
            d) needs and resources

e) response to dying person and impact on client

b. Goals, Plans/Implementation, and Evaluation

Goal 1 (Stage 1): (Content between the asterisks is adapted from M. Neal et al. *Nursing Care Planning Guides, Set 1*, 2nd Ed. "Dealing with Impending Death," No. 1:27. Baltimore: Williams & Wilkins, 1980. Used with permission.): *Client will use denial and isolation to begin to deal with impending death.

Plan/Implementation
- know that client may have a feeling of "the need to protect others," to "fight the battle alone;" be available to spend at least 10 minutes with client daily either conversing or just being with him
- assist client to realize that denial and isolation are normal reactions to the news of the impending loss of life
- allow client to use denial for a period of time until adequate defenses have been mobilized to deal with the impact of the diagnosis and prognosis
- answer questions about life, death, and treatment honestly; clients don't want you to be harsh in your honesty, but they also don't want to be fooled; leave room in your answers for clients to maintain hope if they choose to do so
- do not reinforce clients' denial of their condition (e.g., when clients make an unrealistic statement, "I'm going to be back to work soon," respond in a realistic manner, "It must be difficult for you right now.")

Evaluation: Client denies and finally acknowledges reality of situation; reality is recognized and reinforced by staff.

Goal 2 (Stage 2): Client will express anger verbally about impending death.

Plan/Implementation
- allow and encourage the verbal expression of anger: remember, client is thinking, "Why does it have to be me?" Often this feeling is displaced on others; it is not personally directed at you but is a coping strategy the client is using
- know that the anger may be self-directed and associated with guilt about not seeking medical attention earlier; allow the client to express these concerns but not ruminate on them
- allow open discussion of alternative treatment and life-style options brought up by the client; assist in consideration of these by giving clear, factual information about any alternatives; remember it is the client's choice
- listen to client express anger about distancing behavior from relatives and friends

Evaluation: Client openly expresses anger about current situation.

Goal 3 (Stage 3): Client will try to utilize bargaining to prolong life.

Plan/Implementation
- allow client to cope by bargaining; client may use phrases such as, "If only..." or "I could do..."
- ask client about the importance of the events being bargained for; in this way, you express your availability to listen to discussion of feelings
- part of the bargaining may include the timing and interval of treatment or lack of such; allow the client the opportunity to make such decisions; be sure client is aware of the risk and consequences but allow him to make the decision
- know that this stage is characterized by magical thinking, which helps the client feel the ability to exercise some control over his situation

Evaluation: Client demonstrates progress through grief and mourning process (i.e., bargains).

Goal 4 (Stage 4): Client will verbally recognize the inevitable and allow self to feel sad and depressed.

Plan/Implementation
- know that the client may express sadness verbally or by crying, silence, or talking; when clients attempt to share sadness, do not try to cheer them up, but acknowledge their feelings
- such questions as, "Am I going to die?" are a test of staff's willingness to listen to the client talk about concerns, sadness, and fears; respond, "Do you feel you are going to die?" then support and discuss responses
- be aware that during this stage clients may be so overwhelmed with sadness that they no longer want to talk or be involved in treatment; they may feel "What difference does it make?" Focus

on the normalcy of feeling sad and ascertain with clients what difference coping with the impending death rather than giving up will make to them
- if clients choose not to move beyond this stage, feeling that if they stay depressed they will not have to make a decision about fighting or accepting death, gently remind them that staying depressed involves making a decision not to make another decision
- offer the client opportunities to talk about the impending loss of all that is of value in his life; in addition, the client must have a chance to express feelings about changes in body image and self-esteem

Evaluation: Client expresses recognition of sad, depressed feelings; begins to talk about inevitable outcome.

Goal 5 (Stage 5): Client will accept the impending death as inevitable.
Plan/Implementation
- acceptance involves the realization that death will occur; in preparation for such, the client has taken care of personal and family matters; is able to say death will occur and stops struggling
- know that often acceptance is not achieved but resignation is the method of resolution; resignation involves realizing that death will occur, but the client does not want it to happen; the struggle continues, and client is not at peace with self
- utilize comfort and security measures as necessary for a peaceful conclusion of the dying process
- let client decide whether he would prefer to be alone for periods of time; restrict visitors to short periods of time as client desires*
- the family may not be at the same level of coping as the client
  - spend time with them discussing their feelings
  - know that families respond to the dying member much as they handled other major crisis situations
  - family's greatest needs may be competent physical care for the ill member and empathy for the difficulty of their situation
  - they appreciate the nurse who helps them with packing, arranges a comfortable place to sleep in the hospital that night, or lets them call at any time to find out how their ill relative is or when they can visit

Evaluation: Client moves through the stages of loss at own rhythm to a comfortable and dignified death; expresses feelings and concerns about impending death; participates in decision making for own ADL for as long as is possible; the family or significant other discuss feelings and concerns about death of loved one.

3. **Application of the Nursing Process to the Dying Child**
   a. **Assessment**
   1) child's level of understanding and reaction/feelings about situation; ability to express self with symbols (e.g., play, stories, drawings)
   2) parents' level of understanding and reaction/feelings about situation; parents' strengths and needs
   3) child's physical condition (e.g., vital signs, pain, hydration, needs for ROM, skin care, comfort or security measures)
   4) staff members' feelings and concerns, need for support
   5) siblings' level of understanding; their responses to behavior and health changes in ill sibling, separation from hospitalized ill sibling
   b. **Goals, Plans/Implementation, and Evaluation**

Goal 1: The child/family will express feelings, fears, anxieties, guilt they may be experiencing; will verbalize their understanding of the physical health status and the terminal process.
Plan/Implementation
- determine what the child knows
- work through own feelings; plan to get support from other staff members
- allow and encourage the parents to express their feelings and accept those expressions in a nonjudgmental manner
- permit child to express anger and hostility, but at the same time, do not be totally permissive regarding unacceptable behavior (child may perceive this permissiveness as total hopelessness and abandonment)
- allow child to draw or play with toys to express feelings

- draw own body
- draw a feeling
- draw family
- play doctor/nurse and act out angry feelings; let nurse be the client
* acknowledge the variety of family responses
  - shock, denial, guilt
  - acceptance, belief in God
  - overprotection
  - encourage interaction/involvement of ill child and siblings
  - help siblings to express their feelings; use drawing, storytelling, play therapy
  - help parents understand that siblings' perceptions/interpretations/reactions may not be as intense as parents'
  - "favorite child" angers other siblings; stress is also on siblings who need a chance to discuss feelings; they, too, may feel they did something to cause sibling to become ill
  - stress on marriage: assist with marital stress by encouraging couple to spend an evening away from the hospital and to call when they feel concerned about their child
* refer family to self-help groups in community

Evaluation: Child/family has expressed some degree of awareness of the terminal process; verbalizes some feelings associated with grief and mourning.

Goal 2: Child will maintain as much independence as possible in ADL; will have minimal pain and discomfort; will ingest adequate food and fluid to meet body needs.

Plan/Implementation
* encourage child's participation in ADL as long as his energy levels are not depleted
* ensure adequate fluid and food; use supplements when necessary and allow child choice of food if possible
* preserve skin integrity by massage, lotions, sheepskin, water mattress
* provide pain medication and comfort measures prn
* use passive and active ROM
* permit toys, music, and special objects to be with child
* allow parents to participate in care; explain procedures to parents/child

Evaluation: Child maintains independence in ADL (e.g., feeds self, ambulates to bathroom alone); has minimal pain and discomfort; ingests food and fluid to meet body needs.

inCompetency is not irreversible

Legal Aspects of Psychiatric Nursing

2 Physician certificate (Psychiatrist)

A. Civil Procedures: the court protects the rights of psychiatric clients utilizing civil procedures. Many persons are referred to psychiatric services through the courts. Psychiatric expert testimony is used by the courts when a person uses insanity as a defense.
  1. Civil Admission Procedures
     a. General Information
        1) The Mental Health Systems Act (1980) provided states with a Recommended Bill of Rights for mentally ill clients
        2) each state has its own mental health code determined by the legislature; it provides guidelines for admission procedures of the mentally ill to hospitals for treatment of mental illness
        3) there is considerable disparity among the states in legal commitment procedures
     b. Voluntary Admission: any person over a certain age can apply for admission to an institution for the cure of the mentally ill
        1) admission implies that the individual agrees to receive treatment and abide by hospital rules
        2) most states require that client give written notice to the hospital if requesting early discharge *(72hr. notice)*
        3) if physician believes this release to be dangerous to client or others, involuntary admission must be arranged through the court *(in 3 DAYS)*
        4) in most states a child under the age of 16 may be admitted if his parents sign the required application form
        5) clients retain all rights with voluntary admission
     c. Involuntary Admission: application for admission is initiated by someone other than the client
        1) requires certification by one or two physicians that person is a danger to self and/or to others
        2) the person has a right to a legal hearing within a certain number of hours or days
        3) commitment or discharge may be determined by the judge or jury
        4) most states limit commitment to 90 days
        5) extended commitment is usually for no longer than 12 months
        6) in most states, client retains the right to consult a lawyer at any time
     d. Emergency Admission: any adult may execute an application for emergency detention of another. If a physician is not available, a magistrate must certify that the person is in risk of harming self or others. Medical or judicial approval is required to detain the person beyond 24 hours.
        1) a person who is hospitalized against his will may force court action for release through a procedure called habeas corpus
        2) the court will determine the sanity and alleged unlawful restraint of the person
  2. Competency Hearings: separate from admission hearings
     a. Admission to mental hospital does not mean a person is <u>incompetent to manage own affairs</u>
     b. Legally, *incompetency* indicates the person is no longer able to make responsible decisions for himself, his dependents, or his property

does not anticipate consequences of own behavior.

LEGAL ASPECTS OF PSYCHIATRIC NURSING 35

c. Person declared incompetent has legal status of a minor, i.e., cannot
   1) vote
   2) make contracts or wills
   3) manage personal property
   4) drive a car
   5) sue or be sued
   6) hold a professional license
d. A guardian is appointed for the incompetent person, and has the power of consent
e. Mentally retarded, chronic alcoholics, senile persons can be found incompetent
f. Procedure can be instituted by state or family

B. **Criminal Procedures:** many persons are referred to psychiatric services through the courts; psychiatric expert testimony is used by the courts when a person uses insanity as a defense
   1. Insanity as a Defense: means a person has been indicted for having committed a crime, will stand trial, and will plead not guilty by reason of insanity
      a. Persons found guilty can be sentenced to prison
      b. Persons found not guilty are committed to a mental hospital until judged sane by staff
      c. When released, person who was found not guilty by reason of insanity usually is free and has no legal ruling against self
   2. Tests of Insanity
      a. Definition: a legal term meaning the person had impaired judgment or did not realize the consequences of his actions because of mental illness
      b. An accused person is not criminally responsible for unlawful act that was result of mental disease or defect
      c. Determined by jury, based on psychiatric expert testimony
   3. Inability to Stand Trial: a person accused of committing a crime is mentally irresponsible at time of trial
      a. The person is unfit to stand trial if he cannot understand the charge against him, or is incapable of cooperating with his own defense
      b. If found unfit to stand trial, must be sent to psychiatric maximum security unit until mentally healthy
      c. Once mentally fit, must stand trial and serve sentence, if convicted

C. **Territories:** of psychiatry and law overlap in many ways because both disciplines deal with human behavior

D. **Judicial Precedents:** some have been set recently that
   1. Give clients the right to treatment
   2. Require institutions to devise specific plans of treatment for their individual clients
   3. Require that the plans of treatment be the least restrictive of clients' liberty their condition allows
   4. Protect civil rights
   5. Ensure confidentiality
   6. Give client right to refuse treatment

E. **Role of the Nurse:** functions as advocate for client
   1. Implements nursing care that meets ANA Standards of Psychiatric-Mental Health Nursing Practice
   2. Knows the mental health code of the state in which she or he practices
   3. Charts to reflect accurate observations and interventions
   4. Maintains confidentiality of client information
   5. Consults a lawyer if clarification is needed
   6. Knows difference between omission and commission
      a. Omission: failing to do what should have been done
      b. Commission: doing what should not have been done
   7. Monitors client's understanding of consent forms for medical/psychiatric procedures, e.g., ECT
   8. Monitors nursing actions relative to client protection to prevent assault or battery
      a. Assault: words or actions that produce genuine fear that action will occur without consent
      b. Battery: unconsented touching or restraining of a person without legitimate rationale

Anxious Behavior

General Concepts

A. Overview
1. Anxiety can be a problem in and of itself, but is also an aspect of all other psychosocial problems. Anxiety is a subjective feeling brought on by a nonspecific threat to self. In mild degrees, it is a normal experience that motivates a person to take constructive action in a situation. As anxiety becomes more severe, it can interfere with perception, judgment, and behavior, and requires outside intervention to help the person to function constructively.
2. Anticipatory anxiety, anxiety, and fear are all accepted official nursing diagnoses with established defining characteristics.
   a. *Anticipatory anxiety:* an increased level of arousal associated with a perceived *future* threat to the self
   b. *Anxiety:* a generalized feeling of dread and apprehension, which is a subjectively painful warning of a threat to the self or to significant relationships
   c. *Fear:* a feeling of dread related to an *indentifiable* source that is perceived as a threat or danger to the self or significant relationships
   d. *Anxious behavior:* a manifestation of a subjective feeling resulting from the experience of anxiety, conflict, fear, or stress. Such response ranges from mild to severe, and represents a usual human reaction to a sense of threat.
3. General Causes
   a. A threat to biologic integrity
   b. A threat to security of self; anxiety is a warning signal requesting the organism to act against the threat
   c. A person's own defenses are not working as well as they usually do
4. In psychoanalytic theory, the term *anxiety* is reserved to describe an intrapsychic experience that arises from unconscious conflict and is brought on by a nonspecific threat to self.

Regardless of the different interpretations of the sources of anxious behavior, its prominence as a human occurrence makes it one of the most common concerns in psychosocial nursing. Recognition of anxious behaviors and the appropriate use of helping interventions are essential nursing skills in any health care setting.

B. Application of the Nursing Process to the Client Exhibiting Anxious Behavior
1. **Assessment**
   a. Physiologic and psychologic signs and symptoms
   b. Cause, if known
   c. Coping Mechanisms: adaptive or destructive
2. **General Nursing Goal, Plan/Implementation, Evaluation**

   Goal: Client will use anxiety as a motivation for change.
   Plan/Implementation
   - help client express feelings about stressful situations, unmet needs
     - assist client to acknowledge or name the feelings being experienced
     - express genuine attitude of interest and concern
   - be nonjudgmental and offer unconditional acceptance
   - offer reassurance by giving appropriate information, correcting misinformation; repeat the process if necessary as client may have reduced hearing perception; use short, concise statements

- work with client to identify anxiety-causing situations that can be avoided
- teach client to recognize how he is manifesting anxiety in his behavior
- help client identify situations that trigger anxiety
- assist client to use stress-reduction techniques (e.g., biofeedback, visualization, talking it out) to cope with anxiety; read reprint, "Stress Management," page 113
- be aware that client and nurse have reciprocal influence on each other
  - anxiety is contagious
  - find constructive ways to control own anxiety, frustration, or anger
- prevent mild anxiety from escalating by intervening early, whenever possible
- provide physical care as needed to severely anxious client

Evaluation: Client expresses feelings; identifies situations that cause anxiety; incorporates at least one stress-reduction technique into daily routine; experiences no more than moderate anxiety.

Selected Health Problems
A. Anxiety
1. **General Information**
   a. Four Levels of Anxiety or anticipatory anxiety: on a continuum from mild to panic, which primarily involves sensory perception and level of functioning
      1) *mild anxiety:* characteristics
         a) more alert than usual, increased questioning
         b) heightened capacity to deal with perception of impending danger
         c) focus of attention on immediate events
         d) person experiences mild discomfort, restlessness
         e) may be a useful motivating force; e.g., if a person experiences mild anxiety during NCLEX, this may help to increase ability to answer questions
      2) *moderate anxiety:* characteristics
         a) narrowed perception
         b) reduced ability to listen and comprehend
         c) selective inattention, focus on one specific thing; "tunnel vision" develops
         d) increased tension; increased discomfort; verbalization about expected danger
         e) decreased ability to function
         f) physical symptoms including, e.g., pacing, hand tremors, diaphoresis, increased heart rate, sleep and/or eating disturbances
      3) *severe anxiety:* characteristics
         a) greatly reduced perception; difficulty attending to, understanding, and processing information
         b) sense of impending doom
         c) increased physical symptoms, e.g., diaphoresis, dizziness, increased muscle tension, pallor
         d) dysfunctional coping
         e) survival response (fight or flight)
      4) *panic:* characteristics
         a) altered perception of and focus on reality
         b) helpless, fearful, panicky feelings
         c) physical symptoms, e.g., tachycardia, hyperventilation
         d) extreme discomfort; extreme measures to decrease anxiety
         e) feeling of personal disintegration
         f) severe hyperactivity
   d. Diagnosis of Anxiety: inferred from three kinds of data: physiologic changes, psychologic changes (see table 2.5), and use of coping or defense mechanisms

Table 2.5 Manifestations of Anxiety

Physiologic	Psychologic
Tachycardia	Tension
Palpitations	Nervousness
Excessive perspiration	Apprehension
Dry mouth	Irritability
Cold, clammy, pale skin	Indecisiveness
Urinary frequency	Oversensitivity
Diarrhea	Tearfulness
Muscle tension	Agitation
Tremors	Dread
Narrowing of focus	Horror
	Panic

1) physiologic changes
   a) involve primarily the autonomic nervous system
   b) physiologic operations tend to be speeded up by mild and moderate anxieties
   c) functioning tends to be slowed down by severe panic; can result in complete functional paralysis and death (in prolonged panic)
   d) knowledge of physical manifestations allows the nurse to intervene prior to the panic stage
   e) during panic, when the physical symptoms are severe, immediate intervention is imperative
2) psychologic changes
   a) psychologic manifestations accelerate as anxiety level increases and can become extremely uncomfortable to the person
   b) maladaptive behaviors are mechanisms used to avoid acceleration of anxiety to the panic state (e.g., rumination, compulsivity)
3) coping mechanisms: may be a defense mechanism or any means used to resolve, or at least delay, the conflict
   a) constructive: client, alerted by warning signal that something is not going as expected, resolves the conflict
   b) destructive or disturbed: client tries to protect self from anxiety without resolving the conflict, which can be expressed in maladaptive or dysfunctional behavior
   c) there is a relationship between level of anxiety and type of coping mechanisms used
      • mild-moderate anxiety
        - tendency to use constructive coping mechanisms
        - if the anxiety does not increase, then coping mechanisms are functional
        - e.g., in a test situation, student uses relaxation techniques, deep breathing and tells self that he knows the material as well as possible; if these activities work and the anxiety does not increase, then the coping mechanisms are functional
      • moderate-severe-panic level
        - tendency to use destructive or disturbed coping mechanisms
        - if anxiety continues to increase, then the person must find new ways to cope and may turn to destructive coping mechanisms
        - e.g., student may run out of the room, try cheating or other methods, take on certain neurotic behaviors
        - development of "neurotic" behavior (e.g., phobia, dissociative reaction) is not conscious

2. **Nursing Process**
   a. **Assessment** (refer to page 36)
      1) level of anxiety (signs and behaviors)
      2) coping mechanisms (constructive and/or destructive)
      3) problematic behavior (e.g., weekly episodes of gastritis indicating moderate anxiety related to work conflict)
      4) support systems and their involvement with client
   b. **Goals, Plans/Implementation, and Evaluation**

   Goal 1: Client will develop an open, trusting relationship with the nurse.
   Plan/Implementation
   • approach client in unhurried way and actively listen to concerns and feelings
   • encourage client to express feelings and concerns about unmet needs or stressful situation
   • be aware of one's feelings and behavior and their impact upon client
   Evaluation: Client expresses his concerns and unmet needs to the nurse (e.g., concern about failure or rejection).

   Goal 2: Client will recognize own behaviors of anxiety and gain insight into cause of problems.
   Plan/Implementation
   • assist client to recognize his anxiety by exploring the feelings that precede his anxious behavior

- utilize the nurse-client relationship to increase the client's ability to gain insight into the cause of his problems
- provide a new perspective on the situation, i.e., help client "redefine" the problem
- utilize biofeedback learning to help client to recognize his own tensions
- teach client to evaluate the threat, expectations, or unmet needs and to assess own capabilities realistically

Evaluation: Client identifies own behaviors that are linked to current anxiety; tells nurse when he is feeling increasingly anxious; can state cause(s) of current anxiety.

Goal 3: Client will learn and demonstrate alternative methods of coping with anxiety.
Plan/Implementation
- examine client's patterns of coping with anxiety
- reinforce effective and constructive coping mechanisms
- teach client alternative methods of coping, e.g., visual imagery, relaxation, talking it out
- know that the client with mild-moderate anxiety is generally not hospitalized for treatment depending upon
  - severity of the symptoms
  - incapacity of function
  - threat to self or others
  - nature of the home environment
- observe physical status and intervene directly as necessary for client's well being

Evaluation: Client learns two new coping mechanisms (e.g., talking about feelings, guided imagery; experiences more control over his anxiety).

Goal 4: Client will be able to cope with severe to panic anxiety and reduce anxiety at least one level.
Plan/Implementation
- understand that a severely anxious client may neglect physical needs, exhaust self, or actually injure self; give physical care and protection as indicated
- remove client from other clients if anxiety is increasing
- anticipate and prevent mild disturbances from developing into severe or panic stage by identifying with client early signs of disturbance
- allow client to determine what stresses he can handle
- know that coping mechanisms keep the anxiety within tolerable limits
- do not attempt to argue, ridicule, or reason with a client regarding his defense mechanisms
- help client to adopt and develop effective, positive coping mechanisms
- when tranquilizing agents are prescribed
  - administer as ordered to provide symptomatic relief of anxiety and

Table 2.6 Minor Tranquilizers

Drug	Dosage	Side Effects	Nursing Implications
Meprobamate (Miltown)* (Equanil)	400 mg TID or QID 800-1,600 mg daily	Skin rash. Itching. Urticaria. Drowsiness.	Gradual withdrawal because of both physical and psychic dependence. Warn about hazardous professions and activities. Causes drowsiness.
Chlordiazepoxide (Librium)	5-25 mg TID or QID daily 15-100 mg PO daily 50-200 mg IM daily	Occasional nausea. Constipation. Skin rash. Drowsiness. Ataxia. Confusion.	Gradual withdrawal of drug. Warn about hazardous professions. Symptomatic treatment for side effects. Suicide factor sometimes present.
Diazepam (Valium)	2-10 mg BID, TID or QID 4-40 mg PO daily	Drowsiness. Dizziness. Vertigo. Syncope.	Causes some liver damage. Blood studies should be done frequently during initial period. See Librium (above).

*Trade names are in parentheses.

tensions and to create stability so client may be more able to participate in process of therapy
- know that drugs have potential for addiction and should be prescribed for only short periods of time; drugs may also rob client of motivation for change
- teach client that minor tranquilizers should not be taken with alcohol, as each affects the CNS and enhances the effect of the other
- teach the client actions and side effects of drugs (a common side effect of tranquilizers is drowsiness; therefore persons taking these drugs should avoid driving or involvement in any potentially dangerous activity)
- when client's anxiety has decreased, negotiate reasonable limits on his anxious behavior
- do not reinforce phobias, rituals, or physical complaints by giving them undue attention
- provide physical protection from repetitive acts; some ritualistic behaviors can cause physical discomfort, e.g., compulsive hand washing
- know that client may not be able to sit and may need to keep moving; if so, nurse should walk with him

Evaluation: Client reduces anxiety to at least a moderate level; does not injure self or others; has a constructive, effective coping mechanism (e.g., talking about feelings, whistling, punching bag).

B. Phobias
1. **General Information**
   a. Definition: intense, irrational, fearful reactions to objects or situations, which may interfere with normal function of the person
   b. Common Phobias
      1) agoraphobia: marked fear and avoidance of being alone or in public places from which escape would be difficult
      2) social phobia: persistent fear and compelling desire to avoid situations in which the person is exposed to scrutiny of others for fear of being humiliated or embarrassed
      3) simple phobia: persistent fear and desire to avoid an object or situation (other than agoraphobia or social phobia)
         a) claustrophobia: fear of closed places
         b) acrophobia: fear of heights
         c) zoophobia: fear of animals
   c. Ego defense mechanism utilized is displacement
   d. General treatment measures include individual or group psychotherapy, progressive relaxation and desensitization, behavior modification, and reciprocal inhibition

2. **Nursing Process**
   a. Assessment
      1) level of anxiety: signs and behaviors may be those of mild-panic, depending on situation
      2) specific fear and fearful situation
      3) constructive behavior or coping mechanisms
      4) problem behaviors or maladaptive coping mechanisms
   b. Goals, Plans/Implementation, and Evaluation

Goal 1: Client will identify and discuss fear.
Plan/Implementation
- allow client to describe the fearful experience and identify physiologic responses that may accompany the fear
- use open-ended questions such as, "What bothers you the most about going into elevators?"
- accept feelings and concerns about fearful experience without agreeing with client; e.g., "This must be hard for you," or, "You have been having a difficult time with this situation."
- attempt to identify the specific source of fear

Evaluation: Client can state situation that caused the fear and talk about the associated feelings.

Goal 2: Client will accept and participate in treatment to reduce phobic responses.
Plan/Implementation
- offer hope that treatment will help reduce phobic response
- utilize interventions for mild-moderate or severe-panic anxiety
- allow client to make independent decisions about activities of daily living in hygiene, exercise, involvement in milieu activities

ANXIOUS BEHAVIOR 41

- utilize desensitization, behavior modification, individual and group psychotherapy to enable client to learn new coping behaviors and gain insight into phobic reactions
- listen to and positively reinforce client's experiences of participation in treatment to reduce phobic responses

Evaluation: Client participates in treatment program, and expresses feelings about own response to group.

C. Dissociative Reactions

1. General Information

a. Definition: hysterical reactions characterized by bizarre behavior in which the individual splits off one portion of his conscious mind from the total when that portion represents some major, otherwise unresolvable, conflict for him

Repression

b. Precipitating Event: catastrophic event; characterized by memory loss of the event when person returns to "normal state"

c. *DSM-III* Classifications
   1) *psychogenic amnesia:* sudden, extensive inability to recall important personal information
   2) *psychogenic fugue:* sudden, unexpected travel away from home or customary workplace with assumption of new identity and inability to recall one's past identity
   3) *multiple personalities:* existence in an individual of two or more distinct personalities, each of which is dominant at specific times
   4) *depersonalization disorder:* loss of sense of one's own reality in the absence of psychosis (e.g., self-estrangement, feeling of unreality)

d. Ego defense mechanism utilized is repression; example
   1) person may not remember a certain, anxiety-provoking period of his life
   2) these clients can be admitted to a psychiatric unit not remembering who they are and where they are from; these are termed "John Doe" admissions
   3) dynamics: in using the mechanism of repression, the person removes from consciousness his identity and the situation that caused the overwhelming anxiety

e. Treatment: hypnosis, group or individual psychotherapy ↓Anxiety

2. Nursing Process

a. Assessment
   1) careful observation and assessment of client's physical condition to help rule out organic causes such as brain tumor
   2) note patterns of dissociative behavior, including
      a) preceding events, duration, frequency
      b) client's reaction to milieu and persons
      c) verbal and nonverbal behaviors
   3) identify fundamental source of anxiety as early as possible

b. Goal, Plan/Implementation, and Evaluation

Goal: Client will be oriented to time, place, and person and will participate in reality-based activities.

Plan/Implementation

- relate to the client within reality of the situation, i.e., call client by name, orient to time and place as needed
- expect client to participate in reality-based milieu activities, i.e., activities of daily living, exercise, group activities
- minimize obvious and alterable sources of stress to keep anxiety contained to a manageable level
- utilize interventions for mild-severe anxiety, depending on behaviors

Evaluation: Client can state own name, where he is, day of the week; participates in group activities (e.g., exercise class, psychotherapy group).

D. Obsessive-Compulsive Disorders

1. General Information

a. Definition: presence of obsession (uncontrollable, recurring thoughts) or compulsion (a ritualistic act done in an attempt to relieve the anxiety related to the thoughts or to make the thoughts go away); considered to be a psychologic conversion reaction to anxiety

b. Ego defense mechanisms utilized are displacement and undoing; the person attempts to displace unconscious, hostile, aggressive impulse into unrelated acts (i.e., hand washing); in so doing, the person attempts to undo or negate the unacceptable impulse

42 SECTION 2: NURSING CARE OF THE CLIENT WITH PSYCHOSOCIAL PROBLEMS

c. Signs and Symptoms: may include ritualistic behaviors, i.e., compulsive hand washing or cleanliness or habitual responses such as extreme thrift, neatness, or insistence on same daily routine, with panic or bizarre behavior if usual routine is broken

d. Treatment: individual, family, or group psychotherapy, desensitization, behavior modification

2. Nursing Process

a. Assessment
1) note patterns of compulsive behaviors including preceding events, and client's reactions to specific situations and persons
2) listen for description of obsessions

b. Goal, Plan/Implementation, and Evaluation

Goal: Client will accept limits on repetitive acts and participate in alternative adaptive activities.

Plan/Implementation
- give client a schedule to follow so that ritualistic/repetitive behaviors are *limited*, but not prohibited
- allow client to have choices in schedule and participate in decisions as to how time and energy will be used
- do not abruptly interrupt the repetitive act, as it is allaying anxiety; interruption allows the anxiety to break through and can cause panic
- set reasonable limits on repetitive behavior; give the client adequate warning that at a certain time another activity will begin
- engage in alternative activities with client; do not expect the client to proceed in another activity alone
- provide physical protection from repetitive acts; some ritualistic behaviors can cause physical discomfort, e.g., compulsive hand washing
- as ritualistic/repetitive behaviors decrease, assist client to express feelings and concerns in socially acceptable ways

Evaluation: Client washes hands (or other compulsive act) fewer times/day compared with admission; is beginning to participate in other activities.

E. Anorexia Nervosa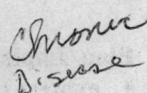

1. General Information

a. Definition: a symptom complex with compulsive resistance to eating, intense fear of being obese, and loss of weight in excess of 25% of recommended body weight

b. Onset: occurs usually in female clients 15–25 years of age

c. Etiology: thought to have origins in the early developmental stages with disturbances in family relationships, ambivalent feelings toward the mother and independence

d. Prognosis: reports of up to 21% of affected youth die from malnutrition, intercurrent infection, or other physical problems such as heart failure

e. *DSM-III* Classification: listed with other eating disorders that are usually first evident in childhood and adolescence, e.g., bulimia (voracious eating from psychologic causes followed by self-induced vomiting) and pica (craving for unnatural foods such as plaster from walls, dirt, clay)

f. Treatment: bed rest, hospitalization for intravenous or oral feedings to restore electrolyte and nutritional balance, psychotherapy, behavior modification, family therapy

2. Nursing Process

a. Assessment
1) weight and percentage of normal body weight lost
2) eating patterns (amount and types of foods taken, time)
3) vomiting after eating, or if food is forced
4) anemia, hypotension, amenorrhea
5) relationships and interactions with parents, friends, staff, other clients
6) feelings about eating, body image, self
7) positive coping mechanisms, strengths, interests

b. Goals, Plans/Implementation, and Evaluation

Goal 1: Client will regain/maintain fluid and electrolyte balance and have adequate nutrition for growth and development.

Plan/Implementation
- express concern and acceptance
- avoid threats, pleas, and health advice
- keep accurate I&O; observe amounts and types of food eaten
- observe for 2 hours after eating, to prevent vomiting/regurgitation
- administer tube feedings/intravenous feedings as ordered
- provide positive reinforcement for weight gain rather than amount of food eaten

Evaluation: Client regains/maintains fluid and electrolyte balance and has adequate nutrition for growth and development.

Goal 2: Client will express feelings and concerns about self and treatment plan; will participate in treatment plan.

Plan/Implementation
- approach with calm, accepting attitude
- assist to express feelings and concerns about self, body image, treatment plan
- verbally recognize and reinforce authentic communication of feelings, concerns, and perceptions
- consistently point out misperceptions
- provide opportunities for choice and decision making in treatment plan and ADL, i.e., time of meal, type of food to be eaten, hygiene, exercise, leisure activities
- know that control issues are an important dynamic; client needs to accept responsibility for self without guilt or ambivalence
- set and maintain firm limits; be clear about limits and consistent with treatment plan
- provide opportunities for staff to meet to ventilate feelings about manipulative and self-destructive behavior

Evaluation: Client expresses feelings and concerns about self/treatment plan; participates in treatment plan (e.g., makes decisions about schedule and activities).

F. Psychosomatic Disorders

1. General Information
a. Definition: psychologically meaningful environmental stimuli are temporarily related to the initiation or exacerbation of a physical condition with demonstrable organic origin or known pathophysiologic process
b. Psychosomatic disorders are sometimes confused with hypochondriasis; the latter is an exaggerated concern with one's physical health and there is no associated organic pathologic condition
c. Reactions: include eczema (skin), migraine headaches (cardiovascular system), backaches (musculoskeletal system), gastrointestinal and respiratory disorders, and psychogenic pain
d. Ego defense mechanism utilized is repression: emotional tension is unconsciously channeled through visceral organs
e. Occurrence: often seen in medical settings and becomes a psychiatric problem when anxiety escalates in spite of physical disorder
f. Possible Secondary Characteristics
1) *dependence:* a person may manifest normal or abnormal dependency needs
    a) inability to make decisions
    b) extreme lack of confidence
    c) a need for more help in meeting problem situations
    d) anxious persons often lack the confidence and living skill to set up a beneficial living situation
2) *secondary gain:* describes an experience of the person resulting from the primary symptom that may be advantageous and/or satisfying to that person
    a) this can be a severe problem, because if the secondary gain is great, recovery may not be chosen by the client; recovery is delayed or prevented
    b) this is an unhealthy way of controlling one's environment rather than doing so in a more socially acceptable way
3) *controlling behavior:* refers to a situation in which a person attempts to exercise a dominating influence over another person
    a) the controlling person feels helpless because of a lack of control over matters pertaining to own self and welfare
    b) fear of this loss generates anxiety and often provokes aggressive, manipulative behaviors

c) controlling behavior includes manipulative techniques to get other persons to do things they would not choose to do (e.g., stay with ill person, feel sorry for person) and generally provokes anger in the manipulated person
4) *self-centeredness:* sometimes referred to as narcissism, is manifested by an undesirable egotism that springs from chronically unsatisfied self-regard and a compensatory need for self-love
   a) the self-centered person uses others to satisfy excessive needs, usually irritates others, and is isolated from the comfort and help of good relationships with others
   b) often believes that any other type of relationship cannot be achieved
   c) low self-esteem leads to belief that needs can be met only through excessive self-attention

2. Nursing Process
a. Assessment
1) signs and symptoms of physical disorder
2) life stressors, perceptions, and reactions to stressors
3) awareness of relationship of stress to symptom
4) secondary, moving-toward behaviors of dependence, secondary gains, control, self-centeredness
5) positive support systems
6) positive coping behaviors and nondisorder-related hobbies, relationships

b. Goals, Plans/Implementation, and Evaluation

Goal 1: Client will express feelings, perceptions, and concerns about symptom and treatment plan; client will participate in treatment plan.

Plan/Implementation
- approach with calm, accepting attitude
- assist to express feelings, perceptions, and concerns about symptoms and treatment plan
- know that physical symptoms are real
- verbally recognize and reinforce authentic communication of feelings, concerns, and perceptions
- involve client in planning and decision making for activities of daily living (ADL) and treatment plan; offer choices in ADL and treatment plan as much as possible
- give appropriate information about medications and treatment
- give verbal and nonverbal reinforcement (smiles, nurse's presence, time) for positive coping mechanisms

Evaluation: Client expresses feelings, perceptions, and concerns about symptom and treatment plan; client participates in treatment plan (e.g., makes decisions about daily schedule, chooses activity group).

Goal 2: Client will perform negotiated self-care activities independently.

Plan/Implementation
- attempt to identify the source of the dependency
  - ongoing lifelong style of coping
  - environmentally stimulated (has the hospitalization decreased and/or removed so much of the client's control that client has turned to dependency as a means of coping?)
- do not criticize or openly acknowledge the dependent behavior
- give frequent, intermittent attention at times other than when the client asks for something
- state when you will be back; return then or send someone else
- praise any independent behaviors
- explain to client that you will not allow him to be so dependent because you respect him and realize that he could do things for himself prior to hospitalization, and that now you do not want to take this independence away
- negotiate areas of self-care and independent activity

Evaluation: Client can verbalize areas of self-care and areas where assistance is needed; can perform self-care without constant attention.

Goal 3: Client will receive treatment for problem of secondary gain; will develop alternatives to primary symptom for coping with anxiety.

Plan/Implementation
- understand unconscious motivation of the behavior and differentiate it from malingering (a deliberate effort to use

an illness to avoid an uncomfortable situation)
- focus intervention on understanding and alleviation of primary symptoms
- encourage exploration with you of the motivation for client's behavior
- explore alternatives to the primary symptom for handling anxiety (e.g., talking directly about the concern, asking for help and support, setting limits with others, saying "no" appropriately)

Evaluation: Client discusses reasons for behavior; develops alternative coping mechanisms (e.g., expressing feelings, asking for help).

Goal 4: Client will accept limits on controlling, manipulative behaviors; will participate in treatment plan.

Plan/Implementation
- recognize person's means of attempting to gain control (negativism, obstinacy, silence, avoidance, increased chatter, crying)
- set limits on controlling/manipulative behaviors; state time limits; make expectations clear; do not impose unnecessary controls
- utilize alternative approaches that allow attainment of the therapeutic goal while permitting the client to retain feeling of control; avoid a battle of wills
- plan daily routine and treatment with client; offer choices in such procedures as timing of medications, baths, hygiene, and decision making relative to activities
- be consistent and support other staff to be consistent
- provide opportunities for staff meetings to ventilate feelings about manipulative behaviors

Evaluation: Client accepts limits on controlling/manipulative behaviors; makes some decisions about own daily schedule, activity groups.

G. Conversion Disorders

1. General Information
a. Definition: hysterical reactions that are manifested by the dysfunction of an organ of special meaning to the person
b. *DSM-III* Classification: a sub-classification of somatoform disorder
c. Conversion disorders differ from hypochondriasis in that in hypochondriasis there is no loss of function. They differ from psychosomatic disorders in that in psychosomatic disorders there is a demonstrable organic origin or known pathophysiologic process; in conversion disorders there is not.
d. Characteristics include
  1) symbolic expression of anxiety (e.g., anxiety about seeing something is controlled by becoming blind, a teacher loses voice)
  2) there is no demonstrable physical lesion
  3) symptoms do not follow motor-nerve paths
  4) the person shows little concern about the incapacity caused by the symptoms (*"la belle indifférence"*)
e. Defense mechanisms utilized are repression and displacement
  1) primary gain: repression keeps anxiety or need out of client's awareness
  2) may have secondary gain of attention; does not have to do work, take care of self

2. Nursing Process
a. Assessment
  1) symptoms of physical disorder and vital signs
  2) client's perceptions of symptoms: *"la belle indifférence"*
  3) stressors, strengths, and positive coping behaviors
b. Goal, Plan/Implementation, and Evaluation

Goal: Client will obtain symptomatic relief from anxiety and physical symptoms; will participate in self-care and therapy process.

Plan/Implementation
- approach in unhurried, calm, accepting manner
- allow client to describe feelings/concerns
- give appropriate information; involve client in decision making in ADL
- do not focus on physical symptoms; assist client to change focus to healthy interests (music, exercise, friends, plans)
- engage in alternative activities with client; do not expect client to proceed in

another activity alone—share it with the client
- monitor responses to drug therapy
- assist with lab tests, x-ray procedures to rule out organic basis for symptoms

Evaluation: Client is relieved of physical symptoms and experiences decreased anxiety; participates in self-care and therapy process.

H. Post-Traumatic Stress Disorders

1. General Information
a. Definition: anxiety neurosis resulting from severe external stress that is beyond what is usual or tolerable for most people
b. Stressors: rape, military combat, natural disasters (e.g., earthquakes), physical accidents involving loss of life of another or loss of body part or its functions (e.g., post accident permanent paralysis), accidental disasters caused by people (e.g., crashes, fires), intentional disasters (e.g., bombing, torture), victims of criminal assaults (e.g., robbery)
c. Characteristics
  1) reexperiencing trauma in at least one of the following ways
    a) recurrent/intrusive recollections of event
    b) recurrent dreams of event
    c) sudden acting out or feeling as if traumatic event were recurring, owing to environmental or ideational stimulus
  2) numbing of responsiveness to or decreased involvement with external world after the trauma
    a) markedly diminished interest in one or more significant activities
    b) feeling of detachment or estrangement from others
    c) constricted affect
  3) at least two of the following symptoms, which were not present before the trauma
    a) hyperalertness or exaggerated startle response
    b) sleep disturbance
    c) guilt about surviving or about behavior required for survival
    d) memory impairment or trouble concentrating
    e) avoidance of activities that arouse recollection of traumatic event
    f) intensification of symptoms by exposure to events that symbolize or resemble traumatic event
d. Related Factors
  1) physical injury may be present because of the nature of the trauma
  2) depression and anxiety are usually present
e. Dynamics: loss of self-esteem and loss of control in the traumatic situation have led to the behavior and feelings described above

2. Nursing Process
a. Assessment
  1) nature of the traumatic event
  2) duration of disorder
  3) degree of impairment
  4) preexistence of problems that may complicate situation (e.g., anxiety, depression)
  5) presence and degree of symptoms
  6) positive support system available
b. Goals, Plans/Implementation, and Evaluation

Goal 1: Client will recount the traumatic event and cope with feelings related to it.

Plan/Implementation
- give client time to describe event in own words (doing so gives client increased sense of control over own thoughts)
- accompany client if there is a need to return to the scene of the trauma
- help client to identify and vent feelings of sadness, loss, guilt, anger, frustration
- be nonjudgmental and matter-of-fact
- acknowledge significance of the traumatic event and the appropriateness of client's feelings
- reinforce that client is worthwhile
- help client to feel safe and secure
- review goals and plans for crisis intervention (page 26), depression, rape (in following pages of this section), and loss (page 30)

Evaluation: Client is able to describe the event and to discuss feelings related to it (e.g., sadness, anger).

Goal 2: Client will resume involvement in external world.

Plan/Implementation
- take measures to prevent the client from becoming isolated
- involve client in a recovering group of people with similar problems (e.g., Victims for Victims)
- gradually increase reinvolvement in pretrauma activities
- discuss feelings about activities
- reinforce client's involvement in activities
- give information about social, financial, or health resources

Evaluation: Client gradually resumes involvement in activities of importance to him.

AIDS affects the brain → organic

Confused Behavior

General Concepts

A. Overview: Confusion can be related to physiologic or psychologic disturbances. It is a bio/psycho/social disorder involving the inability to comprehend and/or integrate words, relationships, or events. It is associated with one or more factors including electrolyte imbalance, infection, chemical or nutritional imbalances, cerebral disease, trauma, and respiratory disturbances.

Confusion can also reflect a combination of physiologic and psychologic interferences with daily functioning. It can be a symptom of other disturbances or a severe disturbance itself. It may be short lived or permanent. Often, confusion is attributed to chronic organic brain syndrome when other physiologic or environmental factors are causative.

B. Application of the Nursing Process to the Client Exhibiting Confused Behavior

Certain physiologic and environmentally induced confused behaviors are short-lived and directly associated with factors that can be controlled, changed, or improved. When the causative factors create permanent or progressive changes, the confusion becomes a chronic state—the selected health problem outlined below.

Selected Health Problem
Chronic Confusion
1. **Definition**
   a. A mental dysfunction related to the response of the brain to disease, damage, or the aging process
   b. Specific Syndromes
      1) Alzheimer's disease: degeneration of the cortex and atrophy of cerebrum; usually begins in persons in their early 60s, death 1-10 years post onset
      2) Korsakoff's syndrome: associated with chronic alcoholism *confabulate — Do not challenge*
      3) trauma-induced confusion, e.g., stroke, residual problems related to neurosurgery
      d. *DSM-III* Classification: chronic organic mental disorder

2. **Nursing Process**
   a. Assessment
      1) onset history
      2) *confused* — orientation to person, time, and place
      3) problems with attention, comprehension, e.g., absentmindedness, inability to understand and follow requests
      4) memory: impairment of recent or remote memory; use of confabulation to cover memory loss
      5) judgment and decision making
      6) speech patterns and social interaction
      7) paranoid ideation
      8) self-care abilities
      9) previous coping mechanisms
      10) feelings and concerns about treatment, impairment
      11) family involvement
      12) physiologic problems: respiratory, skin, cardiac, nutrition, rest and activity
   b. **Goals, Plans/Implementation, and Evaluation**

Goal 1: Client will maintain or improve self-care activities to maintain optimal physiologic functioning.
Plan/Implementation
- arrange for client to have needed eyeglasses, hearing aid, false teeth, and other assistive devices for activities of daily living (ADL)
- plan ADL schedule based on client's established patterns; allow client to

make schedule and activities decisions as appropriate
- give client specific, simple directions for ADL; provide assistance only if client cannot function alone; allow sufficient time for client to perform ADL
- provide range-of-motion (ROM) exercises at least once daily; assist with ambulation as necessary
- schedule rest periods during the day as needed
- follow client's established bedtime routine; avoid use of sedatives, which may increase confusion
- offer 6 small feedings daily of nutritionally balanced foods and fluids
- keep skin clean, dry, and free from surface irritants or pressure that impedes circulation
- supervise medication consumption (kind, time, amount); know side effects of drugs given and carefully observe and record client responses to all medications and treatments
- record vital signs and I&O daily

Evaluation: Client performs some ADL with assistance; attains and maintains ambulation with assistance as required; sleeps six hours nightly; maintains adequate nutritional intake; maintains skin integrity.

Goal 2: Client will regain and maintain contact with reality.
Plan/Implementation
- establish routine; avoid changes in routine or environment
- provide hourly orientation to time/place/person; use clocks, calendars, signs, pictures, and written reminders
- put client's picture and name (big letters) on the door to room and on the bed
- use concrete symbols (photographs, tangible creations) of client's past to strengthen and reassure client's sense of continuity of the self (now threatened with brain deterioration)
- answer questions repeatedly as needed, using short, simple sentences; demonstrate nonverbally to reinforce verbal communications; build on the reality-based statements of the client to strengthen conversation; talk about familiar subjects; establish eye contact when addressing client
- assist client to use previously successful coping mechanisms
- provide adequate sensory stimulation; avoid both sensory deprivation and overload
- utilize touch: back rub, skin care, hold hands as you/client are comfortable doing so
- respect client's privacy (space, time, possessions)
- avoid physical restraints or environmental confinement, which increase helplessness
- obtain necessary orders and administer appropriate symptomatic chemotherapy; observe and record behavioral changes
- help the family and friends, so they will not withdraw from the client
  - discuss client's behavior, memory loss, and confusion; recognize and help them to work through their own feelings of helplessness, anger, depression, love, and guilt; discuss importance of continued interaction for client's self-esteem
  - help them prepare for client's continuing care by raising questions, considering solutions, exploring alternatives, and deciding on a goal and plan of action that meets their needs as well as the client's

Evaluation: Client is oriented as to person, time, and place; interacts with others appropriately; family and friends maintain interaction with client; client and family make reasonable plans for client's continuing care.

Elated-Depressive Behavior

General Concepts
A. Overview
1. Affective disorders are a variety of states and syndromes. They include extremes in mood and affect such as depressive or manic behavior and unresolved grief.
2. Affective states may be viewed as a mood state or a clinical syndrome. For example, the mood state of depression may occur in a normal person, in a client with a psychiatric syndrome, or in a medical client.
3. Management Modalities (Treatment): depends on the severity of the symptoms and includes psychotherapy, chemotherapy, convulsive therapy (electroshock), and milieu therapy in a hospital setting or on an ambulatory basis
   a. Chemotherapy consists of antidepressant drugs (see table 2.7, reprints)
   b. Psychotherapy is aimed toward achieving insight into the underlying depression, acknowledging feelings of worthlessness, and increasing self-esteem
   c. Milieu therapy in the hospital offers client a safe emotional and physical environment
      1) requirements for treating elation or depression in hospital include
         a) protection from self-harm
         b) removal from unbearable pressures encountered outside the hospital
         c) need for problem solving in a sheltered, supportive environment with access to other therapies, reliable atmosphere
         d) staff attitudes that demonstrate interest and a desire to offer the help needed
      2) staff reaction to elated or depressed clients is often characterized by a feeling of ineffectiveness
         a) this can lead to avoidance of client, request for assignment change
         b) engenders further feelings of worthlessness in client, creating further withdrawal
         c) the feelings must be dealt with to ensure a therapeutic milieu
         d) staff must recognize potential for this rejection cycle and avoid it; the staff can support each other in treating client
         e) avoid becoming defensive with manic clients
            - clients have uncanny sensitivity to others' weaknesses and inadequacies; they constantly point these out
            - staff must tolerate criticisms without becoming defensive
            - defensiveness fuels attack and is counterproductive
   d. Electroconvulsive Therapy (ECT)
      1) only form of shock (convulsive) therapy still in use
      2) one of the chief benefits is that it often makes a client more accessible to psychotherapy
      3) electric shock is delivered to brain through electrodes on temples
         a) produces immediate unconsciousness
         b) produces a cerebral seizure
         c) effective in reducing symptoms

B. Application of the Nursing Process to the Client with an Affective Disorder
1. Assessment
   a. Behavioral Changes
      1) combativeness
      2) yelling or screaming
   b. Emotional Changes
      1) anger
      2) anxiety

ELATED-DEPRESSIVE BEHAVIOR 51

Table 2.7 Antidepressants

Generic Name (Trade Name)	Dosage	Side Effects	Nursing Implications
MAO Inhibitors (Mono-amine-oxidase)			
Isocarboxazid (Marplan)	Initially 30 mg daily; then 10-20 mg daily	Headache. Dizziness. Blurred vision. Dry mouth. Postural hypotension. Increased appetite. Dermatitis. Hepatitis. Euphoria. Activates latent schizophrenia.	Potentiates action of many drugs • narcotics • barbiturates • sedatives • atropine derivatives May cause severe headaches. Hypertension with natural foods (e.g., aged cheese) and alcoholic beverages (e.g., beer and wine).
Tricyclic Antidepressants			
Amitriptyline HCl (Elavil, Endep)	10-25 mg TID PO	Dizziness. Nausea. Excitement. Hypotension. Anorexia.	Observe client for side effects and treat symptomatically.
Imipramine HCl (Tofranil)	50-200 mg daily	Dizziness. Weight gain. Skin rash. Hypotension.	Not to be given with MAO inhibitors or immediately following treatment with MAO inhibitors.
Others			
Lithium carbonate	300 mg QID PO Blood level: 0.6-1.0 mEq/l. Toxic blood level: 2.0 mEq/l or greater. Acute mania: 600 mg QID	GI discomfort • nausea • vomiting • stomach pain Thirst. Dazed feeling. Drowsiness. Hand tremor.	Remind client to take medicine. *Frequent blood work needed to assess level of drug.* Client requires careful supervision. Risk of suicide. Monitor salt intake.
Chlordiazepoxide-amitriptyline (Limbitrol)	*5-12.5 PO TID, QID †10-25.0 PO TID, QID	Same as Elavil.	Same as Elavil. Indicated for moderate to severe depression associated with moderate to severe anxiety.

*5.0 mg of chlordiazepoxide, 12.5 mg of amitriptyline
†10 mg of chlordiazepoxide, 25 mg of amitriptyline

3) delusions
4) guilt
5) hostility
6) impaired concentration

c. Physical Changes
1) eating disorders
2) sleep disturbances (too much or too little)
3) interest in sex (increase or decrease)

2. **Goal, Plan/Implementation, and Evaluation**

Goal: The elated or depressed client will demonstrate increased ability to cope with painful feelings by accepting nurse's presence, sharing feelings with nurse and others, and will explore ways to cope with feelings.

Plan/Implementation
- build rapport and relationship by spending time with client at least twice daily; start with 5-10 minutes, and increase time as you and client can tolerate it; encourage client to identify and share feelings with you, accepting what is said; use silence, just the presence of a caring person is helpful when one is learning to cope with painful feelings; *avoid* reassurance
- focus on client's feelings; allow ventilation in ways that seem

- comfortable to the client; share with client that the only way to get through feelings is to stay with them and experience them
- help client explore ways to cope with feelings; talk about alternate ways to express them (e.g., to express anger, try handball, racketball, hitting a punching bag or mattress, shouting, singing, confronting with words, swearing, using batacus, tearing up phone books, throwing sponges or bean bags)
- know that most often anger is directed inward in form of low self-esteem and worthlessness; when directed outward, may seem unprovoked and excessive
- urge client to identify angry feelings
- encourage client to explore sources of anger and to express anger verbally
- avoid arguments, involvement in client's set of rules, and avoid discussions that involve moral values
- prevent punishment that extends to self-mutilation (remove sharp objects, matches, cigarettes)
- involve client in minimal tasks and activities
- know that guilt is related to feelings of repressed hostility, accompanies most depressions, and leads to self-condemnation: client sets up punishing set of rules and regulations
- acknowledge client's view of guilt but show that this is client's view, not nurse's
- assist client to express guilt: explore situation and persons with whom the client experiences guilt, "I feel guilty when I..."; have client try to replace the word "guilt" with "resentment;" explore feelings about this; most situations that involve guilt also involve feelings of anger and resentment; work on these feelings with client
- explore with client the identity of persons in his life with whom he is willing to share feelings; if there is no one, explore with him how this came about and his feelings about this situation; if client expresses dissatisfaction with having no one to share feelings with, explore ways to change situations; practice using role-playing or psychodrama to try alternative ways to initiate sharing of feelings
- explore with client how he feels about listening to others' feelings; often people who have problems tolerating their own feelings tend to feel overwhelmed with others' feelings; practice sharing feelings of being overwhelmed and setting limits on listening to problems; if other clients are willing and available, practice reciprocal sharing of feelings, with discussion of how to set limits and keep relationship
- listen to client focus on meaning of loss, somatic symptoms, feelings tone, "It seems like it just isn't worth it." "You've had a hard time lately, and you're learning to deal with your feelings." "You've lost someone you loved, and you're going through grief and mourning." "Sounds like you remember the good parts and the rough parts of this relationship, and you're beginning to be ready to risk again."
- give positive reinforcement to reality-oriented behavior and realistic expectations

Evaluation: Client demonstrates increased ability to cope with painful feelings (e.g., identifies and expresses the anger, guilt); shares feelings and concerns with nurse and others.

Selected Health Problems

A. Depression

1. **General Information**
   a. Definitions
      1) a disorder of mood or affect characterized by feelings of dejection, sadness, and hopelessness
      2) operational definition: gratification is received from a love object; loss of love object leads to frustration, anxiety, grief, guilt, and hostility; this results in loss of self-esteem and depression
   b. Precipitating Factors
      1) loss of a loved one through separation or death is the most common precipitant; the loss must be significant to the person
      2) threats to self-esteem: disruption in the interpersonal and intrapersonal input of love, respect, and approval results in decreased self-esteem
      3) success: paradoxically, one may become depressed upon achieving

success; this is due to the anticipation of loss of self-esteem if one does not live up to the expectations implied by the success
4) somatic syndromes: depression is often superimposed on other types of psychiatric illness, e.g., gastrointestinal problems, which are really depression in disguise; these are called somatic equivalents of depression
5) physical illness: depression is interrelated with many physical illnesses because of real or anticipated loss of function, independence, role of well person
6) self-image: changes in perception of self as a result of physical, emotional, or life-style changes including role changes, body changes

c. States of Depression: depression may be felt to some degree by anyone; in terms of severity of disruption, there are four kinds of depression
   1) *transitory depression*
      a) seldom seen as presenting problem
      b) mild physiologic problems
      c) symptoms: careful observation reveals a quiet, restrained, inhibited, unhappy person; may appear self-depreciative, may express feelings of hopelessness or have difficulty making decisions, or both; the person may feel trapped and inadequate and be overconcerned with personal problems
      d) short-lived; person institutes own cure
   2) *reactive depression* (exogenous)
      a) *DSM-III* classification: uncomplicated bereavement
      b) related to precipitating environmental or physiologic stress or personal loss (e.g., death of someone close)
      c) initial response is one of numbness followed by yearning and suffering; during this period the person can be withdrawn, apathetic, and angry
      d) likely to experience serious impairment of activities, personal derogation, suicidal thoughts, domestic disturbances
      e) this is followed by a period of preoccupation with the lost person or stressor during which time the experiences, meanings, and emotional significance of the relationship or event are reviewed
      f) resolution involves taking in certain qualities derived from the relationship or event and resignation to the loss
      g) the crisis period takes about 6 weeks; complete resolution is usually achieved in 6–12 months; grief is normal reactive depression
      h) intervention in the grief process involves allowing persons to work through the process, allowing them to ventilate their emotions, and reassuring them that these are normal responses
      i) minimal cognitive changes present
      j) mild physiologic disturbances (e.g., weight loss or gain of less than 10 lb, feels worse as day progresses)
   3) *neurotic depression*
      a) *DSM-III* classification: dysthymic disorder
      b) cognitive changes much greater and may be long-standing
      c) negative self-image derived from years of disappointments and inability to get love from others
      d) negative world view accentuated by disappointing relationships through the years
      e) lack of supportive past experiences causes client to be pessimistic about the future
      f) symptoms seem excessive to overt situations
      g) may have somatic symptoms, usually mild
      h) client in complete contact with reality and is generally able to continue working, going to school, etc.
      i) responds to environmental stimuli
   4) *psychotic depression* (endogenous)
      a) *DSM-III* classification
         • major depressive episode with psychotic features including severe impairment of reality testing and physiologic disturbances

- manic episode with psychotic features
b) depression brought on by severe environmental blows to security; mobilization of extreme guilt; may have biochemical/genetic causes
c) marked cognitive changes
d) vegetative signs (e.g., anorexia, weight loss of more than 10 lb; constipation; insomnia; morning-evening variations of mood; amenorrhea/impotency)
e) delusions of worthlessness, poverty, sinfulness
f) client loses contact with reality, does not respond to environmental stimuli
g) hostility plays greater role than in other depressions
h) with severe symptoms, client needs attention to physical needs
  - *agitated depression:* anxious, tense, extremely restless; pacing, hand wringing, skin picking, poor eating and sleeping
  - *retarded depression:* general physical and cognitive slowness, sitting idly, hanging head, looking haggard; indecisive and uncooperative
  - *bipolar depression (manic-depression):* characterized by attacks of well-defined, self-limiting mania or depression, usually in repeating cycles, with or without an interval of normalcy
    - person usually recovers completely from both phases, but there is a tendency for recurrence
    - a given person may experience only the depressive phase, only the manic phase, or both at different times in life
      * the depressed phase is characterized by depressions of mood, and retardation and inhibition of thinking and physical activity
      * manic phase is characterized by elation, overtalkativeness, extremely rapid ideation (flight of ideas), and increased motor activity

2. **Nursing Process**
   a. **Assessment**
      1) signs and symptoms (refer to page 50)
         a) behavioral changes
            - crying
            - withdrawal
            - psychomotor retardation or agitation
         b) emotional changes: sadness
         c) physical changes
            - nonspecific somatic complaints, (e.g., stomach problem, dizziness)
            - constipation
            - weakness and fatigability
            - menstrual irregularity or perhaps even cessation
            - impotence
         d) cognitive changes
            - the cognitive triad (the emotional, physical, and behavioral changes are *not* specific for depression, but the cognitive changes are)
              - negative view of self (expressed as low self-esteem)
              - negative view of the world
              - negative expectations for the future
            - signs of cognitive changes
              - helplessness and hopelessness
              - self-blame
              - indecisiveness
              - worthlessness
              - memory loss
            - the key to dealing with depression relates to identifying the aspects of cognitive changes that are factors with the client; the less severe the disruptions in this realm, the less debilitating will be the depression
      2) severity and level of depression (refer to "States of Depression" page 53)
      3) priorities for care
         a) client safety (1st priority): assessment of suicidal intent is a very important part of care and must be dealt with initially as well as throughout treatment course
            - potential for suicide always present

- related to negative self-esteem
- depression may cause the person to feel need for punishment
- negative views of world and future can cause person to give up all hope

b) suicide potential; the following must be considered
- presence of a plan: client is at high risk if plan is ready for implementation, likely to be lethal, or cause severe impairment if attempt is unsuccessful (see table 2.8, "Suicide Methods")
- change in behavior, e.g., calmness: may mean person has worked out a plan; as depression lifts, client may have energy to carry out plan
- giving away valued things: saying good-bye, making amends, asking medical questions
- suicidal risk: persons at high risk for suicide include
  - adolescents and people over 50 years old
  - single males
  - black males
  - alcoholics, isolated and unhappy persons
  - depressed persons
  - hallucinating persons responding to voice commands
  - those with a history of family suicide
  - persons experiencing a maturational or situational crisis or a chronic or painful illness
- ambivalent feelings
  - coexistence of opposing emotions in client (i.e., wants to live/die, experiences love and hate toward deceased or absent person)
  - has inability to express anger and hostility toward another person and so may turn hate and aggression inward toward self, leading to self-destructive thoughts/actions
  - feelings of ambivalence are common in severely depressed clients, particularly when the depression is related to the loss of a person important to them

c) physical needs (2nd priority): reduced self-esteem and psychomotor retardation may cause neglect of physical needs, especially adequate nutrition and proper elimination

d) self-esteem (3rd priority): other psychologic and emotional problems associated with low self-esteem (e.g., hopelessness and helplessness, feelings of worthlessness)

b. Goals, Plans/Implementation, and Evaluation

Goal 1: Client will be protected from suicidal gestures; will share feelings of loneliness, helplessness, and concerns about self and situation.

Plan/Implementation
- assume responsibility for safety of client; inspect unit for dangerous items such as sharp items (scissors, nail files, razor blades), pills; remove from client area
- restrict client to observable areas; observe closely for suicidal ideation/gestures
- utilize open questioning about suicidal plans and ideas

Table 2.8   Suicide Methods

Lower Lethality	Higher Lethality
Cutting wrists.	Slashing jugular.
Tranquilizers.	Barbiturates/sedatives.
Inhaling gas.	Carbon monoxide.
Swallowing caustic substances.	Aspirin.
	Medications combined with alcohol.
	Jumping.
	Drowning.
	Hanging.
	Setting self on fire.
	Explosives.
	Automobile crash.
	Shooting self.

- allow client to express feelings of hopelessness and helplessness
- stress client's capabilities/strengths
- involve client in activities that ensure success, e.g., attaining small goals in activities of daily living (ADL), exercise
- provide realistic reassurance; convey attitude that client will succeed
- set limits on repetition of story
- know that client's dependency and demands may cause nurse to feel overburdened and angry; staff needs to meet daily for mutual support and planning
- assess client's abilities realistically and provide only the help needed; irrational demands should be discussed openly and refused
- establish nurse-client relationship that shows nurse as respectful, knowledgeable, able to help solve problems; nurse's attitude should reflect firmness and confidence
- work with client to prepare list of problems and corresponding solutions; use all resources available, including family and community resources
- give client sense that problems are manageable
- utilize emergency methods to counteract suicidal attempts (e.g., lavage, one-to-one observation)
- if suicide attempt occurs, assist client/family to share and work through feelings and concerns
- acknowledge the coexistence of opposing (ambivalent) emotions in the client and family
- do not withdraw when ambivalence is directed toward nursing staff; continue to offer listening and socialization
- review and evaluate interventions

Evaluation: Client demonstrates increased ability to control self-destructive impulses; is protected from suicidal gestures; shares feelings and concerns about self and situation (e.g., hopelessness, helplessness, suicidal ideation).

Goal 2 (Content between asterisks is adapted from M. Neal et al. *Nursing Care Planning Guides, Set 3*, 2nd Ed. "The Patient Experiencing Depression [Psychiatric]." No. 3:35. Baltimore: Williams & Wilkins, 1983. Used with permission.):

*Client will ingest adequate foods and fluids; will achieve an adequate sleep-rest-activity pattern; will resume self-care in grooming.

Plan/Implementation
- assess ADL and vegetative signs
- identify problem areas and work out alternatives with client and health team; take care to consider personal preferences and needs; help client do things for self (many depressed clients become dependent on others, but activity usually helps them to feel better)
- assess areas in which client is making own decisions and give positive reinforcement to self-enhancing ones; assist with decision making when client is profoundly depressed; as depression lifts, expect client to make own decisions, with support
- weigh weekly (continued loss of weight may indicate deepening depression; weight gain may indicate decreased depression)
- work with client to plan ADL in areas of
  - *personal appearance:* help client establish routine for bathing, care of hair, skin, nails, clothes; give positive reinforcement to any care of self
  - *food intake:* work with client to find acceptable eating pattern; if client is anorexic and apathetic to food, find out when this lessens; could you leave a Thermos of hot chocolate, oatmeal cookies, crackers and cheese, 7-Up, etc., at bedside for small snacks at night or during day?
  - *sleeping habits:* help client establish a bedtime routine to promote rest and sleep; without enough sleep, exhaustion may occur and the mental state deteriorate; some depressed persons seem to sleep continuously during the day and do not rest at night; work with client to mobilize self during day to enable rest at night; insomnia increases fatigue and fatigue increases depression; since sedatives are generally ineffective, other nursing measures must be used (e.g., warm milk, snacks, backrub, warm bath)
  - *work assignment* (daily responsibility for ward-maintenance tasks helps to

renew a sense of self-worth and purposefulness): simple tasks, such as emptying ashtrays, staightening chairs, putting away cards, games, or crafts equipment—with supervision—may be appropriate for deeply depressed clients; more difficult tasks can be gradually assigned as client tolerates
- *hobbies and pastimes:* assess previous ones that client enjoyed (often depressed persons have few hobbies and haven't participated in recreational or crafts groups since school days); simple crafts that can be finished in one sitting give the client a therapeutic sense of accomplishment; encourage group singing, poetry reading, painting, working with clay, to assist client to become more comfortable in groups and to establish community and group socialization; client may need nurse's presence to tolerate group activities at first; simple exercises, walks, may progress to group sports
- *bowel habits:* work with client to choose foods for roughage and sufficient fluids if constipated (often resumption of exercise and previous eating habits solves a constipation problem)
- *client's knowledge of morning-evening variations in mood and depression:* for clients with endogenous depression, teach that most clients feel low in the morning and better as the day progresses, especially if they mobilize themselves into activity; for clients with reactive depression, teach that their fatigue level affects their depression, so that as day progresses, they may become tired and feel more depressed; if so, they may need to rest in middle of day and do group work in the morning, when they feel less depressed; when clients are agitated, above nursing actions may help to rechannel their energy

Evaluation: Client ingests adequate food and fluids; achieves adequate sleep-activity pattern; dresses and grooms self daily; participates in planning daily schedule and hobbies.*

Goal 3: Client will strengthen ability to relate to others by increasing social interaction with staff and other clients.
Plan/Implementation
- assist client to identify, define, and problem solve difficult areas in social relationships (e.g., client who is hypercritical of self and others can discuss and practice a softer, more accepting approach)
- help client to look at situations where he may push others away out of fear of rejection (i.e., reject them before being rejected)
- practice social skills, use role-playing
- go with client to group activities, choosing short, simple group activities that client identifies as least threatening (exercise, sports, music)
- involve client in activity that provides chance for success (e.g., simple occupational therapy activities)

Evaluation: Client spends increasing time with staff and other clients; identifies problems in social relationships; practices new social skills with staff and other clients.

Goal 4: Client receiving ECT will be free from preventable injury.
Plan/Implementation
- prep client as if going to OR
- have client sign a consent form
- arrange for spine x-ray, if required
- keep client on regimen of nothing PO
- remove dentures, hairpins, etc.
- give medications as ordered (muscle relaxant)
- sit with client before treatment to provide support
- after treatment, check client's pulse and respirations; observe reaction upon awakening
- orient client to place and to the fact that treatment has been administered (temporary memory loss and confusion are the most distressing side-effects following ECT)
- stay with client through recovery period (about 30 minutes)

Evaluation: Client recovers from ECT safely; is oriented to time, place, and person.

B. Elation and Hyperactive Behavior

1. **General Information**
   a. Definition: elation is a seemingly pleasurable affect that is characterized by an air of happiness and self-confidence as well as extreme motor activity
   b. Precipitating Factors
      1) results from a real or threatened loss of self-esteem
      2) massive denial of depression
      3) may develop from early childhood
         a) child first begins to be independent of mother
         b) mother is threatened by this; responds as if this independence is bad
         c) child fears loss of mother's love
         d) child attempts to meet expectations for compliance
   c. Levels
      1) *mild:* euphoric state of mind, mild exhilaration
         a) person feels happy, unconcerned, uninhibited
         b) mood can change rapidly to irritability and anger
         c) person is very active, but activity is sometimes inappropriate for age and place
         d) relationships are usually superficial
         e) exhibits life-of-the-party type of mood
      2) *acute:* moderate degree of mania called hypomania
         a) extreme emotional lability ranging from wild euphoria to fury
         b) thought disorders: flight of ideas, delusions of grandeur, short attention span, pressure of speech
         c) little sleep, fatigue, very uninhibited, possibly sexually indiscreet
         d) psychomotor activity is extremely exaggerated
         e) often requires hospitalization
      3) *delirium* or *delirious mania:* maximum intensity of reaction
         a) disorganized, seriously delusional
         b) disoriented, incoherent, agitated
         c) prone to self-injury, burn-out, and dehydration
         d) immediate intervention is necessary to meet physical needs (medication, seclusion, restraint)
   d. Prognosis: for a person with manic-depressive episode, it is good, even without treatment, provided that the person does not suffer from complete physical exhaustion in manic phase or commit suicide in depressed phase

2. **Nursing Process**
   a. Assessment
      1) physical needs: neglected because of euphoria and hyperactivity (e.g., little sleep, little eating, dehydration, constant motion)
      2) aggression: frequent; creates problems in management; threatens staff and disturbs other clients
      3) denial of depression: low self-esteem is masked with seeming self-confidence and pseudo-independence
      4) other problems: they may take priority, depending on client's behavior and speech (e.g., delusions, disorientation, disorganization, agitation, emotional lability, manipulation/acting out)
   b. Goals, Plans/Implementation, and Evaluation

   Goal 1: Client will experience decreased sensory stimulation; will be protected from injury; will receive adequate sleep, rest, and nutrition.

   Plan/Implementation
   - provide nourishing liquids and finger foods that can be eaten on the run; note amount of food and fluids that client ingests
   - provide medication to induce sleep and rest
   - reduce stimuli in environment, to help calm client
   - watch for physical symptoms that client may ignore (e.g., exaggerated use of cosmetics and clothing, dehydration, agitation, weight loss, constipation)
   - assist client to do own personal hygiene
   - be alert to client's wishes to leave hospital; physical or chemical restraint may be necessary in acute phases

   Evaluation: Client experiences decreased sensory stimuli; receives adequate sleep and rest; ingests appropriate amounts of food and fluids; remains free from injury.

   Goal 2: Client will cope adaptively with feelings of anger, hostility, and aggression.

Plan/Implementation
- know that manic clients are readily provoked by harmless remarks, can seem to forgive and forget, and may be easily provoked a short time later
- may have furious reaction (e.g., scream, curse, abuse, become violent) to unintentional provocation, then calm down quickly (in contrast to angry paranoid); irritability is expression of anxiety as well as hostile impulses
- recognize behaviors of increased excitement: agitation, irritability, verbal/motor hyperactivity
- utilize measures to prevent overt aggression, i.e., distraction, reduction of environmental stimuli; avoid competitive games
- set limits on behavior; constant fairness and honesty from staff are essential
- discuss feelings surrounding acting out, manipulative, or angry behavior
- assist to identify and cope adaptively with angry feelings
- do not hurry manic clients; hurrying them will result in more anger and hostility
- utilizing quiet persuasion is most effective; involve client in planning ADL

Evaluation: Client participates in quiet activities; discusses triggers to and feelings about angry outbursts.

Goal 3: Client will demonstrate realistic independence in ADL; will develop ability to problem solve, make requests appropriately, and negotiate.

Plan/Implementation
- know that client may have a false sense of independence and self-confidence (pseudo-independence) demonstrated by loud commands to staff and attempts to order staff about
- recognize that underneath demands, client is feeling dependence, inability to cope, overwhelmed
- do not discuss grandiose ideas/plans
- assess client's abilities realistically
- give help only when client is incapable
- discuss capabilities calmly with client
- involve client in planning ADL
- inform client that staff will not comply with unreasonable demands
- assist to develop alternate behavior; teach client to use assertion, problem solving, negotiation

Evaluation: Client does own self-care (showers, wears clean clothes, brushes hair, cleans teeth); makes requests in a quiet voice.

Goal 4: Client will accept limits on manipulative or acting out behaviors.

Plan/Implementation
- avoid impatience and anger if client is manipulative or acts out
- inform client of behaviors expected in short, clear sentences
- set firm, definite limits on client's behavior; consistently enforce limits
- teach client that it is the manipulative behavior that is being rejected, not him
- avoid arguments or displaying disapproval of vulgarity, profanity, or overt sexual behavior resulting from extreme euphoria
- remove client from public places when this behavior could embarrass client or family
- protect other clients from sexual overtures

Evaluation: Client displays manipulative or acting out behaviors less frequently than on admission.

Socially Maladaptive/Acting Out Behavior

General Concepts

A. Overview: socially maladaptive or acting out behavior includes a great many different problem behaviors and conditions. All human beings live within a social system and each social system has values and rules by which to live with other human beings. When an individual copes with tension and anxiety by acting out against the social system's values and rules, society considers the individual to be socially maladapted.

Societies utilize many different ways to deal with socially maladaptive/acting out behavior. Courts, jails, and prisons may be used if laws are broken. Psychotherapy may be used; it facilitates the reentry into society of such persons and helps them to change maladaptive behaviors to adaptive, healthy behaviors.

A society will provide social structure, which minimizes stress, social disorder, and upheaval through promotion of a healthy environment and through the provision of services essential to physical and mental health. These services include health care, schools, religious institutions, the justice system, recreational facilities, and welfare services.

When the structure and expectations of society are stable forces, the family and individual will decrease acting out behavior. Social unrest, economic stress, health care inequities, moral decay, or dysfunctional families may precipitate or perpetuate stress and anger.

B. Application of the Nursing Process to the Client Exhibiting Maladaptive Behavior
1. **Assessment**
   a. Immediate events that precipitated socially maladaptive/acting out behavior: characteristics and frequency
   b. Physiologic changes that accompany angry feelings
   c. Coping behavior that client uses to handle stress and anger: adaptive and maladaptive
   d. Defense mechanisms used to cope with angry feelings
2. **General Nursing Goal, Plan/Implementation, and Evaluation**
   Goal: The socially maladaptive acting-out client will decrease unacceptable behavior; will utilize assertive behaviors as a means of expressing independence and control.
   Plan/Implementation
   - stress to staff the importance of not chastising client or rejecting client's efforts to cope by using aggressive behavior; rather, provide structure and set limits on behavior that is physically destructive
   - teach client the difference between assertive (asking for what one wants, standing up for rights) and aggressive behavior (getting what one wants at the expense of others)
   - reinforce positive (assertive) approaches utilized by the client ("I would like..." versus "Do this...")
   - do not allow client to be destructive to others
     - set firm and definite limits on behavior
     - consistently enforce limits; inconsistent limit setting merely serves to increase the person's belief that manipulative behavior is productive
   - give the opportunity to plan and do things the client likes to do, e.g., sleeping late, knitting, reading
   - praise the efforts of the family/significant others in their attempts to assist the client in coping
   - teach client to use stress-reduction techniques (e.g., imagery, relaxation)

- be sensitive to your own nonverbal behavior and what it says to client; try not to look defensive or act aggressively

Evaluation: Client reduces frequency of unacceptable behavior; can describe the difference between assertion and aggression; can demonstrate at least one assertive behavior; uses positive coping mechanisms to handle stress (e.g., relaxation).

Selected Health Problems

A. Violence in the Family

1. **General Information**
    a. Definitions
       1) violence is the expression of the aggressive drive, normally present, in a destructive manner
       2) a learned behavior, learned either through exposure and imitation or indirectly when an individual is unable to channel aggressive impulses constructively
    b. Some violent persons feel guilty about their behavior, and others do not. Behaving violently, either with or without feeling guilty, can cause a mental health problem for the person or those dependent upon him.
    c. Victims of abuse generally are persons who are dependent on others for their physical, financial, and emotional care; their abuser is often their caretaker. Victims can include
       1) children
       2) spouses
       3) elderly parents or other adults
       4) children or adults in long-term care settings
    d. Characteristics of Abuse (Violence) in the Family
       1) victims have little capacity to defend themselves; may be weaker or younger (child, weak woman or man)
       2) the abuser is physically stronger than the abused
       3) the dynamics of abuse need to be viewed in terms of the following aspects
          a) intrapersonal: internal psychodynamics of those involved
          b) interpersonal: socializing framework of beliefs and values and interaction of individual with others
          c) sociocultural: power structure and belief system of the family or institution
       4) the victims of abuse (child or adult) often believe that they have done something to warrant the abuse; they have low self-esteem; they may feel a need for punishment
       5) abused adults (e.g., battered women) often believe they could not survive outside the home setting without the abusing person and thus are emotionally, if not physically, trapped
       6) abused persons fear the consequences of telling someone outside the family of their treatment; they also feel ashamed and for that reason may not tell health care personnel
       7) abused persons often include the elderly, who are physically, financially, and emotionally dependent on family or other adults
    d. Multidisciplinary Treatment
       1) case finding: health care personnel are often the ones who have the opportunity to assess children and adults for possible abuse, especially when they are seen for injuries
          a) be alert for abuse cases, especially in emergency rooms, pediatrics, ambulatory clinics
          b) carefully document bruises, cuts, etc., size, and location; also document interaction patterns of client and significant other; these become evidence
          c) all suspected child abuse cases must be reported and will be investigated by the state child welfare agency; in some states elder abuse is also reportable
          d) medical personnel cannot be charged with defamation of character if they report an abuse that does not check out as such
          e) assess both the abuser and abused; documentation of behaviors, symptoms, is important for legal aspects
          f) help both to receive emotional treatment if they are willing
       2) community services: numerous branches of the health care system respond to client abuse situations

a) treatment and intervention by child welfare agencies may include alternative living situations for the abused
b) various community agencies provide classes on parenting, dealing with older parents, problem-solving skills, and appropriate expression of emotion, e.g., Parents Anonymous (a self-help group for actual or potential child abusers)

2. Nursing Process
  a. Assessment
    1) the victim: assess for
      a) presence of injuries that do not fit the description of the accident
      b) evidence of multiple bruises, chipped front teeth, or burns, particularly of the type inflicted by a cigarette
      c) x-ray reports that indicate old healed fractures
      d) retarded growth and/or development of the child with no history of pathologic conditions (e.g., walks late, cannot feed self, underweight)
      e) child's clothing inappropriate in relation to weather conditions
      f) evidence of poor hygiene
      g) no immunization appropriate to the child's age
      h) child wary of adults or caretaker from the referring facility
      i) child adapts to hospital unit quickly
      j) child does not seek out parents for comfort or affection
      k) child does not cry when parents leave
      l) grabbing behavior/lap hunger exhibited by the young child
      m) child shows provocative behavior that generates anger in others
      n) delinquent or runaway behavior; teenage pregnancy
      o) adult victim reluctant to talk about injuries, particularly if spouse, parent, adult child, or caretaker from the referring facility is present
    2) the abuser: assess for
      a) denial of abuse; an abuser may or may not see self as such
      b) history of child abuse in family; abusive parents themselves were often abused as children and have learned that pattern of expressing anger
      c) perception of victim; abusers may view the victim as "bad," as someone who tries to make them angry and does things on purpose to irritate or upset them; they view the victim this way regardless of developmental or social inabilities of the victim (e.g., a one-year-old child is viewed as breaking something on purpose to upset them)
      d) knowledge of normal growth and development; abusers often have unrealistic expectations for child's age
      e) guilt or remorse may be absent or abuser may feel guilt or remorse but be unable to stop; abusers who cannot stop—without remorse—include alcoholic or drug abusers as well as other persons
      f) evidence of dysfunctional attachment process in new parent; withdrawal from the child; expresses fears that he will hurt the child
      g) extreme overprotectiveness
      h) defensiveness about behavior with child
      i) evidence of psychosis
      j) alcohol and/or drug abuse
      k) low self-esteem; low self-acceptance
      l) hostility, depression
      m) hypochondriacal complaints
      n) impulsiveness in decision making
      o) seductive behavior toward child
      p) explains need for physical punishment due to "badness" in victim
    3) family or caretaker dynamics: assess for
      a) behavior expected of abused child is not appropriate to child's age
      b) describes abused child as "difficult" or "hateful"
      c) ascribes a special, negatively perceived characteristic to the abused person

d) lack of knowledge of normal growth and development, including the aging process
e) divorce, separation, abandonment, death of spouse
f) financial, housing, or personal crisis; severe stress
g) behavior toward crying/injured child is aloof, not comforting or affectionate
h) expectations that child should give and be "grateful" to parents
i) family refuses to allow diagnostic procedures
j) parents withdraw from hospitalized child
k) parents or caretaker complains of difficulty in coping with the abused person and/or own life
l) impaired communications, low self-image
m) evidence of misuse of defense mechanisms, i.e., projection, scapegoating, denial
n) emotionally cut off from families of origin
o) parents or care taker gives history of being physically abused as child
p) family or care taker has been experiencing chronic sustained anxiety or recent loss

b. Goals, Plans/Implementation, and Evaluation

Goal 1 (Content within the asterisks is adapted from M. Neal et al. *Nursing Care Planning Guides, Set 4*, 2nd Ed. "The Child: Battered-Child Syndrome," No. 4:20. Baltimore: Williams & Wilkins, 1983. Used with permission.): *The abuser will relate to at least one nurse with trust, accept her offer to listen and to help with open discussion of problems and needs.

Plan/Implementation
- be aware of your own nonverbal messages and feelings; demonstrate caring; maintain composure and compassion, refraining from even implied criticism or rejection
- be honest with yourself and if you are uncomfortable with the victim and/or family, admit it and ask for assistance or to be relieved of this assignment
- consider asking abuser to keep a daily diary of feelings and situations that create stress, triggers that set off a chain of events; use the diary as a method to talk through feelings, discuss the need for new coping strategies, and lay plans to participate in family therapy*
- be in touch with own feelings about the abuser and abused and recognize the needs of both (often nurses feel extremely angry with the abuser and very sympathetic with the victim, especially in child-abuse cases)
- remember that the abuser may not view self as such, may want to stop but can't; the abuser may have a very low self-image and needs help and support
  - assist abuser or caretakers to become aware of the importance of their own need-fulfillment feelings and thoughts and how to meet those needs more effectively; treatment measures can help them to look at this and begin to take care of their own needs and not expect those in their care to do it

Evaluation: Parents, adult children, or caretakers begin to talk about their feelings, anxieties, frustrations.

Goal 2: *Victim will have maximum healing, recovery, and protection from further injury after hospitalization.

Plan/Implementation
- follow nursing care plan for specific type of injury (head injury, fracture, burn, etc.)
- monitor visitors discreetly; friendly visits with caretakers can provide acceptance and defuse hostility
- make referral to hospital social service department or your local department of social service, community mental health center, or abuse-prevention center
- allow child to play with dolls/doll house, stuffed animals
- provide drawing materials, as children often depict their feelings in this way; gently ask about meanings of drawings but do not probe
- encourage victim to talk about how she or he feels; be a warm, quiet listener; avoid judgmental comment
- provide for the victim's physical comfort with analgesics prn and attention to physical needs
- give comfort by holding, rocking, stroking gently, hugging; note child's reactions/tolerance

Evaluation: Victim experiences relief of physical and emotional pain; recovers in a safe environment.

Goal 3: Abuser will develop an improved relationship with victim; will find support services to assist with caretaking or other needs.

Plan/Implementation
- develop the abuser's communication skills; help the person to
  - acknowledge emotional problems when they occur; some parents were abused as children
  - learn how to provide good physical care to victim; many abusers do not know how
  - develop new ways to vent anger and to obtain support; emotional therapy can be very effective; have parents explore their own childhood and remember how they felt as children
  - develop effective problem-solving skills
  - *enjoy their child; teach them play skills with children that enhance enjoyment
  - enjoy the pleasure of reading to the child, being careful to select materials that will be of interest to the parent who does the reading as well as to the child
  - join the child in simple games, doll play, drawing and painting experiences*
  - learn about normal expectations of growth and development; parents can learn what can realistically be expected of children at various ages
  - *understand how limits can be set and enforced, how discipline can be given with consistency and fairness and without physical manifestations of anger
  - reinforce with praise and encouragement any attempts to nurture, comfort, or express affection to the child*
  - find ways of socializing or incorporating older parent into new life-style while maintaining independence for involved family members
  - find resources in the community (e.g., Parents Anonymous) to help abusive parents get together and discuss feelings and problems and share solutions

Evaluation: *Abuser can identify at least two new coping mechanisms that will help reduce or eliminate episodes of abuse and handle effectively situations likely to induce it; knows about and has written down the Parents Anonymous's toll-free 24-hour telephone number; has a referral for family and/or individual therapy. Victim accepts placement in a temporary foster home or facility (if conditions at home make this desirable, even necessary, for safety).*

B. Hostile, Aggressive, and Assaultive Behavior

1. **General Information**
   a. Definitions
      1) aggression is a defensive response to anxiety and loss of self-esteem and power
      2) *passive-aggressive behavior*: resistance to demands for adequate performance in both occupational and social functioning are met by timidity, sullenness, stubbornness, forgetfulness, and obstruction
         a) if the behavior is characteristic of the person, it may be considered a personality disorder (*DSM-III* classification)
         b) the person is acting out anger in very indirect ways, e.g., always late, forgetting to do things that are important to another person
         c) the anger of the other person provides the passive-aggressive person with attention and release for anger
      3) *active aggression:* a forceful goal-directed action that may be verbal or physical; the motor counterpart of the affect of rage, anger, and hostility
         a) can be constructive when it is problem solving and appropriate as a defense against realistic attack
         b) can become healthy when channeled through appropriate ways of expression, i.e., assertiveness
         c) is pathologic when it is unrealistic, self-destructive, non-problem

solving and the outcome of unresolved emotional conflict
- d) it is unhealthy when out of control of the person, beyond the problem-solving level, and results in harm, physically or emotionally, to others

b. Dynamics (Content between the asterisks is adapted from M. Neal et al. *Nursing Care Planning Guides, Set 4*, 2nd Ed. "The Patient who is Violent," No. 4:40. Pacific Palisades, CA: Nurseco, 1983. Used with permission.)
1) *theoretically, violence is a response to feelings of impotence and helplessness in the face of a perceived threat
2) the threat may come at the time of admission to a mental health facility; the client may feel that his worst fear has come true, for he has lost control of his behavior, is "crazy," and is being locked up
3) this may be accompanied by a marked increase in anxiety behaviors as he realizes that he must obey the rules or take the consequences
4) with a threat from within and a threat from without, a client may respond with fight, flight, or freeze responses; he is not allowed to leave the hospital, may flee to his room, which he must share with other clients, and he feels increasingly impotent
5) as anxiety and stress increase, the ability to reason decreases, and the client responds more to isolated stimuli and less to the content of the situation

c. Principles and procedures for control of aggression, acting out, and violence should be a part of every mental health facility's routine inservice training
1) therapeutic milieu adequately staffed by well-trained and caring health care workers can prevent most violence
2) each violent incident should be reviewed with a goal of improving client care by identifying situations that contribute to violence and by evaluating and revising interventions
3) interventions that decrease perceived threat and diminish feelings of impotence in the client are usually most successful

2. **Nursing Process**
   a. Assessment
   1) refer to Assessment page 60
   2) behaviors of aggression
      a) overt, constant demands
      b) constant, self-directed anger
      c) refusal to listen to staff
      d) constant or intermittent attempts at changing the plan of care
      e) abusive language
      f) constant or intermittent nonadherence to physician's orders*
   3) level of aggression
      a) is client able to participate in discussion? if so, can client be helped to identify feelings and look at alternatives?
      b) clients can become so angry that they do not think rationally and are unable to label feelings and look for alternative ways of expressing their anger; these clients require external controls through medications and seclusion

   b. Goals, Plans/Implementation, and Evaluation

   Goal 1: *The client will limit or stop aggressive behavior.
   Plan/Implementation
   - refer to General Nursing Goal page 60
   - intervene while client is amenable to discussion and rational thinking
   - set limits on physically harmful behavior and explain to the client why you are doing so
   - always prepare the client (physically and verbally) for what you are going to do, even if you consider it a daily and/or usual activity
   - encourage the client to express the feelings regarding the deprivation caused by the hospitalization and illness; sit down and listen; use open-ended questions
   - recognize that the client's verbal aggression may be in response to fear, increased dependency, and/or anxiety; therefore, do not attempt to defend yourself, the staff, or the agency; listen to what the client is saying and assist him to understand his own method of coping
   - avoid positive reinforcement of negative behaviors

Evaluation: Client limits or stops aggressive behavior; expresses feelings in healthy way.*

Goal 2: Client will stop violent behavior; will verbalize angry feelings.

Plan/Implementation
- be aware of precursory signs of violence (agitation, threatening verbalizations, gestures and other body-language manifestations, changes in behavior)
- reduce stimuli by removing any object or person that appears to frighten client; get client into an area where there are fewer persons and less noise, light, activity, etc.
- assure client by explaining what is happening, telling that he will be safe and asking whether he has any questions; express an attitude of helpfulness and calm
- if a client expresses a fear of committing a violent act, estimate the seriousness of the danger and initiate steps to avert it by decreasing the perceived threat and diminishing feelings of impotence; remove weapons or objects that could be used in a destructive fashion
- whenever a client shows signs of impending assaultive behavior, every effort should be made to find the cause and correct it
- potentially violent clients generally sense when they are about to lose control and seek reassurance that they can be controlled
- offer alternatives to restraints and seclusion
  - identify the anxiety: comment to client, "It seems as though you are upset. Tell me what is going on."
  - provide alternatives: "Let's sit down and talk it over. How about a cup of coffee?"
  - encourage verbalization rather than acting out: "Now what happened to make you so angry?"
  - talk calmly and normally; don't show own agitation
  - give client space; don't crowd him
  - try to keep things quiet; don't make any sudden moves toward the client
  - offer medication; tell client he is getting out of control and if he doesn't take medications, he will have to be restrained; offer choice whenever appropriate
  - know that clients respond quickly to IM doses of major tranquilizers; slow-acting barbiturates are sometimes given
  - restraints should be the very last resort in calming the client

Evaluation: Client stops violent behavior; verbalizes angry feelings.

Goal 3: *The client will tolerate physical restraints if necessary as a last resort to prevent physical violence.

Plan/Implementation
- know institutional policy and state law re use of restraints
- assemble equipment and staff; 4 staff members are necessary to restrain average-sized client; if time available, staff members should remove glasses or pens or other potentially harmful articles from their persons; a blanket or sheet and soft-leather, arm and leg restraints may be needed
- prepare a private room that contains a bed with a metal frame to which restraints can be secured; clear this room of any potentially dangerous items; hallway to room should be cleared of other clients and visitors
- explain to client: "We are concerned about this behavior and we are going to help you control it now, so that you won't hurt yourself or others."
- distract the client with blanket or sheet as if you were about to wrap him totally with it; during this attempt to distract, each staff member should take an arm or leg, raise client off his feet, and place him face down on floor so that he loses his base of support for physically assaultive behavior; use good body mechanics and be aware of client's body alignment to prevent injuries to staff members and client
- transport client to his own room (each limb still carried by a staff member, carrying the legs by placing the support above the client's knees); if necessary for control, carry client face down, protecting his head; if necessary, one staff member can carry both legs
- follow facility procedure for application of restraints; care should be taken to

SOCIALLY MALADAPTIVE/ACTING OUT BEHAVIOR 67

ensure that the restraints do not impair circulation or cause pressure on underlying nerves; A CLIENT IN RESTRAINTS SHOULD NEVER BE LEFT ALONE; stay with client and encourage expression of thoughts and feelings about the incident; explore the situation that caused the client to experience increased anxiety and loss of control
- remove all items from client's clothing, especially potentially dangerous, sharp items and matches
- obtain physician's order for restraints prior to or immediately after emergency situation; if physician orders a parenteral medication, it may be given to client either at site of loss of control or after transporting to room
- take BP and pulse q30min and check extremities for signs of lack of circulation or pressure; offer snacks and fluids; give mouth care as necessary
- remove restraints as soon as possible, when acute agitation has subsided
- allow other clients who may have observed restraining and transporting to ventilate their feelings and concerns about client or their own potential loss of control

Evaluation: Client tolerates short-term use of physical restraints; expresses thoughts and feelings about episode of aggression and restraint.*

C. Acting Out

1. General Information
a. Definition: angry, aggressive behavior (usually nonverbal) short of violence; it is the expression of emotions resulting from unconscious feelings, wishes, or conflicts; includes verbal and nonverbal threats
b. Characteristic of
   1) persons with a bipolar disorder (manic-depressive psychosis), paranoid conditions, and organic mental disorders
   2) persons with character disorders and drug-dependent persons who use impulsive assault in order to get their basic needs met

c. Dynamics
   1) can be a method to express a variety of feelings such as guilt, love, fear; however, it is most frequently an expression of anger
   2) designed to attract other people's attention and usually represents feelings or conflicts the person is experiencing
   3) usually believed to be uncontrollable until the person understands the reasons for the behavior or learns alternative methods of expression
   4) may be related to alterations in biochemistry and therefore responsive to chemotherapeutic agents

2. Nursing Process
a. Assessment
   1) refer to Assessment page 60
   2) signs
      a) elation, restlessness, or agitation; demands constant attention from everyone
      b) impulsive behavior (e.g., suicide, homicide, running away)
      c) inappropriate behavior for age or place
      d) sarcastic, teasing behavior
      e) vulgar and profane conversation
      f) limited attention span
      g) problems with authority
b. Goal, Plan/Implementation, and Evaluation

Goal: Client will participate in self-care and treatment plan.
Plan/Implementation
- Refer to General Nursing Goal page 60
- indicate when, where, how, and to whom acting out behavior is related
- recognize impending violent behavior without total rejection of client as person
- know that nurse and client must believe that client can control this behavior
- encourage communication: remember, you are dealing with the client's actions, rather than personality; listen, but don't take provocative remarks or abusive language personally
- do not use complex ideas or involved explanations; speak in short sentences

- do not feel obligated to explain decisions; nurses sometimes fall into the trap of feeling as though they must explain their decision; the client may take more time refuting the explanation than acting on the decision
- focus on client; let client know you are giving your complete attention

Evaluation: Client decreases acting out behaviors; begins to accept limits and rules; participates in self-care and treatment plan (e.g., group activities).

D. Sexual Acting Out

1. General Information
  a. Definitions
  1) includes sex acts with partners who are legally unable to consent, such as children (pedophilia), with persons who choose not to consent, sex acts accompanied by force or violence (rape), and invasion of other people's privacy without their knowledge (e.g., voyeurism)
  2) voyeurism: the person repeatedly observes other people's naked bodies without their knowledge or consent in order to obtain sexual gratification
  3) exhibitionism: a person exposes his sexual organs when it is socially inappropriate
  4) sadomasochism: obtaining sexual pleasure from having pain inflicted upon oneself or others; may be part of a rape incident or may also be part of other sexual encounter
  5) rape: legal definitions of rape vary from state to state, but most include sexual intercourse without the consent of the other person; statutory rape is the seduction of a minor, even though the minor consented
  b. Profile of a Rapist
  1) rape is not an act of sexual passion; it is an act of aggression and a crime of violence and power
  2) rapists act for the purpose of venting anger and hostility and exercising control and power
  3) many rapes are planned, and the rapist is in some way acquainted with the victim in over 50% of cases
  c. The Victim of Rape (Content within asterisks is adapted from M. Neal et al. *Nursing Care Planning Guides, Set 4*, 2nd Ed. "The Victim of Rape/Sexual Assault," No. 4:39. Baltimore: Williams & Wilkins, 1983. Used with permission.)
  1) *the rape victim may be a woman, man, or child; most rapes and sexual assaults are committed by men against women
  2) only about 10% of rapes are reported
  3) the result of rape for the victim
     a) disruption of physical, emotional, social, and sexual equilibrium
     b) the rape is a situational hazard, and a true emotional crisis may or may not occur, depending upon the victim's coping mechanisms and available sources of support
     c) the psychologic impact is severe; may be long lasting, and is significantly affected by the type of immediate care the victim receives
     d) the emergency room (ER) experience can be either a calming, supportive one or one in which the victim experiences further injustice from the ER staff if they have professional insensitivity and an unhelpful attitude
       - ER staff often question, "Was she *really* raped?" and put blame and responsibility on the victim
       - frequently this is because the staff person is made aware of own vulnerability to rape when confronted with a victim, and the situation is understandably anxiety producing
       - research shows that typical reactions of rape victims in ER are either "expressed" (such as crying, laughing, showing nervousness) or "controlled" (outward calm); if a victim is exhibiting the latter behavior, there is a tendency among ER staff to feel the victim has not been raped, or is dealing with it well and needs no help*
     e) rape should be suspected when a man has been violently assaulted, particularly by a group of men;

may seem sullen and reluctant to describe the assault; needs to be given an opportunity to express feelings
d. *Sexual Assaults on Children
  1) usually grouped into two categories
    a) forced rape, most frequently an isolated, traumatic event, with physical injury, generating fear and pain in the child; child is more upset over the pain and violence than the sexual activity
    b) accessory-to-sex, usually involving exposure, statutory rape, incest, molestation, but not force; recurring episodes may extend over a period of time
       • offenders in accessory-to-sex assaults are usually an adult the child knows, most frequently a family member or relative, sometimes a neighbor of caretaker
         - the offender usually bribes the child with money, candy, etc.
         - threats, authority, and domination are often used by the offender to generate fear in the child and thus maintain secrecy of the assault(s)
         - child may not tell anyone of the assault(s) for fear of being punished, blamed, or disbelieved, but may develop somatic and behavioral symptoms
         - sexually abused children often feel guilty, because they think they did something to cause the sexual abuse or because they may have felt some enjoyment; they may continue to participate if they feel it will "hold the parents together"
    c) the major traumatic impact on the child is psychologic rather than physical
       • the child will react to the family/significant other's reaction more than to the assault itself
       • the child views the event far differently from an adult; when the event is dealt with calmly by significant others, it will usually leave no long-term psychologic scars
    d) the ER nurse's responsibilities are to
       • believe what the child says
       • provide basic crisis intervention techniques for both child and family or significant others
       • assist with medical treatment
       • collect and prepare physical evidence
       • refer child, family, or significant others for follow-up physical and mental health treatment

2. Nursing Process
  a. Assessment
    1) victim's ability to cope: what is victim's level of anxiety? perception of what occurred? are family or significant others outside the hospital? what is victim's emotional response?
    2) signs of assault, bruises, scratches, etc., on victim's body
    3) significant others' coping; often they are the ones to go into crisis and need a mental health referral for themselves
    4) victim's equilibrium after seeing family or significant other and their response to the event
    5) need for information for protection from pregnancy and venereal disease
  b. Goals, Plans/Implementation, and Evaluation

  Goal 1: The adult victim will receive situational support from staff and be allowed to cope with situation in own way; will regain a measure of control over life space; will receive appropriate medical treatment.
  Plan/Implementation
  • always provide a private examining room
  • listen to what the victim is saying (this will help victim regain control) and believe what is said; judgmental comments are destructive to rape victim
  • acknowledge the assault, encourage victim to talk and be supportive ("It must have been a terrifying ordeal for

you."); reflect warmth, interest, respect, and a nonjudgmental attitude
- encourage open ventilation of feelings, especially anger at the rapist; be aware that this anger may be directed at staff
- ask her what is the most difficult thing for her right now and discuss it with her, *refraining* from giving advice or "You should have...," or "Why did you...?" (such statements will not be helpful); provide whatever victim wants and needs to help lower her stress (e.g., information, privacy, Kleenex, warm covers, coffee, etc.)
- if victim says "It was my fault," or, "I should have...," reinforce that the attack was *not* her fault, but the fault of the rapist and that she did what she was forced to do in order to save her life (many victims "pay" the rapist for their life with the sexual act, then feel guilty, unclean, ashamed, self-critical)
- encourage victim to talk about her feelings of the experience (usually of *overwhelming* terror) but do not dwell on the sexual aspects unless she needs to talk about the experience
- victim may not wish to talk and/or may look undisturbed or seem to be coping extremely well; may be denying or minimizing the attack; if any of these, allow her to cope in this way but tell her that at a later date she may experience feelings of anger, fear, or sadness, and that this would be a usual reaction
- do all interviewing sensitively and with consideration for victim's feelings; while it will be necessary (for court records) to know the explicit sexual acts involved, only *one* person, and only once, needs to ask for this information (either doctor or nurse)
- have a female staff member be with female victim at all times, to be her advocate, especially during any examination or assessment; if your hospital has a rape team, a member may fulfill this function; if victim asks for a female police officer, make all attempts to facilitate this request
- express your belief in victim's ability to deal with problems or decisions to be faced in next few days; be sure victim is permitted to take an active role in making and carrying out plans (e.g., reporting to police, returning to work, etc.)
- assist with collection of physical evidence (e.g., vaginal and anal swabs, clothes, foreign materials); follow established protocol and document findings
- if victim is alone and she consents, assist her to call her family/significant other; ask them to bring a change of clothes; if she has no one to call, develop a safety plan for her, e.g., transportation home
- provide victim with information about available counseling services, options, rights, and follow-up treatments (e.g., VD, pregnancy protection); assist and encourage her to call rape crisis center
- male victims need many of the same services as females, i.e., support, acceptance, protection from VD, and referral for further help
- encourage a male victim to talk about the ordeal with a male staff member

Evaluation: The adult victim receives medical treatment; copes with situation in own way (e.g., expresses anger); leaves ER with a family member or friend.

Goal 2: Family/significant others will verbalize an understanding of what victim has experienced; will give client situational support.

Plan/Implementation
- assess family/significant other's reaction to the victim's situation
  - be aware that they often tend to blame the victim, to be nonsupportive, and to isolate her
  - reinforce to them that the attack was not the victim's fault or responsibility and that it was a terrifying experience in which she was afraid she would be killed, that whatever her response to the rapist was, it was a decision made to try to save her life or prevent bodily harm to herself and/or to her children
- family/significant others may feel they are responsible because they weren't there to protect victim and thus feel guilty and vulnerable; again, emphasize that the responsibility lies with the attacker
- discuss with them ways they can be supportive to victim, e.g., by listening

to and believing what victim says, encouraging and allowing victim to talk, helping victim to resume usual life activities, not overprotecting victim, supporting the victim's decision to prosecute or not, not dwelling on the sexual part of the rape but on the victim's *feelings*; stress that victim needs to be held and stroked just as she would in any stressful situation and not to withhold touch (otherwise, they may reinforce victim's feelings of being unclean, ruined)
- share with them that it is typical that rape victims will have increasing fear and anxiety during next 48 hours and may want to talk at length about the experience, that victims may then "seem" to adjust but may reexperience the feelings of the attack at a later date
- tell them that victim may not want to talk about the assault, and if so, they should not press her but continue to provide caring and support
- tell them to work out with victim ways for her to be and feel safe, e.g., locks on windows, new lights, not walking alone at night, etc.; some action may be needed immediately, e.g., changing locks

Evaluation: The family or significant other gives victim situational support (e.g., believes what she says; goes home with her); verbalizes accepting/understanding attitude toward victim.

Goal 3: The child victim will receive situational support from ER staff; will be allowed to cope with situation in own way; will experience protection and relief from pain, injury, fear, or physical abuse.

Plan/Implementation
- encourage the child to talk about the experience and to ventilate feelings but do not dwell on the sexual aspects; suggest drawing a picture of what happened and talking about the drawing (often easier for children to do than just talk); do not minimize child's feelings or try to talk them away, but acknowledge them
- know that these children are often misbelieved; let child know you believe what she or he says, thinks, feels
- use a calm, soothing approach to child, showing your caring, warmth, and interest in the child as a person
- reinforce to child victims that it was not their fault, that they will not be punished by you, and that they are not bad children
- explain to child all procedures before they are carried out; medical procedures may be more frightening to the child than the sexual assault; ensure that a woman (staff member, police, family) stays with female child at all times

Evaluation: Child is free from acute pain; receives situational support from ER staff (e.g., blanket, a woman to stay at all times, listening); copes with situation in own way.

Goal 4: Family/significant others will state they feel less anxious and able to cope with situation; will verbalize an understanding of what child has experienced; will provide situational support for child.

Plan/Implementation
- talk to family separately away from child in order to help them sort out feelings of anger, anxiety, fear, etc.; encourage them to ventilate to you rather than to the child, which could make child feel guilty for having upset the family
- know that the family/significant others may vent anger at the offender or may direct it at the agency/staff or even the child, especially if the offender is someone they know and have liked
- assess their level of coping; do they seem able to cope with situation? are they hysterical? crying? in control? if they are hysterical, be very firm, to calm them down; provide general support (listening, acknowledging feelings) to enhance their own coping ability
- help them focus on the needs of the child right now, rather than on the attacker; point out that the child needs loving, stroking, holding, caring, to feel she or he is not bad, was not at fault
- reinforce that the responsibility for the assault lies with the offender, not the child; family/significant others may be confused, disbelieving, especially if offender is a family member, friend, or neighbor
- if they talk of the child's being "ruined" or "violated" or "she's no longer my little girl," point out that she is indeed still a little girl, the same child

who now has a great need for support, love, reassurance, and protection
- tell them the child may or may not want to talk about the assault and that they should let the child set the pace, not forcing or criticizing in any way
- inform family that the child will be very sensitive to their reactions and will respond to them more than to the assault
- stress the importance of returning to usual family activities as soon as possible; discuss the benefits of family mental health counseling and provide community referrals as necessary

Evaluation: Family/significant others state they feel in control of situation and have plans to protect child from further assaults; have a referral for follow-up physical and mental health care.*

E. Antisocial Behavior

1. **General Information** (Content within the asterisks is adapted from M. Neal et al. *Nursing Care Planning Guides, Set 4*, 2nd Ed. "The Patient with an Antisocial Personality," No. 4:36. Baltimore: Williams & Wilkins, 1983. Used with Permission.)
   a. *Definition: a cluster of personality characteristics manifested by deeply ingrained, basically unsocialized behavior, i.e., continuous and chronic violation of the rights of others; formerly known as sociopathic or psychopathic personality
   b. Characteristics
      1) does not tolerate frustration
      2) feels little guilt
      3) does not change behavior because of punishment
      4) often has an outwardly pleasing, charming personality, but is loyal only to self
      5) has no close personal relationships
      6) "uses" or manipulates other persons and events for own motives; there is a tendency to ascribe the same motivation and behavior to others
      7) has never learned to give, only to take
      8) does not see self as mentally ill and only infrequently does one find such persons presenting themselves for treatment
      9) usually hospitalized for treatment of other disorders, such as to withdraw from alcohol or drugs, or as result of a court order for psychiatric evaluation or treatment
      10) described as selfish, irresponsible, impulsive, and callous
      11) repeatedly in conflict with society, and often with the law*
      12) behaviors differ from psychotics in that they do not exhibit ego disintegration, impaired thought processes, or poor reality testing
      13) behaviors differ from neurotics in that they do not have fixed and exaggerated psychologic defenses
      14) defective personalities predispose them to a disregard for accepted social behavior
   c. Diagnostic Category: these clients show patterns of chronic, lifelong maladaptive behaviors; collectively these behaviors are called personality disorders (*DSM-III* classification)
   d. Treatment: usually consists of applying external controls to limit the acting out behavior
      1) antisocial behavior patterns are difficult to alter and respond poorly to treatment
      2) long-term psychotherapy has had the most success in changing behavior patterns, but relatively few clients remain in psychotherapy because of expense, time involved, poor motivation, and lack of insight

2. **Nursing Process**
   a. Assessment
      1) characteristics of personality disorders
         a) persistent and inappropriately motivated antisocial behavior
         b) persistent pattern of self-defeat and failure to follow any life plan
         c) absence of anxiety
         d) reluctance to accept rules and regulations
         e) poor judgment and failure to learn by experience
         f) poor interpersonal relations
         g) minimal insight and poor impulse control
         h) history of a childhood in which no clear authority, guidelines, or

controls on the child were established and in which the antisocial behavior of the child was accepted and encouraged with a guilty permissiveness by parents
  i) suspiciousness, emotional lability/rigidity
  j) inability to feel or express emotion
  k) poor concentration and motivation
 2) behavior: manipulation, impulsiveness, seductiveness, demanding, acting out, histrionics, violence

b. Goals, Plans/Implementation, and Evaluation

Goal 1: *Client will recognize and observe limits in interactions with others.

Plan/Implementation
- be aware that staff commonly experience uncomfortable feelings of anger, helplessness, frustration, defensiveness, etc., when working with these clients; openly discussing and acknowledging these feelings with other staff members can lead to control of them, thus making one less susceptible to being manipulated; *immature behaviors require firm and consistent limit setting; limits must be consistently applied by individual nurses and staff as group; this type of approach takes a good deal of staff planning and communication to be effective; inconsistent application of this approach is ineffective in changing behavior
- *observe closely client's behavior and interactions with staff and other clients; assess the meaning and understanding of the behavior to the client and validate with client and other staff; hold a staff conference to discuss, set, and inform all staff of approaches and limits for this client; written care plans will provide the best means for consistency of approach
- be aware of other clients who could easily be affected by this client (used, hurt) and intervene as necessary; work with both clients on appropriate ways to respond to each other; if antisocial client refuses to cooperate, separate from rest of unit for time out; state firmly that limits will be set on behavior and that other persons and situations will not be used for one person's ends; make contract with client that states specific cause and effect, such as, "If you take Mr. H's cigarettes, you will not be allowed in the day room when he is there;" follow through on contract on all shifts; be consistent
- review requests made by client with other staff before permission is granted or denied; do not make on-the-spot decisions if delay is possible; remember that this client is often an expert at pitting one staff member against another (re-creating the family triangle and being in the center of attention); staff must present a united front
- give attention to client when he is not manipulating; reinforce positive behavior (often the only attention client gets occurs after he has acted out or manipulated); set reasonable goals with client; reinforce positive efforts to reach them
- explanations, discussions should be short and simple; long, complex ones can provide opportunities for manipulation
- be aware that client may use tears, lies, threats to get own way; limits must be followed by all staff members and may be lifted after client has shown ability to handle responsibility
- know that client's demands may be endless; be firm, and most important of all, be consistent

Evaluation: Client observes limits in interaction with staff and others.

Goal 2: Client will strengthen ability to relate to others in socially acceptable ways.

Plan/Implementation
- help client define problem areas in social relationships (e.g., blames others, lack of concern for others)
- encourage client to discuss this problem area in group therapy and to ask others why they reject him (if they do)
- help client practice social skills; use role-playing; give positive reinforcement for positive behavior*
- avoid responding with hostility or moral judgment
- set rules for client's behavior on the unit, including verbal expression
- respond to infractions of rules with withdrawal of privileges

- know that frequently these clients are rude and sarcastic to other clients; they may be especially biting in their remarks about the habits of neurotic clients and the apathy of psychotics

Evaluation: *Client can cite some limits to interactions with others; demonstrates ability to comply with social mores and to behave within socially acceptable limits at least part of the time (an increasing amount); indicates a willingness to continue mental health therapy in some form that is presently available and potentially helpful.*

Suspicious Behavior

General Concepts

A. Overview: suspicious behavior occurs when a person is overly sensitive to and preoccupied with the behavior and motivations of others. In mild forms, such behavior may include taking protective precautions to avoid becoming the victim of a truly dangerous person (e.g., putting new locks on doors, not being alone, rape prevention). In severe forms, such behavior results from abnormal and unwarranted distrust of others and results in extreme efforts to protect self (e.g., disruptive social and marital relationships, aggressive behavior).

Suspicious behavior may be an aspect of a particular disorder, such as organic mental disorder or schizophrenic disorder, or it may be the predominant problem as in paranoid disorders or paranoid personality disorders.

B. Application of the Nursing Process to the Client Exhibiting Suspicious Behavior
All adults have some level of sensitivity and preoccupation with the behavior and motivation of others. When this behavior becomes exaggerated, it is paranoia, the selected health problem discussed below.

Selected Health Problem

Paranoia [*exaggerated Paranoia*]

1. **General Information**
   a. Definition: behavior characterized by hostility and mistrust of others resulting from grandiose and/or persecutory delusions not due to any other mental disorder such as schizophrenia, affective disorder, or organic mental disorder
   b. Types
      1) paranoia: an insidious development with permanent well-organized, well-defined, unshakable delusional system; chronic; seen less frequently than paranoid schizophrenia [*often chronic*]
      2) acute paranoid disorder: this is the sudden onset in individuals who have experienced drastic environmental changes (e.g., immigrants, POWs); rarely becomes chronic [*< 6 mo.*] [*does eventually go away*]
   c. Characteristics
      1) suspiciousness
      2) grandiose and/or persecutory delusions
      3) no hallucinations
      4) haughty, superior manner
      5) tendency toward hostility, anger, and aggression
      6) no impairment of intellectual or occupational functioning
      7) often severe impairment of social and marital functioning with progressive estrangement from others
      8) duration of at least one week
      9) rarely seek help themselves; brought in by associates or relatives for help
   d. Dynamics
      1) lack of trust
      2) low self-esteem
      3) poor reality testing in area related to delusions
   e. *DSM-III* Classification: paranoid disorder [*> 6 mo.*]

2. **Nursing Process**
   a. Assessment
      1) duration: at least 1 week; chronic if over 6 months; acute if less than 6 months
      2) delusions
      3) problematic behavior
         a) superiority
         b) expression of hostility, anger, or aggression
         c) social and/or marital impairment
      4) self-esteem

b. Goals, Plans/Implementation, and Evaluation

Goal 1: Client will develop a trusting relationship with a staff member.

Plan/Implementation
- establish regular times and places for meetings; keep appointments or notify in advance of cancellation
- be honest and accurate in communication
- make mutual expectations and promises clear and abide by them
- be accepting and nonjudgmental

Evaluation: Client develops a trusting relationship with a staff member as evidenced by a willingness to confide in staff member.

Goal 2: Client will learn to define and test reality regarding the delusional system.

Plan/Implementation
- help client to recognize delusions as signs of anxiety and poor self-esteem
- do not argue about content of delusions, but focus on reality
- limit discussion of delusions
- acknowledge client's feelings and beliefs, but point out that these are not shared
- be honest and reliable
- reassure client that delusions will disappear when client gives them less attention and description
- focus on the here and now

Evaluation: Client gives up delusion; expresses feelings of anxiety.

Goal 3: Client will demonstrate improved self-esteem.

Plan/Implementation
- identify strengths: encourage client to focus on them
- assist client in developing a relationship with another client
- assist client in gradually developing relationships within groups
- intervene with problematic behavior (e.g., superiority, hostility and anger, aggression; refer to those behaviors in *Socially Maladaptive/Acting Out Behavior*)

Evaluation: Client is able to begin a relationship with other clients and groups; controls problematic behavior.

Goal 4: Client will improve social and marital functioning.

Plan/Implementation
- encourage client to discontinue behavior that disrupts social and marital relationships (e.g., accusations, letter writing, threats)
- identify feelings that lead to problematic behavior
- find constructive outlets for the feelings (e.g., relaxation techniques, physical exercise, public service); avoid aggressive, competitive activities
- help client to establish or reestablish trusting, supporting relationship with family members (e.g., promote open, direct communication and involvement in mutually agreed upon activities)
- assist family to explore their feelings about client's behavior; provide information about client's status; help family to examine ways to respond to client

Evaluation: Client improves social and marital relationships; communicates feelings, needs, and wants to family; family members state they feel comfortable around client.

Withdrawn Behavior

General Concepts
A. Overview
1. Definition: an individual responds to stress by retreating from interactions with people and environment. In extreme situations, the person withdraws from reality.
2. Behavioral Continuum
   a. Healthy; temporary pulling back from a stressful situation and focusing psychic energy internally
      1) to remove self from stressful situations, to think, and to take a temporary retreat is a healthy and sometimes necessary response
      2) the individual who plunges forward without thinking can cause undue pain to self and others; each person needs solitary time to think, to plan, to reflect, and to regroup before acting
   b. Unhealthy: isolating oneself from others and the world to the extent that relationships and the ability to function in society are seriously impaired
      1) the person may retreat to avoid facing important social situations; social skills are not learned and a cyclical pattern of withdrawal results
      2) examples of unhealthy uses of withdrawal include
         a) excessive fantasizing that keeps the person from having to deal with day-to-day problems of living
         b) excessive TV watching or involvement in only solitary activities to avoid social encounters
      3) schizophrenia is the most severe form of withdrawal; the person's thought patterns, communications, and relationships with others prevent functioning in a productive manner
3. Withdrawn Behaviors: though withdrawn behaviors occur on a continuum, this section focuses primarily on the most severe form of withdrawal, i.e., schizophrenic disorder
   a. Etiologic Factors: no consensus about cause; various theories
      1) biologic: genetic or physical defect is the cause
      2) psychologic: internal dynamics related to difficulties in thought process, affect, and behavior are the cause
      3) sociologic: family relationships and rigid social expectations are the cause; schizophrenic behavior is learned, i.e., communication patterns, response to double-bind communication are learned from parents
   b. Dynamics: the person views the world as so threatening that withdrawal from interpersonal relationships, social situations, and reality is seen unconsciously as the only alternative
   c. Behavioral, Psychologic, and Sociologic Manifestations
      1) behavioral manifestations: the behaviors of schizophrenic withdrawal are manifested in varying ways and degrees of severity
         a) *affect* (feeling tone or mood) of the withdrawn client is often diagnostic of the status of his illness
            - a specific criterion in judgment is the appropriateness of the affect; that is, the degree to which it is in keeping with the situation at hand, both quantitatively and qualitatively
            - responses may be excessive, or they may be inappropriately

minimal, often referred to as "flat." A flat affect is demonstrated by a blunt or dull emotional tone of expression; it is a generalized impoverishment of emotional reactivity
- inappropriate affect is that which is incongruent with the situation or the content of thought
  b) *behavior disorganization*, in which the client reacts to stress in an unpredictable or bizarre manner (e.g., pacing, rigid posturing)
  c) *disregard of hygiene and grooming* can range from looking unkempt to bizarre clothing and makeup or disregard for bodily care
  d) *disregard of physical safety* includes not being concerned about placing self in dangerous situations, such as walking in a busy street or causing self-inflicted wounds; these persons need close observation
  e) *nutrition deficits* because of poor eating habits
  f) *regression*, in which the client returns to behavior patterns exhibited at an earlier stage of development (e.g., thumb sucking, baby talk, fetal position)
     - main defense mechanism used in schizophrenia
     - allows the person to be dependent and to return to the predictable behavior experienced in childhood
2) psychologic manifestations: these refer to the interpersonal dynamics of the person
  a) *autism:* extreme withdrawal from real world and preoccupation with idiosyncratic thoughts and fantasies
     - a common characteristic of schizophrenic behavior
     - this persistent tendency to withdraw from involvement with the external world and to become preoccupied with ideas and fantasies that are egocentric and illogical causes autistic clients to be unresponsive

- it is difficult to establish communication with them; they may be mute; their conversations may be irrelevant or lack coherence
  b) *hallucinations:* an imagined sensory perception that occurs without an external stimulus
     - can be auditory, visual, or tactile
     - usually occurs in psychotic disorders but can occur in both chronic and acute organic brain disorders
     - auditory hallucinations are the most common form occurring in clients with schizophrenia, although visual, tactile, olfactory, and gustatory hallucinations may be experienced
       - some clients describe the experience as very definite; others describe it with an element of vagueness
       - the auditory hallucinations are often threatening and aggressive, and the client's response to them may account for acts of violence
       - hallucinations temporarily lessen anxiety, because they offer a substitute for interaction with real persons whom the client fears; such experiences are therefore counterproductive and conducive to further withdrawal from reality; when the client becomes aware that others see that he is hallucinating, he becomes ashamed and embarrassed, and this increases his anxiety and the loneliness he feels
  c) *delusion:* a false belief or opinion that is unreasonable and causes distortion in judgment
     - delusion of grandeur is a false, grandiose, or expansive belief that one is a very important or powerful person or entity (e.g., sees self as royalty or as Jesus)
     - delusion of persecution is a false belief that one is victim of

others' hostility and aggressiveness (e.g., "The FBI is after me.")
- although delusions represent a withdrawal from reality into fantasy, their function is to secure the client's identity
- this function makes these belief systems rigid and inaccessible to reason, permitting no modification; any attempt to correct the client's beliefs makes the nurse seem to be an enemy
- trying to reason the client out of his false beliefs will make him work harder to improve the delusion, thus reinforcing it and making it more entrenched

d) *depersonalization:* feelings of unreality or strangeness concerning either the environment or the self, or both
- a common phenomenon in the schizophrenic process and results from the client's poor self-concept
- client treats self as an object
- client seems to have resigned not only from the world of reality but also from himself; this leads to extreme social isolation

e) *associative looseness:* one experience or idea reminds the client of a completely different experience, which is interpreted in an autistic manner
- associative looseness is manifested in the thought process of withdrawn schizophrenic clients
- it is the tendency of the thought process to lose its continuity so that thinking and expression become confused, bizarre, incorrect, and abrupt
- the client's communication is disconnected, follows no logical sequence, and is confusing to the listener

f) *ambivalence:* the coexistence of two opposing feelings toward another person, object, or idea (e.g., love-hate, pleasure-pain, like-dislike)
- occurs normally, from time to time, in all persons and is popularly known as "mixed feelings"
- is one of the classical behaviors in schizophrenia and characterizes the stormy relationships the schizophrenic has with relatives, friends, and associates
- because of the ambivalence felt toward significant others, minor difficulties can lead to disruption of these relationships, which are generally chaotic

3) sociologic manifestations
   a) poor social skills: difficulty with conversation and even physical closeness
   b) retreat from social situations
   c) few or no friends: often has no friends, or relationships are considered to be friendships in spite of minimal contact
   d) pathologic family relationships: often severe communication problems
   e) erratic employment history
   f) difficulty maintaining an independent living situation: unable to care for self, will not pay rent regularly or take care of physical needs; some can do the caretaking tasks but tend to isolate themselves

d. Management: long-term management with continuing follow-up is frequently necessary
   1) medications: major tranquilizers (see table 2.9)
      a) actions: modify intense anxiety, tension, and psychomotor excitement; alleviate delusions and hallucinations
      b) benefits: allow the client to participate in other forms of therapy
      c) side effects: these drugs are not addictive but do have troublesome and occasionally dangerous side effects; see table 2.10, "Side Effects of Major Tranquilizers"
      d) nursing role: administer the medications, observe client response, intervene to prevent

Table 2.9 Major Tranquilizers

Generic Name (Trade Name)	Dosage	Major Nursing Implications for Each Category
Phenothiazines		
Aliphatic Subgroup		
Chlorpromazine (Thorazine)	100-1,000 mg PO daily	Observe for skin reaction.
		Check BP prior to administration.
Promazine (Sparine)	10-200 mg PO q4-6 hr.	Have client remain in lying position 30-60 mins after a IM/(deep IM) dose. Advise client to rise slowly from a sitting or lying position.
		Do periodic liver function tests.
		Warn client that drowsiness may occur until a drug tolerance is reached. Advise against driving a car or operating machinery.
		Notify physician when client complains of sore throat or other signs of infection.
		In case of pseudoparkinsonism, inform client about what is occurring; administer the antiparkinsonian drug.
Piperazine Subgroup		
Prochlorperazine (Compazine)	15-40 mg PO, usually not to exceed 75 mg daily	
Trifluoperazine (Stelazine)	4-10 mg; may be slowly increased to 15-20 mg	Do not give IV.
Fluphenazine HCl, decanoate or enanthate (Prolixin, Permitil)	0.5-10 mg PO daily, not to exceed 20 mg; 12.5-25 mg q2 weeks IM	May mask signs of intestinal disorders, brain tumors, head injuries, poisoning.
Piperidine Subgroup		
Thioridazine HCl (Mellaril)	20-800 mg daily.	Observe for orthostatic hypotension, dryness of the mouth, visual or retinal changes, rash, and gastric irritation.
		Warn client that drowsiness may occur until a drug tolerance is reached.
		Advise against driving a car or operating machinery.
Butyrophenones		
Haloperidol (Haldol)	1.5-6 mg daily; 6-15 mg, up to 100 mg to achieve control	Advise appropriate diet and exercise.
		Observe carefully for regular bowel movement in client too disoriented to do so (client may need laxatives).
		Observe for parkinsonian side effects.
Thioxanthenes		
Chlorprothixene (Taractan)	100-600 mg	Advise client and family of potential side effects.
		Observe for orthostatic hypotension.
Thiothixene (Navane)	6 mg daily, slowly increase to 20-30 mg; rarely exceeds 60 mg	

Table 2.10 Side Effects of Major Tranquilizers

Parkinsonian-type
- pseudoparkinsonism
- dystonia
- akathisia.

Hypotension.
Photosensitivity.
Agranulocytosis.
Jaundice.
Increased restlessness.
Drowsiness.
Weight gain and constipation.
Potentiates narcotics, alcohol, barbiturates, and anesthetics.
Menstrual changes and libido changes.

---

complications related to drug side effects, and teach client and family about the drug, e.g., action, side effects, and need to take on long-term basis
- it is of utmost importance that the nurse be completely familiar with dosage and side effects of these drugs, and that the client be carefully observed when such drugs are prescribed
- the nurse may have difficulty getting the client to take the prescribed drug, e.g., the client may think he is being poisoned, and the nurse may need to use ingenuity in order to get the client to take it
- it is the nurse's responsibility to record and report any side effects or problems to the nurse in charge or to the physician

2) milieu therapy
 a) a form of therapy that is utilized to increase the effectiveness of other psychiatric treatment methods
 b) promotes a positive living environment for each client
 c) uses the interactions within the social context as an opportunity to assess client and implement treatment
 d) uses the inpatient hospital setting as a therapeutic environment
 e) many conditions of client's experience may require hospitalization or at least make it advantageous (e.g., a tendency toward violence directed toward self or others, or an inadequate or negative provision for meeting immediate emotional needs at home)
 f) milieu therapy manipulates both physical and emotional properties of the hospital ward, taking into account the specific needs of individual clients and groups of clients in an effort to promote a positive living experience for each client and the maximum of positive, behavioral change
 g) the therapeutic milieu takes into account the stimuli in the environment (it can be increased or decreased), limit setting, protection, and activities
 h) nurses—on the unit at all times—are in a position to make the greatest contribution to milieu therapy; they can
  - provide a positive role model of care and concern for others
  - note and report the kinds of interactions among clients, clients and staff
  - provide the flexibility to promote opportunity for the client's behavioral experimentation and growth
 i) planned interactions within the milieu designed to promote independence and develop social skills are
  - *government:* clients elect officers to run meetings, negotiate with staff, and administer the various unit activities (e.g., kitchen cleanup, dayroom cleanup); clients report to the president of the government
  - *self-care:* clients may be required to change their own bed linen, do their own laundry, and keep their rooms clean; these activities help clients to maintain or learn independence even while hospitalized

- *assessment of group skills:* several activities are done in groups; clients are able to attend and participate according to their ability
- *occupational therapy:* has long been a useful adjunct in psychiatry
  - generally, occupational therapy is carried on in a room off the nursing unit, assigned for that special purpose
  - although nurses are sometimes involved in the activities of that department, generally registered occupational therapists and student occupational therapists plan and conduct the program for the clients in accordance with specific orders of the psychiatrists
  - gives the client an opportunity
    * to keep occupied
    * to express self nonverbally if communication is a problem
    * to follow activities prescribed to achieve specific psychologic results
- *activity therapy:* includes art, music, and recreation as a planned activity, therapeutically designed, and carried out generally within the unit setting
  - in some situations, the activities are carried out by regular unit personnel
  - in other situations, therapists with special training direct activities
  - nurses are often involved and assume some of the functions of the activity therapists; this is a good way for the nurse to stay involved with the schizophrenic client and avoid mutual withdrawal (i.e., both client and nurse use withdrawal as a coping mechanism)

3) nurse-client relationship
  a) purpose: to assist the client to function as independently as possible, to deal with problems amenable to nursing intervention, and to complement the medical treatment
  b) development of trust
  - therapeutic nursing interventions necessitate the development of a relationship of trust that will stand as a model for relationships with others, in contrast with those client has experienced thus far
  - schizophrenics develop relationships slowly if at all and use their ambivalence to push others away; therefore, the orientation phase of the relationship is the most difficult for them

B. **Application of the Nursing Process to a Client Exhibiting Withdrawn Behavior**
  1. **Assessment**
      a. Suicide Potential
          1) logic, content of thought and general feeling tone: autistic thinking; aggressive/hostile voices; a confused, depressed mood increases suicide risk
          2) refer to *Elated-Depressive Behavior* page 50
      b. Behavioral, psychologic, and sociologic manifestations (refer to page 77)
  2. **General Nursing Goals, Plans/Implementation, and Evaluation**
      (see table 2.11, "Selected Problem Behaviors and Interventions")

  Goal 1: Client will remain physically safe.
  Plan/Implementation
  - keep harmful objects away from impulsive clients
  - observe client at frequent intervals
  - observe for physical problems (e.g., infection, constipation) that may be outside client's awareness
  - know and observe for side effects of drugs; see reprint section
  - monitor rest and sleep; use comfort measures such as pillows, snacks, warm baths to induce sleep

  Evaluation: Client does not injure self; experiences only minimal side effects of drugs; has adequate rest and sleep.

  Goal 2: Client maintains adequate nutrition and fluid and electrolyte balance.

Table 2.11 Selected Problem Behaviors and Interventions

Behavior	Interventions
Aggression	Prevention—early recognition of increased excitement. Encourage verbal expression of feelings surrounding behavior. Reduce stimuli. Avoid reinforcement, e.g., competitive games. Provide distraction. Set limits. Protect other clients.
Anger	Acknowledge or name feeling. Explore sources. Encourage to express verbally. Explore appropriate outlets. Avoid arguing.
Anxiousness	Acknowledge or name the behavior or feeling. Explore sources. Encourage appropriate expression. Give reassurance. Recognize that anxiety in nurse increases client's anxiety.
Associative looseness (thought disorder)	Relate in a concrete manner. Focus on immediate situation. Point out reality.
Autism	Accept at stage client is in; don't push. Give ample time for responses. Do not reinforce dependency.
Controlling behavior	Recognize means of controlling: negativism, obstruction, silence, avoidance, insults, yelling, increased chatter, crying. Do not impose unnecessary controls. Allow client some control. Develop trust: security in giving up control.
Delusions	Avoid arguing. Avoid arousing suspicion. Be honest and reliable. Be consistent. Acknowledge client's feelings. Point out reality: client's beliefs are not shared.
Dependence	Assess abilities and capabilities. Provide only help needed. Encourage to solve problems and make decisions. Display attitude of firmness and confidence. Discourage reliance beyond actual need. Encourage successful participation.
Hallucinations	Help to recognize as manifestation of anxiety. Encourage to give up hallucinations. Help to relate with real persons. Do not give attention to content.
Hopelessness, helplessness	Structure small successes. Give encouragement. Exhibit expectation that client will succeed.
Hostility	Avoid arguing with the client. Acknowledge and name feelings. Explore the source of hostility with client. Encourage to express hostility verbally, rather than resort to physical aggression. Explore appropriate outlets for hostility (e.g., physical activities).
Low self-esteem, feeling worthless	Prevent isolation. Acknowledge client's view. Avoid system of shoulds and should nots and discussions regarding moral judgments. Avoid power struggles. Give minimal tasks and grade them to manageable size. Prevent self-mutilation.
Manipulation/acting out	Spell out acceptable and unacceptable behavior. Set firm and definite limits. Consistently enforce limits. Avoid involvement in intellectualization; i.e., responsibility for behavior rests with client. Treat infractions with withdrawal of privileges. Ensure that staff is united, firm, and consistent. Maintain sense of authority.
Ritualistic behaviors	Don't interrupt repetitive act: could lead to panic. Set limits on repetitive behavior. Engage in alternative activities with client. Provide physical protection from repetitive acts.
Secondary gain	Understand unconscious motivation of the behavior and differentiate it from malingering. Understand and alleviate primary symptoms. Encourage client to explore the motivation of the behavior. Explore alternatives to the primary symptom for handling anxiety.
Somatic behaviors	Don't focus on physical symptoms. Give appropriate information regarding somatic complaints. Point out reality, i.e., correct misinformation.
Superiority	Suggest solitary activities for client. Put client in charge of things, not people. Give client activities at which client can succeed.

Plan/Implementation
- observe for signs of dehydration (e.g., dry skin, lips); encourage to drink fluids
- if client is not eating, assess the reasons (e.g., delusions about food being poisoned, too agitated to sit for meals, unaware of poor eating habits)
- assist client to find methods for increasing food intake (e.g., permit food from home if client fears hospital food is poisoned; provide finger foods client can eat while walking)
- provide positive reinforcement for good eating habits
- teach about nutrition as needed

Evaluation: Client maintains adequate food and fluid intake; skin is hydrated.

Goal 3: Client demonstrates improved hygiene and grooming.

Plan/Implementation
- identify specific client needs for assistance (e.g., with severe withdrawal, client may need nurse to provide care; client with poor reality orientation or attention span may need assistance; more self-sufficient client may only need encouragement)
- use gentle firmness and consistent interest in client's needs
- provide matter-of-fact positive reinforcement for appropriate grooming and cleanliness
- be sure equipment for physical care is available to client

Evaluation: Client does self-care for hygiene (hair, nails, clothing, bathing).

Goal 4: Client will develop a trusting relationship with staff member; will demonstrate increased ability in social interaction.

Plan/Implementation
- know that staff reactions can be the crucial element negating or facilitating attainment of the therapeutic goal for the client
  - often the client's behavior provokes feelings of frustration, helplessness, and incompetence among staff
  - staff members may find themselves withdrawing from the client, because this disorder is often chronic and the prognosis is pessimistic
  - this withdrawal on the part of the staff reinforces the client's past experiences of rejection and feelings of low self-esteem
  - in his own defense, the client will withdraw further into his world of fantasy, negating progress towards the therapeutic goal planned for him
  - in addition, the client may test staff involvement with him by trying to push staff away
  - offer support and encouragement to other staff members; meet regularly to provide support
- use consistent, predictable behavior with client
- persevere even though client may be unreliable or rejecting
- meet for short intervals at regularly scheduled times to increase trust
- use silence; share that you are willing to spend time without talking if client so chooses
- allow ample time for response if client very regressed; use general comments that do not push client for answer
- allow client to set the pace of the relationship
- accept the client where he is in his illness; if communication with him is to be restored, the nurse must understand that he is frightened and both wants and fears contact from others, that he makes responses slowly, and that he needs ample time to trust her sincerity and her interest
- listen in nonjudgmental way to client's thoughts/feelings
- know that autistic clients are extremely sensitive to the feeling tones of others; they pick up negative clues from the nurse, who may be unaware of them
- role-model socially appropriate behavior
- as client begins to accept the nurse, he may become very dependent; a therapeutic goal requires that the nurse maintain contact on a professional level and not reinforce the dependency
- observe verbal and nonverbal behaviors that may indicate any interest in activities; give support to any expression of interest

Evaluation: Client develops a relationship with one staff member; begins to interact with other clients.

Goal 5: Client will define and test reality; will dismiss internal voices/hallucinations.

Plan/Implementation
- recognize disorientation as manifestation of severe withdrawal related to anxiety and frustration
- be meticulously honest and reliable, especially with the suspicious client
- do not give attention to content of hallucinations or delusions (gives them legitimacy): avoid arguing about content
- acknowledge client's feelings and beliefs; point out that these are not shared
- relate to client in a realistic and concrete manner, focusing on the immediate situation; it is helpful for the nurse to point out reality to the client by saying that she doesn't understand and asking for clarification as needed
- encourage to give up hallucinations or delusions; help to recognize hallucinations as sign of anxiety
- reassure that hallucinations and delusions do go away and can be dismissed by client as he focuses on real people and situations
- help client to relate with real persons
- assist client who has depersonalization to discuss his feelings of estrangement with trusted individuals
  - first with a nurse in whom he has developed a trusting relationship
  - as client's condition permits, in group therapy sessions or similar groups involving other persons who may recount similar experiences
  - sharing these disturbing thoughts and feelings of depersonalization is often quite profitable
- focus on reality of the client's body and environment during these discussions

Evaluation: Client dismisses internal voices/hallucinations; increases ability to relate to real persons and situations.

Goal 6: Client increases communication with family members.
Plan/Implementation
- accept client's feelings and thoughts and help client do the same
- explore present family patterns with client; family assessment and intervention during the client's hospitalization may be done
- help client identify feelings associated with family interactions
- help client view self as unique person with values and beliefs that are sometimes different from family's
- practice social skills to use with family members; use role playing, assertion techniques

Evaluation: Client increases adaptive communication with family members.

Goal 7: Client will increase successful decision-making skills.
Plan/Implementation
- relate in a concrete manner; focus on the immediate situation
- encourage decision making at level of client's ability; use therapeutic milieu as tolerated by client
- increase complexity of decisions as tolerated
- provide with tasks of increasing complexity
- do not reinforce unneeded dependency

Evaluation: Client increases ability to make decisions.

Goal 8: Client will demonstrate social skills in individual and group settings.
Plan/Implementation
- be a role model of appropriate social interaction
- role-play social situation with client
- assist client to develop a relationship with one other client
- encourage client to relate to others during activities
- take care not to push client beyond present abilities; may need encouragement to begin developing social skills
- help client to relate to others in more complex situations, slowly as tolerated

Evaluation: Client behaves appropriately in individual and group settings; interacts with other clients; demonstrates fewer problem behaviors.

Goal 9: Client will develop ability to be as self-supporting as possible.
Plan/Implementation
- support client in finding a healthy living situation; may be at home, a halfway house, or in own apartment depending on client's social skills and ability to be self-motivating
- support client in finding employment as appropriate; employment history and assessment of skills in occupational

86 SECTION 2: NURSING CARE OF THE CLIENT WITH PSYCHOSOCIAL PROBLEMS

therapy can help in developing employment plan

Evaluation: Client finds healthy living situation; develops a plan to be self-supporting.

Selected Health Problems

A. Paranoid Schizophrenia

1. **General Information**
   a. Paranoid or grandiose delusions, often accompanied by hallucinations
   b. Behavior tends to be consistent with delusions experienced
   c. Uses defense mechanism of projection
   d. Retreats into fantasy world and attributes to others his emotions and feelings and thus believes that everyone is out to get him or that everyone thinks he is special
   e. Displays a hostile/aggressive/superior attitude
   f. Increased sensitivity
   g. Ideas of reference (a detection of personal reference in insignificant remarks, objects, or events)

2. **Nursing Process**
   a. Assessment
      1) potential for aggression
      2) refer to Assessment page 50
   b. Goal, Plan/Implementation, and Evaluation

   Goal: Client will display decreased hostile/aggressive behavior; will begin to interact with staff and other clients.

   Plan/Implementation
   - *hostility*
     - avoid arguing with the client, as arguing is interpreted by him as antagonism toward him and adds to his fantasized list of enemies
     - assist client to acknowledge and name the feeling
     - explore the source of the hostility with client
     - encourage client to express hostility verbally rather than to resort to physical aggression
     - explore appropriate outlets for the hostility (e.g., physical activities, exercise, sports)
   - *superiority:* these clients usually decline invitations to join in group activities
     - initially, suggest choice of solitary activities for client; after establishing a relationship of trust, suggest activities that involve the client and nurse
     - know that ability for group participation comes slowly, if at all; when these clients do work up to group participation, they should be put in charge of things (not people) as their air of superiority tends to alienate others
     - to deal with the underlying inferiority, give the client activities at which he can succeed; when this is done, the "superior" behaviors tend to decrease
   - *aggression*
     - protect the safety of other clients
     - take preventive measures: observe client's behavior patterns to recognize increased excitement and predict experiences that might provoke aggressive outbursts
     - reduce the stimuli when client shows signs of excitement
     - initiate control measures if the client cannot control himself
     - utilize distraction to deflate aggression
     - encourage client to express feelings verbally rather than physically
     - avoid reinforcing the behavior (e.g., shouting at the client, playing competitive games)

   Evaluation: Client decreases hostile/aggressive behaviors; begins to interact with the staff and other clients.

B. Catatonic Schizophrenia

1. **General Information**
   a. Very severe form of withdrawal; marked regression
   b. Catatonic stupor characterized by
      1) waxy flexibility, in which the client holds a physical position he is placed in for a long time
      2) neglect of bodily needs
      3) impervious to fluctuations in temperature
         a) may expose self to danger of overheating or freezing, or to serious infections
         b) disagreements are in evidence among the caring professions as to

whether the client has an awareness during such periods
4) negativism: the client interprets himself and his environment in a negative manner
5) client may be mute
c. Catatonic excitement characterized by
1) severe agitation
2) grimacing, bizarre gestures and postures, echolalia, echopraxia
3) negativism

2. Nursing Process
a. Assessment (refer to page 50)
b. Goal, Plan/Implementation, and Evaluation

Goal: Client will be physically safe; will be observed for side effects of drugs.

Plan/Implementation
- provide a structured environment
- identify signs of increasing agitation and intervene prior to client's loss of control
- observe for infection, skin breakdown related to immobility, urinary and fecal incontinence
- provide adequate nutrition (refer to General Nursing Goals page 50)

Evaluation: Client remains free from physical injury.

C. Undifferentiated Schizophrenia

1. General Information
a. Undifferentiated schizophrenia and paranoid schizophrenia are most common types
b. The diagnosis is meant for a category of clients who show mixed schizophrenic symptoms over a long period of time: they present definite schizophrenic thought, affect, and behavior and a mixture of symptoms from the other categories

2. Nursing Process
a. Assessment (refer to page 50)
b. Goals, Plans/Implementation, and Evaluation (refer to page 50)

D. Childhood Schizophrenia

1. General Information
a. Has raised a great deal of controversy in the caring professions over etiology and categorization
b. *DSM-III* Classification: pervasive developmental disorder
c. May be genetic or environmental in origin
d. May be a single disease or a complication
e. Symptoms do not include hallucinations or delusions
f. Characterized by withdrawal, impairment in social relationships, disturbance in affect, ritualism, self-mutilation, increased or decreased sensitivity to sensory stimulation
g. At present, using behavior modifications in conjunction with chemotherapy, family therapy, psychotherapy, and therapeutic milieu is the major treatment modality

2. Nursing Process
a. Assessment (refer to page 50)
b. Goal, Plan/Implementation, and Evaluation

Goal: Client will decrease ritualistic and self-mutilating behaviors.

Plan/Implementation
- judiciously ignore these behaviors without compromising client's safety
- provide a structurally consistent environment
- identify behaviors early and divert client to other activities
- provide positive reinforcement for adaptive behaviors

Evaluation: Client does not injure self; decreases ritualism.

Refer to General Concepts for Plans/Interventions aimed at building trust, self-care, communication, etc.

E. Psychotic Disorders not Elsewhere Classified: Schizophreniform Disorder, Brief Reactive Psychosis, Schizoaffective Disorder, Atypical Psychosis (*DSM-III* Classification)

1. General Information
a. While not classified as schizophrenic disorders, these conditions by and large share a similar symptomatology.
b. The major distinguishing factors are
1) sudden onset
2) short duration (less than 6 months)
3) prognosis is more positive than for other psychotic disorders
4) residual defects, minimal or nonexistent
5) usually no history of disturbed interpersonal relationships prior to onset
6) intervention usually not necessary after symptoms subside

2. **Nursing Process**
   a. **Assessment**
      1) duration of onset
      2) stability of interpersonal relationships
      3) refer to page 50
   b. **Goals, Plans/Implementation, and Evaluation**
      1) similar to those discussed in General Concepts (refer to page 50)
      2) continuing, long-term intervention not necessary

Substance Use Disorders

General Concepts
A. Overview
1. Definitions
   a. Substance Use Disorder: "...maladaptive behavior associated with more or less regular use of the substances." (*DSM III*)
   b. Polydrug Abuse: mixing drugs and alcohol in varying degrees (particularly dangerous because of potentiating and toxic interactions of drugs and alcohol)
2. Etiology: not known, but thought to be an interplay of physiologic, psychologic, and sociocultural factors
3. Interaction Variables
   a. The Person
      1) no specific personality type identified
      2) most frequently, the person shows signs of immaturity, low tolerance for frustration, low self-esteem, environmental deprivation, conflicts over parental upbringing, and conflict of values
      3) it is not known if substance abuse fosters development of these characteristics or if the characteristics trigger the abuse
      4) major psychiatric disorders generally associated with substance abuse are antisocial personality and affective disorders
   b. The Family: substance abuse may relate to overall anxiety level in family as well as in individual
   c. The Environment: social aspects and peer pressure may lead the person into drug culture and antisocial acts
   d. The Substance: which substance the person uses depends on the cultural group, availability, costs, and federal regulation of the item (alcohol and/or drug substances other than alcohol)
4. Substance abuse is associated with behavior changes related to more or less regular use of a substance that affects the central nervous system acutely or chronically. Three criteria distinguish substance *abuse* from substance *use*
   a. Pattern of Pathologic Use: depending on the substance, client manifests inability to cut down or stop use despite physical problems; needs daily use for adequate functioning; intoxication throughout the day; episodes of a complication of substance intoxication, e.g., alcoholic blackouts
   b. Impairment of Social or Occupational Functions: legal and economic difficulties because of cost, procurement, or complications of intoxication, e.g., auto accident
   c. Duration of Abuse: disturbance of at least a month
5. Substance Dependence
   a. Definition: a more severe form of substance use disorder than substance abuse
   b. Manifestations
      1) a physiologic need for a substance evidenced by withdrawal or tolerance
      2) almost always, a pathologic use pattern occurs that causes impairment in social or occupational functioning
      3) rarely, manifestations are limited to physiologic dependence
      4) alcohol or cannabis dependence requires evidence of occupational or social impairment; diagnosis of other substance-dependence categories requires only evidence of withdrawal or tolerance

c. Length of Dependence: regular maladaptive use for over six months qualifies as "continuous dependence"
d. Social Complications: although accessibility, chance, peer pressure, and curiosity play a part in who will ingest a drug and who will not, they do not account for the fact that one person becomes addicted and another does not
e. Physiologic Dependence: an altered physiologic state produced by the repeated administration of the drug, which necessitates its continued administration to prevent a withdrawal syndrome
f. Addiction: the compulsive use of a chemical substance with physiologic and psychologic dependence
g. Habituation: repeated use of a substance that results in psychologic dependence
h. Tolerance: markedly increased amounts of the substance are required to achieve the desired effect, or there is a markedly diminished effect with regular use of the same dose
i. Withdrawal: a substance-specific syndrome following cessation or reduction of intake
j. Lethality: the amount of a substance that constitutes a fatal dose
k. Potentiation: two or more substances combined have a greater effect than simple summation (1 + 1 = 3)

6. Substance use disorders in health professionals is a serious problem
   a. Narcotic addiction by physicians estimated at 1%-2%, or 30 times greater than in general population
   b. Estimated 40,000 alcoholic nurses in US
   c. Problems with impaired health professionals' job performance result in danger to clients and the professionals themselves and compromise teamwork
   d. It is the responsibility of health professionals to report concerns about a colleague to supervisor, and for supervisor to take appropriate actions
   e. Professionals are helping, not harming, a substance-abusing colleague by bringing problems to attention of someone qualified to help.

B. **Application of the Nursing Process to a Client with a Substance Use Disorder**
   1. **Assessment**
      a. Substance Use History (Substance abusers are well-known for denying use or seriously understating extent of use. To increase likelihood of accurate history, ask questions in a logical and nonthreatening manner.)
         1) history of recent prescription and nonprescription drug use
         2) drugs doctor prescribed for client in last few months
         3) nonprescription drugs taken in last two months, e.g., for a minor ailment or cold
         4) drugs client has prescribed for self, e.g., nicotine, alcohol, cocaine, marijuana
      b. Work Performance
         1) excessive use of sick time
         2) decreasing productivity or "job shrinkage"
         3) decreasing ability to meet schedules and deadlines
         4) sloppy or illogical work
         5) frequent errors in judgment; in drug-addicted nurses, medication errors, incorrect controlled-drug wastage, or incorrect narcotic counts
      c. Blood levels of suspected substance of abuse
      d. Level of consciousness, reality orientation, mental status exam
   2. **General Nursing Goals, Plans/Implementation, and Evaluation**

   Goal 1: Client will withdraw from substance that is abused or creating dependency.
   Plans/Implementation
   - it is important *not* to do any of the following
     - scold, argue, moralize, blame, or threaten
     - lose one's temper
     - enable person to cover up consequences of actions
     - be overly sympathetic
     - give lesser assignment or do person's work for her/him
     - put off facing problem
   - control symptoms via prn medication; take vital signs q2h and report elevations to physician

- assess potential for violence
- if client is agitated, confused, assaultive, belligerent, stay with him; reassure that current symptoms are only the result of his body's responding to the abused substance, and that they are temporary; tell him he will regain control; use restraints as necessary (follow hospital policy carefully)
- deal with hallucinations by reinforcing reality; speak to client slowly in a calm voice; provide a quiet environment; stay with client until the frightening symptoms have decreased
- provide physical care advocated for additional diseases/conditions that client may have
- keep client ambulatory as much as possible; if necessary, walk with client several times a day; help to bathroom, rather than providing bedpan or urinal

Evaluation: Client withdraws from abused substance, free from complications.

Goal 2: Client will obtain treatment necessary to abstain from substance abuse or dependence.

Plans/Implementation
- sit and talk with client at least twice daily; your presence will say he is not being rejected; be aware of your own nonverbal distancing maneuvers; establish good eye contact
- do not punish or reprimand client for failures or nonresponse to your suggestions/interventions (punishment serves only to give client fuel for continuing to deal with failure or rejection by drinking or taking drugs); ignore it, but do praise *any* positive responses
- have client make decisions about daily care in hospital; involve in some type of occupational therapy, anything in which he can achieve some measure of success (helps increase self-confidence and self-esteem)
- provide opportunities to decrease social isolation and improve social skills (mealtimes, groups, recreation periods); calmly, gently, point out unacceptable behavior such as manipulative acts; reinforce positive social behaviors (e.g., initiating friendly conversations); praise all efforts at participation in activities

Evaluation: Client participates in prescribed treatment.

Goal 3: Client will develop a positive lifestyle that is free from substance use, abuse, or dependence.

Plans/Implementation
- help the client to gradually become aware of the denial by poking holes in denial process; encourage client's assessment of how denial serves client, including delineation of the self-defeating aspects
- help client look at alternative coping methods and deal with abstinence one day (or one morning, one evening) at a time
- work with client to develop sound discharge planning regarding employment counseling, ongoing support via outpatient counseling, or long-term inpatient treatment
- arrange for client and family to attend group counseling sessions, if available in hospital, to discuss feelings, problems, changing behaviors, pressures, sources of support, etc.
- provide information about other types of therapy available, e.g., stress-reduction programs, employee assistance, aftercare programs, and local mental health clinics

Evaluation: Client's approach to daily living is positive and free from substance abuse or dependence.

Selected Health Problems

A. Alcohol

1. **General Information**
   a. Definitions
      1) *alcohol* is a mind- and mood-altering substance classified as a central nervous system depressant
      2) *alcoholism (alcohol dependence)*
         a) no precise agreement on definition, but most refer to these clinical features: chronicity; preoccupation with drinking; loss of control over drinking; damage to health, relationships, and/or work; using alcohol as a solution to most problems
         b) the World Health Organization defines alcoholism as a chronic

disease or disorder of behavior characterized by alcohol consumption that exceeds customary use and interferes with the drinker's health, interpersonal relations, or economic functioning
- c) in some settings may be further defined as alcoholism with no evidence of any preexisting major psychiatric problem (primary alcoholism) or alcoholism occurring after the onset of a major psychiatric disorder (secondary alcoholism)

b. Effects
1) at low levels of consumption, there is little apparent effect on the drinker; moderate levels may produce euphoria; and in large amounts, alcohol acts as a sedative
2) alcohol depresses higher cortical functions, acts as a disinhibitor and tranquilizer, and serves to reduce anxiety rapidly (excessive drinking is often the way a person copes with anxiety)

c. Scope of Alcohol Abuse and Dependence
1) estimates
   a) one-third of general hospital clients, but these clients are rarely admitted with alcoholism diagnosis
   b) one out of 10 Americans who drinks is an alcoholic
   c) 6.6 million adults in US are alcoholic
   d) one in 10 alcoholics is diagnosed and treated
2) occurrence: alcoholism and related problems are widespread among
   a) city residents
   b) minorities
   c) poor men under 25 years of age
   d) persons who have experienced childhood disruptions, e.g., broken homes, alcoholic parents
   e) rural or small-town persons who have moved to urban areas
   f) people of Swedish, Polish, Irish, northern French, and Russian origin

d. Characteristics: common but not exclusive to alcoholics are
1) low self-esteem
2) feelings of isolation
3) emotional immaturity
4) anger over dependence
5) highly anxious in interpersonal relationships
6) inability to express emotions adequately
7) ambivalence toward authority
8) grandiosity
9) compulsiveness, perfectionism
10) sexual-role confusion

e. Withdrawal from Alcohol and Detoxification
1) symptoms develop when there is a physiologic dependence and the intake of alcohol is interrupted or decreased without substitution of other sedation
2) complete cessation of use of alcohol is not necessary for the development of withdrawal symptoms; the beginning of withdrawal can be a reflection of diminished use in those who have developed a marked tolerance and physical dependence
3) monitored detoxification for withdrawal is the top priority need of the alcoholic client
4) withdrawal syndrome has four major manifestations: tremulousness, hallucinations, convulsive seizures, and delirium tremens; this is a progressive process and involves four stages
   a) stage 1: 8 hours plus after cessation: symptoms include mild tremors, nausea, nervousness, tachycardia, increased blood pressure, diaphoresis
   b) stage 2: symptoms include profound confusion, gross tremors, nervousness and hyperactivity, insomnia, anorexia, general weakness, disorientation, illusions, nightmares; auditory and visual hallucinations begin
   c) stage 3: 12–48 hours after cessation: symptoms include all those of stages 1 and 2, as well as severe hallucinations and grand mal seizures ("rum" fits)
   c) stage 4: occurs 3–5 days after cessation: symptoms include initial and continuing delirium tremens (DTs), which are characterized by confusion, severe psychomotor activity, agitation, sleeplessness,

hallucinations, and at onset, uncontrolled and unexplained tachycardia; DTs are a medical emergency (fatality rate is 20% even with treatment)
f. Prognosis: motivation and recognition of the problem are necessary for the elimination of alcohol use; the person experiences fluctuations of sobriety, during which acknowledgement of illness and movement toward a new way of life are punctuated by relapse, shock, and denial; alcoholics are considered as recovering, not cured
g. Treatment: approaches used in all alcohol treatment models
   1) general measures include vitamin and nutritional therapy, sedatives, tranquilizers, and/or disulfiram (Antabuse); avoid drugs containing alcohol, e.g., elixirs, cough syrups, mouth washes
   2) detoxification: the acute phase of treatment
      a) usually occurs in a well-controlled environment such as a hospital
      b) frequently, a 7-day program may include medical treatment and supportive services
      c) magnesium sulfate 50% solution and high doses of chlordiazepoxide (Librium) are used in decreasing doses for anticonvulsant effect
      d) education and group process are frequently used after detoxification when client is able to understand instructions
   3) rehabilitation
      a) aim is to build treatment motivation and overcome denial in clients and significant others
      b) the alcoholic has to learn to give up alcohol forever
      c) the person is helped to learn new ways of problem solving and living a satisfying life without alcohol; this is enhanced by a therapeutic relationship that increases the alcoholic's self-confidence, feelings of self-worth, and attempts to become more independent
   4) major models of treatment
      a) chronic disease model
         • views alcoholism as a primary, physiologic, incurable disease
         • views psychosocial problems as result of drinking
         • includes a maintenance program of recovery
         • emphasis is on self-diagnosis by the alcoholic
      b) psychiatric model
         • focus on unique needs as defined by psychiatric perspective
         • varying psychotherapeutic treatment regimen depends on individual
      c) family systems model
         • views family relationships as a contributing factor
         • examines childhood development of alcoholic, such as drinking patterns of parents, ethnic attitudes, and socialization process regarding drinking behaviors
         • identifies how present family relations recreate old patterns of avoidance or dependence
         • utilizes family commitment and caring to promote recovery
         • integrates recovering alcoholic into revised family structure
   5) Alcoholics Anonymous is a self-help group of recovering alcoholics
      a) 12-step program to achieve sobriety, which members do at their own pace
      b) run entirely by sober alcoholics
      c) requires members to devote themselves completely to mutual help
      d) remarkable success with chronic alcoholism
      e) has member groups for families of alcoholics
         • Al-Anon is an organization of spouses
         • Alateen is an organization of teenage children of alcoholics
         • the emphasis is on education, guidance in relating to the alcoholic family member, the sharing of problems and experiences, and support
   6) long-term treatment may also take place in the controlled environment

of a private or public facility and in an outpatient setting
- a) depending on particular model used, emphasis varies among group process, education, psychotherapy, family therapy, and AA
- b) AA is the backbone to maintain sobriety; some clients attend daily

h. Preventive Measures: include helping the client learn to
1) tolerate psychologic stress
2) do advance planning for anticipated painful events (surgery, separation from a loved one)
3) reduce social isolation

2. Nursing Process
a. Assessment
1) physical assessment/history: conduct as you would for any client with special attention to
- a) skin: spider angiomata, jaundice, acne rosacea, multiple bruises, age of bruises (purple, yellow), oven burns on forearms, mahogany finger stains
- b) orthopedic system: vaguely explained fractures, moderate muscle wasting of proximal muscle groups of lower and upper extremities
- c) cardiovascular system: a first episode of paroxysmal atrial tachycardia as adult, ventricular premature contractions, paroxysmal atrial fibrillation, erratic hypertensive course (alcohol elevates blood pressure)
- d) gastrointestinal system: early tooth losses, esophagitis, gastritis, pancreatitis, palpable liver, peptic ulcer, gastrectomy scar
- e) neurologic system: shakes that worsen with movement, vertigo and nystagmus that clear during the day, vaguely described memory lapses (blackouts), insomnia, development of seizures as an adult
- f) genitourinary system: mild proteinuria, impotence
- g) indications of fluid and electrolyte imbalance

2) psychologic assessment
- a) suicide potential
- b) extent of cognitive disturbance
- c) mental status exam
- d) occurence of signs and symptoms related to major psychiatric disorders

3) other: although not diagnostic in themselves, the following raise possibilities and should be explored further
- a) numerous transient medical symptoms in various organ systems without mention of drinking
- b) unwarranted complaints and signing out against medical advice (hospitalized clients)
- c) functioning at lower job level than intelligence and education would indicate; changing jobs frequently
- d) alcoholism in close relatives (parental alcoholism increases likelihood fivefold)
- e) child or spouse abuse

4) stage of alcoholism and related symptoms (dependent on amount of consumption and the physical makeup of the person)
- a) *early:* 5–10 years of controlled social drinking with some tolerance symptoms
  - signs: dependence on alcohol; without it the person is irritable, has insomnia and tremors; has need for a morning drink; is defensive and tries to conceal his drinking problem
- b) *middle:* symptomatic; dependence increases and tolerance decreases
  - signs and symptoms: blackouts, periods of amnesia; life centered on drinking; social, recreational, and occupational activities affected
  - physical changes: chronic gastritis, fatty infiltration of the liver; all organs can be affected
- c) *late or chronic:* damage to the central nervous system
  - signs: organic brain syndrome, Wernicke's syndrome/Korsakoff's syndrome, pancreatitis, cirrhosis of the liver, nutritional deficiencies
  - withdrawal signs: gross tremors, excessive perspiration, nausea, vomiting, anorexia, restlessness, hallucinations, convulsions

- delirium tremens occur 24–72 hours after the last drink
- signs and symptoms: fear, confusion, profuse sweating, vomiting, constant body motion

5) strengths and stressors, coping mechanisms
6) beliefs, attitudes, feelings, concerns about alcohol consumption

b. Goals, Plans/Implementation, and Evaluation

Goal 1 (Content between asterisks is adapted from M. Neal et al. *Nursing Care Planning Guides, Set 2*, 2nd Ed. "The Patient with Alcoholism," No. 2:01. Baltimore: Williams & Wilkins, 1980. Used with permission.): *Client will withdraw from alcohol, free from the complications of dehydration, electrolyte imbalance, nutritional imbalance; will verbally recognize and discuss his alcoholism as the cause of the withdrawal.

Plan/Implementation
- know that the severity of withdrawal symptoms is related to the length and extent of drinking that preceded the withdrawal period
- institute seizure precautions according to hospital policy
- observe for withdrawal symptoms as early as 8 hours after cessation of drinking
- remove hazardous articles, e.g., razor, glasses (high correlation between alcoholism and suicide)
- report results of electrolyte tests to physician
- monitor for signs of dehydration related to diarrhea and vomiting
- record I&O, weight for several days; check bladder for distention
- ensure a daily fluid intake of at least 2,500 ml orally, unless contraindicated (check with physician); offer favorite juices q2h during waking hours; prevent excessive coffee or tea intake, as caffeine increases tremors (some hospitals allow only decaffeinated coffee)
- identify client's food preferences; provide frequent small feedings or between-meal snacks of high-protein foods; involve client in food-related planning; give multivitamin and mineral supplements as ordered

Evaluation: Client withdraws from alcohol, free from preventable complications; remains calm.

Goal 2: Client will discuss and develop the use of coping mechanisms other than alcohol to deal with the stress and strain of daily life.

Plan/Implementation
- discuss your observations of client's behavior with him, helping him develop insight regarding its relation to alcohol intake
- in an accepting, nonjudgmental way, discuss client's use of alcohol with him; provide information as he wants and asks for it
- recognize and share with client your knowledge that a life-style without alcohol is a major loss to him; anticipate what this may mean and help him plan adaptive ways to compensate for the loss
- if client on disulfiram (Antabuse) therapy, read literature and then explain effects that develop after ingestion of alcohol (severe nausea and vomiting, flushed face, rapid pulse and respirations, drop in BP)
- discuss AA, Al-Anon, Alateen with client and family or other support system; offer to arrange for an AA member to come and see client; encourage him to accept; if client agrees, coordinate referral, treatment, and aftercare with AA

Evaluation: Client begins to explore new coping mechanisms (e.g., increases social skills, talks of going to AA); participates in group activities.

Goal 3: Client will accept the support of others; will discuss with them how they can help him live without alcohol.

Plan/Implementation
- hold weekly conferences of health team to discuss aspects of alcoholism, to share feelings about and responses to caring for an alcoholic client and to coordinate care; explain that it is normal for staff to feel frustrated (angry, guilty, rejecting, anxious) when caring for alcoholic client; staff often feel they have failed if a client is readmitted in an inebriated state after they had discharged him as "improved"
- permit family to express their anger at client's exacerbations of client's

condition; listen to and support them; put family in touch with a community group where consistent support and help are available, e.g., Al-Anon (family group of AA)
- invite a member of AA and/or Al-Anon to a staff conference to share their aims, approaches, etc., or go to a meeting with a colleague

Evaluation: Client/family/significant other has been in contact with AA, Al-Anon and/or other community mental health group; verbalizes an understanding of and expects to participate in a daily program of balanced food and fluid intake, rest, exercise, and recreation; can state the actions and side effects of current medications; has an adequate supply to take with him; has at least one plan to help decrease social isolation and strengthen new behaviors.*

B. Drugs Other than Alcohol

1. **General Information**
   a. Opiates and Opiate Derivatives, Synthetic Opiates (e.g., morphine, Demerol, dilaudid, codeine, heroin): chronic abuse results in tolerance, physical dependence, habituation, and addiction
      1) psychologically, most opiate addicts show a similarity to alcoholics in some aspects of their personality; they are emotionally immature, dependent, hostile, aggressive; and they take drugs to relieve inner tensions
      2) opiate addicts sometimes differ from alcoholics in that they prefer to handle feelings of aggression, dependence, and hostility passively, by avoidance rather than by acting out; choosing drugs (opiates) seems to suppress these inner tensions and thus permits the user to make a passive adaptation
      3) availability, curiosity, and peer pressure play a role in the use of opiates; social factors, such as urban versus rural differences and social class, also play a role; social factors seem related largely to availability of the drug and opportunity for the initiation of use
      4) cultural values regarding the use of opiates may play a role in the rates of addiction
         a) Asian countries, in which opiate addiction has been tolerated, have a high rate
         b) Western European countries, where opiate addiction is treated as a medical rather than a legal problem, have low rates
   b. Barbiturates and Other Sedative Drugs (e.g., Equanil, Librium, Doriden, Placidyl, Valium): if compulsively and chronically abused, cause tolerance, habituation, addiction, and physical dependence
      1) there is a general depressant, withdrawal syndrome associated with all of these drugs
      2) in contrast to the situation with opiate use, many users of the sedative drugs began with a physician's prescription; prescription drugs are considered socially acceptable in western society for the relief of tension and insomnia
      3) persons who become chronic and compulsive users of these drugs have a variety of underlying psychologic difficulties; they may be
         a) anxious or insecure
         b) trying to relieve hostile and aggressive impulses
         c) trying to escape tension through the drug's intoxicating effect
   c. Amphetamines and Cocaine: they have a stimulating effect upon the user
      1) when these drugs are chronically and compulsively abused, they result in tolerance and habituation
      2) when the drug is withdrawn, general fatigue and depression occur along with changes in the sleep EEG; these symptoms are not considered a clinical withdrawal syndrome, and physical dependence is not associated with the abuse of these drugs
      3) chronic use can result also in a toxic psychosis, characterized by vivid hallucinations and persecutory delusions
      4) social, cultural, and psychologic factors have all been cited as causative: family history of alcoholism and psychopathology,

availability, peer pressure, curiosity, and physician prescription; the use of these drugs by persons who are overweight or depressed is more socially acceptable than by those who take them for thrills
5) many amphetamine or cocaine addicts are also compulsive users of barbiturates, alcohol, or morphine
d. Hallucinogens (e.g., lysergic acid diethylamide [LSD], mescaline, PCP [angel dust], STP): produce tolerance, and in some persons, habituation
1) these agents do not produce physical dependence with its concomitant withdrawal syndrome or addiction
2) may produce acute panic and anxiety states and toxic psychosis, characterized by hallucinations and persecutory delusions
3) historically, these drugs were used in connection with religious practices of American and Mexican Indians
4) recently they have been used by persons who wish to explore their own feelings in altered states of drug-induced intoxication
5) persons who compulsively abuse these drugs are thought to be psychologically insecure, dependent, hostile, and immature
6) social class seems to be a factor in the use of hallucinogens, with those in the middle or upper class being more frequent users

2. **Nursing Process**
   a. **Assessment**
   1) physiologic problems: respiratory, circulatory, neurologic problems associated with withdrawal symptoms (priority)
   2) after emergency treatment, assess for problems arising from
      a) consequences of drugs, e.g.,
         • potential seizures (cocaine, barbiturate withdrawal)
         • tolerance
      b) sepsis associated with drug injection
         • abscesses of skin and subcutaneous fat deposits
         • hepatitis
      c) neglect of nutritional needs
         • malnutrition
         • loss of teeth, dental caries
         • respiratory infections
   3) behavior problems: a multiplicity of behaviors are common among drug abusers, e.g.,
      a) denial and/or underreporting of use
      b) somatic complaints
      c) blaming others
      d) anger, hostility, self-pity
      e) family, social, employment, and financial problems
      f) low frustration tolerance
   b. **Goals, Plans/Implementation, and Evaluation**
   Goal 1: Client will withdraw from drug, free from respiratory failure, shock, toxic psychosis.
   Plan/Implementation
   • intervene in respiratory failure: maintain a patent airway, give oxygen
   • administer IV fluids for shock, as ordered
   • assess the level of coma or stupor
   • administer drugs, as ordered to suppress withdrawal or to counter a toxic psychosis
   • give antibiotics as ordered
   • restrain client as necessary for safety
   Evaluation: Client withdraws from drug; breathes adequately, has patent airway; no signs of shock or toxic psychosis.

   Goal 2: Client will decrease purposive drug seeking, manipulative and acting out behavior.
   Plan/Implementation
   • set firm and consistent limits
   • clearly define acceptable and unacceptable behavior
   • client often will complain that nurse who doesn't cooperate doesn't trust him
   • client may plead, cry, ask for money, steal, simulate drug withdrawal syndrome to obtain drugs
   • entire staff needs to adopt consistent approach to client's behavior
   Evaluation: Client decreases purposeful drug seeking and manipulative/acting out behavior; accepts limits of unit.

   Goal 3: Client will decrease intellectualization; will focus on problem solving and ADL.

Plan/Implementation
- client may exhibit dependency behaviors, blame parents, society, world conditions for drug-taking behaviors; be aware that client may try to involve nurse in intellectual discussion about the above, but do not discuss these with client (not therapeutic)
- instead keep focus on client's responsibility for own behavior; do not plead or exhort
- focus on problems in ADL and possible solutions

Evaluation: Client discusses living problems and develops some solutions.

Goal 4: Client decreases denial and superficiality; explores alternative coping mechanisms; verbalizes some awareness of consequences of own actions.

Plan/Implementation
- confront the client face to face with facts about himself that he blatantly or subtly attempts to avoid; use only after foundation of trust and acceptance has been laid or when group relationship is cohesive
- avoid discussions of "why" client abuses drugs
- avoid nagging client to promise total rehabilitation; realistic approach to possibilities of success must be taken
- know that 90% of drug abusers relapse
  - few of the efforts in psychiatry, drug therapy, or psychotherapy have been successful with drug abusers
  - the most effective treatment to date has been that given by former abusers; having been in the situation, these persons are familiar with the demanding behaviors, manipulations, rationalizations, intellectualizations, and denial of drug abusers, and are able to handle them with firmness and with supportive concern; clients are less likely to "put one over" on them
- do not make moral judgments
- many nurses experience rescue, angry, or hostile feelings toward drug abusers; be aware of these feelings and try to control your reactivity in client's presence

Evaluation: Client decreases use of denial; begins to explore alternative coping; visits postdischarge treatment facility; decreases number and frequency of drug-abuse incidents.

Glossary
Terms Common to Psychiatric Nursing
by J. H. Flaskerud

Addiction: The compulsive use and procurement of chemical substances on which the individual has become dependent; has a high tendency to relapse after withdrawal.

Affect: The mood or emotion an individual shows in response to a given situation. Affect can be described, according to its expression, as appropriate, blunted, blocked, flat, inappropriate, or displaced.

Ambivalence: The coexistence of two opposing feelings toward another person, object, or idea (examples: love-hate, pleasure-pain, like-dislike).

Anxiety: Apprehension, tension, or uneasiness that stems from the anticipation of danger, the source of which is largely unknown or unrecognized. Primarily of intrapsychic origin, in distinction to fear, which is the emotional response to a consciously recognized and usually external threat or danger. Anxiety and fear are accompanied by similar physiologic changes. May be regarded as pathologic when present to such an extent as to interfere with effectiveness in living, achievement of desired goals or satisfactions, or reasonable emotional comfort.

Autism: Extreme withdrawal from the real world and preoccupation with idiosyncratic thoughts and fantasies.

Commitment Procedure: The legal procedure for admission to a psychiatric hospital. This procedure can be voluntary, compulsory, or emergency.

Confabulation: A symptom that is usually in organic psychotic disorders, e.g., Korsakoff's psychosis. The individual defensively attempts to fill in details about the past, which he cannot recall because of memory loss. Imaginary experiences are often related in a detailed and plausible fashion.

Conflict: In psychoanalytic terms, it describes the mental struggle that occurs when there are opposing impulses, drives, and demands of the id, ego, and superego.

Conjoint Therapy: The psychotherapy of couples or entire families treated together at the same time by the same therapist.

Countertransference: In Freudian theory, the arousal in the therapist of reactions toward the client based on unconscious feelings and attitudes.

Covert: Implies secrecy or hidden reasons for conscious actions or behavior.

Crisis Intervention Therapy: A type of brief psychiatric treatment in which individuals (and/or families) are assisted in their efforts to cope and problem solve in crisis situations. The treatment approach is immediate, supportive, and direct.

Delirium Tremens (DTs): Generally thought to be a withdrawal syndrome precipitated in chronic alcoholics deprived of alcohol. It is associated with metabolic and nutritional disturbances; early signs include restlessness, irritability, fear, and apprehension. Progression is to confusion, disorientation, illusions, hallucinations, and convulsions.

Delusion: A false belief or opinion that is unreasonable and causes distortion in judgment
 a. delusion of grandeur: a false, grandiose, or expansive belief that one is a very important or powerful person or entity;
 b. delusion of persecution: a false belief that one is victim of others' hostility and aggressiveness.

Depersonalization: Feelings of unreality or strangeness concerning either the environment or the self or both.

Double Bind: A type of interaction, generally associated with schizophrenic families, in which one individual demands a response to a message containing mutually contradictory signals, while the other is unable to respond or comment on the inconsistent and incongruous message. Best characterized by the "damned if you do, damned if you don't" situation.

Dyad: The relationship between any two persons; dyadic pair can be husband and wife, parent and child, sibling and sibling.

Ego: The part of the personality, according to Freudian theory, that mediates between the primitive, pleasure-seeking instinctual drives of the id and the self-critical, prohibitive, restraining forces of the superego. The compromises worked out, on an unconscious level, help to resolve intrapsychic conflict by keeping thoughts, interpretations, judgments, and behavior practical and efficient. The ego is directed by the reality principle, meaning it is the contact with the real world, as well as by the id and superego. The ego develops as the individual grows.

Extrapyramidal Reaction: The usually reversible side effect of some major psychotropic drugs on the extrapyramidal system of the CNS. Characterized by a variety of physical signs and symptoms (similar to those seen in clients with Parkinson's disease) including muscular rigidity, tremors, drooling, restlessness, shuffling gait, blurred vision, and other neurologic disturbances.

Family Therapy: Treatment of more than one member of the family simultaneously in the same session. The treatment may be supportive, directive, or interpretive. The assumption is that a mental disorder in one member of a family may be a manifestation of a disorder in other members and in their interrelationships and functioning as a total group.

Flight of Ideas: A disturbance in the progression of thought characterized by an increased associative activity, a rapid digression from one idea to another with no progress toward the goal idea.

Group Therapy: Application of psychotherapeutic techniques by one or more therapists to a group of persons who have similar problems and are in reasonably good contact with reality. The optimal size of a group is 6-10 members. As a therapy procedure, it is popular because it is versatile, economical, and generally successful.

Hallucination: An imagined sensory perception that occurs without an external stimulus. It can be auditory, visual, or tactile. Usually occurs in psychotic disorders but can occur in both chronic and acute organic brain disorders.

Id: In Freudian theory, the id is identified as the reservoir of psychic energy. It is guided by the pleasure principle, curbed by the ego, and is unconscious. The id wants what it wants when it wants it. Babies are born with an id.

Identified Client: The designation by the family unit of one member who is "sick" and who is identified as the client in need of treatment. In family therapy, the sick member of the family system who exhibits symptoms of psychopathology is regarded as a symptom of family pathology.

Illusion: A misinterpretation of the sensory stimuli, usually auditory or visual, of a real experience.

Insight: The ability of a person to understand himself and the basis for his emotions, attitudes, and behavior.

Interpersonal: All that occurs between persons, e.g., spoken words, gestures, looks, changes in body positions, expressions of emotion such as laughing, crying, etc. In psychiatric nursing, it refers most frequently to what occurs between closely related persons.

Intrapsychic: All that takes place within the mind (psyche).

Latent: Adjective used to describe feelings, drives, and emotions that influence behavior but remain repressed, outside of conscious thought or action.

Limit Setting: A clear enunciation of the rules of behavior and social relationships and the point beyond which going is forbidden, and a consistent enforcement of the rules.

Manipulation: A skillful handling, control, or management of others' behavior or of a situation for one's own purposes.

Milieu: The immediate environment, both physical and social.

Narcissism: Self-love; excessive interest in one's own appearance, comfort, importance, abilities, etc. In Freudian theory, arrest at the first stage of development in which the self is the object of all attention and pleasure.

Neologism: A new word that is invented or made up by condensing other words into a new one; used typically in schizophrenia.

Neurosis: An impairment of personality development and growth that is characterized by excessive use of energy for unproductive purposes. The chief symptom in neurotic disorders is anxiety, which is either felt directly or controlled by various psychologic mechanisms to produce other, subjectively distressing symptoms. Although in some of its forms and degrees it is incapacitating, it does not interfere with the person's contact with reality. Psychosis implies flight from reality; neurosis, an attempt to come to terms with it.

Overt: Open, conscious, and unhidden actions, behavior, and emotions.

Paradoxical Communications: The typical patterns of verbal and nonverbal communication between individuals and within families involving incongruent but consistent contradiction, qualification, or denial of previously made statements and actions. It results in distrust, confusion, and ultimately, meaningless communications.

Paranoid: An adjective describing unwarranted suspiciousness and distrust of others.

Personality: The characteristic way in which a person behaves; the deeply ingrained pattern of behavior that each person evolves, both consciously and unconsciously, as a style of life or way of being in adapting to the environment.

Phenothiazines: The major group of psychotropic drugs used in the treatment of mental illness, chiefly the psychoses. Their chemical action is on the CNS.

Phobia: An irrational, persistent, obsessive, intense fear of an object or situation, which results in increased anxiety and tension and interference with the person's normal functioning.

Psychoanalysis: A form of psychotherapy developed by Freud, based on his theories of personality development and disorder, generally requiring basic commitments from the client (analysand) to the therapist (analyst) of time, money, and procedure. The technique of psychoanalysis involves an examination of the free associations of a client and the interpretation of his dreams, emotions, and behavior. Its focus is mainly on the way the ego handles the id tensions. Psychoanalysis is a lengthy, costly, esoteric treatment approach and is concerned only with the intrapsychic processes of the individual analysand. In psychoanalysis, success is measured by the degree of insight the client is able to gain into the unconscious motivations of his or her behavior.

Psychodrama: A form of group psychotherapy, developed by Moreno, in which clients dramatize their emotional problems. By assuming roles in order to act out their conflicts, they reveal repressed feelings that have been disturbing to them.

Psychodynamics: The usually unconscious forces that are presumed to be at work in a person that result in particular behaviors.

Psychogenic: Implies the causative factors of a symptom or illness are mental rather than organic.

Psychosis: A major mental illness characterized by any of the following symptoms: loss of contact with or a denial of reality, bizarre thinking and behavior, delusions, hallucination, regression, and disorientation. Intrapsychically, it results from the unconscious becoming conscious and taking over control of the person. In psychosis, the ego is overwhelmed by the id and the superego.

Psychotherapy: The treatment of mental disorders or psychosomatic conditions by psychologic methods using a variety of approaches including psychoanalysis, group therapy, family therapy, psychodrama, hypnotism, simple counseling, and suggestion.

Reality: The way things actually are.

Reality-Oriented Therapy: Any therapeutic approach that focuses on helping the client to define his reality, to improve his ability to adjust, and to function productively and satisfactorily within his real situation.

Schizophrenogenic: An adjective used to describe the object or situation that is thought to be causative in the development of schizophrenia.

Significant Others: The meaningful persons in one's life, usually parents and siblings, spouse, guardians, extended family, close friends.

Superego: In Freudian personality theory, the third part of the psyche. It guides and restrains, criticizes and punishes, just as the parents did when the individual was a child. It is unconscious and it is learned. Like the id, the superego also wants its own way. It has a conscious component called the conscience.

Symbiosis: In family therapy, this refers to a pathogenic relationship between the parent (usually the mother) and child that is characterized by retarded ego development and overdependence in the child.

Therapist: Refers to a person who, by reason of his/her training and experience and knowledge, is able and willing to use his/her skills to assist clients in the recovery and maintenance of health.

Transference: In Freudian theory, a carrying over and attaching to the therapist of unconscious feelings and attitudes that the client has toward his family or significant others.

Triad: In contrast to dyad, refers to relationships among three persons.

Unconscious: The repository of those mental processes of which the individual is unaware. The repressed feelings and their energy are stored in the unconscious and directly influence the individual's behavior.

Word Salad: A jumbled mixture of words and phrases that have no meaning and are illogical in their sequence. Seen most often in schizophrenia, e.g., "backter dyce tonked up snorfel blend."

Glossary References

American Psychiatric Association. *A Psychiatric Glossary*. Washington, DC: The Association, 1980.

Morgan, A. and Moreno, J. *The Practice of Mental Health Nursing: A Community Approach*. Philadelphia: Lippincott, 1973.

References

Beck, C., Rawlins, M., and Williams, S. *Mental Health-Psychiatric Nursing: A Holistic Life-Cycle Approach*. St. Louis: Mosby, 1984.

Billings, C. "Emotional First Aid." *American Journal of Nursing*. November 1980:2006-2009.

Brodsley, L. "Avoiding a Crisis: The Assessment." *American Journal of Nursing*. December 1982:1865-1871.

Burgess, A. and Lazare, A. *Psychiatric Nursing in the Hospital and the Community*, 3rd Ed. Englewood Cliffs, NJ: Prentice-Hall, 1981.

Burnside, I. *Nursing and the Aged*. New York: McGraw-Hill, 1981.

Campbell, J. and Humphries, J. *Nursing Care of Victims of Family Violence*. Reston, VA: Reston, 1984.

Carpenito, L. *Nursing Diagnosis; Application to Clinical Practice*. Philadelphia: Lippincott, 1983.

Cohn, L. "The Hidden Diagnosis." *American Journal of Nursing*. December 1982:1862-1865.

Crovella, A. "When Your Patient's an Alcoholic." *RN*. February 1984:50-53.

Davis, M., Eshelman, R., and McKay, M. *The Relaxation and Stress Reduction Workbook*. Richmond, CA: New Harbinger, 1980.

*DeGennaro, M. et al. "Antidepressant Drug Therapy." *American Journal of Nursing*. July 1980:1304-1310.

DeLuca, J. *4th Special Report to US Congress on Alcohol and Health from Secretary of Health and Human Services*. Rockville, MD: National Institute on Alcohol Abuse and Alcoholism, 1981.

*DiMotto, J. "Relaxation." *American Journal of Nursing*. June 1984:754-758.

Ewalt, J. and Crawford, D. "Posttraumatic Stress Syndrome." *Current Psychiatric Therapies*. 1981:145-153.

Goldsborough, J. "On Becoming Non-judgmental." *American Journal of Nursing*. November 1970:2340-2343.

Haber, J., Leach, A., Schudy, S., and Sidelau, B. *Comprehensive Psychiatric Nursing*, 2nd Ed. New York: McGraw-Hill, 1983.

*Hardiman, M. "Interviewing? or Social Chit-Chat?" *American Journal of Nursing*. July 1971:1379-1381.

*Harris, E. "Antipsychotic Medications." *American Journal of Nursing*. July 1981:1316-1323.

*_____. "Lithium." *American Journal of Nursing.* July 1981:1310-1315.

*_____. "Extrapyramidal Side Effects of Antipsychotic Medications." *American Journal of Nursing.* July 1981:1324-1328.

*_____. "Sedative-Hypnotic Drugs." *American Journal of Nursing.* July 1981:1329-1334.

Hoff, L. *People in Crisis: Understanding and Helping.* Reading, MA: Addison-Wesley, 1978.

Jaffe, S. "Help for the Helper: First-Hand Views of Recovery." *American Journal of Nursing.* April 1982:578-579.

Jefferson, L. and Ensor, B. "Help for the Helper: Confronting a Chemically-Impaired Colleague." *American Journal of Nursing.* April 1982:574-577.

Kline, N. and Davis, J. "Psychotropic Drugs." *American Journal of Nursing*, January 1973:54-62.

Leporati, N. "How You Can *Really* Help the Drug-Abusing Patient." *Nursing 82.* June 1982:47-49.

Marks, V. "Health Teaching for Recovering Alcoholic Patients." *American Journal of Nursing.* November 1980:2058-2061.

Mittleman, R., Goldberg, H. and Waksman, D. "Preserving Evidence in the Emergency Department." *American Journal of Nursing.* December 1983:1652-1656.

Murray, R. and Huelskoetter, M. *Psychiatric/Mental Health Nursing: Giving Emotional Care.* Englewood Cliffs. NJ: Prentice-Hall, 1983.

Neal, M. Cohen, P., and Cooper, P. *Nursing Care Planning Guides, Set 1*, 2nd Ed. Baltimore: Williams & Wilkins, 1980.

_____. *Nursing Care Planning Guides, Set 2*, 2nd Ed. Baltimore: Williams & Wilkins, 1980.

Neal, M., Cohen, P., and Reighley, J. *Nursing Care Planning Guides, Set 3*, 2nd Ed. Baltimore: Williams & Wilkins, 1983.

_____. *Nursing Care Planning Guides, Set 4*, 2nd Ed. Baltimore: Williams & Wilkins, 1983.

Pajk, M. "Alzheimer's Disease: Inpatient Care." *American Journal of Nursing.* February 1984:215-222.

Pasquali, E., Alesi, E., Arnold, H., and De Basio, N. *Mental Health Nursing: A Bio-Psycho-Cultural Approach.* St. Louis: Mosby, 1981.

Payne, D. and Clunn, P. *Psychiatric Mental Health Nursing*, 2nd Ed. Garden City, NY: Medical Examination Publishing, 1977.

Peterson, M. "Understanding Defense Mechanisms" (Programmed Instruction). *American Journal of Nursing.* September 1972:(Supp)1-24.

Platt-Koch, L. "Borderline Personality Disorder: A Therapeutic Approach." *American Journal of Nursing.* December 1983:1666-1670.

Potts, N. "Eating Disorders: The Secret Pattern of Binge/Purge." *American Journal of Nursing.* January 1984:33-35.

Robinson, L. *Psychiatric Nursing as a Human Experience*, 3rd Ed. Philadelphia: Saunders, 1983.

Sanger, E. and Cassino, T. "Eating Disorders: Avoiding the Power Struggle." *American Journal of Nursing.* January 1984:30-33.

Schuckit, M. *Drug and Alcohol Abuse: A Clinical Guide to Diagnosis and Treatment.* New York: Plenum, 1979.

Sideleau, B. "The Abusive Family." in J. Haber et al., Eds. *Comprehensive Psychiatric Nursing.* New York: McGraw-Hill, 1978:603-618.

Sundeen, S. and Stuart, G. *Principles and Practice of Psychiatric Nursing*, 2nd Ed. St. Louis: Mosby, 1983.

*Westercamp, J. "Suicide." *American Journal of Nursing*, February 1975:260-262.

Wilson, H. and Kneisl, C. *Psychiatric Nursing*, 2nd Ed. Menlo Park, CA: Addison-Wesley, 1983.

Zamora, L. "The Client who Generates Anger," in J. Haber et al., Eds. *Comprehensive Psychiatric Nursing.* New York: McGraw-Hill, 1978:280-305.

*See Reprint section

Notes

Reprints
Nursing Care of the Client with Psychosocial Problems

Hardiman, M. "Interviewing? Or Social Chit-Chat?" 107
Neal, M. et al. "Assessment of Mental Status." 110
———. "Stress Management." 112
DiMotto, J. "Relaxation." 114
Neal, M. Et al. "Behavior Modification." 119
Westercamp, T. "Suicide." 121
Harris, E. "Sedative-Hypnotic Drugs." 124
DeGennaro, M. et al. "Antidepressant Drug Therapy." 130
Harris, E. "Lithium." 136
———. "Antipsychotic Medications." 142
———. "Extrapyramidal Side Effects of Antipsychotic Medications." 150

Reprinted from American Journal of Nursing, July 1971

Interviewing? Or Social Chit-Chat?

It wasn't an easy lesson to learn, but this student did learn that encouraging a patient to ventilate was far from an intrusive "raking up of painful things about which you can do nothing."

MARGARET A. HARDIMAN

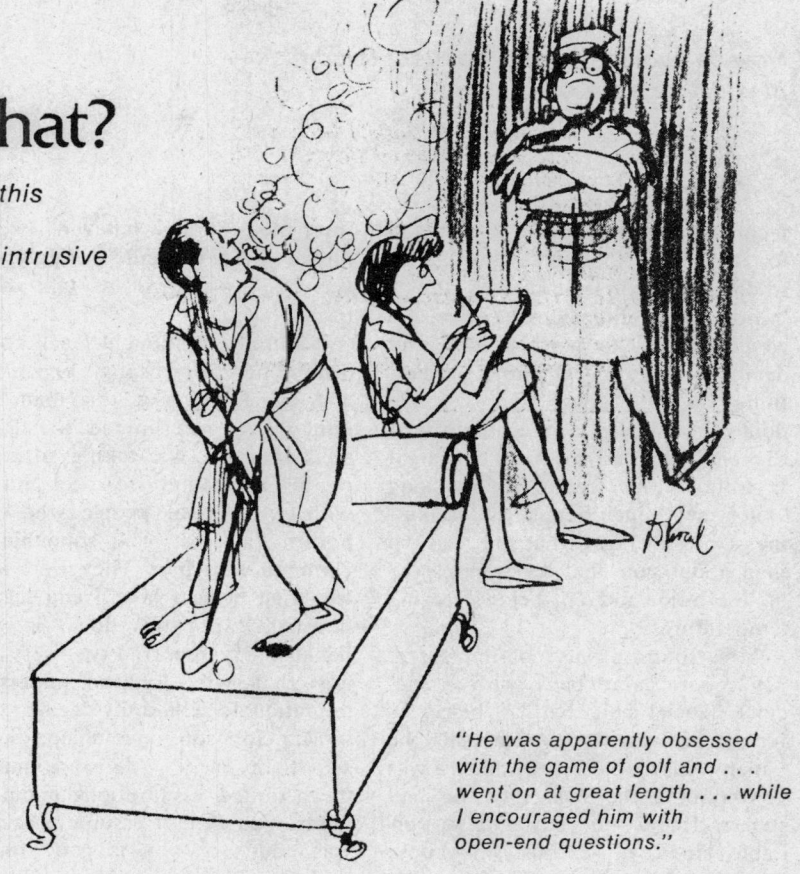

"He was apparently obsessed with the game of golf and . . . went on at great length . . . while I encouraged him with open-end questions."

When I became a nursing student at the age of 40, I had already acquired certain preconceptions and opinions about the role of the nurse. Having borne three children and undergone two operations, I felt that I knew exactly what a patient required and expected of a nurse—good physical care, given promptly, willingly, and graciously.

At my last hospitalization for minor surgery, the policy of the nurses seemed to be what I called "inspired neglect." They gave us good care, were always there when we needed or wanted them, and otherwise left us to our own devices. We often sat up until midnight in the lounge, drinking ginger ale and talking. I found the atmosphere very friendly, and I actually enjoyed my hospital stay. The other patients seemed to feel the same way about it, and there was constant visiting from room to room, luncheon "dates" in one room or another, and a general atmosphere of being very much at home. I intended to try to make my patients' hospital experience as pleasant as my own had been.

But it was immediately apparent that I was not to be allowed to formulate my own plans for nursing care and hospital routine. As community college students, we did not have as much clinical experience as a student in a diploma school would

MRS. HARDIMAN is a student at Nassau Community College, Garden City, N.Y.

have, and my clinical instructor, Mrs. Johnson, was determined to make every minute count. Our classroom lectures were to be applied in the hospital setting, and nothing less than perfection would do. Of course, I thoroughly endorsed these high standards for patient care.

It was when we began learning interviewing techniques that I had problems. None of this fit in with my concept of "inspired neglect"; certainly no nurse in my experience had ever made any attempt to discuss my problems with me or to encourage me to talk about them. It was all new to me, and I felt that it was, somehow, an invasion of privacy.

"But," said Mrs. Johnson summarily, "you are missing the point, Margaret. Read up on the subject. Work at it."

I read everything I could find on interviewing, but I could not shake the idea that encouraging the patient to talk about his fears and worries, without, in most cases, being able to do anything about them, was not only intrusive but unkind. Still, I was a student, and I would do my best.

My very first patient was a man of 42 who had had a prostatectomy with no complications and who was being discharged the next day. He was ambulatory, there was very little physical care to be given, so I decided to work on my interviewing techniques. I didn't know quite where to start, but there is always the age-old cliché about the weather; that was certainly all that was needed to get him started. He was apparently obsessed with golf, and mention of the weather naturally brought the game to mind. He went on at great length, and with tremendous enthusiasm, about his golf game, while I encouraged him with open-end sentences and all the other

How can you persuade a patient to confide in you if he does not want to?

techniques I could think of. I began to think that interviewing was not so difficult or unpleasant after all.

For every clinical experience, we were required to write a long and detailed report, explaining everything we had done, why we had done it, and our own evaluation of the care we had given. That night I wrote out my report on my long "interview," including the fascinating (to me) fact that he was so mad about golf that he even played in the rain and in below-freezing temperatures.

Mrs. Johnson was not impressed. My report came back with a succinct "Social chit-chat!" I began to feel a bit resentful. After all, the patient was not critically ill, he was going home the next day, he had spoken freely—indeed, with a veritable flood of enthusiasm—about something that interested him very much, and he had obviously enjoyed the experience. Wasn't that good therapy for anyone?

My next patient was a fairly young man, still in his thirties, who had been paralyzed from the waist down in an accident a year earlier. His present hospitalization was for a possible kidney stone—not uncommon with paraplegics. Since an aide had bathed him and helped him into his wheelchair before I arrived, I found myself with little to do but to make the bed and follow the doctor's orders about forcing fluids, straining the urine, taking vital signs, and so on—all of which took very little time.

Once again, I decided to practice interviewing, but this patient was reluctant to talk at all, socially or otherwise—at least to me. While I was still busy making the bed, he took off in his wheelchair to visit some fellow patients down the hall. Each time I brought him back to his room for any reason—blood pressure, medication, whatever—he submitted politely and willingly, but was soon off again to talk to his friends.

Naturally, I thought back to my own congenial hospital experiences and concluded that this man, who quite likely had limited social contacts at home, was taking advantage of this opportunity to meet and talk with a group of people who, temporarily at least, had something in common with him. They were all in less than perfect health and all in a hospital. I put this down in great detail in my report; I was very anxious that Mrs. Johnson understand the rationale behind my decisions.

Mrs. Johnson, once again, did not see it my way. "You are making unwarranted assumptions about patients; you cannot assume that what was good for you is good for all patients. Each one is an individual with his own needs and feelings. A nurse should attempt to serve these needs, but how can she if she doesn't know what they are? That is where interviewing comes in. This patient —young, married, with children to support, and confined to a wheelchair for life—must have great problems to deal with. Don't you think he may have needed a bit more than casual conversation with his fellow patients?"

Of course, I could see that only too well. What I could not see was how I could persuade him to confide in me if he did not want to and, even more, how I could possibly help him if he did. Assuming that he was attempting to escape from reality by intensive socializing, was it right to deny him this? How could I, a student, or even a nurse for that matter, know what the patient's needs were at any given moment? Since students seldom saw the same patient twice, there was little time to get well enough acquainted with him to be able to make a considered judgment. My decision with regard to Mr. G. had been influenced almost exclusively by his own behavior. I resolved to keep working at this problem, but secretly I began to think that Mrs. Johnson was being more than a little unreasonable.

Otherwise, things went smoothly. Nursing was hard work, but I didn't mind that. It was what I had always wanted to do, and I was happy and grateful for the opportunity. The one cloud continued to be my problem with interviewing. I began to feel somewhat oppressed. No matter what I did, it was never right, or, at least, never quite good enough.

Then, one day toward the end of the semester, I had for a patient a 65-year-old woman who had been stricken suddenly with a serious and rare form of anemia which left her extremely weak. Mrs. K. was nevertheless bright, cheerful, and optimistic, a great talker who needed no encouragement to tell me at length about her life before her illness. Apparently she had always been extremely active and had done a lot of traveling.

"No one would believe that I was in the hospital," she said. "They all said, 'Oh, no, not Annie. She's much too healthy.' Do you know, this is the first time in my life that I've been in a hospital. I even gave birth to my daughter at home. I always said they'd never get me into a hospital, but here I am. Actually, it's not as bad as I expected, but there's no place like home."

Mention of home must have reminded her of her daughter, and she asked me to get her on the bedside phone. While she talked, I chatted with the other patient in the room, an elderly woman who was about to be discharged. When Mrs. K. had finished her call, she joined in the conversation, which was interrupted by the arrival of two men, wearing the uniform of a local nursing home and pushing a stretcher. Apparently Mrs. S. was not going home; she was being transferred to a nursing home. We bade her cheerful good-byes while she was being strapped on the stretcher and trundled out of the room.

For some reason, I was shocked by this cold, impersonal procedure. I knew, of course, that many elderly patients went to nursing homes after leaving the hospital, but I had never before witnessed the actual departure. It seemed to me that there ought to be a more humane way to make the transfer.

However, I did not intend to let Mrs. K. see that I was disturbed. Turning to her brightly, ready to continue our interrupted conversation, I was startled to see tears running down her cheeks. My cheerful patient had suddenly become a tearful, frightened, elderly woman who was seriously ill and knew it. "I don't want to go to a nursing home," she whispered, clutching my hand. "I want to be able to walk again, so I can go to my daughter's house. If I can't walk, they may send me to a nursing home, and I'm so afraid."

What could I say? I knew that it would be wrong and dangerous to give false hope or reassurance. I also knew something that Mrs. K. did not know as yet; she was, indeed, going to a nursing home as soon as there was an available place. Her daughter had already signed the papers. Under the circumstances, the best thing to do would be to try to help her to overcome her fears so that she would be better able to face whatever was in store for her.

Frantically, I tried to remember all Mrs. Johnson had taught us about "giving support, listening, helping the patient to help himself," for here was a patient who had stopped running and was preparing to face reality. Whether she managed it as painlessly as possible depended to a large extent on me, and I felt terribly inadequate to the job. Interviewing was certainly not one of my best talents, according to Mrs. Johnson, but nevertheless, it was all I had to work with now.

Referring to the patient who had just left, I asked Mrs. K. whether Mrs. S. had shared her fear of nursing homes.

"No, she didn't seem to mind at all," she said, "but, of course, she is a lot older than I am, and she had a stroke and needs a lot of care that she can't get at home. It's different for me; I just need to get my strength back. If they'll just give me time...."

"Have you ever visited a nursing home, Mrs. K.?"

"Oh, no," she said, horrified, "I would never go near one. But I've heard about them from a lot of

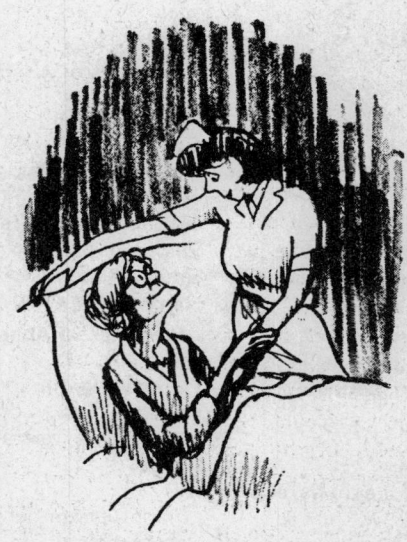

"And so I found out ... the comfort of having somebody really listen to you ... the relief of being able to give expression to your dark thoughts...."

other people, and I know they send you there if you're going to die. If you're going to get well, they send you home."

It was clear that Mrs. K. had a deep-seated fear of nursing homes, based largely on ignorance. I told her about a nursing home I had once visited, very modern and beautiful, and by no means confined to chronically ill, elderly patients. Many of the patients were quite young and were there for convalescence or therapy. I reminded her that she had been afraid of hospitals too, but had found this one much nicer than she had expected. She agreed that it was so, and I added, "We all want to help you as much as we can. Would you like to tell me everything you've heard about nursing homes—and hospitals, too? Maybe talking about it will help us both to understand what is worrying you."

Mrs. K. talked for the rest of the morning, and I listened. She was afraid, but not just of nursing homes. She was afraid of growing old, of being lonely, of being rejected—all human fears which most people have at some time or other, but in her case exaggerated by her illness. As she talked, she grew more relaxed and the tears stopped. When it was time for me to leave, she pressed my hand, and said simply, "Thank you. You've done me so much good. I really feel that I can face things much better now."

And so I found out what Mrs. Johnson meant by interviewing. I had thought of it as an invasion of privacy, an intrusion to no good purpose, a raking up of painful things about which you can do nothing. I hadn't considered the comfort of having someone really listen to you, the value of attention and warmth and acceptance when you feel particularly unworthy and unattractive, the relief of being able to give expression to your secret dark thoughts without having them brushed aside or dismissed as "nonsense."

The policy of inspired neglect may be all right for healthy 30-year-olds, although it may not always be the best course to follow even then. I know now that the really sick person needs a great deal more. I take comfort from the thought that the patient who loved golf really enjoyed his morning of "social chit-chat," but I shall always regret that the only help I gave to the patient who perhaps was trying to escape from an unbearable fact was to collaborate in that escape. It was a mistake I hope never to make again. △

Assessment of Mental Status

Definition: An assessment of observable aspects of the patient/client's psychologic functioning.

General Considerations:
- **The mental status assessment** is a *method* of organizing clinical observations that provides a baseline for the patient's psychologic state; it also provides specific information to assist in establishing diagnoses, planning goals, interventions, and subsequent evaluation.
- In the practice of psychiatric nursing, the mental status is an integral part of the initial assessment. The complete psychiatric examination includes a physical and neurologic study by the physician, as well as a psychiatric history, which includes the statement of the problem, a careful identification of the present episode with the reason why the patient came in at this particular time, a personal history, and a family history.
- The mental status is a useful assessment tool in all areas of nursing practice. Additions to the initial assessment are made by daily observations in inpatient and day treatment facilities, as well as other community settings.
- The nurse may be the first to pick up symptoms of organic brain disease, alcohol or drug use, suicidal ideation, and inappropriate speech activity or behaviors; the patient can then be referred for a thorough medical and psychiatric examination by a physician.
- **The mental status examination** usually includes areas of (1) *appearance and behavior*, (2) *consciousness*, (3) *speech activity*, and (4) *thought process, content, and perceptions*.

Components of Assessment
Appearance & Behavior
Observe for *dress, grooming, & personal hygiene*; colors, makeup, condition of clothes; skin color & condition.

Describe posture: erect, seated, horizontal.
Describe gait
Describe motor behavior: ability to relax, level & pattern of activity, relationship to topics of discussion or activities & people around area.

Components of Assessment
Appearance & Behavior
Describe affect—facial expression & mobility: sad, serious, smiling, immobile, flat (no expression)
Examine for scars & other marks.

Note prostheses: eyeglasses, contact lenses, cane, dentures, etc.
Note culture, growth & development tasks.

Consciousness
Determine orientation to time, place, & person by asking questions about the time of day, date, year, duration of hospitalization.
Use direct questioning if appropriate: "What day is today?" or "How long have you been here?"
Note sensorium: if patient is aware of his surroundings, his sensorium is said to be clear.

Speech Activity
Describe quality: loudness, clarity, pitch, tone, inflection
Note quantity: pace, volume
Assess organization: coherence, relevance, circumstantiality

Thought Processes and Content, Perceptions
Assess feelings by verbal questioning such as: "How are your spirits? How are you managing? Do you get pretty depressed (discouraged, blue)? How do you feel about that? How low do you feel? How do you feel right now? What do you see for yourself in the future?

Examples of Abnormalities

Inappropriate to age or place; condition of clothes unusual; unkempt appearance, unshaven, body odor; pediculosis or other unusual skin condition
Stooped, slumped; note open or closed posture
Shuffles, limps, fast, slow, akathisia
Signs of anxiety: moist hands, restlessness or retarded movement, dilated pupils, carotid pulses visibly noticeable or bounding, pacing

Examples of Abnormalities

Grimacing, tremors, Parkinsonism, & bizarre movements of head & neck in phenothiazine reactions
Birthmarks, operative scars, needle marks, wounds, trauma on wrist, etc.

Inappropriate behaviors for culture, stage of growth & development.

Disoriented to time, place, or person; stuporous, confused, clouded, unconscious

Unaware of surroundings

Slow, monotonous, flight of ideas; incoherent, circumstantial speech with neologisms (self-coined words); slurred speech, speech defect

Important to assess for depression & suicidal risk; see NCPGs #3:35, "The Patient Experiencing Depression (Psychiatric)," #3:36, "The Patient with Manic-Depressive Psychosis", & #3:38, "The Patient who is Suicidal (on a Psychiatric Unit)."
Note evasiveness, hostility, anger, elation, tearfulness, distrustfulness, resentment, apathy, lack of openness & approachability.

Components of Assessment
Thought Processes and Content, Perceptions
Observe the way patient describes own history, symptoms, feelings; follow leads provided by patient's own words.
Ask appropriate questions such as: "What do you think about at times like this?" "Sometimes when people get upset, things seem unreal. Is this happening now to you?

Inquire about feelings of unreality, depersonalization (a sense that one's self is different, changed, unreal, has lost identity), feelings of persecution (a sense that the patient is disliked, persecuted, being plotted against), feelings of influence (a sense that others are controlling or manipulating patient), feelings of reference (a sense that outside events such as TV or radio are related to patient, communicating to patient, or about patient).
Assess for memory of recent events by asking about events in recent past; assess for retention & recall by giving the patient several consecutive numbers and asking him to repeat them.
Ask patient to give a chronological account of his life to assess past memory. Ask about birthdays, anniversaries.
Assess for attention & concentration: tell patient you want to test his ability to concentrate. Read a series of digits, starting with the shortest set and enunciating each number clearly at a rate of 1 per second; ask patient to repeat them back to you. If the patient makes a mistake, give a second try with a different series, such as: 8,5,6,3, or 3,5,6,8,2; or 9,7,6,6,3,2.

Components of Assessment
Thought Processes and Content, Perceptions
Ask patient to repeat digits to you backwards. Ask patient to count backwards from 100 by 5s; note effort required, speed and accuracy of the responses.
Assess judgment: ask about daily life of patient; note ability to compare thoughts, events, relationships, & draw solid conclusions. Ask "What should you do if you are stopped for a traffic/speeding ticket?" "What should you do if you miss the bus?
Assess abstract thinking: ask the patient to interpret simple proverbs such as, "A rolling stone gathers no moss," or "Don't cross your bridges until you get to them."
Assess insight: as assessment interview progresses, does patient show understanding of his present situation? How does he describe his problems or the cause of his present state?

Examples of Abnormalities

Incoherent, disorganized thoughts; blocking, irrelevance, loose associations, talkative, silent, aphasic
Note indications of compulsions (repetitive acts that the patient feels driven to do), obsessions (recurrent, uncontrollable thoughts), doubting & indecision, phobias (irrational fears), free-floating anxieties (feelings of dread or impending doom; ill-defined dread).
Feelings of unreality, depersonalization, persecution, influence, reference, delusions (false, fixed beliefs), illusions (misinterpretation of sensory stimuli), hallucinations (subjective sensory perceptions); assumes listening or watchful posture; attitude may indicate hallucinations.

Poor recent memory in organic brain disease or high anxiety state
Poor retention and recall

Poor performance of digit span is characteristic of organic brain disease; performance is also limited by mental retardation

Unable to repeat at least 5 to 8 digits forward, or 4 to 6 backwards (the usual number).

Examples of Abnormalities

Unable to make comparisons of thought & events, understand the relationships, draw valid conclusions.

Concrete responses may indicate organic brain disorder, schizophrenia, low intelligence.

Unaware of current problems or present situation; unaware of mental illness or abnormal behaviors. Unable to link cause & effect (these are associated with neurotic disorders.)

© 1985 by Williams & Wilkins.
© 1983 by Margo Creighton Neal.
Guide No. 4:41 from *Nursing Care Planning Guides, Set 4*, 2nd Ed. Baltimore: Williams & Wilkins, 1983. Used by permission.

Stress Management

Definition: *Stress* is a generalized, non-specific response of the body to any demand or change, whether positive or negative. *Stressors* are the demands or changes and may be real or anticipated. *Distress* is damaging or unpleasant stress.

GOAL: The patient will maintain homeostasis or optimal adaptive coping by preventing, or recognizing promptly, excessive levels of stress and by utilizing effective measures to manage it.

General Considerations:
- The human body constantly interacts with the environment to maintain physiological and psychosocial homeostasis (optimal adaptive coping).
- **The stress syndrome** is described by Hans Selye as the General Adaptation Syndrome (or GAS). It consists of three stages: the alarm stage, the resistance stage, and the exhaustion stage:
  1) *The alarm stage* is the initial response of the body to stressors. It serves to protect the body from events that threaten homeostasis. Responses are generalized throughout the body and include increased heart rate and respiration, elevation in blood sugar level, increase in perspiration, dilated pupils, slowed digestion, increased activity and alertness, constriction of the blood vessels of the skin, and increased clotting ability of the blood.
  2) *The resistance stage:* the body's defenses, both physiological and psychological, are mobilized to resist the stress. The body adapts to the stress as best it can and repairs any damage resulting from it. When resistance is successful, the characteristic responses of the alarm stage virtually disappear.
  3) *The exhaustion stage* occurs when the body's finite store of adaptive energy is used up (usually after a prolonged period of time); the body's defenses are insufficient to cope with the stress and stressors. If this stage continues long enough, the individual may develop one of the "diseases of stress" such as migraine or tension headaches, hypertension, heart irregularity, peptic ulcer, or others. Continued exposure to stressors during this stage causes the body to run out of adaptive energy, and may even stop functioning. Chronic stress causes chronic disease and can lower the body's resistance to infectious disease.
- **Stress is an ongoing part of life;** a certain amount of stress is essential for survival and allows the individual to function at an alert, efficient level — excessive levels are unhealthful. Each person has a unique optimal level of stress and can learn to cope with stress adaptively.
- **Distress** causes the body to constantly readjust or adapt. Signs of distress include:
  - irritability
  - emotional tension
  - emotional instability
  - impulsive behavior
  - inability to concentrate
  - chronic fatigue
  - accident proneness
  - sweating
  - frequent urination
  - diarrhea or constipation
  - insomnia
  - decrease or increase of appetite
  - alcohol and drug abuse
  - neurotic or psychotic behaviors
  - increased smoking
  - nightmares
  - headache
  - pain in neck or back
  - grinding of teeth
  - stuttering
  - sexual problems
- **Nursing responsibilities** include assessing for signs of distress and maladaptive responses to change, identifying stressors and stage of stress syndrome, and prescribing interventions to promote homeostasis and adaptive coping with stress and stressors. Patient education is vital to promote and maintain optimal adaptive coping.

General Suggestions for Managing Stress Adaptively:
1) **Exercise** daily. Physical activity allows an outlet for mental stress as well as developing flexibility, muscular strength and endurance, and increasing efficiency of body system functioning. Walking, running, dancing, swimming, gardening, participating in sports or body movement exercises, and yoga are examples of methods to reduce stress through exercise. Many community gyms, health clubs, and YMCAs have regular group exercise programs that are fun and enjoyable as well as healthy. Consult personal physician for contraindications to exercise program.
2) **Develop alternative ways to relax.** Choose activities you really enjoy and plan to devote at least an hour a day pursuing them. Allow yourself to explore creative activities such as drawing, pottery, carpentry, writing, musical activities, or photography; let yourself read a good book, watch the sunset, listen to music, take a bubble bath, or cultivate the fine art of short naps. Let yourself remember ways you have relaxed in the past (sports, music) and experience these old ways again. Try something new and different; check out various community activities available through recreation departments, adult education programs, community colleges.
3) **Learn mental exercises** to create a sense of peace and tranquility and to relax muscles. Examples include:
   - *Progressive relaxation:* concentrate on relaxing successive sets of muscles from the tips of your toes to the top of your head; this may include tightening one set of muscles and then letting go of the muscles to a count of six. For example, "I'm

holding tight the muscles in my hand and arm — 1, 2, 3, 4, 5, 6: I'm letting go of the muscles in my hand and arm — 1, 2, 3, 4, 5, 6, with the holding lasting for 15-30 seconds and the letting go lasting an equal amount of time. An alternative way to do progressive relaxation is to focus by saying, "My feet are becoming relaxed and warm; my ankles are becoming relaxed and warm," and progressivily focusing on each successive part of the body.

- *Autogenic training exercises:* repeat verbal formulas with passive concentration and relaxed posture; examples: "My body is becoming warm and relaxed. I am beginning to feel quiet and relaxed. My right arm is warm and relaxed. My heart beat is calm and regular. My lungs breathe for me. My forehead is cool. My jaw is relaxed and easy."
- *Imagery:* use your imagination to daydream, to reminisce, or to remember positive experiences. Focus on your favorite vacation spot and let yourself see, hear, smell, taste, and feel the breeze of that relaxed, pleasurable experience. Concentrate on a beautiful drawing or photograph; let yourself drift off in your imagination to become part of the picture. Listen to music and allow yourself to imagine scenes and pleasurable experiences that the music evokes. Imagine yourself as healthy, effective, graceful, flexible, relaxed . . . whatever you would like to be; be aware of negative thoughts or images, and replace them with positive ones.
- *Positive affirmations:* create positive, active, new statements about yourself as you would like to be: "I am relaxed. I am learning to express my feelings. I am expressing anger in a positive way. I am becoming more assertive. I am making realistic goals for myself. I am relaxing on my lunch break." Write out the statements and place them on your mirror, steering wheel, refrigerator, desk, or any place where they will catch your eye; repeat the statements to yourself several times daily. Be specific, positive, and brief.

4) **Learn Diaphragmatic breathing.** The diaphragm is the primary muscle involved in breathing. Most people waste effort by overusing muscles in the shoulders and chest to breathe. To practice diaphragmatic breathing, sit or recline in a comfortable position with legs uncrossed; place one hand on the chest and the other hand on the diaphragm, approximately two inches below the bottom center of the breastbone. Now practice breathing so that when you inhale the diaphragm expands; the hand covering the diaphragm moves out while the other hand remains almost still. As you exhale, the diaphragm relaxes and the hand covering it moves inward. Focus on *allowing* diaphragmatic breathing to occur rather than *trying*.

5) **Concentrate on allowing yourself (vs. trying) to cope with stress** and to relax; *trying* causes tension and can be avoided by an attitude of *letting* yourself relax, *allowing* yourself to be aware of your needs and wants, and by giving tender loving care to yourself.

6) **Seek work or tasks that you enjoy,** are capable of doing or learning, and which other people appreciate.

7) **Balance work and recreation**; learn to take relaxation breaks.

8) **Share feelings and concerns** with trusted friends, family members, or a counselor; let yourself become more aware of your feelings and express them to others in a positive way.

9) **Be a creative problem solver**; see NCPG #5:47, "Problem Solving."

10) **Avoid self-medication.** The ability to cope with stress comes from within you, not from the outside.

11) **Be aware of own energy and nutrition requirements.** Plan food intake to achieve and maintain ideal body weight with a well-balanced diet; see NCPG #5:41, "Diet: Weight Control."

12) **Learn to listen to your body** for messages of distress. Respond to early warning signals of tension or distress, using relaxation and creative problem solving.

13) **Set priorities;** take one thing at a time. Set limits in an assertive way; learn to say "no."

Teaching Objectives/Outcomes

1) Patient can identify own stress, stressors, and signs of distress.
2) Can describe stress syndrome and the relationship between chronic stress and chronic disease.
3) Can describe a plan to cope with stress in an adaptive way, including plan for exercise, relaxation, nutrition, problem solving, sharing feelings and concerns with trusted friend, family member, or counselor, and giving self tender loving care.

© 1985 by Williams & Wilkins.
© 1981 by Margo Creighton Neal.
Guide No. 5:49 from *Nursing Care Planning Guides, Set 5.*
Baltimore: Williams & Wilkins, 1981. Used by permission.

RELAX

Six techniques you can teach to patients, incorporate into your care, and use yourself—even when you just have ten seconds to spare.

Relaxation, an effective adjunct to the treatment of a variety of ailments, can be achieved through simple techniques that can easily be taught to patients. Patients requiring minor invasive procedures—such as the drawing of blood, or insertion of intravenous catheters—can reduce their anxiety levels by following any one of a number of routes to relaxation. Those with asthma can learn to use these techniques when they anticipate attacks. Relaxation can relieve headaches and menstrual cramps and reduce both acute and chronic pain by alleviating tension in rigidly held muscles surrounding painful areas.

Several characteristics are common to all relaxation methods:

Rhythmic breathing. Most relaxation techniques start with slow deep breathing. As a person becomes relaxed, he consumes less oxygen; so breathing becomes slower and shallower. Although the rate and depth of breathing changes, the rhythm becomes constant. Thus, rhythmicity itself characterizes relaxation. (See chart, next page, for other physiologic changes brought about by relaxation.)

Reduced muscle tension. Some people relax so thoroughly that they can't move their arms or legs. Whether or not such profound relaxation is

Jean Wouters DiMotto, RN, MSN, is a psychophysiologist and educator. She is currently completing law school at Marquette Univerity, Milwaukee, WI.

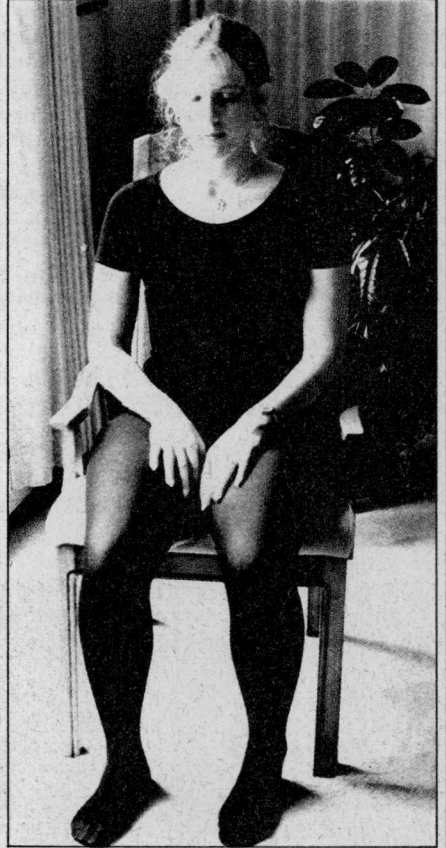

attained, almost any relaxation method will significantly ease muscle tension.

An altered state of consciousness. Your state of consciousness corresponds to your brain waves. The waking, alert state is called beta. During relaxation, you move to a level of consciousness called alpha(1). In the alpha state, which falls between full consciousness and unconsciousness, thought processes become less logical and more associative and creative. Your sense of time and body may be distorted: A 15-minute relaxation exercise may seem to last two minutes or two hours; your body might feel very large or very small; you might feel a heavy, or a light, floating feeling; or, you might experience your body as boundless, at one with the surrounding environment(2).

You have a heightened ability to focus on one idea or image. Focus may be on breathing, sensory experiences, or tension(3). Or, you might concentrate on a particular image, thought, or problem. Alpha state and focused mental activity are the major reasons why mental imagery is so effectively paired with relaxation. Although clients are seldom aware of moving from the beta to the alpha state, when relaxation is finished and they return to the beta level of consciousness they are aware of feeling more alert.

Clinical experience suggests there are individual differences in people's experiences of relaxation. Not everyone will demonstrate all characteristics of a relaxed psychophysiologic state.

RELAXATION TECHNIQUES

Full-body relaxation. A common type of relaxation, this 15-minute method—involves paying attention to different parts of your body, noting any ten-

RELAXATION

BY JEAN WOUTERS DiMOTTO

Reprinted from American Journal of Nursing, June 1984

sion, and replacing it with warmth and relaxation.

If the patient is willing, this is a good relaxation technique to use while giving a bed bath. While preparing the patient for her bath, give the breathing instructions (see chart, p. 758). As you wash each part of her body, ask her to notice any tension in that part. For example, you could say, "As I wash your arm, notice any tightness or tension in it." As you rinse her arm say, "Breathe in warmth and relaxation to this arm and exhale the tension." Dry her arm with slower motions than you used to wash or rinse, saying, "Notice the warmth and relaxation you now feel in this arm." Repeat these instructions as you wash each body part, dealing with her hands independently of her arms, her arms separately from her shoulders, her neck from her face, and her feet from her calves. The bath is likely to take about 20 to 30 minutes, so keep the water warm; cold water inhibits relaxation.

As is true of most relaxation exercises, it is fairly easy for patients to do the exercise themselves once you have done it with them a few times.

Modified autogenic relaxation. This method can be useful in the treatment of asthma, hyperventilation, high blood pressure, cold hands or feet, headache, and ulcers(4). Relaxation is attained through a series of statements—or autosuggestions—about various bodily functions. After assuming a relaxing position, breathe in slowly and deeply, then slowly exhale, repeating to yourself the phrases shown in the chart on p. 0000. Inhale as you identify the parts of your body and exhale as you describe how relaxed you feel.

People enjoy this method and use it because the calming results are so obvious. After a while, subsequent use relaxes them more thoroughly and quickly. For some, just thinking the first statement produces relaxation.

Sensory pacing. While your uncon-

WHAT HAPPENS WHEN WE RELAX?

Physiologic manifestations	Cognitive manifestations	Behavioral manifestations
decreased pulse	altered state of consciousness, usually alpha level	lack of attention to and concern for environmental stimuli
decreased blood pressure	heightened concentration on single mental image or idea	no verbal interaction
decreased respirations	receptivity to positive suggestion	no voluntary change of position
decreased oxygen consumption		passive movement easy
decreased carbon dioxide production and elimination		
decreased muscle tension		
decreased metabolic rate		
pupil constriction		
peripheral vasodilation		
increased peripheral temperature		

Adapted from: Graves, H.H., & Thompson, E.A., "Anxiety: A Mental Health Vital Sign." In: Longo, D.C. and Williams, R.A. (Eds.), Clinical Practice in Psychosocial Nursing: Assessment and Intervention, N.Y., Appleton-Century-Crofts, 1978.

BODY POSTURES FOR RELAXATION

Sitting, reclining, or lying down are all postures conducive to relaxing. In each of these positions, the body should be well supported by a chair, bed, or couch. It is important that your primary position be balanced. Crossing your legs, dropping your head to one side, or leaning your upper body over a table will strain the affected muscles after ten to twenty minutes. Not only will these muscles remain tense, the discomfort will interfere with your attaining or remaining in alpha-level consciousness(5).

Sitting. Sit all the way back resting against the entire back of the chair. Place your feet flat on the floor. (If you're wearing high heels, remove your shoes.) Separate your legs so they're not touching each other. You can hang your arms by your sides or rest them on chair arms. Or, you can place each of your hands flat on each of your thighs. A fourth possibility is to rest your palms on your thighs, letting your fingers hang loosely between your legs.

Align your head with your spine. You can hold it comfortably straight, tilt it slightly forward, or rest your chin on your upper chest. If you choose to hold your head straight, you may unknowingly drop it forward as you relax. This is fine, since your head remains aligned with your spine.

You are now in a balanced, sitting position. Complete your preparation by loosening any tight clothing and making sure you are moderately warm.

Reclining and lying down. Many of the positioning principles for sitting apply. Separate your legs and point your toes slightly outward. Rest your arms at your sides without touching your sides. Keep your head aligned with your spine. You can lie flat or place a small, thin pillow under your head. Thick, large pillows will cause neck and back strain.

You will be able to maintain these postures for as long as you choose, without straining any muscle group. The only problem with reclining or lying down is that it's easy to fall asleep in these positions. In a recent study showing that relaxation training produces prolonged reduction of blood pressure, the author noted that the individual needs to remain awake to obtain maximum benefit from relaxation training(6). If, on the other hand, your purpose for relaxing is to induce sleep, then of course, reclining or lying down are the preferred positions.

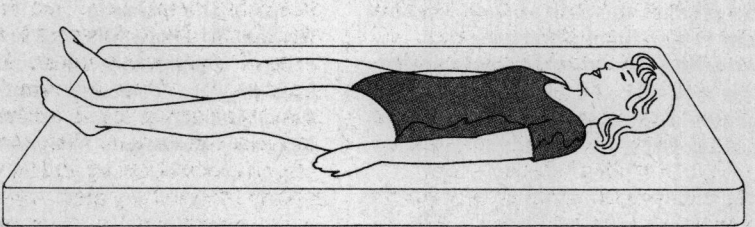

correct

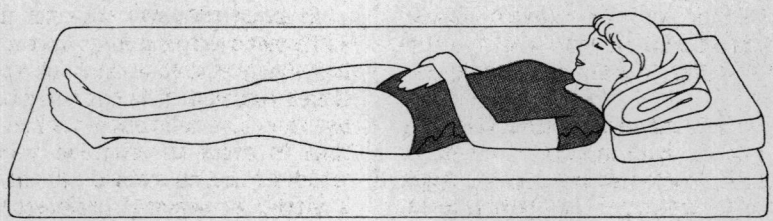

incorrect

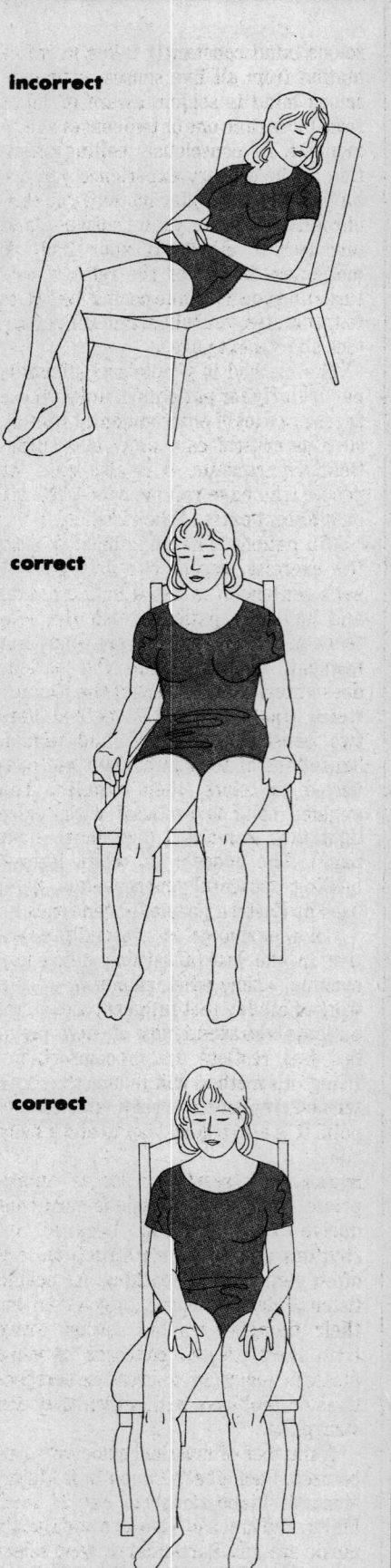

scious mind constantly takes in information from all five senses, your conscious mind is seldom aware of input from more than one or two senses at any moment. By consciously calling attention to the sensory experience you are having at a particular instant, you synchronize, or pace, your conscious and unconscious minds. If your body is motionless in one of the relaxed postures and you continue pacing for two to four minutes, you will attain relaxation (see chart, next page).

The method is simple and effective, particularly for patients in units where there are a lot of environmental stimuli, such as critical care units and outpatient departments. It is also good for people who have trouble concentrating on different parts of their bodies.

If a patient is having difficulty with the exercise, repeat the first part of each sentence (as listed in the chart) and have the patient finish the sentence with what he is aware of at that moment. If at the end the patient doesn't feel relaxed, repeat the pacing.

Color exchange. This method uses two senses—kinesthetic and visual. Sensations of tension or pain are converted to colors, then exhaled. The exhaled color is replaced with white light that is inhaled (see chart, next page). The concept of white light—healing, peaceful energy—has been used by Eastern people for centuries.

Color exchange is especially effective in the late afternoon and early evening, a time when people who have worked all day feel fatigued, and when patients who spend most of their day in bed feel restless and uncomfortable. Using this method will reduce the day's tension, replenish energy, and relieve pain. It is also a good way to end a back rub.

Music. Any restful music is appropriate, but classical music is most conducive to relaxation because its rhythms and harmonic structures are often perceived as soothing. As people listen to classical music, they tend to let their thoughts wander, either away from their present concerns to more pleasant topics, or to creative perspectives on problems with which they are struggling.

A number of classical selections can be used. Pachelbel's Canon in D Major, Mozart's Piano Concerto No. 21 in C Major, and much of Vivaldi's and Bach's music are apt. Particularly, good selections from Vivaldi include *The Four Seasons*, the concerti for mandolin, the baroque guitar concerti, and the six flute concerti (Opus 10). Relaxing selections from Bach include the *Goldberg Variations*, and the six concerti after Vivaldi.

The adagio, larghetto, and largo movements of Vivaldi and Bach have rhythms similar to the human heartbeat. When they listen to these movements, people's pulse rates and other biological rhythms tend to synchronize themselves with the beat of the music. This is particularly true with the largo movement's slow, stately, restful rhythm. The result is deeper, more efficient relaxation(7).

Another excellent choice is Halpern's *Soundscapes*. These are meditative collections of sounds without any familiar rhythm that are designed to relax, balance, and attune the listener(8). Similar selections include Horn's *Inside* albums, Andrew's *Kuthumi* and *The Violet Flame*, and Scott's and Yuize's *Music for Zen Meditations*.

Music can also serve as background accompaniment while using other relaxation methods. Recordings or tapes of environmental sounds (i.e., streams of water, soft rain, wind) are particularly helpful. You can create relaxation tapes for yourself or your patients.

Ten-second relaxation techniques. Even a short exercise can lower pulse and respiration rates, although using stimulants such as caffeine shortly before relaxing interferes with a person's ability to slow physiologic processes.

Two relaxation techniques take only 10 seconds. Both are useful when, for example, postoperative patients begin to feel incisional pain and become tense, as when ambulating or changing positions.

You yourself can use these techniques during a busy day when there is no opportunity to take a break. While walking to a patient's room, taking an elevator, using the restroom, or sitting down to chart, you can lower your tension level with a 10-second exercise: Eyes open, let your lower jaw drop as if you were starting to yawn. Rest your tongue on the bottom of your mouth behind your lower teeth. Breathe slowly and rhythmically through your mouth: inhale, exhale, then rest. Do not form or even think words.

Research on patients who used this technique showed they felt significantly less incisional pain and bodily tension than those who didn't use the technique, and that they used fewer narcotics in the first 24 hours after surgery(9).

The second technique is done while sitting or standing. Close your eyes. Focus on a tiny imaginary star one inch in front of the tip of your nose. Take four deep breaths slowly through your mouth while continuing to focus on the star. This brief exercise requires intense concentration, and is especially helpful when you want to clear your mind as well as relax.

Ending relaxation techniques. The simplest and most comfortable way to end an exercise is to gradually open your eyes and stretch as though you were coming out of a deep sleep. Stretching helps move you from the alpha level of consciousness to the beta level of alert wakefulness. Although some people advocate jerking or contracting an arm or leg, it is more abrupt and less comfortable than stretching. After stretching, get up and move about a bit to become fully alert, especially if you are going to drive or operate medical machinery.

The more often you relax, the easier and faster you relax; relaxation becomes a conditioned response. Simply slowing your breathing, or performing a 10-second relaxation technique, or thinking of a phrase such as "relax," or "down you go," will trigger relaxation.

Relaxing regularly does not necessarily mean relaxing daily. Once a week is probably enough to establish a conditioned response. It is not necessary to use the same relaxation method each time in order to condition yourself; which relaxation method you choose is a matter of personal preference. Patients will also have preferences, so it is usually a good idea to teach them at least two methods.

> **Postop patients who use relaxing techniques feel less pain and tension, and use fewer narcotics.**

USING RELAXATION TECHNIQUES

Relaxation by Sensory Pacing
Assume a relaxing position and slowly repeat and finish each of the following sentences, either in a low voice or to yourself.
Now I am aware of seeing . . .
Now I am aware of feeling . . .
Now I am aware of hearing . . .

Start with your eyes open, allowing them to close when they feel heavy. Begin by repeating and finishing each sentence four times. Then repeat and finish each sentence three times, then two times, then one time. Once your eyes are closed, what you see will be in your mind's eye.

Reference: Carter, P. and Gilligan, S. Personal Communication, 1980.

Full Body Relaxation
Assume a relaxing position. Note your breathing. Is it fast, slow, even or uneven, deep or shallow? Now, change your breathing to slow, abdominal breathing, breathing all the way in, down to your navel. Count to 4, inhaling on 1 and 2, exhaling on 3 and 4. Continue this.

Become aware of your face, your jaws, and your neck. Notice any tightness or tension in these parts. Breathe in warmth and relaxation. Exhale the tension.

Become aware of your shoulders, your arms, your hands and fingers. Notice any tightness or tension. Again, breathe in warmth and relaxation. Exhale the tension.

Become aware of your back—from your shoulders to your tailbone. Notice tightness or tension anywhere in your back. Breathe in, relaxing your back. Exhale the tension.

If you're feeling warm, you're relaxing.

Move to your chest and abdomen. Relax your abdominal muscles. Notice any tightness or tension. Breathe in warmth and relaxation. Exhale the tension.

You may notice that some parts of your body are tingling. It means you're relaxing.

Now move to your pelvic area and buttocks. Notice any tightness or tension in these parts. Breathe in warmth and relaxation to these areas and exhale the tension.

You may feel very heavy, as though you could sink deeply into your chair or bed. Or, you may feel light enough to float on a cloud or sit on a flower. Either way is fine. It means you're relaxing.

Move to your thighs. Notice any tightness or tension in those muscles. Breathe in warmth and exhale tension.

Move to your knees, then your calves, ankles, and feet. Notice any tightness or tension. Breathe in, relaxing all the way down to the tips of your toes. Exhale the tension.

Take time now to enjoy the peace you feel. When you're ready to end the relaxation period, count to ten, slowly open your eyes, wriggle your fingers and toes, and stretch as if you are just waking up.

Modified Autogenic Relaxation
Assume a relaxing position.
Slowly take in a very deep breath. Exhale very slowly.
Repeat each of the following phrases to yourself four times. Say the first part of the phrase as you breathe in for 2 to 3 seconds. Hold your breath in for 2 to 3 seconds. Then say the last part of the phrase as you breathe out for 2 to 3 seconds. Hold your breath out for 2 to 3 seconds.

Breathe in	Breathe out
1. I am	relaxed.
2. My arms and legs	are heavy and warm.
3. My heartbeat	is calm and regular.
4. My breathing	is free and easy.
5. My abdomen	is loose and warm.
6. My forehead	is cool.
7. My mind	is quiet and still.

References: Bauman, Edward, and others. The Holistic Health Handbook. Berkeley, And/Or Press, 1978.
Pelletier, Kenneth R. Mind as Healer, Mind as Slayer. New York, Dell, 1977.

Relaxation by Color Exchange
Assume a relaxing position. Concentrate on your breathing as you slowly take four deep breaths.

Notice any body tension, tightness, aches, or pains. Give the tension or discomfort a color, the first color you think of.

Now breathe in pure white light from the universe. Send the light to the tight or painful place in your body. Surround the color of your discomfort with the white light.

Exhale the color of your discomfort and inhale white light to take its place. Continue breathing in white light and exhaling the color of your discomfort.

Now, continue breathing in white light until your entire body is filled with the light and you have a sense of peace, well being, and energy.

Reference: Radtke, Dawn, D. Personal communication, 1980.

You may find that the more often you teach relaxation techniques to patients, the faster and more deeply you relax when you do an exercise yourself—one way the caregiver benefits directly from the care given.

For years, women preparing for childbirth have learned various breathing patterns and relaxation techniques in order to give birth without tranquilizers or analgesics. New mothers breastfeeding their babies can relax before feeding to increase the flow of milk. They are also more likely to feel at ease and to enjoy the experience.

Relaxation is useful preoperatively not only to help people sleep but to reduce their anxiety about upcoming surgery. Postoperatively, relaxation can be used to relieve pain. And, people can use relaxation to reduce the stress in their lives and to achieve even better health. In whatever nursing setting you choose to practice, there will be numerous indications for teaching relaxation to your patients.

REFERENCES
1. Wallace, R. K., and others. A wakeful hypometabolic physiologic state. *Am.J.Physiol.* 221:795-799, Sept. 1971.
2. Trygstad, Louise. Simple new ways to help anxious patients. *RN* 43:28-32, Dec. 1980.
3. McCaffery, Margo. *Nursing Management of the Patient with Pain.* 2nd ed. Philadelphia, J.B. Lippincott Co., 1979.
4. Davis, Martha, and others. *The Relaxation and Stress Reduction Workbook.* 2nd ed. Richmond, CA, New Harbinger, 1982.
5. Guyton, A. C. *Textbook of Medical Physiology.* 5th ed. Philadelphia, W.B. Saunders Co., 1976.
6. Agras, W.S. Relaxation therapy in hypertension. *Hosp. Prac.* May 1983, p. 134.
7. Ostrander, Sheila, and others. *Superlearning.* New York, Delacorte Press, 1979.
8. Halpern, Steven. *Tuning the Human Instrument.* Belmont, CA, Spectrum Research Institute, 1978.
9. Flaherty, G. G., and Fitzpatrick, J. J. Relaxation technique to increase comfort level of postoperative patients: a preliminary study. *Nurs.Res.* 27:352-355, Nov.-Dec. 1978.

Behavior Modification

Definitions:
- **Behavior modification** is a teaching technique for dealing with behavioral problems; the purpose is to assist individuals to modify behavior that stands in the way of health and well-being.
- **Target behaviors** are those observable and measurable behaviors that have been identified as behavior problems.
- **Terminal behaviors** are the desired new behaviors to be learned.
- **Contingency** is a term that refers to the relationship between a behavior and the events that follow the behavior.
- **Positive reinforcement** means a desired response or behavior is followed by a positive or desired consequence; reinforcement works best when applied immediately.
- **Aversive consequences** are undesirable consequences and can be used to decrease occurrence of behavior.
- **Shaping** is the breaking down of desired terminal behaviors into a sequence of steps and rewarding each successive approximation of the steps.
- **Generalization** is the transfer of an already learned response to another situation.
- **Behavioral objectives** describe in a measurable way the behavior that the learner tries to learn; they permit an ongoing evaluation of the treatment goals (see NCPG #1:48, "Steps in Writing a Nursing Care Plan," Step 3). Example: The patient will swim or walk briskly 15 minutes every day.

General Considerations:
- **Behavioral theory** indicates that both positive and negative behaviors are learned and that behavior can be modified. Behavior modification includes principles of teaching and learning. The basic tenet of behavioral theory is: *behavior that is reinforced tends to be repeated.* Reinforcement should be given *each time* the behavior occurs; *after* the behavior is established, intermittent reinforcement (e.g. every 2–3 times) maintains the behavior *better* than reinforcement every time.
- The patient should be involved in setting goals and objectives and agree to cooperate with the plan; if the patient has limited capacity to understand this procedure, discuss the information with him in simple terms which he can understand.
- Involving the patient encourages participation, self-motivation, self-care, and limits threats to personal freedom and infringement on human rights. (See NCPG #1:49, "Teaching Patients.")
- **Nursing responsibilities** include assessing the patient for behavioral problems that interfere with health and well-being, and contracting with patient to set goals and objectives for behavior modification.
- **Behavior modification consists of six steps:**
    Step 1 Define the behavior to be modified.
    1.1 Identify problem behavior which needs intervention; behavior should be observable and measurable. This behavior is called the *target* behavior.
    1.2 Determine how this behavior interferes with care, health, and the patient's well-being. Example: Patient is 50 pounds overweight, has erratic diet habits, and wants to lose weight as part of treatment plan to decrease blood pressure.
    Step 2 Measure the behavior to be modified.
    2.1 Gather baseline data, i.e., how many times does the behavior occur in a specific time period? Example: Instruct patient to keep diet diary and write down everything s/he eats for one week.
    2.2 Observe sequence and pattern of behavior; example: Patient's weight is 190 lbs; daily diet diary indicates no breakfast, a high calorie 10 AM snack, a sandwich and malt for lunch, peanuts and wine at 5 PM, and a large dinner with dessert at 8 PM.
    Step 3 Analyse current contingencies that maintain problem behavior or lack of ability, knowledge, or experience.
    3.1 Assess for events that precede and follow behavior; pay attention to feelings as well as to who, what, when, how, and why.
    3.2 Involve the patient and family in this analysis; encourage the patient to count and keep track of behavior and feelings that accompany it by keeping a journal, diary, or chart.
    3.3 Assess for deficits in behavioral repertoire; these may be skills and abilities which the patient has not learned or is not currently using. Example: Patient eats to give self treat; does not know how to nurture self in other ways. Gets up too late for breakfast and eats lunch out because there is nothing in the house to take for lunch. Eats dinner late to eat with husband. Snacks to cope with anxiety and depression. Willing to work on anxiety and depression by learning new ways to cope.
    Step 4 Construct program to change behavior in desired directions.
    4.1 Set and write out behavioral objectives to modify the target behavior to the desired terminal behavior; include the setting or conditions under which the desired behavior is expected to occur, the specific desired behavior that can be observed and measured, and the criterion for how and when the behavior will be performed.
    4.2 Include the patient in setting goals and planning program; the patient can help select appropriate positive reinforcers and suitable aversive consequences.
    4.3 Nursing behaviors for positive reinforcement should include spending time with patient, verbal praise and encouragement, smiling, showing interest in discussion of specific subjects, providing opportunity for patient to have special experiences or treats.

4.4 Aversive consequences could include discontinuing special experiences or treats, participation in chores that are disliked by patient, or nursing behaviors of disinterest, frowning, turning face away, or spending less time with patient.

4.5 Teach patient that all behavior has consequences and that each individual can choose among many alternative actions and resulting consequences.

4.6 Set a specific time for trial run of program and agree to evaluate effectiveness at that time. Example: Patient will reduce diet intake to ingest 1200 calories a day, which will include 3 meals plus two snacks and a well-balanced diet. Patient will weigh in once a week and will be able to plan and have a non-food treat (flowers, music, new clothes, perfume) each time s/he loses 5 pounds. Patient will swim or walk 15 minutes daily. If no weight lost or if weight gained, patient agrees to clean out garage or wash down walls for neighbor.

Step 5 Use therapeutic instructions (expectancy).

5.1 Offer specific plan to practice modified behavior; encourage attitude of positive and matter-of-fact expectance that modified behavior will occur. Example: Plan acceptable diet and snacks with some unusual low-calorie treats; plan shopping to include items for breakfast and lunch.

5.2 Break behavior into small steps in a sequence pattern; plan practice of small steps.

5.3 Include some known desired behaviors that cannot be done simultaneously with target behavior. Example: Play guitar or flute instead of snacking; chew gum while cooking dinner instead of tasting food; folk dance or swim instead of drinking alcohol.

Step 6 Practice desired behavior, step by step.

6.1 Begin with known steps and then attempt unknown or new steps; choose simple, unthreatening situations and then gradually include more complex and difficult ones.

6.2 Instruct patient to keep diary or journal of practice, including log of new steps and modified behavior, plus feelings and concerns. Steps might include: Buy low-calorie acceptable food, prepare lunch the night before, get up early to eat breakfast, take guitar/flute lessons, prepare and eat low-calorie, well-balanced meals, keep a journal of all food ingested plus feelings and concerns.

Step 7 Reinforce small, discrete steps in adaptive direction (shaping).

7.1 Provide information of behavior change to patient, verbally and with charts.

7.2 Reinforce progress, using plan of positive reinforcement; ensure that each step taken toward the terminal/expected behavior

7.3 Involve family and friends in giving feedback and encouragement for steps in adaptive direction. Appreciation is not only much appreciated at this point, but also helps shape the desired behavior.

7.4 Involve patient in keeping own record or chart of desired terminal behavior, thus increasing awareness of own behavior and allowing for increased intrinsic motivation. Example: Patient can keep own weight chart and could negotiate with husband, friend, or co-worker to give verbal encouragement. Nurse can give praise and encouragement plus listen attentively to concerns, read patient's journal, and discuss patterns.

Step 8 Generalize terminal behavior to natural environment using natural reinforcers.

8.1 Assist patient to transfer modified behavior to other similar situations and environments by role playing and using problem-solving method.

8.2 Explore and anticipate with patient the natural positive reinforcement that could be expected or planned for with modified behavior. Example: Anticipate and role play dining out situations in which patient asks for fresh fruit or vegetable substitute for high-calorie item. Anticipate camping trip or vacationing with 1200 calorie diet. Encourage patient to imagine self buying smaller sized vacation clothes and having more energy and lower blood pressure.

© 1985 by Williams & Wilkins.
© 1981 by Margo Creighton Neal.
Guide No. 5:49 from *Nursing Care Planning Guides, Set 5*.
Baltimore: Williams & Wilkins, 1981. Used by permission.

Reprinted from American Journal of Nursing, February 1975

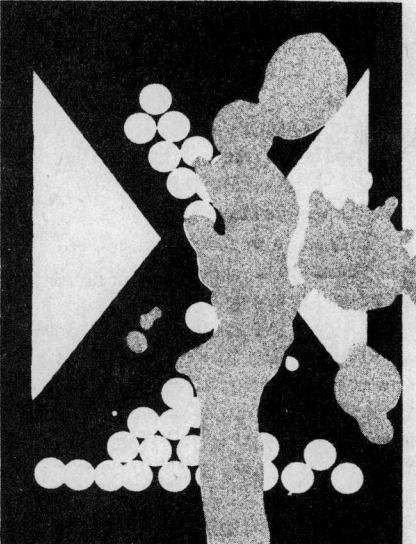

SUICIDE

Why does a person take his own life? Is it because of societal pressure, interpersonal conflict, hopelessness, anger—or all of these?

TWILLA M. WESTERCAMP

Suicide is a major human problem that is not restricted to a certain population or geographical area. The nurse is bound to be faced with the problem at some point in her professional career. Self-destruction seems so out of keeping with the instinctual love of life that one may wonder why anyone should want to kill himself. We all have difficult times in our lives. What is it that makes one person decide to live and another decide to die?"

Suicide is a social phenomenon which is, at the same time, a personal act. The character, personality, temperament, and emotional stability of an individual, the society around him and how it affects him, must all be considered.

First to be considered are the so-

MS. WESTERCAMP received her B.S.N. degree from the University of Iowa, Iowa City, Iowa. She has been a staff nurse at the University of Nebraska Hospital, Omaha, Neb., and is currently working on cancer research and detection, Department of Preventive Medicine and Public Health, Creighton University, Omaha, Nebraska.

cial theories. In his famous work, *Le Suicide,* Durkheim concludes that to understand suicide one must look to dynamic social factors rather than isolated individual motives. The suicidal tendency, which exists everywhere, is the result of collective forces. The common factor in all suicides is increasing alienation between the person and the social group he belongs to. The basic element, which Durkheim calls anomie, is a psychological isolation that occurs whenever the links that unite groups are weakened. "Egoistic" suicide results from a lack of integration of the individual with other members of the group, and "altruistic" suicide results from insufficient individualization. The remedy, he concludes, is to make the social group more consistent and more coherent, to help its members realize their mutual interdependence, and to aim toward creating a society that fulfills the needs of each member(1).

Another theory, symbolic interaction, suggests that a person evaluates himself in much the same way he thinks he is evaluated by others. The person acts, others assess his actions, and he evaluates himself according to his estimation of others' assessment. Suicide, then, is related to disrupted social relations stemming from social rejection(2).

The field theory argues that the social environment outside the individual as well as the needs, urges, drives, and impulses inside him are part of the "field" of forces which determine behavior. Kobler and Stotland extend this perspective to suicide. They hypothesize that the social response to suicidal symptoms determines whether suicide will follow. They think that for suicide to take place, certain conditions must prevail. An individual feels that his future is devoid of hope. He, or someone else, brings the alternative of suicide into his field. The individual tries to communicate his hopelessness to others in an effort to gain assurance that some hope still exists. The character of the response is crucial in determining whether suicide will take place. Those who have committed suicide, according to this theory, found their worlds pervaded by anxiety about suicide and by hopelessness. No person in the immediate environment was hopeful and confident immediately prior to the suicide(3).

Psychoanalytic theories focus almost exclusively on the individual. According to Rushing, Freud believed in a universal death instinct. This death instinct, based on the repetition-compulsion cycle, is always present and precedes the other instincts, but its discharge is circuitous, by way of the subconscious. When the self-preservation instincts which condition this circuitous route are suspended or dulled, the death instinct finds a natural, direct outlet that is suicide. Menninger states that there is a fine edge between love and hate. When the love instinct is frustrated, the hate impulse takes over. The result is the desire to kill, followed by the desire to be killed, which grows to the point where the individual wishes to kill himself(4).

In the psychoanalytic theories, external events are viewed as mere precipitants. An interesting synthesis of social and psychoanalytical theories has been proposed by Farber, who says that suicide is basically a running away from or bursting out of an unbearable situation rather than a hopeful embrace of something prospectively attractive. The suicidal person is one who despairs more easily concerning his ability to cope. This decrease in the ability to sustain hope is based on an impaired feeling of competence. The sense of competence is connected with another person. If that other person cannot supply what is needed, frustration occurs and the individual experiences rage and aggression. Since the significant person is usually very important to the individual, he cannot or will not harm that person, so his anger and frustration turn inward. The suicide is precipitated by some psychic blow. The precipitating event renders life harder to cope with and closes off any possibility of improvement in the situation(5).

Dublin sets forth a crisis theory

which states that everyone at some time finds himself in crisis as he wrestles with problems that are temporarily beyond his capacity to solve. Emotional disequilibrium occurs. The usual coping mechanisms do not help. The person experiences distress and attempts to come to terms with it through various conscious and unconscious searches for coping techniques. The solutions are varied and suicide is just one possibility. The difficulty, according to this theory, lies with the individual's capacity to master the crisis, relate to others, and find useful ways to deal with the problem. When the person cannot or does not relate or communicate his needs adequately, he tends to isolate himself and suicide becomes a distinct possibility(6).

I agree that external conditions and group patterns certainly operate as inhibiting or encouraging forces, but it seems to me that suicide is essentially a personal reaction. The terminal act is the decision of the individual; the final response to his own needs, desires, and circumstances. Suicide, as I define it, is a process of turning anger inward, which results in self-inflicted, destructive action. The steps in this process are:

1. The individual feels a frustration of personal needs.
2. Anger results from the frustration.
3. The individual turns anger inward, which causes feelings of guilt, inadequacy, despair, depression, or hopelessness.
4. A stressful situation develops.
5. The individual perceives the event or series of events as unbearable.
6. The individual tries to communicate his hopelessness to others.
7. The individual is unable to mobilize hope by himself or through others.
8. The individual decides to terminate his life.
9. The individual develops a plan to carry out the decision.
10. The individual takes some self-induced, destructive action that he knows will end his life.

One afternoon I observed a 19-year-old patient, A.E., sitting alone in the dayroom. I knew she had been transferred the night before from a general hospital following a drug overdose.

I asked, "Things must have really piled up on you—gotten to be too much?"

A.E. replied, "No, it wasn't that, I just suddenly realized what my

---

WEEPING WILLOW

I ran away
  but there was no place to go
I looked for a friend
  but there was no one near—
    so
I climbed a tree and looked around—
  there was nothing to see;
  because all was abandoned and lonely.
I wanted to stay invisible in my tree forever; but still
I needed to be with someone, because I was afraid
  of the aloneness I felt—
    so
I began to climb down from the sheltering tree,
  but could find no one to help me descend—
I started to cry, but could summon no tears—
  there was only that sadness I could not explain.
I found myself shrouded in a sense of emptiness and futility
that made me want to fly
  out of my hiding place
    out into space
      and disappear forever....

B.B.

---

whole problem was and I could see no way out of it, so death seemed like it was the best alternative."

"Would you like to tell me?

"I want to tell someone. I'd been on West Ward, and after I was discharged I kept going to this group therapy session. The other day one of the guys put his arm around me and gave me a hug. I suddenly realized that I had never in my life known affection and that is what I wanted—affection, someone to love and care about me, someone I could trust. For the first time I had felt affection. I went home and thought about it but could see no way I'd ever find it. My folks took care of me but never cared, really. It looked so hopeless—a life without affection looked so hopeless. So . . ."

"So you took the pills?"

"Yeah, but first I called Dr. R. She was my psychiatrist on West. I wanted to tell her my feelings and what I planned to do, but I was told she couldn't come to the phone right then. So I hung up and swallowed the pills fast."

"Things must have looked very bleak to you."

"They looked hopeless! But now I want to live. I want something to live for. I want to be happy. I still don't see how, but I want help."

Bodie identifies eight needs expressed by many suicidal individuals as 1) the need to trust; 2) to be accepted; 3) to succeed and break the failure pattern; 4) to increase one's self-esteem; 5) to broaden one's horizon for pleasure; 6) to integrate into group activities; 7) to improve one's masculine or feminine identity, and 8) to increase one's independence and autonomy(7).

In telling of her own struggles and feelings, A.E. expressed many of these needs. In working therapeutically with the suicidal person, it seems most important to keep these basic needs in mind and to strive in all ways possible to help the person learn to fulfill these needs. Another implication I drew from this interaction was the need for serious consideration and awareness of every hint of suicide. Most individuals who are intent on killing themselves still wish very much to be rescued(8). The wish usually is expressed in hints or clues that suicide is being considered. During one session of an adolescent discussion group I was co-leading, the adolescents were discussing their similarities and discovered that each of them had tried to commit suicide at some point. All admitted that they didn't really want to die but just wanted help, and the suicide attempt seemed the most effective way to communicate this.

A close friend of mine, B.B., attempted suicide several times during a stressful time in her life. Before

SUICIDE

each attempt, B.B. told me, she made a desperate call to someone for help. "The response I received to the call for help determined whether I went through with the actual attempt. I wanted help, so if someone responded with genuine interest and genuine caring, even if they couldn't solve the problem, I might change my mind about what I wanted to do."

According to Schneidman, the first clues to an impending suicide may be verbal clues—direct, indirect, or coded. Direct clues would be such statements as "I'm going to kill myself," or "I want to die." Indirect communications might be "Farewell," or "I can't stand it any longer." Coded verbal communication is more subtle; it often has to be "decoded." A remark that "I won't be around much longer for you to put up with" or "I won't be here when you get back," should strike a spark of suspicion in the observant nurse's mind. Individuals may also seek suicide prevention information for a "friend" when actually inquiring for themselves(8).

Behavioral clues can also be identified, the most direct being the "practice run" or the actual suicide attempt. Any use of instruments conventionally associated with suicide—razors, ropes, pills, and so on—should be interpreted as a behavioral cry for help and indicates a severe suicidal potential. Indirect behavioral communications might include such actions as taking a long trip or putting one's affairs in order prematurely. Buying a casket at the time of a friend's or relative's funeral and giving away prized possessions may also be clues to a self-destructive act(8).

Finally, physical and emotional symptoms must be recognized as suicide clues. Feelings of hopelessness, decreasing interest in everyone and everything, loss of sex drive, insomnia, and poor appetite are often evident. Irritability over the slightest disappointment, gentlest criticism or imagined neglect; constant brooding, and feelings of overwhelming guilt are also quite often prominent(9).

Schneidman suggests that most suicides related to depression occur within a few days to three months after the individual has apparently gotten better, for it is then that he has the energy to commit the act. Any significant change in behavior should be assessed as a possible prodrome of suicide(8).

Nurses are in a special position to pick up the hints. Identification of the suicide potential is the basic step in suicide intervention. However, adverse reactions of nurses and physicians to suicidal behavior are probably more common than we realize. In a medical intensive care unit where many people who attempt suicide are admitted, I have seen much anger displayed toward them and heard many insensitive comments. Perhaps I, too, have been guilty at times. When we are fighting desperately to save their lives and they are fighting to die, it is difficult to understand the horrible fear, hurt, and frustration these patients are experiencing. The suicidal individual tends to make nurses, doctors, friends, and family downright angry or perhaps afraid that they themselves or someone they love won't be able to handle a situation and will take the same drastic measures. Perhaps the care givers are feeling frustrated at not really knowing how to help. But it is our responsibility as nurses to recognize our feelings and try to understand those of our patients. Each patient's specific conflicts and highly individualized needs must be kept in mind.

My friend, B.B., is now a successful college student and has developed the unique insight into the real feelings of the suicidal individual that comes only from first-hand experience. She shared many of these feelings with me, to quote,

When a person like me arrives at the point of desiring to kill herself, it is because there seems to be no other alternative. Attempts at making one's problems known have been practically useless, because often there is no clear-cut problem that the person can spot. It's like being trapped in a box with no escape, so that eventually you feel compelled to end your life—like being swept along on a tidal wave. When I locked myself in the bathroom, it was as if I was doing something perfectly natural—and there was nothing else to do. I was in such a state of total submission to my fate that I didn't even feel the knife blade cutting my flesh. It was only as the blood began streaming onto the floor that I was released from my death penalty and realized that I actually didn't want to die. I probably had never really wanted to die—it was just that I felt so totally frustrated and confused that not existing was preferable to existing in that state.

Knowing B.B. has made me even more determined to understand the suicide ideation more fully, to show I care, I help sort out the confusion, and to help someone believe that life *is* worth living. Suicide is a very special sort of tragedy. It causes much suffering both for the individual and for his family and friends. The most tragic part is that most suicides and suicide attempts are preventable if help can be found. Each of us has the ability to be a lifesaver, a preventer of the tragedy.

References

1. DURKHEIM, EMILE. *Suicide*, translated by J. A. Spaulding and George Simpson. New York, Free Press of Glencoe, 1951.
2. BREED, WARREN. Suicide and loss in social interaction. IN *Essays in Self-Destruction*, ed. by E. S. Shneidman. New York, Science House, 1967, pp. 188-203.
3. KOBLER, A. L., AND STOTLAND, EZRA. *The End of Hope: A Social-Clinical Study of Suicide*. New York, Free Press, 1964.
4. RUSHING, W. A. Individual behavior and suicide. IN *Suicide*, ed. by J. P. Gibbs. New York, Harper & Row, 1968, pp. 96-121.
5. FARBER, M. L. *A Theory of Suicide*. New York, Funk and Wagnalls, 1968, pp. 25-60.
6. DUBLIN, L. I. *Suicide: A Sociological and Statistical Study*. New York, Ronald Press, 1963, pp. 164-167.
7. BODIE, M. K. When a patient threatens suicide. *Perspect. Psychiatr. Care* 6(2):76-79, 1968.
8. SHNEIDMAN, E. S. Preventing suicide. *Am.J.Nurs.* 65:111-116, May 1965.
9. IOWA UNIVERSITY COLLEGE OF NURSING, PSYCHIATRIC NURSING DEPARTMENT. *Psychiatric Nursing Syllabus 96:52 and 96:54*. Iowa City, Iowa, The Department, Fall 1973, p. 148.

Sedative-Hypnotic Drugs

Reprinted from American Journal of Nursing, July 1981

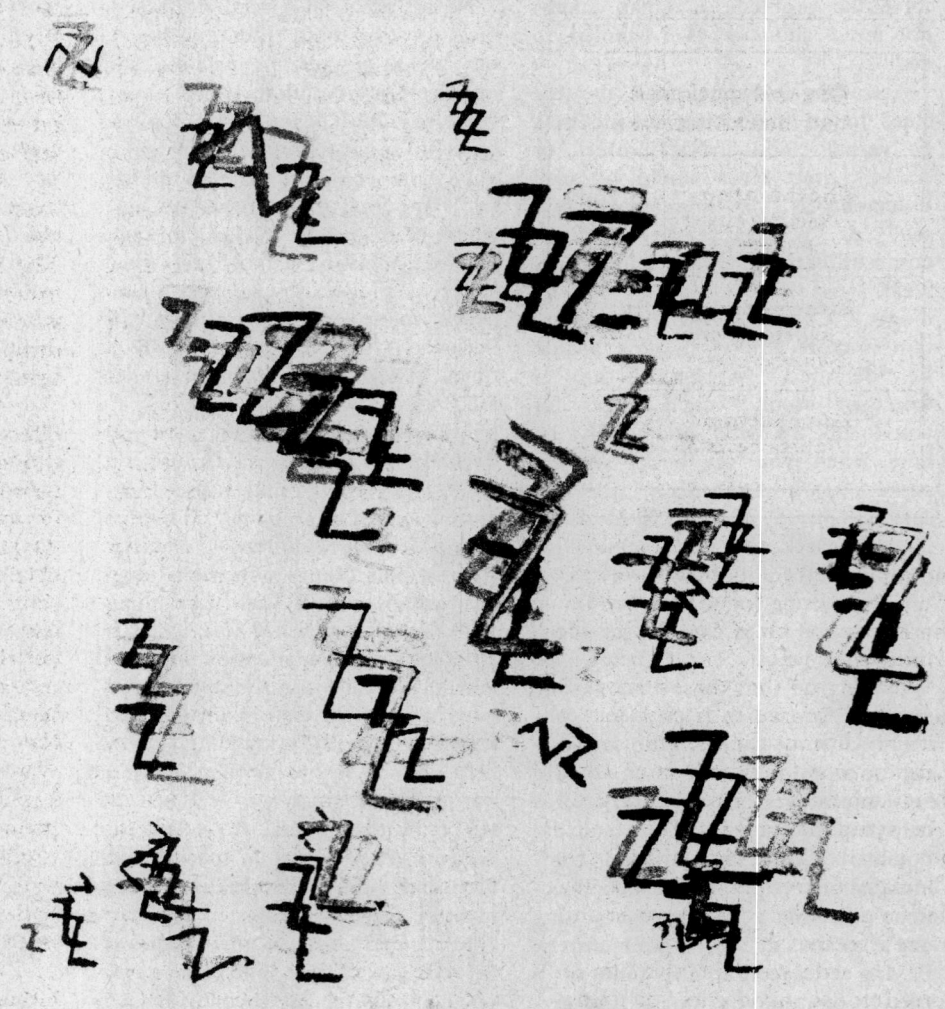

By Elizabeth Harris

The sedative-hypnotics are among the most widely used drugs. But, many authorities maintain, these drugs also are the most widely misused.

Sedative-hypnotics are used to treat anxiety and sleep disturbances, which occur often in both sick and well individuals and can be attributed to a great many causes. They may be symptoms of other conditions. For example, sleep disturbance is a symptom of depression, and anxiety can be due to hyperthyroidism. If so, it is the underlying condition that needs to be treated. But, if the anxiety and sleeplessness a.e severe or intolerable to the patient, or if they adversely affect his health, and particularly when they seem to be temporary, the use of a sedative-hypnotic may be in order.

Each time a patient presents with anxiety or sleep disturbance, it is important to assess carefully the circumstances around the development of the symptom and to exam-

Classification of the Sedative-Hypnotics

I. Barbiturates
II. Nonbarbiturates
　A. Benzodiazepines
　B. Nonbenzodiazepines
　　1. Propanediols
　　2. Quinazolines
　　3. Acetylinic alcohols
　　4. Piperidinedione derivatives
　　5. Chloral derivatives
　　6. Monoureides

Classification of the Barbiturates

Short acting
secobarbital
pentobarbital

Intermediate acting
butabarbital
amobarbital

Long acting
phenobarbital

ine the patient to discover the cause. If a cause can be found and treated, there may be no need to treat the symptom alone.

It may be that these drugs are best used sporadically to treat a patient during the height of his symptoms. Administration of these drugs should be seen as an adjunctive, symptomatic treatment that is not curative, but only a means to alleviate distress, so that the underlying problem can be worked on more effectively.

The sedative-hypnotics, also referred to as anxiolytics, or minor tranquilizers, have been classified in two different ways. One scheme divides them into two classes: the sedatives produce a calming, quieting effect, and the hypnotics induce sleep. In practice, however, it is impossible to place these drugs with certainty into one or the other of these two classes. In fact, all of these drugs in small amounts will produce sedation and in large amounts will induce sleep. It is true that some drugs are preferred for one effect or the other; however, the sedative-hypnotic division is somewhat arbitrary.

A better system is to classify the drugs according to their chemical structure. (See chart, page 1333.) Two other classes of drugs are also used for their sedative-hypnotic effects: the antihistamines and the beta-adrenergic blockers. Because these drugs are so different from other sedative-hypnotics, they will be considered separately.

The sedative-hypnotics are central nervous system (CNS) depressants. In small doses (sedative doses), they create a calming, relaxing effect—an anxiolytic effect. In larger doses, the CNS depression is greater, and the patient will show signs of intoxication, similar to alcohol intoxication, including slurred speech, ataxia, silliness, dizziness, diplopia, and blurred vision. If the patient at this point is provided a quiet, comfortable environment, he will fall asleep—the hypnotic effect. Still larger doses can lead to coma or death.

Tolerance develops with all these drugs, usually within several days. The patient finds that a dose of the drug that relieved his symptoms a few days earlier no longer works as well. The patient may then resort to increasing doses of the drug to produce the desired effect. It is worth noting that a cross-tolerance also develops with all these drugs, so that switching periodically from one drug to another does not help (1,2).

All of these drugs, if taken in large enough doses or long enough, can lead to physical and emotional dependence. Once physical dependence has developed, there are characteristic signs of withdrawal if the drug is abruptly discontinued. Shortly after the last dose (about 24 hours to 2 weeks, depending on the half-life of the drug), the patient will exhibit some or all of the following signs: insomnia, weakness, muscle tremors, anxiety, irritability, sweating, anorexia, fever, nausea and vomiting, headache, incoordination, and restlessness. After a few days, if the patient continues to abstain from the drug, he may develop postural hypotension, tinnitis, incoherence, delirium, psychosis, convulsions, and, eventually, status epilepticus, cardiovascular collapse, or loss of the temperature-regulating mechanism.

The severity of the withdrawal syndrome will depend on the drug, its dose, and the duration of its administration(3,4). It is important to be aware of the symptoms of withdrawal and intoxication, since either may occur in a patient who takes these drugs.

The Barbiturates

The barbiturates are a large, fairly old and well-known group of drugs that are derived from barbituric acid. Phenobarbital is the barbiturate most commonly prescribed(5).

All barbiturates are metabolized into inactive metabolites by the hepatic microsomal enzymes. The inactive metabolites are then excreted in the urine. Phenobarbital is unusual in that 50 percent of the drug is excreted unchanged in the urine(6).

All the barbiturates are equally effective as sedative-hypnotics. Traditionally, the choice of a particular compound depends on the duration of action required. For these purposes, barbiturates are divided according to their half-lives into the short, intermediate, and long-acting compounds. In practice, it has not yet been proven that there are noticeable clinical differences in onset of duration of action, but the system of classification persists(7). The only noticeable clinical difference based on duration of action is that phenobarbital, a long-acting barbiturate, can accumulate in the body to toxic levels if it used repeatedly in patients who have trouble metabolizing it.

All the barbiturates can be used either for daytime sedation or for sleep. The hypnotic dose is generally three or four times the sedative dose. When used as hypnotics, there is conclusive evidence that the barbiturates are useful for no longer than 7 to 14 consecutive nights (8,9).

One advantage of the barbiturates is that they are less expensive than the other sedative-hypnotics. However, their disadvantages far outweigh this advantage.

Disadvantages. When used as

hypnotics, all barbiturates suppress REM (rapid eye movement) or dreaming sleep. It is unclear what the clinical effects of REM suppression are, but what is clear is that after the barbiturate is discontinued the patient can have a rebound effect, with restless sleep, frequent and intense dreaming, or nightmares, for a number of nights or weeks(10).

When used as sedatives or anxiolytics, the barbiturates can cause daytime drowsiness and somnolence. After just a single dose, the patient can have a "hangover" the next day with irritability or excitement and impairment of judgment and fine motor skills(11).

Barbiturates have a narrow margin of safety, particularly as tolerance develops and the effective dose approaches the lethal dose. Barbiturates are often used successfully alone or in combination with other CNS depressants as instruments of suicide. Doses as low as 10 to 15 times the therapeutic dose have been lethal(12).

Tolerance occurs in 7 to 14 days, and there is a high potential for physical dependence with a month or more of use. The long-acting phenobarbital is the only barbiturate that is rarely abused because it has less tendency to produce intoxication or euphoria(13,14).

Barbiturates activate or induce the hepatic microsomal enzymes, which cause more rapid than usual metabolism of a number of drugs, including the barbiturates themselves (this is part of the explanation for tolerance), coumarin derivatives, MAO inhibitor antidepressants, tricyclic antidepressants, phenothiazines, phenytoin, systemic steroids including oral contraceptives, griseofulvin, and rifampicin (15).

Because of these serious drawbacks, barbiturates are seldom indicated for use as oral antianxiety agents and many authorities believe they should be used as hypnotics only for intractable insomnia(16).

The National Institute for Drug Abuse recommends only the following uses for barbiturates:
• thiopental as an anesthetic agent
• phenobarbital, because of its selective anticonvulsant effect, as a first-line drug for treatment of grand mal or cortical focal seizures; other barbiturates, including pentobarbital, amobarbital, or thiopental, given intravenously, are recommended for emergency treatment of seizures
• amobarbital, intravenously, for narcotherapy or intramuscularly, for rapid sedation in patients who are psychotic, manic, or enraged; when used in psychosis, amobarbital is combined with an antipsychotic.
• pentobarbital and secobarbital, as preoperative sedatives(17).

Some drugs, such as Tuinal, combine two barbiturates. Use of these combination drugs is strongly discouraged by most authorities because of the increased risk of abuse and dependence.

Benzodiazepines

The benzodiazepines, chlordiazepoxide (Librium) and diazepam (Valium), are among the most frequently prescribed drugs.

The benzodiazepines offer a number of advantages over the barbiturates. First, they produce less daytime sedation and mental cloudiness while still affording at least an equal antianxiety effect.

Second, they have a higher therapeutic index, so that they rarely are agents for successful suicide. Just as the therapeutic dose is far less, proportionally, than a toxic dose, so also is the difference between the sedative and hypnotic dose greater than for barbiturates (18).

Third, because the benzodiazepines do not activate the hepatic microsomal enzymes significantly, they do not interfere with the metabolism of other drugs.

Fourth, the risk of physical dependence is lower than for any of the other sedative-hypnotics.

Fifth, some studies report greater, more consistent efficacy than with barbiturates and a wider range of usefulness. Others report no significant difference in efficacy (19-21).

As a result of these five factors, it can be said that benzodiazepines may be somewhat more effective as sedative-anxiolytics or hypnotics, and that they are definitely safer than barbiturates. There is overwhelming support in the literature for the use of benzodiazepines in preference to barbiturates, except for the specific indications listed for the barbiturates.

The benzodiazepines also have several disadvantages. All, except the short-acting forms (lorazepam and oxazepam), are converted in the liver to active metabolites with long half-lives. These metabolites are eventually excreted in the urine. This means that the long-acting benzodiazepines can accumulate to a toxic level over several days of continuous use. This can be a particular hazard in the elderly or in patients with liver disease. Such patients are better treated with lorazepam or oxazepam, which have no active metabolites and are quickly excreted(22).

Another effect of the breakdown into active metabolites with long half-lives is that the withdrawal syndrome due to the long-acting benzodiazepines can be prolonged. In fact, the syndrome may not even appear until up to two weeks after the last dose is taken(23).

Tolerance to the benzodiazepines develops, but less quickly than with barbiturates. Dependence is a lesser risk, though there are recent reports that dependence and withdrawal can occur, even when the drugs are taken at therapeutic doses. Oxazepam appears to have the least potential for abuse(24,25).

Another disadvantage is that the intramuscular forms of diazepam and chlordiazepoxide are absorbed slowly, irregularly, and incompletely. Lorazepam, however, is available in an intramuscular form that is well absorbed. Although the benzodiazepines do suppress REM sleep in adequate dosage, there is no evidence of a rebound effect after the drug is discontinued(26).

The benzodiazepines are all equally effective as sedative-hypnotics and differ from each other only in duration of action and pharmacokinetics. They can be divided by duration of action: lorazepam and oxazepam are short acting, and the others are relatively long acting. One resulting consideration is that the short-acting agents must be given in divided doses, whereas the long-acting agents can be given once daily at bedtime after an initial week of divided doses.

There are some specific uses for benzodiazepines in addition to their general use as sedative-hypnotics. Flurazepam may have more potent hypnotic effects and is recommended for use as a hypnotic. As such, it is effective for up to 28 consecutive nights. Chlordiazepoxide and diazepam are often used to detoxify patients who are physically dependent on alcohol. This is possible because of the cross-tolerance that develops.

Benzodiazepines are particularly effective in treating anticipatory anxiety and have been shown to be effective in treating anxiety associated with physical illness. Klein favors using benzodiazepines with tricyclic antidepressants to treat panic disorders. The benzodiazepine treats the anticipatory anxiety (the anxiety of anticipating a panic attack) and the tricyclic treats the panic attacks themselves(27).

Baldessarini suggests using them for agitation during the lag period before antidepressants become effective, and Klein recommends their use in the residual phase of psychosis when the patient is anxious and demoralized and needs the help of an anxiolytic to engage in new activities that will help raise self-esteem(28,29).

Benzodiazepines are also used as preoperative medications. Diazepam is often prescribed as a muscle relaxant, although controlled studies show that it is no more effective than aspirin or placebo. In fact, all CNS depressants have some muscle relaxation effects. Diazepam is used intravenously for emergency treatment of status epilepticus, and clonazepam has been approved for use as an anticonvulsant(30,31). Chlordiazepoxide is the only benzodiazepine available generically at reduced cost.

Nonbarbiturate, Nonbenzodiazepine Compounds

This is another large group of fairly old drugs that are being prescribed less and less since the advent of the benzodiazepines. The National Institute of Drug Abuse reports that although these drugs are equally as effective as other sedative-hypnotics, they offer no advantage over barbiturates or benzodiazepines and may lead to serious toxicity. The disadvantages of this group are many. They present a high risk of abuse and physical dependence; they have a narrow margin of safety; they suppress REM sleep; and with the exception of chloral hydrate, they activate the hepatic microsomal enzymes. Shader argues against the use of meprobamate and other propanediols, but one propanediol, tybamate, produces few withdrawal symptoms and may, therefore, have an advantage(32,33). Chloral hydrate causes distressing GI side effects and can displace and therefore potentiate other protein-bound drugs(34). Methaqualone has been widely abused for years. Paraldehyde, once thought to be a very safe drug, has some major problems. It has a very low therapeutic index, a strong aromatic odor, and a burning, disagreeable taste. It also decomposes on exposure to light and air, and reacts rapidly with some plastics. When given IM it should be given in a glass syringe. Paraldehyde also causes aseptic necrosis when given IM and may cause pulmonary edema. Glutethimide, methyprylon, and ethchlorvynol have pronounced anticholinergic properties and are erratically absorbed from the GI tract. This makes management of overdoses of these drugs especially difficult.

Guidelines for Use

There is overwhelming agreement among psychopharmacologists that when any of these agents are used to treat anxiety or sleep disorder, the course of treatment should be brief and/or intermittent. None of these agents has been shown to be helpful as a hypnotic for any longer than 28 nights. Most are helpful only for 7 to 14 consecutive nights. When used as sedatives, the drugs produce tolerance fairly quickly, so that a higher dose is needed for a therapeutic effect. If this continues unabated, physical dependence develops. Yet, there are times of stress when these agents are indicated for severe anxiety or sleeplessness.

When a patient complains of anxiety or sleeplessness, and an underlying cause is not apparent, it would be wise to try such conservative measures as listening to the complaint, providing reassurance where appropriate, or teaching relaxation techniques, yoga, or meditation. Patients who suffer from sleep disturbance can be helped to create a relaxing routine before bedtime and to increase exercise and decrease caffeine intake during the day. These measures alone may be successful. If not, a sedative-hypnotic may provide the only humane treatment.

Side Effects

Daytime sedation is the most common side effect of sedative-hypnotics. It occurs slightly less with benzodiazepines than with other sedative-hypnotics(35). Paradoxical excitement can occur as a side effect of any of these drugs. This is similar to the disinhibition that can occur with alcohol and can appear as excitement, hostility, rage, confusion, depersonalization, or hyperactivity.

Other rare side effects include blood dyscrasias, rash, photosensitivity, nonthrombocytopenic purpura, menstrual irregularities, GI discomfort, nausea, and vomiting(36).

As is true with many other kinds of drugs, the elderly experience more side effects from the sedative-hypnotics. Elderly patients are more prone to daytime sedation and to the paradoxical excitement effect. Because they have a diminished capacity to metabolize and eliminate these drugs, older patients are more prone to toxic accumulation over time. For this reason, the shorter-acting drugs should be used.

Finally, because elderly patients are often on a variety of medications, special attention must be paid to possible drug interactions.

Contraindications

Absolute contraindications include severe respiratory compromise, known hypersensitivity to individual compounds, and acute intermittent porphyria(37,38).

These drugs should be avoided

The Sedative-Hypnotics

Generic name	Trade name	Hypnotic dose	Sedative dose (total daily dose)	Half-life (hr.)
Barbiturates				
secobarbital	Seconal	100-200 mg.	90-200 mg.	19-34
pentobarbital	Nembutal	100-200 mg.	60-80 mg.	15-48
amobarbital	Amytal	100-200 mg.	60-150 mg.	8-42
butabarbital	Butisol	100-200 mg.	20-200 mg.	34-42
phenobarbital	Luminal and others	100-200 mg.	30-90 mg.	24-140
thiopental	Pentothal	Used for anesthesia		
methohexital	Brevital	Used for anesthesia for ECT only		
Nonbarbiturates				
Benzodiazepines				
flurazepam	Dalmane	15-30 mg.		24-100
nitrazepam	Mogadon	5-10 mg.	Not available in U.S.	18-34
chlordiazepoxide	Librium and others	25	15-80 mg.	6-30
diazepam	Valium	10	6-40 mg.	20-90
oxazepam	Serax	10-30	30-60 mg.	3-21
clorazepate	Tranxene and others		15-60 mg.	40-200
prazepam	Verstran	10-20	20-60 mg.	24-200
lorazepam	Ativan	2-4	2-6 mg.	10-20
Nonbenzodiazepines				
Propanediols				
meprobamate	Equanil Miltown and others	800	0.4-1.2 gm.	10
tybamate	Solacen Tybatran		500-1,500 mg.	
Quinazolines				
methaqualone	Quaalude Parest Optimil Sopor and others	150-300 mg.	250-300 mg.	10-42
Acetylinic alcohols				
ethchlorvynol	Placidyl	0.5-1 gm.	200-600 mg.	10-25
Piperidinedione derivatives				
glutethimide	Doriden	250-500	125-750 mg.	5-22
methyprylon	Noludar	200-400 mg.	150-400 mg.	
Chloral derivatives				
chloral hydrate	Noctec Somnos and others	0.5-2 gm.		
chloral betaine	Beta-Chlor	870 mg.-1 gm.		
triclofos	Triclos	750 mg.-1.5 gm.		
Monoureides				
paraldehyde	Paral	3-8 gm.		

whenever possible in patients with a history of drug or alcohol abuse or suicide attempts by overdose because of the increased risk of abuse. Patients with a history of peptic ulcers should avoid chloral hydrate because of its irritation of the GI tract. In patients with uremia or hepatic insufficiency, hypnotics can precipitate coma due to inadequate metabolism and excretion of the drugs. Patients with renal or hepatic disease can be treated with smaller doses or short-acting compounds. Patients in pain should not receive these drugs unless their pain is controlled, or their discomfort will increase.

The safe use of these compounds in pregnancy and breastfeeding has not been established. There is some evidence of an increased incidence of cleft lip and palate after diazepam use in the first trimester, but there is no other evidence of sequelae of first trimester use(39). However, when barbiturates or benzodiazepines are used in the last trimester of pregnancy, there have been reports of physical dependence in the fetus or neonatal depression, accompanied by poor sucking, hypotonia, and hypothermia. In addition, barbiturates and benzodiazepines are excreted in small amounts in human breast milk and can cause lethargy and weight loss in the breast-fed infant. Most authorities agree that sedative-hyp-

Antihistamines		
Generic name	Trade name	Average daily dose
diphenhydramine	Benadryl	25-100 mg.
hydroxyzine	Atarax	25-200 mg.
	Vistaril	
promethazine	Phenergan	50-200 mg.

notics should be avoided whenever possible during pregnancy and breast-feeding (40,41).

As with any other drug, patients must be told the expected course of treatment, and the name, dose, and schedule of the drug. In addition patients using these drugs should be warned of the risk of tolerance and dependence and told how these risks will be minimized. They should be told not to increase their dosage without contacting the health care provider and not to take an extra tablet or more when their symptoms are not immediately ameliorated with the prescribed dose.

Patients should also be informed that these drugs will not treat the cause of the anxiety or sleeplessness but will only treat the symptoms.

Patients should be advised not to use alcohol or other CNS depressants while taking these medications because of the additive effect. They should be advised against operating cars or any dangerous machinery that requires muscular coordination and mental alertness.

Because of the possible drug interactions with many of these agents, patients should be asked to notify all health care providers when they are taking these drugs.

If the patient lives with children, he should be advised to keep the tablets or capsules in a safe place where children cannot find them and mistake them for candy.

Beta-blockers

The most commonly studied drug in the beta-blocker group is propranolol (Inderal). Propranolol is a beta-adrenergic blocking agent that is used primarily to treat cardiac arrhythmias, angina, and hypertension. Recently, it has also been used experimentally to treat such peripheral autonomic symptoms of anxiety as trembling, tachycardia, palpitations, diaphoresis, and hyperventilation.

The medication does not allay the inner feeling of anxiety; it only removes the outward manifestations. It seems particularly useful for patients whose anxiety appears in specific, highly stressful situations where the possible sedation and mental clouding of the sedative-hypnotics are undesirable—for example, public speaking, musical recitals, acting, or job interviews. Propranolol may also be helpful to patients who focus on the somatic symptoms of anxiety. It is not helpful, however, in treating anticipatory anxiety.

The mechanism of action is thought to be a peripheral beta-adrenergic blockade, although there may also be some central effects. Dosages recommended are 30 to 120 mg. per day in three or four divided doses.

There can be troubling side effects, such as insomnia, hallucinations, impairment of metabolism of other drugs, lethargy or depression, GI distress, or rash. Inderal is contraindicated in some cardiac and pulmonary diseases. The use of propranolol as an antianxiety agent is not FDA approved.

Antihistamines

These drugs can be prescribed to treat sleep disturbance or anxiety states, although these are not the primary uses of the antihistamines. They are less effective sedative-anxiolytics than the sedative-hypnotics and tend to create daytime sedation. When used as hypnotics, they are less powerful than the sedative-hypnotics and are often ineffective. In addition, they can create unwanted and sometimes dangerous anticholinergic side effects. Yet they are effective for some people and are fairly commonly used.

References

1. Baldessarini, R. J. Chemotherapy in Psychiatry. Cambridge, Mass., Harvard University Press, 1977, p. 132.
2. U. S. National Institute of Drug Abuse. Sedative-Hypnotic Drugs, Risks and Benefits, ed. by J. R. Cooper. Washington, D.C., U. S. Government Printing Office, 1977, p. 15.
3. Ibid., p. 16.
4. Gilman, A. G., and others, eds. Goodman and Gilman's The Pharmacological Basis of Therapeutics. 6th ed. New York, Macmillian Publishing Co., 1980, p. 339-375.
5. National Institute of Drug Abuse, op.cit., p. 60.
6. Gilman and others, op.cit., p. 357.
7. Greenblatt, D. J., and Shader, R. I. Psychotropic drugs in the general hospital. In Manual of Psychiatric Therapeutics, ed. by R. I Shader. Boston, Little, Brown & Co., 1975, p. 5.
8. Gilman and others, op.cit., p. 353.
9. National Institute of Drug Abuse, op.cit., p. 15.
10. Ibid., p. 6.
11. Gilman and others, op.cit., p. 358.
12. National Institute of Drug Abuse, op.cit., p. 9.
13. Koch-Weser, J., and Greenblatt, D. J. The archaic barbiturate hypnotics. N.Engl.J.Med. 291:790-791, Oct. 10, 1974.
14. Solomon, F., and others. Sleeping pills, insomnia and medical practice. N.Engl.J.Med. 300:803-808, Apr. 5, 1979.
15. Committee on the Review of Medicines. Recommendations on barbiturate preparations. Br.Med.J. 2:719-720, Sept. 22, 1979.
16. Ibid.
17. National Institute of Drug Abuse, op.cit., p. 106.
18. Klein, D. F., and others, eds. Diagnosis and Drug Treatment of Psychiatric Disorders: Adults and Children. 2d ed. Baltimore, Md., Williams & Wilkins Co., 1980, p. 547.
19. Shader and Greenblatt, op.cit., p. 35.
20. Klein and others, op.cit., p. 526.
21. National Institute of Drug Abuse, op.cit., p. 8.
22. Hoyumpa, A. M. Jr. Disposition and elimination of minor tranquilizers in the aged and in patients with liver disease. South Med.J. 71 (Suppl):23-28, Aug. 1978.
23. Baldessarini, op.cit., p. 144.
24. FDA Bull. Prescribing of minor tranquilizers Feb., 1980.
25. _____ Binding, A. The abuse potential of benzodiazepines, with special attention to oxazepam. Acta Psychiatr.Scand. 274:111-116, 1978.
26. Feinberg, I., and others. Flurazepam effects on sleep EEG. Arch.Gen.Psychiatry 36:95-102, Jan. 1979.
27. Klein and others, op.cit., p. 564.
28. Baldessarini, op.cit., p. 135.
29. Klein and others, op.cit., p. 547.
30. Gilman and others, op.cit., p. 466-467.
31. Anderson, G. D. Benzodiazepines. Nurse Pract. 5:47, 50-51, 60, Jan.-Feb. 1980.
32. Shader and Greenblatt, op.cit., p. 33.
33. Klein and others, op.cit., p. 546.
34. Greenblatt and Shader, op.cit., p. 4.
35. Baldessarini, op.cit., p. 140.
36. Appleton and Davis, op.cit., p. 158.
37. National Institute of Drug Abuse, op.cit., p. 12.
38. Gilman and others, op.cit., p. 358.
39. Goldberg, H. L., and DiMascio, A. Psychotropic drugs in pregnancy. In Psychopharmacology: A Generation of Progress, ed. by M. A. Morris and others. New York, Raven Press, 1978, p. 1051.
40. Committee on the Review of Medicines, op.cit.
41. Goldberg and DiMascio, op.cit.

Reprinted from American Journal of Nursing, July 1981

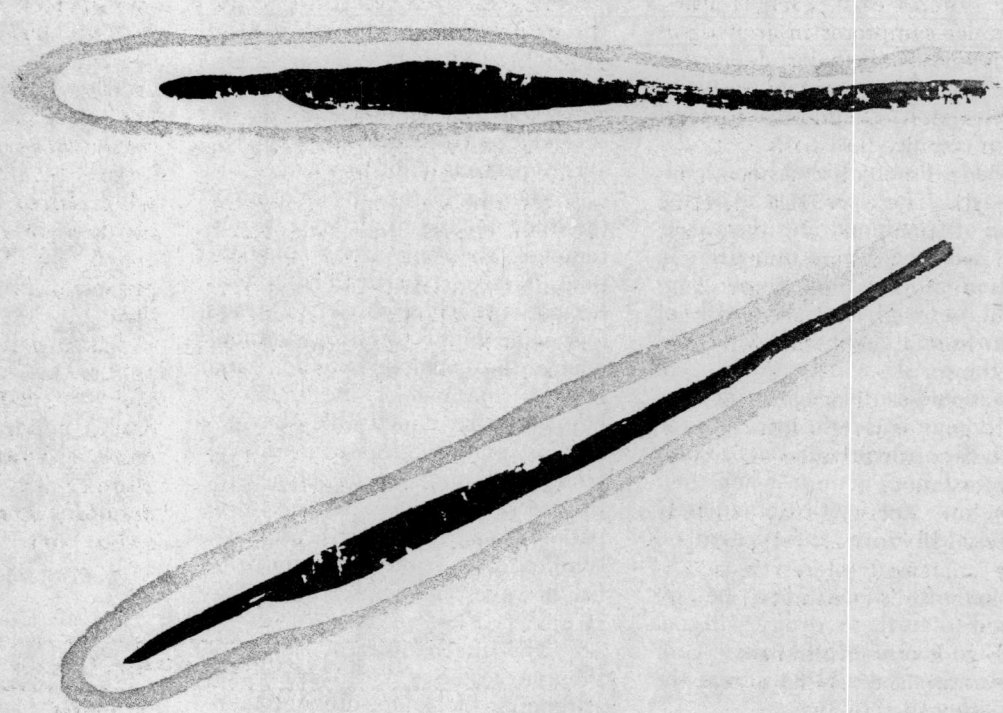

Antidepressant Drug Therapy

By Marion D. DeGennaro
Robyn Hymen
Alice Maltbie Crannell
Peter A. Mansky

Depression, the most common psychiatric disorder, affects an estimated 10 to 16 percent of adults in the United States (1). Numerous theories regarding the etiology of depression have been developed over the years and have been used as a basis for predicting treatment response(2).

Depressive disorders have generally been categorized as endogenous—those depressions thought to arise from biochemical or physiological factors—or exogenous/reactive—those associated with a clear precipitating event or stressor. In the past, it was thought that physiologically based endogenous depressions followed specific symptom patterns that responded best to drug treatment and that reactive exogenous depressions could best be treated with psychotherapy.

Today, however, the distinction between endogenous and exogenous depression is less clear, and the choice of treatment based on etiology is less strict. While depressive symptomatology in certain individuals may be associated with such precipitants as life changes or stress, these factors have been found to have little, if any, effect in predicting response to medication. It is thought that such stresses as marital discord or job problems may actually be a result of early stages of depression and, thus, may follow rather than precede depression. If they do precede depression, it is thought that such stresses may, in fact, play a role in altering central nervous system functioning, thereby causing physiologically based depression (3,4,5).

The diagnosis of *major depressive disorder* is made on the basis of the clinical interview. Several diagnostic systems exist, each focusing on similar symptoms in arriving at the diagnosis of major depressive disorders(6,7). The system we use is the Research Diagnostic Criteria (which forms the basis for the American Psychiatric Association's DSM-III). These criteria describe *major depression* as dysphoric mood present for a minimum of two weeks (depressed, blue, despondent, fearful, worried) and accompanied by at least five of the following symptoms:

• appetite disturbance—either weight gain or weight loss

• sleep disturbance—insomnia or hypersomnia

• low energy—may include decreased libido, easy fatigability

• decreased interest in activities—anhedonia (inability to feel pleasure)

• guilt or worthlessness

• diminished ability to concentrate—slowed thinking

• psychomotor agitation or retardation

• suicidal ideation or behavior, ranging from thoughts that life is not worth living to plans for or actual suicide attempts.

Other symptoms often present with a major depression include feelings of helplessness, hopelessness, dependency, pessimism, difficulty in decision making, irritability, and poor social judgment. There is often a variation in mood, with

---

MARION D. DEGENNARO, R.N., B.S.N., is a psychiatric research nurse, Department of Psychiatry, Albany Medical College, Albany, N.Y.

ROBYN HYMEN, B.A., is research coordinator, Department of Psychiatry, Albany Medical College.

ALICE MALTBIE CRANNELL, R.N., B.S.N., is a community health and research nurse, Capital District Psychiatric Center, Albany, N.Y.

PETER A. MANSKY, M.D., is associate professor of psychiatry, director of the Psychopharmacology Unit at Albany Medical College, and director of Capital District Psychiatric Center in Albany.

---

increased dysphoric feelings in the morning. This symptom is a good prognosticator of a favorable response to drug treatment. Major depression may exist, however, in the absence of diurnal variation or with the reverse variation. A positive family history of depression, suicide, and/or alcoholism may assist the clinician in confirming a diagnosis of depression.

Subtypes of major depression. According to the Research Diagnostic Criteria, major depression may be divided into three subtypes:

• Unipolar—single or recurrent episodes of major depression with no history of mania or hypomania (mania and hypomania refer to mood elevation or irritability accompanied by increased activity and a constellation of other symptoms).

• Bipolar—single or recurrent episodes of depression with a history of mania (true manic-depressive illness).

• Bipolar II—single or recurrent episodes of depression with a history of hypomania (maniclike episodes that are not of sufficient intensity or duration to meet full criteria for mania).

In formulating the diagnosis of major depression, the distinction should be made between primary and secondary depression. (This distinction, however, does not affect the choice of antidepressant.) Depressive symptoms may be considered secondary if they occur as a consequence of a preexisting nonaffective psychiatric illness, such as schizophrenia or alcoholism, or if the depressive symptoms follow the course of a life-threatening or incapacitating illness or surgical procedure.

The presence of other neuropsychiatric disorders, such as profound mental retardation; organic brain syndrome; schizophrenia; neurotic disorders, such as Briquet's disorder, anxiety, phobic, or panic disorder, obsessive-compulsive disorder, and labile or cyclothymic

---

Antidepressant Drugs

Generic name	Trade names	Usual daily dose (mg.)	Maximum daily dose (mg.)
Tricyclics			
imipramine	Imavate, Janimine, Presamine, SK-Pramine, Tofranil	100-200	300
desipramine	Norpramin, Pertofrane	100-200	300
amitriptyline	Amitril, Elavil, Endep	75-200	300
nortriptyline	Aventyl, Pamelor	75-150	150
doxepin	Adapin, Sinequan	75-150	300
protriptyline	Vivactil	15-40	60
trimipramine	Surmontil	75-200	400
Monoamine Oxidase Inhibitors			
isocarboxazid	Marplan	10-30	30
phenelzine	Nardil	15-30	90
tranylcypromine	Parnate	20-30	30
Tetracyclics			
maprotiline	Ludiomil	75-300	300
Others			
amoxapine	Asendin	150-300	400

personality; and chronic alcoholism and/or drug dependency, must be considered in arriving at the diagnosis of primary major depression. For some individuals, however, another psychiatric disorder—most frequently heavy alcohol use and/or anxiety—may be present only during depressive episodes and, as such, may be considered secondary to the depressive disorder. Careful clinical interview and history review are helpful in making this type of determination and differential diagnosis.

Biochemical Theories of Depression

The role of neurotransmitters in depressive illness forms the basis for the major biochemical theories involved in the treatment of depression. These theories aid the clinician in planning and selecting drug treatment.

To date, the most widely used drug treatments, all based to some extent on the role of the neurotransmitter in depression, have included the tricyclic antidepressants, monoamine oxidase inhibitors, the psychostimulants and, just recently, the tetracyclic antidepressants.

Nearly a century ago, the concept of the neurotransmitter and its significance in the transmission of impulses was first introduced. This concept led to the identification of norepinephrine and later to several other specific neurotransmitters.

The neurotransmitter is viewed as the biochemical vehicle of impulse transmission and is stored within the nerve cell in storage vesicles. An impulse is propagated by electrical stimulation of the presynaptic neuron, which causes the release of the neurotransmitter from storage at that site. The neurotransmitter then crosses the synaptic cleft, binds briefly to its postsynaptic receptor, and is released back into the synaptic cleft. About 80 percent of the neurotransmitter is reabsorbed into the presynaptic neuron (reuptake) with the remainder being metabolized by one of two enzymes, either monoamine oxidase or catechol-o-methyl transferase.

If there is an inadequate amount of neurotransmitter in storage vesicles at the presynaptic site, then electrical stimulation will not have sufficient effect on the postsynaptic receptor to produce transmission of a neuronal impulse(8). The dysfunction of a particular neurotransmitter does not appear to be correlated with specific signs or symptoms of depression, and therefore, the implicated neurotransmitter cannot be ascertained through clinical interview. Also, there exist at this time no sophisticated and practical biochemical determinants that can be routinely used to uncover the dysfunctional neurotransmitter. Specific neurotransmitters that have been implicated in depression include norepinephrine and serotonin, and, to a lesser extent, acetylcholine.

Tricyclic Antidepressants

Recent studies have shown that 70 percent of individuals diagnosed as having a depressive disorder respond favorably to tricyclic antidepressants(1). Symptomatic relief, however, is not usually achieved until two to four weeks after this therapy has been started.

Some Common Side Effects of

Side Effect	Intervention
Anticholinergic	
Dry mouth	Encourage frequent sips of water. Suggest lemon juice and glycerine mouth swabs, dietetic or nonsucrose sour ball candies, or a commercial oral lubricant.
Constipation	Encourage intake of bran, fresh fruits and vegetables, and prunes. Maintain adequate fluid intake. Suggest stool softeners or laxatives. Withhold medication and advise physician, as urecholine may be needed to prevent paralytic ileus when constipation is severe.
Urinary retention and delayed micturition	Monitor intake and output. Check for abdominal distention. Withhold medication and advise physician if patient unable to void; catheterization and/or urecholine may be required.
Blurred vision	Assure patient that this is temporary. Suggest eye consult if this persists beyond medication adjustment period (about 3 weeks).
Diaphoresis	Encourage adequate fluid intake (preferably noncaloric) to replace lost fluid. Observe for symptoms of electrolyte imbalance.
Atropine psychosis	Withhold medication and advise physician, as medication must be discontinued.
Cardiovascular	
Tachycardia	Monitor pulse for rate and arrhythmias. Withhold medication and notify physician if resting pulse rate >120.
Orthostatic hypotension	Record blood pressure with patient sitting and standing; withhold medication and notify physician if systolic blood pressure drops more than 20 to 30 mm.
Arrhythmias and T-wave abnormalities	Monitor pulse for irregularities. Provide for routine electrocardiogram (ECG) and serial ECGs if patient has history of conduction defects.

Antidepressant Medications

Side Effect	Intervention
Psychiatric	
Anxiety, restlessness, irritability	Advise physician, as dose may need to be decreased or increased or time of administration changed; medication may need to be changed to one that produces more sedation, such as amitriptyline; sedatives and or antipsychotics may be required.
Hypomania	Withhold medication and inform physician as antidepressant may be unmasking a bipolar disorder.
Mental confusion, psychotic behavior	Discontinue drug; physostigmine (antidote for severe anticholinergic side effects).
Neurologic	
Drowsiness	Advise patient initially not to operate hazardous machinery.
	Administer medication at bedtime.
	If persistent, advise physician, as medication may need to be changed to a less sedative antidepressant, such as imipramine.
Lowering of seizure threshold	Observe seizure precautions during initial treatment.
	Advise physician if seizure occurs, as adjustment of anticonvulsant in patients with seizure disorders and/or discontinuation of antidepressant may be warranted.
Fine tremor and/or ataxia	If severe, withhold medication and advise physician, as change in dose and/or medication may be needed.
Endocrinologic/ Metabolic	
Decreased or increased libido	Assure patient that this is usually transitory.
	If persistent or interfering with compliance, advise physician, as change in medication and/or dose may be indicated.
Ejaculatory and erection disturbances	Advise physician if this interferes with compliance, as medication and/or dose may need to be changed.
Weight gain	Monitor weight.
	Counsel patient to eat well-balanced nutritionally adequate diet.

The tricyclic antidepressants act by blocking the reuptake of the neurotransmitter into the presynaptic neuron, resulting in an increase in neurotransmitter concentration in the synapse. Specific tricyclics selectively affect the neurotransmitters either individually or in combination. If response to the initial tricyclic is partial or minimal, a second tricyclic may be prescribed, based upon either its specificity or its degree of neurotransmitter effect.

With the tricyclic antidepressant nortriptyline—Aventyl, Pamelor, there is evidence that a "therapeutic window" exists. The term "therapeutic window" refers to the fact that there is a small range of serum plasma levels at which the drug is effective. Above or below this window there is not optimal response. Steady state plasma levels are usually reached within 7 to 21 days of repetitive administration of a constant dose of tricyclic. For each patient, the mean steady state plasma level is linearly related to dose; however, intersubject variation can be quite large. Current research is being undertaken to determine if clinical response can be correlated with a specific range of blood levels. Definitive findings regarding the association between clinical response and steady state plasma levels will provide a more accurate indicator of the therapeutic dose required for the treatment of each patient(9,10).

Due to the effect of tricyclic antidepressant medications on body systems, especially the autonomic nervous system, an accurate assessment of a patient's current physical status is imperative prior to prescribing any of these drugs. Because of the anticholinergic activity of these drugs, cardiovascular conditions warrant close monitoring with periodic electrocardiographic evaluations. Treatment with tricyclic antidepressants for those patients who have left bundle branch block is contraindicated. Other conditions that require caution for treatment with tricyclic antidepressants are: narrow angle glaucoma, history of urinary retention, benign prostatic hypertrophy, seizure disorders, and impaired liver function.

Concomitant use of tricyclic antidepressants and monoamine oxidase (MAO) inhibitors in the treatment of depression is generally contraindicated, although some clinicians consider the combination to be effective.

Monoamine Oxidase Inhibitors

The MAO inhibitors' mode of action is distinctly different from that of the tricyclic antidepressants. Monoamine oxidase, located in the mitochondria of the nerve cell, metabolizes norepinephrine and serotonin during the reuptake process. MAO inhibitors act by blocking the metabolism of these neurotransmitters, resulting in an increase in the concentration of these neurotransmitters within the presynaptic neuron. This increase is then available for release following stimulation of the presynaptic neuron.

The MAO inhibitors have not been widely used in the United States, although their use is increasing. In part, this is due to the effectiveness of the tricyclics, but is also related to concern over the potential occurrence of hypertensive crisis after administration of MAO inhibitors. The incidence of hypertensive crisis is associated with the concurrent use of the MAO inhibitors with tyramine-containing foods and/or medications containing sympathomimetics.

MAO inhibitors, due to their high toxicity, are usually prescribed only when tricyclic compounds are ineffective. Contraindications for use of MAO inhibitors are liver disease, pheochromocytoma, glaucoma, impaired renal function, hyperthyroidism, epilepsy, arteriosclerosis, paranoid schizophrenia, hypertension, and cardiovascular disease.

Psychostimulants

The psychostimulants (amphetamines and methylphenidate) have several actions on the nerve terminal. There is evidence that they facilitate release of neurotransmitters into the synapse, thereby increasing concentration, and that they inhibit reuptake activity in a way similar to the tricyclics(11-14). They have, in the past, been widely used in the treatment of depression. Currently, these agents are not considered to be the treatment of choice because they act as stimulants rather than relieving depression and because of the appreciable abuse potential and possible toxic psychosis associated with their use.

Newer Antidepressants

Among the newer antidepressant drugs are the tetracyclic compounds and a variety of compounds unrelated structurally to the tricyclics, tetracyclics, or the MAO inhibitors. Some are available in the United States and some have not yet received FDA approval. Examples are myanserin, amoxapine (Asendin), maprotiline (Ludiomil), and trazadone. The relative potency and neurotransmitter effects of these drugs are not yet fully established. Some of these medications may represent a definite gain in the treatment of depression. As the body of knowledge regarding these drugs increases, their effects may become more important.

The advantages of many of the newer antidepressants are earlier onset of therapeutic effect and less severe and fewer anticholinergic effects than with older antidepressants. Symptomatic relief is usually experienced earlier and, in some patients, may be within one week. Cardiovascular reactions are reported to be less frequently encountered. Lower initial dosages are recommended for the elderly.

Nursing Interventions

Many side effects of antidepressants can be minimized or avoided by gradual dosage increase to the optimum or therapeutic level for the individual patient. Side effects that do arise may be alleviated by nursing interventions, thereby increasing patient compliance with the medication schedule and ensuring therapeutic response to the prescribed drug. Careful observations for assessment of side effects and their severity enable the physician and nurse to work cooperatively in the care of the patient.

The more severe side effects, such as paralytic ileus or serious arrhythmias, can often be averted by alert, frequent evaluation of the patient's progress and by education of the patient with regard to reporting prodromal signs and symptoms of severe side effects. The nurse can play an important role in the treatment of depression by conveying confidence in the medication as well as by being empathic to the mildly annoying side effects that

Antidepressants: Old Drugs, New Uses

By Elizabeth Harris

Antidepressant drugs, used in the treatment of depression for over 20 years, are being used experimentally today for a number of conditions other than depression. Many of these uses are controversial, and some are not yet FDA approved.

Atypical depression. The MAO inhibitors have regained some of the popularity they once had because they appear to be effective in treating patients who have atypical depression(1,2). In these patients, there is a good premorbid history with a fluctuating dysphoric mood.

Symptoms of atypical depression can include fatigue, chronic anxiety, overreactivity of mood, phobias, somatic symptoms or preoccupations, overeating with weight gain, and hypersomnia. Patients with atypical depression may respond better to the MAO inhibitors than they do to the tricyclics(3). The anxiety of atypical depression is better relieved by MAO inhibitors because of the innate antianxiety action of these drugs. The more "typical" depression has symptoms of decreased appetite with weight loss, motor and speech retardation, diurnal mood variation (improvement of mood in the evening), and sleep disturbance with early morning awakening, and responds better to tricyclics.

It is generally believed that either form of depression should be treated first with tricyclics. If a three-week trial with a tricyclic fails to produce results in a patient with an atypical depression, an MAO inhibitor often will produce results.

Some clinicians believe that depression in patients who have an underlying bipolar affective disorder (formerly called manic-depressive illness) responds better to MAO inhibitors(4,5).

Phobias and panic attacks. Phobias, with panic attacks and free-floating anxiety attacks, have been shown to respond to phenelzine (Nardil), an MAO inhibitor, or imipramine (Tofranil), a tricyclic antidepressant(6,7). A panic attack is a sudden, spontaneous, unexplained feeling of helplessness, terror, or impending disaster, accom-

are often initially present. This attitude of support and confidence can help the patient in weighing the risk-benefit ratio of side effects of drug treatment versus depression.

We have categorized side effects of antidepressant medications into anticholinergic, cardiovascular, psychiatric, neurological, and endocrine/metabolic. (The side effects and nursing interventions associated with them are described in the chart, page 1306-1307.)

The anticholinergic side effects are the most commonly encountered. The caricature of a person suffering a severe anticholinergic response (atropine psychosis) has been described as: "*Blind* as a bat. *Red* as a beet. *Mad* as a hatter *Dry* as a bone."

The concommitant use of other drugs with anticholinergic effects, such as antihistamines, atropine, and benztropine (Cogentin), can increase the risk of anticholinergic side effects in patients receiving tricyclic antidepressants. The concomitant use of guanethidine (Ismelin) or methyldopa (Aldomet) for hypertension is also contraindicated with the tricyclic and tetracyclic antidepressants. Propranolol (Inderal) is the drug of choice for treatment of hypertension for patients on tricyclic antidepressants, as its action is not adversely affected by the tricyclics.

Tricyclic antidepressants may be additive to or potentiate CNS depressants, such as alcohol, sedatives, and hypnotics. Generally, simultaneous use of MAO inhibitors and tricyclic antidepressants is contraindicated, due to the danger of hyperpyrexia and other side effects(15,16).

The MAO inhibitors potentiate the action and toxic effects of a wide assortment of medications, especially sympathomimetic drugs such as ephedrine, amphetamine, phenylpropanolamine, and many nonprescription cold remedies. As a result, hypertensive crisis accompanied by intracranial hemorrhage, hyperpyrexia, convulsions, coma, and death may occur. Propranolol

panied by a flight response and autonomic manifestations of anxiety, such as a smothering or choking feeling, dizziness, faintness, difficulty breathing, paresthesias, trembling, feelings of unreality, hot or cold flashes, chest pain, nausea, or fear of imminent death(8). The symptoms can occur in response to specific feared objects or situations—such as a crowded or public place, shopping in stores, or a train—or they can occur spontaneously with no apparent precipitant. They can last minutes or, rarely, hours and, in some patients, occur periodically over several months or years. The action of the drug is to block the panic symptoms.

Obsessive-compulsive disorder. There are recent reports that clomipramine, a tricyclic, is moderately effective in treating severe obsessive-compulsive disorders(9). The drug, however, is not yet released for use in the United States by the FDA.

Hysteroid dysphoria. This is a chronic character disorder with fluctuating moods that is thought to respond to phenelzine; tricyclics have a known adverse affect(10). Patients with this condition have a shallow, brittle mood that changes abruptly from euphoria and elation to desperate unhappiness, depending on external sources of admiration and approval. When these patients are deprived of immediate support and love from their environment, they are likely to search desperately for some means of alleviating their dysphoria. They may abuse drugs or alcohol, plunge into ill-fated love affairs, threaten suicide to gain affirmations of caring, or involve themselves in a variety of other self-destructive situations. Phenelzine helps these patients by moderating the severe dysphoria, so that they are less likely to engage in dangerous or life-threatening activities.

Childhood enuresis. The tricyclics, particularly, imipramine, have been used successfully to treat childhood enuresis.

Hyperactivity. Imipramine and amitriptyline have both been used successfully to treat hyperactivity in children. They are used as an adjunct to other drugs used to treat this condition(11).

Pain. Tricyclics are occasionally useful in some pain syndromes, such as diabetic neuropathy, migraine, and cancer(12-16).

References

1. Stern, and others. Toward a rational pharmacotherapy of depression. *Am.J.Psych.* 137:545-552, May, 1980.
2. Klein, D. F., and others. *Diagnosis and Drug Treatment of Psychiatric Disorders: Adults and Children.* 2d ed. Baltimore, Md., Williams & Wilkins Co., 1980, pp. 309, 323.
3. Gilman, A. G., and others, eds. *Goodman and Gilman's Pharmacological Basis of Therapeutics.* 6th ed. New York, Macmillan Publishing Co., 1980, p. 427.
4. Klein and others, *op.cit.*, p. 345.
5. Kupfer, D. J., and Detre, T. P. Tricyclic and monoamine inhibitor antidepressants overdose. In *Handbook of Psychopharmacology, Volume 14: Affective Disorders: Drug Actions in Animals and Man,* ed. by L. L. Iverson and others. New York, Plenum Publishing Co., 1978.
6. Klein and others, *op.cit.*, p. 557.
7. Sheehan, D. V., and others. Treatment of endogenous anxiety with phobic, hysterical and hypochondriacal symptoms. *Arch.Gen.Psychiatry* 37:51-59, Jan. 1980.
8. Klein and others, *op.cit.*, p. 500
9. Thoren, Peter, and others. Clomipramine treatment of obsessive-compulsive disorder. *Arch. Gen.Psychiatry* 37:1281-1285, Nov. 1980.
10. Klein and others, *op.cit.*, pp. 243, 440.
11. *Ibid.*, pp. 642-645.
12. Davis, J. L., and others. Peripheral diabetic neuropathy treated with amitriptyline and fluphenazine. *JAMA* 238:2291-2292, Nov. 1977.
13. Tofanetti, O., and others. Enhancement of propoxyphene-induced analgesia by doxepin. *Psychopharmacology* 51:213-215, Jan. 31, 1977.
14. Carasso, R. L., and others. Clomipramine and amitriptyline in the treatment of severe pain. *Int.J.Neurosci.* 9(3):191-194, 1979.
15. Couch, J. R., and Hassanein, R. S. Amitriptyline in migraine prophylaxis. *Arch.Neurol.* 36:695-699, Nov. 1979.
16. Shimm, D. S., and others. Medical management of chronic cancer pain. *JAMA* 241:2408-2412, June 1, 1979.

(Inderal) should be avoided in the treatment of hypertension in those patients also receiving an MAO inhibitor, due to the severe side effects that may be potentiated. A minimum of a two-week interval between the discontinuation of the MAO inhibitor and the initial use of Inderal should be observed.

In general, the less severe side effects of the MAO inhibitors resulting from the effects on the autonomic nervous system resemble those of the tricyclic antidepressants. Thus, the nursing interventions to assist the patient in adjusting to the MAO inhibitor are similar to those effective with the tricyclics.

References

1. Kontos, P. G., and Steinhilber, R. M. Using antidepressants effectively. *Postgrad.Med.* 64:55-56, Aug. 1979.
2. Beck, A. T. *Depression: Clinical, Experimental, and Therapeutical Aspects.* New York, Harper & Row Publishers, 1967, pp. 243-252.
3. Mansky, P. A. Treatment of depression. IN *Psychiatric Medicine Update*, ed. by T. C. Manschreck. New York, Elsevier Press, 1981, pp.47-64.
4. _____, and others. Diagnosis and treatment of depression. IN *Psychiatric Medicine Update*, ed. by T. C. Manschreck. New York, Elsevier Press, 1981, pp.11-29.
5. Neu, C., and Mansky, P. A. Diagnosis of depression. IN *Psychiatric Medicine Update*, ed. by T. C. Manshreck. New York, Elsevier Press, 1981, pp.31-46.
6. Spitzer, R. L., and others. *Research Diagnostic Criteria.* Washington, D.C., Program on the Psychobiology of Depression, Clinical Research Branch Collaborative, National Institute of Mental Health, 1977.
7. American Psychiatric Association. *Diagnostic and Statistical Manual of Mental Disorders.* 3d ed. Washington, D.C., The Association, 1980.
8. Axelrod, J. Biogenic amines and their impact in psychiatry. *Sem.Psychiatry* 4:100-210, 1972.
9. Amsterdam, J., and others. The clinical application of tricyclic antidepressant pharmacokinetics and plasma levels. *Am.J.Psychiatry* 137: 653-662, June 1980.
10. Hanson, L. C. Evidence that the central action of (+)-amphetamine is mediated via catecholamines. *Psychopharmacologia* (Berlin) 10:289-297, 1967.
11. Fawcett, J., and Maas, J. W. Depression and MHPG excretion. Response to dextroamphetamine and tricyclic antidepressants. *Arch.Gen.Psychiatry* 26:246-251, Mar. 1972.
12. Rutledge, C. O. The mechanism by which amphetamine inhibits oxidative deamination of norepinephrine in brain. *J.Pharmacol.Exp.Ther.* 171:188-195, Feb. 1970.
13. Maas, J. W. Biogenic amines and depression. Biochemical and pharmacological separation of two types of depression. *Arch.Gen.Psychiatry* 32: 1357-1361, Nov. 1975.
14. Hollister, L. E. Tricyclic antidepressants (first of two parts). *N.Engl.J.Med.* 229:1106-1109, Nov. 16, 1978.
15. Tricyclic antidepressants (second of two parts). *N.Engl.J.Med.* 229:1168-1172, Nov. 23, 1978.
16. Rosenbaum, A. H., and others. Series on pharmacology in practice: 1. Drugs that alter mood; Part 1. *Mayo Clin.Proc.* 54:335-344, May 1979.

Lithium

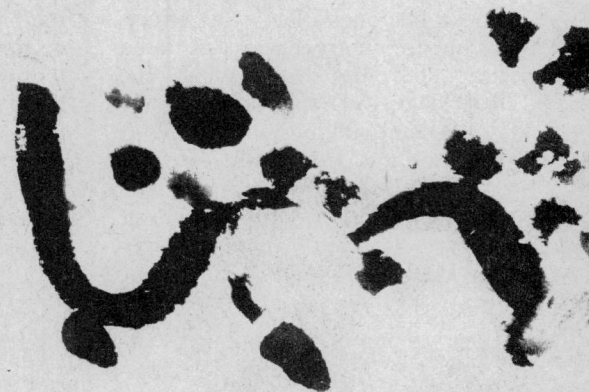

*Reprinted from
American Journal of Nursing,
July 1981*

By Elizabeth Harris

Lithium is the treatment of choice for the short-term management of the manic phase of bipolar disorder (DSM III terminology for what was formerly called manic-depressive illness), and for long-term prophylaxis for bipolar disorder. Lithium is approved by the FDA for only these two uses.

The drug is dramatically effective when it works, and does not produce the sedation or "chemical straitjacket" effect of the antipsychotics. In addition, it causes no known long-range harm as do the antipsychotics.

Lithium is the lightest known solid element. It exists in its natural form as a salt and is also manufactured for patient use as a salt. It is easily absorbed after oral adminis-

ELIZABETH HARRIS, R.N., M.A., is a head nurse at the Payne Whitney Psychiatric Clinic of the New York Hospital-Cornell Medical Center, New York, N.Y.

tration, reaching peak serum levels in one to three hours. The body does not metabolize lithium: it exists in the body as an ion and is distributed evenly throughout the total body water compartment. It is not bound to protein. Lithium is excreted by the kidneys, where it competes with sodium for reabsorption in the proximal tubules. The mechanism of therapeutic action is, as yet, unknown, but there are many theories currently under investigation.

In patients with bipolar disorder, lithium is 80 percent effective in treating the manic phase. When used prophylactically, it decreases the frequency or diminishes the intensity of the manic relapses. It is slightly less effective in preventing depressive relapses, so that often tricyclic or MAO inhibitor antidepressants must be added to the patient's regimen. Patients who have rapid cycling (four or more episodes per year) are less likely to respond favorably to lithium.

For patients who have recurrent episodes of depression without intervening episodes of mania or hypomania (unipolar depressed patients), the treatments of choice are antidepressants or ECT. But, from recent studies, statistics show that lithium may be equally effective. Depressed patients with the following characteristics are thought to be as likely to respond to lithium as to antidepressants or ECT:

- history of mild hypomania
- family history of bipolar disorder
- cyclothymic personality (a chronic mood disturbance with numerous periods of mild depression and hypomania)
- history of postpartal depression
- hypersomnia or hyperphagia
- early age of onset of illness with recurrent cyclical depressions that are not related to environmental events
- endogenous symptom patterns associated with one or more of the above.

Schizoaffective disorder is a nonspecific DSM III term for conditions with some features of schizophrenia and some features of affective illness. Patients with this diagnosis do less well with lithium than patients with a clear-cut bipolar disorder, but enough respond that these patients are often given a trial with lithium.

Studies with alcoholic patients have shown lithium to be useful in some who are primarily depressed and may drink to alleviate their depression. Lithium, however, has not been shown to be useful in alcoholic patients who are not primarily depressed.

Several investigators have reported that violent acting-out behavior decreases significantly when patients who exhibit these behavioral disorders receive lithium. These studies suggest that lithium maintenance may help certain nonpsychotic patients with the following characteristics:

- extreme, rapid reactions to slight provocation with anger or violence
- inability to reflect on actions before acting
- inability to control rage once it has erupted.

In 1972, Rifkin reported that patients with emotionally unstable character disorder respond to lithium maintenance. These are adolescent patients with chronic maladaptive behavior patterns, such as poor acceptance of reasonable authority, truancy, poor work history, and manipulativeness. The core problem seems to be brief mood swings from depression to hypomania that last hours to days. These mood swings are not usually related to environmental or interpersonal events, but seem to occur on their own schedule. In these patients, lithium is thought to stabilize mood and, therefore, decrease the need for maladaptive behavior in response to the mood swings.

Guidelines for Use

Because of its narrow therapeutic index, lithium is considered a potentially dangerous drug. The amount of drug that is therapeutic is only slightly less than the amount that produces toxicity. This is compounded by the fact that no two patients respond alike to lithium or absorb or excrete it at exactly the same rate. The dose requirement for one patient may be two times the lethal dose for another. The dosage is adjusted by measuring serum levels and by observing for clinical signs of toxicity. Before a patient receives lithium, he should have baseline studies of renal, thyroid, cardiac, and electrolyte status.

Lithium is available in the United States as tablets or capsules of 300 mg. of lithium carbonate (Lithane, Lithonate, Lithotabs, Eskalith). It is also available in liquid form as lithium citrate. In this form, 5 cc. equals 8 mEq., which is the equivalent of 300 mg. of lithium carbonate. This form is useful for patients who cannot swallow tablets or capsules. There is no parenteral form.

Because lithium is rapidly absorbed, with peak effects in one to three hours and a narrow therapeutic index, it must be given in at least two divided doses daily. There are some long-acting or slow-release forms available, but so far these have been shown to offer no advantage over the short-acting forms(1).

Patients are usually started on

900 to 1,200 mg. per day in divided doses. Geriatric patients receive lower doses. Dosages are raised slowly in increments of 300 mg. until symptoms remit or toxicity occurs. During this time, serum lithium levels are tested two or three times a week until the blood level is stable. Patients' symptoms usually respond at levels of 0.8 mEq./l. to 1.5 mEq./l. (toward the high end of the range in mania), though this is quite variable. Some patients have responded best at 0.4 mEq./l., while others do not respond until they are over 1.5 mEq./l.

Blood for serum levels is always drawn in the morning, 10 to 14 hours after the last dose of lithium, to standardize measurement. If blood is drawn at any other time, or if the patient mistakenly takes his morning dose before his blood is drawn, the level will be erroneous and must be reported as such.

Once a therapeutic serum level is attained, it takes 7 to 10 days for a clinical response. If the patient is unmanageable during this lag period, it is usual practice to treat the patient with an antipsychotic drug until the lithium begins to take effect. After the initial clinical response, it takes another week or two for the patient to return to his normal mood state. If the manic patient shows no clinical response to the lithium after three weeks with adequate blood levels, he is then considered to be refractory to lithium.

Once the patient's symptoms are in control and he has returned to a normal mood state, he may be continued on lithium maintenance. Patients with bipolar or unipolar disorder are usually not maintained unless they have had at least two major affective episodes. It is only patients with recurrent, disruptive, cyclical relapses who should be subjected to the cost, inconvenience, and risks of long-term chemotherapy. If the decision is made to maintain a patient, his serum level is usually dropped to somewhere between 0.7 and 1.0 mEq./l. (approximately 600 to 1,500 mg. of lithium carbonate), where his psychiatric symptoms are controlled, and few side effects are present.

Manic patients usually require a considerably lower dose once their mania is controlled. If the dose is not reduced as soon as the symptoms remit, the patient will often begin to show signs of toxicity, as his lithium level rises in response to his decreasing tolerance for it. Once the patient is on a stable maintenance dose, serum levels are tested less frequently, and finally tested every three months. Some patients maintained on lithium continue to have episodes of depression or, less often, of mania, but the episodes are less frequent and less intense. Only 20 percent of compliant patients show no change in severity over time. Patients who do respond will find that their response is better the longer they take lithium. Relapses become very infrequent or cease altogether.

There are no clear guidelines about how long to continue maintenance treatment, but some clinicians suggest that a patient who remains symptom free for three to five years should be given a trial off lithium.

Side Effects and Toxicity of Lithium

Mild below 1.5 mEq./l.	metallic taste in the mouth fine hand tremor (resting) nausea polyuria polydipsia diarrhea or loose stools muscular weakness or fatigue
Moderate 1.5-2.5 mEq./l.	severe diarrhea nausea and vomiting mild to moderate ataxia incoordination dizziness, sluggishness, giddiness, vertigo slurred speech tinnitus blurred vision increasing tremor muscle irritability or twitching asymmetrical deep tendon reflexes increased muscle tone
Toxicity 2.5-7.0 mEq./l.	nystagmus coarse tremor dysarthria fasciculations visual or tactile hallucinations oliguria, anuria confusion impaired consciousness dyskinesias—chorea, athetoid movements grand mal convulsions coma death

Side Effects and Toxicity

Most patients will experience side effects. They include a fine resting tremor of the hands; nausea or slight abdominal discomfort; polyuria; thirst; mild diarrhea; muscle weakness or fatigue; and edema of the feet, hands, abdominal wall, or face. These may begin as early as two hours after the first dose and usually occur as isolated symptoms. Most side effects occur at therapeutic serum levels, and most subside in the first few weeks of treatment; some will resolve only to recur periodically throughout the course of treatment.

All side effects are reversible and fairly innocuous, though they may be quite distressing to the patient. Most of these effects are best treated with the reassurance that they will probably stop after a few weeks. If the effects persist, they can be treated by decreasing the lithium dose, by omitting several doses, or by temporarily discontinuing the drug. If nausea is the main problem, it can usually be treated by giving the drug with meals. If the polyuria is severe, but less than three liters per day, it should be considered within normal limits. If the tremors persist, and the patient must have fine motor coordination for his work, he may respond to propranolol (Inderal), 20 to 120 mg./day in divided doses.

If the patient's side effects begin to occur in clusters or gradually progress, this may be a sign of developing toxicity. Fortunately, when toxicity occurs, it usually occurs in a progressive fashion, so that it can often be detected before it becomes harmful to the patient (see table, at left). Certainly, if the patient complains of one or more of these symptoms, it is wise to inquire about them and examine the patient for the full range of symptoms.

Toxicity can occur for many reasons. An increased intake of lithium by a medication error on the part of the patient or staff or by an intentional overdose will cause toxicity. Hemoconcentration, caused by fever, dehydration, excess sweating, diarrhea, or vomiting, can raise the lithium level to a toxic degree. Diminished excretion of lithium secondary to renal disease or a low-salt diet can also raise serum levels.

When toxicity is suspected, it is wise to rely on clinical judgment rather than serum levels. The most recent serum level may not reflect a more recent change in clinical status, and it may be impossible to get a stat sample that is accurate, that is, after a 10-to 14-hour lithium fast. If, upon questioning and examination, the patient shows signs of toxicity, withhold the lithium and inform the patient's physician. For mild or moderate toxicity, the lithium dose is usually lowered or held until the patient's symptoms remit and an accurate level can be drawn. Lithium has an average serum half-life of 24 hours; serum will gradually clear if no more lithium is given.

In more severe toxicity, the lithium is discontinued and the patient is given supportive care and monitored until the lithium is cleared from his body. Blood pressure and intake and output are monitored, and fluid and electrolytes are replaced as necessary. Stronger measures can include osmotic diuresis with mannitol or urea or diuresis with I.V. theophylline. If the lithium level exceeds 3.0 mEq./l., many clinicians suggest starting hemodialysis or, when unavailable, peritoneal dialysis.

Most patients recover gradually as their serum lithium level decreases. Those patients who have died had serum levels above 5 mEq./l.(2). Death is usually caused by complications of coma, such as pneumonia, or by shock or cardiac arrest. If the patient survives after reaching a serum level greater than 5.0 mEq./l., there may be such permanent aftereffects as dementia or cerebellar ataxia.

Long-Term Effects

Now that a number of patients have been receiving lithium maintenance for over 10 years, some long-term effects are being seen. These are, for the most part, innocuous and reversible.

The effect that has received the most attention is renal toxicity. There were some initial reports of structural kidney damage that raised quite a stir. The current thought is that data collected until now indicate that 10 to 15 years of continuous lithium treatment does not lead to marked progressive impairment of glomerular filtration rate with risk of terminal azotemia. In a certain proportion of patients, the treatment leads to impairment of renal concentrating ability, which may be fully reversible, partially reversible, and perhaps in some patients, irreversible(3). The latter problem, the progressive inability to concentrate urine due to a suppression of ADH, can progress in a minority of patients to a nephrogenic diabetes insipidus. A basic rule is that if a patient's 24-hour urine volume is more than three l./day, more specific tests of urine concentrating ability should be performed. If present, diabetes insipidus will sometimes respond to a thiazide diuretic.

Some elderly patients develop organic brain syndrome (OBS) without other signs of toxicity after several years of maintenance. If the OBS is attributable to the lithium, it will reverse when the lithium is discontinued. Some patients develop goiters or chemical hypothyroidism after several years. If the lithium is discontinued, the patient becomes euthyroid in approximately six weeks. If it is essential that the patient continue to receive lithium, the hypothyroidism can be treated with thyroxine (Synthroid). It is extremely rare for patients to develop clinical symptoms of hypothyroidism or myxedema.

Two other long-term side effects reported are weight gain and, less frequently, cogwheel rigidity. In order to evaluate these long-term side effects, periodic laboratory and physical examinations should be performed.

Drug Interactions

Lithium is often used in combination with other drugs. Some combinations have been found to be safe, while others are potentially harmful.

Antipsychotics. Lithium is most often used in combination with an antipsychotic for treatment of acute manic episodes. Lithium is clearly the treatment of choice for acute mania, but there is a lag period between initial administration of lithium and symptom reduction. During this time the patient may be acutely and floridly manic to the point of being dangerous to himself or others and unmanageable even in an inpatient psychiatric setting. In these circumstances, an antipsychotic will dampen the patient's behavior. Below the surface, the mania will continue until the lithium takes effect, but the patient's behavior will be more manageable. Antipsychotics most often used in this way are chlorpromazine (Thorazine) and haloperidol (Haldol). Often, very high doses are needed. Once the mania is under control with lithium, the antipsychotic can be tapered and discontinued. It is worth bearing in mind that the antiemetic properties of the antipsychotics will mask nausea and vomiting as signs of lithium toxicity. There are no other precautions with this drug combination.

Antidepressants. These are also commonly used in combination with lithium. Patients on lithium maintenance are more likely to have depressive relapses than manic relapses. Patients who do continue to suffer depressive relapses may be treated with a combination of lithium plus a tricyclic or MAO inhibitor antidepressant. Either class of antidepressant combines safely with lithium.

Diuretics. Any class of diuretics may decrease lithium excretion. If diuretics are administered, monitor lithium levels and clinical status more frequently.

Nephrotoxins. Lithium toxicity has been precipitated by the tetracyclines and by spectinomycin (Trobicin).

Antiinflamatory agents. Lithium retention and toxicity have been reported with indomethacin (Indocin) and phenylbutazone (Butazolidin).

Antihypertensives. When first started, these can cause a transient decrease in renal function that can lead to lithium retention.

Digoxin. Lithium can potentiate digoxin toxicity by decreasing intracellular potassium. The combination can cause severe nodal bradycardia and slow atrial fibrillation. The combination of lithium, digoxin, and a thiazide diuretic is especially dangerous.

Psychostimulants. Lithium can antagonize the highs of cocaine and amphetamines.

Alcohol. Alcohol intoxication with lithium can cause clouding of consciousness, ataxia, tremor, and incoordination. Lithium can be given safely in combination with disulfiram (Antabuse).

Analgesics. Lithium may potentiate the effects of morphine.

Muscle relaxants and anesthetics. Lithium can prolong neuromuscular blockade of succinylcholine (Anectine) and pancuronium (Pavulon). For patients having surgery, lithium should be discontinued 48 to 72 hours before surgery and restarted on the postoperative return of bowel sounds. Patients having ECT should be monitored closely postanesthetic. Because of reports of neurotoxicity in patients taking lithium and having ECT, these two treatments should probably not be combined(4).

Patient Teaching

All patients should have knowledge of their disease, the alternatives of treatment for their condition, and the risks and benefits of all the treatment alternatives. For patients receiving lithium, this includes teaching about lithium's risks and benefits.

Patients on maintenance will be required to see their health care provider for periodic physicals and lab exams. They will need to obtain and self-administer lithium at least twice daily for at least several years. They may have to tolerate some uncomfortable side effects, and not a day will go by that they will not be reminded that they have a chronic illness. Some patients whose hypomanic periods were pleasurable or even profitable in some business or personal way may miss their "up" periods. In many ways, patients on lithium maintenance have the same problems as other patients with chronic diseases. They have a great many adjustments to make.

The nurse can help these patients by discussing the chronic nature of their problem and the adjustments they must make to it. She can help by fully exploring the risk-benefit ratio so that the patient can better decide about his treatment. It is often helpful to introduce the patient to another patient on lithi-

Contraindications

	Absolute Contraindications
Renal failure / Renal tubular disease	Since Lithium (Li) is excreted via the kidneys, these conditions make treatment difficult or hazardous; these patients should be treated only in the hospital.
Acute MI	Li toxicity can cause arrhythmias and cardiac failure in patients with preexisting heart disease.
Myasthenia gravis	Symptoms are aggravated by Li. Li interferes with the release of acetylcholine and with depolarization and repolarization of motor endplates.
First trimester pregnancy	Studies have shown an increased incidence of cardiac defects in the fetus.
Breast-feeding	Human breast milk has 30-100% the Li serum concentration of the mother; it can cause Li toxicity or hypothyroidism in the infant.
Myeloid leukemia	Li causes reversible leukocytosis at therapeutic serum levels in most patients.
Children under 12 years	FDA recommendation.
	Relative Contraindications
Organic brain syndrome or dementia	Li can exacerbate preexisting OBS or dementia.
Seizure disorders	Li therapy can worsen preexisting complex partial seizures; it can be used in other forms of epilepsy with EEG and clinical monitoring.
Cardiac conduction defects	Even at therapeutic levels, Li can aggravate preexisting arrhythmias and conduction defects; these patients should be treated only in the hospital with ECG monitoring.

The Use of Lithium

Parkinson's disease	Li can aggravate preexisting Parkinson's disease.
2nd and 3rd trimester pregnancy	If it is necessary to treat pregnant patients, keep the dose as low as possible and divide doses throughout the day.
Delivery	Li renal clearance drops 50% after delivery; discontinue Li 2 weeks before delivery and resume 1/2 the former dose after delivery.
Controlled cardiac failure	Li can accumulate with fluid and increase the risk of toxicity.
Tardive dyskinesia	This syndrome is reported to be either improved or aggravated by Li.
Cerebellar disorders	These disorders can mask the symptoms of toxicity.
Diabetes mellitus	Li can increase or decrease glucose tolerance; watch for signs either way.
Ulcerative colitis; ileostomy	GI disease may be aggravated, since Li can cause diarrhea.
Psoriasis; acne	These skin conditions are frequently aggravated by use of Li.
Senile cataracts	Li may increase the speed of development of cataracts.
Electrolyte imbalance; dehydration	Li increases the risk of toxicity.
Acute neurological disorders	These disorders can mask the symptoms of toxicity.
Goiter or hypothyroidism	These conditions can be aggravated by the use of Li; when they occur during Li treatment, they respond to the use of thyroxine.
Low-salt diet	Li is more likely to reach toxic levels.
Suicidal or impulsive patients	Li overdose can be fatal.

um with whom he can share information and problems.

The patient and his family will need to be able to list the side effects and signs of toxicity and should know how to contact their health care provider in the event that toxicity develops. The patient and his family should be able to recognize the signs of recurrence of mania, including euphoria, decreased sleep, increased talkativeness, increased motor activity, grandiosity, and upsurge of sexual interest, distractability, spending sprees, or racing thoughts. These are signs of relapse and should be reported immediately. They should also recognize and report such symptoms of depression as anhedonia, psychomotor retardation, loss of appetite, crying, and hopelessness. It is especially important to teach the patient's family and/or friends, since the manic patient may lack the good judgment to report his symptoms, and a depressed patient may not have the energy.

Women of childbearing age should practice effective birth control. If the patient is considering having children, she and her mate should be advised about the risks to the fetus of her continuing lithium versus the risks to her and her family of discontinuing it.

The patient will need to know his schedule for follow-up. He will need a clear schedule for administering lithium. It may increase compliance to link the taking of doses with mealtimes and bedtime. Reinforce the need for divided doses. If a patient forgets one dose, tell him to skip it rather than double up on the next dose. Doubling up on a dose may cause a brief toxic reaction. Advise the patient to tell other health care providers that he is taking lithium and to keep the physician prescribing his lithium abreast of any other health problems. Advise him of the possible precipitants of toxic reactions: fever, weight-loss diets, profuse sweating, decreased fluid or salt intake, loss of appetite, vomiting, and diarrhea. Advise that he limit alcohol consumption to one drink per day. If your patient has polydipsia, advise against quenching his thirst with high-calorie drinks that might cause weight gain.

Most importantly, give your patient a realistic picture of what lithium can and cannot do. Some patients feel lithium will take away all their problems. It clearly will not do that. What it may do is take away the extreme mood states of depression and mania. To some patients this may make life seem dull and colorless, but it probably will also make it less disrupted by severe episodes of illness and hospitalization. Patients also may need encouragement not to despair if they continue to have minor relapses. In fact, there are only a small number of bipolar patients who remain without relapses from the beginning of treatment. Most have recurrences that stop in the first few months or year of treatment. These are considered good responders. Some have recurrences beyond the first year, but the episodes are shorter and less disruptive. And, some 20 percent, the lithium nonresponders, continue to suffer recurrences of undiminished severity.

References

1. Klein, D. F., and others. *Diagnosis and Drug Treatment of Psychiatric Disorders: Adults and Children.* 2d ed. Baltimore, Md., Williams & Wilkins Co., 1980, p. 426.
2. Shou, M. The recognition and management of lithium toxicity. In *Handbook of Lithium Therapy,* ed. by F. N. Johnson. Baltimore, Md., University Park Press, 1980, p. 399.
3. Vestergaard, Per. Renal side effects of lithium. In *Handbook of Lithium Therapy,* ed. by F. N. Johnson. Baltimore, Md., University Park Press, 1980, p. 354.
4. Tyrer, Stephen, and Shopsin, Baron. Neural and neuromuscular side effects of lithium. In *Handbook of Lithium Therapy,* ed. by F. N. Johnson. Baltimore, Md., University Park Press, 1980, p. 297.

Reprinted from American Journal of Nursing, July 1981

Antipsychotic Medications

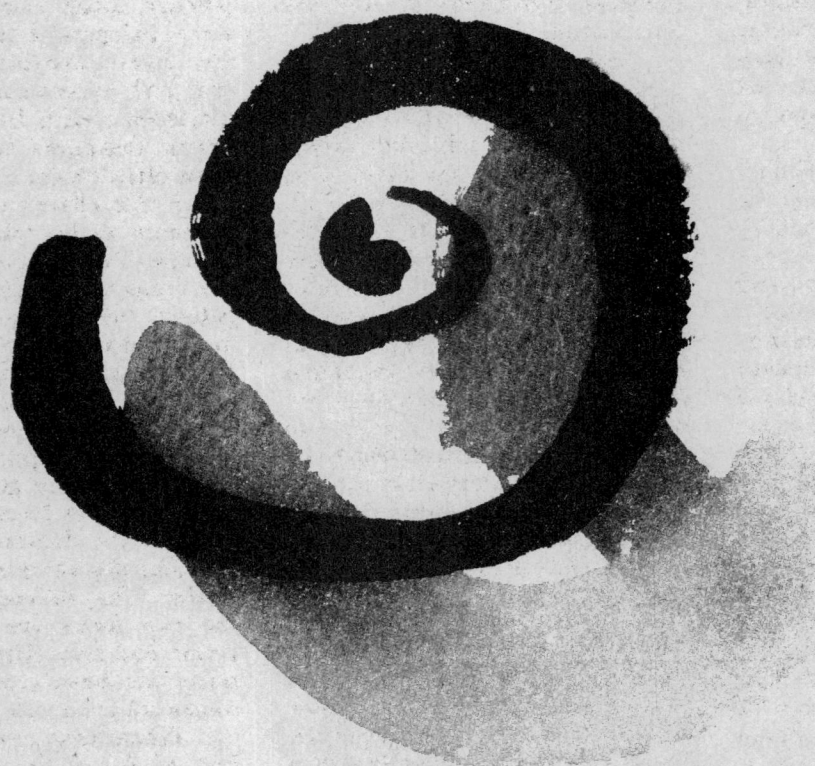

By Elizabeth Harris

Many people mistakenly believe that only patients with schizophrenia take antipsychotic medications (also called neuroleptics, or major tranquilizers). This, however, is not the case.

The antipsychotics are used in the treatment of psychotic conditions that may be caused by schizophrenia, mania, agitated psychotic depression, paranoid disorders, involutional or senile psychosis, a psychotic reaction to amphetamines, organic dementia, and acute brain syndromes(1). Antipsychotics are used to treat the acute psychotic symptoms of these conditions. They are also used prophylactically to prevent psychotic relapse in patients with schizophrenia.

There is also some confusion as to which symptoms these drugs alleviate and which symptoms they do not. The symptoms that respond to antipsychotics are agitation, rage, overreactivity to sensory stimuli, hallucinations, delusions, paranoia, combativeness, insomnia (when this is a symptom of the psychosis), hostility, negativism, and thought disorder. These drugs, however, do not correct poor judgment, poor insight, or social and interpersonal disabilities; they also cannot change an individual's personality(2).

The antipsychotics are also used in treating disorders other than psychosis. They have antiemetic properties and can be used specifically for this purpose(3). Antipsychotics have also been used to treat intractable hiccoughs(4). Haloperidol is used to treat Gilles de la Tourette syndrome(5). Finally, these drugs have been used in combination with other drugs for pain control(3-6).

There are six major classes of antipsychotics grouped according to their chemical structure. The phenothiazine class is further divided into three subclasses (see chart, page 1319). The phenothiazines, the first widely used antipsychotics, were first used in this country in the mid-

1950s. Chlorpromazine was the first phenothiazine and is the prototype of this class.

Another commonly used method of classifying these drugs divides the antipsychotics into two classes—high potency and low potency. The high-potency drugs, such as haloperidol and fluphenazine, are given in low milligram doses and exert a greater antipsychotic effect per milligram. The low-potency drugs, such as chlorpromazine and thioridazine, have higher milligram doses and exert a lesser antipsychotic effect per milligram. This classification scheme is used primarily to discuss side effects, since the low-potency drugs have side effects that differ from those of the high-potency drugs.

All antipsychotics are thought to exert their effect by blocking the dopamine receptors in the brain(7). This is the mechanism of action for both their antipsychotic action and also their neurological side effects. These drugs also have anticholinergic properties that are not thought to contribute to their antipsychotic effect, but which are responsible for some of their side effects.

General Properties

The antipsychotics are rapidly absorbed after oral or intramuscular administration. After oral administration, clinical effects are apparent in 30 to 60 minutes. Following IM administration, effects are seen in about 10 minutes. Antipsychotics are highly lipophilic, so that most of the drug that is absorbed is bound to proteins or membranes(8). The remaining free or unbound drug is available to the central nervous system and, thus, active.

Metabolism of the antipsychotics occurs largely through oxidation by the hepatic microsomal enzymes(9). The serum half-life is fairly short (about 24 hours), yet varying amounts of the drug will linger in the body for weeks or even months after a drug is discontinued.

The antipsychotics and their metabolites begin to accumulate in body tissues, particularly in fatty tissues, from the first dose. As the patient continues to receive these drugs, the tissues take on greater amounts until a saturation point is reached. When the drug is discontinued, the body tissues slowly release their accumulation back into the bloodstream where it can be metabolized and excreted. Therefore, patients who stop their medications after a course of treatment often stay protected from relapse for some time, as their body continues to free small amounts of the medication. For this same reason, patients may experience side effects for weeks after receiving their last dose. Traces of drugs or their metabolites have been found in urine two or three months after discontinuation of the drug(10).

Antipsychotics have a high therapeutic index; they can be given at very high doses with minimal risk. They are not addicting, do not produce euphoria, and there is no tolerance to their antipsychotic effects. However, patients show considerable accommodation to many of their side effects(11). The antipsychotic effect occurs anywhere from several hours to three weeks after the first dose. After the initial antipsychotic effects are seen, it can take anywhere from weeks to months for full improvement to be apparent(12). It is important to make patients aware of this lag period to prevent discouragement when there is no immediate favorable response.

Selection of a Drug

All six classes of antipsychotics have the same antipsychotic effect. None of the newer drugs have been found to be more effective than chlorpromazine(13).

The choice of a drug for a specific patient depends on several factors. If a patient or one of his relatives has responded favorably in the past to one particular drug, then the chances are greater that he will respond well to that same drug. In patients (or relatives) who have had a severe unfavorable reaction, that particular drug is best avoided. For a patient who is acutely disturbed and requires parenteral medication, the choice is limited to the drugs that have injectable forms. For a patient who will need high doses of medication, it would be best to avoid thioridazine, which is the only antipsychotic that has an absolute upper limit to the dose range (800 mg.). For some patients, cost of the drug may be a factor. Some newer drugs are several times more expensive than the older ones.

After all these considerations are taken into account, the choice of drug will depend largely on the different side effects of each drug. For example, the low-potency drugs, such as chlorpromazine and thioridazine, have a higher incidence of the side effects of hypotension and sedation but fewer extrapyramidal symptoms (EPS).

On the other hand, the high-potency drugs, such as fluphenazine, haloperidol, and trifluoperazine, have a low incidence of sedation and hypotension but a high incidence of EPS because they are potent dopamine blockers. Clinicians often choose a drug based on which side effect they believe will be more easily tolerated by the patient. Two long-acting, injectable drugs are available for use in patients who have a history of noncompliance with medication: fluphenazine enanthate and fluphenazine decanoate. Both are long-acting depot injections with a slow, even absorption. The enanthate form can be given in dosages of 12.5 mg. to 50 mg. every 3 to 14 days. The decanoate is given in the same dosages every two to four weeks. The differences between the two forms are in length of action and side effects. The decanoate has been reported to have somewhat fewer side effects(14).

When these medications were first developed, they were thought to provide the answer to the problem of noncompliance and subsequent relapse. Obviously, it seems to be easier to ensure patient compliance when a professional administers the drug by injection every two weeks or so than when the patient is relied on to take oral doses once a day or more often without supervision.

Unfortunately, the early promise of these drugs to greatly reduce relapse in schizophrenia has not proven itself. The use of these drugs has been somewhat limited by the incidence of EPS. Like other piperazine phenothiazines, depot fluphenazines often induce EPS. In addition, there have been disappointing findings regarding their ability to prevent relapse. Results of the recent National Institute of Mental Health Collaborative Fluphenazine Study show that depot fluphenazine markedly improves compliance by 20 to 50 percent over the use of oral fluphenazine. But, despite this increased compliance, the relapse rate after 12 months is equal to that of the oral drugs. This raises doubt about any real advantage of these drugs (15). Nonetheless, these drugs are an important part of the armamentarium and preferred by some patients who do not want the responsibility for taking oral medications on a daily basis.

There is considerable evidence against using more than one antipsychotic at a time. This is reasonable, considering that each has equal antipsychotic effect, and all have the same mechanism of action. Another reason to avoid using more than one antipsychotic is that if the patient responds, it will be unclear to which drug he responded. Likewise, if he has severe side effects, it would be impossible to know which drug caused them.

Contraindications

Antipsychotic drugs should never be used in treating patients who have severe CNS depression or who are in coma as a result of alcohol or barbiturate use or from excessive use of narcotics. These patients are at risk for a synergistic effect that can lead to respiratory paralysis or circulatory collapse. Patients in coma or with severe CNS depression from brain damage or trauma are also at risk for respiratory paralysis.

There are a number of relative contraindications to the use of antipsychotics. Patients who have a known sensitivity or severe allergic response to one of these drugs are at risk for another allergic response if treated with the same drug. If these patients are given a drug from another class of antipsychotic, they should be carefully observed for a sensitivity reaction(16). Patients who have Parkinson's disease may have a recrudescence of symptoms when treated with these drugs due to increased dopamine blockade. This may occur whether or not the patient is being treated pharmacologically for the Parkinson's disease(17).

Patients with a history of a blood dyscrasia are more likely to develop a dyscrasia as a side effect to these drugs than will someone with no such history. Those with a history of liver damage or dysfunction may be more at risk to develop obstructive jaundice when treated with antipsychotics, and those with severe liver damage may not be able to detoxify and inactivate these drugs adequately(18). The anticholinergic properties of the drugs may result in increased intraocular pressure in patients with acute narrow angle glaucoma. Patients with chronic wide angle glaucoma can usually be safely treated with these drugs if the glaucoma is treated with cholinergic eyedrops throughout the course of treatment with antipsychotics(19). Men who have prostatic hypertrophy are more at risk for urinary hesitancy or retention when they are treated with these drugs because of their anticholinergic properties.

Pregnant women should be treated with these drugs only when necessary, especially during the first trimester of pregnancy. Antipsychotics have not conclusively been shown to be teratogenic, but they do pass the blood-placenta barrier and can cause extrapyramidal symptoms or a postnatal depression syndrome, followed by agitation, in newborns delivered from mothers treated with antipsychotics. Antipsychotics are also secreted in human milk in small quantities, and should probably be avoided by nursing mothers.

When a pregnant woman is in need of these drugs, it is necessary to weigh the risks to mother and child of allowing the psychotic symptoms to continue untreated, versus the risks of possible, but unproven, risks to the fetus. In some cases it is a greater risk to allow psychotic symptoms to go untreated(20).

Guidelines for Use

There is wide variation in the way antipsychotics are instituted, the doses used, and the length of the course of treatment. All these factors depend on the patient's age, size, and weight and his history, symptoms, and behavior.

The dosage ranges are wide because of the high therapeutic index. In general, there does seem to be a low limit of effectiveness, below which there is no appreciable antipsychotic effect. This level is 300 mg. of chlorpromazine or its equivalent for any other drug(21). Above this minimum level, there is tremendous variability in the effective dose. Several studies have shown that most patients do as well at doses of less than 1,500 mg. of chlorpromazine or its equivalent than they do at a higher dose(22). However, some patients who do not respond at lower doses do respond at very high doses. Studies report the use of up to 7,000 mg. of chlorpromazine, 1,500 mg. fluphenazine, 1,000 mg. haloperidol, or 600 mg. trifluoperazine(23). At these doses, there are few reports of side effects that are any more intense than those reported at lower doses. Since few patients seem to need such high doses, most patients receive daily doses of somewhere between 300 and 1,600 mg. of chlorpromazine or its equivalent. In the last several years, serum level assays of antipsychotics have become available, but they are of little value in judging when a dose is adequate, since serum levels have not been correlated with antipsychotic effect.

Antipsychotics are usually prescribed as follows: The patient is first given a small test dose to rule out severe hypotension, sedation, or severe allergic response. This test dose is usually about 50 mg. of chlorpromazine or its equivalent. If the patient has no untoward reaction, he is usually started on a schedule of small, daily, divided doses in the range of 600 to 1,200 mg. of chlorpromazine or its equivalent. In patients who are over 40 years of age or who are less acutely ill, the dosage range is 300 to 600 mg. of chlorpromazine or its equivalent. Doses are gradually increased until a dose is reached at which the side effects are unacceptable, or at which clinical improvement occurs(24). At this point, the dose is reduced carefully to the highest

The Antipsychotics			
Generic name	Trade name	Approximate potency relative to chlorpromazine	IM Form
Phenothiazines			
Aliphatics			
chlorpromazine	Thorazine	100 mg.	yes
triflupromazine	Vesprin	25-50 mg.	yes
Piperidines			
thioridazine	Mellaril	100 mg.	no
mesoridazine	Serentil	25-50 mg.	yes
piperacetazine	Quide	10-15 mg.	no
Piperazines			
trifluoperazine	Stelazine	5 mg.	yes
acetophenazine	Tindal	20 mg.	no
fluphenazine	Prolixin	1-4 mg.	yes
fluphenazine enanthate	Prolixin Enanthate	no reliable correlation	yes
fluphenazine decanoate	Prolixin Decanoate	no reliable correlation	yes
perphenazine	Trilafon	8-12 mg.	yes
prochlorperazine	Compazine	15-50 mg.	yes
butaperazine	Repoise	10-15 mg.	no
carphenazine	Proketazine	25-50 mg.	no
Thioxanthenes			
chlorprothixene	Taractan	50-100 mg.	yes
thiothixene	Navane	2-10 mg.	yes
Butyrophenones			
haloperidol	Haldol	1.6-2 mg.	yes
Dihydroindolones			
molindone	Lidone Moban	10-15 mg.	no
Dibenzoxapines			
loxapine	Loxitane Daxolin	10-20 mg.	no
Diphenylbutyl piperidines			
penfluridol pimozide	both are experimental		

dose at which there is clinical improvement of symptoms with minimal side effects.

After 5 or 10 days, when the patient's symptoms are in control and tolerance has developed to the acute side effects, the patient can have his dosage schedule rearranged so he gets the same total dose but divided into one or two doses instead of three or four(25). Patients tend to prefer one dose at bedtime, as it is easier to carry out a simple regimen that does not call for carrying medication during the day. If there are side effects, they will be more likely to occur at night when the patient is asleep. It is also less expensive to buy fewer tablets or capsules of larger doses than to buy more of the smaller dose tablets or capsules.

The patient continues on his dose for a full drug trial of three to six weeks(26). If at that time there has been no improvement, one must question if the patient is actually taking his medicine. Often, lack of response is a result of noncompliance. If the patient continues to be symptomatic and you are fairly certain he is taking his medication, he may require a drug from a different class or subclass.

Even after a full trial of a second drug, there will be some patients who do not respond. There are several alternatives. They can be given a trial of a third antipsychotic, or these patients can be given intramuscular medications with the hope that their nonresponse is due to inadequate absorption in the gut. Occasionally, a nonresponder to oral medications will respond to an IM dose(27). Another alternative for the nonresponder (this comprises 10 to 20 percent of patients with schizophrenia) is electroconvulsive treatment (ECT)(28).

Once the acute phase of the illness is past (usually in 4 to 12 weeks), the dose can be very slowly lowered to a maintenance dose that is often one-half to one-fifth the highest dose used to control the psychotic symptoms(29).

How long a patient remains on maintenance medication will depend on the likelihood that he will have a recurrence of symptoms. A patient having a first psychotic episode, unless it was so severe that it was life threatening, will not require long-term maintenance. Even after a second psychotic episode, there is no need for maintenance medication if the episodes are mild or separated in time by several years. Long-term maintenance is used for patients who have a history of recurring psychotic episodes (usually patients with schizophrenia) where there is a high probability of future relapse. Patients who are continued on long-term maintenance run a risk of developing tardive dyskinesia (see the next article).

Whenever antipsychotics are discontinued, they should be gradually tapered. If chlorpromazine or thioridazine is abruptly withdrawn, the patient may experience such symptoms as nausea, vomiting, and diarrhea within 48 hours of withdrawal. With abrupt discontinuation of high doses of high-potency drugs, there may be withdrawal dyskinesias that should diminish over time(30,31).

Rapid Neuroleptization

There are times when the usual method of treating patients with these drugs is inadequate. When a patient is acutely psychotic and in severe psychic pain, or when he is combative or assaultive or in imminent danger of harming himself or others, rapid neuroleptization may be required.

Before proceeding to medicate such an acutely disturbed patient, it is important to perform a brief physical exam first. This may be difficult because of the patient's inability to cooperate. However, it is imperative to at least check the patient's neurological and cardiovascular status to rule out intracranial tumor, hypertension, hypotension, head injury, or toxic delirium. A brief history, particularly for drug use in the preceding week, is important.

Once the patient has been examined and the above conditions ruled out, antipsychotics are begun orally or intramuscularly. (See table above). The patient is given an initial dose. Then, depending on his response, the same dose is repeated every 30 to 60 minutes until the patient is sedated or falls asleep or until the acute psychotic symptoms (severe anxiety, hallucinations, delusions, suspiciousness, aggressiveness, grandiosity) abate. Before each dose, the patient should have his blood pressure and pulse taken, lying down and standing, to test for orthostatic hypotension, and a brief mental status examination should be performed.

High-potency drugs may reduce the risk of sedation, hypotension, and cardiovascular side effects. However, in practice, some clinicians prefer chlorpromazine because of its sedating properties(32,33).

Most patients will respond favorably to such a regimen after 2 to 10 consecutive doses. When a response occurs, the patient can be changed to a daily oral dose equal to one to one and one-half times the effective IM dose required in the first 24 hours.

As a general rule, geriatric patients have diminished absorption, distribution, metabolism, and excretion of all drugs. Antipsychotics are no exception. Because the elderly are more sensitive to the anticholinergic effects of the antipsychotics, these patients are more likely to experience side effects at a lower dose and can more quickly develop toxic reactions with symptoms of confusion, disorientation, lethargy, restlessness, delirium, or agitation. Elderly patients may experience severe orthostatic hypotension that can result in falls and trauma. They are also more prone to the sedative effects of chlorpromazine and thioridazine, which have the greatest anticholinergic activity. Elderly men with prostate enlargement are more likely to develop urinary hesitancy or retention, and older patients of both sexes are more prone to constipation and bowel obstruction as side effects.

Because they are the least anticholinergic and, thus, have a lesser incidence of sedation and hypotension, such high-potency drugs as haloperidol are recommended for elderly patients(34). Doses of antipsychotics for the elderly are often one-third to one-half those of younger adults, but usually not below the minimum effective dose of 300 mg. of chlorpromazine or its equivalent(35). Doses are raised slowly with careful monitoring of side effects.

Antipsychotic medications are used in children for the same indications as in adults. Smaller doses are often used because of the smaller body size. Doses are 20 to 50 percent of adult doses(36).

Side Effects

Although some side effects are fairly common with these drugs, they are usually not severe or dangerous. They are, however, uncomfortable and sometimes frightening to many patients. When they are recognized and dealt with appropriately, the patient can have a significantly more comfortable course of treatment.

Many of the side effects will diminish after several days or weeks of therapy. Many side effects, however, can be treated by a reduction in dose, and all side effects are reversible, with the exception of some cases of tardive dyskinesia (see the article beginning on page 1324).

Some drugs have a greater in-

Drugs Used for Rapid Neuroleptization

Drug	Dose range for single dose IM
loxapine	5-10 mg.
perphenazine	4-30 mg.
trifluoperazine	1-10 mg.
fluphenazine	1-25 mg.
haloperidol	1-10 mg.
thiothixene	4-30 mg.
chlorpromazine	25-100 mg.

Drug Interactions with the Antipsychotics

Agent	Effect
Alcohol and/or barbiturates	Speeds the action of liver microsomal enzymes so antipsychotic is metabolized more quickly; potentiates CNS depressant effect
Tricyclic antidepressants	Can lead to severe anticholinergic side effects; antipsychotics can raise the plasma level of the antidepressant, probably by inhibiting metabolism of the antidepressant
Hydrochlorthiazide and hydralazine	Can produce severe hypotension
Guanethidine	Antihypertensive effect is blocked by chlorpromazine, haloperidol, and thiothixene
Cigarettes	Heavy consumption requires larger doses of antipsychotic
Meperidine	Respiratory depression is enhanced by chlorpromazine
Anticonvulsants	Seizure threshold may be lowered by antipsychotic requiring adjustment of anticonvulsant
Levodopa	Antiparkinsonian effect may be inhibited by antipsychotics
General anesthesia	Antipsychotic may potentiate effect of anesthetic

cidence of certain specific side effects. In general, it is true that any side effect can occur with any of these drugs. No two patients will have exactly the same side effects with the same drug, and often a patient who experiences a particular side effect on one drug will not experience the same symptoms with another drug.

Sedation. This effect is most common with chlorpromazine, but it can occur with the other drugs. Accommodation to this side effect usually occurs a week or two after the dose has been stabilized. If the sedation is severe, a reduction in the dose should alleviate the symptom. If sedation is mild, it can be treated by encouraging the patient to get up in the morning and get moving in an effort to fight the sedation. Reassure the patient that the symptom will pass with time. For patients with sleep disturbance, sedation will afford the patient a good night's sleep.

Orthostatic hypotension. This effect results from alpha-adrenergic blockade and is more common with low-potency antipsychotics, though it can occur with high-potency drugs as well. Orthostatic hypotension usually occurs early in the course of treatment and usually disappears one or two weeks after the dose is stabilized. The patient experiences this side effect as dizziness or light-headedness, especially in the morning when getting out of bed. The patient often reports accompanying tachycardia or palpitations as his heart rate increases to compensate for the hypotension. To validate these symptoms, the patient's blood pressure and pulse should be taken lying and standing. A fall in systolic blood pressure of 30 mm. Hg or greater is significant.

When this side effect is mild, reassure the patient that the symptom will pass in a week or two. Advise him to get out of bed slowly in the morning, sitting at the side of the bed for a full minute before standing. Likewise, throughout the day, he should rise from sitting positions slowly. Surgical elastic stockings can help in mild cases to prevent venous pooling. When more severe, especially in elderly patients, orthostatic hypotension can result in falls that can lead to fractures or other injuries. If severe, it can be treated by reducing the dosage or by changing to a high-potency drug with a lower incidence of this side effect. Occasionally, the orthostatic drop can be so severe that it can cause fatal cardiac arrest(37).

Alterations in sexual functioning. All antipsychotics can diminish sex drive. This can be beneficial for patients who are hypersexual. For others, this side effect can be distressing. When a patient reports this as a problem, bear in mind that a reduced sex drive can have any number of causes other than medication. It may result from the patient's illness or from current conflicts with the sexual partner(s).

Thioridazine has caused ejaculatory difficulty in males. Patients with this side effect can achieve erection, but they are either unable to ejaculate or they have retrograde ejaculations(38).

Depression of hypothalamic functions. This can lead to a variety of symptoms. Appetite can be increased, leading to weight gain. This is fairly common, particularly for patients taking chlorpromazine, and it is best treated with diet and exercise. Molindone, however, is purported to prevent weight gain and even cause weight loss in obese patients(39).

Occasionally, women will become amenorrheic. When this occurs, bear in mind that the cause of the amenorrhea may be pregnancy or simply the stresses concomitant with the patient's illness. Occasionally, women may also develop galactorrhea. When mild, patients will often tolerate this side effect and wear small breast pads in their bra. When severe, it is best treated by reducing the dose of drug or changing to another drug. Women can have false-positive pregnancy tests while taking antipsychotics.

Male patients can develop gynecomastia. This is usually intolerable to the patient and calls for a change in the drug.

Seizures. All the antipsychotic medications lower the seizure threshold. Patients with a preexisting seizure disorder may need an increase in prophylactic antiepileptic medication. Patients with no history of seizure disorder may have grand mal seizures if given high doses of antipsychotics or if given rapidly increasing doses. This, however, is a rare occurrence. Such patients are not protected from further seizures by the addition of an antiepileptic drug and are best treated by reducing the dose of the antipsychotic(40).

Decreased tolerance to alcohol. Warn patients who plan to drink alcoholic beverages to take a smaller amount than usual and observe their response before proceeding. They may feel intoxicated by a much smaller amount of alcohol than they are accustomed to.

Anticholinergic side effects. These symptoms include nasal congestion, dry mouth, blurred near vision, constipation, and urinary hesitancy or retention. Chlorpromazine and thioridazine are the most anticholinergic of these drugs, and haloperidol and the piperazine phenothiazines are the least(41). Nasal congestion can be relieved temporarily by nasal decongestants but probably is best tolerated until the body adjusts. Dry mouth is best relieved by frequent rinsing or sucking on hard candies or chewing gum. Sugarless gum and candies are preferred, since the sugar in regular candies can foster monilial infections.

Blurred near vision usually abates in a week or two after the dose of medication is adjusted. Patients should be discouraged from getting new glasses unless the blurring continues for more than two weeks after the dose is stabilized.

Constipation, when mild, can be treated by encouraging the patient to increase his intake of bran, fluids, and fresh fruits and vegetables. A mild laxative will also help. When severe, constipation has been known to cause intestinal obstruction.

Urinary hesitancy can lead to urinary retention. This can be treated acutely with catheterization and with the addition of a cholinergic medication such as bethanechol(42). A reduction in antipsychotic dose will also help, or the offending medication can be discontinued and replaced with one that is less anticholinergic.

When antipsychotics are used in combination with other drugs that have anticholinergic properties, such as antiparkinsonian drugs or tricyclic antidepressants, the risk of severe anticholinergic side effects is increased. Some patients, commonly the elderly or those taking several drugs with anticholinergic properties, can develop a psychotic picture with the following symptoms: purposeless overactivity; agitation; confusion; disorientation; dry, flushed skin; tachycardia; sluggish, dilated pupils; bowel hypomotility; dysarthria; and memory impairment. The treatment of this syndrome, often called "atropine psychosis," is discontinuation of the medication(s). IM or I.V. physostigmine may be used in severe cases (43).

Allergic symptoms. The most common allergic response is a pruritic maculopapular rash. It usually appears on the face, neck, and chest about 2 to 10 weeks after the drug is first administered(44). This side effect is most common with chlorpromazine. If the rash is mild, it needs no treatment and will often clear on its own. If it is severe, the medication can be discontinued until the rash clears. A second trial on the same drug may not cause another rash(45). If the patient is acutely disturbed and cannot do without medication, a different drug can be started immediately. Those administering these drugs can develop contact dermatitis from contact with the liquid concentrate or tablets.

Phototoxicity. This is most common with chlorpromazine and rare with high-potency drugs(46). It consists of an extreme sensitivity of the skin to sunlight, such that brief exposure can cause sunburn. Patients should be advised to test for this reaction with a brief exposure to the sun. If they are sensitive, they can wear protective clothing or use a sunscreening lotion containing para-amino benzoic acid.

Cholestatic jaundice. This is a rare side effect of the phenothiazines(47). Early symptoms include malaise, fever, nausea, and abdominal pain. In another week after these symptoms appear, the patient develops itching and jaundice. This side effect is reversible and is usually benign and self-limiting. It is treated by discontinuing the drug, bed rest, and a high-protein, high-carbohydrate diet. It is most common with chlorpromazine and usually occurs in the first month of treatment. If a patient is acutely psychotic, he can be immediately started on a different antipsychotic(48).

Agranulocytosis. This is another rare side effect that occurs in the first eight weeks of treatment. It is most common in older women and most often occurs with low-potency phenothiazines and thioxanthenes(49). It develops abruptly with sore throat, fever, malaise, and sores in the mouth. If these symptoms develop in a patient started on antipsychotics in the past two months, a complete blood count should be drawn immediately, as leukopenia confirms the diagnosis. This should be considered to be an extreme emergency, and is treated by stopping the drug and initiating reverse isolation. If the initial phase of the illness is not fatal, the leukocyte count will return to normal in 7 to 10 days, with rapid recovery. Other blood dyscrasias reported include eosinophilia, thrombocytopenia, anemia, aplastic anemia, and pancytopenia.

Pigmentation of the skin and eyes. This can occur with long-term treatment with low-potency phenothiazines or with thioxanthenes (50). Pigmentation begins as a golden brown coloration, which can progress to slate gray, metallic blue, or purple. It occurs in skin surfaces often exposed to sunlight and is caused by deposition of pigment granules similar to melanin. Pigment can also be deposited in the conjunctiva, sclera, lens, and cornea. These eye changes are usually of no functional significance and do not impair vision(51). The pigment is reabsorbed after the drugs are discontinued.

Pigmentary retinopathy. This has been reported in patients taking thioridazine in doses higher than 800 mg. a day(51). It can cause blindness. Thus, thioridazine is never prescribed in amounts greater than 800 mg. per day.

Hypothalamic crisis. This is a rare but serious side effect(52). Some patients have only one symptom—hyperpyrexia. Other patients have additional symptoms of diaphoresis, drooling, tachycardia, dyspnea, seizures, and unstable blood pressure. This side effect is treated by stopping the drug and treating the individual symptoms.

Hyperglycemia. Occasionally, the side effect of hyperglycemia will unmask a previously undiagnosed case of mild diabetes mellitus. Patients previously diagnosed as having diabetes may need some alteration in insulin dose or diet to compensate(53).

Cardiac changes. These are usually mild and result from the anticholinergic action of the antipsychotics. They consist of mild ECG changes that are due to altered repolarization rather than to myocardial damage(54). In patients with preexisting cardiovascular disease, an ECG should be done before starting antipsychotic medications, and a cardiology consult should be obtained. The best drugs for patients with cardiac disease are those with low anticholinergic effects, such as haloperidol and the piperazine phenothiazines(55).

Gastrointestinal distress. Although many antipsychotics have antiemetic properties, heartburn or nausea can occur. Patients who have gastrointestinal distress usually respond to taking their medications at mealtimes or with a glass of milk.

This comprehensive list of side effects may seem overwhelming; however, in practice, side effects are usually mild. Even so, they can be annoying to the patient and should be recognized and treated. We should encourage patients to continue their medications despite the discomforts of the mild side effects until the maximum therapeutic effect is obtained. Only at that point can the patient decide whether the favorable effects of the drug outweigh whatever discomforts it brings.

Patients and their families often have a variety of misconceptions and fears about antipsychotic drugs. Many believe that these drugs are addictive. This is clearly not true, and the belief should be immediately dispelled. Many people argue against taking their drugs because they feel they are unnatural. The truth is that they are no more unnatural than the psychosis they are designed to treat. What these drugs do, when they are effective, is to return a very disturbed person to his more "natural" or usual state of mind.

Another common misconception is that patients who take high doses are "crazier" than patients who take low doses. Nurses often overhear patients comparing their dosage levels. Explain to patients with this fear that the dose depends on a number of individual factors, such as age, weight, and metabolism, and there is no relationship between number of milligrams and severity of illness.

When patients are started on these drugs, it is important that they be told what the drug will do and what it will not do. For example, a socially isolated, unemployed woman with auditory hallucinations and disorganized thinking can be told that the drug will help stop the hallucinations and help clear up her thinking but will not get her a job and find her friends. It is important that patients have a realistic notion of what to expect. Many hold the mistaken belief that antipsychotics will solve all their problems. In fact, they will only treat the psychosis and thereby free the patient to work on his other problems.

When patients are started on these medications, they should also be given a clear idea of what their course of treatment will be—low doses at first, then gradually increasing doses until the drug takes effect. The patient should be informed that it often takes several days, weeks, or even months to see a complete response. He should be informed of the most common early side effects, such as dystonias, parkinsonism, and sedation and be asked to inform the staff of any unusual symptoms. Patients who will be on maintenance for some months should be told about the risk of tardive dyskinesia and should be taught the early symptoms and the importance of early detection.

Patients leaving the hospital and all outpatients, as well as their families, should know the name of the drug being taken and the exact dose, the number of tablets or capsules, and the exact dose schedule. They should be taught that failure to continue medications when they are prescribed for long-term maintenance has been proven to increase greatly the risk of relapse. And, patients and their families should be taught to recognize the symptoms of relapse and told to report to their health care provider immediately if these symptoms appear.

The symptoms of relapse are somewhat different in different patients, but can include difficulty concentrating, loss of appetite, trouble sleeping, restlessness, preoccupation with one or two thoughts, social withdrawal, paranoia, hallucinations, religious preoccupation, delusions, and many other symptoms. The patient and his family can usually tell you about the particular symptoms of relapse by thinking back to the time just before treatment began.

Outpatients should be told what to do if they forget or skip a dose. If the patient is taking divided doses, he should add the missed dose to the next dose. If he takes only one dose per day, he should skip the missed dose. Patients should be told that they may feel, at times, like stopping or changing the schedule for their medications but that they should check with their health care provider first. They should be warned of a possible decrease in tolerance to alcohol. If they are on a sedating drug, they should be warned about the danger of operating cars or dangerous machinery before their body has had time to adjust to the sedating properties.

When antipsychotic medications are used properly and patients are monitored carefully for side effects, the treatment of acute and painful psychotic episodes can be humane and expeditious.

References

1. Baldessarini, R.J. Chemotherapy in Psychiatry. Cambridge, Mass., Harvard University Press, 1977, p. 31.
2. Ibid., p. 32.
3. Bergersen, B. S. Pharmacology in Nursing. St. Louis, C. V. Mosby Co., 1976, p. 677.
4. Appleton, W. S., and Davis, J. M. Practical Clinical Psychopharmacology. 2d ed. Baltimore, Md., Williams & Wilkins, 1980, p. 60.
5. Gilman, A.G., and others, eds. Goodman and Gilman's The Pharmacological Basis of Therapeutics. 6th ed. New York, Macmillan Publishing Co., 1980, p. 418.
6. Irons, P. D. Psychotropic Drugs and Nursing Intervention. New York, McGraw-Hill Book Co., 1978, p. 15.
7. Snyder, S. H. The dopamine hypothesis of schizophrenia: focus on the dopamine receptor. Am.J.Psychiatry 122:197-202, Feb. 1976.
8. Gilman, A. G., and others, eds. Goodman and Gilman's The Pharmacological Basis of Therapeutics. 6th ed. New York, Macmillan Publishing Co., 1980, p. 404.
9. Ibid., p. 405.
10. Baldessarini, op.cit., p. 23.
11. Ibid., p. 24.
12. Appleton and Davis, op.cit., p. 30.
13. Baldessarini, op.cit., p. 60.
14. Klein, Donald F., and others. Diagnosis and Drug Treatment of Psychiatric Disorders: Adults and Children. 2d ed. Baltimore, Md., Williams & Wilkins Co., 1980, p. 101.
15. Schooler, N. R., and others. Depot fluphenazine in the prevention of relapse in schizophrenia. Psychopharmacol.Bull. 15:44-47, Apr. 1979.
16. Klein and others, op.cit., p. 47.
17. Gilman and others, op.cit., p. 481.
18. Ibid., p. 404.
19. Baldessarini, op.cit., p. 50.
20. Lipton, M. A. and others, eds. Psychopharmacology: A Generation of Progress, New York, Raven Press, 1978, p. 1047.
21. Baldessarini, op.cit., p. 28.
22. Appleton and Davis, op.cit., p. 32.
23. Aubree, J. C., and Loder, M. H. High and very high dosage antipsychotics: a critical review. J.Clin.Psychiatry 41:341-350, Oct. 1980.
24. Shader, R. I., and Jackson, A. H. Approaches to schizophrenia. In Manual of Psychiatric Therapeutics, ed. by R. I. Shader. Boston, Little, Brown & Co., 1975, p. 87.
25. Ibid., p. 88.
26. Gilman and others, op.cit., p. 415.
27. Klein and others, op.cit., p. 109.
28. Salzman, Carl. Electroconvulsive therapy. In Manual of Psychiatric Therapeutics, ed. by R. I. Shader. Boston, Little, Brown & Co., 1975, p. 116.
29. Appleton and Davis, op.cit., p. 39.
30. Appleton and Davis, op.cit., p. 61.
31. Baldessarini, op.cit., p. 45.
32. Appleton and Davis, op.cit., p. 29.
33. Klein and others, op.cit., p. 92.
34. Appleton and Davis, op.cit., p. 56.
35. Salzman, Carl, and others. Psychopharmacology and the geriatric patient. In Manual of Psychiatric Therapeutics, ed. by R. I. Shader. Boston, Little, Brown & Co., 1975, p. 173.
36. Baldessarini, op.cit., p. 40.
37. Shader and Jackson, op.cit., p. 91.
38. Appleton and Davis, op.cit., p. 66.
39. Gardos, G., and Cole, J. O. Weight reduction in schizophrenics by molindone. Am.J.Psychiatry 134:302-304, Mar. 1977.
40. Klein and others, op.cit., p. 198.
41. Baldessarini, op.cit., p. 103.
42. Appleton and Davis, op.cit., p. 74.
43. Baldessarini, op.cit., p. 49.
44. Appleton and Davis, op.cit., p. 67.
45. Gilman and others, op.cit., p. 413.
46. Klein and others, op.cit., p. 192.
47. Ibid., p. 195.
48. Ibid., p. 196.
49. Baldessarini, op.cit., p. 53.
50. Ibid., p. 50.
51. Klein and others, op.cit., p. 193.
52. Baldessarini, op.cit., pp. 48-49.
53. Appleton and Davis, op.cit., p. 69.
54. Klein and others, op.cit., p. 184.
55. Gilman and others, op.cit., p. 404.

Extrapyramidal Side Effects

Reprinted from American Journal of Nursing, July 1981

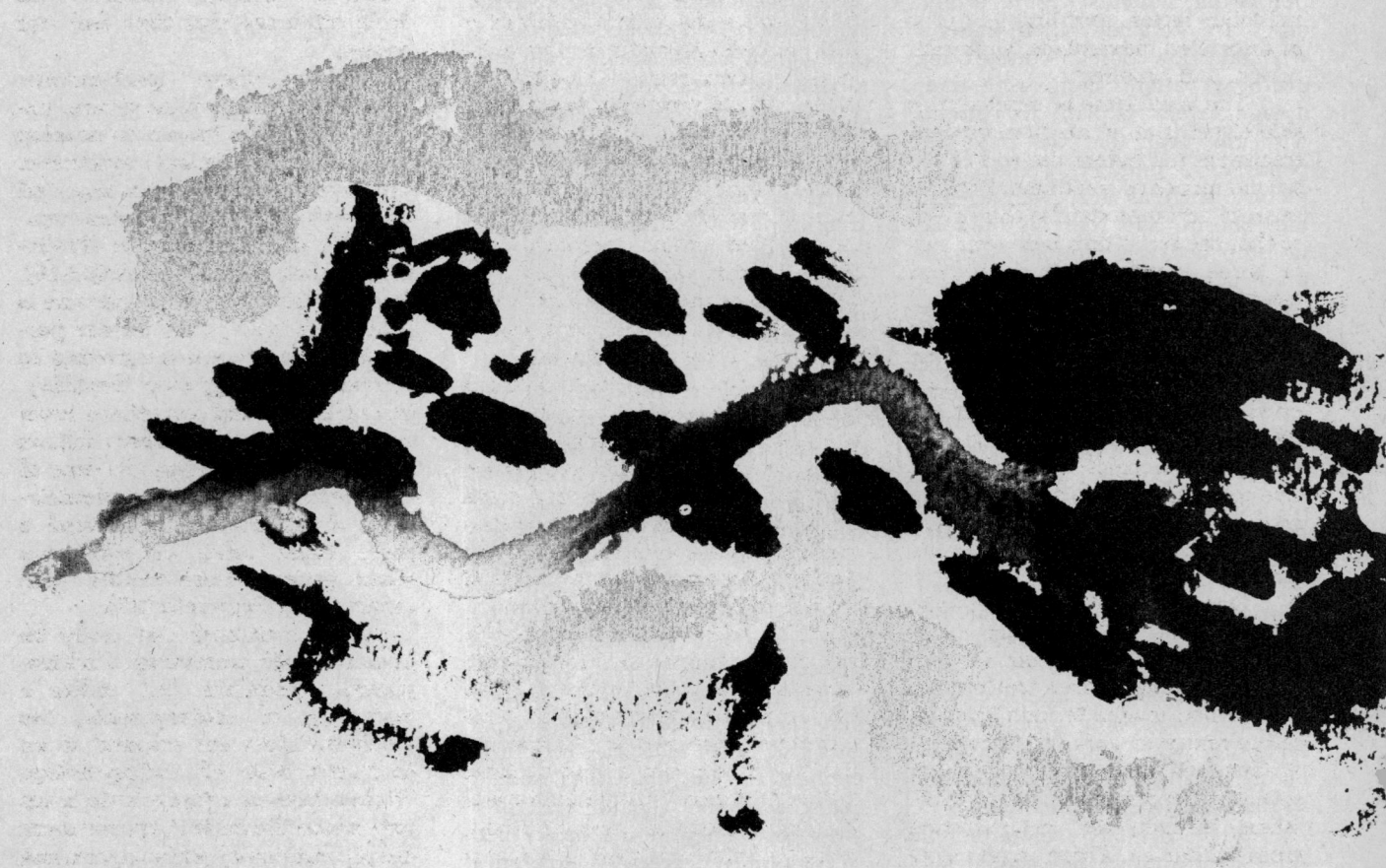

By Elizabeth Harris

The extrapyramidal side effects of antipsychotic drugs are often confusing, frightening, uncomfortable, and embarrassing for patients. About one-third of all patients taking antipsychotic medications will experience EPS[1]. While these side effects are difficult to prevent, they are fairly easily controlled when accurately diagnosed and treated.

Untreated EPS can be so distressing that patients will stop taking their medications in order to alleviate the symptoms. Van Puten found that most patients with schizophrenia who refuse to take their drugs upon discharge from the hospital do so because of discomfort from EPS[2].

Unless health care professionals are knowledgeable about antipsychotic drugs, the symptoms of EPS may be misdiagnosed as any of the following conditions: epilepsy, meningitis, encephalitis, poliomyelitis, tetanus, malingering, hysteria, stroke, joint dislocation, calcium deficiency, or depression. In fact, EPS have been improperly treated with such aggressive measures as hospitalization, lumbar puncture, and tracheotomy[3-5].

These are four general classes of EPS:
- parkinsonism
- dyskinesias and dystonias
- akathisia
- tardive dyskinesia.

Parkinsonism. Drug-induced parkinsonism is a syndrome similar

# of Antipsychotic Medications

in appearance to the naturally occurring Parkinson's disease. This syndrome is thought to be caused by the dopamine blockade created by the antipsychotics. The syndrome consists of akinesia, muscular rigidity, alterations of posture, tremor, masklike facies, shuffling gait, loss of associated movements, hypersalivation, and drooling.

The usual time of onset of this side effect is after the first week of treatment but before the end of the second month of treatment. Patients seem to accommodate to this effect, so that the symptoms fade over two or three months with or without treatment.

Akinesia is often experienced as fatigue, lack of interest, slowness, heaviness, lack of drive or ambition, or vague bodily discomforts. If severe, it can interfere with the patient's psychosocial and rehabilitative activities. Akinesia can often be confused with depression, demoralization, schizophrenic inertia, or negativism.

One patient I cared for who had chronic schizophrenia spent several weeks lying mute in bed. Her psychosis had been treated, but she seemed unable to mobilize herself to return to work. We incorrectly assumed that she was either severely depressed or negativistic, when, in fact, she was suffering from akinesia. Three days after treatment for akinesia was started, she returned to work.

Akinesia should be suspected when patients say they feel weak, less spontaneous, less interested in conversation, generally apathetic, and less inclined to initiate usual activities. To the observer, the patient seems anergic, with fewer gestures and diminished spontaneity. Test the patient's strength in both hands. The patient with akinesia will have decreased muscle strength. Ask the patient if he feels slowed down; the patient with akinesia will almost always answer yes.

Rigidity is a plastic hypertonicity that affects both axial and limb musculature; it is often mistaken for tension or anxiety. Rigidity is most easily tested for by holding a patient's elbow in the palm of your hand with your thumb positioned over the flexor tendons. Flex and extend the arm with your other hand, asking the patient to relax the arm and allow you to do the moving. You may find a smooth resistance to movement, known as "lead-pipe" rigidity, or a ratchet-like phenomenon, known as "cogwheel" rigidity. Either finding is evidence of drug-induced rigidity, rather than simple increased tension. Rigidity will most likely be seen three or four days to two weeks after therapy is started, with a peak incidence at two to four weeks.

Patients with drug-induced parkinsonism tend to have a stooping posture and a festinating, or shuffling and somewhat propulsive, gait. Their tremor is faster and more irregular than that seen in true Parkinson's disease and can be present during movement or at rest at speeds of about 5 cycles/second.

The tremor usually begins in one or both upper extremities and, when severe, involves the tongue, jaw, and lower extremities(6). This symptom is first seen at a half week, peaks at 2 to 6 weeks, and declines at 8 to 16 weeks. This symptom will be most difficult for patients whose work or hobby calls for fine motor coordination.

The masklike facies of parkinsonism can be mistaken for the flat affect of schizophrenia. The difference is that the patient with masklike facies will employ means other than facial gestures to indicate a wider range of affect.

The loss of associated movements is most easily seen in the decreased or absent arm swing. The patient with this symptom will often walk with the forearms perpendicular to the trunk. Patients frequently describe themselves as looking like a puppy begging for a bone, or like a kangaroo. Hypersalivation and drooling are present only in severe cases of parkinsonism.

Patients often describe their parkinsonian symptoms in graphic ways. One patient described her slowness (akinesia) as a feeling of being under water. Many describe the akinesia by saying they feel like robots or zombies. Patients who drool often say that they feel like babies.

When these parkinsonian symptoms become most severe, patients have been known to develop neuroleptic malignant syndrome. This syndrome has been reported only with high doses of potent neuroleptics like fluphenazine (Prolixin) and haloperidol (Haldol)(7-10). Neuroleptic malignant syndrome is gradual in onset, with milder parkinsonian symptoms progressing to mutism, posturing, waxy flexibility, incontinence, and sometimes fever and coma. Improvement follows slowly after decreasing the dose of neuroleptic or adding an anticholinergic drug. One study showed a more rapid relief of symptoms when patients were treated with amantadine (Symmetrel)(7).

This syndrome can easily be confused with worsening of schizophrenic symptoms, but, unlike a worsening of schizophrenia, the syndrome does not respond to an increased dose of antipsychotics. Higher doses of antipsychotic drugs only make the patient appear more deeply catatonic, while decreasing the dose will ameliorate the catatonialike symptoms. One patient with this reaction to haloperidol was transferred to the neurology service to rule out encephalitis. Her symptoms resolved gradually when all her antipsychotic medications were discontinued.

Neuroleptic-induced parkinsonism is easily controlled. Some of the symptoms can usually be eliminated by decreasing the dose of neuroleptic or by changing to another drug with a lesser incidence of this syndrome. If these measures are ineffective or if they are impractical for clinical reasons, the antiparkinsonian agents are commonly administered. (See chart, next page.)

If one of these drugs is unsuccessful, another agent should be tried. Sometimes, if side effects do not respond to one medication, they will respond to another.

Amantadine (Symmetrel) and benztropine mesylate (Cogentin) have long serum half-lives and, therefore, can be given on a once- or twice-a-day schedule. These drugs are, however, slightly more expensive than the others. The other antiparkinsonian drugs have shorter half-lives and should be given in divided doses throughout the day. Amantadine's effectiveness may diminish over time, necessitating a change to another antiparkinsonian drug.

Since drug-induced parkinsonism usually abates in a month or two, with or without treatment, the dose of antiparkinsonian medications should be reduced gradually over two or three months and then discontinued. There is often no recurrence of parkinsonism.

Dyskinesias and dystonias. Dyskinesias are coordinated, involuntary, stereotyped, rhythmic movements of the limbs and trunk that are seen more commonly in males(11).

The dystonias are uncoordinated, bizarre, jerking or spastic movements of the neck, face, eyes, tongue, torso, arm, or leg muscles; backward rolling of the eyes in the sockets (oculogyric crisis); sideways twisting of the neck (torticollis); protrusion of the tongue; or spasms of the back muscles (opisthotonus). These symptoms occur suddenly and dramatically. They are extremely frightening to patients and staff and are often painful as well.

These symptoms are sometimes so severe as to lead to respiratory distress or difficulty talking or swallowing. In fact, the nurse will sometimes become aware of an acute dystonic reaction when a patient approaches with a look of terror, pointing to his sharply twisted jaw, but unable to speak, even to ask for help. Some patients first become aware of this symptom when they find it difficult to chew or swallow food. Other patients will present with a complaint that their eyes keep rolling up in their heads against their will. What at first sounds like it may be a delusion turns out to be an oculogyric crisis. If untreated, these symptoms wax and wane and remit spontaneously in about a week(12). If treated, they remit almost immediately and usually do not recur.

Dystonias may be seen anytime after administration of the first dose of an antipsychotic agent. The incidence peaks in a week and declines in two weeks. The duration of an episode ranges from a few minutes to several hours. Dystonias are twice as common in males and occur more often in younger people(11-13). Patients usually welcome treatment for these painful and frightening symptoms.

Severe, acute dystonic reactions can be treated with parenteral diphenhydramine (Benadryl). Doses of 25 to 100 mg., given intravenously, should be effective in one minute. The same dosage given IM should work in 15 minutes, and an oral dose should work in one hour. Another useful drug is benztropine (Cogentin) 2 mg. I.V. or IM(6). Any of the antiparkinsonian drugs can be administered orally, but the oral route is painfully slow for a patient in an acute crisis. After the acute symptoms have subsided, it is common to give a maintenance dose of antiparkinsonian medications for two or three months to prevent a recurrence.

It is important to treat these reactions quickly because they are so frightening to patients. Reassure the patient that he is experiencing a common side effect of his medication. Tell him how you will be treating the symptoms, and depending on the drug and route used, tell him how long he can expect to wait before feeling relief. It is a good safeguard when a patient is begun on an antipsychotic medication to request that the physician also write a PRN order to give IM diphenhydramine or benztropine in the event of an acute dystonic reaction.

Akathisia. Akathisia is the symptom that most often leads to noncompliance(2). Akathisia is a very discomforting feeling of restlessness and agitation. One patient called it the "walkies and the talkies." The patient finds he is unable to lie down, to sleep, or to sit still. If forced to sit, the patient often shifts his posture, taps his feet, or squirms and fidgets in the chair. Often he cannot resist the compulsion to stand up and walk around. In a situation where a long period of sitting is required, such as in a movie or a therapy session, the patient will sit and stand repeatedly with an obvious inability to stop himself. He thus finds it difficult to perform such activities as reading books,

Drugs Used as Antiparkinsonian Agents

Generic name	Trade name	Usual daily dose (mg.)
Anticholinergics		
benztropine mesylate	Cogentin	1-6
trihexyphenidyl hydrochloride	Artane (and others)	2-15
procyclidine hydrochloride	Kemadrin	5-20
cycrimine hydrochloride	Pagitane	3.75-15.0
biperiden hydrochloride	Akineton	2-6
ethopropazine hydrochloride	Parsidol	50-600
Antihistamines		
diphenhydramine hydrochloride	Benadryl (and others)	25-200
chlorphenoxamine hydrochloride	Phenoxene	150-400
orphenadrine hydrochloride	Disipal	50-250
Others		
amantadine hydrochloride	Symmetrel	100-300

watching television, sewing, or knitting. When standing still, the patient often rocks and shifts his weight. The more severe the akathisia, the more desperate the patient becomes. Occasionally, he experiences the feeling as sexual excitement. More often, the affects he experiences are terror, fright, anger, or rage. In desperation, the patient may become suicidal, violent, or homicidal.

Akathisia is often mistaken for psychomotor agitation. If it is treated with an increase in the dose of the antipsychotic medication, the akathisia becomes worse. In contrast, one or two doses of an antiparkinsonian medication will sometimes relieve it.

Likewise, the patient often erroneously attributes akathisia to a psychological cause. It is important that we clearly explain that the restlessness the patient is experiencing is a side effect of the medication rather than an emotional state.

To differentiate akathisia from anxiety or agitation, several questions can be asked. Ask if the patient ever felt like this before taking his medication. A no answer suggests akathisia. Ask, "Do you feel restless inside? Do you feel more comfortable standing up or walking around than you do sitting or lying down?" If the answers are yes, the patient is likely to be suffering from akathisia. In addition, the patient almost always experiences the symptoms as ego-alien and may feel it is more difficult to endure the akathisia than his original symptoms.

Akathisia is first seen after two weeks of drug treatment. The peak incidence is at 6 to 10 weeks, with a decline at 12 to 16 weeks. It is more common in women and in middle age. The symptoms tend to appear and disappear spontaneously, but accommodation does not develop as it does with parkinsonism. Over half of patients with akathisia also have other extrapyramidal side effects (7,11,12,14).

Akathisia is the EPS most refractory to treatment with antiparkinsonian medications. The first attempt at treatment of akathisia is to reduce the dose of antipsychotic or to change to a drug with a lower incidence of akathisia (see chart at left). If neither of these measures are successful, an antiparkinsonian agent can be tried. If the first trial is unsuccessful, a second trial with another antiparkinsonian drug may succeed. If all else fails, akathisia can be treated with diazepam (Valium). The symptoms should subside in three days if the diazepam is effective(15).

Tardive dyskinesia. If detected early, this syndrome is frequently reversible. Symptoms consist of coordinated, rhythmic, stereotyped, abnormal, involuntary sucking, chewing, licking, and pursing movements of the tongue and mouth. Sometimes, choreiform movements of the extremities are seen. Grimacing, blinking, and frowning are common. Also seen are tongue protrusion and rocking. The symptoms may occur after long-term use of high doses of antipsychotic drugs, often first appearing after the dosage is decreased or the medication discontinued. More recently, cases have been reported following short-term use of moderate doses.

Two of the earliest signs of tardive dyskinesia (TD) are excessive blinking and fine, vermiform movements of the tongue. The symptoms then progress with a fluctuating course until, finally, they interfere with activities of daily living, such as bathing, dressing, or even eating. The symptoms can be suppressed by intense, voluntary effort and are absent during sleep. They are embarrassing to most patients.

It is reported by the APA task force on late neurological effects of antipsychotic drugs that 10 to 20 percent of patients receiving antipsychotic drugs for a year or more develop tardive dyskinesia. Possible predisposing factors are age, being female, presence of organic brain disease, use of antiparkinsonian drugs, use of high-potency neuroleptics, presence of dementia, history of ECT or leucotomy, or a history of tricyclic antidepressant use(16).

Much research is being done to find a cure for tardive dyskinesia. So far, none has been found. There are, however, some guidelines for prevention. Antipsychotics should be used for as short a time as possible, always taking into consideration the balance between the need for the antipsychotic and the risk of tardive dyskinesia. One study showed that only 40 percent of patients, when taken off antipsychotics after six months, require reinstitution of the drug because of exacerbation of symptoms(17). Antiparkinsonian agents should be used only when indicated and, when possible, should be discontinued no later than three months after institution of treatment.

All patients on antipsychotics should be screened for tardive dyskinesia at least every three months. A common tool for this purpose is the AIMS test (Abnormal Involuntary Movement Scale). If any symptoms of tardive dyskinesia are noted, the antipsychotic should be discontinued if clinically possible. In some cases, ECT is then used to treat the patient's acute psychotic symptoms. In the difficult situation where there is no satisfactory alternative to continuing antipsychotic medication, the patient and family should be advised of the patient's condition and of the risks involved in further treatment with antipsychotics. Only if the patient understands the risks involved and is willing to proceed, should antipsychotics be continued. Some institutions require the patient's written consent.

Principles of Treating EPS

The most obvious way to prevent EPS is to use the least amount of antipsychotic medications for the shortest time possible. One study suggests that all patients should have a drug-free trial after six months of treatment, with reinstitution of medications only if there is an exacerbation of symptoms. Fully half of such patients should be able to function well without reinstitution of chemotherapy(17). Others suggest a drug-free trial for all patients at 6 to 12 months after institution of drug treatment(15).

When antipsychotics are used, they are best used initially in divided doses to increase the sedative, hypnotic, and motor-inhibiting properties during the patient's acute psychosis. After a few days, when control is satisfactory, the patient should be put on a once- or twice-a-day schedule. Clinical benefit from the antipsychotic is the same, but on a less frequent dosage schedule, the patient will experience fewer side effects(17). The usual practice is to schedule a single dose for bedtime or arrange a BID schedule, with the larger portion of the total dose at bedtime. It is important to remember that many EPS can be treated by decreasing the dose of the antipsychotic or by changing antipsychotics.

Basically, all antipsychotic drugs produce equal improvement, yet, at times, some will work when others fail. All produce the same range of side effects, though one drug may produce more of one side effect and less of others. For example, high-potency drugs, such as haloperiold (Haldol), trifluoperazine (Stelazine), fluphenazine (Prolixin), and perphenazine (Trilafon), have the greatest incidence of parkinsonism, dystonias, and akathisia. Thioridazine (Mellaril) has the least incidence of EPS, but it has the disadvantages of creating ejaculatory disturbances in a small percentage of males and of having an upper dosage limit of 800 mg. Chlorpromazine and thioridazine commonly cause sedation and orthostatic hypotension. The long-acting injectables, fluphenazine decanoate and enanthate, cause EPS more quickly than other dose forms—within 12 hours to 5 days of injection.

Because EPS are so uncomfortable and frightening to patients and because they often lead to drug resistance, some clinicians believe it is best to treat all patients on antipsychotics with prophylactic doses of antiparkinsonian medications. This would seem to be a very sensible approach. Yet, there are some very good reasons why prophylactic use of antiparkinsonian (AP) drugs is unwise. They include the following:

• Prophylactic AP medications have not been shown to prevent all EPS.

• Not all patients develop EPS.

• Excess doses of AP drugs can cause atropine psychosis.

• Use of AP medications may decrease the blood level of antipsychotics by interfering with absorption.

• AP medications may worsen the symptoms of TD or may add to the risk of developing TD.

• AP medications have their own side effects.

• AP medications add to the patient's expense.

When administering AP medications, watch for the following side effects: paralysis of bladder or bowel; confusion; burred vision; dry mouth; lethargy; dizziness; GI disturbance; dry, flushed skin; and dilated pupils. These are more likely to occur with high doses in young or middle-aged patients or with moderate or low doses in elderly patients.

Nursing Implications

The nurse's approach to extrapyramidal side effects and to their treatment is also important for the patient. When patients are begun on antipsychotic medications, they and their friends or family should be taught about the side effects that may be dangerous.

When a patient experiences EPS, he often attributes his discomfort to emotional distress, to some fault of his own, or to a sinister outside force. Explain to the patient that he is having a side effect of his medication. Validate for the patient that other people with the same symptom find it uncomfortable, unpleasant, or even painful. Tell him that the side effect is usually treatable and that everything possible will be done to treat it quickly. Inform the patient's physician of your findings and discuss the appropriate treatment.

After treatment begins, it is important to monitor the course of the symptoms to evaluate any necessary changes in treatment. It seems to be a great relief to our patients when they see we are familiar with their distress and know how to help them with it.

There is a misconception that there is a relationship between EPS and drug efficacy. There have been no conclusive studies that show antipsychotic drugs to be more effective when the patient experiences EPS. When a patient is stiff or drooling, you know that he has swallowed and absorbed some of his medication, but this does not increase the likelihood that the medication will work to treat his psychosis.

A second common misconception is that EPS are constant in strength and appearance. A nurse who observes that a patient's symptoms occur only in the presence of other people or that they disappear when a patient is alone, will sometimes conclude that the patient is malingering or manipulating. Similarly, a patient whose drug-induced restlessness interferes with sitting still more in group therapy than during a card game will often be accused of copping out. On the contrary, EPS are known to wax and wane over time or with the patient's affective state and level of anxiety(6). The nurse should expect to see EPS occur more often or to be more pronounced in stressful situations.

References

1. Newton, M., and others. How you can improve the effectiveness of psychotropic drug therapy. Nurs. '78 8:46-55, July 1978.
2. Van Putten, T. Why do schizophrenic patients refuse to take their drugs? Arch.Gen.Psychiatry 31:67-72, July 1974.
3. Mills, J. Dystonic reactions to phenothiazines. JEN 4:43-46, Nov.-Dec. 1978.
4. Cavenar, J. O., Jr., and others. Misdiagnosis of severe dystonia. Psychosomatics 20:209-210, Mar. 1979.
5. Baldessarini, R. J. Chemotherapy in Psychiatry. Cambridge, Mass., Harvard University Press, 1977, p. 41.
6. Lipton, M. A., and others. Psychopharmacology: A Generation of Progress. New York, Raven Press, 1978, p. 1021.
7. Baldessarini, op. cit., p. 36.
8. Grunhaus, L., and others. Neuroleptic malignant syndrome due to depot fluphenazine. J.Clin.Psychiatry 40:99-100, Feb. 1979.
9. Baldessarini, R. J. The "neuroleptic" antipsychotic drugs. Part 2. Neurologic side effects. Postgrad.Med. 65:123-128, Apr. 1979.
10. Gelenberg, A. J., and Mandel, M. R. Catatonic reactions to high-potency neuroleptic drugs. Arch.Gen.Psychiatry 34:947-950, Aug. 1977.
11. Klein, D. F., and Davis, J. M. Diagnosis and Drug Treatment of Psychiatric Disorders. Baltimore, Williams & Wilkins Co., 1969, p. 98.
12. Murphy, J. E., and Stewart, R. B. Efficacy of antiparkinson agents in preventing antipsychotic-induced extrapyramidal symptoms. Am.J.Hosp.Pharm. 36:641-644, May 1979.
13. Shader, R. L., and DiMascio, Albert. Psychotropic Drug Side Effects: Clinical and Theoretical Perspectives. Baltimore, Williams & Wilkins Co., 1970, p. 93.
14. Van Putten, T. The many faces of akathisia. Compr.Psychiatry 16:43-47, Jan.-Feb. 1975.
15. Gelenberg, A. J. Treating the outpatient schizophrenic. Postgrad.Med. 64:48-56, Nov. 1978.
16. Schwartz, H. J. Tardive dyskinesia and the long-term patient. Hosp.Community Psychiatry 30:465-467, July 1979.
17. Gardos, G., and Cole, J. O. Maintenance antipsychotic therapy: is the cure worse than the disease? Am.J.Psychiatry 133:32-36, Jan. 1976.
18. McAfee, H. A. Tardive dyskinesia. Am.J.Nurs. 78:359-367, Mar. 1978.

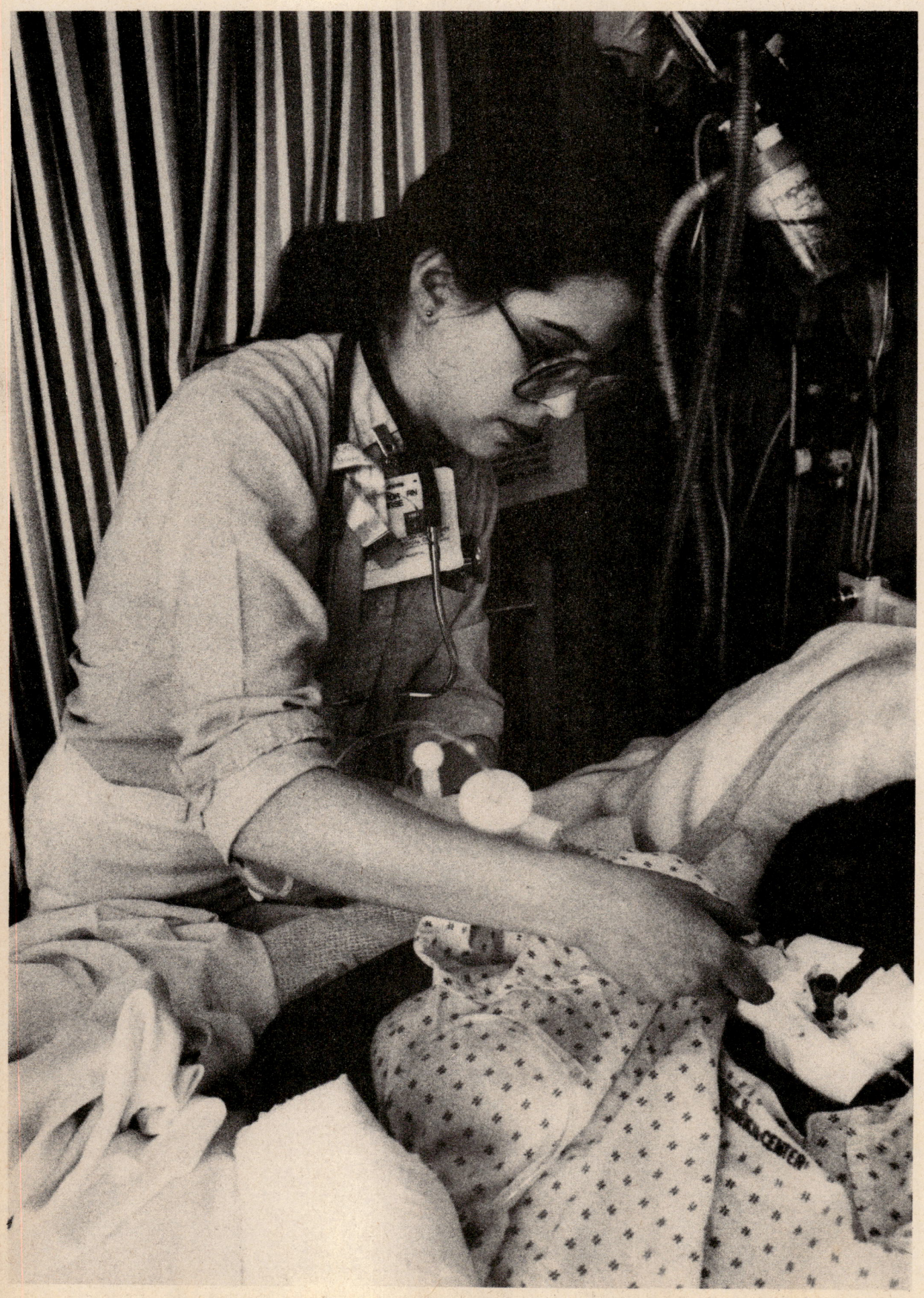

Section 3
Nursing Care of the Adult

Patricia E. Downing, RN, MN, Co-coordinator
Edwina A. McConnell, RN, MS, Co-coordinator

Ida M. Androwich, RN, MS
Kay Bensing, RN, MA
Suzette Cardin, RN, MS, CCRN
Virginia L. Cassmeyer, RN, MSN
Olivian De Souza, RN, MSN
Anne C. Holland, RN, MSN
Karen Krejci, RN, MN
Alma Joel Labunski, RN, MSN
Esther Matassarin-Jacobs, RN, MEd, MSN
Jerry R. Myhan, RN, MSN
Paulette D. Rollant, RN, MSN, CCRN
Judith K. Sands, RN, EdD
Ann M. Schofield, RN, MS

Section 3: Nursing Care of the Adult

THE HEALTHY ADULT 159

SURGERY 164
Overview 164
Perioperative Period 164
Discharge 167

OXYGENATION 170
General Concepts 170
  Overview 170
  Application of the Nursing Process to the Client with
  Oxygenation Problems 172
Selected Health Problems 176
  A. Cardiopulmonary Arrest 176
  B. Shock 178
  C. Angina Pectoris 179
  D. Myocardial Infarction 181
  E. Dysrhythmias 185
  F. Congestive Heart Failure 188
  G. Hypertension 191
  H. Peripheral Vascular Disease 193
  I. Chronic Obstructive Pulmonary Disease (COPD) or
     Chronic Obstructive Lung Disease (COLD) 196
  J. Pneumonia 199
  K. Tuberculosis 201
  L. Chest Tubes and Chest Surgery 203
  M. Cancer of the Lung 205

NUTRITION AND METABOLISM 208

PART ONE: THE DIGESTIVE TRACT 208
General Concepts 208
  Overview 208
  Application of the Nursing Process to the Client with
  Digestive Tract Problems 210
Selected Health Problems 217
  A. Hiatus Hernia 217
  B. Gastritis 217
  C. Peptic Ulcer Disease 218
  D. Diverticulosis/Diverticulitis 224
  E. Appendicitis 225
  F. Cholecystitis with Cholelithiasis 225
  G. Pancreatitis 226
  H. Hepatitis 227
  I. Cirrhosis 229
  J. Complications of Liver Disease: Esophageal Varices,
     Ascites, Hepatic Encephalopathy 231

PART TWO: THE ENDOCRINE SYSTEM 233
General Concepts 233
  Overview 233
  Application of the Nursing Process to the Client with
  Endocrine System Problems 235
Selected Health Problems 236
  A. Hyperpituitarism 236
  B. Hypopituitarism 236
  C. Hyperthyroidism 237
  D. Hypothyroidism 238
  E. Hyperparathyroidism 239
  F. Hypoparathyroidism 240
  G. Hyperfunction of the Adrenal Glands 240
  H. Hyposecretion of the Adrenal Glands 241
  I. Hypofunction of the Pancreas: Diabetes Mellitus 243

ELIMINATION 250

PART ONE: THE KIDNEYS 250
General Concepts 250
  Overview 250
  Application of the Nursing Process to the Client with
  Kidney Problems 252
Selected Health Problems 257
  A. Cystitis/Pyelonephritis 257
  B. Urinary Calculi 258
  C. Cancer of the Bladder 259
  D. Acute Renal Failure 260
  E. Chronic Renal Failure 262
  F. Dialysis 264
  G. Kidney Transplantation 270
  H. Benign Prostatic Hypertrophy 271
  I. Cancer of the Prostate 273

PART TWO: THE LARGE BOWEL 274
General Concepts 274
  Overview 274
  Application of the Nursing Process to the Client with Large
  Bowel Problems 274
Selected Health Problems 276
  A. Alteration in Normal Bowel Evacuation 276
  B. Inflammatory Bowel Disease (Regional Enteritis,
     Crohn's Disease, Ulcerative Colitis) 277
  C. Total Colectomy with Ileostomy 280
  D. Mechanical Obstruction of the Colon 281
  E. Cancer of the Colon 282
  F. Hemorrhoids or Anal Fissure 282

SAFETY AND SECURITY 285
General Concepts 285
  Overview 285
  Application of the Nursing Process to the Client with Safety
  and Security Problems 288
Selected Health Problems of the Nervous System 293
  A. Acute Head Injury 293
  B. Intracranial Surgery 294
  C. Cerebrovascular Accident 295
  D. Meningitis 296
  E. Spinal Cord Injuries 297
  F. Parkinson's Disease (Parkinsonism) 299
  G. Multiple Sclerosis 300
  H. Epilepsy 302
  I. Myasthenia Gravis 304
Selected Health Problems of the Sensory System 306
  A. Cataracts 306
  B. Retinal Detachment 307
  C. Glaucoma 308
  D. Nasal Problems Requiring Surgery 309
  E. Epistaxis 309
  F. Cancer of the Larynx 310

ACTIVITY AND REST 313
General Concepts 313
  Overview 313
  Application of the Nursing Process to the Client with
  Activity and Rest Problems 314
Selected Health Problems 315
  A. Fractures 315
  B. Fractured Hip (Proximal End of Femur) 317
  C. Amputation 318
  D. Arthritis 319
  E. Collagen Disease 322
  F. Herniated Nucleus Pulposus 323

CELLULAR ABERRATION 326
General Concepts 326
  Overview 326
  Application of the Nursing Process to the Client with
  Cancer 327
Selected Health Problems 332
  A. Cancer of the Lung 332
  B. Cancer of the Bladder 332
  C. Cancer of the Prostate 332
  D. Cancer of the Colon 332
  E. Cancer of the Larynx 332
  F. Cancer of the Cervix 332
  G. Cancer of the Breast 333

REPRINTS 337

The Healthy Adult

A. **Health**
  1. Definition
     a. None universally accepted
     b. Defined by the World Health Organization in 1946 as "a state of complete physical, mental, and social well being and not just the absence of disease or infirmity . . . fundamental right of every human being."
     c. Defined by the American Nurses Association (ANA) in 1980 as "a dynamic state of being in which the developmental and behavioral potential of an individual is realized to the fullest extent possible. Each human being possesses various strengths and limitations, resulting from the interaction of hereditary and environmental factors. The relative dominance of the strengths and limitations determines an individual's place on the health continuum; it determines the person's biological and behavioral integrity, his wholeness."
  2. Characteristics
     a. Dynamic state, dependent upon individual's ability to adapt to changing internal and external environment
     b. Continuous spectrum extending from obvious disease through absence of discernible disease, to a state of optimal functioning
     c. Involves social, emotional, and physical aspects
     d. Norms change with age
  3. Duration of Life
     a. Life Span
        1) constant, genetically determined
        2) average appears fixed at 85 years old, with maximum of 115
     b. Life Expectancy (United States)
        1) changes with advances in disease control and treatment
        2) born in 1900: 47 years old; born in 1981: 74.2 years old
  4. Levels of Health Promotion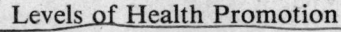
     a. Primary: prevention of disease; promotion of health
     b. Secondary: early diagnosis; prompt treatment
     c. Tertiary: prevention of complications of disease
  5. Health Assessment
     a. Purpose: to identify client's current health status and deviations from optimum status
     b. Factors that Promote Health
        1) nutrition
        2) mental hygiene
        3) adequate housing
        4) moderate/balanced personal habits, e.g., hygiene, rest, exercise
        5) useful, productive role in society
        6) safe, healthy work environment
        7) recreation to balance work
        8) sense of personal security
        9) education

B. **Physiologic Characteristics of the Healthy Adult**
  1. Young and Middle Adult Years (20–65)
     a. General
        1) growth and development appropriate for age
        2) symmetrical body
        3) no pain with motion
        4) balanced sleep patterns (decreases for the young and middle-aged)
     b. Integument
        1) skin
           a) clean, intact, smooth, warm, dry
           b) normal turgor and texture
           c) odorless
           d) no lesions
           e) normal color (no abnormal color changes, jaundice, cyanosis)

2) mucous membranes
    a) pink, intact, hydrated (gloved finger should slide over membrane easily)
    b) no lesions
3) hair
    a) evenly distributed, uniform texture
    b) no dandruff, scales
4) nails
    a) pink nail beds
    b) rapid capillary filling of nail beds after compression
    c) no clubbing of fingers
c. Neck
    1) trachea in midline
    2) no masses
d. Eyes
    1) symmetrical placement
    2) white sclera
    3) pink conjunctiva
    4) PERRLA (*p*upils *e*qual, *r*ound, *r*eact to *l*ight and *a*ccommodation)
    5) visual acuity 20/20 with or without correction
e. Ears
    1) symmetrical placement
    2) auditory acuity (hearing) normal (i.e., can distinguish whispered words at 20 feet)
    3) no drainage from external auditory canal
    4) equilibrium maintained (no vertigo)
f. Thorax and Lungs
    1) open, unobstructed airway
    2) respirations (eupnic)
        a) effortless, noiseless, odorless
        b) rhythmical, normal depth
        c) rate: 12–20/min at rest
    3) bronchovesicular and vesicular breath sounds present in appropriate areas
    4) no adventitious breath sounds
    5) no cough, sputum
    6) thorax: normal anterior-posterior diameter (i.e., AP diameter less than lateral to lateral diameter)
g. Cardiovascular
    1) normal sinus rhythm (NSR)
    2) rate: 60–80/min at rest
    3) blood pressure approximately 120/80 at rest
    4) no chest pain
    5) no palpitations
    6) normal palpable arterial pulses in the extremities (radial, brachial, femoral, popliteal, tibial, dorsalis pedis)
    7) absence of abnormal color changes (e.g., cyanosis, increased pigmentation, redness, etc.)
    8) no peripheral edema
    9) no varicosities/ulcerations of extremities
    10) extremities equally warm
h. Abdomen
    1) no palpable masses
    2) soft, nontender
    3) flat, no distention
    4) normal, active bowel sounds in all quadrants
    5) no organomegaly
i. Gastrointestinal/Nutrition
    1) normal weight for height
    2) normal appetite (i.e., no nausea, weight loss or gain, no change)
    3) balanced, adequate diet (basic four food groups)
    4) normal digestion (i.e., no food intolerance, indigestion, etc.)
    5) well nourished
    6) teeth present, in good repair
    7) normal mastication (i.e., no difficulty or pain with chewing)
    8) no difficulty swallowing
    9) regular bowel habits, stools brown and formed
j. Musculoskeletal
    1) good posture and body alignment
    2) body movements coordinated (no tremors or involuntary movements)
    3) muscles: firm, symmetrical, strong, normal tone (no spasms, contractures, weakness, atrophy, or paralysis), equal size and strength
    4) normal gait (foot strikes heel to toe, normal base of support, arms swing in coordination with leg movements)
    5) joints
        a) no deformities
        b) nontender, not swollen, no crepitation
        c) full, unimpaired range of motion
k. Neurologic
    1) mental status/cognitive functioning
        a) oriented to person, place, time
        b) alert, conscious
        c) memory intact: short- and long-term

           d) capable of abstract thinking
           e) articulates without difficulty
           f) dress/behavior/mood appropriate (no excessive aggression, violence, withdrawal, depression, or mood swings)
        2) sensory
           a) pain perception intact
           b) light touch, temperature, pressure, vibration, position sense, hearing, taste, smell intact
        3) motor
           a) coordinated movement
           b) normal gait
           c) no tremors or involuntary movements
           d) no atrophy of muscles
           e) normal reflexes intact (including deep tendon reflexes)
           f) absence of pathologic reflexes
    l. Genitourinary
        1) no sexual dysfunction (impotency, premature ejaculation, orgasmic dysfunction)
        2) genitals
           a) good hygiene
           b) no lesions, abnormal discharge
        3) breasts
           a) symmetrical size and placement
           b) no masses
           c) no abnormal discharge from nipples
        4) micturition (urination)
           a) nonpainful
           b) voluntary control
           c) no difficulty controlling stream
           d) no frequency or urgency
           e) bladder empty after voiding
           f) approximately 300 ml/voiding
           g) urine: amber, clear
2. Elderly (Over 65)
    a. General: process of slow degeneration
        1) general tissue desiccation and slowed cell division
        2) slowed, weakened speed of response to stimuli
        3) slowed rate of tissue repair
        4) decreased metabolism
        5) mechanisms of homeostasis less rapid and less efficient
        6) rate of change is individual, influenced by factors such as heredity and stress
        7) normal physiologic changes (vs abnormal pathologic changes) have not been completely identified
        8) high incidence of health problems, e.g., CHF, pneumonia, cataracts
    b. Integument
        1) skin
           a) dry, wrinkled, loss of elasticity
           b) decreased perspiration and sebum
           c) fragile, easily injured
           d) decreased subcutaneous tissue
           e) decreased skin turgor
           f) increased sensitivity to cold
        2) hair
           a) decreased number of hair follicles, generalized loss
           b) scant, fine, greying
           c) hirsutism of the woman
           d) possible hereditary baldness
        3) nails
           a) dry
           b) thick
           c) brittle
    c. Eyes
        1) slowed accommodation to light changes
        2) decreased visual acuity
           a) presbyopia (slow lens accommodation)
           b) narrowed field of vision (tunnel)
        3) decreased ability to distinguish colors
        4) night driving may become difficult
    d. Ears
        1) rigidity of bones of middle ear reduces conduction
        2) sensorineural hearing deficit (gradual loss of high and low tones)
        3) decreased acuity to locate or identify sounds or understand group conversation
    e. Thorax and Lungs
        1) decreased lung capacity
        2) decreased elasticity of tissue
        3) increased anterior and posterior diameter of thorax
    f. Cardiovascular
        1) decreased vascular elasticity
        2) increased systolic BP
        3) decreased cardiac output
        4) less tolerance to position change
    g. Gastrointestinal/Nutrition
        1) redistribution of body fat: increased fat in trunk, especially in the abdomen

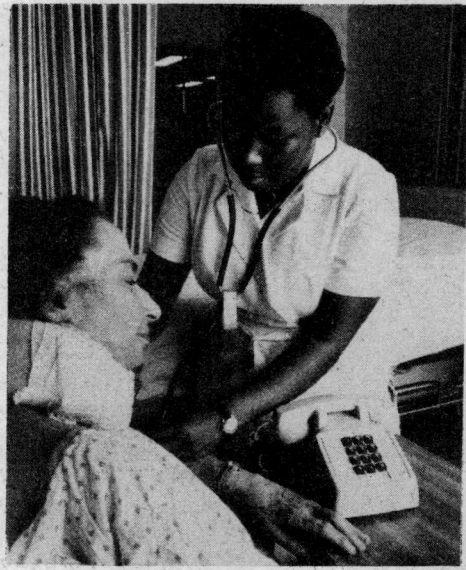

2) teeth and gum problems may require dietary modification
3) change in taste and smell
4) slowed digestion; increased food intolerances
5) decreased metabolism: caloric requirement per day decreases 7.5% for each decade after the age of 25 years
6) atonic constipation common

h. Musculoskeletal
1) tires easily, less stamina
2) symmetrical decrease in muscle bulk
3) decreased muscle strength and tone
4) stiffening of joints
5) generalized loss of from 6–10 cm in stature resulting from
 a) flexion of knee and hip joints
 b) narrowing of intervertebral discs
6) osteoporosis common (especially in vertebral bodies and neck of femur)
7) body takes on bony, angular appearance

i. Neurologic
1) general
 a) progressive decrease in number of functioning neurons in CNS and sense organs
 b) slowed speed of impulse transmission
 c) normal neurologic functioning possible because of tremendous reserve of numbers of neurons
2) mental/cognitive function
 a) altered capacity to retain new information and learn new tasks
 b) some impaired memory and mental endurance
3) sensory
 a) some impaired sensory perception (hearing, smell, sight, taste, touch, temperature, pain)
 b) gradual decrease of visual and auditory acuity
4) motor
 a) slowed reaction to stimuli; lengthening of reaction time
 b) decreased coordination and balance

j. Genitourinary
1) decreased renal capacity to concentrate urine at night
2) nocturia
3) ability to function sexually may continue well into older years

C. **Psychosocial Characteristics of the Healthy Adult**
(see *Nursing Care of the Client with Psychosocial Problems page 15*).

References

Barker, J., Stokes, L., and Billings, D. *Adult and Child Care*. St. Louis: Mosby, 1977.

Beland, I. and Passos, J. *Clinical Nursing*, 3rd Ed. New York: Macmillan, 1975.

Block, G., Nolan, J., and Dempsey, M. *Health Assessment for Professional Nursing: A Development Approach*. New York: Appleton-Century-Crofts, 1981.

Brunner, L. and Suddarth, D. *Textbook of Medical Surgical Nursing*, 4th Ed. Philadelphia: Lippincott, 1980.

Bullough, V. and Bullough, B. *Health Care for the Other Americans*. New York: Appleton-Century-Crofts, 1982.

Caird, F. and Judge, T. *Assessment of the Elderly Patient*. Bath, England: Pitman Press, 1979.

Chambers, C. *Mental Health Aspects of Community Health Nursing*. New York: McGraw-Hill, 1978.

Freiberg, K. *Human Development: A Life Span Approach*. North Scituate, MA: Duxbury Press, 1979.

Mayfield, P., Bond, M., Browning, M., and Evans, J. *Health Assessment*. New York: McGraw-Hill, 1980.

Mezey, M., Rauckhorst, L., and Stikes, S. *Health Assessment of the Older Individual*. New York: Springer, 1980.

Phipps, W., Long, B., and Woods, N. *Shafer's Medical-Surgical Nursing*. St. Louis: Mosby, 1980.

†Roznoy, M. "Taking a Sexual History." *American Journal of Nursing*. August 1976: 1279-1282.

Schmidt, G. "Physical Assessment," in F. Bower, Ed., *Nursing Assessment*. New York: Wiley, 1977.

†"Sensory Changes in the Elderly" (Programmed Instruction). *American Journal of Nursing*. October 1981:1851-1880.

Sorensen, K. and Luckmann, J. *Basic Nursing: A Psychophysiologic Approach*. Philadelphia: Saunders, 1979.

Spector, R. *Cultural Diversity in Health and Illness*. New York: Appleton-Century-Crofts, 1979.

Sullivan, J. *Directions in Community Health Nursing*. Boston: Blackwell, 1984.

† Highly Recommended

Surgery

(The nursing care presented in this unit concerns problems in the care of *adult* clients undergoing surgery.)

A. **Overview**
  1. Surgery is a stressful event.
  2. General Considerations
     a. Dangers are always present for all surgery clients
     b. One complication usually leads to another
     c. Close monitoring is needed
  3. Most Common Types of Complications
     a. Respiratory
        1) atelectasis (air blockage to portion of lung leading to collapse)
        2) hypostatic pneumonia
     b. Circulatory
        1) thrombophlebitis and phlebothrombosis (refer to "Peripheral Vascular Disease" page 193) *[Homan's Sign - calf]*
        2) shock; cardiovascular collapse (refer to "Shock" page 178)
     c. Wound
        1) infection *5-7 days after surgery*
        2) dehiscence (wound separation)
        3) evisceration (separation with protrusion of contents through incision)
        4) hemorrhage
     d. Urinary
        1) retention
        2) oliguria
     e. Gastrointestinal
        1) paralytic ileus (neurogenic disruption of intestine, decreased autonomic innervation, absent peristalsis)
        2) singultus (hiccoughs)
     f. Negative Nitrogen Balance: greater nitrogen excretion than amount ingested
  4. Factors affecting client's response to surgery and development of complications
     a. Age: very old and very young are less able to tolerate stress of surgery
     b. Nutritional status: malnutrition and/or obesity increase risk of poor wound healing
     c. Presence of chronic illnesses
        1) COPD increases risk of pulmonary problems
        2) cardiovascular disease decreases ability to deal with stress of surgery
        3) renal disease increases risk of fluid and electrolyte problems
        4) diabetes mellitus increases risk of poor wound healing
     d. Prolonged immobility after surgery increases risk of thrombophlebitis, abdominal distention, urinary retention, and pulmonary complications
     e. Type of operation: some operations are more frequently associated with complications, e.g., atelectasis after gallbladder surgery.
  5. Each institution has basic admission, preoperative, intraoperative, and postoperative routines. The following content stresses general principles of care that apply to all situations.

B. **Perioperative Period**
  1. General Information
     a. Preoperative care may need to be completed within 1 or 2 hours in an emergency situation or may be given over a longer period for elective surgery.
     b. Postoperative care may be given in recovery room, ICU, or general floor.
     c. Adequate physiologic and psychologic preparation and care are extremely important to the client's successful recovery.
  2. Nursing Process
     a. Assessment
        1) total health status of the client and activities of daily living preoperatively

2) general physical exam preoperatively as described for the healthy adult (if time is limited, focus on cardiovascular, pulmonary, neurologic, renal)
3) postoperative assessment focuses on systems affected by potential complications and surgery
4) diagnostic tests
   a) every client
      - CBC
      - electrolytes
      - urinalysis
      - ECG *over 40*
   b) special considerations
      - type and crossmatch (as necessary)
      - prothrombin time, partial thromboplastin time (PTT), bleeding time and/or clotting time
        – underlying bleeding or coagulation problem
        – receiving anticoagulants or to receive anticoagulants during surgery
        – liver problems or jaundice
      - blood gases and pulmonary function tests (if pulmonary problem is present or pulmonary-cardiovascular surgery is planned)
5) diagnostic tests (post-op) will vary with type of surgery

b. Goals, Plans/Implementation, and Evaluation

Goal 1: Client and significant others will be prepared for surgery.
Plan/Implementation
Day before surgery
- assess learning needs and expectations of surgery
- clarify expectations of surgery
- explain pre-op procedures, post-op routine to client and significant others
- ensure diagnostic tests completed
- evaluate nutritional status
- do skin prep and bowel prep if required
- ensure adequate rest the night before surgery; sedate prn

Day of surgery
- monitor vital signs and report immediately if different from admission vital signs
- have client shower
- remove hairpins, jewelry, medals to avoid loss, injury
- remove prosthetic devices, i.e., dentures, artificial body parts
- apply antithrombosis stockings (TED) as ordered
- have client void immediately before the administration of premedications
- premedicate as ordered
- put side rails up following premedication
- provide quiet environment

Evaluation: Client and significant other can explain surgery; client demonstrates coughing, rests well before surgery; has skin prepared without cuts or scrapes; completed all diagnostic tests.

Goal 2: Client will experience a safe environment in the operating room.
Plan/Implementation
- prepare skin as appropriate
- maintain sterility of equipment and operating team
- prevent static electricity by proper attire, safety of electrical equipment, proper grounding
- position client appropriately
- maintain contact with client during induction (see table 3.1 for types of general anesthetic agents, table 3.2 for regional anesthetic agents, and table 3.3 for stages of anesthesia)
- attend to client during extubation; be prepared to assist as necessary
- promote hemostasis and have appropriate equipment, supplies available (hemostats, ligatures, electrocoagulation, bone wax, styptics, gelatin sponges, cryoprobe, laser beam, saline packs)
- monitor sponge usage; weigh sponges for blood loss as indicated
- measure content of suction bottles; subtract irrigation fluid to approximate blood loss

Evaluation: Client is positioned appropriately; enters operative stage of anesthesia without difficulty; remains stable throughout surgical procedure; is transported to recovery room in stable condition; does not develop any disturbance in circulation (e.g., excess blood loss, signs of shock).

Goal 3: Postoperatively, client's respiratory, circulatory, fluid and

Table 3.1 General Anesthesia

Types	Agents
Inhalation	Gas: oxygen, carbon dioxide, nitrous oxide, cyclopropane Liquid: ethyl ether, halothane (Fluothane), trichloroethylene (Trilene)
Intravenous Adjuncts	• thiopental sodium (Pentothal): CNS depressant • fentanyl & droperidol (Innovar): neuroleptic • ketamine (Ketalar): tranquility and detachment • fentanyl (Sublimaze): analgesic • morphine sulfate, meperidine (Demerol): narcotics • succinylcholine chloride (Anectine): muscular relaxation, depolarizing blocking agent • pancuronium (Pavulon): nondepolarizing agent • neostigmine, edrophonium (Tensilon): antagonistics of nondepolarizing blocking agents

Table 3.2 Regional Anesthesia

Types	Agents

Topical
  blocks peripheral nerves at surface of incised site
Local
  blocks peripheral nerves in subcutaneous tissue at incised site
Field block
  blocks area around incision
Nerve block
  blocks nerves in which conductivity is to be cut off
Spinal
  blocks area beneath diaphragm (anesthetic agents injected into subarachnoid space at 2nd-3rd lumbar space); results in vasodilation (autonomic block), anesthesia (sensory block), muscle paralysis (motor block)
Saddle
  similar to spinal, but area anesthesized is more limited (injection at 3rd-4th lumbar space)
Epidural
  blocks area below the diaphragm (anesthetic injected extradurally)
	• cocaine
	• procaine (Novocain)
	• lidocaine (Xylocaine)
	• mepivacaine (Carbocaine)
	• tetracaine (Pontocaine)
	• bupivacaine (Marcaine)

Table 3.3 Stages of General Anesthesia

Stage	Duration	Manifestations
I	Beginning of induction to loss of consciousness	Loss of judgment powers. Hearing acute.
II	Loss of consciousness to onset of regular breathing	Cerebral or voluntary control lost. Hypersensitive to incoming impulses. Hearing acute.
III	Onset of regular automatic breathing (machinelike), surgery performed during this stage.	Functions of medulla retained.
IV		Respiratory paralysis. Cardiac failure. Death.

Calculation IV Drip →

SURGERY 167

electrolyte, and neurologic status will be optimal.

Plan/Implementation
- monitor vital signs, I&O, IV infusion, electrolytes, drainage tubes, neurologic status, and surgical wound dressing
- report changes to physician
- begin turning, coughing, deep-breathing exercises qh after airway is removed
- monitor respiratory rate, character with vital signs
- suction nasopharynx as needed
- administer respiratory-assistance drugs as ordered
- use blow bottles, inspiratory spirometer as indicated
- give IV therapy, drugs as ordered (see table 3.4 for calculating IV rates)
- use voiding-inducement techniques as necessary
- start oral fluids when appropriate
- keep side rails up until client's neurologic status is normal
- use restraints as necessary

Evaluation: Client's breath sounds are clear; client coughs well; BP remains stable; skin is warm and dry; nail beds blanch briskly; I&O is in balance; IV is infusing appropriately; client is responding appropriately; surgical dressing is dry and intact.

Goal 4: Client will be free from discomfort during the postoperative period.

Plan/Implementation
- position comfortably; turn q2h; begin ROM exercise as appropriate; ambulate to prevent abdominal distention as appropriate
- relieve pain
  - assess
    * source of discomfort
    * location, character, intensity, and duration of pain
    * level of anxiety
    * factors that intensify or decrease discomfort
    * type of anesthetic administered
    * vital signs before and after administration of medication
  - give analgesics as appropriate (see table 3.5 for common analgesics)
  - utilize comfort measures, relaxation, distraction
  - observe client's response to pain-relief measures, e.g., amount, onset, and duration of relief
- prevent nausea and vomiting
  - assess rationale for occurrence (e.g., type of anesthesia, surgery)
  - give antiemetics prn as ordered
  - give frequent oral hygiene

Evaluation: Client's pain is relieved; offers no complaints of nausea.

C. Discharge
1. **General Information:** discharge planning starts at admission
2. **Nursing Process**
   a. Assessment
      1) client's ability to do self-care at home
      2) significant others
      3) home situation
   b. Goal, Plan/Implementation, and Evaluation

Goal: Client and significant others are prepared for client's discharge.

Plan/Implementation
- determine discharge date with consultation with physician
- teach client and significant other as appropriate re: medications, return appointment, treatments, activity, diet
- refer to appropriate community health agency

Evaluation: Client can state time of return appointment, medicines to take and how.

Table 3.4 Calculating IV Rates

$$\frac{\text{amount of IV fluid (ml)}}{\text{time to infuse (min)}} \times \text{drip factor (gtt/ml)} = \text{IV rate (gtt/min)}$$

Example: The order is for 1,000 ml D_5W to run for 10 hours. The drip factor is 15 gtt/ml.

$$\frac{1,000 \text{ ml}}{600 \text{ min} \ (60 \times 10)} \times \frac{15 \text{ gtt}}{1 \text{ ml}} = \text{IV rate of 25 gtt/min}$$

Table 3.5 Analgesics

Nonnarcotic

Description	Drugs that act to decrease pain, often through antiinflammatory actions, without the side effects of narcotics. The major drugs are either salicylates (aspirin) or para-aminophenols (acetaminophen)
Uses	Relief of mild to moderate pain
Side Effects	*Salicylates:* salicylism (headache, nausea, vomiting, palpitations, hyperventilation), hypersensitivity reaction, GI distress and bleeding, anticoagulant effect, liver damage *Acetaminophen:* hypersensitivity, CNS stimulation, liver damage, renal damage, palpitations
Nursing Implications	Avoid use of salicylates in clients with GI disorders, antiinflammatory or anticoagulant therapy, or history of aspirin sensitivity; avoid overuse; keep supply away from children; monitor liver and renal function; warn client to avoid over-the-counter medicines that contain "hidden" aspirin.
Types and Examples	*Salicylates:* acetylsalicylic acid (aspirin) *Para-aminophenols:* acetaminophen (Tylenol, Datril, Anacin-3) *Others:* naproxen (Anaprox), ibuprofen (Motrin)

Narcotic

Description	Drugs that act to decrease pain by inhibiting the transmission of pain impulses, reducing cortical responses to pain stimuli, or altering activity in the pain-perception areas of the brain
Uses	Treatment of moderate to severe pain
Side Effects	Drowsiness, dizziness or lightheadedness, euphoria, respiratory depression, constipation, urinary retention, hypersensitivity reactions, hypotension
Nursing Implications	Monitor effectiveness of analgesia; watch for hypotension and respiratory depression; monitor I&O, bowel movements; prevent respiratory depression; watch for possible tolerance and dependence.
Examples	Morphine, oxymorphone (Numorphan), meperidine HCl (Demerol), codeine, methadone (Dolophine), butorphanol tartrate (Stadol), propoxyphene hydrochloride (Darvon)

References

Bushong, M. "Principles of Post Anesthetic Management: Criteria for Patient Discharge." *Current Reviews for Recovery Room Nurses.* 1979:73-80.

DiBlasi, M. and Washburn, C. "The Management of Pain; Using Analgesics Effectively." *American Journal of Nursing.* January 1979:74-78.

Dziuurbejko, M. and Larkin, J. "Including the Family in Preoperative Teaching." *American Journal of Nursing.* November 1978:1892-1894.

*Heidrich, G., Perry, S. "Helping the Patient in Pain." *American Journal of Nursing.* December 1983:1828-1833.

Long, B., Gowon, C., and Bushong, M. "Surgical Intervention." In Phipps, W. et al, *Medical-Surgical Nursing: Concepts and Clinical Practice*, 2nd Ed. St. Louis: Mosby, 1983:401-462.

Marcinek, M. "Stress in the Surgical Patient." *American Journal of Nursing.* October 1977:1809-1811.

* See reprint section

McConnell, E. "Be Prepared for Double Trouble if your Surgical Patient's a Diabetic." *Nursing 81*. November 1981:118-123.

Metheny, N. and Shirley, W. "Perioperative Fluids and Electrolytes." *American Journal of Nursing*. May 1978:840-845.

Nursing Grand Rounds. "Postoperative: How to Help the Patient When Everything Goes Wrong." *Nursing 81*. March 1981:50-55.

Patras, A. "The Operation's Over but the Danger's Not." *Nursing 82*. September 1982:50-56.

Steele, B. "Test Your Knowledge of Postoperative Pain Management." *Nursing 80*. March 1980:76-78.

Schuman, P. "How to Help Wound Healing in Your Abdominal Surgery Patient." *Nursing 80*. April 1980:34-40.

ABG's → *Central venous pressure —, 0*

Oxygenation

(The nursing care presented in this unit concerns selected health problems related to disturbances in the cardiovascular and respiratory systems.)

General Concepts
A. Overview
1. The cardinal purpose of the cardiovascular and respiratory systems is to provide adequate oxygenation to the body as a whole
   a. Respiratory system: responsible for the intake of oxygen (O_2), elimination of carbon dioxide (CO_2); plays a major role in maintaining acid-base balance
   b. Cardiovascular system: responsible for the transport of O_2, CO_2, nutrients, and waste products
2. The heart is a high-energy pump, which forcefully ejects blood with enough pressure to profuse the pulmonary and peripheral capillary beds
3. Flow of blood through the heart: inferior and superior vena cava → right atrium → tricuspid valve → right ventricle → pulmonic valve → pulmonary arteries → lungs → pulmonary veins → left atrium → mitral valve → left ventricle → aortic valve → aorta → systemic circulation
4. Blood returning to the right side of the heart is unoxygenated, venous blood. Blood ejected into the systemic circulation from the left side of the heart is oxygenated, arterial blood.
5. The heart is surrounded by a sac of fibrous tissue known as the pericardium. Between the pericardium and epicardium there is a small space that contains a few drops of fluid that lubricate the heart surface.
6. The heart itself is composed of three layers
   a. Epicardium: outer layer; coronary arteries lie on this surface (this layer is structurally the same as the visceral pericardium)
   b. Myocardium: middle layer; cardiac muscle activity originates here
   c. Endocardium: inner layer; lines the valves, chordae tendineae, and papillary muscles
7. The cardiac impulse originates in the sinoatrial (SA) node, then travels to the right and left atria → atria contract. The impulse reaches the atrioventricular (AV) node and accelerates through the bundle of His, bundle branches, and Purkinje's fibers. These fibers distribute the impulse rapidly and evenly over the ventricles → ventricles contract. The conduction process is controlled by the autonomic nervous system
   a. sympathetic stimulation increases the heart rate
   b. parasympathetic or vagal stimulation decreases the heart rate
8. Adequate blood flow through the vital organs must be maintained at all times. The mean arterial blood pressure is the driving force for blood flow through all the organs.
9. Mean Arterial Pressure = Cardiac Output x Total Peripheral Resistance
   Cardiac Output = Stroke Volume (amount of blood ejected/beat) x Heart Rate
   Arterial pressure can be increased by increasing cardiac output (either stroke volume, heart rate, or both), or by increasing total peripheral resistance. Both cardiac output and total peripheral resistance are influenced by a variety of

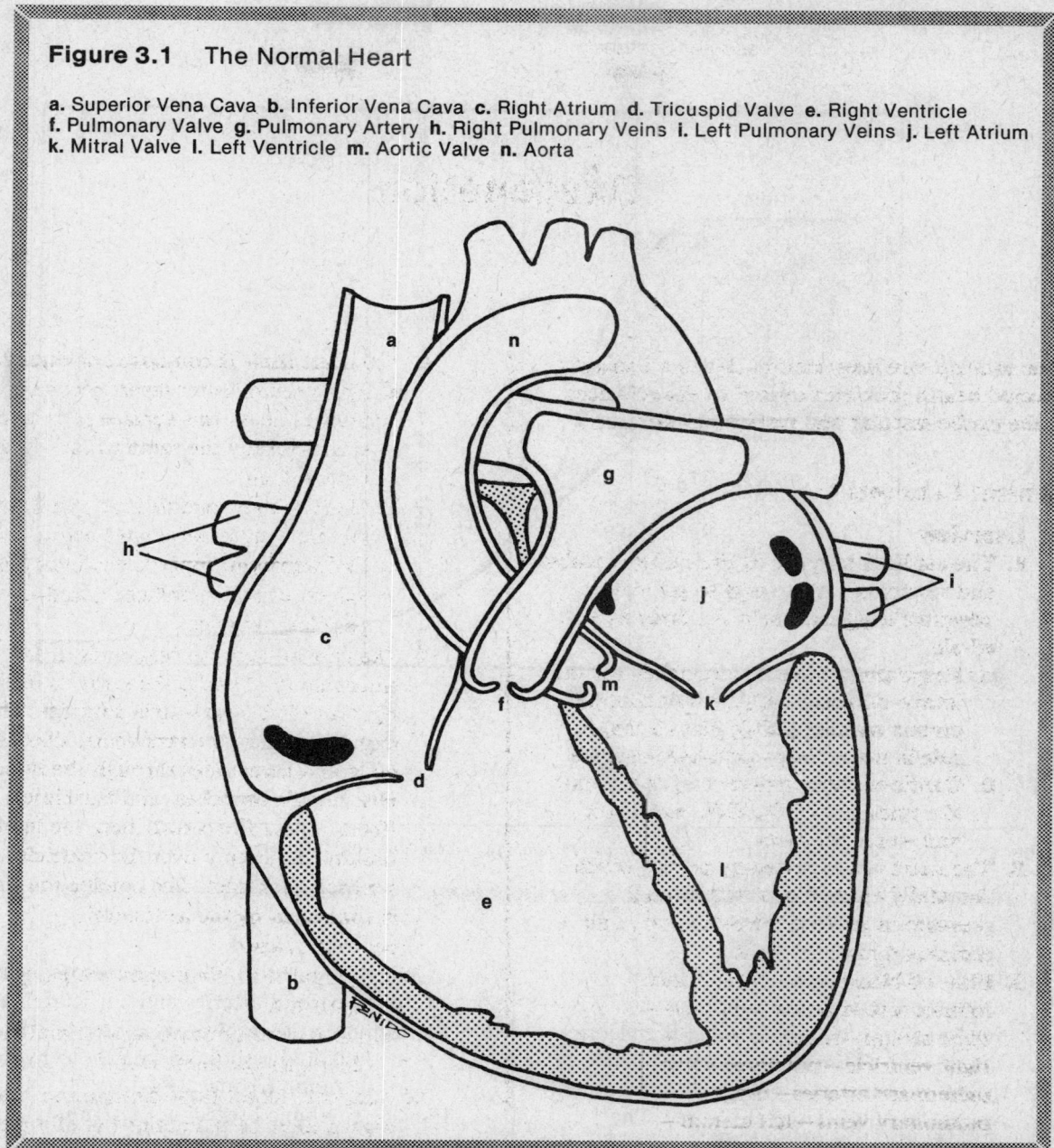

Figure 3.1 The Normal Heart

a. Superior Vena Cava b. Inferior Vena Cava c. Right Atrium d. Tricuspid Valve e. Right Ventricle
f. Pulmonary Valve g. Pulmonary Artery h. Right Pulmonary Veins i. Left Pulmonary Veins j. Left Atrium
k. Mitral Valve l. Left Ventricle m. Aortic Valve n. Aorta

factors, particularly the activity of the sympathetic nervous system, which can increase heart rate, stroke volume, and total peripheral resistance.

10. The blood pressure varies throughout the circulation: greatest in the arterial system; lowest in the venous portion (see figure 3.2). Central venous pressure (CVP) is the pressure within the right atrium; normal: 4–10 mm Hg.

11. The respiratory system is composed of upper and lower airway structures

　　a. The upper airway consists of the nose and nasopharynx, mouth, oropharynx, and the larynx
　　b. The lower airway is composed of the trachea, mainstem bronchi, bronchioles, alveolar ducts, and terminal alveoli
　　c. The airways not only provide a passageway for air but also serve to filter, warm, and humidify inspired air

12. The lungs lie in and are protected by the thoracic cavity. This bony cage is composed of sternum and ribs anteriorly,

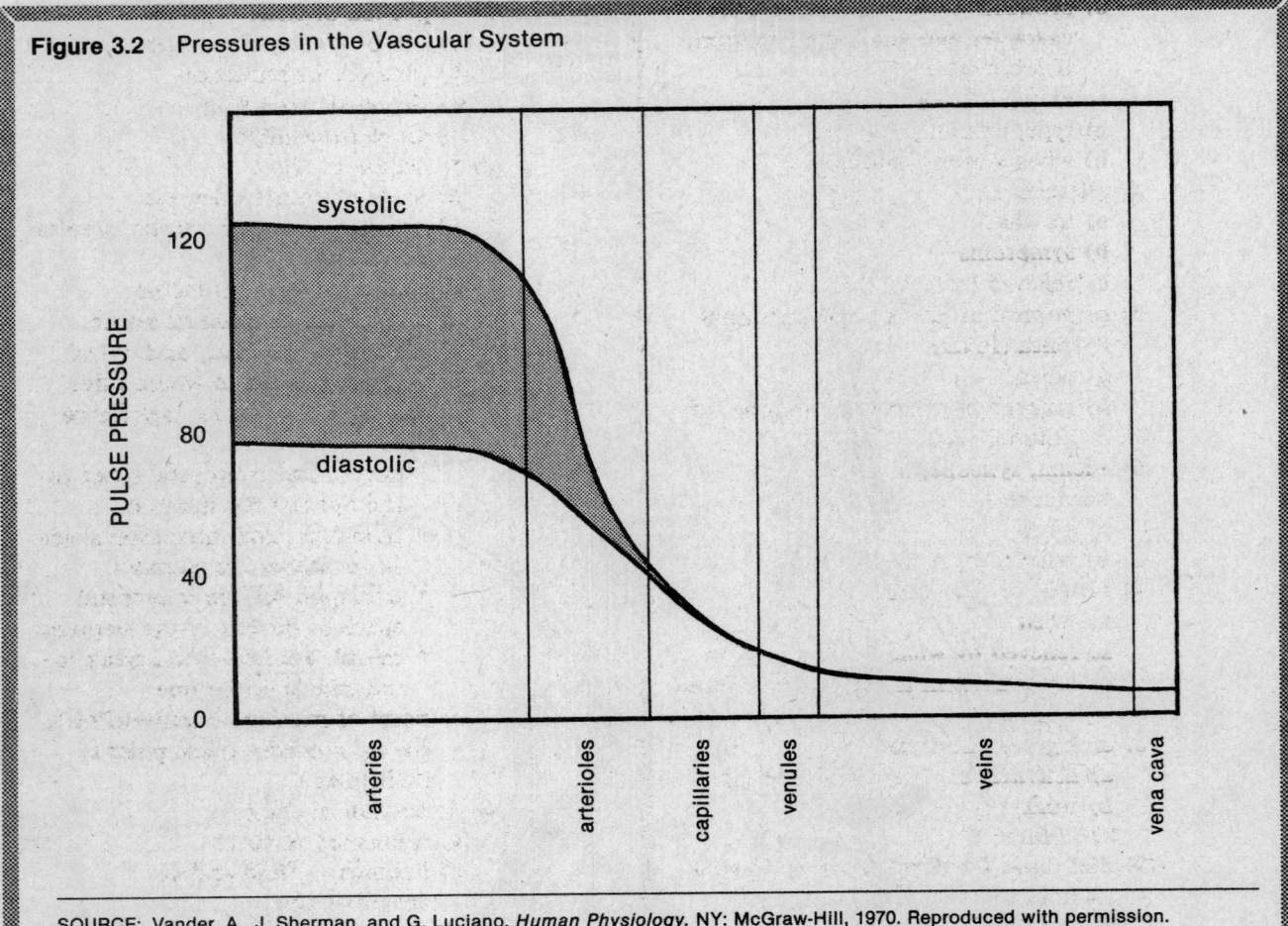

Figure 3.2 Pressures in the Vascular System

SOURCE: Vander, A., J. Sherman, and G. Luciano, *Human Physiology*. NY: McGraw-Hill, 1970. Reproduced with permission.

and the ribs, scapulae, and vertebral column posteriorly. The thoracic cavity is lined with a serous membrane, the pleura; one surface of the pleura lines the inside of the rib cage (parietal pleura) and the other covers the lungs (visceral pleura). The pleural space (which is really a potential space) exists between the surfaces of the two pleurae. Subatmospheric pressure in the pleural space is responsible for the continued expansion of the lungs.

13. The basic gas-exchange unit of the respiratory system is the alveolus. Pulmonary capillaries lie adjacent to each alveolus; through the process of diffusion, the exchange of O_2 and CO_2 takes place across the alveolar-capillary membrane.

14. The neural control of respirations is located in the medulla. Under normal conditions, this center is stimulated directly or reflexly by the concentration of CO_2 in the blood (Pco_2). Chemoreceptors located in the carotid arteries and aortic arch also stimulate the respiratory center of the medulla and respond primarily to hypoxia in the blood (reduced Po_2).

15. The rhythmic breathing pattern is dependent on the cyclical excitation of the respiratory muscles by the phrenic nerve (to the diaphragm) and the intercostal nerves (to the intercostal muscles).

B. Application of the Nursing Process to the Client with Oxygenation Problems
   1. Assessment
      a. Health History
         1) dyspnea or chest pain/discomfort
            a) when (e.g., rest, activity)
            b) relieved by what
         2) cough
            a) when

b) productive/nonproductive; note character and amount of sputum, if productive
3) smoking
   a) type, amount, duration
   b) when stopped, duration
4) allergies
   a) to what?
   b) symptoms
   c) relieved by what
5) orthopnea or paroxysmal nocturnal dyspnea (PND)
   a) when
   b) relieved by what (e.g., number of pillows, rest)
6) edema, syncope, dizziness, or headache
   a) when
   b) relieved by what
7) fatigue or weakness
   a) when
   b) relieved by what
   c) compare with client's normal level of exercise
8) changes in life-style
   a) activities of daily living (ADL)
   b) work
   c) leisure
9) diet (have the client describe previous 24-hour intake)
   a) restrictions (e.g., sodium, cholesterol)
   b) difficulties complying with prescribed diet
   c) alcohol intake
   d) food preferences/intolerances
   e) who shops/prepares meals
10) medications (prescription and nonprescription)
   a) dose
   b) side effects
   c) effectiveness
11) personal or family history
   a) pulmonary problems (e.g., tuberculosis, pneumonia, asthma)
   b) cardiac problems (e.g., angina, myocardial infarction, hypertension)

b. Physical examination
  1) vital signs
   a) blood pressure: lying/sitting/standing, and in both arms
   b) pulse: rate and rhythm
   c) respirations: rate, depth, effort
   d) temperature

2) inspection of chest
   a) use of accessory muscles
   b) presence of retraction
   c) degree of excursion
   d) chest deformity
3) palpation of chest
   a) areas of pain/tenderness
   b) presence of carotid thrills, atypical pulsation
   c) change in tactile fremitus
   d) anatomical landmarks: aortic, pulmonic, tricuspid, and mitral area correspond to where valve closing is the loudest (see figure 3.3)
     • aortic: 2nd intercostal space to the right of the sternum
     • pulmonic: 2nd intercostal space to the left of the sternum
     • tricuspid: 4th-5th intercostal space to the left of the sternum
     • mitral: 5th intercostal space in the midclavicular line
   e) point of maximal impulse (PMI); for most clients apical pulse is their PMI
4) percussion of chest:
   a) resonance = air
   b) dullness = fluid and/or consolidation

Figure 3.3 Areas of Auscultation of Heart Valves

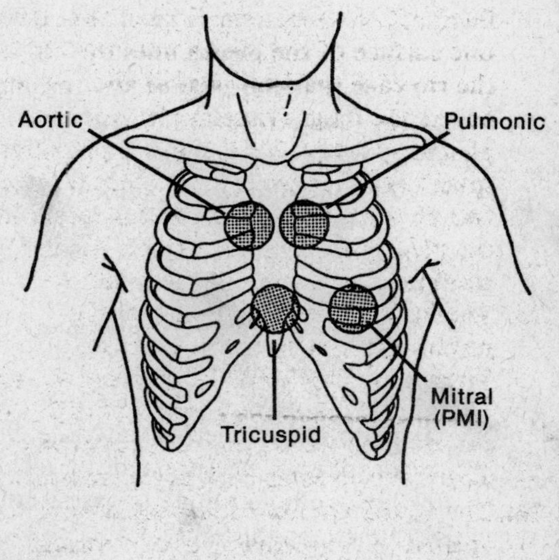

174 SECTION 3: NURSING CARE OF THE ADULT

5) auscultation of the lungs
   a) normal breath sounds
   b) abnormal breath sounds
      - rales
        - high-pitched crackling
        - caused by air passing through abnormal secretions in alveoli
      - rhonchi
        - loud, coarse gurgling
        - caused by air passing through abnormal secretions in bronchi
      - wheezing
        - high-pitched whistling
        - caused by air passing through narrowed bronchi
6) auscultation of the heart
   a) apical pulse (see figure 3.3)
      - rate and rhythm
      - pulse deficit = apical minus radial pulse (*NOTE:* the two pulses must be taken at the same time by *two* practitioners)
   b) normal heart sounds
      - S₁ (lub)
        - closing of mitral and tricuspid valves
        - at onset of ventricular systole
      - S₂ (dub)
        - closing of aortic and pulmonary valves
        - at onset of ventricular diastole
   c) extra heart sounds
      - S₃, S₄
        - abnormal in adults
        - sometimes normal in children and young adults
      - murmurs: caused by turbulent blood flow
7) skin and extremities
   a) skin color, e.g., pallor, cyanosis, rubor
   b) skin temperature
   c) edema
   d) peripheral pulses: presence, strength, equality

c. Diagnostic Tests
   1) pulmonary function tests: the direct or indirect measurement of various lung volumes; done to assess lung function; see figure 3.4
      a) *tidal volume* (TV): volume of gas inspired and expired with a quiet normal breath (500 cc)
      b) *inspiratory reserve volume* (IRV) maximal volume that can be inspired at the end of a normal inspiration (3,100 cc)
      c) *expiratory reserve volume* (ERV): maximal volume that can be forcefully exhaled after a normal expiration (1,200 cc)
      d) *residual volume* (RV): volume of gas left in lung after maximal expiration (1,200 cc)
      e) *minute volume* (MV): volume of gas inspired and expired in 1 minute of normal breathing (6 liters per minute)
      f) *vital capacity* (VC) maximal amount of air that can be expired after a maximal inspiration (TV + IRV + ERV) (4,800 cc)
   2) sputum specimens
      a) examinations
         - culture and sensitivity
         - cytology
      b) nursing care
         - collect specimen in morning
         - collect sterile specimen
         - collect sputum, not saliva
   3) chest x-rays/tomograms
   4) lung scan: following injection of radioactive material, lung is scanned for presence of obstruction or areas that are poorly perfused
   5) bronchoscopy
      a) insertion of a rigid or flexible fiberoptic bronchoscope through the oral cavity into the bronchus in order to visualize the area; bronchial brushing, biopsy, or bronchogram may be done during the procedure
      b) nursing care
         - preparation
           - explain procedure
           - NPO 6–12 hours
           - oral hygiene
           - remove dentures
           - premedicate
         - postprocedure
           - NPO until gag reflex returns
           - observe respirations
           - observe hoarseness, dysphagia
           - observe for subcutaneous emphysema (crackling under the skin when pressed, caused by air from perforated airway)

OXYGENATION **175**

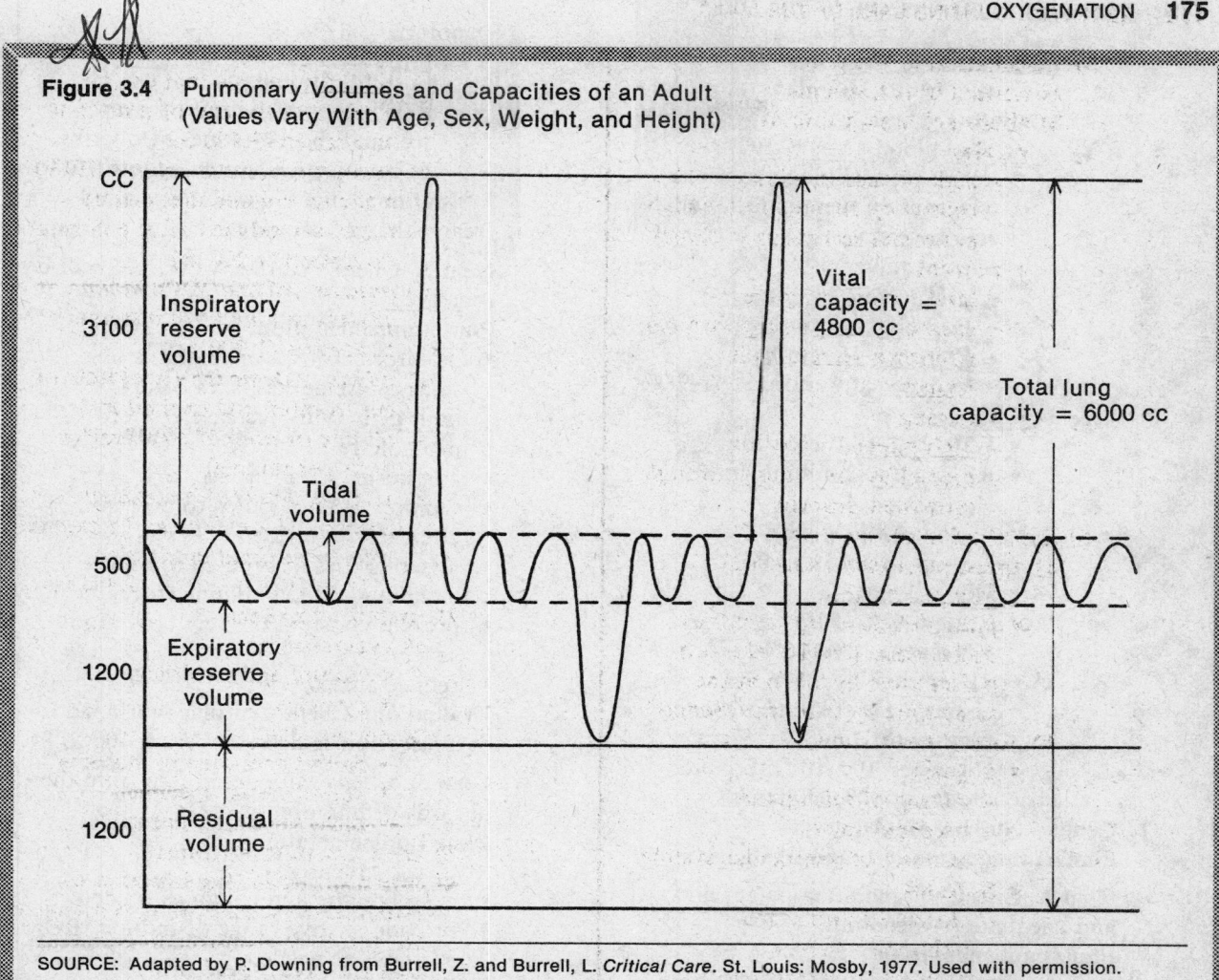

Figure 3.4 Pulmonary Volumes and Capacities of an Adult (Values Vary With Age, Sex, Weight, and Height)

SOURCE: Adapted by P. Downing from Burrell, Z. and Burrell, L. *Critical Care*. St. Louis: Mosby, 1977. Used with permission.

- bloody sputum normal after biopsy
6) myocardial scan: following injection of radioactive thallium, heart is scanned to detect areas of the myocardium that are poorly perfused
7) ECG
   a) resting-12-lead
   b) exercise (stress test)
      - treadmill or bicycle
      - ECG shows cardiac function during exercise
8) echocardiography: cardiac wall motion is visualized by ultrasound
9) cardiac catheterization/angiography
   a) under local anesthesia and fluoroscopy, catheters are inserted into the femoral or brachial artery. The injection of radiopaque dye permits visualization of the coronary arteries, ventricular contractility, and patency of the valves; pressures are also recorded.
   b) nursing care
      - preparation
        - explain procedure
        - NPO 6–12 hours
        - take and record pulses/temperature of all extremities
        - check for allergy to iodine
      - postprocedure
        - monitor pulse/temperature in area below catheterization site (spasms/emboli can cause these to diminish or disappear; emboli formation requires immediate intervention)
        - prevent stress on incision line (no bending, no ambulation for 12–24 hours if femoral site)
        - use pressure dressing

postural drainage

176 SECTION 3: NURSING CARE OF THE ADULT

10) hematologic studies: normal values will vary slightly from laboratory to laboratory
   a) arterial blood gases (ABG)
      - test of arterial blood to assess oxygenation, ventilation, and acid-base status
      - normal values
        - pH: 7.35–7.45
        - Po_2: 80–100 mm Hg
        - Pco_2: 35–45 mm Hg
        - % Hgb saturation: 95%–98%
   b) CBC
      - WBC: 5,000–10,000/mm³
      - RBC: 4.2–6.2 million/mm³
      - Hgb
        - men: 14–18 g/dl
        - women: 12–16 g/dl
      - Hct
        - men: 42%–54%
        - women: 38%–46%
   c) electrolytes
      - sodium: 135–145 mEq/liter
      - potassium: 3.8–5.5 mEq/liter
      - chlorides: 100–108 mEq/liter
   d) cholesterol: 120–330 mg/dl

2. **General Nursing Goals, Plans/Implementation, and Evaluation**

Goal 1: Client will maintain patent airway and adequate oxygenation.
Plan/Implementation
- monitor respiratory status (e.g., vital signs, breath sounds, skin color)
- reduce anxiety
- limit/space activities to decrease O_2 need
- turn frequently if on bed rest
- place in Fowler's position to increase air exchange
- humidify air
- administer O_2 as needed
- cough and deep breath frequently
- avoid sedatives that depress respirations and cough reflex (e.g., narcotics)
- force fluids to liquefy secretions
- suction as needed; provide hyperventilation before and after suctioning to decrease chances of hypoxia
- carry out postural drainage, clapping, and vibration if needed
  - give humidified air or bronchodilators 10–15 minutes before
  - no longer than 15 minutes at one time
  - clapping/vibration can be done with postural drainage
  - avoid clapping/vibrating over sternum, breast tissue, below ribs
  - to be effective, coughing must follow

Evaluation: Client is well oxygenated (Po_2 greater than 60 mm Hg).

Goal 2: Client's cardiac work load will be decreased.
Plan/Implementation
- monitor cardiovascular status (e.g., vital signs, pulse deficit, skin color)
- limit activity to decrease O_2 need
- promote rest
- administer O_2 as needed
- monitor I&O of fluids to prevent circulatory overload
- give diuretics as ordered to reduce circulating blood volume (see table 3.16)
- prevent constipation (e.g., use stool softeners)
- reduce anxiety

Evaluation: Client's cardiac workload is decreased; pulse decreases from 100 to 84.

Goal 3: Client will remain free from the hazards of immobility.
Plan/Implementation
- turn frequently
- deep breathe and cough as needed
- provide passive range-of-motion (ROM) exercises as needed
- teach client ankle flexion/extension exercises
- give good back care
- apply T.E.D. hose
- give anticoagulants if ordered

Evaluation: Client remains free from thrombophlebitis, decubitus ulcers, pulmonary consolidation.

Selected Health Problems Resulting in Interference with Oxygenation

A. Cardiopulmonary Arrest   *ABC's*

1. **General Information**
   a. Definition: complete failure of the heart and lungs to adequately perfuse and ventilate; it is a medical emergency
   b. Classification: medical emergency

2. **Nursing Process**
   a. **Assessment**
      1) *a*irway
      2) *b*reathing, respiratory effort
      3) *c*irculation: carotid or femoral pulse

b. Goals, Plans/Implementation, and Evaluation

Goal 1: Client will have an open airway and receive adequate ventilation.

Plan/Implementation
- clear airway of foreign matter if present
- hyperextend neck to open airway
- watch for breathing
- give 4 quick, full breaths, if not breathing
- use Heimlich's maneuver to clear airway, if unable to ventilate
- ventilate mouth to mouth
- rate: 12/minute if carotid pulse present
- if available
  - use airway and Ambu bag
  - administer O_2

Evaluation: Client is well oxygenated (e.g., has normal skin color; Po_2 and Pco_2 within normal limits).

Goal 2: Client will circulate adequately oxygenated blood.

Plan/Implementation
- check carotid pulse
- begin cardiac massage, if carotid pulse absent
- depress sternum 1½–2 inches
- compression rate: 60/minute
- 1 person: 15 compressions/2 ventilations; 2 persons: 5 compressions/1 ventilation
- continue CPR until spontaneous respirations and pulse return
- if available
  - monitor ECG
  - defibrillation if needed

Evaluation: Client has carotid pulsation with each compression; maintains BP of at least 100 systolic.

Goal 3: Client will receive appropriate emergency drugs.

Plan/Implementation
- obtain cart with emergency drugs
- insert IV for drug administration
- administer emergency drugs as needed (see table 3.6 for common emergency drugs)
- record accurately all drugs given

Table 3.6 Emergency Drugs*

Name	Indications
Atropine sulfate	Bradycardia.
Bretylium tosylate (Bretylol)	Ventricular dysrhythmias unresponsive to lidocaine.
Calcium chloride	Asystole and electromechanical dissociation; to counteract the effects of hyperkalemia on the heart.
Dobutamine HCl (Dobutrex)	To increase cardiac contractility.
Dopamine HCl (Intropin)	To increase BP; in small doses improves renal perfusion.
Epinephrine	Asystole and ventricular fibrillation; to increase heart rate, cardiac output, and BP (beta- and alpha-receptor stimulant).
Isoproterenol HCl (Isuprel)	To increase heart rate and thus BP (beta-receptor stimulant).
Lidocaine HCl (Xylocaine)	PVCs and ventricular tachycardia.
Procainamide HCl (Pronestyl)	PVCs and ventricular fibrillation when lidocaine is not effective.
Sodium bicarbonate	To reverse metabolic acidosis during cardiac arrest.
Verapamil (Calan)	Supraventricular tachydysrhythmias (calcium blocker).

*Drugs that should be readily available for all emergencies

178 SECTION 3: NURSING CARE OF THE ADULT

Evaluation: Client received appropriate doses of ordered drugs; cumulative totals were accurately recorded.

B. Shock

1. **General Information**
   a. Definition: a syndrome associated with abnormal cellular metabolism; the common pathology in all shock is failure of perfusion of O_2 and nutrients at the cellular level
   b. Causes
      1) hemodynamic disturbances of the
         a) heart
         b) blood vessels
         c) blood volume
      2) disturbances within cells
   c. Etiologic Classifications
      1) hypovolemic (decreased volume)
      2) cardiogenic (inadequate pump)
      3) neurogenic (pooling due to vasodilation)
      4) septic (infective organisms cause impairment of the cell membrane, thus preventing uptake of nutrients, O_2, etc.; release of toxins may cause vasoconstriction of precapillary sphincters and shunting of blood around capillary beds; a relative hypovolemia, resulting from the leakage of fluids and plasma into injected or inflamed areas, may be present in some clients)
      5) anaphylactic (release of histamine and related substances causing massive capillary vasodilation)
   d. Precipitating Factors
      1) anaphylactic reactions
      2) infections, particularly gram negative
      3) spinal anesthesia
      4) spinal cord trauma
      5) myocardial infarction
      6) pulmonary emboli
      7) dysrhythmias
      8) hemorrhage
      9) burns
      10) GI loss of fluid and electrolytes
   e. Body's Response to Shock
      1) stimulation of the adrenal medulla by the sympathetic nervous system
         a) tachycardia
         b) tachypnea leading to respiratory alkalosis
         c) vasoconstriction
         d) redistribution of blood
         e) thirst; cool, clammy skin; oliguria; decreased bowel sounds
      2) stimulation of renin-angiotensin-aldosterone system and ADH
         a) decreased urine volume
         b) increased concentration of urine
      3) stimulation of cortisol and growth hormone secretion
         a) increased glucose metabolism
         b) increased fat mobilization

2. **Nursing Process**
   a. Assessment
      1) identify high-risk client: very young or old, clients with GU infections who undergo cystoscopy, post-MI with severe dysrhythmias and/or no pain control, adrenocortical problems, severe GI loss, hemorrhage (recent postoperative GI bleeding), burns, known allergic reactions, massive or overwhelming infections
      2) vital signs: tachycardia, tachypnea; early BP may be normal due to compensatory mechanisms but will decrease later
      3) mental status: restless, early increased alertness but as hypoxia occurs → decreased alertness → lethargy, coma
      4) skin changes
         a) cool, clammy skin seen early if hypovolemia and/or cardiac dysfunction are present
         b) flushed, cool if vasodilation present (as in neurogenic shock)
         c) flushed, warm in early septic shock and then cool, clammy
      5) fluid status: check skin turgor, I&O, urine specific gravity, CVP
   b. **Goals, Plans/Implementation, and Evaluation**

Goal 1: Client will remain free from any undetected change in cellular perfusion.
Plan/Implementation (high-risk client)
- assess vital signs q4h; more frequently if unstable
- measure I&O at least q8h; qh if unstable
- note skin turgor, temperature, color q8h
- monitor ECG if dysrhythmias present
- obtain blood work as appropriate (CBC, electrolytes, BUN, creatinine, blood gases)

Evaluation: Client maintains stable vital signs, fluid balance; no signs of impending shock.

Goal 2: Client will have adequate perfusion.
Plan/Implementation
- monitor blood pressure (mean should be at least 80), pulse, respiration
- note and report any dysrhythmias
- monitor CVP (normal = 4–10 cm H₂O); measure the same way each time
- maintain output at least at 30 ml/h min. and equal to intake
- monitor mental status
- monitor GI function
- administer fluids as ordered: blood, colloid fluids, or electrolyte solutions as necessary (until CVP = 16–19 cm H₂O)
- administer drugs only after client's circulating volume is returned to normal (table 3.6)
    - vasopressors/adrenergic stimulants (epinephrine, dopamine, dobutamine, norepinephrine [Levophed], isoproterenol [Isuprel]) cause vasoconstriction and/or increase heart rate to increase perfusion
        * administer with a controlled-volume regulator
        * monitor BP q15min continually
        * wean off drugs as soon as possible
        * know that some of these drugs cause severe vasoconstriction and can worsen organ damage (renal failure, hepatic failure)
        * watch for extravasation of vasopressors (if Levophed extravasates, infiltrate around area with regitine)
        * titrate drug infusion to keep BP at a mean of 80, or as ordered
    - since vasopressors cause severe vasoconstriction, some clinicians use vasodilators (nitroprusside, hydralazine) with vasopressors
    - when using vasopressors and vasodilators together
        * if BP drops, decrease vasodilator first; then increase vasopressor
        * if BP increases, decrease vasopressor and then increase vasodilator
    - administer other drugs if ordered, e.g., cardiac glycosides to enhance cardiac contractility (see table 3.15)
- position in modified Trendelenburg's (feet up 45° and head flat or Fowler's, if client unable to tolerate flat bed)

Evaluation: Client's BP is maintained at a mean of 80 mm Hg.

Goal 3: Client will have adequate O₂/CO₂ levels. O₂ – 80–100 CO₂ – 35–45
Plan/Implementation
- see General Nursing Goals page 176
- provide comfort measures (*NOTE*: if giving pain medications, do not use IM or subcutaneous route since medications may accumulate and not be absorbed; when perfusion improves, client may get overdose)
- temperature: keep room warm, not hot or cold (heat causes sweating; cold causes shivering)

Evaluation: Client is well oxygenated (Po₂ greater than 60 mm Hg; no air hunger or cyanosis).

Goal 4: Client will be protected from injury, complications.
Plan/Implementation
- keep side rails up; if client confused, watch carefully, avoid restraints
- apply T.E.D. stockings to prevent venous stasis
- turn frequently to prevent decubitus ulcers, pulmonary problems
- use sterile technique with all procedures (changing IVs, suctioning) since client has decreased resistance to infection

Evaluation: Client is free from preventable complications (e.g., falls, infections).

C. Angina Pectoris

1. **General Information**
    a. Definition: chest pain caused by temporary ischemia of the myocardium
    b. Risk Factors (coronary artery disease)
        1) *hypertension:* increased arterial resistance makes the heart work harder
        2) *hyperlipidemia:* increased lipid levels in the blood increase chances of plaque formation
        3) *smoking:* nicotine causes spasms of the arteries
        4) *obesity:* increases workload of the heart
        5) *diabetes:* causes premature arteriosclerosis
        6) *high stress:* stimulation of sympathetic nervous system resulting in spasms of arteries

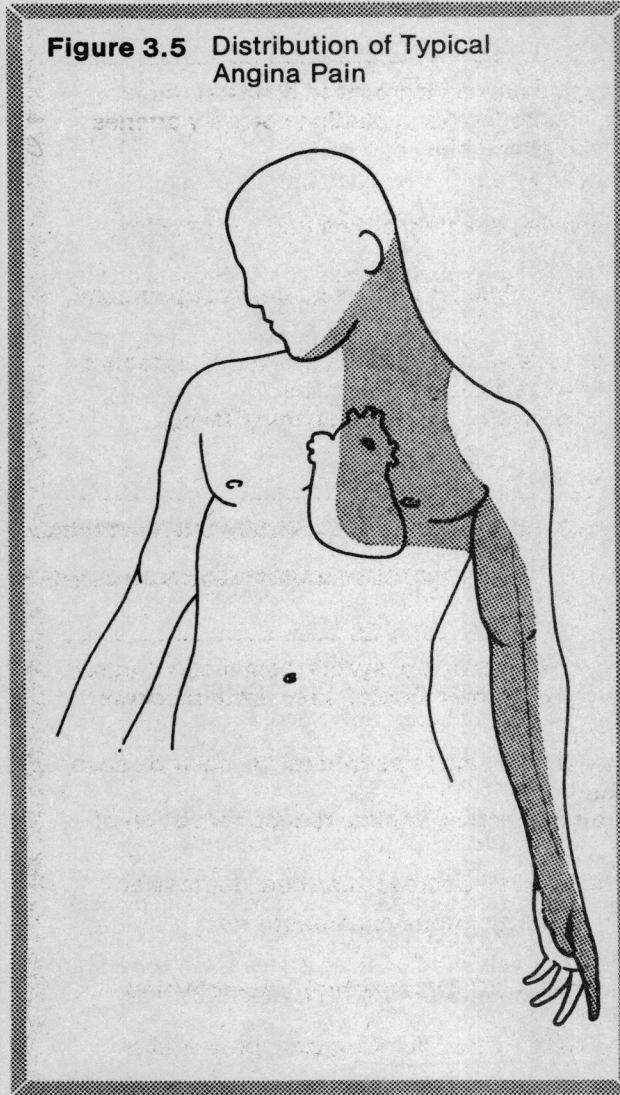

Figure 3.5 Distribution of Typical Angina Pain

7) *sedentary life-style:* heart is not conditioned; nor is there development of collateral circulation
8) *family history* (risk factor that cannot be modified)
9) *sex:* male (risk factor that cannot be modified)

c. Precipitating Factors (immediate): five "E"s
  1) *exercise*
  2) *exertion:* arteries are able to provide blood to myocardium at rest, but an increased demand on coronary circulation cannot be met temporarily
  3) *emotions:* stimulate sympathetic nervous system→increased demand on heart
  4) *eating a heavy meal:* increased perfusion of the gastrointestinal tract for digestion; pressure from full stomach against diaphragm
  5) *exposure to cold*

2. Nursing Process
   a. Assessment
     1) precipitating factor(s)
     2) pain
       a) pattern varies with each individual, but is usually the same for a specific person
       b) usually retrosternal
       c) tends to radiate into neck, jaw, shoulder, and down inner aspect of left arm
       d) short duration
       e) usually relieved by rest, immobility, relief of stress, increased warmth, and nitroglycerin
     3) ECG changes (if any): ST segment depression and T wave inversion on stress ECG
   b. Goals, Plans/Implementation, and Evaluation

   Goal 1: Client will have improved perfusion of the myocardium.
   Plan/Implementation
   - give coronary vasodilating drugs (see table 3.7)
   - know side effects of these drugs, e.g., generalized vasodilation

   Evaluation: Client is able to do daily activities without pain by spacing activities or by taking nitroglycerin tablet prior to bathing, eating, taking daily walks, or taking part in conferences.

   Goal 2: Client will learn methods to prevent attacks and be able to state what he should do.
   Plan/Implementation
   - teach client
     - to recognize symptoms; client's own pattern
     - to take medications and cope with side effects
       - when to take medications (e.g., before activity)
     - to avoid precipitating factors if possible
     - to change life-style to decrease risk factors, e.g., diet, smoking
     - to reduce cholesterol and fats to prevent further atherosclerosis (see table 3.13)

Table 3.7 Coronary Vasodilators

Description	Drugs that act on blood vessels to cause an increase in diameter, thereby improving blood flow. They are most effective in dilating coronary arteries and less effective dilating peripheral vessels.
Uses	Antianginal (most common)
Side Effects	Generalized vasodilatation (headache, flushing, orthostatic hypotension, tachycardia)
Nursing Implications	Know correct route and schedule of administration, e.g., prn vs regular, oral, sublingual, or transdermal.
Types and Examples	*Nitrites/Nitrates:* amyl nitrate (Vaporade), nitroglycerin (Nitro-Bid), isosorbide dinitrate (Isordil SL); pentaerythritol tetranitrate (Peritrate) *Calcium Channel Blockers:* nifedipine (Procardia), verapamil (Calan), diatiazem (Cardizem) *Peripheral Vasodilators:* papaverine HCl (Pavabid)

Table 3.8 Adrenergic Blockers

Description	Drugs that act as antagonists to the actions of sympathomimetic drugs. Alpha-blockers act on postsynaptic alpha-receptor sites. Beta-blockers act on the beta-receptor sites.
Uses	*Alpha blockers:* hypertension, vasospasms in peripheral vascular disease, diagnose pheochromocytomas *Beta-blockers:* hypertension, dysrhythmias, angina, reduce formation of aqueous humor (timolol)
Side Effects	Hypotension, dizziness, bradycardia, GI distress, diarrhea, depression
Nursing Implications	Monitor for side effects; warn about hypotension; monitor for bronchospasm in asthmatics.
Examples	*Alpha-Blockers:* phenoxybenzamine HCl (Dibenzyline), phentolamine (Regitine), tolazoline (Priscoline) *Beta-Blockers:* metoprolol (Lopressor), nadolol (Corgard), propranolol (Inderal), timolol (Timoptic)

- define activity level (space and eliminate activities that might precipitate angina, e.g., mowing grass, shoveling snow)
- help client list strategies for modifying/avoiding precipitating factors

Evaluation: Client is able to explain medications, dosage, time schedule, side effects; has a tentative schedule for rest and activities.

Goal 3: Client will be able to state what to do if symptoms change.

Plan/Implementation
- teach client to describe pain pattern
- teach client to recognize change in pain and to notify physician of change

Evaluation: Client is able to explain ways of dealing with a change in anginal pain.

D. Myocardial Infarction

1. **General Information**
   a. Definition: occlusion of one or more coronary arteries causing death to a portion of the myocardial tissue (infarct); see figures 3.6 and 3.7
   b. Incidence
      1) leading cause of death in the United States
      2) more common in men; rate in women rises after menopause
   c. Risk Factors (see risk factors for angina pectoris page 179)

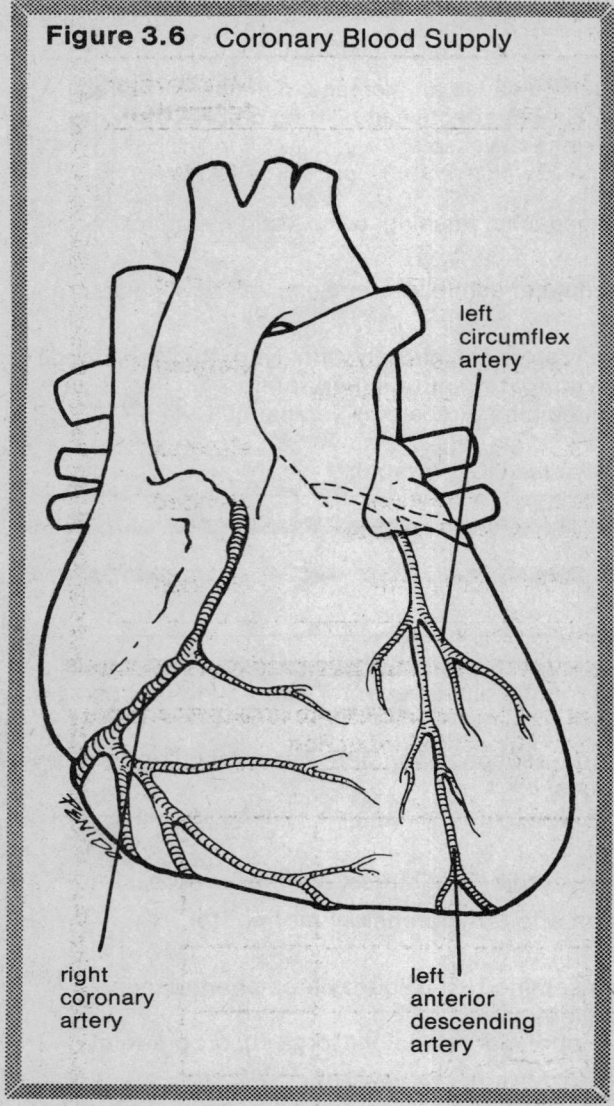

Figure 3.6 Coronary Blood Supply

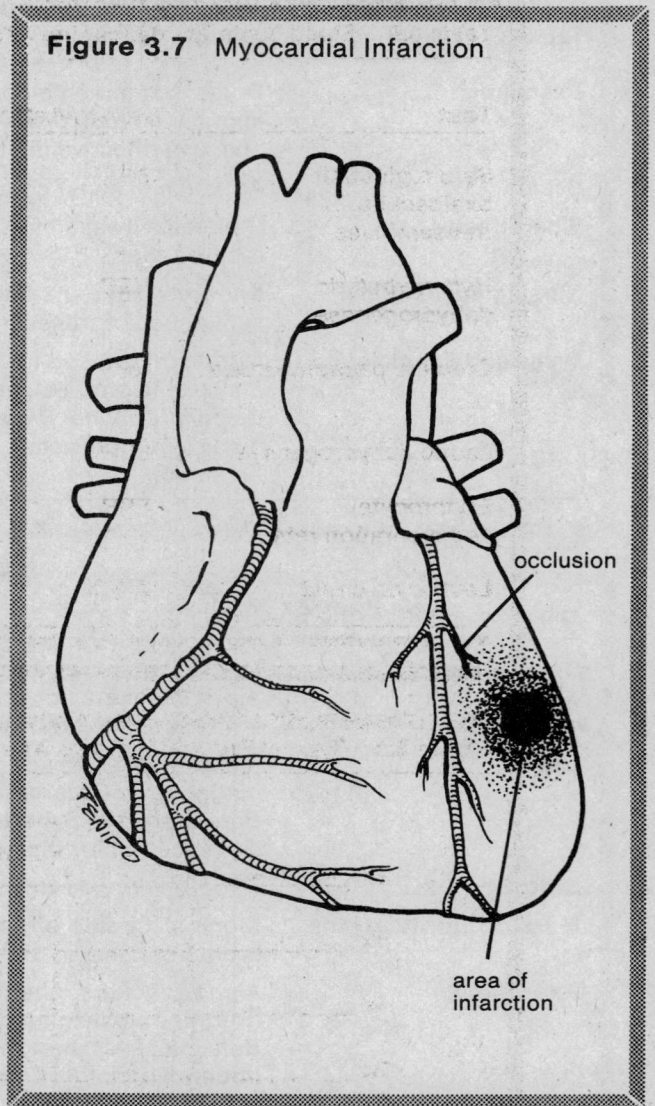

Figure 3.7 Myocardial Infarction

2. **Nursing Process**
   a. **Assessment**
      1) chest pain
         a) intense, crushing, substernal
         b) not relieved by rest or nitroglycerin
      2) ECG changes: elevation or depression of ST segment; T wave inversion; Q wave changes
      3) blood-tests (see table 3.9 and figure 3.8)
   b. **Goals, Plans/Implementation, and Evaluation**

Goal 1: Client's chest pain will be controlled.
Plan/Implementation
- give analgesics (e.g., IV morphine sulfate) until pain is relieved
- administer O_2
- give sedatives prn to promote rest

Evaluation: Client states pain was relieved.

Goal 2: Client's cardiac workload will be decreased.
Plan/Implementation
- see General Nursing Goal 2 page 176
- tell client to avoid Valsalva maneuver (increases intrathoracic pressure and causes sudden temporary increase in work load)
- keep accurate I&O

Evaluation: Client's cardiac work load is reduced as evidenced by heart rate of 68.

Goal 3: Client will remain free from new blood vessel occlusions.

OXYGENATION 183

Table 3.9 Blood Tests for Myocardial Infarction

Test	Abbreviation	Normal Values	Myocardial Infarction
Serum glutamic-oxaloacetic transaminase	SGOT	8–20 units/liter	elevated
Hydroxybutyric dehydrogenase	HBD	114–290 units/ml	elevated
Creatine phosphokinase	CPK	men: 23–99 units/liter women: 15–57 units/liter	elevated
Lactic dehydrogenase	LDH	48–115 IU/liter	elevated
Erythrocyte sedimentation rate	ESR	men: 0–10 mm/hour women: 0–20 mm/hour	elevated
Leukocyte count	WBC	4,100–10,000 μ liter	elevated

Note: Normal values will vary somewhat depending on the laboratory doing the tests.

Figure 3.8 Typical Enzyme Patterns After an Acute Myocardial Infarction

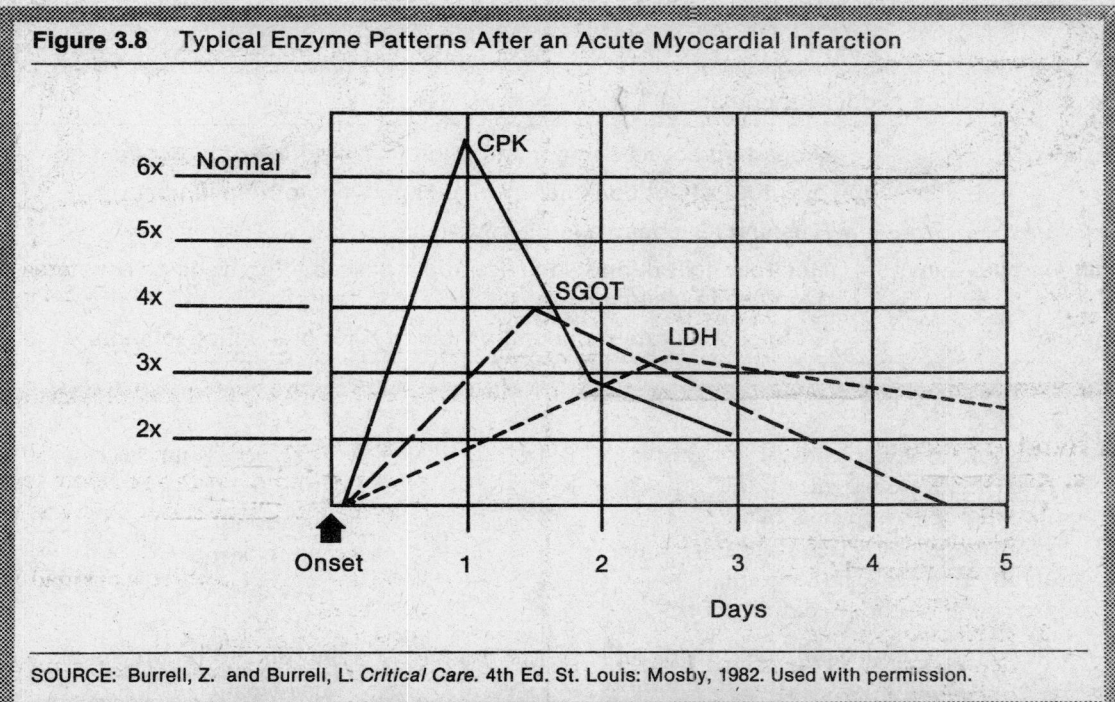

SOURCE: Burrell, Z. and Burrell, L. *Critical Care.* 4th Ed. St. Louis: Mosby, 1982. Used with permission.

Plan/Implementation
- administer anticoagulants as ordered (see table 3.10)
- apply T.E.D. hose
- teach client ankle flexion/extension exercises

Evaluation: Client's condition remains stable; no signs of further occlusions.

Goal 4: Client will remain free from complications.   K+ 3.5–5.5

Plan/Implementation
- monitor ECG for dysrhythmias
- monitor lab reports (enzymes and electrolytes)
- monitor for symptoms of cardiogenic shock (see page 178)

Table 3.10 Anticoagulants

Description	Drugs that interfere with blood clotting. *Heparin* prevents the formation of thrombin from prothrombin. *Coumadin* and *dicumarol* block the hepatic synthesis of prothrombin and the other vitamin K-dependent clotting factors. Neither form has any effect on existing thrombi.
Onset/Duration of Action	*Heparin:* almost immediate effect, lasts 4 hours. *Oral:* Slow onset (2–3 days), cumulative effect lasts 7–9 days after last dose.
Uses	Prevention and treatment of thromboses throughout the body. The parenteral drugs can also be used to prevent clotting of blood outside the body (e.g., extracorporeal circulation, transfusions).
Side Effects	Hemorrhage
Nursing Implications	Avoid use of any other product that increases anticoagulation or causes bleeding (e.g., aspirin); teach client safety precautions to avoid bleeding (e.g., soft toothbrush, electric razor). Monitor lab tests • parenteral: partial thromboplastin time (PTT) • oral: prothrombin time (PT)
Types and Examples	*Parenteral:* heparin *Oral:* bishydroxycoumarin, called also dicumarol; warfarin (Coumadin); phenindione (Hedulin)

Table 3.11 Anticoagulant Antagonists

Description	Drugs that act as antagonists to block the action of anticoagulants
Uses	Overdose of anticoagulants; bleeding; hypoprothrombinemia
Side Effects	Flushing, GI upset, allergic reactions
Nursing Implications	Monitor client during administration; assess effectiveness by noting a decrease in bleeding.
Examples	Protamine sulfate for heparin; vitamin K for oral anticoagulants

- monitor for symptoms of congestive heart failure (see page 189)
- monitor for symptoms of thrombophlebitis (see page 194)

Evaluation: Client shows gradual improvement without complications.

Goal 5: Client and significant others will be able to explain care during acute and recovery phase, and care that will follow discharge.

Plan/Implementation
- teach
  - level of activity
  - diet
    * reducing calories if client is obese
    * sodium restricted (see table 3.12)
    * cholesterol and fat restricted (see table 3.13)
    * high potassium necessary (see table 3.17)
  - medications
    * administration
    * schedule
    * side effects
  - symptoms to report immediately
    * chest pain
    * dyspnea
    * fluid retention
  - sexual activity: following an uncomplicated MI, may resume sexual intercourse in 6–8 weeks

Evaluation: Client can explain own activity; can plan menu for a sodium-restricted diet; knows what symptoms to report to physician immediately.

OXYGENATION 185

Na+ Restriction

Table 3.12 Approximate Sodium Content in Selected Food Items*

Food items	Portion	Sodium Content in mg
Breads and cereals		
White bread	1 slice	200
Regular Corn Flakes	1 oz	260
Dairy Products		
Milk	8 oz	130
American cheese	1 slice	238
Cottage cheese, low fat	4 oz	435
Fish and shellfish		
Flounder, broiled filet	2 oz	355
Scallops	3½ oz	265
Fruits and vegetables		
Tomato juice	6 oz	275
Peas, canned	5¼ oz	349
Meats and poultry		
Chicken, roasted	2 pieces	57
Bacon	1 slice	101
Bologna	1 slice	226
Beef	3 oz	381
Miscellaneous food items		
Olives	1	130
Catsup	1 tbsp	154
Peanut butter	2 tbsp	167
Potato chips	14 chips	191
Italian salad dressing	1 tbsp	315
Chocolate pudding, instant	½ cup	404
Dill pickle	1 large	1,137
Beef broth	1 cube	1,152
Salt	1 tsp	2,400

*Exact amount of sodium varies with brands of food items.

Teaching guidelines for sodium restricted diets.

a. Discuss salt, sodium chloride, and other sodium-containing compounds.
b. Explain relationship of sodium to high blood pressure, rationale for eliminating sodium from diet.
c. Stress avoidance of foods and medications that contain multiple sodium compounds; read labels carefully.
d. Eat 3 well-balanced meals a day with foods naturally low in sodium.
e. Add no salt while preparing food and add no salt at table.
f. If sodium intake is limited to only 2 gm, food can be salted lightly during preparation, but no additional salt added at table.
g. Season food without using sodium-containing compounds.
h. Seek advice from physician concerning salt substitutes.

E. Dysrhythmias Possible complication

1. General Information
   a. Definition: disturbance of rate and/or rhythm of the heartbeat
   b. Normal Cardiac Conduction: normal sinus rhythm (NSR) (refer to General Concepts page 170)
   c. Common Dysrhythmias
      1) *sinus or atrial dysrhythmias*
         a) sinus tachycardia: normal conduction pathways with rapid rate (100–180/minute)
         b) sinus bradycardia: normal conduction with rate under 60/minute
         c) other atrial dysrhythmias: an ectopic focus in the atrium (other than SA node) may stimulate heart, e.g., wandering atrial

Table 3.13 Cholesterol and Saturated Fat Content in Selected Food Items*

Food Items	Serving	Cholesterol (mg)	Saturated Fat (gm)
Dairy Products			
Milk, skim	8 oz	0	0
Yogurt, low fat	8 oz	11	1.8
American cheese	1 oz	27	5.6
Butter	1 tbs	31	7.1
Milk, whole	8 oz	33	5.1
Ice cream	8 oz	59	8.9
Fish and Shellfish			
Clams	3 oz	50	0.4
Fish, lean	3 oz	59	0.3
Shrimp	3 oz	126	0.5
Meats and Poultry			
Beef liver	3 oz	372	2.5
Egg	1 whole	274	1.7
Beef, lean	3 oz	56	2.4
Chicken breast	3 oz	63	1.3
Fruits and Vegetables			
All fruits		No cholesterol and generally no saturated fats	
All vegetables		(see vegetable oils below for exceptions)	
Vegetable Oils			
Coconut oil	1 tbs	0	11.8
Palm oil	1 tbs	0	6.7
Olive oil	1 tbs	0	1.8
Corn oil	1 tbs	0	1.7
Safflower oil	1 tbs	0	1.2

*Exact amount of cholesterol and saturated fat varies with brands of food items.

pacemaker (*NOTE*: In cardiac conduction, fastest foci pace the heart; cardiac tissue has property of autoelectricity, so foci from anywhere in heart can initiate cardiac cycle. Under normal conditions this does not occur, because junctional foci have slower rate than atrial foci [40–60]; ventricular foci are the slowest [30–40].)

  d) sinus arrest: SA node ceases firing
  e) premature atrial contraction (PAC): atrial foci other than SA nodes fire prior to anticipated next beat
  f) paroxysmal atrial tachycardia (PAT): rapid run of PACs, each stimulating a ventricular response (rate = 160–250/minute)
  g) atrial flutter: rapid atrial rhythm with ventricles responding periodically at a ratio of 2:1–6:1
  h) atrial fibrillation: multiple ectopic foci discharge 300–500 times/minute; ventricular response varies but is generally over 90/minute; one of most common atrial dysrhythmias

2) *junctional dysrhythmias*: ectopic focus in AV nodal area
3) *ventricular dysrhythmias*: most dangerous dysrhythmias
  a) ventricular tachycardia
- ventricles contract at rate of 140–220/minute
- often paroxysmal
- indicates severe myocardial irritability

  b) premature ventricular contraction or beat (PVC): an ectopic focus in ventricle stimulates a contraction
  c) ventricular fibrillation
- most serious
- not consistent with life

- multiple foci stimulate rapid and ineffective ventricular contractions
4) *conduction defects* (heart blocks)
   a) bundle branch block
   b) incomplete heart block: may be 1st or 2nd degree
   c) complete heart block
d. Medical Treatment
   1) medical intervention
      a) sinus dysrhythmias: generally respond to reduction in anxiety, pain, or elimination of caffeine, nicotine
      b) atrial fibrillation/atrial flutter: may require cardioversion to restore NSR
      c) ventricular dysrhythmias: frequent monitoring; drug administration (lidocaine) for PVCs; electric countershock for tachycardia or fibrillation
      d) heart blocks: may require pacemaker implantation
   2) surgical intervention: pacemaker
      a) external (temporary)
      b) internal (permanent)
         - fixed (continuously fires at a preset rate)
         - demand (fires only if heart rate drops below given rate)

2. **Nursing Process**
   a. **Assessment**
      1) rate, rhythm, and quality of all pulses
      2) ECG: alterations in P wave, PR interval, QRS and T complexes
      3) lab tests
         a) electrolytes
         b) serum digoxin levels
   b. **Goals, Plans/Implementation, and Evaluation**

   Goal 1: Client will remain free from undetected dysrhythmias.
   Plan/Implementation
   - monitor with oscilloscope; ensure electrodes are properly placed and monitor alarm is functional
   - note quality and rate of pulse in clients at high risk for dysrhythmias
   - be alert to altered electrolyte levels, serum levels of pharmacotherapeutic agents
   - instruct client to report syncope, pain, dyspnea, palpitation, restlessness, nausea and vomiting

   Evaluation: Client's dysrhythmias are immediately detected.

   Goal 2: Client's dysrythmias will revert to NSR.
   Plan/Implementation
   - know that attempts will be made to convert client's dysrhythmia to NSR whenever possible
   - carefully report and document episodes of dysrhythmias as well as client's responses
   - administer antidysrhythymic drugs as ordered; assess and record client's response
   - institute measures to reduce client's anxiety
   - maintain IV at a "keep open" rate for emergency use
   - ensure that emergency drugs and equipment are readily available and that equipment is in good working order
   - ensure all members of health care team are acquainted with respective responsibilities in emergency situation

   Evaluation: Client receives all antidysrhythmic drugs on time; converts to and maintains NSR.

   Goal 3: Client will remain free from hazards of cardioversion or electric countershock.
   Plan/Implementation
   - administer sedation (diazepam [Valium]) as ordered, prior to procedure
   - observe and record LOC and respirations during and after procedure

   Evaluation: Client's vital signs remained stable during cardioversion.

   Goal 4: Client will undergo pacemaker implantation free from preventable complications.
   Plan/Implementation
   - postimplantation
     - monitor for changes in pulse rate and rhythm
     - keep insertion site clean; inspect for signs of infection
     - monitor for temperature elevation
     - support extremity on which pacemaker attached (external pacemaker)
   - teach client with permanent pacemaker
     - level of activity

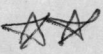

- take own pulse daily
- symptoms of pacemaker failure: vertigo, syncope, palpitations, hiccoughs, bradycardia
- avoid improperly grounded electrical appliances, e.g., some power tools
- avoid sources of high frequency signals, e.g., microwave ovens, radio stations
- schedule for battery replacement
- carry card
- importance of follow-up care

Evaluation: Postimplantation, client maintains a regular, normal heart rate.

F. Congestive Heart Failure (CHF)

1. **General Information**
   a. Definition: state in which cardiac output is inadequate to meet the metabolic needs of the body; characterized by circulatory congestion.
   b. Etiology: one or more of the following
      1) inflow of blood to heart greatly increased (e.g., excessive IV fluids, sodium and water retention)
      2) outflow of blood from heart obstructed (e.g., damaged valves, narrowed arteries)
      3) functional capacity of myocardium decreased; (e.g., myocardial infarction, dysrhythmias)
      4) metabolic needs of body accelerated (e.g., fever, pregnancy)
   c. Cardiac Compensation
      1) mechanisms
         a) *myocardial hypertrophy*: fibers of myocardium increase in length and diameter; heart beats more forcibly
         b) *ventricular dilation*: increases volume in chambers
         c) *tachycardia*
      2) terminology
         a) *compensated CHF*: compensatory changes maintain adequate cardiac output   adq circ.
         b) *decompensated CHF*: compensatory changes unable to maintain adequate cardiac output; CHF becomes symptomatic   inadq circ
   d. Left-sided Congestive Heart Failure: left ventricle cannot eject all blood from left atrium; therefore left atrium cannot accept all blood from pulmonary bed
      1) etiology
         a) hypertension
         b) mitral and/or aortic valvular disease
         c) ischemic heart disease: damage or infarction of the myocardium of the left ventricle
      2) pathophysiology: blood backs up in pulmonary bed (see table 3.14 for results and symptoms)
   e. Right-sided Congestive Heart Failure: right ventricle cannot eject all blood

---

Table 3.14   Congestive Heart Failure

Results	Symptoms
Left-Sided Pathophysiology: Blood backs up from left ventricle to pulmonary bed.	
Pulmonary congestion. Pulmonary edema.	Dyspnea. Orthopnea. Rales. Paroxysmal nocturnal dyspnea (PND). Decreased vital capacity. Cyanosis.
Cerebral anoxia.	Irritability. Restlessness. Confusion.
Decreased O_2 to cells.	Extreme weakness. Fatigue. Oliguria.
Right-Sided Pathophysiology: Blood backs up from right ventricle to systemic circulation.	
Increased hydrostatic pressure in systemic circulation.	Peripheral edema. Dependent edema: sacrum, ankles.
Elevated venous pressure.	Distended neck veins.
Congestion in kidneys, retention of sodium.	Oliguria.
Venous congestion in extremities.	Cool and cyanotic legs.
Congestion in GI tract.	Anorexia. Nausea. Bloating.

from right atrium, therefore right atrium cannot accept all blood from systemic circulation
1) etiology
   a) pulmonary disease
   b) tricuspid and pulmonic valvular disease
   c) ischemic heart disease: damage or infarction of the myocardium of the right ventricle
2) pathophysiology: blood backs up in systemic circulation (see table 3.14 for results and symptoms)

2. **Nursing Process**
   a. Assessment
      1) left-sided CHF
         a) arterial blood gas studies showing decreased Po$_2$, i.e., less than 80 mm Hg
         b) abnormal breath sounds
      2) right-sided CHF
         a) elevated central venous pressure
         b) distended neck veins
         c) hepatomegaly (enlargement of the liver)
         d) abnormal liver function (hepatic congestion)
         e) peripheral edema
      3) both right- and left-sided congestive heart failure (CHF)
         a) cardiac enlargement; point of maximum intensity (PMI) displacement
         b) decreased urinary output
         c) weight gain
         d) tachycardia
   b. Goals, Plans/Implementation, and Evaluation

   Goal 1: Client will experience increased force and strength of the ventricles.
   Plan/Implementation
   - administer cardiac glycosides as ordered (see table 3.15)
   - monitor vital signs closely

   Evaluation: Client's heart rate is stable at 80 beats/minute.

   Goal 2: Client will eliminate excess fluid.
   Plan/Implementation
   - give diuretics as ordered (see tables 3.16 and 3.40)
   - keep accurate I&O
   - weigh daily
   - restrict sodium intake
   - apply T.E.D. hose

   Evaluation: Client's weight decreases to pre-CHF level.

   Goal 3: Client's cardiac workload will be decreased.
   Plan/Implementation
   - see General Nursing Goal 2 page 176

   Evaluation: Client's cardiac workload is decreased as evidenced by reduction of heart rate from 96 to 80.

   Goal 4: Client will remain free from the hazards of immobility.
   Plan/Implementation
   - see General Nursing Goal 3 page 176

Table 3.15   Cardiac Glycosides

Description	Drugs that act directly on myocardium to increase force of contraction. Cardiac output is increased while heart rate is slowed.
Uses	CHF, dysrhythmias (especially those with increased rate), cardiogenic shock with pulmonary edema
Side Effects	GI upset, visual disturbances, dysrhythmias, heart block.
Nursing Implications	Take pulse prior to administration; if above 120 or below 60, hold medication and notify physician; monitor for toxicity and hypokalemia if client is taking diuretics; teach client to monitor pulse rate at home, eat high potassium diet if taking diuretics.
Examples	Lanatoside C (Cedilanid D), ouabain (G-strophanthin), digitoxin (Crystodigin), digoxin (Lanoxin), digitalis

190 SECTION 3: NURSING CARE OF THE ADULT

Goal 5: Client will remain free from pulmonary edema.
Plan/Implementation
- monitor closely for symptoms
  - severe dyspnea
  - audible rales
  - frothy, blood-tinged sputum
  - extreme anxiety
- institute therapy *immediately* if pulmonary edema develops
  - place in Fowler's position
  - give O₂ by positive pressure if available (increases O₂ and helps to push fluid from alveolar space)
  - apply rotating tourniquets (see figure 3.9) to reduce circulating blood volume by obstructing *venous* flow in 3 extremities
    * rotate one tourniquet every 15 minutes in *one* direction
    * remove one at a time when edema is controlled
  - give morphine sulfate IV (relieves anxiety and dilates pulmonary vascular bed)
  - administer cardiac glycosides (see table 3.15) as ordered
  - give diuretic as ordered, e.g., furosemide (see table 3.16)
  - give aminophylline IV (see table 3.19)

Evaluation: Client's respirations are 16/minute; lung fields are clear on auscultation.

Goal 6: Client and significant others will be able to explain need for care after discharge.
Plan/Implementation
- teach
  - to balance between activity and rest
  - diet

Figure 3.9 Pattern for Rotating Tourniquets

Rotate *one* tourniquet every 15 min. in the *same* direction.

9:00   9:15   9:30   9:45

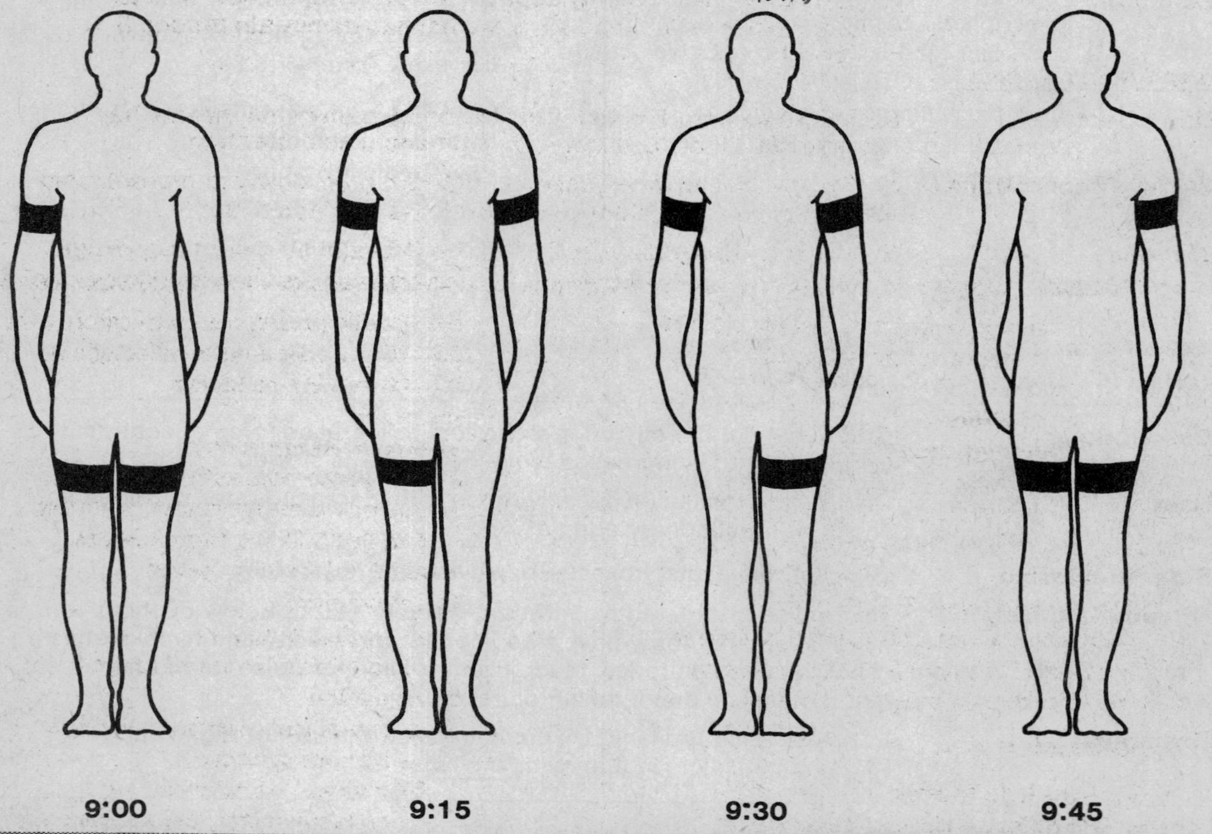

OXYGENATION 191

Table 3.16 Antihypertensives

Description	Drugs that act to reduce the blood pressure through a wide variety of mechanisms
Uses	Control of moderate to severe hypertension

Thiazide Diuretics

Side Effects	Hypokalemia, hyponatremia, hyperuricemia, hyperglycemia, orthostatic hypotension
Nursing Implications	Maintain K^+ level, teach high K^+, Na^+-restricted diet; monitor I&O, BP.
Examples	Chlorothiazide (Diuril), hydrochlorothiazide (Hydrodiuril, Oretic, Esidrix), furosemide (Lasix)

Potassium-Sparing Diuretics

Side Effects	Hyponatremia, hyperkalemia, GI disturbances, allergic reaction
Nursing Implications	Monitor K^+ intake to ensure excess not ingested; monitor I&O, BP.
Examples	Spironolactone (Aldactone), triamterene (Dyrenium)

Sympathetic-Inhibiting Agents

Side Effects	Orthostatic hypotension, depression, drowsiness, GI disturbances, impotence (methyldopa, guanethidine sulfate), bradycardia, sodium and water retention
Nursing Implications	Caution client to change position slowly, monitor for side effects, maintain Na^+-restricted diet, restrict alcohol use (may exacerbate hypotension).
Examples	Reserpine (Serpasil), methyldopa (Aldomet), guanethidine sulfate (Ismelin), propranolol (Inderal), trimethaphan camsylate (Arfonad)

Vasodilating Agents

Side Effects	Excess vasodilatation with flushing and hypotension, headache, tachycardia, GI disturbances, sodium and water retention
Nursing Implications	Monitor BP closely when used IV, withdraw drug slowly to prevent rapid rise in pressure, monitor I&O, maintain Na^+-restricted diet
Examples	Hydralazine (Apresoline), nitroprusside (Nipride) (IV emergency drug)

- * sodium restricted (see table 3.12)
- * high potassium as necessary (see table 3.17)
- medications
  - * administration
  - * schedule
  - * side effects
- to weigh daily to monitor fluid balance
- how to apply T.E.D. hose

Evaluation: Client can correctly describe care needs for home (e.g., drug therapy, how to take own pulse).

G. Hypertension

1. **General Information**
   a. Definition: a chronic elevation of systemic arterial blood pressure in which the systolic pressure is consistently over 150–160 mm Hg and the diastolic is 90–100 mm Hg or higher
   b. Incidence
      1) affects all age groups
      2) prevalence rises with age
      3) one of the major causes of illness and death in the United States
   c. Blood Pressure Physiology
      1) determinants
         a) cardiac output
         b) total peripheral resistance
      2) regulation
         a) neural stimulation: autonomic nervous system
         b) humoral stimulation, e.g., catecholamines, aldosterone, angiotensin

Table 3.17 Foods High in Potassium

Food	Portion	Potassium mEq
Whole milk	1 cup	9.0
Broiled meat	3 oz	9.6
Apricots (canned)	4 halves	7.9
Banana	1 small	9.5
Honeydew melon	⅛ medium	9.6
Fresh orange	1 medium	9.5
Dried prunes	4 large	12.0
Watermelon	½ slice–1" thick	15.3
Baked potato	1 medium	12.9
Dried lima beans	½ cup cooked	14.5
Soybeans	½ cup cooked	13.8
Winter squash	½ cup cooked	10.0
Dried white beans	½ cup cooked	10.6

d. Pathophysiology
   1) no obvious early pathologic changes in blood vessels and organs
   2) large vessels (aorta, coronary arteries, basilar artery to brain, peripheral vessels in limbs) eventually become sclerosed and tortuous
   3) lumens narrow resulting in decreased blood flow to heart, brain, and lower extremities
   4) vessels become completely occluded or hemorrhage may occur
   5) damage to the intima of small vessels causes local edema and intravascular clotting
   6) decreased blood supply to tissues of heart, brain, kidneys results in dysfunction of these organs
e. Types
   1) primary (essential) approximately 90% of all cases; etiology unknown; types include
      a) benign: slowly progressive
      b) malignant: rapidly accelerating
   2) secondary: approximately 10%–15% of all cases; caused by an identifiable primary disease
      a) adrenal causes, e.g., pheochromocytoma (large amounts of catecholamines excreted)
      b) coarctation of the aorta
      c) kidney disease, e.g., narrowing of the renal artery
f. Predisposing Factors
   1) stress
   2) familial history
   3) obesity

2. Nursing Process
   a. Assessment
      1) blood pressure elevated on at least three different occasions
      2) headache, change in vision (hemorrhages in retina, blurred vision)
      3) epistaxis
      4) personality change: forgetful and irritable
   b. Goals, Plans/Implementation, and Evaluation

   Goal 1: Client's blood pressure will decrease to safe level and permanent damage will be prevented.
   Plan/Implementation
   • monitor BP
   • modify life-style to reduce stress
   • modify diet
     – reduced calories if client is obese
     – sodium restricted (see table 3.12)
     – high potassium if needed (see table 3.17)
   • exercise in a regular, planned program
   • avoid smoking
   • administer antihypertensive medications (see table 3.16)
     – diuretics
     – sympathetic inhibitors
     – vasodilating agents
   Evaluation: Client's blood pressure is reduced to 140/90; client is free from heart disease.

   Goal 2: Client will be able to carry out self care activities after discharge.

Plan/Implementation
- teach client
  - take own BP
  - modify life-style
  - institute exercise program
  - manage diet (sodium restricted, high potassium as necessary) (see tables 3.12 and 3.17)
  - medications (see table 3.16)
    * administration
    * schedule
    * side effects
    * importance of compliance
  - stop smoking, caffeine
  - importance of follow-up care

Evaluation: Client knows all components of therapeutic regimen; has an appointment for return visit.

H. Peripheral Vascular Disease

1. General Information
a. Definition: changes in blood vessels peripheral to the heart; types: arterial and venous

b. Types of Arterial Problems
  1) *arteriosclerosis obliterans*: atherosclerotic plaque formation that involves arteries of lower extremities; occurs in men aged 50–70 and women after menopause
  2) *Raynaud's disease*: intermittent constricting spasms of superficial vessels of digits and arteries of extremities, resulting in pain and cyanosis
  3) *Buerger's disease* (thromboangitis obliterans): disease of arteries and veins of extremities characterized by diffuse, inflammatory, proliferative changes in arteries and veins

c. Types of Venous Problems
  1) *varicose veins*: dilated, tortuous superficial veins; incompetent valves cause dilation; increased pressure causes tortuosity; increased capillary pressure results in edema
  2) *varicose ulcers*: ulcers resulting from circulatory insufficiency
  3) *thrombophlebitis*: inflammation of vessel with thrombus formation
  4) *phlebothrombosis*: thrombus formation in a vein without inflammation

Do not dislodge thrombus — Don't massage

2. Nursing Process: Arterial Problems
a. **Assessment:** symptoms of impaired peripheral arterial circulation (see figure 3.10)

b. **Goals, Plans/Implementation, and Evaluation**

Goal 1: Client will have adequate arterial blood flow to extremities.
Plan/Implementation
- teach client to eliminate/avoid
  - tobacco
  - exposure to temperature extremes
  - trauma
    * tissue injury and infections
    * maintain good foot care
  - excessive exercise
  - vasospastic drugs, e.g., epinephrine
  - constrictive clothing
- institute dietary modifications
  - low cholesterol
  - moderate fat
  - reduced calories if client is obese
- give anticoagulants if indicated (see table 3.10)

Evaluation: Client's extremities are warm; has peripheral pulses of good quality.

Goal 2: Client will have minimal discomfort.
Plan/Implementation
- rest when pain occurs
- administer vasodilator adrenergic medications as ordered, e.g., Vasodilan (see table 3.18)

Evaluation: Client has developed schedule of activities that keeps pain under control.

Goal 3: Client will be able to explain when surgery might be used; will be free from preventable complications.
Plan/Implementation
- know that bypass surgery may be used if client has localized occlusion with arteriosclerosis obliterans; that infrequently sympathectomy may be used to treat Buerger's disease; that amputation is the treatment for gangrene
- provide post-op care: avoid strain on incision (do not bend joint over which graft passes), monitor for hemorrhage resulting from disruption of graft or occlusion of graft, administer anticoagulants as ordered (see table 3.10)

Figure 3.10 Common Manifestations of Chronic Arterial and Venous Peripheral Vascular Disease

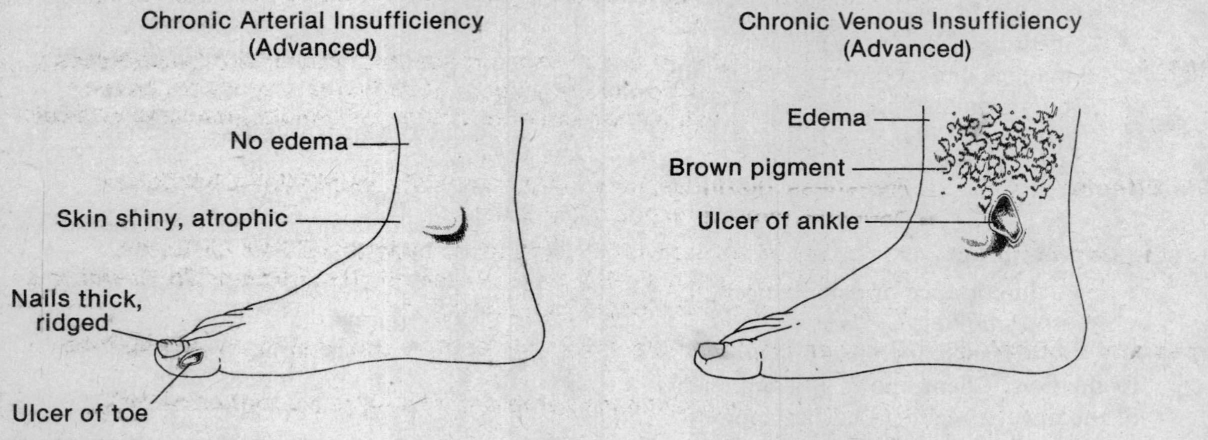

Chronic Arterial Insufficiency (Advanced)
- No edema
- Skin shiny, atrophic
- Nails thick, ridged
- Ulcer of toe

Chronic Venous Insufficiency (Advanced)
- Edema
- Brown pigment
- Ulcer of ankle

Symptoms	Chronic Advanced Arterial Insufficiency	Chronic Advanced Venous Insufficiency
Pain	Severe ischemic pain (e.g., intermittent claudication)	Crampy pain; Thrombophlebitis: Inflammatory pain—Homans'
Skin changes	Thin, shiny, atrophic skin; loss of hair over foot and toes; nails thickened and ridged	May show brown pigmentation around ankles
Temperature	Cool	Normal to cool
Color	Pale, especially on elevation; dusky red on dependency, cyanotic	Normal, or cyanotic on dependency
Pulses	Decreased or absent	Normal, though may be difficult to feel through edema
Edema	Absent or mild	Present, often marked; decreased by elevation
Ulceration	If present, involves toes or points of trauma on feet	If present, develops at sides of ankles (i.e., lower 1/3 of leg); not painful
Gangrene	May develop	Does not develop

SOURCE: Adapted from Bates, B. *A Guide to Physical Assessment.* 3rd ed. Philadelphia: Lippincott, 1983. Used with permission.

Evaluation: Client explains the type of surgery that he may receive; is free from complications postoperatively (e.g., split incision, frank hemorrhage).

3. **Nursing Process: Venous Problems**
   a. **Assessment:** symptoms of impaired venous circulation (see figure 3.10)
   b. **Goals, Plans/Implementation, and Evaluation**

   Goal 1: Client will have adequate venous blood flow to extremities.

   Plan/Implementation
   - teach client to avoid
     - tobacco
     - injury and infections
     - constrictive clothing, e.g., garters
     - standing or sitting for long periods
     - crossing legs at knee
   - teach client to
     - wear T.E.D. hose
     - elevate legs
     - do ankle push-ups when standing (promotes venous return)

Table 3.18 Adrenergics

Description	Drugs that mimic the action of the sympathetic nervous system. There are many types of specific drugs that exert more or less influence on the adrenergic system.
Uses	Symptomatic relief of anaphylactic reactions, hypotension (vaspressors); bronchodilation and pulmonary decongestion; restoration of cardiac rhythm after arrest; management of acute open-angle glaucoma; topical hemostasis
Side Effects	Weakness, dizziness, nervousness, anxiety, palpitations, headache, insomnia, hypertension, tachycardia
Nursing Implications	Avoid use in clients with hypertension, hyperthyroidism, diabetes, Parkinson's disease, COPD, benign prostatic hypertrophy, Tb, or with the elderly; monitor BP closely; monitor I&O.
Types and Examples	*Endogenous catecholamines:* epinephrine (Adrenalin), norepinephrine, dopamine *Synthetic catecholamines:* isoproterenol (Isuprel), dobutamine HCl (Dobutrex) *Vasopressor amines:* metaraminol (Aramine), mephentermine (Wyamine) *Nasal decongestants:* phenylephrine (Neo-Synephrine), ephedrine (Tedral), tetrahydrozaline (Tyzine) *Ophthalmic decongestants:* epinephrine (Adrenalin), naphazoline HCl (Privine HCl), phenylephrine (Neo-Synephrine) *Bronchodilators (beta-adrenergic):* albuterol (Proventil), ephedrine (Bronkaid), metaproterenol (Alupent), terbutaline (Brethine) *Vasodilators:* isoxsuprine HCl (Vasodilan), nylidrin HCl (Arlidin) *CNS stimulants and anorexiants:* amphetamine (Benzedrine)

Aminophylin tox → seizures.

Evaluation: Client's feet are warm; client is free from ankle edema.

Goal 2: Client with thrombophlebitis will be protected from dislodgement of thrombus.
Plan/Implementation
- maintain bed rest 7–10 days
- elevate legs
- apply T.E.D. hose
- apply warm, moist packs to involved site (prevent burns)
- do not rub legs
- give anticoagulant therapy as ordered (see table 3.10)

Evaluation: Client is free from any signs of movement of thrombus.

Goal 3: Client's ulcers will heal.
Plan/Implementation
- ensure bed rest with leg elevated when ulcer is acute
- monitor and report needs for debridement
- monitor for signs of cellulitis and report immediately
- give antibiotics as ordered if infected
- know and inform client that skin grafting may be necessary
- discuss with client the long-term nature of treatment

Evaluation: Ulcer remains clean, uninfected, and is healing well.

Goal 4: Client with varicose veins will be able to describe surgical procedure and postoperative care.
Plan/Implementation
- teach client regarding planned surgical procedure
- elevate legs
- apply T.E.D. hose
- monitor for bleeding, thrombosis postoperatively
- teach client to move about when out of bed and not to stand still

Evaluation: Client can describe surgical procedure; applies T.E.D. hose; states rest and activity restrictions.

I. Chronic Obstructive Pulmonary Disease (COPD) or Chronic Obstructive Lung Disease (COLD)

1. **General Information**
   a. Definition: chronic respiratory disorders that involve a persistent obstruction of bronchial air flow
   b. Incidence
      1) fastest growing cause of death in the US
      2) occurs in adults and children
   c. Predisposing factors
      1) smoking
      2) environmental factors: smoke, coal, hay, asbestos, air pollution
      3) allergic factors
      4) chronic, recurrent respiratory infections
      5) genetic factors (possibly)
   d. Pathophysiology
      1) reduced thoracic excursion due to bronchial obstruction, air trapping, and thoracic overdistention; possible inflammatory reaction in airways causing bronchial spasm and increased secretions
      2) tidal volume, vital capacity, and inspiratory reserve necessary for effective coughing are decreased by reduced thoracic excursion
      3) to breathe, client employs accessory muscles of respiration, shoulder girdle, abdominal muscles; purses lips to maintain open bronchioles with expiration
      4) bronchial obstruction, air trapping leads to destruction of lung, permanently reduced alveolar ventilation, and CO_2 retention
      5) increased susceptibility to infections, especially pulmonary type, i.e., acute bronchitis, pneumonia, and other complications
      6) respiratory alkalosis may occur if there is hyperventilation
      7) respiratory acidosis may result from airway obstruction
   e. Hypoxemia
      1) definition: deficient oxygenation of the blood
      2) frequently chronic, possibly acute
      3) characterized by
         a) subtle changes in mentation such as restlessness, agitation, headache, drowsiness, and confusion (due to less O_2 to the brain and stimulation of the sympathetic nervous system)
         b) tachycardia, hyperventilation will be seen early in hypoxia; possibly followed by bradycardia and hypoventilation
         c) hypertension due to tachycardia may be present early with hypoxia
   f. Hypercapnia
      1) definition: excess of CO_2 in blood
      2) can occur with hypoxemia; may be chronic or acute
      3) characterized by
         a) CNS depression: drowsiness, inability to concentrate, progressive loss of consciousness
         b) early behavioral changes: irritability, inability to get along with others, discontentment with food, care, etc., inability to sleep
         c) headache
         d) tremors, dizziness, cardiac dysrhythmias
   g. Common examples of COPD
      1) *bronchial asthma:* a chronic disease characterized by episodic attacks of respiratory distress due to constriction of the bronchi and bronchioles (refer to *Nursing Care of the Child* page 536)
      2) *chronic bronchitis*
         a) definition: chronic inflammation of the bronchi with production of large amount of sputum that results in bronchial obstruction
         b) predisposing factors
            • smoking
            • occupational hazards: smoke, coal, hay, asbestos, air pollution
            • chronic respiratory infections
         c) etiology and pathophysiology: air pollution or smoking causes inflammatory reaction of mucosa of the bronchi with resulting edema and increased production of mucus; also predisposes person to recurrent respiratory infections by slowing down ciliary and phagocytic activity in the bronchi
      3) *emphysema*
         a) definition: chronic lung condition characterized by abnormal enlargement of alveoli and

OXYGENATION

[handwritten margin: get air out of lungs. pursed lip + Diaphramic]

   alveolar ducts with destruction of alveolar walls
   b) incidence: highest in men over age 50
   c) etiology: exact cause not identified
   d) pathophysiology: air trapped behind partially obstructed bronchioles produces overdistention and destruction of alveoli; loss of elastic recoil of lungs reduces expiratory flow; barrel chest develops

2. **Nursing Process**
   a. Assessment
      1) respiratory distress (dyspnea on exertion progressing to dyspnea at rest)
      2) apprehension
      3) cough (productive)
      4) lethargy (results from hypoxemia)
      5) use of accessary muscles
      6) abnormal breath sounds (rales, rhonchi, wheezing, decreased breath sounds)
      7) weight loss
      8) skin color
         a) flushed (hypercapnia)
         b) cyanosis (hypoxemia)
      9) abnormal pulmonary function tests, e.g., decreased expiratory and inspiratory volumes, increased residual volume
      10) blood gases
         a) at first Po_2 decreased only with activity, then continuously
         b) Pco_2 increases as disease worsens
      11) respiratory acidosis, compensated (from chronic CO_2 retention)
      12) frequent respiratory infections (decreased resistance)
   b. Goals, Plans/Implementation, and Evaluation

   Goal 1: Client will maintain a Po_2 of at least 60 mm Hg and a Pco_2 of 35–40 mm Hg; airway will be clear, sputum will be thin and clear.

   Plan/Implementation
   - see General Nursing Goal 1 page 176
   - administer bronchodilators as ordered (see table 3.19)
   - administer expectorants (see table 3.20) as ordered
   - administer IPPB as ordered
     - bronchodilators (see table 3.19)
     - mucolytics (see table 3.21)
   - teach relaxation techniques and breathing exercises (e.g., pursed-lip breathing) *[handwritten: Diaphramic breathing]*
   - administer low concentrations of humidified O_2 (1–2 liters/min); *CAUTION:* high O_2 flow may precipitate respiratory failure in presence of hypercapnia and hypoxia *[handwritten: 24%]*
   - give emotional support to client and family
   - encourage activity to tolerance
   - if client must be confined to bed for any period of time (usually infection or asthma attack)
     - semi-Fowler's or Fowler's position
     - turn frequently

[handwritten: barrel chest — loss of lung elasticity extension of alveoli]

Table 3.19	Bronchodilators (Xanthine Derivatives)
Description	Drugs that relax bronchial smooth muscle and inhibit the release of histamine and slow release substance A (SRS-A) from most cells. They are mild diuretics and cardiac stimulants.
Uses	Symptomatic relief of asthma, bronchial spasms
Side Effects	GI upset, nausea, nervousness, frequency, diarrhea, insomnia, tachycardia, palpitations
Nursing Implications	Use with care in clients with hypertension, hypoxemia, glaucoma, hyperthyroidism, benign prostatic hypertrophy, and diabetes; monitor for CNS symptoms; give with food to decrease GI upset; prohibit smoking.
Examples:	Aminophylline (Aminodur), theophylline (Theo-Dur), oxtriphylline (Choledyl)

[handwritten: tox. seizures]

Don't give Inderal to COPD'er.

198 SECTION 3: NURSING CARE OF THE ADULT

Table 3.20 Expectorants *AM given*

Description	Drugs that facilitate removal of thick mucus from lungs and act as soothing demulcent by stimulating secretion of a lubricant. (May be no more effective at liquefying secretions than high fluid intake and humidification.)
Uses	Facilitate productive cough
Side Effects	Nausea/vomiting, GI irritation, drowsiness
Nursing Implications	Instruct client not to use these preparations more than 1 week without seeing physician and to use additional measures (high fluid intake and humidity) to help cough; don't follow administration with water (except potassium iodide).
Examples	Ammonium chloride, guaifenesin (Robitussin), potassium iodide (SSKI)

Table 3.21 Mucolytics *PM*

Description	Drugs that act by disrupting the molecular structure of mucous secretions. They liquefy secretions throughout the tracheobronchial tree.
Uses	To liquefy thick secretions and minimize bronchiolar obstruction
Side Effects	Nausea/vomiting, rhinorrhea, hypersensitivity reaction, bronchial spasms
Nursing Implications	Watch asthmatic clients closely; ensure that client either expectorates secretions or is suctioned; monitor client for nausea and vomiting.
Examples	Acetylcysteine (Mucomyst)

- encourage to take frequent deep breaths and to breathe out slowly and completely
- active ROM exercises (passive if client too weak to do active exercises)
- employ diversional activities to avoid napping during the day so as to prevent insomnia and nocturnal restlessness
- *NOTE: avoid bed rest if at all possible to prevent hypoventilation, stasis of secretions, weakened ventilatory muscles, weakness of other muscles, and decreased cough reflex*
- give diet as tolerated, e.g., small amounts of soft food 4–5 times/day

Evaluation: Client's Po_2 remains greater than 60 mm Hg; Pco_2 remains between 35 and 45 mm Hg; sputum is clear and thin.

Goal 2: Client will be protected from any injuries.

Plan/Implementation
- know that if client has hypoxia, hypercapnia, or uncompensated respiratory acidosis, he may be lethargic, confused, or in coma
- use side rails, pad if necessary
- keep bed low to floor
- avoid restraints, sedatives, or tranquilizers
- if client is confused, have someone stay with him
- maintain quiet environment
- speak in low, calm, soothing tone

Evaluation: Client is free from injury.

Goal 3: Client will be protected from CO_2 narcosis. *due too much O_2 often*

Plan/Implementation
- know that uncontrolled O_2 delivery will eliminate hypoxic drive of respirations
- administer O_2 at low concentrations (1–2 liters/minute)
- observe for symptoms of narcosis with O_2 therapy
  - decreased respiratory rate and depth
  - headache
  - skin changes (flushing)
  - behavioral changes: confusion→coma

- blood gases
  - * increased P_{CO_2}
  - * *increased* P_{O_2}
- respiratory failure
- assist ventilation when needed

Evaluation: Client maintains spontaneous respirations.

Goal 4: Client and significant others will be able to explain home preventive measures and how to maintain adequate O_2 and CO_2 levels.

Plan/Implementation
- teach client
  - balance of activity and rest
  - breathing/relaxation exercises
  - effective coughing
  - postural drainage
  - diet
    - * small, frequent meals
    - * adequate fluids
  - medications
    - * administration
    - * side effects
  - use of O_2 equipment
  - preventive health habits
    - * stop smoking
    - * avoid respiratory infections
    - * seek treatment for respiratory infections *early*
    - * avoid factors that precipitate bronchospasms: (e.g., pollens, air pollutants)

Evaluation: Client has developed a schedule that allows activities of daily living, work obligations, and social activities.

J. Pneumonia

1. **General Information**
   a. Definition: acute inflammation of the alveolar spaces of the lung
   b. Etiology
      1) microorganisms
         a) bacteria
         b) viruses
         c) fungi
      2) chemicals
         a) inhalation (e.g., smoke)
         b) aspiration (e.g., vomitus)
   c. Predisposing Factors
      1) decreased immunity (e.g., COPD)
      2) debility (e.g., malnutrition)
      3) immobility (e.g., postsurgery)
   d. Pathophysiology
      1) causative agent is inhaled
      2) alveoli become inflamed and edematous
      3) alveolar spaces fill with exudate
      4) diffusion of O_2 and CO_2 is obstructed
      5) involved lung tissue becomes consolidated

2. **Nursing Process**
   a. Assessment
      1) chills, fever, malaise [post-op 1st 24°]
      2) chest pain (limits chest excursion)
      3) respirations: rapid, shallow, dyspneic
      4) tachycardia
      5) productive cough
      6) sputum
         a) viscid, tenacious — should not be bright blood
         b) rusty → yellow
         c) positive for causative microorganism
      7) breath sounds (diminished over involved areas, rales, and pleural friction rub)
      8) dehydration (if fever unchecked)
      9) leukocytosis
      10) cyanosis with advanced hypoxia
   b. Goals, Plans/Implementation, and Evaluation

Goal 1: Client's pulmonary ventilation will improve.
Plan/Implementation
- see General Nursing Goal 1 page 176
- administer organism-specific antibiotics (refer table 3.22)
- administer expectorants prn (see table 3.20)
- care for tracheostomy if present (see tracheostomy care page 310)
- administer analgesics for chest pain
- provide good oral hygiene

Evaluation: Client has decreased dyspnea.

Goal 2: Client will remain free from atelectasis. [O_2 + CO_2 exchange will not occur]
Plan/Implementation
- assess client status q2-4h for atelectasis (area of lung that is collapsed, airless, and shrunken)
- suction when necessary
- position client on unaffected side [expand lung]
- perform chest physical therapy (see General Nursing Goal 1 page 176)
- encourage coughing and deep breathing
- check pulse rate

Evaluation: Client has clear lungs on auscultation; breathes easily.

Table 3.22 Antibiotics

Description	A group of drugs that are either bacteriostatic (inhibiting or arresting the growth of microorganisms) or bacteriocidal (killing of microorganisms). The terms antibacterial, antimicrobial, antiinfective, and antiseptic are often used synonymously with antibiotic.

Penicillins

Uses	Treatment of common infections caused by penicillin-sensitive microorganisms
Side Effects	Allergic reactions including anaphylaxis; diarrhea; development of resistant organisms; superinfection; GI distress
Nursing Implications	Watch closely for rash or early signs of allergic reaction; check all clients for allergy before giving drug; obtain appropriate culture and sensitivity before starting drug; teach client to take full course of medicines as ordered.
Examples	Penicillin G (Wycillin); penicillin V (Pen-Vee K); oxacillin (Prostaphlin); ampicillin (Polycillin); ticarcillin (Ticar); nafcillin (Unipen)

Aminoglycosides

Uses	Treatment of gram-negative infections (often nosocomial or iatrogenic); effective in treating serious, systemic, gram-negative infections
Side Effects	Ototoxicity, nephrotoxicity, superinfections; allergic potential is small.
Nursing Implications	Monitor closely for hearing changes; monitor kidney function; watch for the development of superinfections.
Examples	Streptomycin, gentamycin (Garamycin), tobramycin (Nebcin), kanamycin (Kantrex), neomycin

Cephalosporins

Uses	Treatment of septicemia and most systemic infections; effective against some penicillin-resistant organisms
Side Effects	Allergic reactions (2/3 of penicillin-sensitive clients are also cephalosporin sensitive), superinfection, nephrotoxicity with higher doses, phlebitis at IV site, diarrhea
Nursing Implications	Monitor known penicillin-sensitive clients closely for allergy; give IV preparations slowly to reduce chances of phlebitis; give oral preparations 1 hour before or 2 hours after meals for maximum effectiveness; monitor for superinfections especially oral or vaginal fungal infections.
Examples	Cephalothin (Keflin), cefazolin (Kefzol), cephalexin (Keflex), cefamandole (Mandol), cefoxitin (Mefoxin)

Tetracyclines

Uses	Effective against a wide variety of pathogens including many of those causing diarrhea and pneumonia; used to control acne
Side Effects	Diarrhea, nausea, vestibular disturbances (minocycline), hypersensitivity reactions, GI upset, permanent discoloration of teeth especially in children, impairment of bone growth, and superinfection
Nursing Implications	Check for symptoms of hypersensitivity; don't give to pregnant women or children under age 8; don't administer with milk or antacids; give with sufficient water; watch for superinfections.
Examples	Tetracycline (Achromycin), chlortetracycline (Aureomycin), doxycycline (Vibramycin), minocycline (Minocin)

OXYGENATION   201

Table 3.22 Continued	
Polypeptides	
Uses	Treatment of superinfections of the skin and mucous membranes; to control some types of diarrhea and urinary tract infections
Side Effects	Pain on IM injection, renal damage, hypersensitivity, superinfection
Nursing Implications	Monitor closely for hypersensitivity; administer IM injections deeply; refrigerate oral suspensions; monitor for superinfections; use care when administering otic and ophthalmic preparations to prevent contamination.
Examples	Bacitracin (Baciguent), colistimethate (Coly-Mycin M), colistin sulfate (Coly-Mycin S), polymyxin B sulfate (Aerosporin)

Goal 3: Client will be able to care for self after discharge.
Plan/Implementation
- teach
  - activity level
  - avoid overfatigue
  - medications
    * administration
    * side effects
  - breathing exercises

Evaluation: Client develops a plan for balanced rest and activity; knows actions and side effects of all prescribed medications.

K. Tuberculosis

1. **General Information**
   a. Definition: a reportable, communicable disease usually affecting the respiratory system
   b. Incidence: an estimated 10% of the United States population is infected; black and Indian populations have higher incidence
   c. Etiology: *Mycobacterium tuberculosis*, an acid-fast bacillus *inhaled*
   d. Predisposing Factors
      1) lowered resistance caused by
         a) overcrowding
         b) poor sanitation
         c) poor nutrition
         d) poorly ventilated living conditions
         e) debilitating diseases
      2) virulence of organisms
      3) length of exposure
   e. Pathophysiology: tuberculosis bacillus is usually inhaled; transmitted by droplet produced by individual with active disease
      1) most common site of implantation is on alveolar surface of lung parenchyma
      2) induces hypersensitivity reaction in host
      3) inflammation occurs, then acute pneumonia develops
      4) caseous nodule (tubercle) is formed around organism
      5) organism never completely disappears but is walled off in lungs
      6) may remain quiescent for long time, but physical and emotional stress can cause organism to become active and multiply (reactivation process)
      7) inflammation can occur and tuberculous process begins again
      8) disease may also spread through lymphatics and vascular system (miliary tuberculosis)
      9) if medical therapy fails, surgical resection of one or more lobes may be advised

2. **Nursing Process**
   a. Assessment   *When stressed can begin to show sym.*
      1) dyspnea
      2) pleuritic pain
      3) rales
      4) fatigue
      5) night sweats
      6) low-grade fever in afternoon
      7) weight loss
      8) anorexia
      9) hemoptysis (late symptom)
      10) abnormal chest x-ray
      11) sputum culture positive for *Mycobacterium tuberculosis*

[Handwritten note at top: BCG vaccine give (+) test for Tuberculin test.]

202 SECTION 3: NURSING CARE OF THE ADULT

(*NOTE*: may take 3–12 weeks to obtain positive result)

12) positive skin testing
   a) OT (old tuberculin) (Mantoux)
   b) PPD (purified protein derivative) is most reliable
   - intradermal injection on inner aspect of forearm
   - negative reaction: absence of erythema and/or induration after 48 hours
   - positive reaction: 8–10 mm *induration* in 48 hours
     - indicates contact with tuberculosis bacillus but not necessarily an active infection
     - do chest x-ray if positive
     - do not repeat skin testing in future (screen with a chest x-ray)
     - prophylactic chemotherapy may be indicated

b. Goals, Plans/Implementation, and Evaluation

Goal 1: Client's active tuberculosis will be arrested.

Plan/Implementation
- administer antituberculous drugs as ordered (see table 3.23)
- provide adequate rest (*not* bedrest)
- institute adequate diet

Evaluation: Client's sputum culture converts to negative after 2 weeks of medications.

Goal 2: Staff, client's family, and others will be protected from infection with tuberculosis.

Plan/Implementation
- maintain appropriate *[handwritten: airborne]* isolation necessary while client has positive sputum smear and culture and/or is coughing
  - discontinue after symptoms disappear (often within 2 weeks after start of treatment)
- prevent the transmission of droplets
  - cover mouth, nose when coughing, sneezing, laughing
  - dispose of tissue by burning
  - careful hand washing when handling sputum
  - adequate air circulation (air changes will dilute number of bacilli in air of isolated client's room)
  - bacilli are killed by direct sunlight in 1–2 hours; boiling temperature of water kills bacilli in 5 minutes
- emphasize the importance of continuing prescribed medication
- refer to public health department for case finding

Evaluation: Client's family does not contract tuberculosis.

Table 3.23	Antituberculous Drugs
Description	Drugs act to inhibit or destroy the tubercle bacillus. They are mainly bacteriostatic (except rifampin and INH, which are bacteriocidal). Combination drug therapy is utilized to potentiate the effects and reduce the chances of microbial resistance. The drugs are divided into first-line drugs (dependable, low toxicity) and second-line drugs (more toxic, used to treat resistant organisms).
Uses	To treat tuberculosis; tuberculosis prophylaxis
Side Effects	Neurotoxicity, visual changes, GI distress, ototoxicity (streptomycin)
Nursing Implications	Know side effects of each specific drug; stress importance of continued therapy to prevent development of resistant bacteria; provide frequent vision, hearing, and neurologic screening; give B_6 (pyridoxine) to block side effects of INH.
Types and Examples	*First-Line Drugs:* isoniazid (INH), ethambutol (Myambutol), rifampin (Rifadin), streptomycin *Second-Line Drugs:* para-aminosalicylic acid (PAS), capreomycin (Capastat), cycloserine (Seromycin), ethionamide (Trecator-SC), pyrazinamide

Goal 3: Client will be able to cope with disease.
Plan/Implementation
- know there is a social stigma associated with tuberculosis
- encourage expression of fears, concerns, questions
- spend time talking with client (refer to table 2.4) *Case finding*

Evaluation: Client verbalizes a desire to practice safe health measures.

Goal 4: Client will be able to care for self at home and will practice health habits that prevent reactivation of infection.
Plan/Implementation
- teach
  - medications
    * administration
    * side effects
    * importance of compliance
  - importance of activity
  - nutritious diet
  - isolation technique if necessary
  - not to swallow sputum
  - importance of follow-up care
  - arrange public health follow-up

Tuberculin rest of life

Evaluation: Client complies with medication regime.

L. Chest Tubes and Chest Surgery

1. **General Information**
   a. Clients who experience open-chest injuries, are surgically treated for lung cancer, or have open-heart surgery require similar care because of the opening of the thoracic cavity and the subsequent presence of chest tubes
   b. Lung Expansion: supported by
      1) visceral and parietal pleura
      2) pressure in pleural space
      3) sucking effect on lung
   c. Disruption of Airtight Thoracic Cavity
      1) spontaneous pneumothorax
      2) stab wound
      3) bullet wound
      4) thoracotomy
      5) tear of pleura by fractured ribs
   d. Tension Pneumothorax
      1) cause: closed chest wound; air is unable to escape on expiration; lung collapses as intrathoracic tension increases
      2) emergency treatment: chest tube if available, otherwise insert a needle to allow air to escape
   e. Chest Tube Drainage
      1) open tube to gravity does not work: atmospheric pressure is greater than intrathoracic pressure→collapsed lung
      2) purpose of water seal: to seal the chest tube so it acts as one-way valve (air and fluid travel down the tube but room air cannot travel up the tube)
      3) 1-, 2-, or 3-bottle system or Pleur-evac (see figures 3.11 and 3.12)
      4) two chest tubes used for client with lobectomy, segmental resection, or hemothorax; one chest tube with pneumothorax, cardiac surgery
         a) placement
            - anterior, upper thoracic area for air removal
            - 2nd tube, if required, in posterior, lower thoracic area for drainage (drainage is heavier than air)
         b) purposes
            - to promote air and/or drainage removal from pleural space and prevent their return
            - to help re-expand remaining lung tissue
            - to prevent shifting of mediastinum and collapsed lung tissue by equalization of pressure
      5) no chest tubes used for client with pneumonectomy
         a) no lung left to re-expand
         b) increased danger of mediastinal shift
      6) application of suction
         a) controlled suction: intermittent positive pressure is used to facilitate removal of secretions and aid in lung expansion
         b) uncontrolled suction: gravity drainage; breaker bottle controls the amount of suction

2. **Nursing Process**
   a. Assessment
      1) fluctuation of water in water-seal bottle
      2) bubbling of water-seal bottle
      3) bubbling in "breaker bottle"
   b. Goals, Plans/Implementation, and Evaluation

204 SECTION 3: NURSING CARE OF THE ADULT

Figure 3.11 Water-Seal Chest Drainage

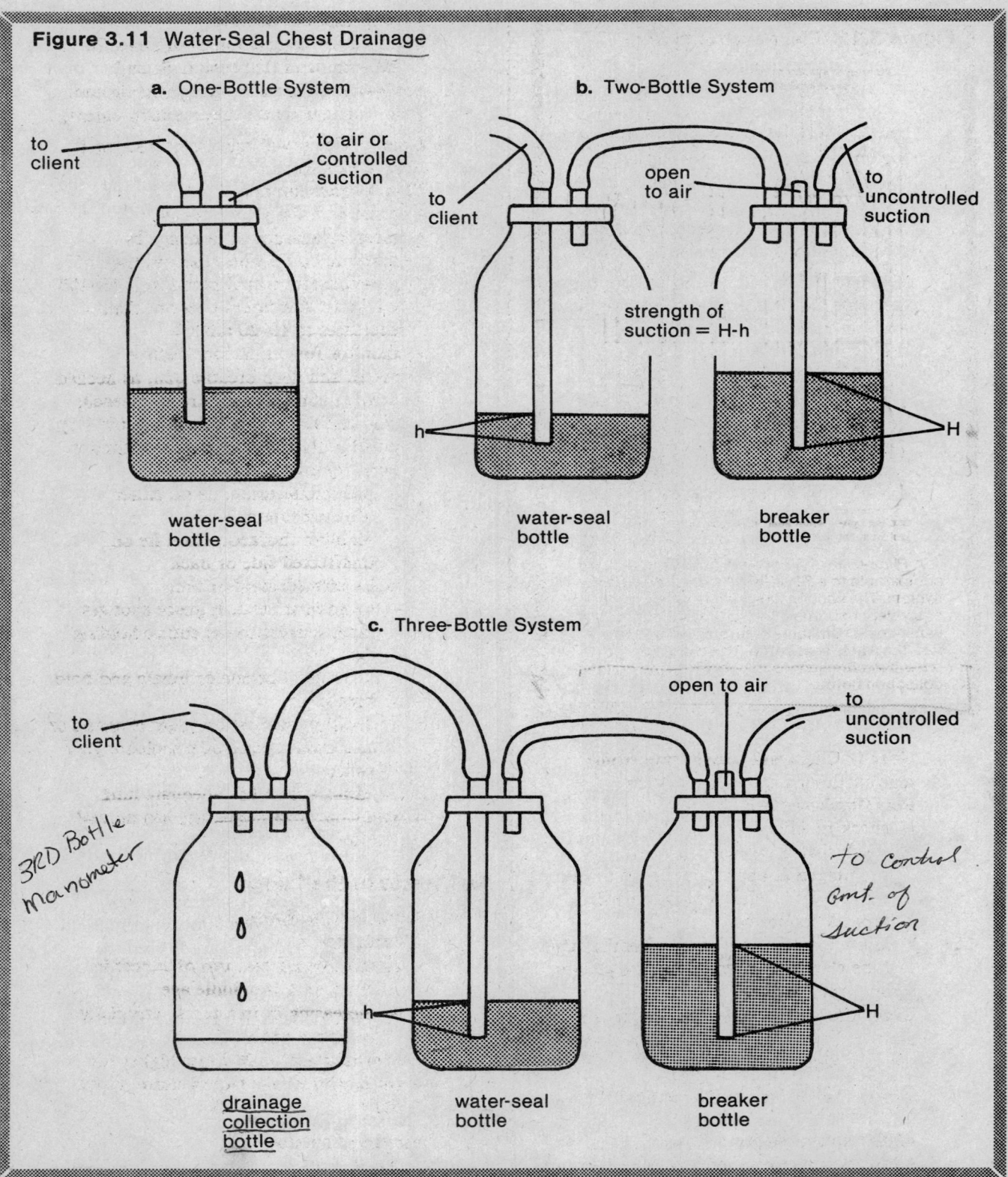

OXYGENATION 205

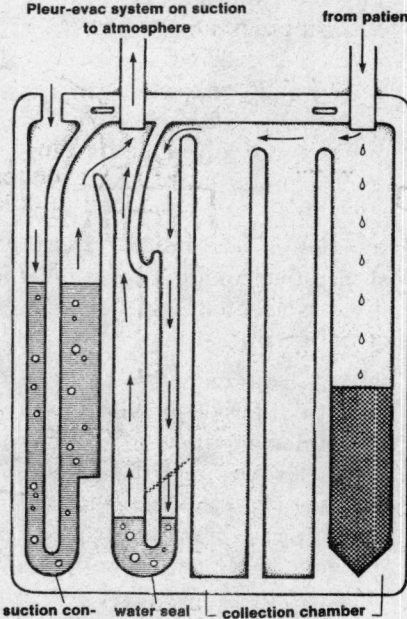

Figure 3.12 Pleur-evac System

A Pleur-evac unit consists of three chambers comparable to a 3-bottle water-seal drainage system. The suction control chamber is equivalent to bottle #3—the breaker bottle. The water-seal chamber is equivalent to bottle #2—the water-seal bottle. The collection chamber corresponds to bottle #1—the drainage collection bottle.

Portable

Goal 1: Client will remain safe from malfunctioning water-seal system.
Plan/Implementation
- check functioning of system
- check that manometer tube is submerged at appropriate level or that water level in Pleur-evac is correct
- tape all connectors
- know what to do if system breaks: have tube clamps at bedside and use clamps appropriately

Evaluation: Client receives prompt and appropriate care if system breaks; water-seal drainage remains intact.

Goal 2: Client will have tube patency maintained.
Plan/Implementation
- position tubes correctly; ensure that they are not kinked
- attach tube to bed linens to prevent it from falling over side and pulling at insertion site
- strip tubes as ordered
- check for fluctuation of drainage in tube (ensures that tube is patent)

Evaluation: Client has adequate air and fluid drainage (chest tubes remain patent).

Goal 3: Client will experience adequate lung re-expansion.
Plan/Implementation
- assist with daily chest x-ray
- measure amount of drainage by marking bottle with tape and time of measurement (usual blood loss: 50–100 ml/hr 1st few hours post-op; then decreases to 10–20 ml/hr)
- monitor for respiratory distress
- cough and deep breathe q2h, as needed
- provide comfort measures as needed; pain medications as ordered (table 3.5)
- position the client to ensure optimum lung expansion
  - pneumonectomy: lie on either affected side or back
  - all other thoracotomies: lie on unaffected side or back
- assist with removal of tube
  - equipment needed: gauze sponges, tape, scissors to cut suture holding the tube
  - have client exhale or inhale and hold breath
  - dressing application: tight dressing of 4x4s over a piece of petroleum jelly gauze

Evaluation: Client has adequate lung reexpansion; breathes easily, has normal skin color.

M. Cancer of the Lung
1. **General Information**
   a. Incidence
      1) most common form of cancer in men; peak in middle age
      2) increasing in frequency, especially among women
   b. Mortality rate is 20 times higher for those who smoke two or more packs daily
2. **Nursing Process**   *Sym appear late*
   a. Assessment
      1) cough: chronic, persistent
      2) abnormal chest x-ray
      3) positive sputum cytology
      4) positive biopsy

5) hemoptysis, weakness, anorexia, weight loss, dyspnea, chest pain: symptoms of advanced disease
6) pleural effusion (peripheral tumors)

b. Goals, Plans/Implementation, and Evaluation

Goal 1: Client and significant others will be able to explain diagnostic tests and postprocedure care.

Plan/Implementation
- assess level of knowledge of client/significant others
- explain procedures (e.g., bronchoscopy, sputum exams, page 174)

Evaluation: Client/significant others know what to expect during and after procedures.

Goal 2: Client and significant others will be able to explain planned medical treatment.

Plan/Implementation
- know that radiation therapy and/or chemotherapy are often given if surgery not possible or pre-op in conjunction with surgery (refer to *Cellular Aberration* page 326)

Evaluation: Client describes expected actions, side effects of planned medical therapy.

Goal 3: Client and significant others will be able to explain preoperative care, postoperative needs, OR-RR-SICU environment, purpose of chest tubes, and pain control for planned surgery.

Plan/Implementation
- assess level of knowledge of client and significant others
- give pre-op instruction (refer to *Surgery* "Perioperative Care" page 165; and chest tube care page 205)
- tour ICU
- assess level of anxiety
- encourage expression of fears
- give emotional support/relieve anxiety (refer to *The Client with Psychosocial Problems* page 13 and table 2.4)

Evaluation: Client can demonstrate adequate coughing and deep breathing; states an awareness of ICU environment.

Goal 4: Postoperatively, client will have adequate respiratory function, stable cardiac function, and adequate pain control.

Plan/Implementation
- cough, deep breathe, turn qh
- monitor vital signs, CVP, I&O
- suction prn
- give O_2 as ordered
- relieve pain, analgesics prn
- monitor chest tubes
- position appropriately for lung expansion (refer to chest tube care page 205)

Evaluation: Client remains free from postoperative complications (breathes easily, has adequate I&O, experiences good control of pain).

Goal 5: Client and significant others will be able to discuss fears and concerns.

Plan/Implementation
- assess level of anxiety and fears of client and significant others
- encourage expression of fears/anxieties
- provide emotional support/relieve anxiety
- maintain hope
- refer to appropriate support groups

Evaluation: Client and significant others discuss fears, ask questions concerning diagnosis.

Goal 6: Client and significant others will be able to explain needs upon discharge.

Plan/Implementation
- teach
  - levels of activity and rest
  - how to prevent respiratory infections (e.g., avoid crowds)
- encourage client to stop smoking
- arrange follow-up appointment

Evaluation: Client knows date for return appointment with physician; states a willingness to comply with restrictions.

References

Armstrong, M., Dickason, E., Howe, J., Jones D., and Snider, M. *McGraw-Hill Handbook of Clinical Nursing*. New York: McGraw-Hill, 1979.

Brunner, L. and Suddarth, D. *Textbook of Medical-Surgical Nursing*. Philadelphia: Lippincott, 1980.

Burrell, Z. and Burrell, L. *Critical Care*. St. Louis: Mosby, 1977.

Cardin, S. "Acid-Base Balance in the Patient with Respiratory Disease." *Nursing Clinics of North America*. September 1980:593-601.

Cavanaugh, A. and Mancini, R. "Drug Interactions and Digitalis Toxicity." *American Journal of Nursing*. December 1980:2170-2171.

Cohen, S. "How to Work with Chest Tubes" (Programmed Instruction). *American Journal of Nursing*. April 1980:685-712.

Cohen, S. "New Concepts in Understanding Congestive Heart Failure" (Programmed Instruction). *American Journal of Nursing*. Part 1, January 1981:119-139; Part 2, February 1981:357-380.

Cohen, S. "Nursing Care of Patients in Shock. Part 1: Pharmacotherapy." *American Journal of Nursing*. June 1982:943-963.

Erickson, R. "Chest Tubes: They're Really Not that Complicated." *Nursing 81*. May 1981:34-43.

Fuller, E. "The Effect of Antianginal Drugs on Myocardial Oxygen Consumption." *American Journal of Nursing*. February 1980:250-255.

Grim, C. "Nursing Assessment of the Patient with High Blood Pressure." *Nursing Clinics of North America*. June 1981:349-364.

Hartshorn, T. "What to do when the Patient's in Hypertensive Crisis." *Nursing 80*. July 1980:32-35.

Hill, M. "Helping the Hypertensive Patient Control Sodium Intake." *American Journal of Nursing*. May 1979:906-909.

Hudgel, D. and Madsen, L. "Acute and Chronic Asthma: A Guide to Intervention." *American Journal of Nursing*. October 1980:1791-1795.

Hutchins, L. "Drug Treatment of High Blood Pressure." *Nursing Clinics of North America*. June 1981:365-376.

Jett, G., Cortese, D., and Fontana, R. "Lung Cancer: Current Concepts and Prospects." *Cancer Journal for Clinicians*. March/April 1983:74-86.

Kaufman, J. and Woody, J. "For Patients with COPD: Better Living through Teaching." *Nursing 1980*. March 1980:57-61.

Kirilloff, L. and Tibbals, S. "Drugs for Asthma: A Complete Guide." *American Journal of Nursing*. January 1983:55-61.

Lesage, J. (Ed). "Symposium on Drugs and the Older Adult." *Nursing Clinics of North America*. June 1982:253-340.

*Long, M., Winslow, E., Scheuhing, M., Callahan, J. "Hypertension: What Patients Need to Know." *American Journal of Nursing*. May 1976:765-770.

Pinney, M. "Pneumonia." *American Journal of Nursing*. March 1981:517-518.

Price, S. and Wilson, L. *Pathophysiology, Clinical Concepts of Disease Processes*. New York: McGraw-Hill, 1982.

Purcell, J. "Shock Drugs: Standardized Guidelines." *American Journal of Nursing*. June 1982:965-974.

Rifas, E. "Teaching Patients to Manage Acute Asthma: The Future is Now." *Nursing 83*. April 1983:77-82.

Robinson, J. (Ed). *Giving Cardiovascular Drugs Safely* (Nursing 78 Skillbook Series). Horsham, PA: Intermed Communications, 1978.

Rokosky, J. "Assessment of the Patient with Altered Respiratory Function." *Nursing Clinics of North America*. June 1981:195-209.

Tannenbaum, R., Sohn, C., Cantwell, R., Rogers, M., and Hollis, R. "The Pain of Angina Pectoris: How to Recognize It, How to Manage It." *Nursing 81*. September 1981:44-51.

Wade, J. *Comprehensive Respiratory Care: Physiology and Technique*. St. Louis: Mosby, 1982.

Waldron, R. "Oxygen Transport." *American Journal of Nursing*. February 1979:272-275.

Wooden, L. "Your Patient with a Pneumothorax: A Patient in Distress." *Nursing 82*. November 1982:50-56.

*See reprint section

Nutrition and Metabolism

(The nursing care presented in this unit concerns selected health problems related to disturbances in the digestive tract and the endocrine system.)

Part One: The Digestive Tract

General Concepts

A. Overview
1. Function: to transfer food and water from the external to the internal environment of the body and transform these substances into a form suitable for distribution to the cells via the circulatory system
2. Anatomy
   a. Upper Gastrointestinal Tract
      1) mouth, teeth, salivary glands
      2) esophagus
      3) stomach
   b. Lower Gastrointestinal Tract
      1) small bowel
      2) large bowel
      3) rectum
      4) anus
   c. Accessory Organs of Digestion
      1) liver
      2) gallbladder
      3) pancreas
3. Processes
   a. Digestion: the process of breaking down proteins, polysaccharides, and fat; accomplished by the action of acid and enzymes secreted into the GI tract
   b. Secretion: the process of elaborating a specific product as a result of glandular activity
      1) saliva (mouth): contains salivary amylase (hydrolyzes starch into maltase)
      2) gastric secretions
         a) mucus: lubricates stomach lining and content
         b) hydrochloric acid (HCl): essential to provide the acid medium necessary for the function of pepsin
         c) pepsin: breaks down proteins to polypeptides, proteoses, and peptones

Table 3.24 Gastrointestinal Hormones

Hormone	Source	How Stimulated	Action
Gastrin	Mucosa of stomach	Distention by food and vagal stimulation.	Stimulates secretion of hydrochloric acid.
Secretin	Duodenal mucosa	Gastric contents entering duodenum.	Stimulates secretion of pancreatic fluid.
Cholecystokinin	Duodenal mucosa	Fat in duodenum.	Contraction of gallbladder. Stimulates secretion of enzyme-rich pancreatic juice.

NUTRITION AND METABOLISM 209

Table 3.25 Digestive Enzymes

Enzymes that Digest	Source	Selected Action and Products
Carbohydrates		
Amylase	Parotid and sub-maxillary glands	Hydrolyzes starch to maltose.
Sucrase, maltase, isomaltase, lactase	Intestinal fluids	Split disaccharides into monosaccharides.
Pancreatic amylase	Pancreas	Splits starches into maltose and isomaltose.
Fats		
Gastric lipase	Gastric mucosa	Digests butterfat.
Intestinal lipase	Intestinal fluids	Splits fats into glycerol and fatty acids.
Pancreatic lipase	Pancreas	Hydrolyzes fat into glycerol and fatty acids.
Protein		
Pepsin	Gastric mucosa	Breaks down dietary protein into proteoses, peptones, and polypeptides.
Peptidases	Intestinal glands	Splits polypeptides into amino acids.
Trypsin	Pancreas	Splits proteins into peptides and amino acids.
Chymotrypsin	Pancreas	Splits proteins into polypeptides.
Carboxypeptidase	Pancreas	Splits polypeptides into smaller peptides.
Other		
Enterokinase	Duodenal mucosa	Activates trypsin.
Nucleases	Pancreas	Splits nucleic acids.

      d) lipase (small amounts): digests butterfat
      e) gastrin: involved in stimulation and release of HCl
   3) small bowel secretions
      a) peptidases: split polypeptides into amino acids
      b) sucrase, maltase, isomaltase, lactase: split disaccharides into monosaccharides
      c) intestinal lipase splits fats into glycerol and fatty acids
      d) secretin and cholecystokinin-pancreozymin stimulate the pancreas and gallbladder
   4) pancreatic secretions
      a) trypsin, chymotrypsin, nucleases, carboxypeptidase, pancreatic lipase, and pancreatic amylase break down protein, fats, carbohydrates
      b) bicarbonate-rich isosmotic electrolyte solution
   5) gallbladder secretes bile
  c. Absorption: the process by which the small molecules that are the result of digestion cross cell membranes of the intestine and enter the blood and lymph
   1) carbohydrates and proteins are absorbed by active transport along with sodium
   2) fatty acids are absorbed by diffusion
   3) water and electrolytes are absorbed in the small and large intestines
   4) synthesis and absorption of vitamin K, thiamine, riboflavin, vitamin B_{12}, folic acid, biotin, and nicotinic acid take place in the large intestine as a result of bacterial activity, primarily *E. Coli*
  d. Motility: the process by which contractions of the smooth muscle lining the walls of the GI tract produce movement of substances through the GI tract while digestion and absorption occur
   1) GI tract contains an intrinsic nerve supply that controls tone and peristaltic action
   2) nerve fibers from both the sympathetic and parasympathetic branches of the autonomic nervous

system supply the intestinal tract and interact with intrinsic nerve supply
3) the vagus nerve (the major autonomic nerve supplying the GI tract) is composed of motor parasympathetic fibers and many sensory fibers; parasympathetic stimulation *increases* motility and secretion; sympathetic stimulation *decreases* motility and secretion
   e. Metabolism
      1) all of the changes or body processes that take place in order to sustain life; the chemical changes that occur allow chemical energy to be changed to other forms of energy so that cellular functions can be maintained
      2) intermediary metabolism includes all the cellular functions in the body's internal environment; this phase of metabolism begins after the ingestion and digestion of foodstuffs from the external environment
      3) two-part process
         a) anabolism: the process of synthesis of smaller molecules to larger molecules; energy is saved
            • building process: proteins from amino acids, fats from fatty acids, polysaccharides from monosaccharides
            • increased during growth, pregnancy, recovery states, or times of increased intake
         b) catabolism: the breaking down of larger molecules into smaller molecules
            • protein, fats, carbohydrates are broken down into units that can be used by the cells
            • excesses in catabolism are seen in starvation, illness, trauma
            • breakdown involves the release of CO_2, water, and urea with amino acid metabolism
      4) adenosine triphosphate (ATP) is the high-energy phosphate that is the major source of energy for cellular function
      5) adenosine diphosphate (ADP) is one of the end products released when energy is used and ATP is broken down
      6) metabolic balance remains unless a change in the internal or external environment produces imbalances (for the balance to be maintained, the rate of catabolism must equal anabolism)
      7) variances in metabolic rate occur with differences in sex, age, hormonal environment, seasonal and environmental temperature changes, culture, activity levels, ingestion of drugs (e.g., caffeine, nicotine, epinephrine)
      8) materials needed for metabolism
         a) nutrients to supply energy and build tissue: glucose, glycerol, fatty acids, amino acids
         b) minerals, electrolytes
         c) materials (primarily proteins) to promote synthesis of enzymes and hormones
         d) vitamins that function as co-enzymes
         e) enzymes and hormones to function as organic cellular catalysts
      9) metabolism governs the activities of muscle contraction, nerve impulse transmission, glandular secretion, absorption, and elimination

B. **Application of the Nursing Process to the Client with Digestive Tract Problems**
   1. Assessment
      a. Health History
         1) normal dietary pattern: changes in appetite
         2) normal weight: changes in weight (how much, time period)
         3) change in energy level: weakness, fatigue, general malaise
         4) stool: changes in frequency, color, character
         5) indigestion: which drugs used, frequency, effectiveness
         6) heartburn: pattern, relief with drugs
         7) difficulty in swallowing: dysphagia with onset by solids or liquids
         8) difficulty tolerating certain foods: allergies
         9) vomiting/nausea: character of vomitus; pattern of nausea; relationship to intake, other events
         10) abdominal pain: presence, location, character, pattern
         11) abdominal distention
         12) abdominal surgery

13) jaundice
14) bruising, bleeding: onset, duration, extent
15) urine: dark, orange color
16) alcohol habits

b. Physical Examination of the Abdomen (*NOTE:* Palpation is done last because it can stimulate bowel sounds)
   1) inspection
      a) skin characteristics: scars, striae, engorged veins, spider angiomata
      b) visible peristalsis
      c) visible pulsations
      d) visible masses
      e) contour: rounded, protuberant, concave, asymmetric
   2) auscultation: listen to all four quadrants
      a) bowel sounds: location, frequency (number per minute), characteristics
         • normal: succession of clicks/gurgles
         • abnormal
           – hyperperistalsis: loud gurgles
           – paralytic ileus: absent or infrequent
           – intestinal obstruction: loud, rushing, high-pitched tinkling proximal to the obstruction
           – air/fluid in stomach: succession of splashes
      b) bruits
   3) percussion
      a) stomach (tympany normal)
      b) liver size (normally dull)
      c) gaseous distention
   4) palpation
      a) pain
      b) masses, especially liver enlargement
      c) skin reflexes
      d) fluid waves

c. Diagnostic Tests
   1) hematologic studies: normal values will vary slightly from laboratory to laboratory
      a) electrolytes
         • sodium: 135–145 mEq/liter
         • potassium: 3.8–5.5 mEq/liter
         • chlorides: 100–108 mEq/liter
      b) CBC
         • WBC: 5,000–10,000/mm³
         • RBC: 4.2–6.2 million/mm³
         • Hgb:
           – men: 14–18 g/dl
           – women: 12–16 g/dl
         • Hct
           – men: 42%–54%
           – women: 38%–46%
      c) serum glutamic-oxaloacetic transaminase (SGOT): 8–20 units/liter
      d) serum glutamic-pyruvic transaminase (SGPT): 6–36 units/liter
      e) bromsulphalein (BSP): less than 10% retention after 45 minutes
      f) alkaline phosphatase: 90–239 units/liter
      g) ammonia levels: less than 50 µg/dl
      h) albumin: 3–4.5 g/dl; globulin: 2.3–3.5 g/dl
      i) lipase: 32–80 units/liter; amylase: 60–180 units/dl; gastrin: less than 300 pg/ml
      j) bilirubin: less than 1 mg/dl
      k) cholesterol: 120–330 mg/dl
      l) glucose levels
         • glucose: 70–100 mg/ml
         • postprandial: less than 145 mg/dl
         • glucose tolerance: peak of 160–180 mg/dl
      m) carcinoembryonic antigen (CEA): less than 5 ng/dl
      n) hepatitis B surface antigen (HB$_S$Ag) and hepatitis B surface antibody (anti-HB$_S$): negative
      o) prothrombin time: comparable to normal control
   2) urine tests
      a) glucose, acetone
      b) urobilinogen
   3) stool tests
      a) ova and parasites (stool must be warm)
      b) occult blood (guaiac)
      c) fecal fat (after a 72-hour collection)
      d) culture
   4) radiographic studies
      a) flat plate of abdomen
      b) upper GI series (often with small bowel follow-through)
         • definition: x-ray of esophagus, stomach, duodenum following oral intake of contrast medium (barium)
         • nursing care pretest: nothing PO for 8 hours prior to test

Table 3.26 Acid-Base Imbalance

Problem	Etiology	Assessment	Compensating Mechanisms	Nursing Interventions

Respiratory Acidosis
• pH <7.35
• PCO_2 >45
• HCO_3 normal
	Hypoventilation
	• acute causes
	  - respiratory infections
	  - CNS depressant overdose
	  - paralysis of respiratory muscles
	  - atelectasis
	  - brain damage
	  - post-op abdominal distention
	• chronic causes
	  - obesity
	  - ascites
	  - pregnancy.
		Hypoventilation.
		Tachycardia, irregular pulse.
		Decreased chest excursion.
		Headache, dizziness.
		Cyanosis.
		Drowsiness leading to coma.
			Kidneys retain and manufacture more bicarbonate leading to
			• pH 7.4
			• PCO_2 >45
			• HCO_3 >28.
				Turn, cough, and deep breathe qh.
				Suction prn.
				Monitor vital signs.
				Give respiratory stimulants as ordered.
				Give bronchodilators.
				Give O_2 cautiously to prevent CO_2 narcosis.

Respiratory Alkalosis • pH >7.45 • PCO_2 <35 • HCO_3 normal	Hyperventilation • emotions, hysteria • O_2 lack • fever • salicylate poisoning • CNS stimulation by drugs/disease.	Hyperventilation • light-headed • tingling of hands and face (tetany). Convulsions. Diaphoresis. Low serum K^+.	Kidneys excrete large amounts of bicarbonate leading to • pH 7.4 • PCO_2 <35 • HCO_3 <23.	Calm client. Slow the rate of ventilation. Use rebreather to increase PCO_2. Administer O_2 as needed.
Metabolic Acidosis • pH <7.35 • PCO_2 normal • HCO_3 <23	Bicarbonate loss • diarrhea • GI fistula. Acid gain • diabetic ketoacidosis • lactic acidosis • renal failure • salicylate intoxication • K^+ excess.	Headache, dizziness. Kussmaul's respiration. Fruity breath odor. Disoriented. Coma. Nausea/vomiting. High serum K^+.	Lungs hyperventilate to blow off CO_2 and reduce plasma carbonic acid content leading to • pH 7.4 • PCO_2 <35 • HCO_3 <23.	Administer sodium bicarbonate as ordered. Give insulin as ordered. Monitor I&O, vital signs. Support client.
Metabolic Alkalosis • pH >7.45 • PCO_2 normal • HCO_3 >28	Acid loss • vomiting or GI suction • steroid therapy • thiazide diuretics. Bicarbonate retention • excess use of bicarbonate (baking soda) as antacid • excess infusion of Ringer's lactate • citrated blood.	Headache. Numbness and tingling leading to tetany and convulsions. Hypoventilation. Confusion and agitation. Low serum K^+.	Lungs hypoventilate to retain CO_2 and increase plasma carbonic acid content leading to • pH 7.4 • PCO_2 >45 • HCO_3 >28.	Give IV ammonium chloride as ordered. Maintain K^+ level with diet or drugs. Teach client high K^+ diet if taking thiazide diuretics. Give acetazolamide (Diamox) as ordered. Maintain calm, quiet environment.

NUTRITION AND METABOLISM

Table 3.27 Fluid Imbalance

Etiology	Assessment	Nursing Interventions
Overhydration		
Renal failure.	Vital signs.	Prevention
Excessive fluid intake.	Weight (increases).	• monitor IV fluids closely.
Excess IVs.	Peripheral edema.	• monitor urine output.
Water intoxication (GU irrigation with hypotonic fluids).	Venous pressure (increases).	• monitor I&O, weight.
	Pulmonary edema.	Treatment
Hypernatremia.	Symptoms of CHF or increased intracranial pressure.	• reduce edema.
		• give diuretics as ordered.
		• limit intake.
		• maintain low sodium intake.
Dehydration		
Nausea & vomiting.	Skin turgor (poor).	Prevention
Increased urinary output.	Thirst.	• monitor I&O.
Diuretics.	Vital signs.	• replace lost fluids.
Insufficient intake (because of age, immobility, etc.).	Urine output.	• patient teaching re excess perspiration.
	Weight.	
Inadequate replacement following excess fluid loss (diaphoresis, diarrhea).	Level of consciousness.	Treatment
		• replace fluids carefully.
		• monitor I&O, weight.

- nursing care post-test
  - laxatives, force fluids to remove barium
  - encourage mobility to stimulate peristalsis
- c) lower GI, barium enema, refer to "Large Bowel" page 274
- d) cholecystogram
  - definition: x-ray visualization of gallbladder and biliary tract following oral ingestion of iodine dye
  - nursing care pretest
    - check for iodine allergies
    - dye (usually Telepaque in form of 6 tablets) given 12 hours before test (give with sufficient water 30 minutes apart since it may cause diarrhea)
    - low fat evening meal the day prior
    - nothing PO for 8 hours prior to test
  - nursing care post-test: no special concerns
- e) cholangiogram (IV, via T-tube, or via common bile duct during surgery)
  - definition: x-ray visualization of gallbladder and biliary tract following injection of iodine dye
  - nursing care pretest
    - check for iodine allergies
    - nothing PO for 8 hours prior to test
    - permit signed if applicable
  - nursing care post-test: force fluids (dye acts as diuretic)
- f) abdominal CAT scan: with or without contrast medium
5) endoscopy
   - a) definition: direct visualization of a part or parts of the GI tract through a lighted scope; may be a treatment modality as well (e.g., polypectomy, remove foreign objects, cauterize GI bleeding sites)
   - b) types
     - esophagoscopy (esophagus)
     - gastroscopy (stomach)
     - duodenoscopy (duodenum)
     - peritoneoscopy (liver, gallbladder, and mesentery)
     - endoscopic retrograde cholangiography (ERCP) (pancreas and biliary tree)
     - sigmoidoscopy (sigmoid colon)
     - colonoscopy (entire colon)
     - proctoscopy (rectosigmoid)
   - c) nursing care pretest
     - nothing PO for 8 hours prior to test

Table 3.28 Electrolyte Imbalances

	Problem	Etiology	Assessments	Nursing Interventions
Sodium	*Hypernatremia* Na+ greater than 145 mEq/L	*Hypersmolar* Sodium increased in relation to water. Water loss without sodium loss. Dehydration.	Increased hemoglobin. Signs of dehydration. Thirst. Decreased BP. Concentrated urine with high specific gravity.	Low sodium diet, restricted fluids. Strict I&O. Prevent shock. Maintain adequate urine output. Monitor serum Na.
		Isotonic Both sodium and water increased. Renal failure. Cirrhosis. Steroid therapy. Aldosterone excess.	Edema. Weight gain. Normal sodium. Hypertension. Symptoms of fluid overload.	Low sodium diet, water restriction. Strict I&O. Monitor for signs of CHF or increased intracranial pressure. Daily weight. Diuretics (Na-wasting) as ordered.
	Hyponatremia Na+ less than 135 mEq/L	*Hypo-osmolar or "dilutional"* Water increased in relation to sodium. Water intoxication. Exercise. IVs without NaCl. Low sodium diet.	Fluid volume excess. Increased urine output with low specific gravity. No thirst. Nausea/vomiting. Weakness/cerebral dysfunction.	Restrict water. Monitor I&O, serum Na. Watch for circulatory overload. Replace Na carefully. Give high Na diet.
		Isotonic Both sodium and water decreased. Diuretics. GI losses. Burns.	Decreased BP. Poor skin turgor. Dehydration/shock. No thirst. Oliguria.	Monitor for shock. Good skin care. Give isotonic fluids. Monitor I&O, serum Na.
Potassium	*Hyperkalemia* K+ greater than 5.0 mEq/L	Severe burns. Crush injuries. Addison's disease. Renal failure. Acidosis. Excessive K intake (oral or IV).	ECG changes (high T wave). Skeletal muscle weakness. Bradycardia, cardiac arrest. Oliguria. Intestinal colic and diarrhea.	Monitor cardiac function, serum K, neurologic signs. Limit K intake. Give D_{50} plus insulin as ordered. Give exchange-resins (sodium polystyrene sulfonate [Kayexalate] po or enemas) as ordered. Give bicarbonate to correct acidosis. Dialysis (renal/peritoneal).
	Hypokalemia K+ less than 3.5 mEq/L	Diuretic therapy (thiazides). Poor intake. GI loss. Ulcerative colitis. Cushing's syndrome. Alkalosis.	Digitalis toxicity. Muscle weakness and decreased reflexes. Flaccid paralysis. Paralytic ileus. CNS depression, lethargy. Hypotension. Anorexia. ECG changes (flattened T wave).	Administer K slowly IV. Monitor ECG. Teach adequate K replacement when taking diuretics. Administer po K drugs/diet.

Table 3.28 Continued

	Problem	Etiology	Assessments	Nursing Interventions
Calcium	*Hypercalcemia* Ca^{++} greater than 11 mg	Immobility. Hyperparathyroidism. Bone metastasis. Excess vitamin D intake. Parathyroid tumor. Osteoporosis. Decreased renal excretion.	Skeletal muscle weakness. Bone pain. Renal calculi. Pathologic fractures. CNS depression, altered LOC. GI (constipation, nausea, vomiting, anorexia). Decreased serum phosphorus.	Limit intake. Patient teaching. Prevent fractures. Give phosphorus. Maintain adequate I&O. Monitor neurologic signs.
	Hypocalcemia Ca^{++} less than 9 mg	Hypoparathyroidism. Low vitamin D in diet. Parathyroidectomy. Pregnancy and lactation. Postthyroidectomy. Rickets. Renal disease.	Tetany, tingling, paresthesias of fingers and around mouth/muscle twitching, cramps. Positive Chvostek's and Trousseau's signs. Laryngospasm. Increased phosphorus.	Give Ca as needed. Monitor for early muscle spasms, neurologic signs. Monitor those at risk. Give phosphate-binding antacids. Monitor serum Ca.
Magnesium	*Hypermagnesemia* Mg^{++} greater than 2.8 mEq/L	Renal insufficiency. Diabetic ketoacidosis. Excess Mg intake (antacids). Dehydration.	CNS and neuro- muscular depression. Hypotension. Sedation. Arrest.	Monitor replacement carefully. Support respiration. Teach client correct antacid intake. Monitor neurologic signs.
	Hypomagnesemia Mg^{++} less than 1.5 mEq/L	Alcoholism. Loss (GI, diuresis). Low intake. Hypercalcemia. Diabetes. Toxemia. Renal disease.	Tremors and neuro- muscular irritability. Disorientation. Positive Chvostek's and Trousseau's signs. Convulsions.	Give Mg cautiously as ordered. Monitor closely for Mg excess. Teach adequate intake. Monitor neurologic signs.

- bowel prep for lower GI endoscopy
- pretest sedation as ordered

d) nursing care post-test
- check vital signs frequently the first 24 hours
- feed when gag reflex returns after upper GI endoscopy
- observe for bleeding (indicated by frequent swallowing/bloody emesis), sharp pain (indicates perforation)
- force fluids as needed

6) hepatic angiography: liver, gall- bladder, pancreas

7) abdominal ultrasound
   a) definition: examination of the abdomen using sound waves
   b) nursing care pretest
      - laxatives and cathartics the evening before
      - nothing PO for 8 hours prior to test
      - have client drink 6–8 glasses of water just prior to test and not void until test is over, or clamp Foley catheter
   c) nursing care post-test: no special concerns
8) analytical studies

a) gastric analysis (with NG tube)
- definition: to determine amount/absence of digestive juices, bacteria, or parasites
- nursing care
  - nothing PO for 8 hours
  - insert nasogastric tube
  - collect fasting specimen
  - collect specimens after gastric secretions have been stimulated by food, alcohol, histamine, insulin, secretin
  - observe for vital-sign changes and anaphylaxsis when histamine, insulin are administered
  - have diphenhydramine (Benadryl) on hand for allergic reactions

b) gastric analysis (without NG tube)
- definition: analysis of stomach pH done with diagnex blue
- nursing care
  - nothing PO for 8 hours
  - have client empty bladder
  - give diagnex blue tablet
  - several hours later, have client empty bladder and send urine to lab (if gastric secretion has pH of 3 or less, the dye will have been excreted)

c) Schilling's test
- definition: assessing vitamin B_{12} absorption to differentiate between intrinsic factor deficiency and absorption problem
- nursing care
  - administer parenteral, saturating dose of nonradioactive B_{12} to a fasting client
  - 1–2 hours later, administer oral radioactive B_{12} test dose
  - start 24-hour urine specimen collection to assess levels of radioactive B_{12} excreted (normal = 8%–40% of injected activity)

9) biopsies
a) excisional
- rectal (done at time of sigmoidoscopy)
- gastric (done at time of gastroscopy)

b) needle (percutaneous liver biopsy)
- definition: needle biopsy of liver tissue to establish a microscopic picture of the liver
- nursing care pretest
  - ensure informed consent is on chart
  - check prothrombin time (if less than 40% test will not be done)
  - instruct client to hold breath while biopsy is being done and not to move during procedure
- nursing care post-test
  - have client lie on right side with pillow or sand bag over the insertion point
  - take frequent vital signs the first 24 hours
  - assess for pain or respiratory difficulty

2. **General Nursing Goals, Plans/Implementation, and Evaluation**

Goal 1: Client will ingest a diet that conforms to prescribed restrictions yet contains all needed nutrients.
Plan/Implementation
- increase or decrease dietary nutrients as ordered
- teach client the rationale for dietary restrictions
- explore with client means of fostering compliance
- provide needed support and encouragement

Evaluation: Client can select appropriate diet from sample menus; verbalizes rationale for restrictions; expresses positive attitude toward diet alteration.

Goal 2: Client will be as comfortable and as pain free as possible.
Plan/Implementation
- administer pain medications as appropriate
- use noninvasive pain-relieving techniques such as positioning, massage, distraction
- teach client and significant others about measures that will minimize pain when client is discharged, e.g., dietary regimen, medications

Evaluation: Client states that he is pain free or experiencing only minimal pain;

verbalizes measures to control pain after discharge.

Goal 3: Client's fluid and electrolyte balance will return to normal.
Plan/Implementation
- institute replacement therapy or restrictions as ordered
- keep accurate I&O
- monitor daily weight

Evaluation: Client's fluid and electrolyte levels are within normal limits.

Goal 4: Client will be knowledgeable about disease process, medications, and the prevention of complications.
Plan/Implementation
- explain disease process
- discuss rationale for ordered treatment regimen
- provide information regarding the administration and side effects of all medications
- help client and significant other to identify factors that might trigger complications of the disease

Evaluation: Client relates medications and the prevention of complications to the disease process.

Goal 5 (if surgery is performed): Client will be free from postoperative complications.
Plan/Implementation
- give standard post-op care, refer to *Surgery* page 165
- client will receive nothing PO for several days or until bowel sounds return post-op (usually 2–3 days); then progress to clear liquids and bland diet as tolerated
- maintain client in semi-Fowler's position (especially for hiatus hernia repairs)
- attach NG tube to suction
  - do not irrigate unless ordered
  - will remain in place at least 5–7 days to permit healing of internal incision
  - record all nasogastric drainage as output
  - bloody drainage→old blood→normal gastric secretions in 24 hours
- if client has chest tubes, refer to *Oxygenation* page 205

Evaluation: Client recovers from surgery free from prior symptoms, respiratory complications, infection, hemorrhage, constipation or diarrhea; tolerates appropriate diet; ambulates with minimal difficulty.

Selected Health Problems Resulting in Problems with Digestion

A. Hiatus Hernia (Diaphragmatic Hernia)

1. **General Information**
   a. Definition: a small opening in the diaphragm allows the esophagus and vagus nerve to pass through. When that opening is enlarged, stomach contents protrude into the thoracic cavity and regurgitation of stomach contents into the esophagus may occur.
   b. Precipitating Factors
      1) congenital or acquired weakness of the diaphragm
      2) obesity
      3) heavy lifting
      4) increased intra-abdominal pressure
      5) pregnancy
   c. Medical Treatment
      1) medical intervention: diet adjustment, change in eating pattern, antacids
      2) surgical intervention: repair of diaphragm through the abdomen or thorax

2. **Nursing Process**
   a. Assessment
      1) symptoms vary from mild to acute
      2) pain and/or heartburn, particularly when in recumbent position
      3) dysphagia
   b. Goal, Plan/Implementation, and Evaluation

Goal: Client will be free from pain/heartburn.
Plan/Implementation
- give small frequent meals, bland diet
- instruct client
  - to sit up for at least 1 hour after meals
  - about the use of antacids
- know that elevating head of bed at night may alleviate symptoms
- have client avoid activities that will increase abdominal pressure, e.g., coughing, lifting
- avoid anticholinergic drugs

Evaluation: Client is free from heartburn; is able to state the foods to be included in diet, meal patterns; can describe the correct use of antacids; can carry out ADL, avoiding strenuous activities.

B. Gastritis

1. **General Information**
   a. Definition: acute or chronic inflammation of the stomach

218 SECTION 3: NURSING CARE OF THE ADULT

b. Precipitating Factors
1) dietary intolerances
2) alcohol
3) drugs: aspirin, steroids
4) uremia
5) certain systemic diseases: hepatitis, typhoid fever
6) ingestion of strong acids or alkalis (corrosive gastritis)

2. **Nursing Process**
   a. Assessment
      1) nausea/vomiting
      2) indigestion
      3) hematemesis
      4) history of onset of pain
      5) history of ingested substances
      6) history of any systemic problems
   b. **Goals, Plans/Implementation, and Evaluation**

   Goal 1: Client will experience relief of nausea, vomiting, and hyperacidity.
   Plan/Implementation
   - identify and remove cause if possible
   - keep NPO until symptoms subside
   - give antacids as ordered
   - introduce bland foods when client is able to take food; monitor tolerance
   - know IV fluids with electrolyte replacement may be given during acute phase

   Evaluation: Client is symptom free in 2–3 days; eating without problems.

   Goal 2: Client will be free from complications.
   Plan/Implementation
   - take emergency measures to prevent scarring/obstruction following ingestion of alkalis or acids
     - neutralize acids with antacids, alkalis with lemon juice or dilute vinegar
     - do not induce vomiting
   - give bland diet, antacids as ordered
   - know that vitamin B_{12} may be indicated for clients with chronic gastritis to prevent pernicious anemia

   Evaluation: Client regains adequate gastric functioning (e.g., no pain, eating well) and tolerating foods (liquids).

C. Peptic Ulcer Disease
1. **General Information**
   a. Definition: sharply defined break in mucosa, which may involve the submucosa and muscular layers of the esophagus,stomach, and duodenum

   b. Incidence (*NOTE:* references differ on incidence)
      1) gastric type: 2 times higher in men, usually over 50 years of age
      2) duodenal type: 4 times higher in men, 25–50 years age range; 80% of all ulcers of the GI tract
   c. Predisposing Factors
      1) smoking
      2) diet (not clearly documented)
      3) economic and social status
      4) high emotional stress
      5) physiologic stress: severe burns, extensive surgery (stress ulcer)
      6) drugs, e.g., salicylates, indomethacin (Indocin), glucocorticoids, caffeine irritate the mucosa and increase its permeability
      7) presence of another disease: pancreatitis, chronic obstructive pulmonary disease, arthritis
      8) genetic predisposition (not clearly documented)
   d. Precipitating Factors: unknown; believed to be influenced by
      1) increased HCl
         a) duodenal ulcers and some prepyloric gastric ulcers are caused by an increased quantity or an increased level of acidity of gastric juices that, in turn, overcome the resistance of the mucosa to the acidity
         b) hypersecretion of acid continues between meals when there is no stimulus for secretion
      2) a breakdown in tissue resistance and defense mechanisms due to inadequate blood supply, inadequate regeneration of epithelial tissue, and inadequate quantities of mucus
      3) heredity, environment, or hormones
   e. Diagnostic Aids
      1) direct visualization (gastroscopy)
      2) upper GI
      3) gastric analysis (amount of HCl)
      4) stool exams (occult blood)
      5) serum gastrin level
   f. Complications of peptic ulcer disease requiring surgery
      1) hemorrhage
      2) perforation and peritonitis
      3) obstruction
      4) intractable pain
   g. Medical Treatment

1) medical intervention
   a) bland diet
   b) drugs: histamine receptor antagonist, e.g., cimetidine (Tagamet), anticholinergic drugs, antacids
   c) rest
   d) decreased stress
   e) removal of possible causes
2) surgical intervention
   a) vagotomy: severing of vagus nerve to eliminate acid-secreting stimulus to gastric cells *(Try to do together)*
   b) pyloroplasty: revision of passage between pyloric region and duodenum to enhance emptying in gastric atony associated with vagotomy
   c) subtotal gastrectomy
      - Billroth I: removal of part of stomach, anastomosis of remaining portion to duodenum
      - Billroth II: resection of distal 2/3 of the stomach; anastomosis of jejunal loop to remaining portion with remaining duodenal stump sutured shut *(Dumping Syndrome)*

2. **Nursing Process**
   a. Assessment
      1) gastric
         a) pain
            - ½–1 hour after meals, rare at night
            - not helped by food ingestion
            - antacids don't help
         b) hematemesis more common than melena
         c) vomiting caused by pyloric obstruction from scarring, edema, and inflammation of the pylorus
         d) weight loss possible
      2) duodenal
         a) pain: caused by action of digestive juices on exposed nerve endings of inflamed mucosa
            - chronic and periodic (occurs 1–4 hours after eating and may occur in middle of night)
            - relieved by the ingestion of some types of food or by antacids
            - located in epigastrium and may radiate around the costal border to the back
            - described by the client as a gnawing, boring, or nagging sensation
         b) melena or occult blood in stools
         c) eructation *burping*
      3) absence of pain: sometimes there will be no manifestations of pain until hemorrhage, perforation, peritonitis, or obstruction occurs *(Pot. compl.)*
         a) hemorrhage
            - excessive hematemesis and/or melena
            - signs and symptoms of shock
         b) perforation/peritonitis: ulcer penetrates entire wall with leakage of GI contents into abdominal cavity
            - sudden onset of epigastric pain
            - vomiting
            - diffuse abdominal tenderness
            - diminished bowel sounds
            - boardlike abdomen with diffuse distention
            - tachycardia, shallow respirations, shock symptoms
         c) obstruction: if ulcer is close to sphincter, edema occurs with irritation
            - scarring
            - projectile vomiting
   b. Goals, Plans/Implementation, and Evaluation

Goal 1: Client will be free from pain.
Plan/Implementation
- give antacid drugs as ordered, to neutralize gastric secretion
- give histamine receptor antagonists as ordered, to reduce acid secretion
- utilize and teach a therapeutic diet to decrease secretory activity
  - bland proteins and fats
  - small, frequent meals
  - no stimulants of gastric secretions (e.g., caffeine, alcohol, spicy foods, smoking)
  - progress to full diet as soon as possible
- assist client to stop smoking

Evaluation: Client can tolerate diet without discomfort; can state or institute measures that will decrease/prevent pain.

Goal 2: Client will have increased rest.
Plan/Implementation
- provide peaceful, calm environment

Antacids 1 hr after meals

220 SECTION 3: NURSING CARE OF THE ADULT

Table 3.29 Drug Therapy for Peptic Ulcer Disease

Description	*Antacids:* act to neutralize hydrochloric acid and provide a protective coating on the lining of the stomach. *Histamine H$_2$ receptor antagonists (cimetidine):* decrease gastric acid secretion, total acidity, and pepsin activity. *Carafute:* forms an adherent acid resistant barrier over an ulcer.
Uses	To treat duodenal ulcers, reduce gastric acid secretion and concentration; prevent stress ulcers; prevent recurrence of ulcers; relieve excess gas (simethicone).
Side Effects	Cimetidine: diarrhea, dizziness, rash, gynecomastia, alopecia, neutropenia, impotence, bradycardia Aluminum Salts: constipation Magnesium Salts: diarrhea
Nursing Implications	Monitor for relief of symptoms; watch for recurrence of ulcer symptoms when discontinued. Do not give cimetidine within 1 hour of antacids; give cimetidine with meals; give antacids 1 hour after meals.
Examples	Cimetidine (Tagamet); aluminum hydroxide (Amphojel, Creamalin); magnesium hydroxide (Maalox, Aludrox); magnesium and aluminum hydroxide with simethicone (Gelusil, Mylanta II)

- use calm and reassuring approach when interacting with client
- provide sedation (e.g., phenobarbital and tranquilizers) prn as ordered
- set limits on activity when necessary

Evaluation: Client rests comfortably throughout most of the day; sleeps at night (or at usual time).

Goal 3: Client will identify and alleviate stressful factors.

Plan/Implementation
- assist client/significant other to identify stressful factors in his life/life-style
- encourage client to express emotions and needs
- teach client relaxation/stress-reduction techniques
- mutually design a balanced work, play, rest schedule

Evaluation: Client can identify stressors on the job and at home; is beginning to express emotions verbally; expresses a willingness to find an outlet to release stress; adheres to a mutually planned schedule of activities while in the hospital and at home.

Goal 4: Client will identify activities to prevent ulcer recurrence.

Plan/Implementation
- teach client to avoid factors that tend to activate ulcer (e.g., diet, stress)
- help client plan to balance work, play, and rest
- clarify dietary restrictions
- encourage elimination of smoking, alcohol
- encourage follow-up health care including periodic x-rays to determine the extent to which the ulcer has healed
- teach regarding medications, side effects; time and method of administration; medications that irritate ulcer (e.g., ASA)

Evaluation: Client can state measures that will reduce the chances of recurrence; follows prescribed diet; takes medication correctly; has a balanced activity schedule; stops or decreases smoking or alcohol ingestion.

Goal 5 (if surgery is required): Client will be free from preventable complications preoperatively.

Plan/Implementation
- institute measures to control bleeding as ordered
  - insert nasogastric tube; irrigate stomach with cool saline until clear; connect to suction
  - give antacids/cimetidine (Tagamet) after acute bleeding has stopped
  - administer IV fluids; type and crossmatch client's blood in order to replace blood loss as ordered
  - offer emotional support
- minimize consequences of perforation
  - give antibiotics as ordered

Table 3.30 Dietary Worksheet.

Directions: Fill in each diet column by selecting the appropriate food for the therapeutic diet from the general diet list on the left. The answers are given in Table 3.31.

	General	Soft/Bland	Full Liquid	Salt Free	Fat Free	Low Residue/ #2 Ulcer	Weighed
BREAKFAST	Orange juice. Puffed rice or oatmeal. Poached egg. Crisp bacon. Orange marmalade or apple jelly. Toast/butter. Milk. Coffee/tea/Sanka. Sugar/salt/pepper.						
LUNCH	Cream tomato soup. Broiled hamburger (bun, catsup) or sliced turkey. French fried potatoes or baked potato. Baby limas or buttered carrots. Coleslaw (mayonnaise or vinegar) or canned fruit in strawberry gelatin. Strawberries with powdered sugar or vanilla ice cream. Bread/butter. Milk. Coffee/tea/Sanka. Sugar/salt/pepper.						
DINNER	Chicken noodle soup or apricot nectar. Fried pork chop/applesauce or lamb chop. Buttered broccoli or buttered peas. Sliced banana in cream or pumpkin pie with Cool Whip. Bread/butter. Milk. Coffee/tea/Sanka. Sugar/salt/pepper.						

Table 3.31 Sample Therapeutic Diets

	General	Soft/Bland	Full Liquid	Salt Free	Fat Free	Low Residue/#2 Ulcer	Weighed
BREAKFAST	Orange juice	Strained orange juice	Orange juice	Orange juice	Orange juice	Strained orange juice (1 oz.)	Orange juice
	Puffed rice or oatmeal	Puffed rice or oatmeal	Strained oatmeal	Puffed rice or salt-free oatmeal	Puffed rice or fat-free oatmeal	Strained oatmeal	Puffed rice or oatmeal
	Poached egg	Poached egg	Meritene with egg	Poached egg	Poached egg	Poached egg	Poached egg
	Crisp bacon	Crisp bacon	—	—	—	—	—
	Orange marmalade or apple jelly	Apple jelly	—	Orange marmalade or apple jelly	Orange marmalade or apple jelly	Apple jelly	—
	Toast/butter	Toast/butter	—	Toast	Toast	Toast/butter	Toast/butter
	Milk	Milk	Milk	Milk (120 cc)	Skim milk	200 cc half & half (ulcer diet only)	Skim milk
	Coffee/tea/Sanka	Coffee/tea/Sanka	Coffee/tea/Sanka	Coffee/tea/Sanka	Coffee/tea/Sanka	Coffee/tea/Sanka (low residue only)	Coffee/tea
	Sugar/salt/pepper	Sugar/salt	Sugar/salt	Sugar/pepper	Sugar/salt/pepper	Sugar/salt	Salt/pepper
LUNCH	Cream tomato soup	Cream tomato soup	Cream tomato soup	Salt-free cream tomato soup	Fat-free tomato broth	Cream pea soup	Tomato broth
	Broiled hamburger (bun, catsup) or sliced turkey	Broiled hamburger (bun) or sliced turkey	—	Salt-free broiled hamburger (salt-free bread or salt-free turkey).	Broiled hamburger (bun, catsup) or sliced turkey	Broiled hamburger (bun) or ground turkey	Broiled hamburger or sliced turkey
	French fried potatoes or baked potato	Baked potato with butter	—	Salt-free buttered baked potato	Baked potato	Baked potato with butter	Baked potato
	Baby limas or buttered carrots	Buttered carrots	—	Salt-free baby limas or carrots	Fat-free baby limas or carrots	Pureed carrots	Lima beans or carrots
	Coleslaw (mayonnaise or vinegar) or canned fruit in strawberry gelatin	Canned fruit in strawberry gelatin	Plain gelatin	Coleslaw (salt-free mayonnaise or vinegar), Knox gelatin with fruit juice/cooked fruit.	Coleslaw (vinegar) or canned fruit in strawberry gelatin	Plain gelatin	Coleslaw (vinegar)

Table 3.31 Continued

	General	Soft/Bland	Full Liquid	Salt Free	Fat Free	Low Residue/#2 Ulcer	Weighed
LUNCH (cont.)	Strawberries with powdered sugar or vanilla ice cream	Vanilla ice cream	Vanilla ice cream	Strawberries with powdered sugar or orange sherbet	Strawberries with powdered sugar or orange sherbet	Vanilla ice cream	Strawberries
	Bread/butter	Bread/butter	—	Salt-free bread/butter	Bread	Bread/butter	Bread/butter
	Milk	Milk	Milk	Milk (120 cc)	Skim milk	200 cc half & half (ulcer diet only)	Skim milk
	Coffee/tea/Sanka	Coffee/tea/Sanka	Coffee/tea/Sanka	Coffee/tea/Sanka	Coffee/tea/Sanka	Coffee/tea/Sanka (low residue diet)	Coffee/tea
	Sugar/salt/pepper	Sugar/salt	Sugar/salt	Sugar/pepper	Sugar/salt/pepper	Sugar/salt	Salt/pepper
DINNER	Chicken noodle soup	Chicken noodle soup or apricot nectar	Cream chicken soup	Salt-free chicken noodle soup or apricot nectar	Fat-free chicken noodle soup or apricot nectar	Cream chicken soup or apricot nectar	Fat-free chicken broth
	Fried pork chop/applesauce or lamb chop	Broiled lamb chops	—	Salt-free fried pork chops/applesauce or salt-free lamb chops	Broiled lamb chops	Ground broiled lamb chop	Broiled lamb chop
	Buttered broccoli or buttered peas	Buttered peas	—	Salt-free buttered broccoli or peas	Fat-free broccoli Fat-free peas	Buttered peas	Fat-free broccoli or peas
	Sliced banana in cream or pumpkin pie with Cool Whip	Sliced banana in cream or pumpkin chiffon pudding/Cool Whip	Banana eggnog or pumpkin chiffon pudding with Cool Whip	Sliced banana in cream or salt-free pumpkin chiffon pudding	Sliced banana or pumpkin chiffon pudding/skim milk	Sliced banana or pumpkin chiffon pudding/skim milk	Sliced banana or orange pudding
	Bread/butter	Bread/butter	—	Salt-free bread/butter	Bread	Bread/butter	Bread/butter
	Milk	Milk	Milk	Milk (120 cc)	Skim milk	200 cc half & half (ulcer diet only)	Skim milk
	Coffee/tea/Sanka	Coffee/tea/Sanka	Coffee/tea/Sanka	Coffee/tea/Sanka	Coffee/tea/Sanka	Coffee/tea/Sanka (low residue diet)	Coffee/tea
	Sugar/salt/pepper	Sugar/salt	Sugar/salt	Sugar/pepper	Sugar/salt/pepper	Sugar/salt	Salt/pepper

224 SECTION 3: NURSING CARE OF THE ADULT

- maintain client in Fowler's position to localize gastric contents to 1 area of peritoneum
- do as much pre-op teaching as time allows; include significant others in discussions of what will happen

Evaluation: Client is physically prepared for immediate surgery (e.g., NG tube in place; vital signs stable).

Goal 6: Client will recover from gastric surgery with minimal anemia.
Plan/Implementation
- know that 20%–50% of clients will experience anemia postresection
  - vitamin B_{12} deficiency (pernicious anemia) if parietal cells of the stomach were removed
  - iron deficiency from blood loss
- give dietary supplements as ordered

Evaluation: Client's postoperative course is free from anemia.

Goal 7: Client will understand dumping syndrome and ways to control it.
Plan/Implementation
- teach client
  - symptoms of *early* dumping syndrome (following subtotal or total gastrectomy: food enters duodenum rapidly; hyperosmolarity of intestinal contents pulls H_2O from vascular bed and stimulates a neuroendocrine response)
    * reaction occurs 30 minutes after eating
    * client feels dizzy, weak
    * pulse increased
    * skin cool, clammy
  - symptoms of *late* dumping syndrome (rapid emptying of stomach contents into the intestine → rapid absorption of glucose → hyperglycemia → pancreas is stimulated to secrete excess of insulin → hypoglycemic reaction)
    * occurs about 2 hours after meal
    * complaints of dizziness, weakness, restlessness
    * pulse increased
    * skin cool, clammy
    * malabsorption results
  - prevention techniques
    * eat small meals that are dry, high in fat, low in carbohydrate (eat complex carbohydrates only)
    * drink liquids between meals only
    * lie down after eating

- know that if the above does not relieve the problem, surgical intervention may be necessary to narrow the opening between stomach and intestine
- know that for some clients malabsorption and dumping syndrome become chronic, unrelieved problems

Evaluation: Client can state symptoms of and methods to prevent dumping syndrome, symptoms of malabsorption syndrome; can identify a plan for work and relaxation; can select appropriate foods from diet list.

Goal 8: Client and significant others will be prepared for discharge.
Plan/Implementation
- refer to Goal 7 above
- help client to continue to modify lifestyle to decrease stress
- encourage client to follow prescribed diet
- encourage regular medical checkups

Evaluation: Client and significant others can describe discharge plan; can carry out all ADL.

D. Diverticulosis/Diverticulitis

1. **General Information**
   a. Definitions
      1) diverticulum: outpouching of the musculature of the intestine
      2) diverticulosis: the condition of being afflicted with diverticulum
      3) diverticulitis: inflammation of the diverticulum
   b. Most common in the sigmoid colon
   c. Risk Factors
      1) diet high in refined and processed foods
      2) age (frequently over 40 years of age)
      3) chronic constipation
   d. Medical Treatment
      1) medical intervention: low residue diet, bulk laxatives, antispasmodics; in acute episodes nothing PO, antibiotics, and IV fluids
      2) surgical intervention: bowel resection with/without a temporary colostomy

2. **Nursing Process**
   a. Assessment
      1) crampy, lower quadrant pain
      2) diarrhea with blood and mucus
      3) weakness
      4) anemia

NUTRITION AND METABOLISM 225

b. **Goals, Plans/Implementation, and Evaluation**

Goal 1: Client's acute episode will subside without complications.

Plan/Implementation
- give antibiotics, IV fluids, electrolytes as ordered
- nothing PO until pain subsides, then advance to clear liquid diet
- conserve energy if anemia is a problem
- observe for complications of perforation/peritonitis (most common complication)

Evaluation: Client remains free from pain complications; has normal bowel function, tolerates diet.

Goal 2: Client will recover from any necessary surgery (e.g., bowel resection, colostomy) without complications (refer to *Elimination* page 281).

Goal 3: Client will take measures to control diverticulosis.

Plan/Implementation
- teach client
  - *[Constipation reversal]* to eat a high residue, high fiber diet
  - to take bulk laxatives, e.g., psyllium hydrophilic (Metamucil), as ordered
  - about use of ordered antispasmodics (e.g., propantheline [Pro-Banthine])
  - ways to decrease stress in life/life-style

Evaluation: Client remains free from symptoms of diverticulitis, tolerates low-residue diet, decreases stress.

E. Appendicitis

1. **General Information**
   a. Definition: inflammation of the appendix
   b. Incidence: most common cause of acute inflammation in right lower quadrant of abdominal cavity; affects men more than women, teenagers more than adults
   c. Usual Treatment: appendectomy

2. **Nursing Process**
   a. **Assessment**
      1) abdominal pain localized in right lower quadrant
      2) rebound tenderness at McBurney's point (halfway between the umbilicus and anterior spine of the ilium)
      3) nausea and vomiting of recent onset
      4) leukocytosis
      5) increased temperature
      6) signs of peritonitis

b. **Goals, Plans/Implementation, and Evaluation**

Goal 1: Client will be prepared for emergency surgery (refer to "Perioperative Period" in *Surgery*, Goals 1 and 2, page 165).

Plan/Implementation
- give nothing PO until diagnosis is made
- know that IV antibiotics may be given pre-op
- give no pain meds until diagnosis confirmed

Evaluation: Client takes nothing PO; can state postoperative routine; has stable vital signs; exhibits minimal anxiety.

Goal 2: Client will recover from surgery free from complications (refer to General Nursing Goals page 217)

Plan/Implementation
- know that if perforation did occur, client will have an NG tube to suction, an abdominal drain, and orders for massive antibiotic therapy *[abd. drain sometimes]*

Evaluation: Client remains afebrile; ambulates early without difficulty; tolerates diet; resumes normal bowel patterns.

F. Cholecystitis with Cholelithiasis

1. **General Information** *[Stones]*
   a. Definition: inflammation of the gallbladder caused by presence of stones (composed of bile pigment, cholesterol, calcium)
   b. Incidence: higher in Caucasian women over age 40, diabetics
   c. Predisposing Factors
      1) obesity
      2) high fat intake
      3) circulatory stasis; chemical stasis
      4) multiple pregnancies, birth control pills

   [5 F's: Fair, FAT, 40, Fertile, Female]

   d. Medical Treatment
      1) medical intervention
         a) low-fat diet
         b) weight reduction
      2) surgical intervention
         a) cholecystostomy: incision and drainage of gallbladder (performed immediately after client's condition has been stabilized)
         b) elective surgery done 4–6 weeks later, after client has been maintained on low fat diet at home

- cholecystectomy (removal of gallbladder and cystic duct): Penrose drain in gallbladder bed
- choledocholithotomy (removal of stones in common bile duct): T-tube inserted into common bile duct
  - common duct exploration always requires T-tube insertion to prevent bile spillage into peritoneum and maintain ductal patency while healing takes place
  - crossbar of T-tube lies in common bile duct; long end is brought out through a stab wound in the abdomen and connected to receptacle for gravity drainage

[margin note: 10 days after cholangiogram → to see if blocked before removing T-tube]

2. Nursing Process

a. Assessment
1) abdominal pain, usually in the right upper quadrant; may radiate to back
2) fullness, eructation, dyspepsia following fat ingestion
3) nausea and vomiting (distention of bile duct initiates stimulation of vomiting center)
4) abnormal cholecystogram, ultrasound
5) jaundice, pruritus with bile duct obstruction
6) clay-colored stools (decreased bilirubin in intestine)
7) dark amber urine (increased levels of serum bilirubin)

b. Goals, Plans/Implementation, and Evaluation

Goal 1: Preoperatively, client will be comfortable and prepared for surgery (refer to "Perioperative Period" in *Surgery*, Goals 1 and 2, page 165).

Plan/Implementation
- relieve pain with analgesics as ordered; meperidine (Demerol) is usually ordered since morphine causes spasms of bile ducts;
- relieve reflex spasms with antispasmodics prn as ordered; nitroglycerin may be used to relax smooth muscle
- relieve vomiting and decrease gastric stimulation with NG tube to suction
- give broad-spectrum antibiotics as ordered (ampicillin, tetracycline, cephalosporins are frequently used)
- relieve pruritus: tepid cornstarch baths, cortisone ointments
- assess for signs of bleeding; administer vitamin K if ordered
- teach about possibility of T-tube

Evaluation: Client states he is pain free without itching, nausea, vomiting; knows a T-tube might be in place post-op.

Goal 2: Client will recover from surgery without complications (refer to General Nursing Goals page 217)

Plan/Implementation
- know that post-op pain is severe
- protect skin; bile from Penrose drain is very irritating
- care for T-tube if present
  - avoid tension and obstruction of tubing
  - measure amount of drainage carefully, record as output (drainage will be 200–500 ml/day for 1st several days; continuing large amounts indicate obstruction)
  - clamp as ordered in 3–4 days during meals to determine tolerance
  - usually removed 10–12 days post-op following T-tube cholangiogram to determine status of duct
- monitor for complications specific to biliary tract: jaundice, increased T-tube drainage; increased temperature; severe abdominal pain indicating possible infection, leakage, or obstruction

[margin note: incision under diaphragm cough & deep breathing cause pain but is needed]

Evaluation: Client recovers from surgery free from skin irritation, diet intolerance, biliary tract complications.

G. Pancreatitis

1. General Information

a. Definition: inflammation of the pancreas resulting in obstruction and edema; autodigestion by the trapped pancreatic enzymes results; regurgitation of bile through the pancreatic duct may occur

b. Types
1) acute: with or without hemorrhage; when hemorrhage occurs, shock and death can occur; pseudocysts can occur following acute attacks

[margin note: No surgery in this phase]

2) <u>chronic</u>: results in hyperglycemia and diabetes caused by degeneration of islet cells
  c. Risk Factors
    1) alcohol abuse
    2) gallbladder disease
    3) trauma
    4) infections (e.g., mumps, hepatitis)
    5) peptic ulcer disease
    6) about 20% of all cases have no identifiable cause
  d. <u>Medical Treatment: generally conservative; surgery is to be avoided if possible</u>

2. Nursing Process
  a. Assessment
    1) history of risk factors, e.g., alcohol abuse, gallbladder disease, infection
    2) extreme epigastric pain extending to back
    3) vomiting
    4) abdominal distention
    5) <u>elevated serum amylase and lipase</u>
    6) <u>elevated urinary amylase</u>
    7) fever
    8) jaundice
    9) hyperglycemia
    10) hyperlipidemia
    11) shock (kinin is a vasodilator activated by trypsin secretion)
    12) hypocalcemia (insoluble calcium salts form because of fat necrosis): mild tetany
  b. Goals, Plans/Implementation, and Evaluation

Goal 1: Client will be free from or have <u>minimal pain</u>.
Plan/Implementation
- give nothing PO until inflammation subsides
- know that <u>meperidine (Demerol) is indicated as narcotic of choice; morphine is contraindicated since it causes spasm of the sphincter of Oddi</u>

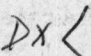

- give anticholinergics such as propantheline (Pro-Banthine) as ordered, to decrease secretions and relax the sphincter
- administer antacids frequently in mild cases

Evaluation: Client states pain is subsiding.

Goal 2: Client will be <u>free from shock</u> in the acute phase (refer to "Shock" in *Oxygenation* page 178).

Goal 3: Client will maintain adequate <u>nutrition</u>.
Plan/Implementation
- give clear liquids or elemental diet such as Vivonex after the inflammation subsides; progress to a bland diet
- teach regarding bland diet, avoiding stimulants, alcohol
- monitor blood sugar, urine sugar and acetone levels
- treat hyperglycemia with insulin prn as ordered
- <u>know that pancreatic enzymes may be given to aid fat digestion in chronic pancreatitis if attack is severe, complete bowel rest with total parenteral nutrition (TPN) may be instituted</u>

Evaluation: Client is free from nutritional deficiencies, digestive problems; ingests and tolerates prescribed diet; has no weight loss; chooses bland foods from diet menu.

Goal 4: Client will institute measures to prevent chronic pancreatitis.
Plan/Implementation
- discuss how client can eliminate the underlying cause when possible
- suggest alcohol rehabilitation programs
- know cholecystectomy will be done, if indicated, to remove biliary reflux as a cause of pancreatitis

Evaluation: Client has no recurrences; has joined and consistently attends Alcoholics Anonymous.

H. Hepatitis
1. **General Information**
  a. Definition: viral, infectious inflammation of the liver
  b. Types
    1) type A
      a) causative agent: infectious hepatitis virus
      b) mode of transmission
        - oral, fecal, or respiratory route
        - blood, serum, or plasma transfusion from an infected person
        - contaminated food (particularly milk and shellfish), polluted water are implicated
        - contaminated syringes and needles
      c) incubation: 3–7 weeks
      d) incidence
        - worldwide prevalence

↑ BUN + Ammonia — fries brain

228 SECTION 3: NURSING CARE OF THE ADULT

- higher during fall and winter months
- higher among children and young adults

2) type B *serum*
  a) causative agent: serum hepatitis virus, homologous serum jaundice
  b) mode of transmission
     - parenteral route
     - blood or blood component transfusions from an infected person
     - contaminated needles and syringes
     - skin puncture with contaminated medical instruments
     - mucosal transmission: dental instruments or venereal contact
  c) incubation: 6 weeks to 6 months (average 2½–3 months)
  d) incidence
     - worldwide prevalence
     - higher among recipients of blood and blood products (e.g., surgical, dialysis clients)

Incubation — longer 6 wks – 6 mos.

3) non-A/non-B: little is known; occurs in clients with multiple blood transfusions; treated similarly to hepatitis B

c. Pathophysiology
  1) elevated serum levels of bilirubin
  2) hyperplasia of Kupffer's cells of liver
  3) bilirubin and urobilinogen excreted in urine *lght. stools*
  4) bile salts accumulate in skin (itching)
  5) stretching of liver capsule because of inflammation (pain)
  6) reduced energy metabolism by the liver (fatigue)
  7) visceral reflexes may reduce peristalsis (nausea)
  8) reduced prothrombin synthesis; reduced production of fat-soluble vitamin K
  9) inflammatory process: release of pyrogens (fever)

2. Nursing Process
   a. Assessment
      1) jaundice
      2) clay-colored stools *lght. stools*
      3) dark urine
      4) pruritus
      5) abdominal pain in right upper quadrant
      6) large, tender liver
      7) anorexia, nausea, vomiting
      8) bleeding tendencies (severe cases)
      9) fever (rare in type B)
      10) abnormal liver function tests
      11) positive hepatitis antigen
      12) fatigue and weakness
      13) signs and symptoms of hepatitis encephalopathy *↑BUN + Ammonia*
   b. Goals, Plan/Implementation, and Evaluation

   Goal 1: Significant others and staff will be protected from the client's infection.
   Plan/Implementation
   - provide a private room with separate toilet facilities
   - use gown, gloves when in contact with client or his blood or excreta
   - use special precautions for handling blood and feces
   - know that respiratory isolation is used either routinely or when client has copious respiratory secretions
   - discard needles and syringes in puncture-resistant containers and incinerate
   - use disposable eating utensils and dishes; incinerate
   - prohibit food sharing with others
   - use good hand-washing techniques
   - double bag linens, label, mark for special handling by laundry
   - teach client and visitors isolation routine
   - disinfect toilet facilities routinely
   - know that if client has positive hepatitis antigen without signs of active disease, isolation is not needed except for precautions with syringes, needles, blood products, respiratory secretions
   - give gamma globulin to those exposed to hepatitis A; give hepatitis B immune globulin to those exposed to hepatitis B
   - hepatitis B vaccine may be given to high-risk persons (e.g., dialysis, cancer clients; medical, dental personnel)

   Evaluation: Staff members and client's significant others remain free from disease.

   Goal 2: Client will have reduced metabolic demand on liver.
   Plan/Implementation
   - place on bed rest; explain reason to client
     - limit activities until symptoms have subsided

NUTRITION AND METABOLISM 229

[handwritten top left: Compazine extremely toxic to liver]

- provide environment for adequate rest
- provide diversionary activities as needed
• monitor liver function tests throughout care *[handwritten: SGOT goal to 7000]*
• control pruritus (refer to "Cholecystitis" Goal 1 page 226)
• avoid administering drugs toxic to the liver; use sedatives and opiates with caution
• administer corticosteroids (anti-inflammatory effects) as ordered
• maintain diet low in fats

Evaluation: Client is resting most of the day; sleeps throughout the night.

Goal 3: Client will have adequate nutrition.

Plan/Implementation

[handwritten left margin: ↑ BUN & Ammonia →]

• encourage high carbohydrate, high vitamin, low fat, normal to high protein diet (restrict proteins if evidence of hepatic encephalopathy is present)
• know that good nutrition is hard to maintain because of anorexia, nausea and vomiting
• encourage antiemetics prior to meals and small frequent feedings rather than 3 large meals
• have food available at client's bedside (e.g., hard candy)

Evaluation: Client's nutritional status appears adequate (no weight loss, intake equals output, normal energy level).

Goal 4: Client will remain free from reinfection.

Plan/Implementation

• health teaching and preventive measures: type A
  - encourage optimal sanitation practices
  - instruct client in good personal hygiene
  - prevent use of blood and blood components taken from infected donors
  - instruct client not to donate blood
  - administer immune serum globulin IM as ordered
  - use disposable needles and syringes and dispose of them carefully
• health teaching and preventive measures: type B
  - reject blood donors who have had serum hepatitis

[handwritten: Never Donate Blood]

  - instruct client not to donate blood
  - administer hepatitis B immune globulin as ordered
  - use disposable needles and syringes; dispose of them carefully
  - test clients with history of drug abuse for hepatitis B antigen/antibody regularly

Evaluation: Client is able to state methods to prevent transmission, recurrence.

I. Cirrhosis

1. **General Information**
   a. Definition: chronic disease with destruction of liver cells followed by cell regeneration and an increase in connective tissue; impaired function of liver and obstruction of venous and sinusoidal channels causing portal hypertension
   b. Incidence: twice as common in men than women, higher in people 40-60 years old
   c. Predisposing/Precipitating Factors
      1) malnutrition; effects of alcohol abuse; poisoning, i.e., chloroform, industrial chemicals, drugs

      [handwritten: anesthetic halophone]

      2) congestive heart failure
      3) viral hepatitis
   d. Pathophysiology
      1) liver cell destruction results in progressive inability of liver to carry out functions
      2) increased resistance to blood flow through the liver (decreased outflow of blood through the hepatic vein, usually with an increase in splanchnic arterial blood flow) resulting in portal hypertension: sustained elevation of pressure in the portal vein above normal (6-12 cm H_2O)
      3) portal hypertension results in splenomegaly, varices of gastric and esophageal veins, hemorrhoids, and ascites

2. **Nursing Process**
   a. **Assessment**
      1) intermittent jaundice
      2) ache or heavy feeling in right upper quadrant (enlarged, hardened liver)
      3) abnormal blood study results
         a) elevated serum enzymes (SGOT, SGPT, LDH, alkaline phosphatase)

b) abnormal albumin/globulin ratio; hypoproteinemia
c) increased prothrombin time (lengthening of the time it takes the blood to clot)
d) decreased platelet count
e) reduced hematocrit
f) decreased leukocytes
g) increased bilirubin, urobilinogen

4) changes resulting from hormonal abnormalities: palmar erythema, amenorrhea, atrophy of testicles, enlarged breasts, parotid hypertrophy, vascular lesions on the skin resembling small spiders
5) frequent infections
6) folic-acid deficiency
7) lower-leg edema
8) emaciation, malnutrition
9) prominent abdominal wall veins *[Spider Angioma's]*
10) hemorrhoids
11) manifestations of hepatitis
12) ascites *[R/T ↑ vascular pressure, ↓ shift H2O + protein in 3RD space]*
13) esophageal varices
14) renal failure
15) hepatic encephalopathy, coma

b. Goals, Plan/Implementation, and Evaluation

Goal 1: Client will be free from hemorrhage.
Plan/Implementation
- observe for bleeding: urine, stool, gums, skin-petechiae *[swabs for mouth]*
- apply pressure to injection sites for a longer than usual time because of increased bleeding tendency
- monitor protime, PTT
- avoid brushing teeth; use cotton swabs; give frequent mouth care
- handle the client gently to avoid bruising
- prevent scratching/bleeding from pruritus *[prevent scratching, cut nails]*

Evaluation: Client remains free from bruises, bleeding gums.

Goal 2: Client will have reduced metabolic demands on liver.
Plan/Implementation
- provide bed rest during periods of acute malfunction
- have client rest before and between activities if anemia becomes worse
- eliminate ingestion of all substances toxic to liver: sedatives and opiates, alcohol *[compazine]*
- arouse client regularly to assess level of consciousness

Evaluation: Client rests quietly most of the day; keeps activities to a minimum; sleeps through the night.

Goal 3: Client will have adequate nutrition and hydration.
Plan/Implementation
- give a high protein/carbohydrate/calorie (over 2,000), sodium-restricted diet when there is no evidence of encephalopathy
- plan small, frequent meals
- administer multiple-vitamin therapy as ordered (higher doses of thiamine and fat-soluble vitamins if there is deficient fat absorption)
- restrict fluids and sodium intake if there is edema and/or ascites
- provide mouth care before meals (foul taste may be present)

Evaluation: Client eats prescribed diet; is adequately hydrated; maintains weight.

Goal 4: Client will be free from infection.
Plan/Implementation
- know that reverse isolation may be necessary with extreme leukopenia
- assess for signs of urinary or respiratory infection *[↓ resp excursion]*
- turn frequently to prevent any skin breakdown

Evaluation: Client has normal temperature; skin remains free from abrasions, inflammation.

Goal 5: Client will learn preventive health measures.
Plan/Implementation
- teach client to balance rest and activity, to avoid fatigue
- instruct client
  - to eat a highly nutritious diet; if finances are a problem, consider diet planning and use of community resources
  - to avoid persons with infections
  - to avoid alcohol or drugs metabolized by liver

Evaluation: Client can state dietary activity and drug needs.

hard to sedate — toxic to liver

Not usually on respirator

J. Complications of Liver Disease: Esophageal Varices, Ascites, Hepatic Encephalopathy

1. **General Information: Esophageal Varices**
   a. Definition: dilation of collateral veins that bypass a scarred liver to carry portal blood to vena cava; may occur in distal esophagus and stomach
   b. Pathophysiology
      1) as liver becomes increasingly cirrhotic, portal hypertension increases,
      2) collateral circulation in the esophagus develops in vessels that are weaker than normal vessels *Bleed easily*
      3) as pressure in collateral vessels increases, they become overdistended and can rupture and bleed
   c. Usually asymptomatic until the varices rupture
   d. Usually associated with cirrhosis
   e. Treatment
      1) medical intervention: Sengstaken-Blakemore tube *several days*
      2) surgical intervention: portacaval shunt (anastomosis between the portal vein and inferior vena cava [has a high mortality rate]) *↓ pressure*

   very anxious — can't be sedated

2. **Nursing Process**
   a. Assessment
      1) active bleeding following
         a) physical activity (increased abdominal venous pressure)
         b) mechanical trauma (abrasions from swallowing poorly chewed food)
         c) esophageal irritation by HCl
      2) hematemesis *bright red*
      3) signs of shock
   b. Goal, Plan/Implementation, and Evaluation
   Goal: Client will have esophageal bleeding detected and treated immediately.
   Plan/Implementation
   - carefully monitor client to detect signs and symptoms of bleeding: restlessness, tachycardia, hypotension, cool skin, pallor
   - if bleeding is detected, perform gastric lavage with ice-cold saline continuously until the returns are clear
   - give blood transfusions as ordered
   - administer vitamin K as ordered, to correct clotting problems
   - maintain patent airway (danger of aspiration when vomiting occurs)
   - administer magnesium sulfate and saline enemas as ordered, to prevent ammonia intoxication and hepatic coma
   - give intestinal antimicrobial agents as ordered, i.e., neomycin enemas to decrease intestinal bacterial action on the blood *↓ Ammonia*
   - institute esophageal tamponade by use of Sengstaken-Blakemore tube as ordered

   Evaluation: Client's esophageal bleeding was detected immediately; physician notified; condition remains stable.

3. **General Information: Ascites**
   a. Definition: an abnormal intraperitoneal accumulation of watery fluid containing small amounts of protein
   b. Pathophysiology
      1) portal hypertension
      2) decreased albumin production in liver; decreased colloidal osmotic pressure
      3) decreased removal of aldosterone by liver: sodium and water retention
      4) transudation of fluid from mesenteric veins and lymphatic seepage
      5) respiratory difficulty as abdomen enlarges and fluid pushes on diaphragm
   c. Precipitating Factors
      1) advanced cirrhosis
      2) metastatic liver disease
   d. Medical Treatment *control fluid*
      1) medical intervention
         a) sodium-restricted diet
         b) diuretics *Aldactone K+ sparing*
         c) paracentesis: removal of fluids from the peritoneal cavity; indicated if respiratory distress is present
      2) surgical intervention: LeVeen Shunt (placement of a catheter to shunt ascites from peritoneum to inferior vena cava)

4. **Nursing Process**
   a. Assessment
      1) respiratory difficulty
      2) enlarged abdominal girth
      3) abdominal pain, discomfort

blood in stomach → broken down to Ammonia.

- 4) daily weight
- 5) I&O
- 6) nutritional status: dehydration, malnutrition
- 7) fatigue
- 8) cause of ascites (i.e., cancer vs cirrhosis)

b. **Goal, Plan/Implementation, and Evaluation**

Goal: Client will be comfortable following a reduction of ascites.

Plan/Implementation
- give sodium-restricted diet
- use "salt" substitutes, i.e., lemon juice, spices; and, if approved by physician, a commercial salt substitute
- restrict fluids
- monitor fluid and electrolyte balance, I&O
- monitor daily weights
- measure abdominal girth at least every shift;
- administer diuretics as ordered; if potassium also excreted, e.g., furosemide (Lasix), give potassium supplement or potassium-sparing diuretics, e.g., spironolactone (Aldactone)
- administer IV albumin for hypoalbuminemia as ordered *[salt poor albumin]*
- maintain high-Fowler's position for maximum respiratory effectiveness and comfort *[high Fowlers]*
- support abdomen with pillows
- assist with paracentesis if performed *[Empty bladder]*
  - have client void before the procedure
  - monitor client during and after the paracentesis for tachycardia, shock, dyspnea, and dizziness
  - take vital signs *before*, then frequently *after* the procedure *[before]*
  - observe puncture wound for leakage, signs of infection *[bacteria up through wound]*

Evaluation: Client is comfortable; undergoes paracentesis without complications; ascites reduced by 2 liters; abdominal girth reduced each day; experiences a reduction of respiratory distress.

5. **General Information: Hepatic Encephalopathy** *[poor prognosis]*
   a. Definition: cerebral dysfunction associated with severe liver disease
   b. Pathophysiology: inability of the liver to detoxify ammonia (convert ammonia to urea); cause is loss of functioning hepatic cells or no filtration of ammonia because blood bypasses liver
   c. Higher incidence among clients who have had a portacaval shunt

6. **Nursing Process**
   a. **Assessment**
      1) mental status, level of consciousness: lethargy→coma
      2) mental changes: dullness, slurred speech
      3) neurologic exam: twitching, muscular incoordination, asterixis (a flapping tremor)
      4) serum ammonia level
      5) history of liver disease, portacaval shunt
      6) bowel function *[a lot bacteria → more ammonia]*
      8) behavioral changes: not interested in appearance
   b. **Goals, Plans/Implementation, and Evaluation**

Goal 1: Client will have decreased ammonia production.

Plan/Implementation
- decrease ammonia formation in the intestine
  - prevent constipation *[↑ Ammonia]*
  - give laxatives, enemas as ordered
  - administer lactulose (Cephulac) and neomycin (oral or rectal) as ordered
- reduce dietary protein to 20–40 gm/day (see table 3.42)

Evaluation: Client's serum ammonia level is within normal limits; client tolerates a low protein diet.

Goal 2: Client will remain free from injury.

Plan/Implementation
- perform general nursing measures for the unconscious client (refer to *Safety and Security* page 292)
- assess mental status frequently

Evaluation: Client regains consciousness free from injury.

Goal 3: Client and significant others will learn to prevent future episodes of encephalopathy.

Plan/Implementation
- obtain nutritionist to counsel client regarding low protein diet

[usually damage too bad to undo it]

- ensure client understands how to avoid and treat constipation
- ensure that client has an appointment for return follow-up care with physician
- teach client to balance activity and rest periods to prevent hypoxia

Evaluation: Client can state measures to ensure proper bowel functioning; can state principles of a low protein diet and planned rest periods.

Part Two: The Endocrine System

General Concepts

A. Overview
1. The endocrine system is a chemical communication system that functions together with the nervous system as the body's communication network
   a. Endocrine glands synthesize and secrete chemical substances (hormones) that control and integrate body functions (see table 3.32)
      1) secreted in minute amounts
      2) circulated in the blood
      3) regulated by
         a) negative feedback systems
         b) changes in the plasma concentration of specific substances
         c) direct autonomic nervous system activity
         d) circadian rhythms
      4) action alters specific physiologic responses
         a) growth and development
         b) reproduction
         c) metabolism
         d) responses to stress and injury
   b. Health problems involving the endocrine system result from hormone imbalances
      1) primary problems: involvement of the target gland of the hormone
      2) secondary problems: involvement of the primary gland of secretion, i.e., pituitary or hypothalamus
2. Glands
   a. Pituitary
      1) anatomy
         a) lies in the sella tursica above the sphenoid at the base of the brain
         b) consists of two lobes connected by the hypothalamus
      2) functions (see table 3.32)
         a) anterior lobe (adenohypophysis) secretes ACTH, MSH, TSH, FSH, GH, and prolactin
         b) posterior lobe (neurohypophysis) secretes ADH and oxytocin
         c) regulates the function of the other endocrine glands through the stimulation of target organs
         d) controlled through the action of releasing and inhibiting factors from the hypothalamus
   b. Thyroid gland
      1) anatomy
         a) located at or below the cricoid cartilage in the neck, anterior to the trachea
         b) consists of two highly vascular lobes
      2) functions (see table 3.32)
         a) controls the rate of body metabolism through the production of thyroxine (T_4) and triiodothyronine (T_3)
         b) produces calcitonin
   c. Parathyroid Glands
      1) anatomy: four small glands located near or imbedded in the thyroid gland
      2) functions: secrete parathyroid hormone (PTH) and control calcium and phosphorus metabolism in the body
   d. Adrenal Glands
      1) anatomy: two small glands lying in the retroperitoneal region, capping each kidney
      2) functions (see table 3.32)
         a) adrenal cortex (outer capsule)
            - secretes the adrenocortical steroids (cortisol, cortisone, corticosterone)
            - secretes the mineralocorticoids (aldosterone)
            - secretes the adrenal sex hormones (androgen, estrogen, progesterone)
         b) adrenal medulla (inner parenchyma of gland)
            - stimulated by the sympathetic nervous system

Table 3.32 Hormones

Gland	Hormone	Action
Hypothalamus	Releasing hormones	Stimulate release of hormones from pituitary gland.
	Inhibiting hormones	Inhibit release of hormones from pituitary gland.
	ADH	See Pituitary, Posterior Lobe.
Pituitary, Anterior Lobe	Growth hormone (GH)	Acts directly on bones and other tissues to stimulate growth.
	Prolactin (LTH)	Stimulates development of mammary tissue and lactation.
	Thyrotropic hormone (TSH)	Stimulates thyroid gland.
	Adrenocorticotropic hormone (ACTH)	Stimulates adrenal cortex.
	Melanocyte-stimulating hormone (MSH)	Stimulates darkening of the skin.
	Luteinizing hormone (LH)	Initiates ovulation and formation of corpus luteum.
	Follicle-stimulating hormone (FSH)	*Women:* stimulates ovarian development of graffian follicle. *Men:* maintains spermatogenesis.
Pituitary, Posterior Lobe	Antidiuretic hormone (ADH): produced in hypothalamus and stored in pituitary	Facilitates reabsorption of H_2O in the kidneys, vasoconstriction in arterioles.
	Oxytocin	Initiates expression of breast milk; stimulates uterine contractions at delivery.
Thyroid	Triiodothyronine (T_3) Thyroxine (T_4)	Control body metabolism and influence physical and mental growth; nervous system activity; protein, fat, carbohydrate metabolism; reproduction.
	Calcitonin	Lowers serum calcium levels, inhibits bone resorption.
Parathyroid	Parathormone (PTH)	Regulates calcium and phosphorus metabolism.
Adrenal Cortex	Glucocorticoids: cortisone, cortisol	Decrease protein synthesis; regulate serum glucose by increasing rate of gluconeogenesis; suppress the inflammatory and immune response; increase fat mobilization; support adaptation during stressful situations.
	Mineralocorticoids: aldosterone	Facilitate reabsorption of Na^+ and elimination of K^+.
	Sex hormones: primarily androgens	Responsible for development of secondary sex characteristics.
Adrenal Medulla	Epinephrine	Initiates stress response.
	Norepinephrine	Causes vasoconstriction.
Pancreas	Insulin	Enables glucose to freely enter cells; helps muscle and tissue oxidation of glucose; promotes storage of glycogen.
	Glucagon	Increases gluconeogenesis in liver.
Ovaries	Estrogen	Responsible for secondary sex characteristics, mammary duct system, growth of graffian follicle in women.
	Progesterone	Prepares corpus luteum; maintains pregnancy.
Testes	Testosterone	Responsible for secondary sex characteristics, normal reproductive functioning in men.

- secretes catecholamines (epinephrine and norepinephrine)
  e. Pancreas
     1) anatomy
        a) long, soft gland that lies retroperitoneally
        b) head of the gland is in the duodenal cavity and the tail lies against the spleen
     2) functions
        a) exocrine function to produce digestive enzymes
        b) endocrine function to control carbohydrate metabolism
           - glucagon secreted by alpha cells
           - insulin secreted by beta cells

B. **Application of the Nursing Process to the Client with Endocrine System Problems**
  1. Assessment
     Hormones have very diverse systemic effects. Hypofunction or hyperfunction can result in dysfunction in a wide variety of organs and organ systems.
     a. Health History
        1) current symptoms
           a) change in client's energy level or stamina
           b) change in personal appearance
              - size of head, hands, or feet
              - weight, skin, or hair
              - secondary sex characteristics
           c) increased sympathetic nervous system activity
           d) change in alertness or personality
           e) change in sexual functioning
        2) past or family history *Genetic*
           a) abnormal progression in growth and development
           b) family history of diabetes, hypertension, infertility, mental illness
     b. Physical Exam
        1) inspection: subtle or dramatic deviations from normal in body size, muscle tone, skin, hair, voice, and sexual characteristics
        2) palpation: limited to the thyroid gland
     c. Diagnostic Tests
        1) measurement of the amounts of hormones present in serum or urine
        2) fluctuations in daily pattern of secretion means random specimens have limited value

  2. **General Nursing Goals, Plans/Implementation, and Evaluation**
     Goal 1: Client will ingest a diet that conforms to prescribed restrictions yet provides all needed nutrients.
     Plan/Implementation
     - increase or decrease dietary nutrients as ordered
     - teach client the rationale for dietary restrictions
     - explore with client means of fostering compliance
     - provide needed support and encouragement

     Evaluation: Client can select appropriate diet from sample menus; verbalizes rationale for restrictions; expresses a positive attitude toward dietary alterations.

     Goal 2: Client will adapt to changes in body image.
     Plan/Implementation
     - encourage client to verbalize concerns
     - provide client with correct information about the degree of symptom reversibility

     Evaluation: Client expresses self-acceptance and engages in usual social activities.

     Goal 3: Client's fluid and electrolyte balance will be restored to normal range.
     Plan/Implementation
     - institute replacement therapy or restrictions as ordered
     - keep strict I&O
     - monitor daily weight

     Evaluation: Client's lab values are within normal ranges; client exhibits no abrupt fluctuations in body weight.

     Goal 4: Client will be knowledgeable about disease process, medications, and the prevention of complications. *Teach*
     Plan/Implementation
     - discuss rationale for ordered treatment regimen
     - provide data concerning the administration and side effects of all medications
     - assist client to identify potential stressors in his life-style that might trigger complications of the disease; discuss appropriate client actions

     Evaluation: Client takes medications as ordered; returns for follow-up care; remains free from preventable complications.

Selected Health Problems

A. Hyperpituitarism

1. **General Information**
   a. Definition: oversecretion of one or more hormones of the pituitary gland, frequently caused by tumors
      1) anterior pituitary→acromegaly or giantism *Growth Hormone*
      2) posterior pituitary→syndrome of inappropriate secretion of ADH (SIADH)
   b. Incidence
      1) acromegaly
         a) insidious onset in middle age
         b) more common in women than men
      2) SIADH
         a) may be triggered by malignancies or the stress of surgery and anesthesia
         b) syndrome is usually self-limiting
   c. Diagnosis
      1) acromegaly
         a) thorough history and inspection
         b) plasma levels of GH
         c) skull x-rays, CAT scan
      2) SIADH
         a) clinical picture of sudden weight gain with decreasing urinary output
         b) serum sodium below 125 mEq/liter
         c) urine osmolality usually higher than plasma osmolality
   d. Medical Treatment
      1) acromegaly: surgical hypophysectomy by transsphenoidal approach if possible
      2) SIADH: strict fluid restriction to less than 1,000 ml/day

2. **Nursing Process**
   a. Assessment
      1) acromegaly
         a) increases in hat, shoe, and glove size
         b) protruding jaw, enlarged nose, jaw, hands, feet
         c) headache
      2) SIADH
         a) falling urine output
         b) sudden weight gain
         c) decreasing level of consciousness
         d) signs of sodium and potassium imbalance (see table 3.28)
   b. Goals, Plans/Implementation, and Evaluation

   Goal 1: Client who has been treated by transsphenoidal hypophysectomy will not experience postoperative pain.
   Plan/Implementation
   - refer to "Intracranial Surgery" in *Safety and Security* page 294
   - note any nasal leakage of cerebrospinal fluid
   - have client avoid coughing, sneezing, straining at stool
   - keep head of bed elevated to 30°
   - monitor signs of diabetes insipidus or adrenal crisis *greater > 300 qº*

   Evaluation: Client remains free from post-op infection or alteration in mental status, maintains stable vital signs and fluid balance.

   Goal 2: Client treated by hypophysectomy will be prepared for knowledgeable self-care.
   Plan/Implementation
   - see General Nursing Goals 2 and 4 page 235
   - provide information about the importance of lifelong replacement therapy with regular medical supervision

   Evaluation: Client follows prescribed medication regimen, experiences minimal fluctuations in hormone levels, expresses self-acceptance.

   Goal 3: Client with SIADH will reestablish normal fluid and electrolyte balance
   Plan/Implementation
   - restrict fluid intake as ordered (less than 1,000 ml/day)
   - maintain accurate I&O and daily weight records
   - monitor for symptoms of Na^+ or K^+ imbalance
   - assess for signs of cerebral edema (refer to *Safety and Security* page 291)

   Vasopressin Drug used for Diuresis

   Evaluation: Client's weight is stable; urinary output is within acceptable limits.

B. Hypopituitarism

1. **General Information**
   a. Definition: undersecretion of one or more of the hormones of the pituitary

gland caused by disease, tumor, postpartum hemorrhage (Sheehan's syndrome), neurologic surgery, or trauma
1) anterior pituitary→failure of GH secretion followed by failure of secretion of other hormones
2) posterior pituitary→diabetes insipidus from failure of secretion of ADH
b. Diagnosis: see "Hyperpituitarism" page 236
c. Medical Treatment: supplementary administration of the deficient pituitary hormones
1) corticosteroids
2) thyroid hormone
3) growth hormone
4) sex hormones
5) vasopressin

2. **Nursing Process**
a. Assessment
1) anterior pituitary hypofunction
a) dwarfism in children (GH)
b) decreased stress tolerance (ACTH)
c) decreased metabolism (TSH)
d) menstrual irregularities, decreased or altered secondary sex characteristics (gonadotropin)
2) posterior pituitary hypofunction: diabetes insipidus
a) excessively high urinary output
b) low urinary specific gravity
c) elevated serum osmolality
d) signs of dehydration and hypernatremia
b. Goals, Plans/Implementation, and Evaluation

Goal 1: Client's hormone levels will be restored and maintained in the normal range.
Plan/Implementation
- provide information about medications (i.e., name, dosage, side effects) and the importance of lifelong replacement with ongoing medical supervision
- teach client the effects of physical and psychologic stress on hormone needs

Evaluation: Client follows prescribed medication regimen and adjusts life-style to maintain hormone balance.

Goal 2: Client with diabetes insipidus will reestablish and maintain normal fluid and electrolyte balance.

Plan/Implementation
- administer replacement fluids as ordered
- keep accurate I&O; monitor daily weight, urine specific gravity
- monitor for signs of hypovolemic shock (refer to "Shock" in *Oxygenation* page 178
- administer vasopressin nasal spray or vasopressin (Pitressin Tannate) IM as ordered
- teach client safe administration of nasal preparation
- teach signs and symptoms of fluid volume excess

Evaluation: Client's fluid balance is within normal limits; client can self-administer replacement medications safely.

C. Hyperthyroidism — GRAVE Disease
1. **General Information**
a. Definition: oversecretion of the thyroid gland; second to diabetes in incidence
b. Grave's Disease
1) a recurrent syndrome
2) most common form of hyperthyroidism
3) occurs primarily in women 30–50 years of age
4) possibly autoimmune in nature
c. Diagnosis — very specific
1) elevated T_3, T_4, PBI, ^{131}I uptake values
2) abnormal findings from thyroid scan
d. Complications
1) thyroid storm or crisis: an extreme physiologic state of life-threatening hypermetabolism
2) cardiovascular disease
3) exophthalmos owing to increased deposits of fat and fluid in the retro-ocular tissue
e. Medical Treatment
1) medications
a) propylthiouricil (PTU): antithyroid drug that depresses the synthesis of thyroid hormone; takes about three months to be completely effective
b) iodine preparations (SSKI): decrease the size and vascularity of the gland
c) radioactive iodine: limits the secretion of hormone by damaging or destroying thyroid tissue

Inderal

238 SECTION 3: NURSING CARE OF THE ADULT

d) propranolol (Inderal): adrenergic antagonist that relieves the adrenergic effects of excess thyroid hormone (e.g., sweating, tachycardia, tremors)
2) surgical intervention (only attempted when client is in a neutral thyroid state) → euthroid state (normal)
   a) subtotal thyroidectomy
   b) total thyroidectomy (if carcinoma present)

2. **Nursing Process**
   a. **Assessment** *(hyperthyroidism / ↑ metabolism)*
      1) cardiovascular: elevated BP, bounding pulse, tachycardia, palpitations
      2) nutrition: weight loss, increased appetite
      3) integument: flushed, moist skin; heat intolerance
      4) musculoskeletal: fatigue, muscle weakness, fine tremors
      5) psychologic: anxiety, insomnia, mood swings, personality changes
      6) other: menstrual irregularities, change in libido
      7) exophthalmos *edematous*
   b. **Goals, Plans/Implementation, Evaluation**

   Goal 1: Client will return to and remain in euthyroid state.
   Plan/Implementation
   - provide calm, restful physical environment with low levels of sensory stimulation *(prevents thyroid storm)*
     - ensure physical comfort; comfortable environmental temperature
     - provide adequate rest
   - provide adequate nutrients
     - high calorie (4,000–5,000), balanced diet
     - increased fluid intake
   - provide eye care if exophthalmos present
     - eye drops, dark glasses, patch eyes if necessary
     - elevate head of bed

   Evaluation: Client enjoys restful sleep, verbalizes decreased discomfort and fatigue, maintains or increases body weight, and is free from corneal damage.

   Goal 2: Client undergoing thyroidectomy will be free from postoperative complications.
   Plan/Implementation
   - prepare client's room prior to return from OR with O_2, suction, tracheostomy set and calcium gluconate at bedside
   - monitor for signs of bleeding or excessive edema
     - elevate head of bed 30°; support head and neck
     - check dressings frequently, assess for constriction
     - check behind the neck for bleeding
   - assess for signs of respiratory distress, hoarseness
   - be alert for the possibility of
     - tetany (owing to hypocalcemia caused by accidental removal of parathyroid glands)
     - thyroid storm: markedly increased temperature and pulse with increasing restlessness and agitation
   - administer food and fluid with care (dysphagia is common)

   Evaluation: Client maintains normal vital signs, experiences no excessive bleeding or respiratory distress, supports head and neck during movement.

   Goal 3: Client will maintain normal levels of thyroid hormone.
   Plan/Implementation
   - provide client with information about prescribed medications, i.e., name, dosage, side effects, and the importance of ongoing medical supervision
     - total thyroidectomy necessitates lifelong replacement medication
     - subtotal thyroidectomy necessitates careful monitoring of the return of thyroid function

   Evaluation: Client follows prescribed medication regimen; is free from hyper- or hypothyroid function.

D. **Hypothyroidism**

1. **General Information**
   a. Definitions: underactive state of the thyroid gland resulting in diminished secretion of thyroid hormone
      1) *cretinism*: deficiency occurring in infancy and childhood
      2) *myxedema*: deficiency occurring in adulthood, usually in the fifth to sixth decade; affects women five times more frequently than men

b. Diagnosis
1) decreased T_3 and T_4
2) elevated TSH and cholesterol
c. Complications
1) cretinism: severe physical and mental retardation
2) myxedema
a) accelerated development of coronary artery disease
b) organic psychosis
c) myxedema coma: rapid development of impaired consciousness and suppression of vital functions
d. Medical Treatment: thyroid replacement
1) levothyroxine (Synthroid) is the drug of choice, if client does not have disabling cardiac involvement
2) dessicated thyroid, thyroglobulin (Proloid)
3) liothyronine (Cytomel) is useful in clients who experience allergic responses to other preparations

2. Nursing Process *met ↓ + drugs are not excreted as fast*
a. Assessment
1) fatigue, weight gain, constipation   *hypo-thyroidism*
2) dry skin, cold intolerance
3) coarse, thinning hair
4) mental sluggishness
5) thick tongue, swollen lips
6) menstrual irregularities, infertility
7) extreme sensitivity to narcotics, barbiturates, anesthetics *nonallergic*
b. Goal, Plan/Implementation, Evaluation

Goal: Client will return to and remain in a euthyroid state.
Plan/Implementation
- provide a warm environment conducive to rest
- avoid use of all sedatives *sm. doses*
- assist client in choosing low calorie diet
- increase intake of fluid and roughage to relieve constipation
- gradually increase physical activity and sensory stimulation as condition improves
- provide information about prescribed medication, i.e., name, dosage, side effects, and the importance of lifelong medical supervision

Evaluation: Client follows prescribed medication regimen; loses weight; experiences increased activity tolerance and alertness

E. **Hyperparathyroidism** *↑PTH*
1. General Information
a. Definition: overactivity of one or more of the parathyroid glands
1) primary: a problem within the gland itself; usually benign adenomas
2) secondary: a compensatory response to other conditions that produce hypocalcemia (e.g., vitamin D deficiency, chronic renal disease, malabsorption)
b. Diagnosis
1) elevated serum calcium, with low serum phosphate
2) x-rays show demineralization of bones, bone cysts
c. Complications
1) renal failure   *↑ Level Ca+*
2) cardiac dysrhythmias   *Kidney stones*
3) bone fractures or collapse
d. Medical Treatment
1) medical intervention
a) hydration with normal saline, plus diuretics
b) calcium-blocking agents
2) surgical intervention: parathyroidectomy leaving any disease-free glands intact   *Remove any 4 of them*

2. Nursing Process
a. Assessment (*NOTE:* some clients are clinically asymptomatic)
1) skeletal pain, weakness, fatigue, backache   *dizzy*
2) vague abdominal pain, nausea and vomiting, constipation
3) depression, mental dullness
4) cardiac dysrhythmias *1st sym. sometimes*
5) renal colic, stones *flank pain*
b. Goal, Plan/Implementation, and Evaluation

Goal: Client undergoing parathyroidectomy will be free from complications.
Plan/Implementation
- provide low calcium diet pre-op; avoid milk and milk products
- encourage high fluid intake pre-op (at least 3,000 ml/day)
- perform general post-op care as for thyroidectomy, and in addition
  - observe carefully for tetany *cramps convulsions*   *rebound affect*
  - institute high calcium diet *muscle twitching*
- encourage ambulation to stimulate bone recalcification

240 SECTION 3: NURSING CARE OF THE ADULT

Evaluation: Client's calcium values are within normal range; client experiences normal muscle functioning.

F. Hypoparathyroidism

1. **General Information**
   a. Definition: failure of the parathyroid glands to produce adequate amounts of parathormone (PTH)
   b. Precipitating Causes
      1) usually surgically induced by thyroidectomy
      2) idiopathic forms, possibly autoimmune in nature *Tumor*
   c. Diagnosis
      1) low serum calcium
      2) elevated serum phosphate
   d. Complications
      1) cardiac dysrhythmias
      2) premature cataract formation
   e. Medical Treatment
      1) oral calcium preparations
      2) high-dose vitamin D
      3) aluminum hydroxide to lower serum phosphate

2. **Nursing Process**
   a. Assessment
      1) signs of tetany
         a) positive Chvostek's and Trousseau's signs
         b) muscle spasms
         c) tingling of fingers and around lips
      2) cardiac dysrhythmias
   b. Goal, Plan/Implementation, and Evaluation

   Goal: Client will be free from the complications of prolonged calcium imbalance.

   Plan/Implementation
   - acute stage
     - assess for symptoms of tetany frequently
     - keep calcium gluconate at bedside
   - chronic stage
     - provide high calcium, low phosphorus diet
     - provide information about prescribed medications, i.e., name, dosage, side effects *Calcium gluconate*
   - teach client symptoms of calcium imbalance

   Evaluation: Client follows prescribed medication and diet regimen; is free from the symptoms of hypocalcemia.

G. Hyperfunction of the Adrenal Glands *Near kidneys*

1. **General Information**
   a. Definition: oversecretion of hormones from either the adrenal cortex or adrenal medulla
      1) Cushing's syndrome: excessive secretion of glucocorticoids and possibly androgens from the adrenal cortex
      2) pheochromocytoma: catecholamine-producing tumor of the adrenal medulla
   b. Incidence
      1) Cushing's syndrome
         a) true Cushing's syndrome is relatively rare, but occurs most frequently in women aged 20–60
         b) can result from adrenal tumors or excessive pituitary secretion of ACTH from any cause
         c) a common result of the chronic use of exogenous steroids
      2) pheochromocytoma *Tumor*
         a) rare disorder; may occur in middle age in either sex
         b) has a familial tendency
   c. Diagnosis
      1) Cushing's syndrome
         a) increased plasma cortisol, blood glucose, urinary 17-hydroxysteroids and 17-ketosteroids; decreased potassium
      2) pheochromocytoma
         a) elevated 24-hour urine vanillymandelic acid (VMA) (*NOTE:* Client must avoid ingestion of fruits, coffee, vanilla, and chocolate prior to this test)
         b) elevated urine metanephrines
   d. Complications
      1) Cushing's syndrome
         a) cardiac problems, e.g., CHF, hypertension★
         b) skeletal fractures
      2) pheochromocytoma *labile BP*
         a) CVA★   *hypertension*
         b) renal damage
         c) blindness
   e. Medical Treatment
      1) Cushing's syndrome
         a) surgical adrenalectomy if tumor is present

b) hypophysectomy for tumor of pituitary
c) drug therapy with cortisol inhibitors
d) alteration in exogenous steroid dose if possible
2) pheochromocytoma
a) surgical adrenalectomy
b) pre-op drug therapy with alpha- and beta-blocking agents

2. Nursing Process
a. Assessment
1) Cushing's syndrome
a) abnormal fat distribution
- weight gain, thick trunk, thin legs
- moon face, buffalo hump (cervical dorsal fat pad)
b) skin changes
- thin skin, red cheeks
- purple striae (stretch marks)
- bruises, acne
c) cardiovascular
- hypertension
- fluid overload, CHF
- sodium and water retention, hypokalemia
d) musculoskeletal
- muscle weakness, decreased muscle mass
- osteoporosis
e) increased susceptibility to infection
f) decreased resistance to stress
g) increased secretion of pepsin and HCl acid
h) hyperglycemia
i) mental changes and mood swings
j) changes in secondary sex characteristics, amenorrhea
2) pheochromocytoma
a) labile hypertension
b) tachycardia, palpitations
c) diaphoresis

b. Goals, Plans/Implementation, and Evaluation

Goal 1: Client with Cushing's syndrome will achieve stabilized symptoms.
Plan/Implementation
- provide diet low in calories and sodium, high in protein, potassium, and calcium
  - offer diet in small, frequent feedings
  - monitor for signs of hyperglycemia, GI bleeding
- protect client from unnecessary exposure to infection
  - monitor vital signs regularly
  - use strict hygiene and asepsis
  - institute reverse isolation if needed
- provide atmosphere conducive to rest; space activities and assist with care as needed
- observe for signs of CHF
- monitor daily weights, I&O, blood and urine glucose measurements
- offer needed support in dealing with changes in body image

Evaluation: Client will maintain or lose weight; will experience increased strength and stamina; will be free from infection, accidental injury, or peptic ulceration; will refer to self in a positive way.

Goal 2: Client treated with adrenalectomy will be free from complications.
Plan/Implementation
- measure urine output accurately and frequently
- monitor vital signs frequently
- watch for signs of adrenal crisis; have IV fluids, pressor drugs, corticosteroids readily available
- prevent thrombotic and respiratory problems
- teach regarding post-discharge self-care (e.g., diet, medications, activity level, follow-up care)

Evaluation: Client maintains stable vital signs, adequate urine output and respiratory gas exchange post-op; can state self-care needs to expect after discharge.

Goal 3: Client with pheochromocytoma will have his BP controlled prior to surgery.
Plan/Implementation
- administer antihypertensives or blocking agents as ordered; monitor vital signs frequently
- provide rest and control anxiety
- provide sedation if needed

Evaluation: Client's BP remains within prescribed parameters; client is free from palpitations or tachycardia.

H. Hyposecretion of the Adrenal Glands

1. General Information
a. Definition (Addison's disease): insufficient secretion of glucocorticoids,

mineralocorticoids, and androgens from the adrenal cortex
  b. Incidence
      1) rare disease occurring in 1 in 100,000; affects both sexes and usually occurs in middle age
      2) true Addison's is usually idiopathic but will occur after surgical removal of the adrenal glands
  c. Diagnosis
      1) low serum cortisol levels
      2) low urinary 17-hydroxysteroids and 17-ketosteroids
      3) low serum sodium and glucose
      4) elevated serum potassium
  d. Complications: adrenal crisis: acute adrenal insufficiency with sudden, marked deprivation of adrenocortical hormones producing cardiovascular collapse → Shock
  e. Medical Intervention: steroid replacement maintained throughout life
      1) glucocorticoids
          a) cortisone usually given for maintenance
          b) diurnal rhythm maintained (e.g., 25 mg in morning, 12.5 mg in evening)
          c) hydrocortisone given in emergencies
          d) dose will need to be increased at any time of increased stress, including illness or surgery
      2) mineralocorticoids: fludrocortisone (Florinef) 0.05–0.2 mg daily (if more needed, long-acting preparation may be given)
      3) periodic testosterone injections to increase protein anabolism

2. Nursing Process
   a. Assessment (*NOTE:* The clinical picture from the history and symptoms is often vague)

Table 3.33 Steroids

Description	Drugs that block the inflammatory, allergic, and immune responses by a variety of processes; include both naturally occurring and synthetic glucocorticoids
Uses	Replacement for primary or secondary adrenocortical insufficiency; to treat a wide variety of inflammatory, allergic/autoimmune disorders including rheumatoid disease, collagen disease, allergic reactions, dermatologic responses, ophthalmic problems, ulcerative colitis, Crohn's disease, neoplasms
Side Effects	Salt and water retention, GI ulceration from increased HCl secretion, hypertension, CHF, hirsutism, striae, impaired wound healing, fatty redistribution, decreased growth in children, protein catabolism, osteoporosis, emotional lability, leukopenia (increased susceptibility to infection), sterility, diabetes, cataracts, hypokalemia
Nursing Implications	Warn client about need to avoid infections and increased need for steroids during times of physical and emotional stress. Monitor decreased response to stress and side effects; help client to minimize side effects as much as possible (e.g., low salt, high potassium, low carbohydrate diet). Give with an antacid; give in morning to mimic normal release; stress need for client to strictly adhere to medication regimen. Offer support to the client experiencing changes in body image. Teach that these drugs cannot be discontinued abruptly. Suggest carrying ID stating client is on steroid regimen.
Examples	Dexamethasone (Decadron), cortisone acetate (Cortistan), hydrocortisone (Cortef, Solu-Cortef), beclomethasone diproprionate (Vanceril), prednisone (Deltasone), betamethasone valerate (Valisone), fluocinonide (Lidex), methylprednisolone acetate (Medrol), triamcinolone acetate (Kenalog)

1) gastrointestinal symptoms: anorexia, nausea, weight loss
2) bronzing of skin (from excess MSH production)
3) orthostatic blood pressure changes
4) weakness

b. Goals, Plans/Implementation, and Evaluation

Goal 1: Client will recover from an adrenal crisis. *Replace Steroids*

Plan/Implementation
- give large doses of glucocorticoids and vasopressors by IV infusion
- encourage complete bed rest; prevent physical activity and emotional stress
- monitor vital signs and fluid and electrolyte balance until condition stabilizes

Evaluation: Client's vital signs remain within normal limits; exercise and activity levels gradually return to normal.

Goal 2: Client with Addison's disease will maintain normal hormonal balance.

Plan/Implementation
- provide information about prescribed medications, i.e., name, dosage, side effects, and the importance of ongoing medical supervision
- teach client the signs and symptoms of under- or overdose of medications, and conditions that will require dosage adjustments

Evaluation: Client is asymptomatic; takes and adjusts medications as indicated; receives ongoing medical care.

I. Hypofunction of the Pancreas: Diabetes Mellitus

1. General Information

a. Definition: a chronic systemic disease producing disorders in carbohydrate, protein, and fat metabolism; results from disturbances in the production, action, or utilization of insulin; eventually produces destructive changes in a wide variety of organs and tissues. The insulin deficiency may be relative or absolute.

b. Incidence
1) most common endocrine disorder; more than 10 million diabetics in the US
2) diabetes and its complications are among the leading causes of death and disability in the US

c. Etiology
1) basic etiology remains unknown
2) considered to be a group of syndromes whose development is influenced by genetic factors, viruses, autoimmunity, and environmental factors such as stress and obesity

d. Types
1) Type 1 (insulin dependent): results from destruction of the beta cells of the pancreas resulting in little or no insulin production; requires daily insulin administration *Child usually but not always*
2) Type 2 (non-insulin dependent): probably results from a disturbance in insulin reception in the cells; most common in middle aged, overweight adults

e. Pathophysiology
1) normally blood-glucose levels are maintained in the homeostatic range of 60–100 mg/100 ml by a series of feedback mechanisms
2) in the absence of insulin, glucose accumulates in blood and urine leading to
   a) hyperglycemia *hunger*
   b) glycosuria
3) glucose is hypertonic and depletes the body of large amounts of water (from extracellular fluid) as it is excreted by the kidneys causing
   a) polyuria
   b) polydipsia
   c) loss of sodium and potassium
4) glucose is then not available for cellular nutrition and this causes polyphagia
5) fat and protein stores are broken down and used for energy; so utilization of these stores is not sufficient, causing *ketones*
   a) ketoacidosis
   b) ketonuria
   c) weakness
6) other metabolic effects
   a) micro- and macrocirculatory changes producing athero- and arteriosclerosis, e.g., coronary artery disease, peripheral vascular disease, retinal and kidney damage
   b) alteration in immune and inflammatory response

- glucose concentration in the skin creates an excellent medium for infection
- glucose inhibits the phagocytic action of leukocytes → decreased resistance

c) alterations in perception and coordination caused by developing neuropathies (a common complication—the cause of which is poorly understood)

f. Medical Treatment
1) drug therapy (see table 3.34)
   a) insulin: short-, intermediate-, and long-acting forms
   b) oral hypoglycemic agents
2) diet: individually planned regimens based on the client's age, sex, weight, and usual life-style (see table 3.35)
   a) diet is manipulated to distribute the nutrient intake appropriately over a 24-hour period
   b) diet is planned using the American Diabetic Association's (ADA) exchange method of meal planning
   c) diet is used to correct obesity when necessary

2. Nursing Process
   a. Assessment
      1) polyphagia, polyuria, polydipsia, weight loss
      2) hyperglycemia, glycosuria, ketonuria
      3) weakness, fatigue
      4) increased susceptibility to infection
      5) alterations in circulation, slow wound healing

Table 3.34 Hypoglycemics

Description	Drugs that act to either stimulate the islet cells in the pancreas to secrete more insulin (oral) or act as insulin replacement when pancreatic function ceases (parenteral)
Uses	Treatment of diabetes mellitus
Side Effects	Hypoglycemic reactions, GI distress, neurologic symptoms, alcohol intolerance (oral preparations), and allergic reactions
Nursing Implications	Know onset and duration of action for each agent and teach to client; monitor for and teach client to monitor for hypoglycemic reaction; stress compliance with total diabetic regimen; check for beef or pork allergy (insulin preparations); teach client self-administration of insulin including proper storage, care of equipment, site rotation, and urine testing for sugar and acetone.

Types and Examples	Peak (hours)	Duration (hours)
Oral agents		
Acetohexamide (Dymelor)		12–24
Chlorpropamide (Diabinese)	3–6	24
Tolbutamide (Orinase)	5–8	6–12
Tolazamide (Tolinase)	10	16
Insulin		
Rapid Acting (onset 1 hour)		
Crystalline zinc	2–4	5–8
Regular	2–4	4–6
Insulin zinc suspension prompt (Semilente)	6–10	12–16
Intermediate Acting (onset 2–4 hours)		
Globin zinc (Iletin)	6–10	18–24
Isophane insulin suspension (NPH)	8–12	28–32
Insulin zinc suspension (Lente)	8–12	28–30
Long Acting (onset 4–6 hours)		
Protamine zinc (PZI)	16–24	24–36
Insulin zinc suspension extended (Ultralente)	16–24	more than 36

Table 3.35 Diabetic Meal Planning with Exchange Lists*

Food Exchange Group	Protein in GM	CHO in GM (per serving)	Fat in GM	Calories
Milk	8	12	trace	80
Vegetable (½ cup) †	2	5	-	25
Fruit	-	10	-	40
Bread	2	15	-	70
Meat	7	-	3	55
Fat	-	-	5	45

*Source: American Diabetes Association, Inc.; American Dietetic Association, *Exchange Lists for Meal Planning*, 1976.
† Some vegetables in the vegetable exchange can be used freely when raw. Starchy vegetables are listed in the bread exchange list.

Examples of Foods in Exchange Lists

Free Foods	List 1 Milk Exchanges	List 2 Vegetable Exchanges	List 3 Fruit Exchanges	List 4 Bread Exchanges	List 5 Meat Exchanges	List 6 Fat Exchanges
Coffee, tea. Clear broth. Gelatin (unsweetened). Pepper and other spices.	Whole milk (omit 2 fat exchanges). Skim milk. Buttermilk made with skim milk.	Asparagus. Beets. Broccoli. Cabbage. Cauliflower. Cucumbers. Chard. Collards. Mushrooms. Onions. Tomatoes. Turnips. Raw Vegetables (List 2) Chicory. Chinese cabbage. Endive. Escarole. Lettuce. Parsley. Radishes. Watercress.	Apple. Apple sauce. Banana. Strawberries. Cantaloupe. Cherries. Grapefruit. Orange juice. Pear. Pineapple. Prunes, dried. Watermelon.	Bread. Cereals. Spaghetti, noodles. Crackers. Beans and peas (dried and cooked). Corn. Potatoes.	Meat and poultry. Cold cuts. Frankfurters. Eggs. Fish. Shrimp. Cheese: cheddar, cottage. Peanut butter.	Butter or margarine. Bacon (crisp). Cream. Mayonnaise. Nuts. Olives.

General Rules (for all clients to know and follow carefully):

1) Eat all meals about the same time daily. Do not skip meals.
2) Eat only those foods, in the amount given, on the diet list.
3) Do not eat between meals UNLESS it is a part of the dietary plan, unless replacing food not eaten at a previous meal, or unless an insulin reaction is "coming on."

Standard Exchange List Procedure for Liquid Diets (for frequent, continuing meal replacement of more than one day's duration and for tube feedings as necessary):

1) List the total number of food exchanges allowed per day in each of the 6 categories (fruit, vegetable, meat, fat, bread, and milk).
2) Substitute fruit juices for the fruit exchanges; puree and strain cooked vegetables and dilute with water for the vegetable exchanges; and select from the suggestions below for the meat, fat, bread, and milk exchanges.
3) Distribute the liquid substitutes in balanced amounts every 1-2 hours through the waking day.

For 1 meat exchange and 1 milk exchange:	Eggnog made of 1 egg and 8 oz whole milk flavored with saccharine and vanilla.
For 1 bread exchange and ½ milk exchange:	Cooked cereal diluted with 4 oz whole milk.
For 1 bread exchange and 2 fat exchanges:	Ice cream, ½ cup.
For 2 meat exchanges, 1 milk exchange, and 1 fat exchange:	Mix 8 oz whole milk with 2 oz melted cheddar cheese and 1 tsp margarine; flavor with celery salt.

246 SECTION 3: NURSING CARE OF THE ADULT

6) altered neurologic functioning
   a) peripheral neuropathies
   b) visual and sexual dysfunction
b. Goals, Plans/Implementation, and Evaluation

Goal 1: Client will demonstrate knowledge of the principles of diet control.
Plan/Implementation
- reinforce teaching of the dietician as needed
- encourage client to use the individualized meal plan
- reinforce the importance of not skipping meals
- measure foods accurately; do not estimate them
- discuss with client the diet modifications needed to compensate for changes in life-style or illness

Evaluation: Client makes appropriate selections from sample menus; maintains normal body weight; maintains fasting blood-sugar levels within normal ranges.

Goal 2: Client will correctly administer insulin.
Plan/Implementation
- teach client preparation of injection, storage of insulin and the principles of site rotation
  - insulin in current use may be stored at room temperature, all others in refrigerator
  - insulin must be at room temperature before administration
  - roll insulin to mix, double-check label concentration
  - if client mixes insulin, he should do so in the same sequence each day
  - rotate sites so that no one site is used more frequently than once a month
  - inject at 90° angle
- provide opportunities for multiple return demonstrations
- teach at least one family member to administer insulin
- teach client factors that influence the body's need for insulin
  - increased need: trauma, infection, fever, severe psychologic or physiologic stress
  - decreased need: active exercise

Evaluation: Client properly administers own insulin; shows no signs of lipodystrophy.

Goal 3: Client will monitor diabetic status regularly and correctly through the use of urine testing and/or finger sticks.
Plan/Implementation
- teach client the principles of urine testing
  - consistent use of one product
  - test before meals and at bedtime
    * fresh urine sample is mandatory
    * double voiding is considered preferable
  - record results in percentages
- teach client about common medications that interfere with urine test results
  - vitamin C and salicylates
  - cephalosporin antibiotics
- teach client proper technique for finger sticks
  - follow product guide carefully for timing results
  - avoid use of the center of tips of fingers
- keep accurate date and time records for both urine and finger-stick testing
- teach client to notify physician if urine tests greater than 1% or finger-stick results are greater than the physician-specified limit

Evaluation: Client demonstrates accurate urine testing and/or finger-stick glucose measurements; correctly interprets the results; maintains consistent, accurate records of the results.

Goal 4: Client will establish and maintain a pattern of regular exercise.
Plan/Implementation
- individualize exercise plan for each client
- perform exercise after meals to ensure an adequate level of blood glucose
  - teach client to carry a rapid-acting source of glucose
  - teach client that excessive or unplanned exercise may trigger hypoglycemia

Evaluation: Client engages in planned regular exercise without experiencing difficulties with hypoglycemia.

Goal 5: Client will practice good personal hygiene and positive health promotion to avoid diabetic complications.
Plan/Implementation
- teach client diabetic foot care
  - daily gentle cleansing and inspection

NUTRITION AND METABOLISM

Table 3.36 Differentiating Hypoglycemia from Ketoacidosis (Hyperglycemia)

	Hypoglycemia (Insulin Reaction)	Ketoacidosis (Diabetic Coma)
Causes	Too much insulin. Not enough food (delayed or missed meals). Excessive exercise or work. Diarrhea. Vomiting. Alcohol. Sudden fear or anger.	Too little insulin. Too much or wrong kind of food. Infection. Illness. Injuries. Pregnancy. Insufficient exercise. Emotional stress.
Onset	Sudden: regular insulin. Gradual: modified insulin or oral hypoglycemic drugs.	Slow (days).
Symptoms:		
(early)	Hunger. Sweating. Pallor. Cold skin. Tremor. Feelings of nervousness, anxiety. Irritable behavior. Decreased spontaneity. Weakness. Lethargy.	Thirst. Increased urination (nocturia). Anorexia. Nausea, vomiting. Dim vision. Headache.
(gradual)	Blurred or double vision. Mentally dull. Change in behavior (negativistic, weepy, aggressive). Fatigue. Confusion. Dizziness. Slurred speech. Slow, uncoordinated movement.	Abdominal pain (cramps due to bloating from gastric atony). Constipation. Drowsiness. Headache. Weakness and fatigue. Listlessness.
Signs	Shallow, rapid respiration. Rapid pulse. Dilated pupils. Tachycardia.	Flushed, dry skin (lack of skin turgor). Fast, labored, deep breathing (air hunger). Weak, rapid pulse. Subnormal temperature. Soft eyeballs. Acetone (fruity) breath odor. Hypotension. Coma.
Urine	Negative for sugar and acetone.	Positive for sugar and acetone.
Blood Glucose	60 mg or less/100 ml.	Greater than 250 mg/100 ml.

Treatment	• Give about 10 gm CHO
	  – 4 oz fruit juice, or
	  – 2 tsp corn syrup, or
	  – 2 tsp honey, or
	  – 5 Life Savers, or
	  – 1 glass soft drink.
	• If client is unable to swallow, squeeze concentrated glucose between gums into mouth (Reactose, Glucose, Cake Mate, a decorating gel).
	• If necessary, IV Glucagon, 1 mg, may be given (can also be given IM or subcutaneously).
	• Obtain blood and urine specimens for lab testing.
	• Notify client's physician re time of reaction, signs and symptoms, what given and response.
	• Give crackers and milk about 1 hour following initial treatment.
		• Keep client flat in bed, and warm.
		• Have client, if conscious, drink sugar-free, hot liquids such as coffee, tea, broth, bouillon.
		• Record I&O.
		• Notify client's physician.
		• Obtain blood and urine specimens for lab testing.
		• Check and record vital signs and level of consciousness.
		• Prepare to administer parenteral fluids under a physician's order.
		• Prepare to administer at least 20-40 units regular insulin with physician's order.
		• Connect to cardiac monitor and observe for potassium imbalance.

Adapted from Neal, M. et al. "Differentiating Hypoglycemia and Ketoacidosis (Hyperglycemia)," *Nursing Care Planning Guides*, Set 1, 2nd Ed., No. 1:35, Baltimore: Williams & Wilkins, 1980.

- properly fitting shoes
- use lanolin cream to prevent dryness and cracking *sparingly Don't over soften*
- avoid going barefoot
- wear socks with shoes
- visit a podiatrist regularly for care of nails, calluses, corns
• teach client interventions to prevent peripheral vascular disease (refer to "PVD" in *Oxygenation* page 193)
• teach client the adjustments that must be made in the event of minor illness (e.g., colds, flu)
  - continue taking insulin or oral hypoglycemic regularly (infection increases the body's need for insulin)
  - maintain fluid intake, replace diet with appropriate semisolid exchanges if unable to eat solid food (see table 3.35)
  - increase the frequency of blood/urine testing
  - contact physician if necessary
• assist client to identify stressful situations in life-style that might interfere with good diabetic control
• encourage regular checkups by dentist and good daily hygiene
• advise regular eye exams
• teach aggressive care for minor skin cuts and abrasions; avoid clothing and activities that cause chafing and irritation

Evaluation: Client's teeth and gums are in good repair; skin is soft and intact; states adjustments that are to be made to maintain control during periods of minor illness.

Goal 6: Client can recognize the signs of hypoglycemia and ketoacidosis and take appropriate actions.

Plan/Implementation
• teach signs of hypoglycemia and the situations that may trigger it (see table 3.36 for symptoms)
  - too much insulin or too little food
  - strenuous unplanned exercise
  - vomiting or diarrhea
  - emotional upsets
• teach client to reverse hypoglycemia if possible with rapid-acting source of glucose (50% glucose is administered IV if client loses consciousness)
• teach client signs of ketoacidosis and situations that may trigger it (see table 3.36 for symptoms)
  - failure to take insulin
  - too much food
  - episode of illness or infection
• teach client that development of ketoacidosis requires immediate transport to a health care facility
  - correct dehydration by administration of IV fluids
  - correct blood sugar level with administration of insulin (usually low-dose insulin infusion)
  - replace electrolytes as ordered
  - record I&O accurately (Foley catheter is usually necessary)
  - monitor urines and finger sticks at frequent intervals
  - assess for decreasing LOC and declining cardiopulmonary status at frequent intervals
• tell client to wear a diabetic alert bracelet or tag at all times.

Evaluation: Client can list the symptoms of hypoglycemia and ketoacidosis and state appropriate actions to take for each; wears a diabetic alert tag.

References

Camunas, C. "Transsphenoidal Hypophysectomy." *American Journal of Nursing*. October 1980:1820-1823.

Dexter, M. "Antacid Therapy." *American Journal of Nursing*. April 1981:788-789.

Fletcher, P. "The Oral Antidiabetic Drugs: Pro and Con." *American Journal of Nursing*. April 1976:596-599.

Fredette, S. "When the Liver Fails." *American Journal of Nursing*, January 1984:64-67.

Gannon, R. and Pickett, K. "Jaundice." *American Journal of Nursing*, March 1983:404-407.

Gever, L. "Anticholinergics." *Nursing 84*, September 1984:64.

Griggs, B. and Hoppe, M. "Update: Nasogastric Tube Feedings." *American Journal of Nursing*. March 1979:481-485.

Jenkins, E. "Living with Thyrotoxicosis." *American Journal of Nursing*. May 1980:956-958.

King, D. "How to Give Your Portal Hypertension Patient a Fighting Chance." *RN*. September 1984:32-37.

Kratzer, J. and Rauschenbergen, D. "What to Teach Your Patient About His Duodenal Ulcer." *Nursing 78*. January 1978:54-56.

Marks, V. "Health Teaching for Recovering Alcoholic Patients." *American Journal of Nursing*. November 1980:2058-2061.

Masoorli, S. and Piercy, S. "A Life Saving Guide to Blood Products." *RN*. September 1984: 32-37.

"Metabolic Alkalosis," in Clinical Insights, *Nursing 84*. August 1984:60-61.

Miller, B. and White, N. "Diabetes Assessment Guide." *American Journal of Nursing*. July 1980:1314-1316.

Miller, P. "Teaching Patients About Adrenal Corticosteroids." *American Journal of Nursing*. January 1981:78-81.

Neal, M., Cohen, P., Cooper, P. *Nursing Care Planning Guides, Set 1*, 2nd Ed. Baltimore: Williams & Wilkins, 1980.

*Neal, M., Cohen, P., Reighley, J. "Hyperalimentation." *Nursing Care Planning Guides, Set 3*, 2nd Ed. Baltimore: Williams & Wilkins, 1983.

Neilsen, L. "Interpreting Arterial Blood Gases." *American Journal of Nursing*. December 1980:2197-2201.

Nursing 81. *Diagnostics*. Springhouse, PA: Intermed Communications, 1981.

Schuman, D. "Disturbances in Glucose Metabolism," in Jones, Dunbar and Juovec, *Medical-Surgical Nursing*. New York: McGraw-Hill, 1978.

Shahinpour, R. "The Adult Patient with Bleeding Esophageal Varices." *Nursing Clinics of North America*. June 1977:331-343.

Strange, J. "An Expert's Guide to Tubes and Drains." *RN*, April 1983:35-42.

Sweet, K. "Hiatal Hernia—What to Guard Against Most in Postop Patients." *Nursing 83*, December 1983:39-45.

Thorpe, C. and Caprin, J. "Gallbladder Disease: Current Trends and Treatments." *American Journal of Nursing*. December 1980:2181-2185.

Wimpsett, J. "Trace Your Patient's Liver Dysfunction." *Nursing 84*, August 1984:56-57.

* See reprint section

Elimination

(The nursing care presented in this unit concerns selected health problems related to disturbances in the kidneys and the large bowel.)

Part One: The Kidneys

General Concepts

A. Overview
1. Kidneys
   a. Location: paired organs that lie in the retroperitoneum at the costovertebral angle (CVA)
      1) upper border: T-12
      2) lower border: L-3
   b. Size: 120–170 gm (4–6 oz) each
   c. Regions
      1) cortex
         a) outer layer
         b) contains glomeruli, proximal and distal tubules
      2) medulla
         a) middle layer
         b) composed of 6–10 renal pyramids, formed by collecting ducts and tubules
         c) deepest part of loop of Henle
      3) pelvis
         a) innermost layer
         b) hollow collection area composed of calyces
         c) papillae move urine into ureter by peristaltic action
   d. Nephron
      1) functional unit of kidney
      2) one million nephrons in each kidney
      3) composition
         a) glomerulus
         b) tubule
            - Bowman's capsule
            - proximal convoluted tubule
            - loop of Henle
              – descending limb
              – ascending limb
            - distal convoluted tubule
            - collecting duct
      4) action: all elements to be excreted or conserved are acted on in the nephron by the processes of filtration, concentration, reabsorption, or secretion
2. Ureters
   a. Join with renal pelvis; distal end implanted in bladder
   b. Composed of smooth muscles that have peristaltic action
   c. Narrow at ureteropelvic junction, bifurcation of iliac vessels and join with bladder
3. Bladder
   a. Stores urine until eliminated
   b. Muscular organ
4. Urethra
   a. Passageway for urine during excretion
   b. Surrounded by prostate gland in men
5. Functions of the Kidney
   a. Fluid and Electrolyte Balance
      1) control of sodium balance
         a) intake in normal diet is usually greater than needed
         b) filtered by glomeruli
         c) reabsorption in tubules is controlled by active and passive processes and by the renin-angiotensin-aldosterone system
      2) control of chloride balance follows sodium
         a) intake in normal diet is usually greater than needed
         b) filtered by the glomeruli
         c) actively transported out of the ascending loop of Henle

ELIMINATION 251

Figure 3.13 Components of the Kidney

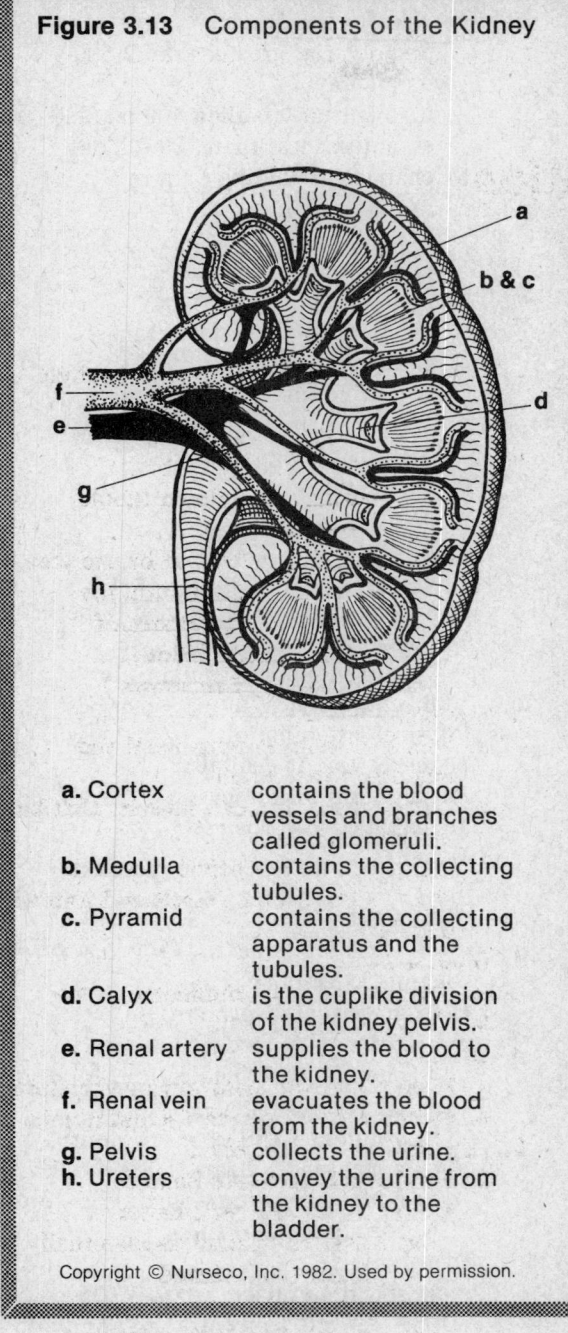

a.	Cortex	contains the blood vessels and branches called glomeruli.
b.	Medulla	contains the collecting tubules.
c.	Pyramid	contains the collecting apparatus and the tubules.
d.	Calyx	is the cuplike division of the kidney pelvis.
e.	Renal artery	supplies the blood to the kidney.
f.	Renal vein	evacuates the blood from the kidney.
g.	Pelvis	collects the urine.
h.	Ureters	convey the urine from the kidney to the bladder.

Copyright © Nurseco, Inc. 1982. Used by permission.

Figure 3.14 Components and Functions of the Nephron

Part of Nephron	Function	Substance
a. Glomeruli	Filtration	H_2O and solute, electrolytes (Na, K, PO_4, Ca, Cl, Mg), urea, creatinine, uric acid, glucose, amino acids
b. Proximal tubules	Reabsorption, secretion	H_2O, electrolytes (Na, K, Mg, Ca, Cl, HCO_3), glucose, amino acids
c. Loop of Henle	Reabsorption	H_2O, electrolytes (Na, K)
d. Distal tubule	Acid-base balance, secretion	Hydrogen ions (H), Na
e. Collecting tubule	Concentration	H_2O

Copyright © Nurseco, Inc. 1982. Used by permission.

3) control of H_2O balance
   a) intake controlled by social habits and thirst
   b) reabsorption controlled by antidiuretic hormone (ADH) concentration in the collecting duct

4) control of potassium balance
   a) intake adequate in normal diet
   b) filtered by glomeruli
   c) almost all filtered potassium is reabsorbed in proximal tubules
   d) secreted into distal tubules and into distal ducts where there is selective secretion or reabsorption
   e) dependent upon hormonal influence
      • increase of aldosterone causes increased potassium secretion

- decrease of aldosterone causes decreased potassium secretion
            f) potassium also lost through GI tract
        b. Control of Acid-Base Balance
          1) excretion of organic acids
            a) HPO_4 buffer system: $H + HPO_4 \rightarrow H_2PO_4$
            b) NH_3 buffer system
              - $NH_3 + H \rightarrow NH_4$
              - $NH_4 + NaCl \rightarrow NH_4Cl + Na$
            c) liberation of free hydrogen ions
          2) conservation of bicarbonate
        c. Excretion of waste products (primarily products of protein metabolism: urea and creatinine)
        d. Production and secretion of erythropoietin in response to hypoxia (stimulates bone marrow to produce hemoglobin)
        e. Manufacture and activation of vitamin D (plays a role in calcium metabolism: active form of vitamin D must be available for parathormone to work).
        f. Regulation of arterial blood pressure: renin and aldosterone
          1) kidneys secrete an enzyme called renin, which acts on plasma protein to cause the release of angiotensin (a vasoconstricting substance)
          2) angiotensin increases total peripheral resistance leading to increased aldosterone secretion by adrenal cortex
          3) increased aldosterone stimulates increased sodium reabsorption
          4) increased sodium reabsorption leads to increased water retention and plasma volume, which increases arterial BP

B. **Application of the Nursing Process to the Client with Kidney Problems**
  1. Assessment
    a. Health History
      1) urinary retention, stasis, e.g., associated with pregnancy, neurogenic bladder, immobility, diabetes
      2) bladder infections: caused by contamination from large intestine (especially young girls)
      3) intrusive procedures: e.g., catheterization, cystoscopy, coitus
      4) bone demineralization
      5) metabolic disease
      6) changes in color, e.g., hematuria
      7) changes in volume
        a) polyuria: greater than 2,500 ml/day
        b) oliguria: less than 400 ml/day
        c) anuria: less than 100 ml/day
      8) changes in voiding pattern
        a) nocturia
        b) frequency
        c) hesitancy
        d) urgency
        e) change in urinary stream
        f) incontinence
          - amount
          - frequency of occurrence
          - dribbling
      9) medications
        a) diuretics
        b) antibiotics
        c) nephrotoxic agents: ASA, acetaminophen, mercaptomerin sodium, phenylbutazone, sulfonomides, gentamycin
        d) cholinergics, anticholinergics
    b. Physical Examination
      1) inspection of genitals
      2) palpation of kidneys
      3) palpation of prostate
      4) pain
        a) back
        b) flank
        c) CVA tenderness ⊃ pylonephritis
    c. Diagnostic Tests
      1) urine (visual inspection)
        a) color: pale to deep amber; changes with medication, food, or disease
        b) volume: 30 ml or more/hour
        c) appearance: clear
        d) odor: strong ammonia after stored for a period of time
      2) urinalysis
        a) specific gravity: 1.002–1.035
          - reflects concentrating ability of kidneys
          - increases (greater than 1.035) with glucosuria and proteinuria
          - decreases (less than 1.002) with distal renal tubular disease and endocrine disorders associated with insufficiency of ADH
          - fixed (1.010) with glomerulonephritis
        b) pH: 4.8–8.0
          - reflects the acid-base balance

Table 3.37 Laboratory Tests Used to Evaluate Renal Function

Test	Normal Range	Usual Range in Renal Disease	What it Measures
Hemoglobin	12–18 gm/100 ml	Lowered	Formation of red blood cells
Blood urea nitrogen (BUN)	8–20 mg/100 ml	Elevated	Renal excretory function
Electrolytes			
Sodium	136–145 mEq/L	Elevated (not necessarily) or lowered	Fluid and electrolyte balance
Potassium	3.5–5 mEq/L	Elevated or lowered	Electrolyte balance
Chloride	90–102 mEq/L	Elevated (not necessarily) or lowered; has partnership with sodium	Fluid and electrolyte balance
Serum creatinine	0.4–1.2 mg/100 ml	Elevated	Renal function
Serum osmolarity	275–295 mOsm/L		Dissolved particles in the blood
Glucose	70–110/100 ml	Slight hyperglycemia	
Blood pH	7.38–7.44	Usually lowered	Acidity vs. alkalinity of blood
Arterial	7.3–7.41		
Venous			
Calcium	4–5 mEq/L	Usually lowered	Renal excretory function
Phosphorus	3.5–5.5 mEq/L	Elevated	Renal excretory function
Albumin	3.2–5.5 g/100 ml	Usually lowered	Albumin, which helps maintain blood's osmotic pressure

SOURCE: Larson, E. "Renal Function Assessment," in Larson, E., Lindbloom, L. and Davis, K., eds., *Development of the Clinical Nephrology Practitioner*. St. Louis: Mosby, 1982. Used with permission.

- greater than 8.0: alkaline; occurs with metabolic alkalosis, overuse of alkalizing medications, in presence of urinary tract infection (UTI)
- less than 4.8: acidic; occurs with metabolic acidosis, uncontrolled diabetes, some medications (e.g., ammonium chloride, high doses of vitamin C)

c) glucose
- normally not present
- may occur after heavy meal, emotional stress, or with infusion of glucose
- occurs abnormally with diabetes mellitus, pancreatic disorders, impaired reabsorption in the proximal tubules

d) ketones
- normally not present
- occur with uncontrolled diabetes, fasting, severe infections accompanied by nausea and vomiting

e) protein
- normally not present
- occurs with serious kidney or proximal tubular disorders, nephrotic syndrome, toxemia
- may occur after heavy protein meal, strenuous exercise, or prolonged standing

f) red blood cells
- normally 0–3/high power field
- increase with kidney malfunction or trauma to urinary tract or tumor or infection in urinary tract

g) white blood cells
- normally 0–4/high power field
- increase with infection within urinary tract system

h) hyaline casts
- normally not present

- indicate acute glomerulo- or pyelonephritis, chronic renal disease, or renal calculi
  i) granular casts
    - normally not present
    - indicates acute renal rejection (transplant), pyelonephritis, or chronic lead poisoning
3) urine culture and sensitivity
   a) voided specimen: bacterial count over 100,000 organisms/ml (if infection is cause)
   b) sterile, catheterized specimen: over 10,000 organisms/ml
4) tests of filtration function
   a) creatinine clearance (the most important test of kidney function)
      - amount of creatinine filtered by glomeruli (since creatinine is not reabsorbed and is only minimally secreted, this test is a measure of glomerular filtration rate)
      - determined by 24-hour urine specimen
      - normal values
        – 115 ± 20 ml/min
        – serum creatinine: 0.4–1.2 mg/100 ml
      - as glomerular filtration rate falls, serum creatinine rises and 24-hour urine creatinine decreases
      - advantage of serum creatinine: independent of protein metabolism
   b) blood urea nitrogen (BUN)
      - normal: 8–20 mg/100 ml
      - urea: end product of protein metabolism
      - increases with decrease in glomerular filtration
      - less reliable measure than serum creatinine because
        – after being filtered, urea is reabsorbed back into renal tubular cells
        – urea production varies according to the state of liver function, and protein intake and breakdown
5) radiologic tests
   a) KUB: kidney, ureters, bladder
      - simple x-ray without contrast medium
      - results indicate size, position, and any radiopaque calcifications
   b) tomography
      - x-ray at different angles: no contrast medium
      - useful for clear picture when colon and other organs block kidney
      - can distinguish solid tumors from cysts
   c) IVP: intravenous pyelogram (excretory urogram)
      - injection of contrast medium that is excreted by kidneys
      - allows visualization of collecting system, calyces, pelvis, ureters, and bladder
      - used to diagnose masses, cysts, obstructions, renal trauma, bladder dysfunction
      - contraindicated in severe renal disease and individuals allergic to shellfish or iodine
      - nursing care
        – pretest
          * check for iodine allergies
          * ensure informed written consent is on the chart
          * tell client that a dye is injected and x-rays are taken at 2-, 5-, 10-, 15-, 20-, 30-, and 60-minute intervals
          * administer strong cathartic, enemas night before
          * nothing PO after midnight
          * have client void immediately prior to test
        – post-test: check for signs and symptoms of allergic reaction to dye and signs of acute renal failure
   d) nephrotomogram
      - techniques of tomography with IVP
      - provides a clearer visualization
   e) retrograde pyelogram
      - catheter is passed through urethra, urinary bladder, and into right or left ureter where contrast medium is injected
      - allows more detailed visualization of the urinary collecting system independent of the status of renal function

[handwritten at top: evacuate bowel before testing — doesn't all visualization of urinary sys.]

- disadvantages: increased chances of trauma (catheter manipulation) and infection
- nursing care
  - pretest
    * check for iodine allergies
    * ensure informed written consent is on the chart
    * teach client concerning procedure
    * administer cathartics, enemas evening before
    * nothing PO after midnight
  - post-test
    * observe amount of urine
    * watch for hematuria
    * watch for signs of urinary sepsis
    * check for signs and symptoms of allergic reaction to dye

f) renal angiography, arteriography
- catheter is introduced through the femoral artery to the renal artery
- contrast medium is injected and 2–3 x-rays are taken at 2-second intervals
- allows visualization of renal arteries, capillaries, and venous system
- used to diagnose renal artery stenosis, renal masses, trauma, thrombosis, and obstructive uropathy
- risks: bleeding, thrombosis, damage to vessels, allergic reaction
- nursing care
  - pretest
    * check for iodine allergies
    * ensure informed written consent is on the chart
    * administer cathartics, enemas evening before
    * ensure that chart contains hematologic evaluation
    * have client void immediately before to test
  - post-test
    * bed rest 12–24 hours; flat, no sitting
    * check insertion site for hematoma formation
    * check pressure dressing on insertion site

[handwritten margin: may cause bleeding — nick tumor]

* monitor post-op vital signs
* check peripheral pulses distal to insertion site
* measure urine output

g) cystography
- a flexible metal tube is inserted into the bladder and a dye is injected; x-rays are taken at 30-minute intervals
- assesses bladder function and explores the possible presence of stones in the bladder
- nursing care: same as retrograde pyelogram

h) cystoscopy
- a cystoscope is inserted into bladder through the urethra
- direct inspection of bladder to treat and resect tumors and diverticuli, to remove stones, cauterize bleeding areas, dilate ureters, and implant radium seeds
- nursing care
  - pretest
    * ensure written informed consent is on the chart
    * administer prep as ordered
    * teach client about procedure, e.g., position (lithotomy), darkened room
    * keep NPO if general anesthesia will be used
    * administer pre-op medication as ordered
  - post-test
    * monitor urine output
    * monitor urine color, blood-tinged is common
    * provide comfort measures (back pain, bladder spasms, feeling of fullness are common), e.g., sitz baths and/or analgesics, e.g., belladonna and opium suppository as ordered
    * check temp and urine for signs of infection

i) renal biopsy
- a specially designed needle is inserted percutaneously to obtain sample of kidney
- determines histology of glomeruli and tubules
- contraindications: a single, functioning kidney; infection;

[handwritten margin: very still if not can puncture vessel → bleed.]

tumors; hydronephrosis; coagulation disorders; or uncooperative client
- risks: uncontrolled bleeding, hematuria, loss of kidney function
- nursing care
  - pretest
    * ensure a written informed consent
    * teach client to hold breath during procedure
  - post-test
    * maintain bed rest for 24 hours with tight dressing or sandbag over insertion site
    * force fluids
    * monitor vital signs frequently
    * monitor hematocrit frequently
    * monitor urine
    * teach client to avoid strenuous activity for approximately two weeks

2. **General Nursing Goals, Plans/Implementation, and Evaluation**

Goal 1: Client will be free from infection.
Plan/Implementation
- collect necessary urine specimen for culture and sensitivity
- teach women proper perineal hygiene
- use and teach client good hand-washing techniques
- use strict sterile technique during catheterization procedures
- provide daily Foley catheter care using good techniques
- administer antibiotics as ordered, for full 10–14 days
- increase fluid intake to 3,000–5,000 ml/day, if not contraindicated by renal or cardiovascular status
- teach client signs and symptoms of URI and importance of seeking early treatment
- acidify urine through acid-ash diet (e.g., meats, eggs, cheese, fish, fowl, whole grains, cranberries, plums, prunes) or by administration of methenamine hypurate (Hiprex) or vitamin C if compatible with antibiotic therapy
- teach good oral-hygiene techniques
- screen client from staff or significant others with URIs; teach client to avoid exposure to persons with infections
- monitor level of potentially nephrotoxic agents (i.e., gentamycin, tetracycline, tobramycin)
- teach client potentially nephrotoxic agents

Evaluation: Client is free from dysuria, frequency, fever and other signs of infection; is able to state procedure for proper perineal hygiene; takes medications as prescribed; I&O is at least 3,000–5,000 ml/day; is able to state signs and symptoms of URI and need for early treatment; can state potentially nephrotoxic agents to avoid in the future.

Goal 2: Client will be free from discomfort.
Plan/Implementation
- administer sitz baths to decrease urethral burning
- administer phenazopyridine HCl (Pyridium) (turns urine rust color) or urinary antispasmodics if ordered
- apply hot water bottle or heating pad to suprapubic region

Evaluation: Client is free from pain, discomfort; reports no burning with urination.

Goal 3: Client's normal urinary function will be maintained.
Plan/Implementation
- measure urine output accurately
- collect urine specimens for routine urinalysis
- encourage adequate fluid intake
- observe for early signs of renal failure

Evaluation: Client's urine output remains equal to or greater than 30 ml/hour; client remains free from symptoms of renal failure.

Goal 4: Client and significant others will receive emotional support.
Plan/Implementation
- provide encouragement when client becomes frustrated with treatment and progression of illness
- explain cause of disease and treatments to client/significant others as necessary
- allow client and significant others to express fears, feelings, and questions
- encourage discussion of diagnosis and ways to cope with problems (e.g., group session for families)
- prepare the client for possibility of hemodialysis or peritoneal dialysis

- refer to social service or pastoral care as needed

  Evaluation: Client/significant others are able to state necessity of treatments; show increasing acceptance of diagnosis and treatment; work through feelings and fears; can discuss altered body image; have plans to alter life-style.

Selected Health Problems Resulting in Alteration in Urinary Elimination

A. Cystitis/Pyelonephritis

1. **General Information**
   a. Definitions
      1) *cystitis*: inflammation of the bladder wall
      2) *pyelonephritis*: inflammation of the kidney caused by a bacterial infection
         a) acute (short course): organisms gain access to the kidney by ascending from the lower urinary tract or via bloodstream; no permanent renal impairment
         b) chronic (slowly progressive): multiple, recurrent, acute attacks that scar the renal parenchyma, damaging tubules, vessels, glomeruli
   b. Incidence: both more common in women
   c. Risks/Predisposing Factors
      1) cystitis
         a) prostatic hypertrophy with urinary retention (men)

Table 3.38 Urinary Antiseptics

Description	Drugs that act as disinfectants within the urinary tract. These drugs are concentrated by the kidneys and reach therapeutic levels only within the urinary tract.
Uses	Treatment of urinary tract infections
Side Effects	Nausea, vomiting, GI upset, diarrhea, hypersensitivity reactions
Nursing Implications	Maintain adequate I&O; keep urinary pH in acid range with vitamin C or cranberry juice; give with food; warn client that drugs may discolor urine; watch for hypersensitivity.
Examples	Cinoxacin (Cinobac); methamine hippurate (Hiprex); nalidixic acid (NegGram); nitrofurantoin (Furadantin, Macrodantin); trimethoprim (Trimpex)

Table 3.39 Sulfonamides

Description	Drugs that are bacteriostatic against both gram-positive and gram-negative organisms. The drugs are excreted unchanged and dissolve well in urine; therefore they are excellent for treating urinary tract infections.
Uses	Urinary tract infections, acute otitis media, ulcerative colitis, chronic bronchitis
Side Effects	GI distress, allergic/hypersensitivity reaction, headache, peripheral neuritis, hearing loss, crystalluria, and hypoglycemia
Nursing Implications	Administer drugs with large amounts of fluid; monitor serum glucose values (may produce false positive glucose on urine tests); monitor for allergic reactions; monitor I&O; maintain alkaline pH in urine since drugs are more soluble in alkaline urine; teach client to take full course of drugs
Examples	Mafenide (Sulfamylon), co-trimoxazole (Bactrim, Septra), sulfasalazine (Azulfidine), sulfisoxazole (Gantrisin)

- b) contamination from large intestine (women)
- c) postintrusive procedures: catheterization, cystoscopy, coitus (women)
- d) gender (women)
- e) atonic bladder (spinal cord injury)
- f) chronic disease (e.g., diabetes)
- g) pregnancy (because of pressure of uterus on bladder and urethra)
- h) chronic stasis (e.g., atonic bladder, immobility and infrequent voiding)

2) pyelonephritis
  - a) anomalies of the kidney
  - b) pregnancy
  - c) calculi
  - d) diabetes mellitus
  - e) neurogenic bladder
  - f) instrumentation (i.e., procedures)
  - g) bacterial infection elsewhere in the body

2. **Nursing Process**
   a. Assessment
      1) cystitis (often asymptomatic)
         - a) burning
         - b) frequency
         - c) urgency
         - d) suprapubic pain
         - e) slight hematuria
      2) pyelonephritis
         - a) symptoms of cystitis may or may not be present
         - b) severe flank pain, CVA tenderness
         - c) hematuria, pyuria
         - d) fever
         - e) chills
      3) diagnostic tests
         - a) urine C&S, urinalysis: midstream urine specimen for evaluation of bacterial content
         - b) CBC: leukocytosis
   b. Goals, Plans/Implementation, and Evaluation (refer to General Nursing Goals 1, 2, and 3 page 256)

B. **Urinary Calculi**
   1. General Information
      a. Types
         1) calcium oxylate: hard, small; alkaline urine
         2) calcium phosphate: large, soft; alkaline urine
         3) cystine: metabolic, familial; acid urine
         4) uric acid: may be accompanied by gout; acid urine
         5) struvite: large, soft; associated with urinary tract infections, alkaline urine
      b. Incidence: can occur at any age
      c. Locations
         1) bladder
         2) ureter (especially at narrow points)
         3) pelvis of the kidney
      d. Risk Factors
         1) supersaturation of urine with poorly soluble crystalloids (calcium, uric acid, cystine)
         2) infection: alkaline urine leads to precipitation of calcium and struvite
         3) increased concentration of urine
         4) stasis
         5) bone demineralization leading to increased calcium phosphate in serum and urine
         6) metabolic diseases: e.g., gout (increased uric acid)
         7) certain medications: e.g., corticosteroids, vitamin D (hypervitaminosis D)
      e. Medical Treatment: surgical intervention
         1) *ureterolithotomy*: incision into ureter through the abdomen to extract stones from lower 2/3 of ureter
            - a) ureteral catheter is inserted to act as splint; ureter not sutured to avoid stricture; catheter is never irrigated to maintain patency
            - b) Penrose drain inserted around ureter to collect any extra drainage
         2) *pyelolithotomy*: removal of a stone from renal pelvis and/or proximal 1/3 of the ureter through a flank incision; Penrose drain inserted outside renal pelvis
         3) *nephrolithotomy*: parenchyma of kidney is cut and stone extracted
            - a) nephrostomy tube placed to divert urine and drain pelvis to allow kidney to heal; never irrigated unless specifically ordered
            - b) Penrose drain inserted
         4) *nephrectomy*: removal of kidney
            - a) may be needed if stone and infection have caused extensive damage to kidney parenchyma
            - b) Penrose drain inserted into renal bed

[Handwritten notes at top:] Electroshock Therapy / Wave Thiotripsy / Obstruct/Complic. / Major → RIT accumulation of sand + lg. particles / 1st Strain all urine / Bruise on back side where shocked.

ELIMINATION 259

2. **Nursing Process**
   a. **Assessment**
      1) pain
         a) renal colic: sudden, sharp, severe; located in deep lumbar region; radiating to side
         b) ureteral colic: same type pain radiating to genitalia and thigh
      2) renointestinal reflex: nausea and vomiting, diarrhea, constipation
      3) hematuria, frequency, altered pH of urine
      4) increased WBC
      5) fever, chills
      6) signs of paralytic ileus with right-sided renal colic
      7) if stone is formed in renal pelvis, may be asymptomatic for years until signs of infection occur
      8) IVP results
      9) urine for mineral precipitate
      10) blood levels of uric acid, calcium, and phosphorus if metabolic problems suspected
   b. **Goals, Plans/Implementation, and Evaluation**

   Goal 1: Client will be free from pain.
   Plan/Implementation
   - administer analgesics as ordered (often morphine is necessary because of severity of pain)
   - administer anticholinergics, propantheline (Pro-Banthine) as ordered, to relax smooth muscles
   - encourage client to ambulate
   - strain all urine for stones

   Evaluation: Client is free from discomfort; able to ambulate; strains all urine for stones.

   Goal 2: Client will be free from infection leading to urinary calculi (refer to General Nursing Goal 1 page 256)

   Goal 3: Client will decrease risk of stone formation.
   Plan/Implementation
   - teach client importance of maintaining adequate fluid intake (3,000 ml/day)
   - teach client about medications and reason for prescription, e.g., to maintain recommended urinary pH
   - teach client about any medication ordered to decrease levels of minerals (e.g., aluminum hydroxide + $PO_3 \rightarrow AlPO_3$, eliminated through the GI tract)
   - teach client how to measure urine pH
   - assess diet for excess intake of substances that contribute to stone formation
   - teach client about dietary restrictions
   - explain advantages of regular exercise and regular elimination habits, e.g., to prevent calculi

   Evaluation: Client can state importance of maintaining large urine output; can state actions and need for medication to maintain recommended pH; demonstrates ability to monitor urinary pH; demonstrates adherence to dietary restrictions.

   Goal 4: Client will be free from postoperative complications.
   Plan/Implementation
   - refer to *Surgery* page 165
   - note urine: amount, color, specific gravity
   - for flank incision: maintain adequate respiratory function
   - encourage early ambulation
   - monitor for
     - hypostatic pneumonia (client may be reluctant to deep breathe and cough because of discomfort)
     - hemorrhage
     - paralytic ileus (from reflex paralysis)
     - severe pain
     - urinary tract infection
   - give urinary antiseptics and anti-infectives as ordered

   Evaluation: Client is resting comfortably; free from signs of UTI (no WBCs, culture less than 100,000 organisms/ml); free from signs of complications of surgery.

   Goal 5: Client will understand home care.
   Plan/Implementation
   - refer to General Nursing Goal 3 page 256
   - teach client how and why to avoid upper respiratory tract infection (strep) which can lead to glomerulonephritis
   - tell client to avoid heavy lifting for 4–8 weeks post-op

   Evaluation: Client can state health measures to institute at home.

C. **Cancer of the Bladder** *[handwritten: often reoccurs]*
   1. **General Information**
      a. **Characteristics**
         1) more than 66% occur in men
         2) most tumors start as benign papillomas or as leukoplakia

[Handwritten at bottom:] roll pt over tachick for bleeding / flank incision - prone to pneumonia

[Handwritten at top: Stoma on abd for urine. Nursing care empty as freq. as possible. Do not want urine to lay on stoma - pdt go back in stoma also. Don't lay on back side to long for drainage → side lying]

260 SECTION 3: NURSING CARE OF THE ADULT

    3) multiple tumors frequent
    4) tumors often recur
  b. Risk Factors: probably a disease of multiple etiologies, not yet specifically identified; industrial carcinogens, smoking, aniline dyes, benzine, asbestos, and alcohol have been implicated
  c. Medical Treatment
    1) surgical intervention
      a) transurethral bladder resection if tumors are of the trigone or posterior bladder wall (85%)
      b) complete cystectomy when cure highly probable
      c) urinary diversion
- ileal conduit: a portion of the ileum becomes a conduit; the ureters are transplanted into one end and the other end becomes an external stoma
- cutaneous ureterostomy: dissection of one or both ureters, bringing them to the skin, forming one or two stomas (for inoperable tumors)

    2) radiation therapy
      a) pre-op irradiation improves survival in clients with high-grade tumors
      b) external or internal radiation therapy for nonoperable tumors or clients who refuse surgery

[Handwritten margin notes left side: remove tumor usually have to remove bladder; using the bowel; no pouch for urine; chemo drug thiothpa; Foley cath lie on back side + rotate 360° 20 min on each side then sit up + go to BR. smells terrible; Urine diversion crya powder in urine + back up in stoma can cause renal damage; crya powder only for bowel; Colostomy Stoma - pouch crya powder protects skin. Clean skin soap + H₂O then Crya then paste then pouch]

[Handwritten middle column notes: Bag placed soon after surgery. Some will come from OR c̄ bag. observe for CVT → pyelonephritis, check output also. pdt for bowel bac to enter ureters. remain pink, will shrink. urine excoriates. Anus → TUC's]

2. **Nursing Process**
  a. Assessment
    1) painless hematuria
    2) abnormal cystogram
    3) abnormal blood and urine studies
    4) cystoscopy, biopsy results
  b. Goals, Plans/Implementation, and Evaluation

Goal 1: Client will be prepared for surgery.
Plan/Implementation
- refer to *Surgery* page 165
- give or arrange for sexual counseling regarding impotence (in men)
- give bowel prep as ordered
- arrange for introduction to diversionary appliance
- ensure stoma site (RLQ) is marked

Evaluation: Client is able to discuss planned surgery and its implications; inspects diversionary appliance.

Goal 2: Client will remain free from postoperative complications.
Plan/Implementation
- refer to *Surgery*, page 165
- check ureteral splints for patency, output and color of urine qh
- record I&O for at least 3 days; encourage up to 3,000 ml fluid intake/day
- offer psychologic support as needed

Evaluation: Client maintains intake of 3,000 ml/day; shows no signs of shock or hemorrhage (e.g., tachycardia, hypotension, apprehension, cold clammy skin, decreased BP, increased pulse).

Goal 3: Client will learn care of urinary diversion appliance and will begin to adjust to alteration in body-image.
Plan/Implementation
- have enterostomal therapist orient client to appliance and its care
- reinforce all teaching regarding skin care, cleanliness, odor control
- allow client an opportunity to express feelings and concerns regarding changed body image
- encourage client to assume full care of appliance as soon as possible

Evaluation: Client is coping adaptively to body-image change (e.g., discussing change, caring for appliance) achieves self-care management of appliance with successful odor control.

D. Acute Renal Failure

1. **General Information**
  a. Definition: a sudden and potentially reversible loss of kidney function
  b. Categories and Causes of Renal Failure
    1) prerenal (outside kidney): poor perfusion, decrease in circulating volume
    2) renal: structural damage to kidney resulting from acute tubular necrosis
    3) postrenal: obstruction within urinary tract
  c. Risk/Predisposing Factors
    1) prerenal
      a) reduction in blood volume (shock)
      b) trauma
      c) septic shock
      d) dehydration
      e) cardiac failure
    2) renal
      a) hypersensitivity (allergic disorders)

b) obstruction of renal vessels (embolism, thrombosis)
c) nephrotoxic agents (bacterial toxins, drugs)
d) mismatched blood transfusion
e) glomerulonephritis
3) postrenal
   a) kidney stones or tumors
   b) benign prostatic hypertrophy or obstruction

2. **Nursing Process**
   a. **Assessment**
      1) oliguric phase (urine volume less than 400 ml/24 hours)
         a) decreased serum sodium and increased potassium; decreased calcium, bicarbonate
         b) increased BUN, creatinine maintaining a 10:1 ratio
         c) increased specific gravity
         d) hypervolemia
      2) diuretic phase (urine volume greater than 3,000 ml/24 hours)
         a) serum sodium and potassium may return to normal, stay elevated, or decrease
         b) increased BUN and serum creatinine
         c) decreased specific gravity of urine
         d) hypovolemia
         e) weight loss
      3) recovery phase: gradual return of normal function over period of 3–12 months
   b. **Goals, Plans/Implementation, and Evaluation**

   Goal 1 (if prerenal failure): Client will experience increased renal blood flow through an increased circulating blood volume.
   Plan/Implementation
   - monitor VS as ordered, especially BP and pulse
   - strict I&O
   - administer IV fluids as ordered
   - treat shock if present
   - administer prescribed medications to increase renal flow (e.g., dopamine 2–5 µg/kg/min)
   - administer prescribed diuretics to increase production of urine (e.g., mannitol, furosemide) if client still has output
   - monitor urinary and cardiovascular status hourly

   Evaluation: Client has adequate circulation (normal BP, palpable pulse with regular rate and rhythm, skin warm, oriented in 3 spheres) urine output is greater than 30 ml/hour.

   Goal 2: Client will maintain fluid, electrolyte, and nitrogen balance.
   Plan/Implementation (oliguric phase)
   - weigh client daily
   - measure I&O carefully
   - administer only enough fluid to replace losses
   - include insensible losses in measurement of output
     - 500 ml/day if less than 5,000 ft above sea level
     - 1,000 ml/day if more than 5,000 ft above sea level
   - observe for edema and electrolyte imbalance
   - monitor serum lab test results
   - administer 50% dextrose with 5–10 units regular insulin as ordered, to drive potassium into cells
   - administer ion-exchange resin Kayexalate enema as ordered, to lower high potassium levels
   - reduce potassium, sodium, phosphorus in diet
   - administer IV sodium bicarbonate for acidosis
   - administer phosphate binders such as aluminum hydroxide (Amphojel) or aluminum carbonate (Basaljel) for hyperphosphatemia
   - reduce protein in diet and teach client rationale; provide high biologic value protein for diet

   Plan/Implementation (diuretic phase)
   - prevent dehydration; balance I&O
   - increase dietary sodium and potassium to normal levels
   - maintain positive nitrogen balance and sufficient calories, prevents body protein from being metabolized
   - prevent infection

   Evaluation: Client maintains approximately equal intake and output and stable weight; remains free from signs of electrolyte imbalance, edema, and dehydration; weight remains stable; I&O is approximately equal; is able to list foods on a low potassium, low protein diet.

   Goal 3: Client will be free from infection and further damage to kidneys (refer to General Nursing Goals 1 page 256)

Table 3.40 Diuretics

Description	Drugs capable of increasing the output of urine, leading to a net loss of body fluid. The mechanism of action varies from drug to drug, but most act primarily by increasing sodium excretion.

Carbonic Anhydrase Inhibitors

Uses	To treat glaucoma, edema not responding well to single drug therapy; adjunctive to anticonvulsant therapy for epilepsy.
Side Effects	Paresthesias, lethargy, anorexia, tinnitus, headache, hypokalemia, hyponatremia, ureteral colic, acidosis
Nursing Implications	Use cautiously in clients with respiratory acidosis, diabetes, and gout; monitor K^+ and Na^+ levels; watch for hypersensitivity reactions; monitor visual improvement.
Examples	Acetazolamide (Diamox), ethoxzolamide (Cardrase), methazolamide (Neptazane), dichlorphenamide (Daranide)

Osmotic Diuretics

Uses	To reduce intraocular pressure in the treatment of glaucoma; to treat cerebral edema and oliguria; to prevent renal failure
Side Effects	Dry mouth, thirst, headache, blurred vision, nausea/vomiting, diuresis, dehydration, electrolyte imbalance, dizziness, hypotension
Nursing Implications	Monitor I&O carefully, watch for electrolyte imbalance and/or dehydration; monitor cardiovascular and renal functions closely.
Examples	Glycerin (Osmoglyn), isosorbide (Ismotic), mannitol (Osmitrol), urea (Ureaphil)

Thiazide Diuretics see Table 3.16

Potent Diuretics

Uses	To control edema associated with kidney disease, ascites, cirrhosis, CHF, lymphedema, hypertension.
Side Effects	Dehydration, electrolyte imbalance, hyperglycemia, hyperuricemia, flushing, orthostatic hypotension, dizziness, blurred vision, weakness, pruritus, dermatitis, hypersensitivity reaction if allergic to sulfonamides, may enhance beta blockers (Inderal).
Nursing Implications	Monitor fluid and electrolytes carefully; instruct client in proper use of medications and possible side effects; monitor for gout and glucose intolerance; check for sulfonamide allergies before administering; monitor BP and pulse if client is taking a beta-blocker; monitor for digitalis toxicity if potassium gets low.
Examples	Ethacrynic acid (Edecrin), Furosemide (Lasix)

Potassium-sparing Diuretics   see Table 3.16

E. Chronic Renal Failure

1. **General Information**
    a. Definition: a progressive, irreversible deterioration of renal function that ends in fatal uremia unless kidney transplant or dialysis is performed
    b. Risk/Predisposing Factors
       1) urinary tract obstruction and infection
       2) infectious diseases that cause hypertension and increased catabolism with retention of metabolites (glomerulonephritis)
       3) metabolic disease (diabetes)
       4) nephrotoxic agents (bacterial toxins, drugs)
       5) acute renal failure
    c. Pathophysiology

renal pt → emollient stool softners → Surfac, Colace

ELIMINATION 263

1) kidneys lose their ability to reabsorb electrolytes
2) urine output is decreased
3) anemia (thought to be caused by inadequate production of erythropoietin, and depression of bone marrow as uremia increases)
4) end products of protein metabolism accumulate in blood (BUN, creatinine)
5) reduced resistance to infection
6) complications: acidosis, pericarditis, and renal osteodystrophy (abnormal calcium metabolism)

2. **Nursing Process**
   a. Assessment
   1) urine output: oliguria, anuria
   2) metabolic indicators
      a) elevated BUN, creatinine
      b) hyperphosphatemia
      c) hyperkalemia *→ cardiac arrhythmias*
      d) metabolic acidosis
      e) elevated, normal, or decreased serum sodium depending on water retention
   3) cardiovascular indicators
      a) hypertension *→ from ↓ prod. Renin.*
      b) congestive heart failure
      c) pericarditis
   4) hematologic indicators
      a) anemia (decreased renal production of erythropoietin)
      b) alteration of platelet function leading to bleeding tendencies
      c) susceptibility to infection (changes in leukocyte function)
   5) respiratory indicators
      a) pulmonary edema
      b) uremic pneumonitis
      c) uremic pleurisy
   6) gastrointestinal indicators *limit fluids*
      a) mucosal irritation in GI tract
      b) ammonia on breath (uremic fetor)
      c) anorexia, nausea, vomiting, hiccoughs
   7) central nervous system indicators
      a) early: mild deficit in mental functioning
      b) late: altered sensorium, slurred speech, generalized seizures, encephalopathy with toxic psychosis, coma
   8) peripheral nervous system indicators
      a) peripheral neuropathy involving all extremities
      b) burning, painful paresthesias

   9) musculoskeletal indicators
      a) renal osteodystrophy
      b) bone pain in feet and legs upon walking and standing, pathologic fractures
   10) dermatologic indicators
      a) pruritus *→ uric acid*
      b) dry skin: caused by atrophy of sweat glands
      c) easy bruising, petechiae, and purpura *↓ platelets*
      d) pallor related to anemia
      e) sallow, yellow-tan color to skin
      f) brittle, dry hair
      g) dry and ridged nails
      h) uremic frost: crystalization of urea on skin *late sym. (very)*
   11) endocrine indicators
      a) hypothyroidism
      b) decreased T₄ level
   12) reproductive indicators
      a) infertility
      b) loss of libido
      c) amenorrhea in women
      d) decreased testosterone, sperm count in men

   b. Goals, Plans/Implementation, and Evaluation

   Goal 1: Client will maintain fluid and electrolyte balance (refer to "Acute Renal Failure," Goals 1 and 2 page 261).

   Supp. IV KVO/rate or heparin locke give just what is needed

   Goal 2: Client will remain free from infection (refer to General Nursing Goal 1 page 256). *Antibiotics*

   Goal 3: Client will maintain adequate caloric intake to prevent muscle wasting and prevent own body stores from being metabolized.
   Plan/Implementation
   • initiate daily calorie count
   • adjust level of protein in diet to client's serum levels of BUN and creatinine *↑BUN ↓Protein*
   • encourage protein of high biologic value (essential amino acids)
   • serve food attractively and at appropriate temperature
   • give medication to control nausea and vomiting before meals
   Evaluation: Client's BUN and creatinine levels remain within normal limits or stable; calorie count is 35–40 calories/kg body weight.

   Goal 4: Client will be protected from self-injury during period of altered sensorium. *due to ↑BUN*

↑Roughage ↑fiber → ↑H₂O content

Table 3.41 Modifications of Food, Fluid, and Electrolyte Intake in Renal Failure

Stage of Renal Failure	Food Intake for Energy	Protein Intake	Fluid Intake	Sodium Intake	Potassium Intake	Phosphorus Intake
Renal insufficiency	Adequate to maintain body weight.	No restriction.	Determined by state of hydration and volume of output.	Determined by state of hydration and B/P.	Determined by blood level.	Determined by blood level.
Moderate renal failure	30-40 cal/kg body weight (adequate to prevent catabolism).	0.6-1.0 gm/kg ideal weight (total average intake: 40-60 gm).	Limited to volume of output in previous day.	Determined by state of hydration and B/P.	Determined by blood level.	Determined by blood level.
Severe renal failure	30-40 cal/kg (adequate to prevent catabolism).	Total average intake: 18-20 gm.	Determined by state of hydration and daily weight.	Determined by state of hydration and B/P.	Determined by blood level.	Determined by blood level.
Renal failure treated by peritoneal dialysis	35-45 cal/kg.	No restriction.	Determined by state of hydration.	No restriction.	Determined by blood level.	Determined by blood level.
Renal failure treated by hemodialysis	30-45 cal/kg.	1-1.5 gm/kg ideal weight.	Limited to 800-1,000 ml plus equivalent of previous day's output.	1,500-2,000 mg.	Determined by blood level.	Determined by blood level.

Plan/Implementation
- restrain, if necessary
- institute seizure precautions
- perform neurologic checks frequently
- monitor BUN and creatinine closely
- teach significant others about cause of altered sensorium

Evaluation: Client is free from injury during periods of confusion; significant others state awareness of relationship between disease process and altered sensorium.

Goal 5: Client will be relieved of itching and maintain skin integrity.
Plan/Implementation
- avoid soap
- use soft cloth
- add oil to bath water
- use tepid bath water (baking soda in water may help)

Evaluation: Client's itching is relieved; skin remains intact.

Goal 6: Client and significant others will be supported emotionally (refer to General Nursing Goal 4 page 256)

Goal 7: Client will adapt to altered sexual functioning.
Plan/Implementation
- teach client and significant other about alterations in sexual functioning
- provide or arrange sexual counseling if necessary
- encourage client and significant other to discuss the problem

Evaluation: Client and significant other discuss change and alteration in sexual expression.

F. Dialysis
1. General Information
   a. Definition: passage of particles (ions) from an area of high concentration to an area of low concentration (diffusion) across a semipermeable membrane;

Table 3.42 Low Protein Diet Sample Menu

	Serving	Gm of Protein
Breakfast		
Orange juice	½ glass	1
Farina	½ cup	1
Margarine	1 tbsp	Trace
Sugar	1 tbsp	—
Low-protein bread	1 slice	1
Jelly	1 tbsp	—
Milk	½ cup	3.5
Coffee		—
Lunch		
Fruit salad:		
Peaches (canned)	1	Trace
Pears (canned)	1	Trace
Apple (fresh)	1	Trace
Low protein bread, toasted	1 slice	1
Margarine	1 tbsp	Trace
Jelly	1 tbsp	—
Sherbet	½ cup	1
Ginger ale with added sugar	1 glass	—
Tea		—
Dinner		
Omelette	2 eggs	13
Asparagus	½ cup	Trace
Carrots	⅔ cup	1
Baked potato	1	3
Margarine	1 tbsp	Trace
Ginger ale with added sugar	1 glass	—
Coffee		—
Cantaloupe	¼	½
	Total	**26 gm**

simultaneously water moves (osmosis) toward the solution in which the solute concentration is greater. When dialysis is used as a substitute for kidney function, the semipermeable membrane used is either the peritoneum (peritoneal dialysis) or an artificial membrane (hemodialysis). The principle of exchange is the same with both methods. The pores in the membrane are large enough to allow the passage of urea, electrolytes, and creatinine, but are too small to allow the passage of blood cells and other protein molecules.

b. Peritoneal Dialysis
　1) definition: placement of catheter through abdominal wall into peritoneal space.
　2) procedure: room temperature dialysate is allowed to flow into the peritoneal cavity by gravity. The solution remains in the abdomen for exchange to occur and then is drained from the peritoneal cavity by gravity. It carries with it waste products and excess electrolytes. Can last from 12–24 hours.
　3) number of cycles: varies according to the client's problems, tolerance, response, and type of solution
　4) types
　　a) intermittent manual
　　b) intermittent automatic
　　c) continuous ambulatory (CAPD)
　　　• advantages
　　　　- lower BP (9 out of 10 clients can come off BP meds)
　　　　- increased Hct and Hgb
　　　　- less expensive
　　　　- greater freedom for client

266 SECTION 3: NURSING CARE OF THE ADULT

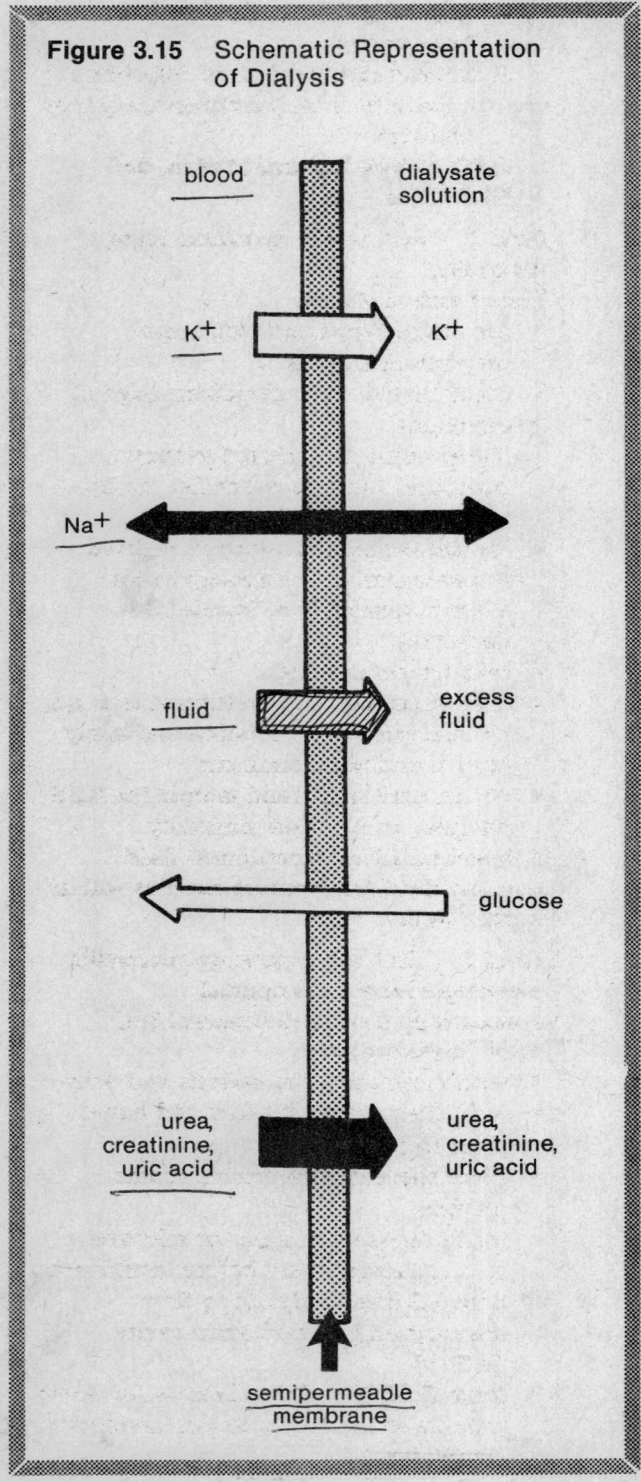

Figure 3.15 Schematic Representation of Dialysis

- weight gain from glucose absorbed from dialysate (later can become a disadvantage)
- **disadvantages and risks**
  - peritonitis
  - infection at catheter exit site → *inward*
  - dialysate leakage
  - hypotension
  - hypoalbuminemia (caused by increased loss of protein from repeated peritonitis and large pores in peritoneum)
  5) peritoneal access, e.g., Tenckhoff peritoneal catheter extends access to the peritoneal cavity for weeks to months

c. **Hemodialysis** — *most effective*
  1) definition: passage of **heparinized** blood from client through a tube consisting of a semipermeable membrane immersed in a dialysate bath composed of all important electrolytes in their ideal concentration. Diffusion and ultrafiltration occur between the client's blood and the dialysate. *(pot. for bleed ↑ their pot for bleeding)*
  2) procedure: fresh dialysate is used continuously until the client's electrolyte and fluid balances are within safe levels.
  3) schedule varies with clinical condition and type of dialyzer
     a) up to 3 times/week
     b) 4–6 hours/day is possible for coil and hollow-fiber dialyzers; 10–12 hours/day is necessary for plate-type dialyzers
  4) access to client's circulation
     a) **arteriovenous (AV) shunt** *not access of choice*
        • external device
          - composed of two non-thrombogenic silastic rubber tubes or cannulas with teflon tips, one sutured in artery, the other in vein
          - between dialysis, the two tubes are joined by Teflon connector
          - most common used vessels are the radial artery and cephalic vein of forearm
        • advantages
          - can be used immediately after insertion
          - use is relatively simple
        • disadvantages
          - clotting
          - infection
          - accidental dislodgement with hemorrhage
          - limited longevity

b) **arteriovenous (AV) fistula**: access of choice for hemodialysis
- internal access
  - created by side-to-side or end-to-end anastomosis between adjacent vein and artery (often radial artery and cephalic vein)
  - creates enlarged superficial vein with easy access for venipuncture
- advantages
  - longevity
  - no danger of disconnection
- disadvantages
  - must be constructed 4–12 weeks in advance
  - needs time to mature
  - complications *clot oss*
    * thrombosis
    * venous hypertension distal to anastomosis
    * ischemia of extremity
    * infection (less frequent than AV shunts)

c) **graft**
- internal access, e.g., piece of bovine carotid artery or Gore-Tex material
- usually done when client's vessels are unsuitable to be used as a fistula
- advantages
  - not dependent on adequate client circulation for placement
  - diameter is predetermined
- disadvantages
  - does not have healing properties, e.g., more chance of bleeding, infection, aneurysm formation
  - cannot be used for several weeks
  - not used for clients awaiting transplants since bovine grafts can be rejected

2. **Nursing Process: Peritoneal Dialysis**
   a. Assessment
      1) temperature, pulse, respirations, and blood pressure
      2) blood chemistries (electrolytes, BUN, creatinine, glucose)
      3) daily I&O
      4) daily weight (after fluid is drained from cavity)
      5) catheter site for signs of infection or leakage (redness, tenderness, pain, or exudate)
   b. Goals, Plans/Implementation, and Evaluation

   Goal 1: Client will be protected from peritonitis.
   Plan/Implementation
   - use scrupulous aseptic technique throughout dialysis
   - check dialysate for cloudiness (sign of infection)
   - if peritonitis is suspected (cloudy peritoneal fluid, fever, chills), notify physician immediately
   - initiate antibiotic therapy as ordered (cephalosporins or aminoglycosides either systemically or instilled into dialysate) *get specimen before*
   - take temperature q4h
   - change catheter site dressing at least qd; cleanse with iodine solution and apply topical antibiotic ointment
   - obtain peritoneal fluid sample for fluid analysis, culture and sensitivity

   Evaluation: Client's peritoneal fluid remains clear; temperature remains within normal limits.

   Goal 2: Client will experience successful dialysis and maintain optimal concentrations of serum electrolytes.
   Plan/Implementation
   - weigh client prior to dialysis and daily
   - have client empty bladder and bowel prior to paracentesis
   - place client in comfortable supine position
   - warm dialysate in water or microwave to room temperature before instilling
   - permit 2 liters dialysate to flow unrestricted into peritoneal cavity (inflow)
   - leave fluid in peritoneal cavity for 30–45 minutes so that solution can equilibrate (dwell time)
   - drain equilibrated fluid from peritoneal cavity
   - record amount of fluid loss or gain; outflow should be approximately 100–200 ml more than inflow; have client turn on sides to localize fluid and promote drainage; if retention continues, notify physician

- repeat cycle as ordered
- perform blood chemistries as ordered
- maintain client comfort during dialysis

Evaluation: Client's weight decreases after each dialysis session; has larger output than inflow.

Goal 3: Client will be free from hypertension.

Plan/Implementation
- monitor BP standing and sitting
- monitor BP during dialysis (should decrease as fluid volume is reduced)
- if hypertension persists, use a more hypertonic dialysate
- restrict fluid and sodium intake
- give antihypertensive medications as ordered
- if symptoms of hypotension occur during procedure, notify physician (treat by administering normal saline directly into the arterial or venous line and slowing the dialyzing procedures)

Evaluation: Client's BP remains within predetermined guidelines.

Goal 4: Client will be successful with CAPD at home if client's condition requires chronic dialysis.

Plan/Implementation
- educate client and significant others in the principles, process, and techniques of CAPD
  - instill 2 liters dialysate
  - leave in peritoneal cavity 4–8 hours
  - go about daily activities
  - drain fluid and discard
  - replace with 2 liters fresh dialysate
  - repeat procedure 4 times/day
  - leave dialysate in peritoneal cavity overnight
- educate re sterile technique and its importance in preventing peritonitis
- have client keep a written record of daily weight and BP
- provide diet instruction to replace lost protein; liberalize protein, potassium, salt, and water intake
- teach the importance of regular medical and nursing follow-up for lab work, catheter change, evaluation of dialysis technique, monitoring of weight and BP, and any other problems

Evaluation: Client uses CAPD at home free from any problems, explains proper diet and the importance of follow-up.

Goal 5: Client will be assisted to cope psychologically with ongoing dialysis treatments (refer to "Hemodialysis," Goal 3 page 269).

3. **Nursing Process: Hemodialysis**
   a. Assessment
      1) vascular access: AV shunt, AV fistula, or graft

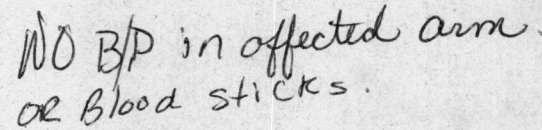

a) monitor site for good arterial flow; color of blood should be bright, cranberry red
b) palpate for thrill
c) listen for bruit
d) check skin temperature and pulses distal to access site
2) check client's temperature and BP
3) check dialysate composition and temperature
4) client's psychologic reaction to dialysis
  a) reaction to physical condition
  b) predialysis personality
  c) family support system
  d) financial status
  e) signs of depression, fear, anxiety, denial, and regression
  f) noncompliance with diet or fluid restrictions
  g) verbalization of self-deprecation
  h) relinquishment of decision making to family or staff
  i) suicidal ideation
  j) reaction to sexual dysfunction
b. **Goals, Plans/Implementation, and Evaluation**

Goal 1: Client will have access site protected from trauma.
Plan/Implementation
- keep extremity elevated several hours after insertion
- instruct client to keep affected arm or leg as straight as possible at all times
- have clamps or tourniquet available at all times to control any severe bleeding from accidental dislodgement
- notify physician immediately of severe bleeding or clotting of cannula
- instruct client to avoid lifting heavy objects with affected arm
- do not use affected arm for BP or venipuncture
- instruct client to avoid constrictive clothing over shunt site
- instruct client to avoid exposing access site to extreme cold

Evaluation: Client's blood flow to access site remains cranberry red with palpable thrill, audible bruit, and warm temperature.

Goal 2: Client will remain free from infection at access site.

Plan/Implementation
- check site frequently for signs of infection (pain, redness, tenderness, or increase of temperature)
- perform suture line care (10–14 days until sutures are removed)
  - remove old dressing
  - clean suture line with povidone-iodine solution
  - apply new sterile dressing
- instruct client not to irritate scabs that form over needle insertion sites
- apply skin softening cream to scabs
- wash the affected limb with antibacterial soap and water daily

Evaluation: Client remains free from pain, redness, and tenderness at site of shunt.

Goal 3: Client will be assisted to cope psychologically with ongoing dialysis treatments.

Plan/Implementation
- encourage client to express concerns, feelings and to ask questions re procedures and life-style adaptations
- educate client concerning treatments and rationale behind restrictions
- give consistent information to client and significant others
- encourage client to maintain as active and productive a life as possible, and to plan daily activities around treatments
- encourage client to be as independent and responsible for care as possible
- encourage significant others to express their feelings
- counsel significant others to avoid unrealistic expectations and overprotectiveness
- assist client to move from depression, despair, and defeat to acceptance of illness by exhibiting hope and planning for realistic goals
- refer for vocational rehabilitation, shelter workshops, or special services as needed (e.g., financial)
- provide marital or sexual counseling
- conduct regular team conferences to discuss care of clients

Evaluation: Client is leading as active and productive a life as possible within the constraints of the illness; shows acceptance of disease by managing care and setting realistic goals.

G. Kidney Transplantation

1. **General Information**
   a. Definition: the surgical implantation of a donated, allogeneic kidney to restore kidney function in a client with end-stage renal failure
   b. Donor
      1) live *better*
      2) cadaver
   c. Rejection of the grafted kidney is a significant problem
      1) attempts to minimize: tissue typing prior to transplantation (must indicate high degree of histocompatibility)
      2) types of rejection
         a) hyperacute: occurs on the operating room table
         b) acute: 1st episode can occur 5–7 days posttransplant; subsequent episodes can occur within the 1st year
         c) chronic: rejection continues despite repeated attempts at immunosuppression
         d) rejection rates
            - 20%–25% of cadaver grafts
            - 5%–10% of live donor grafts *(if good match)*
            - greatly increased by the presence of diabetes
   d. Immunosuppressive drugs are given to all transplant recipients (azathioprine [Imuran]; corticosteroids [prednisone]; Cyclosporin A) ***

2. **Nursing Process**
   a. Assessment
      1) metabolic state
      2) tissue histocompatibility
      3) immunologic defense status
      4) psychologic and emotional status
      5) potential sources of post-op infection (carious teeth, infected donor kidneys) since client will be immunosuppressed
      6) age; desires of the client regarding this risk-filled procedure
   b. Goals, Plans/Implementation, and Evaluation

   Goal 1: Client will be adequately prepared preoperatively to maximize the chances of a successful outcome.
   Plan/Implementation
   - refer to *Surgery* page 165

   Dialysis prior to surgery

   - maintain accurate I&O; adhere to fluid restriction
   - know that the client may need to undergo pre-op hemodialysis to achieve an optimal metabolic state
   - protect client from possible sources of infection

   Evaluation: Client is able to describe the postoperative routine.

   Goal 2: Client will be psychologically prepared for the surgery.
   Plan/Implementation
   - refer to *Surgery* page 165
   - allow client the opportunity to discuss feelings and concerns regarding the surgery and its chances of success
   - answer client's questions as honestly and completely as possible
   - *Discuss feelings* allow client an opportunity to discuss any ambivalent feelings about the donor (may be a very close relative)
   - know that significant others also need support and information

   Evaluation: Client's preoperative anxiety level is moderate; expresses realistic hope regarding outcome of transplant.

   Goal 3: Client will be free from postoperative complications.
   Plan/Implementation
   - refer to *Surgery* page 165
   - assess fluid and electrolyte balance carefully
     - measure urine output (may range from massive diuresis [live donor] to aneuresis [cadaver donor])
     - may require hemodialysis

     too much or little fluid will damage kidney

   - protect client from infection
     - give Foley care
     - may be in reverse isolation
     - monitor temperature
   - observe for signs of acute rejection of transplant

     - fever
     - increased blood pressure
     - swollen, tender kidney (in pelvic area)
     - decreased urine volume
     - flu symptoms
   - maintain integrity of venous access (refer to "Dialysis" page 264)

   Evaluation: Client's vital signs are within normal limits; output is equivalent to fluid intake; remains free from infection.

Goal 4: Client will learn to take medications.
Plan/Implementation
- teach client that immunosuppressive drugs are the main defense against transplant rejection
- teach side effects and complications of these drugs and that withdrawal (if it is ever appropriate) must be done gradually
- tell client that he is more susceptible to infection while taking these drugs and to notify physician at the 1st sign of a cold or infection
- teach client how to avoid or at least decrease exposure to sources of infection

Evaluation: Client can list side effects of all drugs; knows when to call physician regarding drug-related problems; states an awareness of administration schedule and importance of maintaining it.

H. Benign Prostatic Hypertrophy (BPH)

1. **General Information**
   a. Incidence: more than 50% of all men over 50
   b. Predisposing Factors: unknown
   c. Medical Treatment: surgical intervention
      1) transurethral resection of prostate (TURP) is most common
      2) suprapubic and retropubic approaches also used

2. **Nursing Process**
   a. Assessment *nocturia, retention, diff starting a stream*
      1) urinary dysfunction
      2) symmetrical, smooth enlargement of prostate
      3) signs and symptoms of hydronephrosis followed by renal failure (late)
   b. Goals, Plans/Implementation, and Evaluation

Goal 1: Client will have adequate urinary flow preoperatively. *Not nurses job*
Plan/Implementation
- insert Foley catheter — *Cuda cath. urologist*
- measure I&O
- know that a suprapubic catheter may be necessary

bleed ↓ obstruc + will need order to manual irrig.

Evaluation: Client's intake and output remain balanced.

urine → @ least 30cc/°

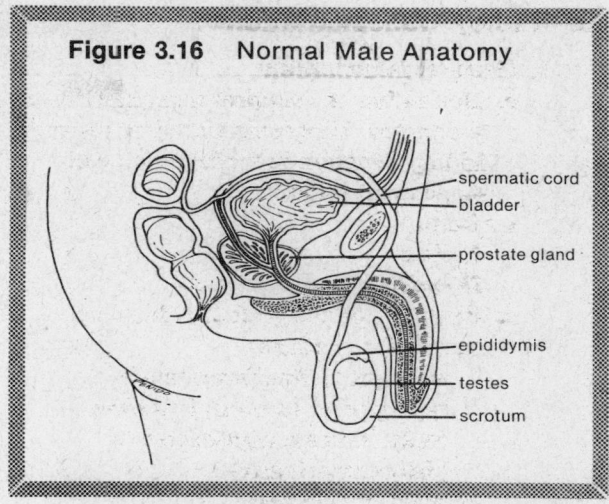

Figure 3.16   Normal Male Anatomy
- spermatic cord
- bladder
- prostate gland
- epididymis
- testes
- scrotum

Goal 2: Client will be able to describe surgical approach and postoperative care (see table 3.43).
Plan/Implementation
- teach client that vasectomy is usually done to reduce chance of epididymitis
- know that all prostatectomies produce retrograde ejaculation and sterility

Evaluation: Client can describe a TURP; knows what to expect postoperatively (e.g., pain and discomfort, ambulation).

Goal 3: Client will have normal urinary drainage, clear to lightly pink-tinged in color; will be free from hemorrhage.
Plan/Implementation
- know that a 3-way Foley catheter with 30cc balloon will be inserted post-op *instill on side + drain off the other irrigation*
- ensure Foley is patent
- apply traction on the Foley for 24 hours (puts pressure on prostatic bed) *↓ bleeding*
- maintain constant bladder irrigation (CBI) *then release 4-5 hr later after lasix given* *H₂O toxication*
- if increased blood seen, increase speed of irrigation; if this is not effective, notify physician
- measure I&O each shift
- monitor for adequate urinary output after Foley is removed (2–3 days)
- if suprapubic prostatectomy done, care for dressing around suprapubic catheter

Evaluation: Client's urine remains clear and amber-colored.

Goal 4: Client will have minimal discomfort from bladder spasms.

constant irrig may be turned up c̄ no order. if blood is seen need order to irrg c̄ saline.

Table 3.43 Prostatectomies

Type	Surgical Approach	Common Problems	Nursing Implications
Transurethral Resection (TUR)	Client in lithotomy position. Gland removed through resecting cystoscope. Most common approach	Not all gland removed.	Explain that benign prostatic hypertrophy can recur.
		Constant bladder irrigation to decrease bleeding.	Ensure catheter patency. Run irrigant at rate to keep urine light pink. Use only isotonic solution to prevent water intoxication.
		May damage internal sphincter leading to incontinence or bladder-neck strictures.	Teach perineal exercises.
		May or may not cause sterility.	Reassure client potency *not* affected.
Suprapubic	Abdominal approach. Bladder is opened. Allows abdominal exploration.	Suprapubic catheter or drain with urinary drainage.	Do frequent dressing changes. Prevent infection or irritation.
		Hemorrhage common; large-balloon Foley with traction is used to stop bleeding.	Watch closely for bleeding. Check catheter patency. Irrigate with saline prn to prevent clots.
		Bladder spasms common.	Reposition client. Give propantheline bromide (Pro-Banthine).
		Causes sterility.	Reassure potency not affected.
Retropubic	Low abdominal incision; no bladder incision. Allows complete, direct removal of gland with less bleeding.	Can be done for cancer or BPH. Causes sterility.	Assure client potency *not* affected.
		Less chance of bleeding. Sometimes constant bladder irrigation is ordered for 24 hours.	Watch for bleeding.
		Few spasms.	Medicate prn.
Perineal, Radical (for Ca)	Incision in perineum between scrotum and rectum.	Causes impotence, sterility, and some incontinence.	Allow expression of feelings. Teach perineal exercises.
		Large perineal wound with risk of infection and bleeding.	Clean well. Check and change dressing prn.
		Straining or rectal trauma may increase bleeding.	Avoid rectal temperatures or tubes. Give stool softeners.
		May be done for castration for carcinoma.	Talk to client. Explain changes.

Plan/Implementation
- know that a large balloon on the Foley can stimulate spasms (more likely to be used with TURP)
- administer narcotics plus anticholinergic drugs as ordered

Evaluation: Client's postoperative bladder spasms are controlled.

Goal 5: Client will remain free from undetected complications
Plan/Implementation
- observe for signs of osteitis pubis after a retropubic prostatectomy
- institute strategies to prevent thrombophlebitis
- know that incisional infection is more frequent with suprapubic prostatectomy
- observe for signs of epididymitis if vasectomy was not done

Evaluation: Client is free from postoperative infections, signs of epididymitis.

Goal 6: Client will be able to explain postdischarge activities allowed.
Plan/Implementation
- tell client to refrain from sexual activity until approximately 6 weeks post-op
- have client avoid heavy lifting, straining, driving car for approximately 6 weeks
- monitor urine: should be continually clear
- teach client to increase fluid intake, i.e, 1 glass of fluid qh
- teach client to avoid alcohol for 6 weeks
- teach client that dribbling may occur after removal of catheter and that perineal exercise can help increase sphincter tone

Evaluation: Client can describe activity restrictions; states he will monitor urine at home.

I. Cancer of the Prostate

1. **General Information**
   a. Incidence
      1) increasing
      2) 2nd most common cancer in men
      3) most frequent in 50+ age group
   b. Predisposing Factors
      1) family tendency
      2) environmental risks and oncogenic virus suspected
   c. Other Information
      1) usually starts in posterior lobe
      2) most commonly adenocarcinoma
   d. Medical Treatment: surgical intervention
      1) radical perineal prostatectomy
      2) radical retropubic prostatectomy
      3) TURP for palliation followed by hormonal manipulation (DES or bilateral orchiectomy)

2. **Nursing Process**
   a. **Assessment:** findings depend on size of tumor
      1) if large, tumor will cause obstruction and findings similar to those in BPH
      2) if small, no findings except hard nodule when prostate palpated rectally
      3) if metastasis occurs, it is usually to spine causing low back and leg pain
      4) positive biopsy
      5) acid phosphatase increased with spread beyond capsule; alkaline phosphatase increased with bony metastasis
   b. **Goals, Plans/Implementation, and Evaluation**

Goal 1: Client will be able to explain the planned surgery and what to expect postoperatively.
Plan/Implementation
- refer to *Surgery* page 165
- counsel client regarding impotence
- include significant others in pre-op discussion

Goal 2: Client's incision will be kept clean and remain intact.
Plan/Implementation
- do not take rectal temperatures or insert rectal tubes
- use T-binder
- give sitz baths after drains removed
- maintain patency of Foley

Evaluation: Client's incision is healing well.

Goal 3: Client will remain free from postoperative complications.
Plan/Implementation
- refer to *Surgery* page 165

Goal 4: Client will regain perineal muscle tone and urinary continence.
Plan/Implementation
- teach perineal and buttock-tightening exercises

stool c̄ alot fat — smells alot

274 SECTION 3: NURSING CARE OF THE ADULT

- institute exercises 48 hours post-op; have client do them qh
- reassure client that some urinary control can be obtained

Evaluation: Client can demonstrate perineal exercises; expresses a positive attitude about regaining continence.

Goal 5: Client will be able to explain alternate ways of sexual expression.

Plan/Implementation

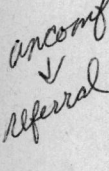
uncomf. → referral

- encourage client to discuss concerns/fears
- encourage client to discuss sexuality with significant other; have them explore different ways to satisfy each other sexually

Evaluation: Client shows a willingness to discuss sexual concerns.

Goal 6: Client and significant other will understand the therapy for advanced disease.

Plan/Implementation
- explain hormonal manipulation and side effects of female hormones
- prepare client for bilateral orchiectomy if indicated
- prepare client for TURP if cancer is causing obstruction but is not surgically treatable

Evaluation: Client is able to describe future care needs.

Part Two: The Large Bowel

General Concepts

A. Overview
1. The large intestine extends from the ileocecal valve to the anus (cecum, ascending colon, transverse colon, descending colon, sigmoid colon, rectum, and anal canal).
2. The major functions of the colon are the absorption of water and electrolytes in the proximal half of the large intestine and storage of feces in the distal half until defecation occurs.
3. Bacterial action in the large bowel not only provides gases to increase the bulk of and propel the feces but also facilitates synthesis of vitamin K, thiamine, riboflavin, vitamin B_{12}, folic acid, biotin, and nicotinic acid.

B. Application of the Nursing Process to the Client with Large Bowel Problems
1. Assessment
   a. Health History
      1) bowel habits: frequency and character of stool patterns
      2) changes in bowel habits: decrease or increase in frequency, change in consistency (more liquid→diarrhea; less liquid→constipation)
      3) presence of blood or change in color of stool *or mucous*
      4) use of laxatives or other methods that affect elimination
      5) effect of dietary habits on elimination
      6) presence of abdominal or rectal pain
      7) altered weight
   b. Physical Examination
      1) inspection
         a) abdomen
            - scars, striae, wounds, fistulas, and/or ostomy
            - engorged veins
            - skin characteristics
            - visible peristalsis and pulsations
            - visible masses and altered contour
         b) anus
            - presence of dilated veins
            - constipation
            - breaks in skin, fissures
      3) auscultation
         a) bowel sounds
         b) bruit
         c) hum and friction rub
      4) percussion
         a) liver size
         b) presence of fluid
      5) palpation
         a) masses
         b) rigidity of abdominal muscles
         c) pain/tenderness
         d) fluid waves
   c. Diagnostic Tests
      1) stool examinations
         a) odor, consistency, color
         b) presence or absence of mucus
         c) occult blood (by guaiac exam)
         d) ova and parasites
      2) barium enema
         a) definition: barium is instilled in the rectum through a rectal catheter; permits x-ray visualization of large intestine

ELIMINATION

b) nursing care
- pretest
  - explain procedure
  - administer cleansing enemas prior to procedure *laxatives*
  - may restrict diet to low-residue foods for 24 hours prior to exam
- post-test
  - administer laxatives following procedure as ordered, to prevent impaction
  - instruct client that stool will remain white for 24–72 hours

3) proctoscopy, sigmoidoscopy, colonoscopy

  a) definition: visualization of inside of colon through a lighted scope
  - proctoscopy: rigid scope
  - colonoscopy: flexible scope

  b) nursing care
  - pretest
    - explain procedure
    - give clear liquids 24 hours prior to exam
    - prepare bowel with laxatives, enemas, or suppositories as ordered
  - post-test
    - observe for hemorrhage, abdominal distention, pain
    - check for return of normal bowel function postprocedure

4) biopsy

  a) definition: removal of polyps or section of the colon through a specialized piece of equipment inserted into the proctoscope or on the end of colonoscope

  b) nursing care
  - same as for proctoscopy
  - monitor carefully for hemorrhage

2. General Nursing Goals, Plans/Implementation, and Evaluation

Goal 1: Client's bowel elimination will follow a normal pattern.

Plan/Implementation
- instruct client how to promote proper bowel function; adjust teaching if client has an ileostomy or colostomy
- teach client to respond to defecation reflex since holding feces can contribute to constipation
- instruct client on the use of foods high in bulk and roughage: skins and fibers of fruits and vegetables
- increase fluid intake if allowed
- encourage regular exercise to aid in elimination
- teach about the relationship of stress to altered bowel function
- prevent diarrhea through proper sanitation and hygiene
- restrict fruit juices and raw fruits and vegetables that contribute to diarrhea
- observe client with diarrhea for signs of fluid and electrolyte imbalance
- administer medication to control diarrhea (e.g., diphenoxylate (Lomotil) or paregoric) as ordered
- encourage intake of electrolyte-containing drinks (e.g., Gatorade)

Evaluation: Client establishes a normal pattern of bowel elimination; can list, and consumes, foods that promote bowel evacuation; has established a pattern of regular exercise; passes stool of normal consistency.

Goal 2: Client's dietary intake will follow prescribed restrictions yet provide all needed nutrients. *malabsorption*

Plan/Implementation
- increase or decrease dietary nutrients as ordered
- teach client rationale for restrictions
- explore with client means of fostering compliance
- provide needed support and encouragement

Evaluation: Client can select appropriate diet from sample menus; verbalizes rationale for restrictions; expresses a positive attitude toward diet alteration.

Goal 3: Client will be knowledgeable about disease process, medications, and the prevention of complications.

Plan/Implementation
- explain disease process and its relationship to medications
- discuss rationale for ordered treatment regimen
- provide data concerning the administration and side effects of all medications
- assist client to identify potential stressors in life-style that might trigger

complications of the disease; discuss appropriate client actions

Evaluation: Client takes medications as ordered, returns for follow-up care; remains free from preventable complications.

Selected Health Problems

A. Alteration in Normal Bowel Evacuation

1. **General Information**
   a. Definitions
      1) *constipation*: difficult or infrequent defecation with passage of unduly hard and dry fecal material
      2) *diarrhea*: frequent passage of abnormally watery bowel movements
      3) normal bowel evacuation: 2–3 movements/day to 2/week; varies in healthy individuals
   b. Precipitating Factors
      1) constipation: worry, anxiety, fear, improper diet, intestinal obstruction, tumors, excessive use of laxatives, use of certain drugs, atony or spasticity of intestinal musculature
      2) diarrhea: diet, inflammation or irritation of intestinal mucosa, GI infections, use of certain drugs, psychogenic factors

2. **Nursing Process**
   a. Assessment
      1) stool consistency, appearance
      2) acute or chronic pain, rebound tenderness
      3) weight loss, malnutrition
      4) dehydration
      5) nausea, vomiting; projectile vomiting
      6) electrolyte imbalance, especially sodium, potassium, chloride
      7) aggravation by certain foods and milk products
      8) drug history
      9) malabsorption of foods
      10) mass in abdomen
      11) low-grade fever
      12) anemia
      13) anorexia
      14) presence of bowel sounds: increased or decreased
      15) abdominal distention
      16) decreased flatus
   b. **Goal, Plan/Implementation, and Evaluation**

   Goal (refer to General Nursing Goal 1 page 275)

Table 3.44 Laxatives

Description	Drugs that facilitate evacuation of the bowel by a wide variety of mechanisms; classified according to action
Uses	Treatment of constipation; preparation for certain GI and renal studies
Side Effects	Abdominal cramping, nausea, diarrhea, fluid and electrolyte imbalance, obstruction, laxative dependence
Nursing Implications	Suggest alternate methods to promote bowel movements: diet, fluid, exercise, etc.; time administration according to length of action so that rest is not disturbed; do not use if obstruction suspected; give adequate fluids.
Types and Examples	*Irritants:* cascara (Cas-Evac), senna (Senokot), castor oil (Alphamul), bisacodyl (Dulcolax) *Bulk Formers:* agar, psyllium (Metamucil) *Saline/Osmotic:* MgOH (milk of magnesia), magnesium citrate, magnesium sulfate (Epsom salt), lactulose (Cephulac) *Emollients:* dioctyl sodium sulfosuccinate (Colace), dioctyl calcium sulfosuccinate (Surfak) *Lubricants:* mineral oil (Petrolagar)

Table 3.45 Antidiarrheals

Description	Drugs that act to reduce the liquidity of feces. Local agents act within the bowel to soothe the intestinal tract and increase the absorption of water, electrolytes, and nutrients; systemic agents act systemically to inhibit the peristaltic reflex and reduce GI motility.
Uses	Treatment of acute and chronic diarrhea
Side Effects	Nausea, vomiting, acute glaucoma (atropine), headache, drowsiness, hypersensitivity reactions, nystagmus
Nursing Implications	Identify cause of diarrhea and intervene if possible; don't use atropine-containing preparations in clients with glaucoma or benign prostatic hypertrophy; avoid overuse; prevent constipation; protect drugs from light and moisture.
Types and Examples	*Local:* kaolin and pectin (Kaopectate), bismuth subsalicylate (Pepto-Bismol) *Systemic:* diphenoxylate hydrochloride with atropine sulfate (Lomotil); loperamide (Imodium); paregoric, formerly called camphorated tincture of opium

B. Inflammatory Bowel Disease (Regional Enteritis, Crohn's Disease, Ulcerative Colitis)

1. **General Information**
   a. Definition: regional enteritis (Crohn's disease) is a segmental transmural inflammatory process that may involve any part of the alimentary tract. Ulcerative colitis is a continuous inflammatory process of the mucosa and, less frequently, the submucosa of the colon and rectum.
   b. Incidence: young people between 20 and 40 years of age
   c. Etiology: unknown; possibly result of infection, stress, and/or autoimmunity; familial tendency
   d. Pathophysiology
      1) regional enteritis presents with marked thickening of the submucosa with lymphedema, hyperplasia, granulomas, ulcerations, and fissures; the longitudinal ulcers and transverse fissure produce a cobblestone effect; in the later stages, full thickness penetration of the intestinal wall results in the formation of fistulas and abscesses; the ileum is the principal site
      2) ulcerative colitis presents with congestion, edema, multiple superficial ulcerations, and crypt abscesses in the rectum and distal colon and spreads upward; mucosal hemorrhage and pus are common; colon is scarred, loses elasticity and absorptive capacity
   e. Diagnostic Tests
      1) stool for blood, fat, and culture
      2) proctosigmoidoscopy with biopsy
      3) barium enema (cathartics are contraindicated as a prep)

2. **Nursing Process**
   a. **Assessment**
      1) rectal bleeding
      2) diarrhea: frequent liquid stools with tenesmas; may contain blood, mucus, or pus
      3) abdominal cramps before bowel movement; colicky cramping with urgency to defecate
      4) pain, usually located in the left lower quadrant, with ulcerative colitis
      5) anorexia, nausea, vomiting
      6) dehydration
      7) electrolyte imbalance, e.g., decreased potassium and sodium, metabolic acidosis
      8) weight loss
      9) weakness, debilitation, malnutrition
      10) anemia
      11) fever

278 SECTION 3: NURSING CARE OF THE ADULT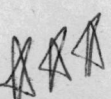

Table 3.46 Comparison of Crohn's Disease and Ulcerative Colitis

Characteristic	Regional Enteritis (Crohn's Disease)	Ulcerative Colitis
Depth of involvement	Transmural (all layers of submucosa)	Mucosa and submucosa
Rectal involvement	50%	95%
Right colon involvement	Frequent	Occasional
Small bowel involvement	Involved	Usually normal
Effect on ileum (if involved)	Narrowed	Widened
Distribution of disease	Segmental	Continuous
Inflammatory mass	Common, chronic, extensive	Rare (acute crypt abscess)
Rectal bleeding	Infrequent	Common (90%–100%)
Anal abscess	Common (75%)	Occasional (10%)
Fistula (abdominal wall and internal)	Common	Rare
Anorectal fissure and fistula	Common (80%)	Rare (10%–20%)
Cobblestone appearance of mucosa	Common	Unusual
Granuloma	Common (67%)	Absent
Mesenteric fat and lymph involvement	Edema and hyperplasia	Not involved
Megacolon, toxic	Occasional	Occasional
Steatorrhea	Frequent	Rare
Malignancy results	Rare	Occasional after 10 years
Nutritional deficit	Common	Frequent
Fibrous stricture	Common	Absent
Course of disease	Usually slowly progressive	Remissions and relapses
Abdominal pain	Colicky (45%)	Predefecation (60%–70%)
Hematochezia	Unusual or absent	Almost always present
Diarrhea	Present but less frequent (65%–85%)	Early and frequent (80%–95%)
Weight loss	Present (60%–70%)	Present (20%–50%)
Fever	Present (35%)	Present (10%)
Vomiting	Present (35%)	Present (15%)

SOURCE: Given, B. and Simmons, S. *Gastroenterology in Clinical Nursing*, 4th ed. St. Louis: Mosby, 1984. Used with permission.

12) emotional concerns, immature and dependent personality
13) dietary habits

b. Goals, Plans/Implementation, and Evaluation

Goal 1: Client will be free from infection.
Plan/Implementation
- prevent and treat secondary infection through use of sulfonamides (sulfasalazine [Azulfidine] sulfathiazole) as ordered
- assist and teach client to turn, cough, and deep breathe q2–4h (during acute stage)
- check temperature q4h, avoid taking rectal temperature if anus is excoriated
- administer oral hygiene as necessary
- provide good skin care

Evaluation: Client remains free from signs of infection (e.g., increased temperature, infiltrate in lungs, or secondary infection in mucous membranes of mouth, skin, or colon).

Goal 2: Client will be well nourished and hydrated.
Plan/Implementation
- weigh client daily
- in acute stage give nothing PO; give parenteral fluids with vitamins and minerals as ordered
- administer total parenteral nutrition (TPN) as ordered

- initiate high-protein, low-residue, high-calorie, bland diet as tolerated
- avoid gas-producing or irritating foods and milk products
- offer small feedings as necessary
- replace deficiency of fat-soluble vitamins (A, D, E, and K)
- record caloric intake
- avoid too hot or too cold foods
- urge up to 3,000 ml fluid intake/day (if not contraindicated); keep I&O (include measurement of liquid stools)
- involve client and significant others with dietitian for proper diet instructions

Evaluation: Client maintains weight; can state meal plan utilizing high-protein, low-residue, high-calorie, bland diet; maintains at least 2,500 ml fluid intake daily.

Goal 3: Client will experience reduced physical and psychologic stress.
Plan/Implementation
- in acute stage, enforce bed rest to decrease intestinal motility
- maintain quiet, comfortable, nonstressful environment
- keep room odorfree
- empty bedpan frequently and have within easy reach of client during acute episodes
- keep perianal area clean and dry, applying lubricant or ointments as necessary
- administer pain medications as ordered
- give sitz baths at least 3 times/day or as needed

Evaluation: Client states relief of pain; rests comfortably.

Goal 4: Client will have fewer bowel movements than when admitted
Plan/Implementation
- administer antidiarrheal medications as ordered
  - opium alkaloids (paragoric)
  - diphenoxylate (Lomotil)
  - anticholinergic drugs (tincture of belladonna, Donnatol)
  - kaolin and pectin (Kaopectate)
- reduce inflammation by administration of
  - azathioprine (Imuran) immunosuppressive agent
  - 6-mercaptopurine
  - corticosteroids as ordered
- check bowel sounds q2-4h; report increase or decrease to physician
- note frequency, color, and amount of stools
- report increase in abdominal distention to physician
- reduce emotional stress (direct influence on course of illness)

Evaluation: Client has a decrease in frequency and amount of stools; has no increase in abdominal distention.

Goal 5: Client will maintain a balance of adequate rest and exercise.
Plan/Implementation
- encourage rest after meals
- do not confine to bed unless very weak
- provide calm, reassuring environment
- give sedation as necessary to provide adequate night's sleep
- initiate ambulation at short, frequent intervals

Table 3.47 Foods to be *Avoided* on Low Residue Diets

Types of Foods	Foods to be Avoided
Beverages	Milk in excess of 2 cups.
Breads and cereals	Whole grain or bran.
Desserts	Any containing fruits and nuts.
Fruits	Any with seeds or skins, raw fruits except bananas.
Meats, fish, poultry, cheese, eggs	Tough meats. Pork. Fried or highly seasoned meats. Fish. Cheese.
Vegetables	Raw vegetables

[Handwritten note at top left: Stoma necrosis — gray or blue]

[Handwritten note at top right: AVOID enteric coated tabs because ā pass through + not be absorbed.]

- allow for frequent rest periods

Evaluation: Client verbalizes that he is receiving adequate rest periods; sleeps through the night; is able to increase periods of ambulation as strength returns.

Goal 6: Client will accept alteration of lifestyle imposed by chronic illness.

Plan/Implementation
- provide teaching regarding
  - how to live with chronic disease
  - factors in environment that aggravate colitis (emotional stress, dietary indiscretion, ingestion of irritants, overfatigue, infections, or pregnancy)
  - how to maintain nutrition
  - importance of medical management of the disease
  - need for biannual sigmoidoscopy and barium enema (increased incidence of carcinoma of large intestines)
- provide emotional counseling and support as needed
- encourage verbalization of anxieties
- provide diversional activities

Evaluation: Client verbalizes acceptance of disease; can list life-style modifications to be initiated.

C. Total Colectomy with Ileostomy

1. **General Information**
   a. Definition: surgical removal of the entire colon, rectum, and anus with the construction of permanent ileostomy to provide for passage of feces
   b. Indications: when medical management fails and constant relapses with intractability occur; occurrence of complications; e.g., perforation, hemorrhage, obstruction, toxic megacolon, abscess and fistula; more effective as a treatment for ulcerative colitis

2. **Nursing Process**
   a. Assessment
      1) physical status
      2) emotional status
      3) acceptance of ostomy
      4) understanding of ostomy function
      5) ability to verbalize feelings
   b. Goals, Plans/Implementation, and Evaluation

Goal 1: Client will be physically and psychologically prepared for surgery.

Plan/Implementation
- refer to *Surgery* page 165
- give TPN as ordered, to improve nutritional status pre-op
- prepare bowel for surgery: low-residue diet, clear liquids, oral antibiotics, cathartics, enema
- obtain help of an enterostomal therapist, if available, to plan site of stoma placement and to introduce client to appliance
- encourage client to express fears and concerns regarding change in body image
- introduce client to concept of ostomy support groups; obtain volunteer if desired

Evaluation: Client views appliances; expresses positive reaction to outcomes of surgery.

Goal 2: Client will remain free from infection and complications postoperatively.

Plan/Implementation
- refer to *Surgery* page 165

Evaluation: Client remains free from any signs of postoperative infection or complications (e.g., has normal temperature, clear lungs).

Goal 3: Client will maintain normal fluid and electrolyte balance.

Plan/Implementation
- monitor I&O, weigh daily, NG tube drainage
- monitor state of hydration (skin turgor and condition of mucous membranes); urine output
- monitor serum electrolyte levels
- monitor ileal output; drainage begins immediately post-op *[handwritten: pouch needed]*
- administer IV fluids as ordered, until client can take oral nourishment

Evaluation: Client's I&O, electrolytes remain within normal limits.

Goal 4: Client will understand dietary restrictions.

Plan/Implementation
- teach client that food ingested will pass through the ileostomy within 4–6 hours
- teach client that each individual has different food tolerances
- provide diet information: most ostomy clients are discharged on a low-residue, high-protein, high-carbohydrate diet

rich in high-potassium foods and low in gas-producing, highly seasoned, or fried foods
- know that vitamin supplements A, D, E, K, and B₁₂ may be necessary
- prepare client for possible weight gain resulting from increased food tolerance post-op
- refer to dietitian as necessary

Evaluation: Client is able to state dietary changes; verbalizes intent to work out a diet plan within the limits of the individual variations.

Goal 5: Client will achieve self-care management.

Plan/Implementation
- instruct client (step by step) and receive return demonstration on stoma care including
  - equipment: type, how to use, and where to purchase
  - skin care: ileostomy drainage is erosive and continuous
  - application of appliance
  - odor control
  - use services of enterostomol therapist if available
- refer to visiting nurses (VNA) for home follow-up or continue following up by enterostomol therapist

Evaluation: Client successfully manages self-care of ileostomy.

Goal 6: Client will successfully cope with altered body image.

Plan/Implementation
- encourage verbalization of concerns
- assure client that major change in lifestyle is not necessary
- encourage involvement in ostomy club
- provide emotional support to the significant other in adjusting to ostomy
- obtain sexual counseling for client, if needed *should be not impotent*

Evaluation: Client is able to discuss altered body image; shows evidence of coping with change and resumption of normal activity.

D. Mechanical Obstruction of the Colon

1. **General Information**
   a. Pathophysiology
   1) obstruction can be partial or complete
   2) emergency situation if blood supply is compromised
   3) if blood supply is not compromised, fluid and electrolyte deficiency becomes the major problem
   4) absorption decreases and fluids and electrolytes accumulate in GI tract
   5) fluid will either stay in GI tract or be lost through vomiting
   6) subsequent decrease in extracellular fluid volume (dehydration)
   7) metabolic acidosis results
   b. Risk Factors/Causative Factors
   1) small intestine: adhesions, hernia, volvulus
   2) large intestine: neoplasm, stricture, diverticulitis
   c. Medical Treatment
   1) medical intervention
      a) decompression with intestinal tubes
      b) fluid and electrolyte replacement
   2) surgical intervention *remove tumor*
      a) colon resection
         - end-to-end anastomosis
         - temporary colostomy
         - permanent colostomy
      b) abdominoperineal resection with permanent colostomy

2. **Nursing Process**
   a. Assessment
   1) abdomen distended; altered bowel habits; most common with large intestine obstruction
   2) projectile vomiting and severe pain, most common with small intestine obstruction
   3) decreased or increased bowel sounds
   4) decreased flatus
   b. Goals, Plans/Implementation, and Evaluation

   Goals 1 through 4: refer to "Total Colectomy with Ileostomy" page 280
   Plan/Implementation
   - know that in addition, the client will undergo pre-op bowel preparation that will include
     - clear liquids several days pre-op; then nothing PO
     - NG tube or intestinal tube (Cantor or Miller-Abbott) to intermittent suction
     - bowel sterilization routine as ordered with neomycin and sulfonamides
     - several enemas and cathartics
   - monitor I&O, urine specific gravity, and gastric output

- give narcotics sparingly (may mask symptoms); avoid morphine (decreases intestinal motility)

Evaluation: Client's bowel is clean and prepared for surgery.

Goal 5: Client will successfully cope with altered body image.

Plan/Implementation
- see "Total Colectomy with Ileostomy" Goal 6 page 281
- instruct client about irrigation and dietary management for regulation of colostomy
- if the colostomy is to be closed at a future date, encourage client to work for that day while at the same time reinforcing the importance of good daily care and adjustment to a temporarily changed body image

Evaluation: Client is able to discuss altered body image; expresses a willingness to adjust and to maintain colostomy until closure can be accomplished.

E. Cancer of the Colon

1. **General Information**
   a. Definition: malignant neoplasm of the large bowel; 70% of cases occur in the rectosigmoid area
   b. Incidence
      1) 2nd most common malignancy in adults
      2) equal in both sexes
      3) occurs after 4th decade; peaks in the 7th decade
      4) most are adenocarcinoma
   c. Risk Factors
      1) family history
      2) history of ulcerative colitis, polyps
      3) possibly related to increased fat in diet, food additives, low-fiber diet, or chronic constipation
   d. Metastasis
      1) lymph nodes
      2) liver via the bloodstream
   e. Diagnostic Tests
      1) rectal exam (almost 50% of these tumors are palpable on digital exam)
      2) sigmoidoscopy, colonoscopy
      3) barium enema
      4) stool exam for occult blood
      5) alkaline phosphatase and SGOT: metastasis to liver
      6) carcinoembryonic antigen (CEA) level: elevated in advanced adenocarcinoma
   f. Medical Treatment
      1) surgical intervention: colon resection
         a) colectomy with anastomosis of the remaining colon or colostomy
         b) abdominal-perineal resection with a permanent colostomy
      2) medical intervention
         a) radiation therapy
         b) chemotherapy

2. **Nursing Process**
   a. Assessment
      1) change in bowel habits; blood in stool (more likely with left colon and rectal involvement)
      2) vague, dull pain (more likely with ascending-colon involvement)
      3) anorexia, weight loss, weakness, and anemia
      4) signs of obstruction
      5) hemorrhage
      6) perforation with peritonitis, abscess and fistula formation
   b. Goals, Plans/Intervention, and Evaluation
      Refer to "Total Colectomy with Ileostomy" page 280.
      Refer to "Mechanical Obstruction of the Colon" page 281.
      Refer to *Cellular Aberration* for information and goals pertinent to chemotherapy and radiation therapy.

F. Hemorrhoids or Anal Fissure

1. **General Information**
   a. Definitions
      1) *hemorrhoids*: dilated veins under the mucous membranes in the anal area; may be either internal or external
      2) *anal fissure:* linear ulceration on the margin of the anus
   b. Predisposing Factors
      1) straining at stool
      2) pregnancy
      3) portal hypertension
      4) congestive heart failure
   c. Complications
      1) bleeding
      2) thrombosis
      3) strangulation
      4) infection
   d. Medical Treatment
      1) medical intervention
         a) high-roughage diet and 6-8 glasses of fluid/day
         b) stool softeners

Handwritten note at top: Teach AVOID Constipation → perineal wound will occur

ELIMINATION 283

c) ointments or suppositories to shrink hemorrhoids
d) warm sitz bath
e) injection of a sclerosing substance into the tissues at the base of the vein
f) rubber band ligation
2) surgical intervention
a) hemorrhoidectomy: excision of dilated veins
b) fissurectomy: excision of fissure

2. **Nursing Process**
   a. **Assessment**
      1) pain and pruritus around anus
      2) character and amount of rectal drainage
      3) usual bowel habits
      4) abdominal distention
      5) urinary retention
      6) anemia caused by chronic bleeding
   b. **Goals, Plans/Implementation, and Evaluation**

Goal 1: Client will remain free from postoperative complications.
Plan/Implementation
- refer to *Surgery* page 165
- avoid sitting for prolonged periods; while sitting, use flotation pad *Never use ring flotation*
- prevent infection *↑ pressure on rectum*
  - initiate procedures as ordered for thorough pre-op bowel cleansing
  - DO NOT take rectal temperature
  - administer perineal care with antiseptic solution after each stool
  - administer sitz baths as necessary to clean incision

Evaluation: Client remains free from complications (e.g., infection).

Goal 2: Client will experience relief of pain.
Plan/Implementation
- give analgesics as ordered
- avoid supine position; if supine position is unavoidable, use flotation pad under buttocks
- apply ice packs or warm, moist compresses if ordered
- do not use rubber rings
- administer topical anesthesia as ordered

Evaluation: Client states pain is controlled; is comfortable in all positions.

Goal 3: Client's bowel function will return to normal.

Plan/Implementation
- give low-residue, soft diet as tolerated for 1st week post-op; then advance diet to include roughage and fresh fruits
- force fluids to 2,500–3,000 ml/day unless contraindicated
- administer stool softener/lubricant or laxative as ordered
- provide support during initial BM, noting presence of blood in stool; be alert for vertigo; and administer analgesic as necessary
- teach client how to avoid constipation after discharge
- watch for and teach client symptoms of anal stricture (and report to physician)
  - increased pain with BM
  - difficulty passing stool

Evaluation: Client passed soft, brown, formed stool on 3rd postoperative day with minimal discomfort; can list ways to prevent constipation; can state signs of anal stricture

References

Arenz, R. "Do It Yourself Dialysis." *RN*. July 1981:57-60.

Ash, S., Wimberly, A., and Mertz, S. "Peritoneal Dialysis for Acute and Chronic Renal Failure: An Update." *Hospital Practice*. January 1983: 179-210.

Ash, S., Wimberly, A., and Mertz, S. "Fear of Floating to a Renal Unit." *Nursing 82*. December 1982:42-43.

Barrett, N. "Continent Vesicostomy: The Dry Urinary Diversion." *American Journal of Nursing*. March 1979:462-464.

Broadwell, D. and Sorrells, S. "Loop Transverse Colostomy." *American Journal of Nursing*. June 1978:1029-1031.

Bromley, B. "Applying Orem's Self-Care Theory in Enterostomal Therapy." *American Journal of Nursing*. February 1980:245-299.

Casadonte, L. "The Patient with a Fistula, a Colostomy, and an Ileal Conduit." *RN*, September 1984:42-46.

Ceccarelli, C. "Hemodialytic Therapy for the Patient with Chronic Renal Failure." *Nursing Clinics of North America*. September 1981: 531-550.

*Chambers, J. "Bowel Management in Dialysis Patients." *American Journal of Nursing*. July 1983:1051-1052.

Given, B. and Simmons, S. *Gastroenterology in Clinical Nursing*, 4th Ed. St. Louis: Mosby, 1984.

Griggs, B. and Hoppe, M. "Update: Nasogastric Tube Feedings." *American Journal of Nursing*. March 1979:481-485.

Hughes, R. "Continuous Ambulatory Peritoneal Dialysis." *Journal of Arkansas Medical Society*. May 1981:521-524.

Juliani, L. "Assessing Renal Function." *Nursing 78*, January 1978:34-35.

Lazarus, J. "Dialytic Therapy: Principle and Clinical Guidelines." *Hospital Practice*. October 1982:111-133.

Leste, G. "Nondialytic Treatment of Established Acute Renal Failure." *Critical Care Quarterly*. September 1978:11-23.

Lewis, S. "Pathophysiology of Chronic Renal Failure."*Nursing Clinics of North America*. September 1981:501-513.

Luke, B. "Nutrition in Renal Disease: The Adult on Dialysis." *American Journal of Nursing*. December 1979:2155-2157.

Metheny, N. "Renal Stones and Urinary pH." *American Journal of Nursing*. September 1982:1372-1375.

Murphy, L. and Cole, M. "Renal Disease: Nutritional Implications." *Nursing Clinics of North America*. March 1983:57-70.

Neal, M., Cohen, P., and Reighley, J. *Nursing Care Planning Guides, Set 3*, 2nd Ed. Baltimore: Williams & Wilkins, 1983.

Oestreich, S. "Rational Nursing Care in Chronic Renal Disease." *American Journal of Nursing*. June 1979:1096-1098.

Orr, M. "Drugs and Renal Disease."*American Journal of Nursing*. May 1981:969-971.

Pickering, L. "Fluid, Electrolyte and Acid-Base Balance in the Renal Patient." *Nursing Clinics of North America*. September 1980:577-592.

Plantemoli, C. "When the Patient has a Foley." *RN*. March 1984:42-43.

Quinlan, M. "UTI: Helping Your Patients Control It Once and For All." *RN*. March 1984:38-42.

Reed, S. "Giving More Than Dialysis." *Nursing 82*. April 1982:58-63.

Roberts, S. "Renal Assessment: A Nursing Point of View." *Heart and Lung*. January/February 1979:105-113.

Sorrels, A. "Peritoneal Dialysis: A Rediscovery." *Nursing Clinics of North America*. September 1981:515-529.

Stahlgren, L. and Morris, N. "Intestinal Obstruction." *American Journal of Nursing*. June 1977:999-1002.

Stark, J. "How to Succeed Against Acute Renal Failure." *Nursing 82*. July 1982:26-33.

Tyndale, G. "Chronic Renal Failure: Past and Future Trends." *Nursing Clinics of North America*. September 1981:489-499.

Wilpizeski, M. "Helping the Ostomate Return to Normal Life." *Nursing 81*. March 1981:62-66.

* See reprint section

Safety and Security

(The nursing care presented in this unit concerns selected health problems related to disturbances in the nervous system, eye, ear, nose, and throat.)

General Concepts
A. Overview
1. Nervous System: like an electrical conductance system; coordinates and controls all activities of the body
   a. Receives stimuli or information from internal and external environments over varied sensory pathways
   b. Communicates information between distant parts of body (periphery) and central nervous system
   c. Computes or processes information received at various reflex (spinal cord) and conscious (higher brain) levels to determine responses appropriate to existing situations
   d. Transmits information rapidly over varied motor pathways to effector organs for body-action control or modification
2. Central Nervous System
   a. Brain
      1) cerebrum or cerebral cortex (see figure 3.20)
         a) frontal lobe: functions
            - personality
            - higher intellectual functions (e.g., learning, problem solving)
            - ethical, social, and moral behavior
            - posterior edge of frontal lobe: center for initiation of motor function
         b) parietal lobe: responsible for interpretation of sensory input
         c) temporal lobe: center for hearing, taste, and smell
         d) occipital lobe: visual center
         e) structure
            - skull
            - meninges: connective tissue covering brain and spinal cord
            - layers of brain
              – duramater
              – extradura
              – epidura
              – inner dura (tentorium)
              – arachnoid
              – pia mater
            - blood-brain barrier
      2) brainstem: contains midbrain, pons, and medulla oblongata
         a) relays impulses from spinal cord to cerebrum
         b) controls basic body functions (cardiac, respiratory, and vasomotor centers [medulla])
      3) cerebellum
         a) orientation of body in space (equilibrium)
         b) coordination and inhibition of movement
         c) control of antigravity muscles
         d) coordination of muscle tone
   b. Spinal cord
      1) 31 segments (do not correspond in name to the vertebral segments)
         a) 8 cervical: supply neck and upper extremities, diaphragm, and intercostals
         b) 12 thoracic: supply thoracic and abdominal areas
         c) 5 lumbar: supply lower extremities
         d) 5 sacral: supply lower extremities; urinary tract and bowel control
         e) 1 coccygeal
      2) anterior portion of cord carries motor information (descending tracts)

3) posterior section of cord carries sensory information (ascending tracts)
4) lateral columns contain preganglionic fibers for autonomic nervous system
3. Peripheral Nervous System
   a. Cranial Nerves (12): classified in order of their arising from the brain (number) and by describing their nature, function, and distribution (name) (see table 3.48)
   b. Spinal Nerves (31 Pairs)
4. Autonomic Nervous System: concerned with the control of involuntary bodily functions; divided into parasympathetic (craniosacral) and sympathetic (thoracolumbar) divisions
   a. Divisions
      1) parasympathetic or craniosacral division controls normal body functioning
      2) sympathetic or thoracolumbar division prepares body for fight or flight
   b. Most effector organs receive innervation from both sympathetic and parasympathetic fibers
   c. Vascular supply of skeletal muscle receives only sympathetic innervation
5. Vision
   a. Major function of eyes is to produce vision: lightwaves → cornea → lens → retina → optic nerve (II) → occipital lobe of brain
   b. Cranial Nerves of the Eye
      1) optic (II): vision
      2) oculomotor (III), trochlear (IV), abducent (VI): external muscles of the eye
      3) oculomotor (III) also controls pupil size
   c. Exterior of Eye
      1) tears secreted by lacrimal glands to lubricate lids and keep corneas moist; excess tears drain through lacrimal ducts into nasal cavity
      2) six extrinsic eye muscles produce movements of eyeball
      3) outer layer of eye
         a) cornea: transparent covering of eye, called "window of the eye"
         b) sclera: opaque, connective tissue covering all of eye except cornea
   d. Interior of Eye (see figure 3.17)
      1) iris: circular muscle that constricts or dilates pupil
      2) lens: focuses image accurately on retina
      3) aqueous humor and vitreous humor: liquids acting along with lens as refracting media
      4) choroid: black, inner surface of eye that prevents scattering of light rays
      5) retina: light-sensitive layer of eye; sensations of vision result from retina's focused response to image

Table 3.48 Cranial Nerves

Number	Name	Type
I	Olfactory	sensory
II	Optic	sensory
III	Oculomotor	motor, parasympathetic
IV	Trochlear	motor
V	Trigeminal	sensory, motor
VI	Abducent	motor
VII	Facial	sensory, motor, parasympathetic
VIII	Acoustic or Auditory	sensory
IX	Glossopharyngeal	sensory, motor, parasympathetic
X	Vagus	sensory, motor, parasympathetic
XI	Accessory	motor
XII	Hypoglossal	motor

Table 3.49 Parasympathetic and Sympathetic Effects

Site	Parasympathetic Effect	Sympathetic Effect
Eye	Pupils constricted. Ciliary muscles excited.	Pupils dilated.
Nasal Mucosa	Thin, copious mucus secreted.	Vasoconstriction in nasal mucosa.
Lungs	Bronchoconstriction.	Bronchodilation.
Heart	Cardiac rate slowed. Contraction force decreased.	Cardiac rate increased. Contraction force increased. Coronary arteries dilate.
Liver		Hepatic glycongenolysis and lipolysis.
Gallbladder	Biliary ducts stimulated.	
Intestine	Peristalsis stimulated.	Peristalsis inhibited.
Urinary Bladder	Detrusor muscle excited. Trigone inhibited. Urinary excretion promoted.	Detrusor muscle inhibited. Trigone excited. Urinary retention promoted.
Adrenal Hormones	Secretion inhibited.	Secretion increased.

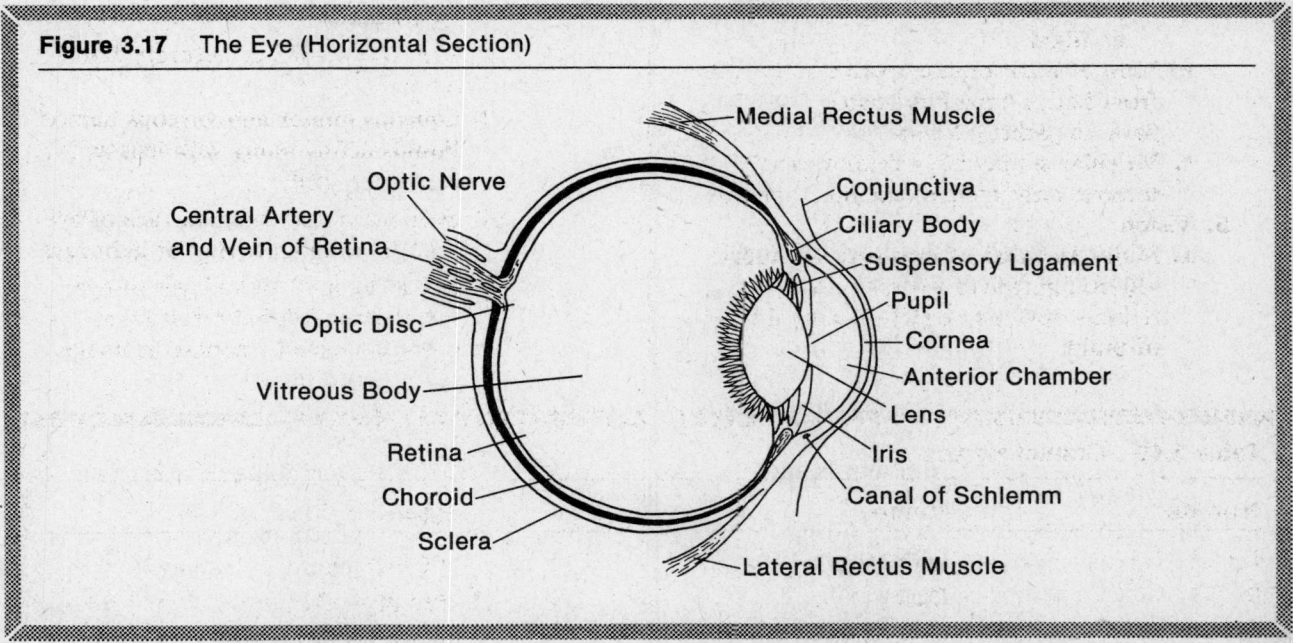

Figure 3.17 The Eye (Horizontal Section)

6) optic disk: entrance of optic nerve into eyeball
7) optic pathway: transmits visual data to occipital lobe of the brain
   e. Cerebrum/Occipital Lobe: interprets visual information
6. Hearing
   a. The major functions of the ears are balance and hearing; hearing pathway: sound waves→pinna→external ear canal→tympanic membrane→ossicles in middle ear→cochlea→auditory nerve (VIII)→auditory cortex in temporal lobe
   b. External Ear
      1) pinna: external flap of cartilage covered with skin that gathers and concentrates sound waves
      2) external ear canal (auditory meatus): cavity in skull lined with skin; ceruminous glands produce cerumen (wax) to assist in protecting the canal from small foreign particles; conveys

sound waves from pinna to tympanic membrane
3) tympanic membrane: flexible membrane that closes distal end of external auditory canal; membrane vibrates in response to sound, transmitting vibrations to middle ear
c. Middle Ear
1) ossicles: malleus, incus, and stapes
2) set into motion by sound waves from tympanic membrane
3) amplifies sound waves and transmits them to inner ear
4) connected with nasopharynx by eustachian tube
d. Inner Ear
1) cochlea: organ of sound perception
2) innervated by the auditory nerve VIII
a) cochlear branch: transmits auditory impulses from the cochlea to auditory cortex of brain
b) vestibular branch: controls balance
e. Auditory Portion of Cerebral Cortex: interprets auditory information (temporal lobe)
7. Nose
a. Air Passageway
b. Contains Sensory Receptors for Smell
c. Lined with Mucosa, Hair
1) secretes mucus
2) filters, warms, and humidifies inspired air
d. Paranasal sinuses drain into nasal cavity
8. Throat
a. Contains pharynx with tonsils and larynx with vocal cords
b. Glottis closes over larynx during swallowing to prevent aspiration
c. Chief function: passageway for air; filters and humidifies air

B. **Application of the Nursing Process to the Client with Safety and Security Problems**
1. **Assessment**
a. Health History
1) family history
2) history of problem: date of onset, precipitating factors, extent, duration or frequency, interventions that have been effective, location, any changes in description
3) headaches
4) seizures
5) medications: prescription and nonprescription
6) recent change in behavior or personality
b. Physical Examination
1) neurologic examination
a) cognitive function
- general behavior, emotional status
- level of consciousness (LOC): major index of client's neurologic status
  - *level 1*: consciousness (oriented to person, place, and time)
  - *level 2*: lethargy, somnolence, drowsiness, or obtundation
  - *level 3*: stupor (can be aroused by verbal stimuli but responds poorly or inappropriately)
  - *level 4*: light coma, semicoma (no response to verbal stimuli but responds to painful stimuli)
  - *level 5*: deep coma (no reaction to painful stimuli)
- attention span
- ability to follow commands
- memory: short and long term
- arithmetic ability
- abstract thinking
- language/speech
  - motor aphasia (expressive): inability to speak or write words
  - sensory aphasia (receptive)
    * visual: inability to comprehend written words
    * auditory: inability to comprehend spoken words
  - dysarthria: difficult speech caused by paralysis of muscles
b) cerebellar function
- balance
- coordination
c) motor function
- muscle size, tone, and strength
- involuntary movements, e.g., tremors
- coordination and accuracy of movement
- motor integration
- bowel and bladder function

d) sensory function
- superficial sensation: touch and pressure
- superficial pain
- sensitivity to temperature and vibration
- deep pressure, pain
- motion and position sense
- vision
  - amount of sight with or without glasses or contact lenses
  - distortion
    * halos around lights
    * difficulty adjusting to dark room
    * diploplia
    * floaters
- hearing
  - amount of hearing
    * use of hearing aid
    * tinnitus or other noises
  - conductive deafness (common causes: otosclerosis, otitis media) *hearing aid*
    * impairment of outer- and middle-ear conduction of sound waves
    * causes problems of perception of volume, not discrimination of sounds
    * can benefit from hearing aid
  - sensorineural deafness (common causes: old age, noise, drug toxicity) *lower voice*
    * impairment of inner-ear nerve conduction
    * causes problems of loss of sensitivity to and discrimination of sounds
    * hearing aid not beneficial
  - combined (conductive and sensorineural)
  - general speech pattern
  - indications of hearing loss
    * says "huh" frequently
    * asks you to repeat what you said
    * does not respond to questions or conversation
    * responds inappropriately to questions or comments
e) reflexes: superficial and deep tendon
f) cranial nerves (see table 3.48)

2) neuro check
  a) LOC: *most reliable indicator of neurologic status* (see cognitive function above)
  b) vital signs
  c) pupils: size and reaction to light
  d) motor function
    - move all extremities
    - muscle strength (grip)
  e) sensory function: response to touch or painful stimuli
  f) seizures
  g) blood or fluid leakage from nose or ear(s)
  h) posturing
    - decorticate posture (corticospinal tract): rigid flexion of head, arms, wrists, and fingers, and extension with internal rotation of legs (see figure 3.18)
    - decerebrate posture (midbrain and pons): rigid extension of head, neck, back, arms, and legs, with hyperpronation of arms and plantar flexion of feet (see figure 3.19)

c. Diagnostic Tests
  1) lumbar puncture (LP)
    a) description
      - collection of cerebrospinal fluid (CSF), measurement of pressure and characteristics of spinal fluid
      - Queckenstedt's test can be done during LP: with manometer still in place, compress jugular veins for 10 seconds
        - normal response: increase in spinal fluid pressure of approximately 100 mm H$_2$O within 10 seconds and return to normal within 30 seconds after compression is removed
        - abnormal response: drop in spinal fluid pressure or no rise in pressure; indicates complete obstruction of flow of spinal fluid
    b) nursing care
      - explain procedure carefully to client prior to procedure

Figure 3.18 Decorticate Posturing

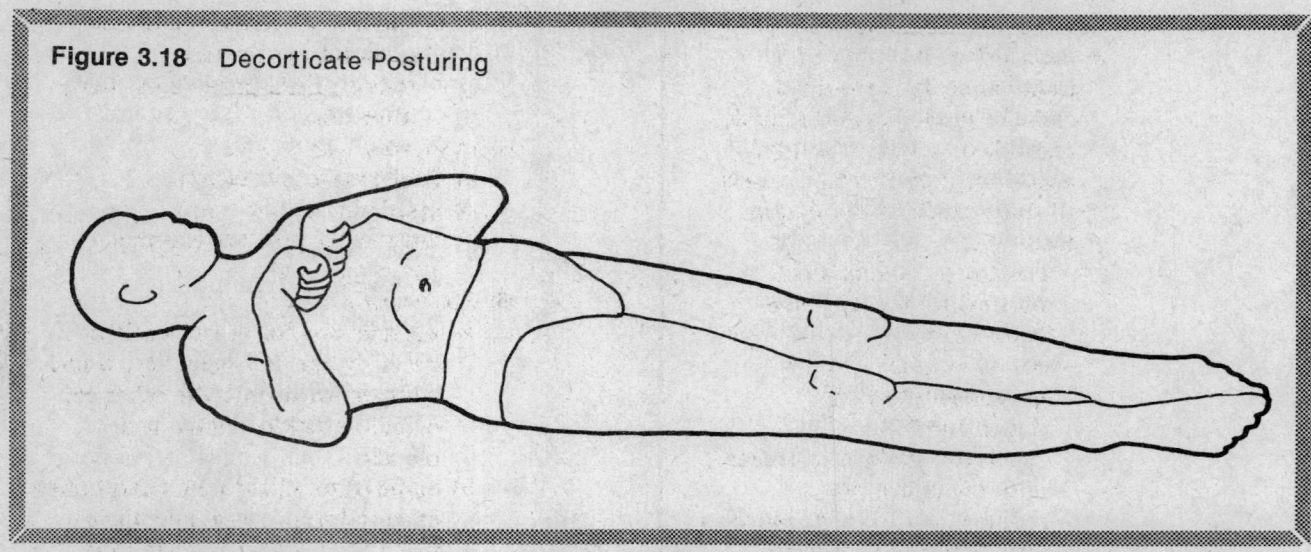

Figure 3.19 Decerebrate Posturing

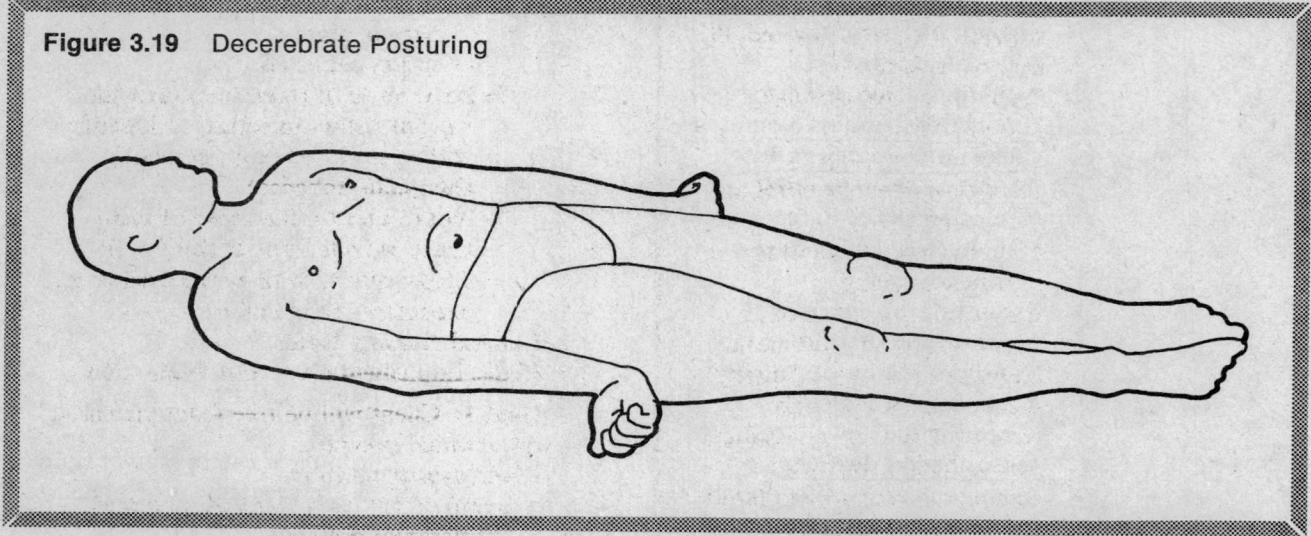

- <u>position client on side with legs flexed onto abdomen and head bent down</u>
- keep client flat in bed up to 24 hours after test to avoid a headache caused by fluid-tension change
- force fluids
- observe for headache
2) radiologic exams
   a) x-rays of skull and spine
   b) computerized axial tomogram (CAT scan)
      - description: 360° photographed view of brain in 1° angles; provides data on integrity of intracranial structures and precise location of abnormalities; used with or without contrast medium
      - nursing care
        - explain procedure to client beforehand
        - client needs to lie still on table for 30–60 minutes
   c) brain scan
      - description: following administration of oral or IV radiopharmaceutical, the head is scanned and uptake of the material is recorded
      - nursing care
        - explain procedure to client
        - reassure about radioactivity

d) cerebral arteriogram
  - description: injection of a radiopaque dye through a catheter inserted into femoral, carotid, or vertebral artery; aortic arch; or brachial vessels to study cerebral circulation
  - nursing care
    - explain procedure and posttest routine to client before test
    - ensure pretest baseline neurologic status is documented
    - check for allergies to iodine and report if present
    - sedate client, remove hairpins and dentures as ordered
    - bed rest 8–24 hours after test with head of bed elevated 30°
    - care of incision
      * check for hemorrhage frequently
      * pressure dressing to incision site if femoral or brachial artery used
      * ice bag may be used to reduce swelling
    - watch for symptoms of sensitivity to dye (urticaria, pallor, respiratory difficulty) and report immediately
    - watch for neurologic changes that indicate emboli in cerebrovascular system (limb weakness or paralysis; facial paralysis; speech difficulty; disorientation; change in level of consciousness) and report immediately
    - observe and record vital signs and neurologic signs per protocol (usually q15min until stable then q1h for several hours, then q4h)
e) ventriculogram
f) pneumoencephalogram
3) electroencephalogram (EEG)
  a) description: study of electrical activity of brain
  b) nursing care
    - give information to client to allay fear of being electrocuted
    - client's hair must be clean before the test
    - client must remain calm and quiet during the test
    - remove EEG paste from hair after test
4) eye tests
  a) Snellen test (eye chart)
  b) ophthalmoscopic exam
  c) intraocular pressure (normal: 12–20 mm Hg)
5) ear/hearing tests
  a) whisper test for gross hearing: cover the ear not being tested and whisper words into the other ear or hold a ticking watch near the ear
  b) audiogram: client wears earphones in soundproof room and signals when tone is heard, when tone disappears, and in which ear the tone is heard
  c) otoscopic exam
6) nose/sense of smell tests: provide various scents for client to identify with eyes closed (e.g., alcohol, chocolate, tobacco)
7) mouth and throat/sense of taste tests: provide various things for client to taste with eyes closed (e.g., chocolate, peppermint)

2. **General Nursing Goals, Plans/Implementation, and Evaluation**

   Goal 1: Client will be free from increased intracranial pressure.
   Plan/Implementation
   - monitor for early signs of increased intracranial pressure
     - changes in level of consciousness
     - vital signs changes
       * BP: widening of pulse pressure
       * rise in temperature
       * bradycardia
       * slow, deep irregular respirations
     - pupils: unequal, progressing to fixed and dilated
     - other clinical signs and symptoms
       * headache (generalized)
       * projectile vomiting
       * papilledema
   - assess at least q15min
   - administer osmotic diuretics (mannitol) as ordered and then monitor urine output qh
   - keep client slightly dehydrated to reduce or prevent cerebral edema

> receptive — can't understand others.
> expressive — can't tell what thinking

- administer corticosteroid therapy, if ordered
- prevent transient increases in intracranial pressure
  - elevate head of bed 15°–30°
  - avoid neck flexion
  - maintain calm environment
  - avoid Valsalva maneuver (straining)
  - administer stool softeners and teach client not to strain with bowel evacuation
  - avoid bending over, coughing, sneezing, or vomiting
  - avoid isometric contraction of muscles, i.e., pushing up in bed on elbows or pressing feet against a footboard

Evaluation: Client's intracranial pressure remains within normal limits (5-10 mm Hg); increase in intracranial pressure is immediately detected.

Goal 2: Client will remain free from complications of unconsciousness.
Plan/Implementation
- prevent contractures and immobile joints, e.g., use range-of-motion exercises
- keep skin clean, dry, and intact
- keep mucous membranes clean, moist, and intact
- maintain adequate bowel and bladder function
- ensure normal respiratory function, e.g., turn client frequently
- provide safe environment, e.g., side rails
- provide adequate nutrition, e.g., tube feedings
- administer feedings per NG tube if in place   *** NG Tube care
  - put client in high-Fowler's position if allowed
  - check to be sure tube is in stomach and not lungs (aspirate stomach contents; inject 5 ml of air while listening with a stethoscope over the gastric area for a swishing sound)
  - give feeding at slow rate
  - observe for regurgitation during and after feeding
  - give feedings at room temperature
  - know that client will probably be given no more than 2 liters/day of a liquid feeding with a concentration of 0.5–1 kilocalorie/ml

- check tissue hydration
- monitor fluid and electrolyte balance
- prevent corneal damage, e.g., use eye patches as needed
- maintain communication with client

Evaluation: Client is free from complications (no contractures, immobile joints, pressure sores, fecal impactions, respiratory distress, injuries, malnutrition, and fluid and electrolyte imbalances).

Goal 3: Client with aphasia will maximize ability to use and understand written and spoken words.
Plan/Implementation
- determine client's level of understanding
- determine client's use of speech or communication skills
- use gestures if client understands that best
- use aids to increase and improve communication: word cards, pictures, slate boards, and audiotapes
- talk slowly, using natural tone (do not abbreviate, reducing sentences to a shorter, incomplete form; it does not help comprehension)
- use simple words and phrases
- allow client time to respond; be patient
- listen and watch carefully when the client attempts to communicate
- keep distractions to a minimum
- maintain a calm, accepting manner
- sit level with client and maintain eye contact
- arrange for referral to speech therapist as needed

Evaluation: Client attempts to communicate using written and spoken words.

Goal 4: Disabled client will become as independent as possible.
Plan/Implementation
- determine client's strengths and deficits
- establish realistic, long-range goals with client and significant other
- devise measures with client to achieve goals
  - institute measures for regaining bowel and bladder control
  - arrange for physical therapy
  - arrange for occupational and recreational therapy
  - encourage client and family to express feelings

Evaluation: Client performs ADL, to extent possible, without assistance.

Goal 5: Client will adapt to blindness.
Plan/Implementation
- call client by name when approaching him
- identify yourself when approaching client
- communicate in usual manner
- teach client
  - how to summon staff
  - where possessions are
  - physical layout of room
  - placement of food on tray
  - arrangement of food on plate
  - use of cane to aid in walking
- provide meaningful sensory input
  - interaction with staff, significant others
  - radio, records, TV
  - physical exercise
- provide safe environment, e.g., remove unnecessary equipment
- refer to appropriate community agencies
- encourage and reinforce client's independence

Evaluation: Client can function in hospital environment without difficulty.

Goal 6: Client will adapt to hearing loss.
Plan/Implementation
- face client when speaking
- keep light on your own face so client can watch your mouth
- speak with normal speech pattern
- allow more time than usual for communication
- assist client to get a hearing aid if appropriate

Evaluation: Client understands conversation.

Selected Health Problems of the Nervous System

A. Acute Head Injury

1. General Information
   a. Clients with acute head trauma need close scrutiny immediately following trauma
   b. Types
      1) concussion: no structural alteration, but immediate and transitory impairment of neurologic function resulting from mechanical force
      2) contusion: structural alteration (bruised cortex) characterized by extravasation of blood
      3) laceration: a tear in brain or blood vessel
      4) hemorrhage
         a) extradural or epidural: arterial blood collects between skull and dura rapidly; usually results from a tear in an artery
            - may lose consciousness and regain it temporarily
            - within few hours, rapid deterioration: lethargy, coma, hemiplegia
         b) subdural: venous bleeding (hematoma) below dura accompanied by manifestations of increased ICP
            - acute: develops within few days after injury; surgical intervention needed
            - subacute: develops between few days to three weeks; surgical intervention follows
            - chronic: develops weeks to months after injury

2. Nursing Process
   a. Assessment: refer to neurologic exam page 288
   b. Goals, Plans/Implementation, and Evaluation

Goal 1: Client will have an open airway at all times.
Plan/Implementation
- establish and maintain airway
- position client for optimum ventilation
- maintain adequate O₂ level through use of respiratory aids as necessary

Evaluation: Client's airway remains unobstructed (color normal; blood gases within normal limits).

Goal 2: Client will be protected from increasing intracranial pressure.
Plan/Implementation: refer to General Nursing Goal 1 page 291.

Goal 3: Client will maintain optimal fluid and electrolyte status.
Plan/Implementation
- monitor and record I&O
- administer IV fluids as ordered (fluids are usually restricted because of fear of increased intracranial pressure)

- give osmotic diuretics (mannitol) as ordered
- monitor serum electrolyte levels

Evaluation: Client's output remains greater than intake.

Goal 4: Client will have any fluid or blood from nose or ears detected.

Plan/Implementation
- observe and record at least qh any leak of blood or clear fluid from nose or ears
- do not pack nose or ear; have fluid drain onto sterile towel or dressing
- report to physician immediately if any drainage is found

Evaluation: Client remains free from fluid or blood leakage from nose and ears.

Goal 5: Client will be free from infection or injuries.

Plan/Implementation
- protect from chilling
- take seizure precautions: padded side rails, nonmetal airway, suction apparatus at bedside
- employ aseptic technique during all invasive procedures
- do not permit visitors with colds

Evaluation: Client remains free from infection; skin and mucous membranes remain free from cuts, ecchymosis, and abrasions.

B. Intracranial Surgery

1. General Information

a. Definitions: surgery performed inside the cranial cavity
  1) craniectomy: removal of part of the skull for the purpose of exposure of the brain to allow surgical procedures. It may be left off immediately after surgery to allow for expansion of cranial contents and replaced at a later time, or it may be replaced at the time of surgery
  2) craniotomy: any operation on the cranium
     a) tentorium: fold of dura mater between cerebellum and occipital lobes
     b) supratentorial: above the cerebellum
     c) infratentorial: posterior cranial fossa
  3) cranioplasty: repair of cranial defect by inserting a bone graft or a plate made of a synthetic substance; protects the brain from trauma

b. Reasons for Surgery
  1) to debride or repair any trauma to the skull and underlying structures
  2) to control intracranial hemorrhage, e.g., aneurysms
  3) to remove space-occupying lesions, e.g., scar tissue, abscess, tumor
  4) intracranial neoplasms
     a) all potentially fatal unless treated, because of lack of space within skull
     b) more than 50% are malignant
     c) types
        - gliomas (within brain substance)
        - meningiomas (external to brain substance)

2. Nursing Process

a. Assessment
  1) establish baseline data (refer to neurologic exam page 288)
  2) client and significant others' knowledge of procedure and expected outcome

b. Goals, Plans/Implementations, and Evaluation

Goal 1: Client and significant others will be able to explain the surgery planned, postoperative care, and OR-RR-ICU environment and care.

Plan/Implementation
- teach regarding type and length of surgery, expected results
- prepare client for the likelihood of periocular edema and photophobia post-op
- explain post-op routine; what the OR-RR-ICU environment looks like

Evaluation: Client and significant others can state type of procedure; can describe postoperative routine.

Goal 2: Client will be physically prepared for surgery.

Plan/Implementation
- refer to *Surgery* page 165
- know that narcotics are contraindicated pre-op
- prepare scalp
  - wash hair
  - cut hair (save according to agency policy); shave scalp

- wash head and cover with clean towel
- carry out any special orders (e.g., insert indwelling Foley catheter, give enemas slowly to avoid straining and increased intracranial pressure)

Evaluation: Client's scalp is prepared for surgery without nicks or cuts.

Goal 3: Client will remain free from respiratory, circulatory, renal, neurologic, or psychologic complications or any infections postoperatively.

Plan/Implementation

(deep breath only)

- refer to *Surgery* page 165
- perform frequent neuro checks; compare with pre-op baseline
- observe for seizures
- monitor breathing; NO COUGHING
- support head when turning client
- position properly and frequently
  - supratentorial craniotomy: do not position on operative site if large tumor was excised; elevate head 45°
  - infratentorial craniotomy: keep head of bed flat and client's head aligned with vertebral column at all times; position on either side for 1st 24 hours, not on back; avoid flexion of neck (danger is brain-stem compression)
- do not suction via nose
- do not use central nervous system depressants, e.g., opiates, sedatives
- check ears, nose, and dressing for drainage (blood/CSF leakage)
- change dressings only when ordered; reinforce as needed
- use strict aseptic technique for all dressings and other procedures
- assess periocular edema; relieve with ice packs
- administer steroids as ordered, e.g., dexamethasone sodium (Decadron) to prevent/relieve cerebral edema
- do not take oral temps
- give passive ROM exercises q8h

Evaluation: Client remains free from complications in the postoperative period.

C. Cerebrovascular Accident (CVA)

1. **General Information**
   a. Definition: severe, sudden decrease in cerebral circulation caused by either a thrombus or hemorrhage resulting in a cerebral infarct (also called a stroke)
   b. Incidence
      1) 3rd leading cause of death in the United States
      2) from 60–69 years: most frequent cause is thrombosis
      3) from 30–60 years: most frequent cause is a ruptured aneurysm with hemorrhage
   c. Symptomology: dependent upon
      1) location of the infarct
      2) amount of collateral circulation to affected area of the brain
   d. Risk Factors
      1) hypertension *majority*
      2) arteriosclerosis/atherosclerosis
      3) intracranial aneurysms
      4) diabetes mellitus
      5) peripheral vascular disease
   e. Etiology
      1) rupture of the wall of a cerebral artery or an aneurysm
      2) trauma to a cerebral artery
      3) severe spasm of the cerebral artery
      4) embolus or thrombus blocking cerebral arterial system

2. **Nursing Process**
   a. Assessment
      1) refer to neurologic exam page 288
      2) hemiplegia (paralysis) or hemiparesis (muscular weakness) of half of body *(contralateral to side of brain)*
      3) aphasia (most common with left cerebral infarct)
      4) ataxia (staggering gait)
      5) nuchal rigidity (with hemorrhage)
      6) perceptual deficit
      7) emotional lability
      8) emotional needs of client/significant others
      9) results of diagnostic studies
         a) CAT scan
         b) lumbar puncture
   b. Goals, Plans/Implementation, and Evaluation

   Goal 1: Client will be free from any additional cerebral damage.

   Plan/Implementation
   - monitor neurologic status frequently until stable
   - do not stimulate cough
   - give passive ROM
   - if thrombus is cause of CVA: administer vasodilators and anticoagulants as ordered

anticoagulants   *BR neuro checks*

Figure 3.20 Areas of the Brain that Control Certain Motor and Sensory Functions

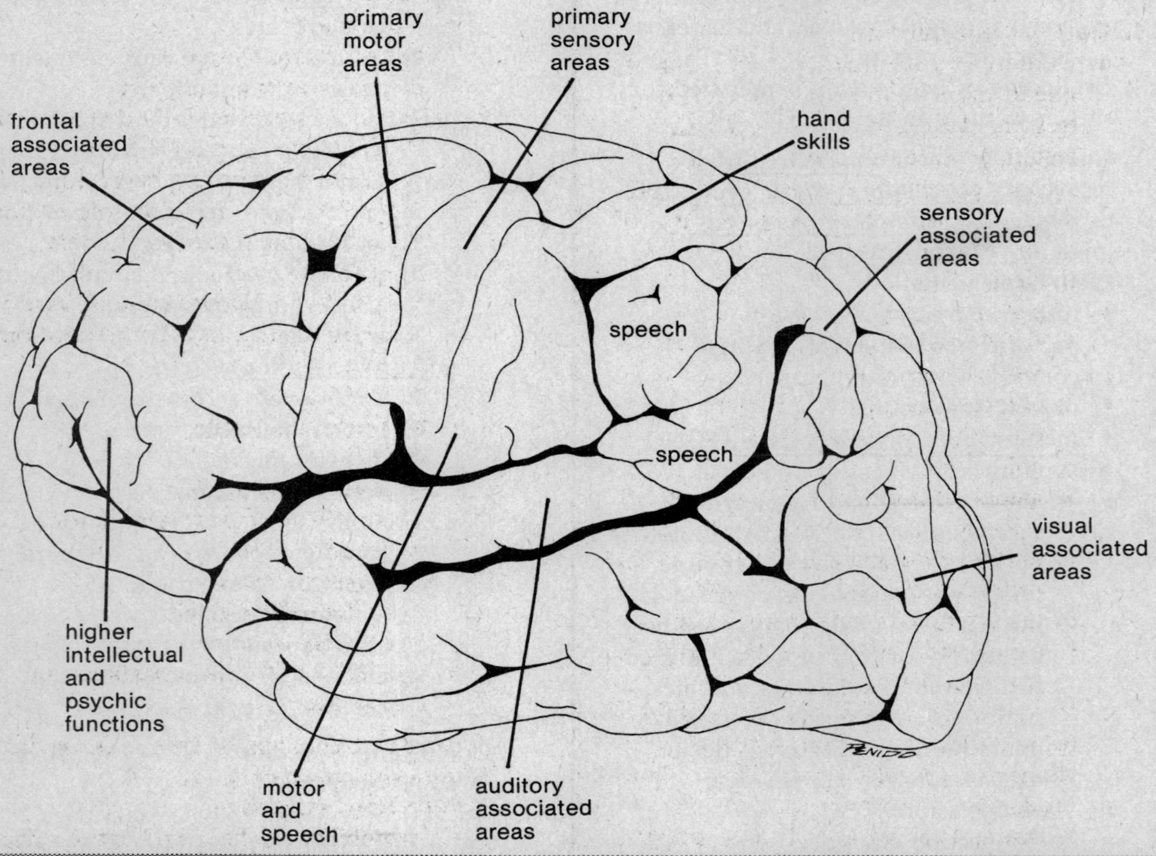

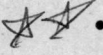

- if hemorrhage is cause of CVA
  - elevate head of bed 30°–45° (to improve venous drainage)
  - turn *gently*
  - decrease environmental stimuli, e.g., keep room semidark
  - maintain complete bed rest until bleeding has been controlled and client's condition is stable

Evaluation: Client's condition remains stable; remains free from additional cerebral damage.

Goal 2: Client will ingest adequate fluids and food.

Plan/Implementation
- help client feed self as needed
- provide adequate fluids to maintain skin turgor and sufficient output
- give small, frequent feedings as indicated (more easily tolerated than 3 large meals)
- administer tube feedings if client is unable to take food and fluids orally (see page 292)
- monitor electrolyte levels

Evaluation: Client's weight remains stable; skin turgor is firm; urinary output is greater than 30 ml/h; urine is clear, straw colored, and free from pus and blood.

Goal 3: If unconscious, client will remain free from complications (refer to General Nursing Goal 2 page 292)

Goal 4: Client will become as independent as possible (refer to General Nursing Goal 4 page 292)

D. Meningitis
(refer to *Nursing Care of the Child* "Safety and Security" page 577)

SAFETY AND SECURITY 297

E. Spinal Cord Injuries
(refer to reprint "The Person with a Spinal Cord Injury" page 354)

1. **General Information**
   a. Definition: fracture or displacement of one or more vertebrae, causing damage to spinal cord and nerve roots with resulting neurologic deficit and altered sensory perception or paralysis or both. There will be total or partial absence of motor and/or sensory function below the level of the injury.
   b. Types of Injuries
      1) fracture of vertebral body (excessive vertical compression)
      2) compression of vertebral body (excessive flexion of vertebral column)
      3) spinal malalignment or vertebral body displacement (rotational injury)
      4) partial or complete dislocation of one vertebra onto another
      5) disruption of intervertebral disk and compressed interspinous ligament (hyperextension injury)
   c. Incidence: an estimated 10,000–20,000 people affected annually; usually a younger age group
   d. Predisposing Factors
      1) trauma: car or motorcycle accidents, falls, or diving accidents
      2) tumors
      3) congenital defects: spina bifida
      4) infectious and degenerative diseases
      5) ruptured intervertebral disks
   e. Immediately after an accident, care must be taken to prevent further damage to the spinal cord while a patent airway and circulation are maintained

2. **Nursing Process**
   a. Assessment
      1) respiratory function
      2) cardiovascular function
      3) loss of sensation in body parts below injury level (see table 3.50)
      4) loss of perspiration below injury level with resultant inability to cool body (autonomic responses become unpredictable)
      5) bowel and bladder control (assess for paralytic ileus and urine retention)
      6) pain
      7) edema
      8) nutritional status
      9) fever
      10) psychologic needs
      11) remaining sensory and motor function
      12) diagnostic tests
         a) neurologic exam
         b) x-ray of spine
   b. Goals, Plans/Implementation, and Evaluation

   Goal 1: Client will be free from further injury to spinal cord.
   Plan/Implementation
   - immobilize the head and entire spine
   - keep client's body and head in even alignment
   - "logroll" if moving client is necessary
   - use specialized equipment for turning: Stryker frame, Foster frame, CircOlectric bed
   - apply cervical traction for cervical lesion

Table 3.50 Spinal Cord

Area of Spinal Cord	Gross Movements Controlled
Upper cervical	Neck and head movement; elevation of the shoulders.
Middle cervical	Movement of the upper arms and forearms; diaphragmatic breathing.
Lower cervical	Movements of fingers and hands.
Thoracic	Intercostal muscles involved in respiration; muscles involved in abdominal contractions.
Upper lumbar	Leg flexion at hip; adduction of thigh.
Lower lumbar	Remaining thigh movements; movements in lower legs.
Sacral	Foot and toe movements; sphincter and perineal muscle contraction.

- know that a laminectomy may be done to prevent further compression of spinal cord
- administer steroids (dexamethasone sodium [Decadron]) or mannitol (osmotic diuretic) IV as ordered, to reduce cerebral edema and edema of spinal cord

Evaluation: Client shows no signs of progression of paralysis; body is maintained in good alignment.

Goal 2: Client will maintain adequate respiratory function.
Plan/Implementation
- observe respirations frequently (client may have spontaneous respirations after an accident but lose them later)
- maintain respiratory function through use of a respirator if necessary
- if respirations are spontaneous, have client deep breathe and cough qh
- care for and suction tracheostomy tube if in place

Evaluation: Client's respirations remain within normal limits; respirator continues to maintain client's respirations.

Goal 3: Client will be free from undetected spinal shock.
Plan/Implementation
- expect spinal shock to develop 30–60 minutes postinjury and to last 2–3 days to 3 months
- observe for
  - hypotension
  - dyspnea
  - flaccid paralysis
  - urinary retention
  - absence of sweating
- administer colloid fluids and analgesics prn as ordered

Evaluation: Client's spinal shock is detected.

Goal 4: Client's fluid and electrolyte balance will remain within desired range.
Plan/Implementation
- observe qh for signs of fluid and electrolyte balance until stable and then q4–8h
- replace fluids and electrolytes as needed

Evaluation: Client's fluid and electrolytes are in desired balance; has had any imbalance detected and corrected immediately.

Goal 5: Client with cervical or high-thoracic injury will remain free from autonomic dysreflexia.
Plan/Implementation
- observe for
  - rapidly increasing BP
  - bradycardia
  - severe headache
  - flushing
  - profuse sweating
  - goose pimples
- prevention
  - prevent bowel and bladder distention (chief causes of this phenomenon)
  - observe urinary drainage from catheter frequently
  - prevent pressure sores, pain in lower extremities, or pressure on penis or testes when client is in prone position
- remedial
  - initiate treatment immediately (medical emergency)
  - remove the cause
  - check the bladder for distention
  - elevate head of bed to lower blood pressure
  - look for sources other than bladder distention (e.g., cold air, drafts, sharp objects pressing on skin below level of injury)
  - administer ganglionic-blocking agents as ordered

Evaluation: Client remains free from signs of autonomic dysreflexia; bowel and bladder functions are maintained.

Goal 6: Client will ingest adequate fluids and nutrition.
Plan/Implementation
- give liquid diet until possibility of paralytic ileus has passed, then diet as tolerated
- administer vitamin supplements as ordered
- encourage fluid intake
- monitor I&O

Evaluation: Client's weight remains within desired range; skin turgor is firm.

Goal 7: Client will be free from urinary tract infection.
Plan/Implementation
- insert Foley catheter or use intermittent catheterization as ordered, using sterile technique
- give aseptic care to Foley catheter

- observe client for signs of bladder infection (e.g., fever; abnormal UA, urine C&S)
- encourage fluid intake to 3 liters/day
- observe odor, appearance, and amount of urine
- monitor I&O carefully

Evaluation: Client's urine remains free from signs of infection; no fever; draining 30 ml urine/hour via Foley catheter.

Goal 8: Client will be free from stress ulcer.

Plan/Implementation
- monitor for complaints of ulcerlike pain
- observe for melena, hematemesis
- administer antacids frequently as ordered, to prevent gastric irritation

Evaluation: Client remains free from signs and symptoms of stress ulcer.

Goal 9: Client will be free from pain in paralyzed limbs.

Plan/Implementation
- handle the affected limbs gently to avoid muscle spasms
- identify and eliminate stimuli that cause spasms
- medicate as ordered, to control spasms and pain

Evaluation: Client experiences relief of pain.

Goal 10: Client will become as independent as possible (refer to General Nursing Goal 4 page 292).

F. Parkinson's Disease (Parkinsonism)

1. **General Information**
   a. Definition: a progressive debilitating disease in which there is degeneration of nerve cells in the basal ganglia that impairs
      1) important centers of coordination, especially control of associated automatic movements
      2) control of muscle tone to produce finely coordinated movements
      3) control of initiation and inhibition of gross, intentional movements
   b. Incidence: one of the major causes of neurologic disability; estimated to affect more than a half-million people in the United States
   c. Onset: usually 50–60 years of age
   d. Etiology
      1) Etiology unknown ↓ Dopamine
      2) it is hypothesized that these clients have a deficiency of dopamine, which is required for normal functioning of the basal ganglia; drug therapy aims at returning dopamine levels to normal to control symptoms of the disease
   e. Precipitating Factors
      1) drug-induced: phenothiazines and Rauwolfia alkaloids
      2) atherosclerosis
      3) trauma, e.g., midbrain compression
      4) encephalitis
      5) toxic poisoning: carbon monoxide

2. **Nursing Process**
   a. Assessment
      1) muscle rigidity
         a) major disability
         b) bradykinesia and akinesia
      2) tremors at rest (nonintentional)
         a) especially of hands (pill rolling), arms, and head
         b) rhythmic: regular and rapid
      3) facial mask
      4) speech difficulty
      5) loss of automatic movements, e.g., blinking of eyes
      6) propulsive gait, shuffling in nature
      7) emotional changes (mood disturbances), depression, and confusion
      8) autonomic nervous system dysfunction
         a) decreased salivation
         b) perspiration
         c) lacrimation
         d) constipation
         e) incontinence
         f) decreased sexual activity
   b. Goals, Plans/Implementation, and Evaluation

Goal 1: Client will have optimal function of muscles and joints.

Plan/Implementation
- arrange for physical therapy
- administer prescribed medications (see table 3.51) Antiparkison.
- observe for side effects of medications
- assist client to remain as active as possible
   - frequent ambulation
   - ADL
   - attention to grooming

Table 3.51 Antiparkinsonian Drugs *loose effectiveness over time*

Description	Drugs that increase the level of dopamine in the CNS. They are often given in conjunction with anticholinergics, since cholinergic activity is increased when a deficit of dopamine exists.
Uses	Control of symptoms of Parkinson's disease
Side Effects	Nausea, vomiting, anorexia, orthostatic hypotension, dry mouth, dysphagia, ataxia, headache, insomnia, anxiety, urinary retention
Nursing Implications	Use cautiously in clients with cardiovascular, respiratory, endocrine, or hepatic disease; peptic ulcers; wide-angle glaucoma; diabetes; psychosis.
Examples	Levodopa (Larodopa), levodopa and carbidopa (Sinemet), amantadine (Symmetrel)

Evaluation: Client maintains movement in muscles and joints; continues to ambulate and participate in ADL.

Goal 2: Client will be free from injury.
Plan/Implementation
- use ambulatory aids such as handrails in all rooms and near bathtub or shower
- instruct client to walk slowly and carefully
- balance activity and rest to avoid fatigue

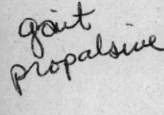
gait propulsive

Evaluation: Client is free from cuts, abrasions, and falls; has balance of activity and rest.

Goal 3: Client will maintain gastrointestinal integrity.
Plan/Implementation
- provide adequate fluid intake
- give high fiber diet
- watch for constipation
- administer stool softeners or laxatives as ordered, prn
- give oral hygiene to relieve dryness of the mouth
- keep urinal and bedpan handy in case client is unable to reach bathroom in time

Evaluation: Client is free from constipation and impactions; has adequate bowel function.

Goal 4: Client will maintain positive body image/self-concept.
Plan/Implementation
- provide assistive devices to make ADL easier
- teach about/provide clothes that are simple and easy to put on
- allow sufficient time for meals
- in general, do *not* hurry client
- supervise and assist in skin care and personal hygiene
- allow expression of depression and hopelessness
- reward attempts at activity that the client makes
- arrange for speech therapy for dysarthria

Evaluation: Client's grooming projects positive self-concept; accepts responsibility for ADL to the extent possible.

Goal 5: Client and significant others will express fears and other feelings about present and future.
Plan/Implementation
- set aside time to talk to client and significant others
- allow them to express feelings and ask questions
- convey that feelings expressed are all right to have, are usual and expected
- explain disease and drug therapy
- clarify misconceptions and lack of information
- explain prognosis

Evaluation: Client and significant others express feelings (e.g., fear, sadness, anger); can state what to expect in the future.

G. Multiple Sclerosis   *Does not occur at equator*

1. **General Information**
   a. Definition: chronic progressive disease of the central nervous system characterized by unpredictable exacerbations and remissions; typically demyelinization of the white matter of

the spinal cord and brain occurs in multiple areas
  b. Incidence
    1) disease of young adults
    2) more common in women
  c. Risk Factors
    1) living in the temperate zone 40°–60° north or south of the equator
    2) higher incidence among higher socioeconomic classes
  d. Etiology
    1) unknown
    2) may be a virus that is latent for months or years before some other factor initiates disease
    3) possibly an autoimmune disorder
    4) mineral deficiency, toxic substances
2. **Nursing Process**
  a. Assessment
    1) at onset: vague symptoms
      a) diplopia
      b) awkwardness in handling articles and frequent dropping of articles
      c) stumbling or falling with no apparent cause
    2) symptoms vary depending on location of myelin or nerve fiber destruction
      a) classic symptoms include
        - nystagmus (rapid, involuntary movements of eyes)
        - intention tremors, absent at rest
        - scanning speech (slow enunciation with tendency to hesitate at beginning of a word or syllable, speech with pauses between syllables)
      b) sensory disorders
        - paresthesias (numbness, tingling, "dead" feeling, "pins and needles")
        - diminished vibration sense
        - impaired proprioception
      c) visual disorders
        - optic neuritis
        - diplopia
        - scotomata (blind spots)
      d) motor disorders: spastic weakness or paralysis of limbs
      e) cerebellar dysfunction: cerebellar ataxia
      f) bowel and bladder dysfunction
        - hesitancy, urgency, frequency
        - retention, incontinence
        - constipation

g) emotional disorders
  - euphoria
  - mood swings
3) long-term effects of progressive disease
  a) spasticity
  b) paraplegia
  c) speech defects
  d) eating difficulties
  e) extreme fatigue
  f) vision difficulties
  g) complete paralysis
  b. Goals, Plans/Implementation, and Evaluation

Goal 1: Client will have optimal function of muscles and joints.
Plan/Implementation
- arrange for physical therapy (muscle stretching and strengthening)
- assist with gait retraining if ataxic
- encourage client to remain active and to do as many ADL as possible

Evaluation: Client's joints and muscles are functioning well; can participate in ADL.

Goal 2: Client will maintain health-promoting habits in daily living.
Plan/Implementation
- determine and encourage optimal activity level
-  promote adequate rest periods to prevent exhaustion
- use safety devices such as hand rails and walkers to prevent falls
- maintain good nutrition and fluid intake
- supply self-help devices for eating, ambulation, reading
- provide pain medication and muscle relaxants as ordered
- attend to incontinence and pressure areas to maintain integrity of skin and mucous membranes
- make referral to community agencies (e.g., VNA, local branch of National Multiple Sclerosis Society) to help client/significant others in long-term management
- educate client/significant others about these aspects of care

Evaluation: Client maintains good personal hygiene; eats a nutritious, well-balanced diet.

Goal 3: Client will maintain positive body image/self-concept.

Plan/Implementation
- provide assistive devices to make ADL easier
- promote as much independence in client as possible; teach significant others to do the same
- encourage hobbies and other pleasurable distractions
- do *not* hurry client
- supervise and assist in skin care and personal hygiene
- reward client's attempts at activity
- encourage and reinforce perseverance and hope
- help client identify realistic goals

Evaluation: Client's grooming projects positive self-image; can perform ADL within own limits.

Goal 4: Client and significant others will express fears about present and future.

Plan/Implementation
- set aside time to talk to client and significant others, together and separately
- encourage expression of feelings
- convey that it is OK to express feelings
- clarify misconceptions and lack of information about present and prognosis
- allow expression of depression and hopelessness
- emphasize what the client can still do

Evaluation: Client and significant others can express fear about the disease; can state what to expect in the future.

Goal 5: Client and significant others will learn to cope with illness-related problems and prevent complications.

Plan/Implementation
- teach client/significant others information discussed in Goals 1 and 2
- evaluate knowledge and skills that client/significant others have and go over areas where they have not retained information
- continue to teach and evaluate knowledge and skills related to Goals 1 and 2

Evaluation: Client and significant others have knowledge of care needed because of disabilities; can explain how to avoid complications related to disabilities.

H. Epilepsy

1. General Information
a. Definition: chronic brain dysfunction manifested by recurrent seizures
b. Incidence
   1) 1 out of every 200 for general population, or 2–4 million in the United States
   2) for 80%–85% of people with epilepsy, condition can be controlled by medication and they can lead normal lives
c. Etiology: in most cases unknown
d. Predisposing Factors
   1) heredity: higher incidence in children of epileptics
   2) birth injury or anoxia
   3) metabolic and chemical imbalance
   4) increased intracranial pressure
   5) age: before 4 and after 60
e. Types of Seizures
   1) *petit mal:* abrupt, brief lapse of consciousness; vacant stare or brief pause in conversation; most common in children
   2) *focal motor or sensory seizures:* arise in motor and/or sensory areas of brain
      - Jacksonian: discharge of impulses in the motor area of the brain that spreads to adjacent areas
      - paresthesias: abnormal sensation, numbness; visual, auditory, olfactory, or gustatory (taste) distortion
   3) *psychomotor seizures (automatisms):* automatic behavior without volition; often associated with temporal lobe dysfunction
   4) *grand mal:* generalized type of seizure characterized by loss of consciousness for several minutes with tonic and clonic types of motor activity
   5) *status epilepticus:* recurrent seizures occurring at such frequency that full consciousness is not regained between seizures

2. Nursing Process
a. Assessment
   1) aura or symptoms that occur before seizures
   2) character of the seizure (grand mal)

a) loss of consciousness that persists for several minutes
b) bilateral tonic contractions with transitory cessation of respiration
c) next follows a series of clonic contractions (muscle groups alternately contract and relax); shallow and irregular breathing returns
d) fecal and urinary incontinence may occur during clonic phase
e) relaxation of muscles, partial consciousness regained, improved color
f) no memory of seizure
g) sleepiness follows seizure
3) history of seizures
4) emotional needs of client and family

b. Goals, Plans/Implementation, and Evaluation

Goal 1: Client will be free from injuries during seizure.

Plan/Implementation
- maintain patent airway; insert padded tongue blade in mouth *before* convulsion begins if possible
- remove dangerous objects that client may fall against
- pad side rails
- have suction equipment available
- observe and chart characteristics of seizure
  - occurrence of aura
  - onset (site of initial movement, head and eye positions, posture of body, chewing movements, LOC)
  - progression of movement through body
  - skin color
  - pupillary changes
  - occurrence of incontinence
  - LOC
  - duration
- observe and chart client's condition during postictal phase
  - duration
  - LOC
  - injuries
  - behavior
- administer anticonvulsant medications, as ordered (see table 3.52)

Evaluation: Client remained free from abrasions, bruises, and tongue injuries.

Goal 2: Client and significant others will learn how to cope with problems commonly associated with epilepsy.

Plan/Implementation
- teach how to take drugs, to take them regularly, and common side effects
- encourage regular ADL: eating, activities, rest and sleep; avoid alcohol, stress
- obtain counseling and vocational rehabilitation for job training: there are

---

Table 3.52 Anticonvulsants

Description	A wide variety of drugs that act to decrease nerve cell excitability in various ways
Uses	Treatment of epilepsy and other seizure disorders
Side Effects	GI irritation, dizziness, apathy, nervousness, ataxia, gum hyperplasia (phenytoin), blurred vision
Nursing Implications	Teach client to comply with consistent medication regimen; avoid use of alcohol; warn about drowsiness or decreased alertness; give with meals to decrease GI distress.
Types and Examples	*Anticonvulsant Barbiturates:* phenobarbital, primidone (Mysoline) *Hydantoins:* phenytoin (Dilantin), mephenytoin (Mesantoin), ethotoin (Peganone) *Oxazolidinediones:* paramethadione (Paradione), trimethadione (Tridione) *Succinimides:* ethosuximide (Zarontin), methsuximide (Celontin), phensuximide (Milontin) *Miscellaneous:* carbamazepine (Tegretol), phenacemide (Phenurone), clonazepam (Clonopin), valproic acid (Depakene), magnesium sulfate

certain jobs the person with idiopathic epilepsy may not be able to carry out
- refer client/significant others to community agencies as needed
  - American Epilepsy Foundation
  - National Epilepsy League
- teach client and significant others what to do if seizure occurs
- have client carry medical ID to inform strangers of what to do if seizure occurs
- assist the person to identify the specific stimuli that precipitate seizures (e.g., illness, emotional stress, physical stress, hyperventilation, sensory stimuli, stimulants like caffeine and amphetamine, flickering lights)
- tell client to report any change in health status to physician (e.g., bleeding gums, jaundice)

Evaluation: Client/significant others can state what to do if seizure occurs; client has obtained a medical ID bracelet.

Goal 3: Client with status epilepticus will maintain respiratory function and adequate ventilation and will have the convulsions brought under control.

Plan/Implementation
- establish airway between seizures
- provide O₂
- monitor vital and neurologic signs
- monitor blood gases (to detect hypoxia of brain) between seizures
- administer IV anticonvulsant medications immediately as ordered

Evaluation: Client's oxygenation is adequate (no cyanosis, nailbeds pink); seizures have ceased.

I. Myasthenia Gravis

1. **General Information**
   a. Definition: a chronic, progressive neuromuscular disorder characterized by rapid exhaustion of voluntary muscles owing to a defect at the myoneural junction
   b. Pathophysiology: transmission of impulse from nerve to muscle is impaired because of inadequate acetylcholine at the myoneural junction; contractions of voluntary muscles become progressively weaker and cease when the muscle is stimulated
   c. Etiology
      1) unknown
      2) possibly an autoimmune disorder
      3) client may have a genetic predisposition

2. **Nursing Process**
   a. Assessment
      1) onset of symptoms insidious and gradual
      2) progressive voluntary-muscle weakness
      3) incapacitating fatigue
      4) ocular symptoms: ptosis, inability to open eyes, diplopia

Table 3.53	Cholinergics
Description	Drugs that mimic the effects of cholinergic nerve stimulation and produce a response similar to acetylcholine
Uses	Glaucoma (miotic), urinary retention, post-op abdominal distention, myasthenia gravis, antidote for curare
Side Effects	Headache, conjunctival hyperemia (ocular preparations only), urinary urgency, severe hypotension, bronchospasm, respiratory paralysis, cholinergic crisis.
Nursing Implications	Administer ophthalmic preparations on time; note CNS irritability; monitor vital signs; have atropine available as antidote; avoid IV or IM use (may cause severe hypotension).
Types and Examples	*Direct-Acting Cholinomimetics:* acetylcholine (Miochol); carbachol, carbacel, bethanechol (Urecholine); pilocarpine (Almocarpine) *Indirect-Acting Cholinomimetics:* physostigmine (Antilirium), demecarium bromide (Humorsol), neostigmine methylsulfate (Prostigmin), endrophonium (Tensilon), pyridostigmine bromide (Mestinon), isoflurophate (Floropryl)

SAFETY AND SECURITY

5) expressionless appearance with facial muscle involvement; characteristic "snarl" when client attempts to smile
6) respiratory distress
7) diagnostic test: positive Tensilon test (anticholinesterase): edrophonium chloride (Tensilon) injected IV produces increase in strength

b. Goals, Plans/Implementation, and Evaluation

Goal 1: Client will have control of voluntary muscles.
Plan/Implementation
- administer anticholinesterase medications to control symptoms, e.g., neostigmine methylsulfate (Prostigmin), pyridostigmine bromide (Mestinon); see table 3.53
- administer medications on individually adjusted schedule

Evaluation: Client has control of voluntary muscles.

Goal 2: Client will remain free from respiratory impairment.
Plan/Implementation
- observe respiratory status
- use postural drainage; turn frequently
- give prophylactic antibiotics to prevent respiratory infections
- instruct client to avoid exposure to people with URIs
- teach client diaphragmatic breathing exercises, to maintain strength with maximum ventilation and minimum energy expenditure
- balance physical activities with rest
- put client in a rocking bed
- know that client may require mechanical ventilation

Evaluation: Client's lungs are clear; no respiratory distress noted.

Goal 3: Client will remain well nourished.
Plan/Implementation
- give anticholinesterase medications, e.g., pyridostigmine bromide (Mestinon) 20–30 minutes before meals for full advantage
- provide small, frequent, semisolid, or fluid meals that are nutritious and high in potassium (adequate serum levels of potassium potentiate anticholinesterase effect)
- provide IV or NG feedings if needed
- have suction equipment available
- allow client to eat meals without rushing
- observe for anorexia, nausea, diarrhea, abdominal cramping (common side effects of anticholinesterase drugs)

Evaluation: Client's weight remains stable.

Goal 4: Client will receive psychologic and rehabilitative support.
Plan/Implementation
- evaluate client and significant others' attitudes toward and knowledge of disease
- provide careful explanations of disorder

Table 3.54 Anticholinergics

Description	Drugs that act as competitive antagonists at cholinergic-receptor sites, thereby blocking the action of acetylcholine
Uses	To produce mydriasis; pre-op to decrease salivation and prevent bradycardia; decrease GI motility; antiparkinsonian; decrease nasopharyngeal and bronchial secretions
Side Effects	Blurred vision, photophobia, urinary hesitancy, increased intraocular pressure, palpitations, flushing, tachycardia, allergic reaction, restlessness
Nursing Implications	Contraindicated in clients with glaucoma, GI obstruction, benign prostatic hypertrophy, renal or hepatic disease; caution client against driving; warn client about usual side effects; monitor vital signs; give 30 minutes before meals.
Examples	Atropine, scopolamine, belladonna extract, benztropine (Cogentin), clidinium bromide (Quarzan), dicyclomine HCl (Bentyl), methantheline bromide (Banthine), oxybutynin chloride (Ditropan), propantheline bromide (Pro-Banthine), trihexyphenidyl HCl (Artane), hyoscyamine sulfate (Cystospaz), phenylephrine (Neo-Synephrine)

306 SECTION 3: NURSING CARE OF THE ADULT

- offer opportunities for expressions of feelings
- promote a balance of rest and activities
- encourage healthy life-style
- refer to Myasthenia Gravis Foundation for information and support

Evaluation: Client expresses positive outlook for future; has a plan for balancing activities with adequate rest periods.

Goal 5: Client remains free from an undetected "cholinergic" crisis.
Plan/Implementation
- know that a "cholinergic crisis" (medical emergency) occurs when client cannot tolerate the dosage of anticholinesterase medications
- carefully monitor vital signs, including pupil checks, of client receiving increasing doses of anticholinesterases
- observe for dramatic increase in myasthenic symptoms accompanied by severe diarrhea, nausea and vomiting, hypersalivation, pallor, lacrimation, miosis, hypotension
- discontinue medications and give IV anticholinergic drug as ordered, e.g., atropine

Evaluation: Client is free from symptoms of cholinergic crisis (no diarrhea, pallor).

Selected Health Problems of the Sensory System

A. Cataracts

1. **General Information**
    a. Definition: total or partial opacity of the normally transparent crystalline lens; the opacity of the lens interferes with light passage through the lens to the retina
    b. Etiology: unknown
    c. Risk Factors
        1) aging: onset usually after age 55
        2) diabetes mellitus
        3) intraocular surgery
        4) previous injury to the eye
        5) prolonged treatment of glaucoma with topical preparations
        6) radiation of the head for cancer
        7) possibly steroid therapy
    d. Medical Treatment: surgical removal of lens
        1) intracapsular extraction most common
        2) extraction by cryosurgery
        3) partial iridectomy done with lens extraction to prevent acute glaucoma
        4) possible lens implantation

2. **Nursing Process**
    a) Assessment
        1) distortion of vision
        2) absence of red reflex (the red reflection seen when the retina is viewed through an ophthalmoscope)
        3) gradual and painless loss of vision
        4) knowledge of treatment modalities
        5) knowledge of posttreatment course of recovery
    b. Goals, Plans/Implementation, and Evaluation

    Goal 1: Client will be able to explain preoperative care, the treatment planned, postoperative care, and the OR-RR environment.
    Plan/Implementation
    - teach client and significant others before surgery
        - about planned surgery
        - type of anesthetic: frequently a local
        - procedure to be followed in OR-RR
        - post-op procedures
            * bed position varies with type of surgery (usually head of bed up 30°)
            * no turning or turn only to unaffected side post-op
            * how to use call bell
            * bed rails up at all times
            * keep hands away from eyes to prevent infection
            * ROM exercise routine
    - review client knowledge
    - continue to explain areas client does not understand

    Evaluation: Client can state plan of treatment and postoperative care; can explain what will happen in OR-RR.

    Goal 2: Client will be able, preoperatively, to explain how to prevent increasing intraocular pressure.
    Plan/Implementation
    - teach client before surgery
        - no straining
        - no coughing or sneezing
        - no bending
        - to prevent vomiting
        - no squeezing shut of eyelids
    - evaluate client knowledge after teaching

- continue to explain areas client does not remember or understand

Evaluation: Client can explain how to prevent increased intraocular pressure.

Goal 3: Client will remain free from postoperative complications.
Plan/Implementation
- refer to *Surgery* "Perioperative Care" page 165
- provide adequate fluids
- deep breathe qh, no coughing
- turn only to *unaffected* side, if turning is permitted
- check dressing frequently for bleeding (q15min for 2h, then qh for 8h)
- prevent increased intraocular pressure
- give antiemetics prn
- observe and report severe eye pain

Evaluation: Client's vital signs are stable; has no complaints of pain; observes postoperative activity restrictions.

Goal 4: Client will know the characteristics of the type of lenses or glasses to be worn for optimal vision.
Plan/Implementation
- teach according to client's situation
  - cataract glasses (wear old glasses until curvature changes are complete: 12–14 weeks post-op)
    * magnify objects 1/3
    * clear vision only through center
  - contact lenses (less vision distortion than glasses; more costly)
  - intraocular lens
    * synthetic lens implanted into eye
    * designed for distance vision
    * for near vision, needs corrective glasses
- discuss with client a plan for obtaining new glasses or lenses

Evaluation: Client can explain type of protective eyewear prescribed.

Goal 5: Client will be discharged with a written rehabilitation plan and a physician's appointment for follow-up.
Plan/Implementation
- develop a plan for client to follow that explains
  - progressively increased exercise
  - return to sexual activity
  - driving
  - bending, stooping, and lifting restrictions
  - dressing changes, eye meds as required

prevent constipation

- instruct significant others in dressing change and medication administration
- secure physician or clinic appointment for client

Evaluation: Client can state activity limitations upon discharge; significant others can administer eye meds correctly.

B. Retinal Detachment

1. **General Information**
   a. Definition: actual splitting of the retina between the rod and cone layers of the retina and the pigment epithelial layer. Partial separation becomes complete (if untreated) with subsequent total loss of vision.
   b. Pathophysiology: vitreous humor seeps through opening and separates retina from pigment epithelium and choroid. Blindness results.
   c. Types
      1) primary: from a break in the continuity of retina
      2) secondary: from intraocular disorders (e.g., post-cataract extraction, perforating injuries, severe myopia)
   d. Early surgical repair imperative to avoid irreparable damage and irreversible blindness

2. **Nursing Process**
   a. Assessment
      1) gradual or sudden onset
      2) sudden flashes of light
      3) blurred vision that becomes progressively worse
      4) loss of portion of visual field
      5) ophthalmologic examination: retina hangs like a grey cloud; one or more tears

   immed. bed rest

   b. Goals, Plans/Implementation, and Evaluation

   Goal 1: Client will be able to explain preoperative preparation, surgical treatment, planned postoperative care, and the OR-RR environment.
   Plan/Implementation
   - apply bilateral eye patches pre-op
   - protect client from injury
   - minimize stress on eye (e.g., avoid sneezing, coughing, sudden jarring)
   - explain surgical procedure
   - instill pre-op meds as ordered (cycloplegics, mydriatics)
   - teach client post-op positions, care

308 SECTION 3: NURSING CARE OF THE ADULT

Evaluation: Client can explain surgical plan, pre- and postoperative care, and the OR-RR environment.

Goal 2: refer to "Cataracts" Goal 2 page 306.

Goal 3: Client will recover free from postoperative complications.
Plan/Implementation
- refer to *Surgery* page 165
- avoid prone position ↑ pressure *[miotics contraindicated]*
- speak before approaching client
- check eye patches frequently
- give antiemetics, analgesics prn

Evaluation: Client's condition is stable; client is free from postoperative complications.

Goal 4: Client will be discharged with a plan for rehabilitation.
Plan/Implementation
- inform client of activities upon discharge
  - may watch television
  - avoid reading for 2–3 weeks
  - continue to avoid straining, injury to head
  - may shave, comb hair, bathe, and ambulate
- if pinhole glasses are prescribed, provide client with instructions for use

Evaluation: Client can state activities and limitations upon discharge.

C. Glaucoma

1. **General Information**
   a. Definition: abnormal increase in intraocular pressure caused by any obstruction of the outflow channels of aqueous humor; uncontrolled glaucoma causes irreversible blindness as a result of atrophy of the optic nerve
   b. Types
      1) *chronic* (wide angle): most common
         a) resistance to flow because of thickening of collecting channels, trabecular network, and canal of Schlemm
         b) insidious onset characterized by a decrease in peripheral vision
      2) *acute* (narrow angle) *[Don't need to know diff.]*
         a) occurs when iris is abnormally structured in an anterior position
         b) exerts pressure on collecting channels and decreases size of anterior chamber
         c) sudden onset characterized by severe eye pain and rapid loss of vision
   c. Risk Factors
      1) heredity
      2) trauma
      3) tumor or inflammation of the eye
      4) vascular disorders
      5) diabetes
      6) prior eye surgery
   d. Other Information
      1) one of leading causes of blindness
      2) early detection is crucial (vision destroyed by optic nerve atrophy cannot be restored)
      3) regular eye exams that include tonometry (measure of intraocular pressure) are recommended for persons over age 35

2. **Nursing Process**
   a. **Assessment**
      1) loss of peripheral vision; loss of central vision with progression
      2) halos around lights
      3) difficulty adjusting to dark rooms
      4) difficulty focusing on close work
      5) increased intraocular pressure (normal = 12–20 mm Hg)
      6) client's support system
      7) client's and significant others' coping mechanisms
   b. **Goals, Plans/Implementation, and Evaluation**

Goal 1: Client's intraocular pressure will remain within normal limits.
Plan/Implementation
- teach client
  - how to instill eyedrops correctly *[goes conjunctiva]*
  - how miotic eyedrops decrease intraocular pressure, e.g., pilocarpine (see table 3.53)
  - that emotional or stressful events can increase intraocular pressure
  - to avoid lifting, shoveling, wearing constrictive clothing around the neck

Evaluation: Client's intraocular pressure remains between 12-20 mm Hg.

Goal 2: Client will be free from further visual impairment.
Plan/Implementation
- impress upon client that ocular damage that has already occurred is not reversible, but further visual impairment can be prevented by compliance with prescribed regimen

- emphasize importance of routine eye exams

Evaluation: Client develops no further visual impairment.

D. **Nasal Problems Requiring Surgery**
   1. **General Information**
      a. Definition: bone and soft tissue deformities requiring corrective surgery (usually under local anesthesia)
      b. Precipitating Factors
         1) fracture
         2) tumor
         3) foreign body
         4) deviated septum
         5) polyps
         6) cosmetic problems
      c. Types of Surgery
         1) submucous resection (rhinoplasty)
         2) reduction of a nasal fracture
         3) removal of polyps, tumors, foreign bodies
   2. **Nursing Process**
      a. Assessment
         1) nasal obstruction
         2) pain (fractures)
         3) nasal congestion
         4) bleeding
         5) allergies
         6) self-concept/body image
      b. Goals, Plans/Implementation, and Evaluation

      Goal 1: Client, significant others will understand planned surgery and postoperative care.
      Plan/Implementation
      - teach client and significant others about
        - mouth breathing post-op
        - local anesthesia
        - no nose blowing
        - Fowler's position
        - post-op appearance (black eyes, dressing)
        - ice packs
      - explain procedure

      Don't blow nose after surgery

      Evaluation: Client and significant others can explain the surgery and postoperative course.

      Goal 2: Client will remain free from any postoperative complications.
      Plan/Implementation
      - refer to *Surgery* page 165
      - provide adequate fluids
      - deep breathe qh
      - medicate for pain prn
      - observe for frequent swallowing (hemorrhage)
      - check dressing frequently for bleeding
      - change gauze pad under nose when saturated and note amount of bleeding
      - apply ice continuously to the area for 1st 24 hours
      - give frequent oral hygiene
      - maintain Fowler's position to prevent aspiration

      Evaluation: Client remains free from complications (vital signs are within normal limits; minimal periorbital edema and discoloration).

E. **Epistaxis** — *Nasal Bleeding*
   1. **General Information**
      a. Definition: nose bleed
      b. Risk Factors
         1) trauma
         2) hypertension
         3) acute sinusitis
         4) deviated nasal septum
         5) nasal surgery
   2. **Nursing Process**
      a. Assessment
         1) bleeding from nose
         2) frequent swallowing
         3) bright red vomitus

         Changes VSS can be drastic.

      b. Goals, Plans/Implementation, and Evaluation

      Goal 1: Client will experience control of epistaxis.
      Plan/Implementation
      - utilize first-aid interventions: direct pressure, Fowler's position, ice pack
      - know that cautery may be used
      - monitor anterior and/or posterior nasal packing (removed in 48–96 hours to prevent infection)
      - give vasoconstrictors as ordered, e.g., topical phenylephrine HCl (Neo-Synephrine)
      - observe frequently for bleeding

      Evaluation: Client remains free from any further bleeding from nose.

      Goal 2: Client will remain free from future attacks.
      Plan/Implementation
      - teach client and significant others first-aid measures in event of future attack
      - demonstrate proper nasal care
      - help client identify precipitating factors
      - monitor BP for hypertension

freq nose bleed → hypertension

Evaluation: Client can state methods to prevent future attacks.

F. Cancer of the Larynx

1. **General Information**
   a. Curable if diagnosed early
   b. Incidence: most common malignancy of upper respiratory tract
   c. Risk Factors
      1) irritants to mucous membranes, e.g., chemicals, allergies
      2) smoking
      3) excessive alcohol intake
      4) familial predisposition
      5) chronic laryngitis
      6) voice abuse
   d. Medical Treatment
      1) surgical intervention
         a) laryngectomy
         b) laryngectomy with modified, radical neck dissection
      2) medical intervention
         a) radiation therapy
         b) chemotherapy not used *not effective*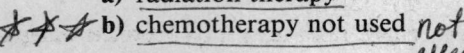

2. **Nursing Process**
   a. Assessment
      1) persistent hoarseness (early symptom)
      2) dysphagia, burning with hot liquids
      3) persistent sore throat
      4) pain in laryngeal prominence
      5) feeling that something is in throat
      6) swelling of the neck
      7) diagnostic tests: abnormal laryngoscopy, biopsy
   b. Goals, Plans/Implementation, and Evaluation

   Goal 1: Client will be physically prepared for surgery; will be able to explain the treatment plan, postoperative care, and the OR-RR environment.
   Plan/Implementation
   - give frequent oral care
   - arrange for good respiratory care
   - have male clients shave
   - promote no smoking, alcohol
   - teach client and significant others about
     - planned surgery
     - what will be experienced in OR-RR
     - post-op procedures
       * presence of drains/HemoVac
       * tracheostomy care and suctioning
       * breathing through tracheostomy tube, inhalation treatments
       * possible IVs, tube feedings
   - discuss communication problems that will result
   - determine methods of post-op communication, e.g., writing pad, picture board, call bell, magic slate, hand signals

   Evaluation: Client can explain course of treatment; client, significant others, and nurse have plan for postoperative communication.

   Goal 2: Client and significant others will begin the process of coping with diagnosis and treatment prior to surgery.
   Plan/Implementation
   - assist client and significant others to discuss feelings and fears about surgery, loss of normal speech, and possibility of dying
   - know that client and significant others will begin a grieving process over the loss of normal speech, health

   Evaluation: Client and significant others have begun discussing feelings and fears related to diagnosis.

   Goal 3: Client will remain free from postoperative complications.
   Plan/Implementation
   - refer to *Surgery* page 165
   - assess frequently post-op
     - presence of patent airway
     - breath sounds, respiratory rate and depth
   - maintain fluid infusion as ordered
   - turn, deep breathe qh; suction as needed
   - check dressing frequently for bleeding (q15min for 2h then qh for 8h)
   - give constant attention and emotional support
   - elevate head of bed 30°–45° (promotes drainage and facilitates respirations)
   - administer humidified oxygen
   - suction tracheostomy frequently
     - sterile suction setup
     - prepare equipment
     - hyperoxygenate client (suctioning can lower Po_2 10–30 mm Hg)
     - lubricate catheter (with H_2O-soluble lubricant) and insert catheter with suction turned off; advance catheter till client coughs
     - withdraw, rotating catheter and applying intermittent suction; suction no longer than 10-15 seconds at one time

Airway Priority

Suction on top of balloon the deflate balloon

- hyperoxygenate client
- repeat procedure allowing client to rest between suctionings
- facilitate entry into mainstem bronchi
  * right bronchus: turn client's head to the left with chest tilted to right
  * left bronchus: turn client's head to the right with chest tilted to left
  NOTE: these procedures may not help; usually catheter enters the right bronchus, which forms a less acute angle with the trachea
- observe cardiac monitor if in use; if bradycardia or dysrhythmias occur, terminate suctioning immediately and hyperoxygenate client

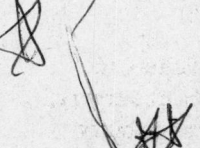

if client has inflated endotracheal or tracheostomy tube in place and you must deflate cuff, use the following procedure
  * suction trachea via tube as outlined above
  * suction oro- and nasopharynx
  * open new sterile setup and then deflate cuff and suction through tube immediately
  * reinflate cuff until air can no longer be heard, being careful not to overinflate the cuff
- give laryngeal-tube care; clean tube at least q8h
- suction nose and tracheostomy using separate sterile catheters
- give frequent oral hygiene
- check drains/HemoVac for neck drainage
- provide calm, restful environment
- organize nursing care to provide rest periods

Evaluation: Client remains free from respiratory distress; vital signs are stable; rests comfortably.

Goal 5: Client will experience relief of pain after surgery.
Plan/Implementation
- give pain medication as ordered (narcotic and nonnarcotic analgesics)
- provide continuous support of the head and neck
- aid relaxation through back and limb rubs and your physical presence
- teach relaxation techniques

Evaluation: Client states he has relief from pain or feels no pain.

Goal 6: Client will have satisfactory communication with staff and significant others in postoperative period.
Plan/Implementation
- institute communication measures decided upon pre-op
- remain with client as often as possible
- explain to client how to summon you; respond promptly when called
- have significant others remain with client
- reassure client that you will not abandon him

Evaluation: Client is able to communicate needs effectively.

Goal 7: Client will receive adequate nutrition.
Plan/Implementation
- give NG tube feedings as ordered
- give vitamin supplements as ordered
- supervise 1st oral intake; know that aspiration is not possible unless a fistula has formed
- check skin turgor to monitor adequate hydration of tissues
- monitor urinary output

Evaluation: Client's weight remains stable; fluid intake approximates output.

Goal 8: Client will demonstrate positive self-concept.
Plan/Implementation
- allow time for client to communicate in the manner determined before surgery
- provide honest answers to questions; clarify misconceptions
- encourage activities, clothes, and makeup that accentuate the positive aspects of the client's appearance
- encourage client to make future plans; assist in realistic goal-setting
- assist family or significant others to provide needed support for the client
- enlist help of role models such as laryngectomees who have been rehabilitated (contact American Cancer Society for a visitor)
- encourage client to utilize self-help groups

Evaluation: Client's grooming and attitude demonstrate a positive self-concept; states intention to attend laryngectomee club meeting.

Goal 9: Client and significant others will continue grieving process after surgery.

Plan/Implementation
- encourage expression of feelings on a continuing basis
- support client's frustration over communication problems
- reinforce and encourage self-care
- focus on goals of rehabilitation, not on loss of normal speech

Evaluation: Client and significant others continue to grieve appropriately; efforts at communication are successful.

Goal 10: Client and significant others will have a written plan to cope with problems related to client's illness upon discharge.

Plan/Implementation
- teach
  - tube care
  - stoma care
  - proper clothing
  - diet
  - activity and recreation
  - bathing
  - oral hygiene
- refer to laryngectomee club (American Cancer Society)
- make referral to speech therapist
- secure appointment at physician's office or clinic

Evaluation: Client has written plan for taking care of tube, stoma; has referral to speech therapist and to American Cancer Society.

References

Agee, B. and Herman, C. "Cervical Logrolling on a Standard Hospital Bed." *American Journal of Nursing*. March 1984:314-318.

Barry, L. "The Patient With Myasthenia Gravis Really Needs You." *Nursing 82*. July 1982:50-53.

Boyd-Monk, H. "Cataract Surgery." *Nursing 77*. June 1977:55-61.

Buchanan, L. "Emergency: First Aid for Spinal Cord Injury." *Nursing 82*. August 1982:68-78.

Callahan, M. "Caring For a Stroke Patient Like Me." *Nursing 84*. May 1984:65-67.

Czaplinski, R. "Test Your Knowledge of Caring for the Stroke Patient." *Nursing 80*. September 1980:68-71.

Fernsebner, W. "Early Diagnosis of Acute Angle-closure Glaucoma." *American Journal of Nursing*. July 1975:1154-1155.

Hanawalt, A. and Troutman, K. "If Your Patient Has a Hearing Aid." *American Journal of Nursing*. July 1984:900-901.

Johnson, L. "If Your Patient Has Intracranial Pressure, Your Goal Should Be: No Surprises." *Nursing 83*. June 1983:58-63.

Kess, R. "Suddenly in Crisis—Unpredictable Myasthenia." *American Journal of Nursing*. August 1984:994-998.

Larsen, G. "Rehabilitation for the Patient with Head and Neck Cancer." *American Journal of Nursing*. January 1982:119-120.

Lazure, L. "Defusing the Dangers of Autonomic Dysreflexia." *Nursing 80*. September 1980:52-53.

Mauso-Clum, N. "Bringing the Unconscious Patient Back Safely." *Nursing 82*. August 1982:34-42.

Meyd, C. "Acute Brain Trauma." *American Journal of Nursing*. January 1978:40-44.

Mizuki, J. "There's No Place Like Home." *American Journal of Nursing*. May 1984:646-648.

Musolf, J. "Chemonucleolysis." *American Journal of Nursing*. June 1983:882-885.

*"The Person with a Spinal Cord Injury" (Continuing Education). *American Journal of Nursing*. August 1977:1319-1336.

Resler, M. and Tumulty, G. "Glaucoma Update." *American Journal of Nursing*. May 1983:752-756.

Tilton, C. and Maloof, M. "Diagnosing the Problems in Stroke." *American Journal of Nursing*. April 1982:596-601.

Trebas, J. "Managing Epilepsy—Don't Forget the Patient." *Nursing 82*. February 1982:62-65.

* See reprint section.

Activity and Rest

(The nursing care presented in this unit concerns selected health problems related to disturbances in the musculoskeletal system.) The nurse plays an important role in maintaining musculoskeletal function by assessment, range-of-motion techniques, exercise, and early progressive ambulation.

General Concepts

A. Overview
1. Musculoskeletal System
   a. Muscles: contract and relax under the control of the nervous system to produce movement of the body as a whole or of its parts
      1) *fascia:* surrounds and divides muscles, main blood vessels, and nerves
      2) *tendons:* fibrous attachment between muscles and bones
      3) *ligaments:* fibrous connective tissue connecting bones, cartilage, and serving as support for or attachment of muscles and fascia
   b. Bones: for support and protection
      1) *joints:* junction between two bones
         a) synovium: lining of joints that secretes fluid to lubricate
         b) bursa: a closed cavity containing a gliding joint
      2) *cartilage:* dense connective tissue covering the ends of bones and at other sites where flexibility is needed
2. Terminology
   a. *Adduction:* movement toward the main axis of the body
   b. *Abduction:* movement away from the main axis of the body
   c. *Flexion:* act of bending
   d. *Extension*: stretching out into a straightened position
   e. *Strain:* trauma to the muscle caused by violent contraction or excessive forcible stretch
   f. *Sprain:* trauma to a joint with some degree of injury to the ligaments
3. Range-of-Motion (ROM) Exercises
   a. Uses
      1) prevent atrophy
      2) prevent weakness
      3) prevent contracture
      4) prevent degeneration of muscles and joints
   b. Types
      1) active — *client does it*
      2) passive — *client-nurse centered activity*
   c. Procedure
      1) stress importance of performing full ROM exercises
      2) perform ROM exercises at least twice daily
      3) breathing should be as normal as possible, e.g., client should not hold breath
      4) perform movements slowly and gently
      5) provide rest between each exercise
      6) perform each exercise same number of times on both sides of body; initially do each exercise three times, then work up to five times
      7) teach significant others to do ROM exercises for client
         a) demonstrate exercises
         b) allow return demonstration
         c) provide written instructions
4. Massage (centripetal: toward the heart)
   a. Uses
      1) increases circulation
      2) reduces edema
      3) relieves spasm
   b. May be used with heat

5. Isometric Exercises (move muscles)
    a. Definition: alternately tightening and relaxing muscles without moving the joints
    b. Uses
        1) maintain muscle tone
        2) increase muscle strength
    c. Procedure
        1) one to five contractions per muscle group
        2) duration of contraction: one to five seconds
        3) two-minute rest period between contractions
    d. Sites of Choice
        1) abdomen
        2) buttocks
        3) thighs
        4) upper arms

B. Application of the Nursing Process to the Client with Activity and Rest Problems
    1. Assessment
        a. Health History
            1) current health status
            2) history of present complaint, e.g., weakness, stiffness, pain, or swelling
            3) usual activities, e.g., work, social, and recreational pursuits
            4) diet and sleep patterns
        b. Physical Examination
            1) general inspection
                a) symmetry of the two sides of the body
                b) presence of spinal deformities, skin lesions, masses
                c) posture
            2) gait and balance: watch for specific gait patterns associated with specific disorders
            3) joints: range-of-motion
            4) muscle strength and bulk
            5) vascular system of extremities
                a) pulses
                b) varicosities
                c) edema
            6) deep tendon reflex testing (do not test in painful or arthritic joints)
                a) upper extremities
                    • biceps
                    • triceps
                    • radial
                b) lower extremities
                    • patellar
                    • Achilles
        c. Diagnostic Tests (know what used for)
            1) radiologic studies
                a) x-rays: detection of bone and soft tissue injury
                b) bone scan: detection of bone tumors
                c) myelogram
                    • inspection of the spinal column
                    • radiopaque medium injected into subarachnoid space of the spine
                    • nursing care
                        – pre test
                            * check for iodine allergy
                            * teach client regarding spinal tap and x-ray procedure
                        – post test
                            * keep flat in bed for 6–8 hours
                            * force fluids
                d) CAT scan
            2) hematologic studies
                a) sedimentation rate: rheumatoid arthritis
                b) C-reactive protein in serum: rheumatoid arthritis
                c) serum uric acid: gouty arthritis
                d) CBC (increased WBC with gouty arthritis)
                e) serum globulin: protein
                f) antinuclear antibodies (ANA): positive with systemic lupus erythematosis (SLE)
                g) LE factor
            3) electromyogram (EMG): a graphic record of the contraction of a muscle as a result of electrical stimulation
    2. General Nursing Goals, Plans/Implementation, and Evaluation

    Goal 1: Client will achieve and maintain maximum physical mobility.
    Plan/Implementation
    • teach client the proper use of assistive devices
    • help client learn proper use of prosthetic devices
    • provide needed support and encouragement
    Evaluation: Client expresses and demonstrates proper use of assistive devices; maintains maximum physical mobility.

    Goal 2: Client will adapt to changes in body image.
    Plan/Implementation
    • encourage client to verbalize concerns

- provide client with correct information about extent of body-image alteration

Evaluation: Client expresses self-acceptance; engages in usual social activities.

Goal 3: Client will be knowledgeable about disease process, medications, and the prevention of complications.

Plan/Implementation
- outline symptoms of disease
- outline progression of disease if applicable
- explain the rationale for ordered treatment regimen
- provide information regarding the administration and side effects of all medications
- discuss interventions that prevent the development of complications, including musculoskeletal damage and deficits

Evaluation: Client takes medications as prescribed, returns for follow-up appointments; remains free from preventable complications.

Goal 4: Client will be free from complications of immobility.

Plan/Implementation
- prevent constipation
  - increase fluid intake, unless contraindicated
  - increase dietary roughage
- prevent urinary calculi with increased fluids
- prevent pressure sores
  - turn q2h
  - gently massage skin
  - keep skin clean and dry
- prevent thrombophlebitis
  - apply antiembolic hose
  - encourage isometric exercises
  - avoid pillows behind the knees
- prevent atelectasis by having client cough and deep breathe

Evaluation: Client remains free from complications of immobility.

Selected Health Problems Resulting in an Interference with Activity and Rest

A. Fractures

1. **General Information**
   a. Types
      1) classified according to severity
         a) *compound:* open
         b) *closed:* simple
         c) *complete*
         d) *comminuted:* fragmented
         e) *compression:* depressed
         f) *stress:* fatigue
         g) *pathologic*
      2) classified according to direction of fracture line
         a) *linear, longitudinal (vertical):* fracture runs parallel to long axis of the bone
         b) *transverse, horizontal:* fracture line runs straight across the bone
         c) *oblique, spiral:* twisted
   b. Risk Factors
      1) old age
      2) active sports
      3) accidents
      4) osteoporosis from disease or steroid therapy
   c. Medical Treatment
      1) closed reduction (external fixation) casts
         a) manual manipulation of bone fragments into anatomic alignment
         b) immobilized in cast
      2) open reduction (internal fixation)
         a) surgical procedure with direct visualization
         b) realignment of fracture fragments and immobilization with metallic device (e.g., plate, intramedullary rod)
         c) advantages: allows early weightbearing
         d) complications include post-op infections and delayed union
      3) ambulation with assistive devices
         a) crutches
            - non-weight bearing: 3-point gait
            - weight bearing
              - 2-point gait
              - 4-point gait
              - swing-to gait
         b) cane carried in hand opposite affected leg for support
         c) walker
         d) sling for arm
      4) traction (refer to *Nursing Care of the Child* page 596)
   d. Emergency Care of Suspected Fractures
      1) control of evident hemorrhage (most important problem); sterile bandage to open wound
      2) immobilize affected part (splint)
      3) do not attempt to reduce fracture

4) apply ice pack to reduce swelling, hematoma, pain
5) transport to medical facility as soon as possible

2. Nursing Process
  a. Assessment
    1) age, developmental considerations
    2) usual activity, recreational needs
    3) circumstances of fracture occurrence (most result from accidents)
    4) concurrent health problems
  b. Goals, Plans/Implementation, and Evaluation

Goal 1: If closed reduction is used, client's cast will dry properly.
Plan/Implementation
- support cast on pillows along length of cast until dry (usually 24 hours)
- know that drying creates heat, which causes cast to harden; heat should be uniform in nature, not felt as isolated hot spots
- use fan to stir air
- *never* use heat lamp or hair dryer on plaster cast
- do not completely cover the cast; when dry it is porous and will allow skin underneath to "breathe"
- do not handle cast when wet, if possible; handle with palms, not fingertips
- do not place on hard surface while drying
- know that x-ray will be taken after cast application to ensure proper alignment

Evaluation: Client's cast has completely dried with fracture in proper alignment.

Goal 2: Client's circulation will be maintained after cast is applied.
Plan/Implementation
- observe circulatory status in exposed fingers or toes frequently during each shift
  - color: normal
  - temperature: warm and dry
  - swelling: minimal or none
  - circulation: good blanching; nail beds fill rapidly; adequate pulses
- observe for neurologic impairment
  - ability to move digits
  - degree of sensation
- avoid pressure areas on extremity
  - position client away from side on which he has a cast
  - support cast on pillow in a nondependent position
  - check for "hot spots" which indicate an area of inflammation beneath them
  - "petal" cast edges to eliminate rough, abrasive edges
- note odor under cast (necrotic tissue will produce malodor)

Evaluation: Client's toes (fingers) are warm, color good, blanch well.

Goal 3: Client's activity level will be safe and maintained to the extent allowed.
Plan/Implementation
- know the instructions client has been given for crutch walking and reinforce teaching
- reinforce the principles of non-weight bearing or use of affected extremity
- instruct client in principles of safe movement (i.e., no hopping around)
- instruct client in isometric, range-of-motion exercises as appropriate

Evaluation: Client uses crutches correctly and safely.

Goal 4: Client will experience relief of pain.
Plan/Implementation
- administer pain medications as ordered
- know that pain may herald problems with the cast (i.e., too tight) or infection of a compound fracture (pain should decrease after fracture is set)
- instruct client to notify nurse of any new pain of any new pain or pain unrelieved by analgesics
- have client on crutches ambulate only with assistance after administration of pain medication

Evaluation: Client states he is free from discomfort.

Goal 5: Client's rehabilitation course will remain free from complications.
Plan/Implementation
- teach client signs and symptoms of complications (e.g., poor circulation, infection)
- teach client principles of cast care
  - keep clean and dry
  - don't put objects (i.e., for scratching) down the cast
- alert client to possible side effects of decreased mobility (e.g., weight gain, constipation)

ACTIVITY AND REST   317

- increase fluids
- readjust diet to include more protein and roughage, fewer carbohydrates

Evaluation: Client can demonstrate methods of cast care; maintains weight; remains free from constipation.

Goal 6: If open reduction with a cast or skeletal traction is utilized, client will be free from postoperative complications.

Plan/Implementation
- observe for post-op bleeding
  - draw circle around evidence of bleeding on cast; mark with date and time
  - check frequently
- apply ice pack if ordered to reduce swelling and pain (protect cast from moisture)
- administer analgesics as ordered
- maintain traction in proper alignment, with correct amount of weight
- prevent complications of immobilization
  - give frequent skin care over bony prominences to prevent decubitus ulcers; use sheepskin or egg-crate mattress
  - perform isometric and ROM exercises on unaffected extremities to prevent contractures, thrombophlebitis, foot drop
  - know that if the fracture occurred in the middle 1/3 of the femur, client may exercise ankle; if fracture is in the lower 1/3, no ankle exercise
  - increase fluids, roughage to prevent constipation, urinary calculi
- observe carefully for post-op wound infection
  - provide pin care q8h
  - if client has a cast, observe for increased pain, swelling, or a malodor coming from cast
- provide bedriden client with age-appropriate diversions/activities, as possible
  - arrange for school work for child/adolescent
  - arrange private time for adult clients and their visitors
- be aware that prolonged bed rest may lead to sleep disturbances, sensory deprivation

Evaluation: Client is free from complications during the recovery phase (maintains proper alignment, skin integrity); performs ROM exercises on unaffected extremities.

B. Fractured Hip (Proximal End of Femur)

1. **General Information**
   a. Definition: "broken hips" include fractures of the femur head (called intracapsular), fractures of the femur neck (extracapsular), and those of the greater or lesser trochanter
   b. Incidence
      1) increases after age 60
      2) more common in women than men
   c. Precipitating Factors
      1) falls associated with osteoporotic and degenerative changes of the bone
      2) age-related physiologic changes in balance and perception
   d. Medical Treatment
      1) medical intervention: closed reduction (rare in older clients)
      2) surgical intervention: open reduction and internal fixation, or a prosthetic head-of-the-femur

2. **Nursing Process**
   a. Assessment

      1) affected leg
         a) shortened
         b) externally rotated
         c) adducted
      2) age of client and circumstances of injury
      3) current health, mental status including degree of orientation
      4) availability of family support mechanisms
   b. Goals, Plans/Implementation, and Evaluation

Goal 1: Preoperatively, client will experience relief of symptoms and be protected from further injury.

Plan/Implementation
- administer analgesics as ordered
- use skin traction (Buck's) to relieve muscle spasms and reduce edema
- turn only 45° to affected side; may turn to unaffected side
- use fracture pan for elimination
- prevent external rotation of affected hip
- assess and monitor coexisting medical problems

Evaluation: Client remains free from pain with affected leg in good alignment, preoperatively.

Goal 2: Postoperatively, client will maintain the proper position for functional healing of the hip.
Plan/Implementation
- prepare client's bed, e.g., firm mattress, bed board, overhead trapeze, adjustable foot board, bed rails, and other decubitus-ulcer-prevention aids
- maintain abduction of affected leg at all times, e.g., use an abductor splint or pillows between legs
- prevent external rotation by placing a trochanter roll along affected side
- "logroll" client to unaffected side q2h, supporting the leg in an abducted position
- prevent acute flexion of hip by keeping head of the bed low, i.e., not higher than 35°- 40°

Evaluation: Client's leg is maintained in good alignment.

Goal 3: Client will remain free from complications of immobility.
Plan/Implementation
- see General Nursing Goal 4

Evaluation: Client's postoperative course is free from complications (e.g., no fever, skin in good condition).

Goal 4: Client will receive progressively increasing activity (depending on type of surgery).
Plan/Implementation
- internal fixation with nails or pins
  - get client up in chair 1-2 days post-op
  - allow only partial weight bearing for 3 months
  - allow full weight bearing in 6 months
- femoral-head prosthesis
  - have client stand at side of bed, starting 2-4 days post-op
  - allow partial weight bearing 4-10 days post-op
  - allow full weight bearing 2-6 months post-op
  - do not use wheelchair for 2 weeks
  - prevent flexion greater than 90°
- consult physician regarding muscle-setting exercises for gluteal and quadriceps muscles, movements of the affected leg, ambulation, and weight bearing on the nonaffected leg
- work with physical therapist to coordinate exercise and mobilization regimen
- perform full ROM exercises at least twice daily on unaffected limbs
- lead with unaffected leg when using transfer techniques

Evaluation: Client ambulates with or without assistance and with or without partial weight bearing, depending on surgical intervention.

Goal 5: Client will remain free from psychosocial complications of hospitalization and immobility.
Plan/Implementation
- refer to *Nursing Care of the Client with Psychosocial Problems,* "Depression" page 52 and "Confusion" page 48.

Evaluation: Client maintains contact with reality; behaves with minimal confusion, disorientation, and/or dependency.

Goal 6: Client will develop a workable plan for long-term convalescence.
Plan/Implementation
- assist client and significant others regarding home care or decide where client will go upon discharge, e.g., home, extended-care facility
- teach client and significant others what they need to know about
  - length of convalescence and progress of weight-bearing ambulation
  - general health measures to be followed, e.g., medications, exercise, diet
  - correct safety precautions for use of cane, walker, or wheelchair
  - persons and agencies who can be contacted for services
- help client and significant others develop a plan to eliminate unsafe environmental conditions that may have contributed to fracture in the first place

Evaluation: Client makes adequate arrangements for long-term convalescence.

C. Amputation
1. **General Information**
   a. Definition: traumatic or surgical removal of an appendage or limb
   b. Indications
      1) certain tumors
      2) severe traumatic injuries (usually affects upper extremities)
      3) problems related to peripheral vascular disease, e.g., gangrene; usually affects lower extremities

ACTIVITY AND REST

2. Nursing Process
   a. Assessment
      1) physical and psychologic strengths of client
      2) support systems, e.g., family and friends
      3) health status, high-risk factors, i.e., smoking habits, cardiovascular disease, diabetes, cancer
      4) condition of affected appendage or limb
         a) color of skin
            - necrotic tissue may be blue or gray-blue
            - turns dark brown or black
         b) presence of infection
            - red streaks along lymphatic channels
            - systemic symptoms
      5) availability of skilled rehabilitation team
   b. Goals, Plans/Implementation, and Evaluation

Goal 1: Client will be physically and emotionally prepared for surgical outcome.
Plan/Implementation
- explain that surgery is performed above level of healthy tissue
- explain that grieving is normal
- allow client and significant others opportunities to express anger and fears
- initiate exercises to develop strength in muscles that will be used in rehabilitation
- prepare client for post-op stump care and prosthesis if appropriate
- give prophylactic antibiotics as ordered

Evaluation: Client is able to express grief over anticipated loss.

Goal 2: Client's stump will remain free from contractures and will be reduced in size.
Plan/Implementation
- elevate stump a maximum of 24 hours (hasten venous return and prevents edema)
- avoid elevation of stump after 1st 24 hours post-op to prevent hip contracture (most common post-op complication)
- keep stump in an extended position; have client with a leg amputation lie prone for short periods daily to prevent flexion contractures
- use "shrinker sock" or elastic bandage applied in a figure-eight fashion to reduce size of stump in preparation for prosthesis; teach client how to apply properly (elastic bandages applied to above-the-knee amputations are also wrapped around the waist)
- know that an immediate prosthetic fit reduces the incidence of post-op complications, particularly incisional pain and phantom limb-sensation

Evaluation: Client applies shrinker sock properly; stump is clean, free from contractures.

Goal 3: Client will recover from surgery free from complications.
Plan/Implementation
- refer to *Surgery* page 165

Goal 4: Client will adapt to altered body image.
Plan/Implementation
- refer to General Nursing Goal 2 page 314

Goal 5: Client will use prescribed prosthetic device.
Plan/Implementation
- see General Nursing Goal 1 page 314.
- know that a good prosthetic fit takes time and adjustments
- reinforce teaching done by the prosthetist
- teach client to observe stump for signs of infection, irritation
- teach client proper skin care: wash and dry daily, avoid use of skin creams
- continue to offer encouragement and support to client and significant others throughout the rehabilitation process
- reinforce client's efforts at maintaining balance and posture, and increasing auxiliary muscle strength
- if prosthesis is not an option, assist client in safe use of wheelchair, transfer techniques

Evaluation: Client is adapting to prosthesis with few problems; can transfer from bed to wheelchair safely.

D. Arthritis
1. **General Information**
   a. **Rheumatoid Arthritis**
      1) definition: a chronic, systemic, diffuse, collagen disease

characterized by inflammatory changes in joints and related structures, resulting in crippling deformities
2) incidence
a) occurs 3 times more frequently in women
b) peak incidence between 30 and 40 years of age
c) primarily affects proximal joints and synovial membranes
3) predisposing factors
a) possibly an autoimmune disorder
b) stress, obesity, aggravation are implicated
4) pathophysiologic sequence: synovitis→pannus formation→fibrous ankylosis→bony ankylosis (frozen joint)
b. Osteoarthritis   Jt. c̄ wear + tear
1) definition: a chronic disease involving the weight-bearing joints; nonsystemic
2) incidence
a) occurs 5 times more frequently in women
b) peak incidence between 50 and 70 years of age
3) predisposing factors
a) aging
b) trauma
c) excessive use of joint (e.g., worker who sews)
d) obesity
4) pathophysiologic sequence: degeneration of articular cartilage→new bone formation: Heberden's nodes (bony nodules or spurs on the dorsolateral aspects of distal joints of fingers)
c. Gouty Arthritis
1) definition: inflammation of a joint caused by gout (uric acid crystals deposited in joint)
2) incidence
a) 19 times more frequent in men
b) peak incidence between 20 and 40 years of age
c) often affects a terminal joint (e.g., great toe)
3) predisposing factors
a) hyperuricemia
b) several metabolic disorders
4) pathophysiology
a) metabolic disorders of purine metabolism
b) urate deposits in and around joints
d. Medical Treatment: surgical interventions for rheumatoid, osteoarthritis
1) tendon transplant: from a normal muscle to another location to assume function of a damaged muscle
2) osteotomy: cutting bone to correct bone or joint deformity
3) synovectomy: removal of synovial membrane; helps prevent recurrent inflammation
4) arthroplasty
a) *hemiarthroplasty:* one part of a joint is replaced, e.g., head of femur
b) *total hip replacement:* head of the femur and the acetabulum are replaced
c) *total knee replacement:* both articular surfaces of the knee are replaced
d) *interphalangeal joint replacement*

2. Nursing Process: Rheumatoid Arthritis and Osteoarthritis
a. Assessment
1) rheumatoid arthritis
a) stiffness, especially in morning
b) proximal joint pain that decreases with use
c) swollen joint
d) limitation of muscle strength and atrophy; functional impairment caused by pain and muscle irritation
e) acute and chronic episodes with remissions and exacerbations
f) systemic symptoms (e.g., anemia, elevated body temperature)
g) elevated sedimentation rate
h) elevated C-reactive protein in serum
2) osteoarthritis
a) stiffness, especially in mornings
b) joint pain that increases with use
c) limitation of joint motion
d) aggravation of symptoms with temperature, humidity change, and weight bearing
b. Goals, Plans/Implementation, and Evaluation

Goal 1: Client will function as comfortably and as normally as possible.

Plan/Implementation

- teach client to balance rest and activity
  - encourage to optimum level of functioning
  - exercise joint to point of pain—never beyond *at least to pt. of pain*
  - PT and OT activities as prescribed
  - during acute phase
    * complete bed rest
    * splints
- apply heat to provide analgesia and relax muscles
- teach client about medications and their side effects, see table 3.55
- assist client to modify environment to accomplish activities easily

Evaluation: Client maintains activity without undue stress; can state side effects of ordered medications.

Goal 2: Client will adjust to the chronicity of the condition.

Plan/Implementation

- allow client to express fear and concerns
- encourage as much activity as possible
- teach client that continuous immobilization may cause increased pain
- teach client to avoid sudden jarring movements of joints
- warn client about "quacks" who promise miracle cures
- encourage continued follow-up to reevaluate progression of disease and efficacy of drug therapy
- counsel client and family regarding the need for a well-balanced diet and, if obesity is a problem, weight reduction

Evaluation: Client states a willingness to continue with therapeutic regimen as prescribed; maintains activity level as possible.

Goal 3: Client will be prepared for surgery.

Plan/Implementation

- refer to *Surgery* page 165

Evaluation: Client knows what to expect in immediate postoperative period.

Goal 4: If surgery is performed on the affected hip, client will remain free from postoperative complications.

Plan/Implementation

- refer to *Surgery* page 165
- turn as allowed, *always* keeping the affected hip abducted
- keep hip abducted at all times regardless of client's position; rapid onset of sharp hip pain may indicate dislocation
- apply a T.E.D. stocking from toes to groin on unaffected leg
- monitor HemoVac drainage; ensure that tubes remain patent

Table 3.55 Anti-Inflammatory Drugs (Nonsteroidal)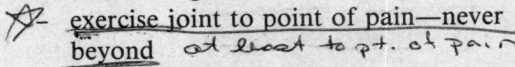

Description	A large group of drugs with antiinflammatory, and often analgesic, properties. They act to reduce the symptoms of inflammation such as redness, swelling, fever, and pain.
Uses	To treat mild to moderate pain due to inflammatory conditions; symptomatic relief of arthritic conditions and gout
Side Effects	GI irritation, ulcers, bleeding; dyspepsia; bone-marrow depression; headache; dizziness; bowel changes; allergic reaction
Nursing Implications	Take with food or antacid to decrease GI distress; monitor blood counts for bone-marrow depression; monitor for GI bleeding; monitor for aspirin allergy; do not administer aspirin and other anti-inflammatory preparations concurrently.
Types and Examples	*Salicylates:* aspirin *Pyrazolones:* phenylbutazone (Butazolidin), oxyphenylbutazone (Tandearil) *Nonsteroids:* ibuprofen (Motrin), indomethacin (Indocin), fenoprofen (Nalfon), naproxen (Naprosyn), sulindac (Clinoril) *Antigout:* colchicine

322 SECTION 3: NURSING CARE OF THE ADULT

- elevate foot of the bed 15°
- ☆ elevate head of bed 45° for meals only

Evaluation: Client is afebrile post-operatively; has minimal pain; leg is maintained in abduction.

Goal 5: Client will regain use of joint to the maximum degree possible.
Plan/Implementation
- get client out of bed as permitted, assisting with transfers
- keep leg abducted and avoid hip flexion *(Don't flex to sit on toilet, use a raiser)*
- have client relax and contract gluteal and quadricep muscles 10 times/hour during the day
- teach client and family about precautions after discharge
  - avoid sleeping on operative side
  - use cane, walker, or crutches for support and partial weight bearing
  - do not cross or twist legs
  - do not lift heavy objects
  - observe carefully for signs of wound infection
- reinforce need for continued exercise and maintenance of normal activities as possible

Evaluation: Client uses rehabilitative measures to enhance recovery; pursues activities within range of ability, age, and level of interest.

3. Nursing Process: Gouty Arthritis
a. Assessment
  1) pain, swelling, and inflammation of affected joint (usually great toe)
  2) increased serum uric acid
  3) increased sedimentation rate
  4) increased WBC count
b. Goals, Plans/Implementation, and Evaluation

Goals 1 and 2: refer back to "Rheumatoid Arthritis"

Goal 3: Client will adjust diet and life-style to prevent future attacks.
Plan/Implementation
- teach client about use of medications and their side effects
- obtain dietary counseling for client; instruct in a low purine diet (i.e., restrict meats, especially organ meats, and legumes)
- encourage daily high intake of fluids to prevent precipitation of uric acid crystals in the kidney
- advise regarding weight control as needed

Evaluation: Client can state foods to be avoided; has a plan for weight reduction.

E. Collagen Disease
1. **General Information**
   a. Definition: a group of diseases characterized by widespread pathologic changes in connective tissue; they are difficult to diagnose, have no cure, and cannot be prevented
   b. Types
      1) Polymyositis: inflammation of striated muscle
      2) Systematic Lupus Erythematosis (SLE): generalized connective tissue disorder
         a) incidence
            - affects women 4 times more frequently than men
            - more likely to occur in young adults and adolescents
         b) etiology and risk factors are unknown; an autoimmune disease
   c. Medical Treatment: aim is temporary remission or slowing of collagen destruction
      1) high doses of steroids
      2) aspirin for pain

2. **Nursing Process**
   a. Assessment
      1) arthritic-like symptoms
      2) sensitivity to sun
      3) presence of erythematous "butterfly" rash across bridge of nose
      4) involvement of other organ systems *(Most die of renal failure)*
         a) renal
         b) cardiovascular
         c) peripheral vascular
         d) nervous
         e) respiratory
      5) diagnostic test results
         a) positive lupus erythematosus (LE) prep
         b) anemia
         c) proteinuria
   b. Goals, Plans/Implementation, and Evaluation

Goal 1: Client will follow correct medication regimen.
Plan/Implementation
- outline plan for steroid therapy

Life stress can cause exacerbation

- minimize side effects through diet modification, time of administration, etc.
- teach client safety precautions for steroid therapy (see table 3.33)

Evaluation: Client can describe medications and their expected side effects.

Goal 2: Client will understand disease and its complications. *watch for infec.*
Plan/Implementation
- see General Nursing Goal 3 page 315

F. Herniated Nucleus Pulposus (Intervertebral Disk)

1. **General Information**
   a. Definition: a protrusion of the gelatinous cushion between the vertebrae (intervertebral disk) through the surrounding cartilage causing pressure on nerve roots with resultant pain
   b. Incidence
      1) more frequent in men
      2) commonly occurs in the space between the 4th and 5th lumbar vertebrae
   c. Predisposing/Risk Factors
      1) sedentary occupations
      2) long-term driving, e.g., truck driver
      3) infrequent physical exercise, certain sports (e.g., bowling, baseball)
   d. Medical Treatment
      1) medical intervention
         a) bed rest on a firm mattress with bed board
         b) skin traction
         c) proper body alignment, e.g., no prone position
         d) medications
            - muscle relaxants
            - analgesics
            - anti-inflammatory agents
            - steroids
         e) physical therapy
            - diathermy
            - back exercises
            - braces
         f) weight reduction as needed
      2) surgical intervention
         a) indications
            - prevention of further nerve damage and deficits
            - severe back and leg pain that does not respond to conservative therapy
            - a totally extruded disk that causes sensory and motor deficits in the lower extremities, bowel, and bladder (an emergency)
         b) procedures
            - laminectomy: removal of herniated portion of intervertebral disk that was causing pressure
            - spinal fusion (for additional stability): bone graft from iliac crest used to fuse two or more vertebrae together
         c) success rate ranges from 50%-90%

2. **Nursing Process**
   a. Assessment
      1) low back pain radiating down posterior thigh (sciatic nerve involvement)
      2) paresthesia of affected nerve roots
      3) muscle weakness, muscle spasm in lumbar region
      4) numbness, weakness, paralysis, or decreased reflexes along affected nerve pathway of leg, ankle, and foot
      5) character of pain
         a) intermittent; more frequent and severe depending on degree of herniation
         b) may be related to a single traumatic event
         c) gets progressively worse
         d) worsened by anterior and lateral flexion of the spine; rotational movements, laughing, sneezing, coughing, straining; straight leg raising to 80° or 90° while supine
      6) client's occupation, exercise routine, physical status
   b. Goals, Plans/Implementation, and Evaluation

Goal 1: Client will be relieved of pain.
Plan/Implementation
- place on bed rest on a firm mattress with bed board, traction as ordered *pelvic*
- administer analgesics, muscle relaxants as ordered, noting client's response
- prevent twisting and straining
- use noninvasive methods to relieve pain, e.g., frequent back rubs, diversion

Evaluation: Client experiences decreased pain; requires infrequent analgesia; maintains bed rest.

Goal 2: Client will remain free from complications of immobility.
Plan/Implementation
- refer to General Nursing Goal 4 page 315

Goal 3: Client will learn how to care for back to prevent future episodes.
Plan/Implementation
- observe and reinforce physical therapy regimens
- give warm bath and muscle relaxants prn prior to exercise sessions
- assist client to apply and wear back supports correctly, observing for any signs of skin irritation
- teach client to use appropriate body mechanics
  - use broad base of support
  - use large body muscles
  - maintain good posture
  - bring object close to the body before moving
  - pull rather than push on object
  - do not lift items
  - squat, do not bend over
- walk rather than than stand, but stand rather than sit

Evaluation: Client can demonstrate back exercises correctly and states a willingness to do them regularly.

Goal 4 (if surgery is required): Client will be physically and psychologically prepared for surgery.
Plan/Implementation
- refer to *Surgery* page 165
- explain importance and demonstrate post-op positioning, "logroll" turning, and body alignment
- explain that if spinal fusion is to be done, a turning frame may be used
- tell client about incision needed for bone graft and HemoVac that may be in place
- obtain pre-op neurologic assessment for post-op comparison

Evaluation: Client verbalizes a positive attitude toward the surgical outcome; demonstrates understanding of planned procedure and immediate postoperative care.

Goal 5: Client will remain free from postoperative complications.

Plan/Implementation
- refer to "Surgery" page 165
- keep client flat in bed for 1st 12 hours; then may raise head of bed to 30°
- know that client will usually get out of bed on 1st or 2nd post-op day (unless spinal fusion done)
- use turning sheet and turn client by "logrolling"
- report numbness or tingling in feet or legs
- give medications for pain and frequent muscle spasms as ordered
- provide laxative to avoid straining
- when client is allowed to be up, have him stand and not sit
- apply TED stockings and have client do leg exercises to prevent thrombophlebitis
- when ambulating, have client wear shoes, not slippers, for better support
- prepare client for 3-6 month use of body cast or brace post-op if fusion was done

Evaluation: Client's postoperative course is uneventful; dressing dry and intact; sensation in toes is adequate; client ambulating frequently with minimal discomfort.

Goal 6: Client and significant others will be adequately prepared for discharge.
Plan/Implementation
- refer to General Nursing Goal 3 page 315
- provide client and significant others with written instructions regarding care of operative site, back-care regimen, and back exercises
- ensure that client knows proper application of back brace, if ordered
- provide client with a list of instructions or a timetable to resume activities such as driving, sexual intercourse, sports, housework, or job responsibilities
- ensure that client knows to report signs of illness, fever, increasing back pain or muscle spasms to physician

Evaluation: Client can state schedule for exercising; applies back brace correctly; knows when to resume additional activities.

References

"Adult Arthritis." *American Journal of Nursing.* February 1983:253-278.

Cohen, S. "Nursing Care of a Patient in Traction." *American Journal of Nursing.*

(Programmed Instruction). October 1979:1771-1797

Krysenyshen, P. and Fischer, D. "External Fixation for Complicated Fractures." *American Journal of Nursing.* February 1980:256-259.

Meador, R. "Learning to Live with a New Leg." *American Journal of Nursing.* August 1979:1393-1395.

Musolf, J. "Chemonucleolysis." *American Journal of Nursing.* June 1983:882-885.

Myers, M., McNelly, R., and Nelson, K. "Total Hip Replacement—a Team Effort." *American Journal of Nursing.* September 1978:1485-1488.

Neal, M., Cohen, P., Cooper, P. *Nursing Care Planning Guides, Set 1,* 2nd Ed. Baltimore: Williams & Wilkins, 1980.

Neal, M., Cohen, P., and Reighley, J. *Nursing Care Planning Guides, Set 3,* 2nd Ed. Baltimore: Williams & Wilkins, 1983.

Neal, M. and Cohen, P. *Nursing Care Planning Guides, Set 4,* 2nd Ed. Baltimore: Williams & Wilkins, 1983.

"Patient Assessment: Examining Joints of the Upper and Lower Extremities." *American Journal of Nursing.* April 1981:763-786.

Walters, J. "Coping with a Leg Amputation." *American Journal of Nursing.* July 1981: 1349-1352.

Cellular Aberration

(The nursing care presented in this unit contains selected health problems related to neoplastic disease.)

General Concepts

A. **Overview**
1. Terms pertaining to neoplasia
   a. *Cancer:* a group of diseases characterized by uncontrolled growth and spread of abnormal cells
   b. *Neoplasm:* neo = new; plasm = formation
   c. *Carcinoma:* a malignant tumor arising from epithelial tissue
   d. *Sarcoma:* a malignant tumor arising from nonepithelial tissue
   e. *Differentiation:* degree to which neoplastic tissue resembles the parent tissue
   f. *Metastasis:* spread of cancer from its original site to other parts of the body
   g. *Adjuvant Therapy:* therapy designed to be adjunctive or supplemental to primary therapy
   h. *Palliation:* relief or alleviation of symptoms without cure
2. Tumors are characterized by tissue of origin
   a. Adeno: glandular tissue
   b. Angio: blood vessels
   c. Basal cell: epithelium, mainly sun-exposed areas
   d. Embryonal: gonads
   e. Fibro: fibrous tissue
   f. Lympho: lymphoid tissue
   g. Melano: pigmented cells of epithelium
   h. Myo: muscle tissue
   i. Osteo: bone
   j. Squamous cell: epithelium
3. Incidence
   a. 2nd leading cause of death in the US
   b. One of every four Americans can expect to develop cancer
   c. Occurs in all age groups; incidence increases with age
4. Etiology: No *single* cause
5. Risk Factors (American Cancer Society)
   a. Tobacco: smoking or chewing
   b. Alcohol: excessive intake
   c. Hormones, e.g., estrogen
   d. Genetic predisposition
   e. Immune deficiency
   f. Age
   g. Occupational: exposure to carcinogens (e.g., asbestos, vinyl chloride)
   h. X-rays: overexposure
   i. Sunlight: long exposure
   j. Diet: high fat and/or high total calories
6. Physiology/Pathophysiology (not a single disease)
   a. Normal Cell Cycle: five phases
      1) G_0 (G means gap): resting phase; minimal biologic activity
      2) G_1 (1st growth period): enzymes, RNA, structural protein are synthesized
      3) S: synthesis of DNA
      4) G_2 (2nd growth period): RNA and protein synthesis
      5) M (mitosis): cell division
   b. Characteristics of Malignant Cells
      1) anaplastic (loss of differentiation)
      2) disorderly division
      3) uncontrolled growth pattern
      4) loss of normal growth-limiting mechanisms
      5) nonencapsulated
      6) tend to metastasize
      7) may be necrotic from poor vascular supply
      8) often recur after treatment
7. Metastasis
   a. Modes
      1) lymphatic
      2) vascular
   b. Site(s)

1) usually determined by the lymph and blood drainage patterns of the original cancer site, e.g., primary tumors entering systemic venous circulation are apt to lodge in the lung
2) most common: lung, liver, bone, and brain

8. Classification
   a. Histologic Classification (grading of tumor appearance and degree of differentiation)
      1) grade 1: most differentiated (resembles parent tissue most closely), best prognosis
      2) grade 2: intermediate differentiation
      3) grade 3: essentially undifferentiated
      4) grade 4: highly undifferentiated (most unlike parent tissue), anaplastic, poorest prognosis
   b. TNM Classification: *t*umor, *n*odes, *m*etastasis
      1) tumor
         a) T_0: no evidence of primary tumor
         b) TIS: carcinoma in situ
         c) T_{1-4}: progressive increase in tumor size and involvement
         d) TX: tumor cannot be assessed
      2) nodes
         a) N_0: regional lymph nodes not demonstrably abnormal
         b) N_{1-3}: increasing degrees of demonstrable abnormality of regional lymph nodes
         c) NX: regional lymph nodes cannot be assessed clinically
      3) metastasis
         a) M_0: no evidence of distant metastasis
         b) M_{1-3}: ascending degrees of distant metastasis, including metastasis to distant lymph nodes

9. Prognosis
   a. Factors
      1) tumor size
      2) nodal involvement
      3) metastasis
   b. 5 year survival: approximately 1 out of 3 persons

B. **Application of the Nursing Process to the Client with Cancer**
   1. Assessment
      a. Health History
         1) seven warning signs (CAUTION)
            a) *c*hange in usual bowel and bladder function
            b) *a* sore that does not heal.
            c) *u*nusual bleeding or discharge: hematuria, tarry stools, ecchymosis, bleeding mole
            d) *t*hickening or a lump in the breast or elsewhere
            e) *i*ndigestion or dysphagia
            f) *o*bvious change in a wart or mole
            g) *n*agging cough or hoarseness
         2) family history
         3) presenting symptoms
            a) appetite
            b) weight loss
            c) energy level
            d) pain (severe pain is *not* a common problem)
      b. Physical Exam
         1) general appearance
         2) percussion
            a) fluid waves (ascites)
            b) chest percussion
         3) palpation
            a) masses
            b) lymph nodes
      c. Diagnostic Tests
         1) lab tests
            a) CBC, platelet count
            b) blood chemistries
            c) CEA (carcinoembryonic antigen)
            d) specific tests depending on suspected site of cancer
         2) cytologic studies (microscopic exam of body secretions for cancer cells), e.g., pap smear
         3) biopsy of mass — most dx tool
         4) radiologic studies
            a) x-rays, e.g., mammogram
            b) CAT scans
            c) radioisotope scanning
            d) ultrasound
            e) thermography
         5) endoscopic examinations, e.g., bronchoscopy, gastroscopy
      d. Medical Treatment
         1) surgery
            a) principles
               • excision/radical excision: tumor plus margin of healthy tissue must be excised
               • often results in some significant defect or loss of function
            b) uses
               • diagnosis
               • cure
               • palliation
                 – remove obstruction

- debulk large unresectable tumors
- control pain, e.g., cordotomies, nerve blocks
- ablative: removal of hormone-producing organs to effect a response in hormone-dependent tumor
2) radiation
   a) definition: the use of ionizing radiation to cause damage and destruction to cancerous growths
   b) effect: radiation causes damage at the cellular level
      - indirectly: water molecules within the cell are ionized
      - directly: causes strand breakage in the double helix of DNA
      - not every cell is damaged beyond repair
   c) uses
      - cure
      - palliation
      - combined with surgery
         - pre-op: to reduce size of the tumor
         - post-op: to retard/control metastasis of tumor cells
      - combined with chemotherapy
   d) administration
      - external, e.g., cobalt
      - internal, e.g., implants
   e) side effects
      - radiation syndrome: effects not related to site treated
         - experienced to one degree or another by most clients receiving radiation therapy
         - symptoms
            * fatigue, malaise
            * headache
            * anorexia, nausea, vomiting
      - specific side effects: related to site treated
         - cranium: transitory or permanent hair loss
         - mouth, rectum: mucositis, stomatitis
         - mouth, head and neck: taste alteration, reduced saliva production, dental caries
         - throat, esophagus: dysphagia
         - GI tract: nausea, vomiting, diarrhea
         - abdomen: malnutrition, anorexia
         - pelvis, long bones, sternum: bone-marrow suppression
            * thrombocytopenia (platelets)→bleeding
            * leukopenia (WBCs)→infection
            * erythropenia (RBCs)→anemia
         - bladder, pelvis: cystitis
         - testicles, ovaries: sterility
         - rectum: proctitis
         - lungs, chest wall: pneumonitis
3) chemotherapy
   a) definition: the use of drugs to retard the growth of or destroy cancerous cells
   b) classification/effect (see table 3.56)
      - antineoplastics
         - cell-cycle specific: attack cells at a specific point in the process of cell division
         - cell-cycle nonspecific: act at one time during cell division
      - hormones
         - alter the hormone balance
         - modify the growth of some hormone-dependent tumors
   c) combination chemotherapy
      - two or more drugs used simultaneously
      - each drug has different effect
      - increases the effectiveness of the destruction/retardation of cancerous cells
   d) uses
      - cure
      - palliation
      - combined with surgery
      - combined with radiation
   e) administration
      - intravenous infusion
         - most common route
         - diffuses drug throughout the entire body
      - arterial infusion
         - drug is introduced through a catheter directly into the tumor via the main artery that supplies it
         - advantage: high proportion of drug is absorbed by tumor before it reaches systemic circulation
      - regional perfusion

Table 3.56 Chemotherapeutic Agents

Antineoplastics

Alkylating Agents

Uses	Leukemias, lymphomas, multiple myeloma
Side Effects	Bone-marrow depression, nausea & vomiting, vesicant action if extravasated, alopecia, hemorrhagic cystitis (cyclophosphamide)
Nursing Implications	Monitor blood counts closely; teach client safety precautions re low WBC, platelet count; avoid extravasation or any contact of drug with skin, hydrate well (cis-platinum)
Examples	Busulfan (Myleran), chlorambucil (Leukeran), cis-platinum (Platinol), cyclophosphamide (Cytoxan), mechlorethamine (nitrogen mustard), triethylene-thiophosphoramide (thiotepa)

Antimetabolites

Uses	Leukemias, testicular and ovarian tumors (cis-platinum), colon and GI tumors (5-FU)
Side Effects	GI ulceration (stomatitis); bone-marrow depression; nephro- and ototoxicity, anaphylaxis (cis-platinum)
Nursing Implications	Give citrovorum factor (leucovorin) as ordered to decrease toxicity of methotrexate; monitor blood counts closely; watch for GI bleeding.
Examples	Methotrexate (Mexate), 6-mercaptopurine (6-MP), 5-fluorouracil (5-FU), cytarabine or cytosine arabinoside (Cytosar)

Antibiotics

Uses	Lymphoma, testicular cancer, breast cancer, Wilms' tumor, head and neck tumors, neuroblastoma
Side Effects	GI ulceration (stomatitis); alopecia; bone-marrow depression; cardiac abnormalities (doxorubicin); pulmonary fibrosis (bleomycin)
Nursing Implications	Monitor blood counts; avoid extravasation and monitor ECGs (doxorubicin); monitor chest x-rays (bleomycin).
Examples	Doxorubicin (Adriamycin), dactinomycin (Cosmegen), bleomycin (Blenoxane), mithramycin (Mithracin), mitomycin C (Mutamycin)

Plant Alkaloids

Uses	Hodgkin's disease, testicular cancer, leukemia, breast cancer
Side Effects	Alopecia, neuropathy; bone-marrow depression; constipation
Nursing Implications	Monitor blood counts; check reflexes frequently; note neuromuscular changes; teach client measures to prevent constipation.
Examples	Vinblastine (Velban), vincristine (Oncovin)

Hormones

Androgens

Uses	Breast cancer
Side Effects	Fluid retention; masculinization
Nursing Implications	Low salt diet, monitor BP, give psychologic support in event of side effects.
Examples	Testosterone (Oreton), fluoxymesterone (Halotestin)

330 SECTION 3: NURSING CARE OF THE ADULT

Table 3.56 Continued

Estrogens

Uses	Prostatic cancer, estrogen-receptor-positive breast cancer in postmenopausal women
Side Effects	Fluid retention, CHF, feminization
Nursing Implications	Low salt diet, monitor BP, give psychologic support in event of side effects.
Examples	Diethylstilbestrol (DES), ethinyl estradiol (Estinyl)

Progestins

Uses	Metastatic endometrial cancer
Side Effects	Dermatitis
Examples	Hydroxyprogesterone (Delalutin), medroxyprogesterone (Provera)

Steroids

Uses	Leukemias, lymphomas, breast cancer, multiple myeloma, cerebral edema caused by brain metastasis (dexamethasone)
Side Effects and Nursing Implications	See table 3.36, "Steroids"
Examples	Prednisone (Colisone), dexamethasone (Decadron)

Antiestrogens

Uses	Premenopausal, estrogen-receptor-positive breast cancer
Side Effects	Dermatitis
Examples	Tamoxifen (Nolvadex)

- one extremity is isolated from the general circulation
- advantage: systemic circulation of drug is diminished, thus systemic toxic effects are reduced
- oral, IM
  f) side effects *chemotherapy*
  - common
    - nausea and vomiting
    - bone-marrow depression
    - alopecia
    - fatigue, anorexia
    - stomatitis
    - menstrual irregularities, aspermatogenesis
  - drug specific (see table 3.56)
  4) supportive, e.g., nutrition, comfort measures
2. **General Nursing Goals, Plans/Implementation, and Evaluation**

   Goal 1: Client will know guidelines for early detection of cancer.
   Plan/Implementation
   - use detection/screening services
   - explain importance of American Cancer Society guidelines for early detection in asymptomatic individuals
     - cancer-related checkup
       * every 3 years ages 20–40
       * every year after age 40
     - breast exam
       * by self (SBE): every month after age 20
       * by physician: every 3 years ages 20–40; every year after 40
       * by mammogram: single baseline x-ray between ages 35–40; every year after age 50
     - uterus
       * pelvic exam: every 3 years ages 20–40; every year after age 40
       * Pap smear: every 3 years after 2 initial negative tests one year apart, from onset of sexual activity throughout life
     - colon and rectum (men and women)
       * digital rectal exam: every year after age 40
       * guaic test: every year after age 55

* proctosigmoidoscopy: every 3–5 years after 2 initial negative exams one year apart, after age 50
- refer client to American Cancer Society for information

Evaluation: Client can state guidelines for early detection of cancer.

Goal 2: Client undergoing cancer surgery will be physically and psychologically prepared for events of the perioperative period

Plan/Implementation
- refer to Surgery page 165
- assist client to deal with body-image changes
- arrange referral to appropriate agency, e.g., Lost Chord, Reach to Recovery

Evaluation: Client is physically and psychologically prepared for events of the perioperative period.

Goal 3: Client and staff will be knowledgeable about planned radiation treatment and how to minimize side effects.

Plan/Implementation
- discuss reasons for radiation therapy and type to be used, e.g., external or internal
- external radiation
  - tell client that while he is alone during the treatment someone will be watching him closely
  - explain that skin markings must not be washed off for duration of therapy
  - teach proper skin care
    * avoid soaps and bathing the area unless approved
    * avoid exposing area to sun and temperature extremes
    * expose area to air
    * wear nonconstrictive clothing
    * do not apply cosmetics, lotions, or powder to area unless directed to do so MAy cause burning
  - maintain or improve client's nutritional status
    * administer antiemetics as needed
    * obtain nutritional counseling
    * observe for signs of mucositis
    * teach good oral hygiene
    * teach use of prescribed medications, e.g., viscous lidocaine (Xylocaine) and oral antibiotics (nystatin [Mycostatin] suspension)
    * advise small, low residue meals if diarrhea develops
    * encourage fluid intake
    * advise sweet foods if taste is altered
  - protect client from bleeding and/or infection
  - help client balance activity with rest
- internal radiation
  - tell client that once the radiation source is removed, the radioactivity is gone
  - protect staff and significant others from exposure to radiation source
    * explain that three factors critical to safe care are *time, distance,* and *shielding*
    * place client in private room
    * mark room with signs regarding radiation therapy
    * restrict visitors to one 15-minute visit/day
    * allow only nonpregnant visitors
    * use long forceps to handle a dislodged implant
    * handle client's body fluids and eating utensils as radioactive, if client has received oral or IV radioactive substances
  - prevent dislodgement of cervical implant
    * maintain strict bed rest
    * reduce residue in diet
    * prevent bladder distention

Evaluation: Client undergoes radiation therapy with minimal side effects.

Goal 4: Client will understand the goals of chemotherapy, names of drugs, anticipated side effects, and treatment of side effects.

Plan/Implementation
- discuss treatment plans with client
- tell client names of drugs prescribed and probable side effects
- maintain integrity of veins   burns
  - use arm veins
  - discontinue infusion at first sign of infiltration
  - know drugs that are vesicants (e.g., nitrogen mustard, doxorubicin)
- avoid prolonged, severe nausea and vomiting
  - use antiemetics

332 SECTION 3: NURSING CARE OF THE ADULT

Table 3.57 Antiemetics *Don't wait until nauseated*

Description	Drugs that act to treat and prevent nausea and vomiting. Most act by inhibiting the chemoreceptor trigger zone (CTZ) or by depressing the vestibular apparatus in the inner ear.
Uses	Treatment of nausea and vomiting, motion sickness
Side Effects	Drowsiness, dry mouth, flushing, hypotension, restlessness, fatigue, extrapyramidal effects (parkinsonism, akathisia, tardive dyskinesia, and dystonia)
Nursing Implications	Monitor I&O, BP; when client is on long-term phenothiazine therapy, monitor for liver disease and extrapyramidal symptoms; warn client about drowsiness; monitor effectiveness.
Types and Examples	*Phenothiazines:* prochlorperazine (Compazine), perphenazine (Trilafon)
	Nonphenothiazines: dimenhydrinate (Dramamine), benzquinamide (Emete-con), diphenidol (Vontrol), phosphated carbohydrate solution (Emetrol), trimethobenzamide (Tigan), thiethylperazine (Torecan)

- advise light food intake before treatments
- avoid dairy products and red meats
- encourage dry, bulky foods, sweet foods, clear fluids, and noncarbonated cola
- prevent infection or bleeding
  - monitor client's bone-marrow function
  - obtain CBC and platelet count before treatments (WBC of at least 3,000 is needed before therapy is started)
- prepare client for possible hair loss
  - explain that all body hair is susceptible to effects of chemotherapy but that the fastest growing hair is most affected
  - advise client to purchase a wig, hats, or scarves before losing hair
  - tell client that hair will grow back after chemotherapy is discontinued, but color and texture may be different
- maintain good oral hygiene
  - teach client good oral hygiene
  - teach client signs and symptoms of stomatitis
  - teach client what to do if stomatitis develops

Selected Health Problems

A. Cancer of the Lung
(refer to *Oxygenation* page 205)

B. Cancer of the Bladder
(refer to *Elimination* page 259)

C. Cancer of the Prostate
(refer to *Elimination* page 273)

D. Cancer of the Colon
(refer to *Elimination* page 282)

E. Cancer of the Larynx
(refer to *Safety and Security* page 310)

F. Cancer of the Cervix
1. General Information 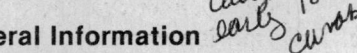 *Caught early 100% curable*
   a. Incidence
      1) second most common cancer location in women
      2) 100% cure if detected early (stage 0)
      3) squamous cell most common cell type
   b. Classification: clinical stages
      1) stage 0: carcinoma in situ
      2) stage I: confined to cervix
      3) stage II: spread from cervix to vagina
      4) stage III: involves lower one-third of vagina and has invaded paracervical tissue to pelvic wall on one or both sides and is associated with palpable lymph nodes in pelvic wall
      5) stage IV: involves bladder and rectum and extends outside true pelvis
   c. Predisposing Factors
      1) early, frequent coital exposure to multiple partners
      2) pregnancy at young age
      3) history of sexually transmitted disease/herpes
   d. Medical Treatment
      1) stage 0: conization of the cervix

2) stage I: hysterectomy or possible conization
3) stage II or III: intracavitary and external beam irradiation; possible radical hysterectomy
4) stage IV: radiation therapy followed by pelvic exenteration when there is persistent disease

2. Nursing Process
a. Assessment
1) menstrual history
2) pain in back, flank, and legs
3) vaginal discharge
4) diagnostic tests: positive cytology; Schiller's test and punch biopsy

b. Goals, Plans/Implementation, and Evaluation

Goals: refer to *Nursing Care of the Childbearing Family* page 442

G. Cancer of the Breast
1. General Information
a. Incidence
1) most common cancer in women
2) can be bilateral
3) highest incidence 40–49 and 65+
4) incidence increasing, especially in women under age 40

b. Predisposing Factors
1) family history
2) chronic irritation; fibrocystic disease
3) menarche before age 11; menopause after age 50
4) no children or 1st child after age 30
5) previous breast cancer
6) uterine cancer

c. Medical Treatment
1) surgical intervention
   a) modified radical mastectomy: breast, axillary contents
      - most commonly performed surgery
      - suitable for palpable, nonfixed tumors
   b) wedge (quadrant) resection of breast
      - a wide local excision
      - suitable for small (less than 1 cm) or nonpalpable tumors
      - usually followed by radiation and chemotherapy, hormonal manipulation
      - often done in combination with axillary lymph node dissection or sampling
      - remains somewhat controversial
   c) Halstead radical mastectomy: breast, axillary contents, pectoralis muscle
      - for advanced, fixed tumors
      - infrequently used

2) adjuvant therapy
   a) chemotherapy: specifics of therapy vary from institution to institution
   b) hormonal manipulation done if tumor is known to be estrogen receptor positive
      - premenopausal women: anti-estrogen therapy
      - postmenopausal women: estrogen therapy

d. Sequence of Surgery
1) one-step: biopsy, frozen section, and mastectomy if positive; one anesthetic
2) two-step: biopsy under local or general anesthetic; client is awakened and when pathology results are available (2–3 days), treatment options are discussed; mastectomy or definitive surgery under a 2nd anesthetic

2. Nursing Process
a. Assessment
1) dimpling of skin
2) retraction of nipple
3) hard lump; not freely movable
4) change in skin color
5) change in skin texture (peau d'orange)
6) alterations of contour of breast
7) discharge from nipple
8) pain
9) diagnostic tests: positive mammography, biopsy, and frozen section
10) ulcerations (late sign)
11) symptoms of bone, lung, and brain involvement (common areas of metastasis)

b. Goals, Plans/Implementation, and Evaluation

Goal 1: Client will be able to explain proposed surgery, effects of surgery, and pre- and postoperative care.

Plan/Implementation
- refer to *Surgery* "Perioperative Care" page 165

334 SECTION 3: NURSING CARE OF THE ADULT

- explore with client her expectations of what surgical site will look like
- discuss skin graft if one is a possibility

Evaluation: Client demonstrates knowledge of treatment options and expresses satisfaction with treatment decision.

Goal 2: Client will remain free from postoperative complications.
Plan/Implementation
- refer to *Surgery* page 165 for common complications
- check under dressing and under client's back for bleeding

Evaluation: Client is free from postoperative complications, evidence of bleeding.

Goal 3: Client will regain use of arm, joint, movement on side of surgery.
Plan/Implementation
- position arm on operative side on a pillow
- encourage hand activity, e.g., squeeze small ball
- have client use arm and hand for daily activities, e.g., brush hair
- consult with physician regarding additional exercises
- instruct client in post-op exercises, e.g., wall climbing

Evaluation: Client demonstrates appropriate postoperative exercises; knows schedule for exercising.

Goal 4: Client will be able to explain incision care, prosthetic devices available.
Plan/Implementation
- encourage client to look at incision
- on discharge, have her wear her own bra with cotton padding or "Reach to Recovery" prosthesis
- discuss with client plans for obtaining a permanent prosthesis
- teach client to wash incision with soft cloth using soap and water

Evaluation: Client has viewed incision, can explain wound care.

Goal 5: Client will be able to describe lymphedema and list ways to prevent it.
Plan/Implementation
- teach client reasons for lymphedema
- have client sleep with arm elevated on pillows
- elevate arm throughout day
- avoid any constriction around arm
- apply elastic bandage, arm TED as needed
- decrease sodium and fluid intake
- obtain an order for a JOBST pressure machine if above methods are ineffective

Evaluation: Client can state measures to prevent lymphedema; keeps arm elevated at rest.

Goal 6: Client will be able to describe precautions necessary to prevent infections in arm on side of surgery.
Plan/Implementation
- avoid BP measurements, injections, blood drawing in affected arm
- wear gloves when gardening, etc.
- attend to any small cut or scrape immediately
- avoid biting, chewing nails
- prevent sunburn and any kind of regular burn
- do not shave axilla on affected side

Evaluation: Client can state measures to avoid arm infection.

Goal 7: Client will demonstrate positive self-concept.
Plan/Implementation
- encourage return to normal activities
- help plan for prosthesis fitting and discuss types of clothes she can wear
- discuss reconstruction possibilities
- encourage client to discuss operation and diagnosis with significant others
- spend time with significant others to allow discussion of concerns and fears, so they can provide support for client's needs
- arrange "Reach to Recovery" visit

Evaluation: Client had "Reach to Recovery" visit; discusses self in positive terms; has plans to obtain prosthesis.

Goal 8: Client will experience normal grieving.
Plan/Implementation
- allow client to cry, withdraw, etc.
- explain that these feelings are usual and expected, that other women in a similar situation feel the same way
- help client focus on future, but discuss loss
- let client know that sometimes grief is delayed 2 or 3 months, and that it is a normal experience nonetheless

Evaluation: Client is expressing grief over loss of breast, diagnosis.

Goal 9: Client and significant other can describe additional treatment when appropriate.
Plan/Implementation
- refer to General Nursing Goal 3

Evaluation: Client can state anticipated side effects of planned adjuvant therapy.

References

Bjeletich, J. and Hickman, R. "The Hickman Indwelling Catheter." *American Journal of Nursing*. January 1980:62-65.

Burns, N. "Cancer Chemotherapy: A Systemic Approach." *Nursing 78*. February 1978:56-63.

Dobittal, S. "Enabling a Patient to Die at Home." *American Journal of Nursing*. August 1980:1448-1450.

Kelly, P. and Tinsley, C. "Planning Care for the Patient Receiving External Radiation." *American Journal of Nursing*. February 1981:338-342.

Mamaril, A. "Preventing Complications After Radical Mastectomy." *American Journal of Nursing*. November 1974:2000-2056.

O'Connor, A. (Ed.) *Nursing: The Oncology Patient*. New York: American Journal of Nursing Company, 1980.

Valentine, A., Steckel, S., and Weintraub, M. "Pain Relief for Cancer Patients." *American Journal of Nursing*. December 1978:2054-2056.

Varricchio, C. "The Patient on Radiation Therapy." *American Journal of Nursing*. February 1981:334-337.

Vredevoe, D., Derdarian, A., Sarna, L., Friel, M., and Shiplacoff, J. *Concepts of Oncology Nursing*. Englewood Cliffs, NJ: Prentice-Hall, 1981.

Woods, M. and Kowalski, J. "Symposium on Oncologic Nursing Practice." *Nursing Clinics of North America*. December 1982.

Reprints
Nursing Care of the Adult

Heidrich, G. et al. "Helping the Patient in Pain." 339
Long, M. et al. "Hypertension: What Patients Need to
   Know." 345
Neal, M. et al. "Hyperalimentation." 351
Chambers, J. "Bowel Management in Dialysis Patients." 352
"The Person with a Spinal Cord Injury." 354

Helping The Patient in Pain

Reprinted from American Journal of Nursing, December 1982.

By George Heidrich
Samuel Perry

When it comes to pain management, you can feel caught between the patient and the physician. The patient is in pain—either the pain medication he received is not strong enough or it is not given often enough. The physician, on the other hand, is being cautious: analgesics may cause oversedation or lead to addiction. What do you do?

There are several approaches to pain management that will eliminate the conflict between what a patient needs and what has been ordered. One approach involves being able to assess a patient's pain and its relief. Another is to administer a prescribed pain medication in the most effective way. Others include using nonpharmacological methods for diminishing pain and reviewing a pain problem with the primary physician when changes in the analgesic regimen are necessary.

How do you assess pain?

How can you determine how much a patient hurts and how well the prescribed analgesics are working? Some nurses do not know how to assess pain and end up relying on their judgment of how much a patient *should* hurt. But subjective judgments about someone else's discomfort may lead to an adversarial rather than a trusting relationship. Further complicating the issue are studies indicating that patients undergoing the same procedure or suffering from the same illness vary widely in the severity of pain they experience and in their response to identical doses of an analgesic[1]. In other words, how much pain a patient experiences is unique to each patient.

Another problem arises when a patient's behavior is taken as the only indicator of the existence or severity of pain. Restlessness, moaning, or grimacing can be misleading. The patient may not be in pain but, rather, disoriented, confused, hypoxic, febrile, or having a medication reaction. The patient who appears to be resting comfortably may be struggling not to show pain or trying not to aggravate the pain by moving. In one study, volunteers were videotaped as they were injected with a solution that causes pain. It was found that nearly half

---

GEORGE HEIDRICH, RN, MA, is program coordinator, analgesic research, University of Wisconsin Hospital and clinics, Dept. of Anesthesiology, Madison. Mr. Heidrich is editor of *PRN forum*, a newsletter for pain research nurses

SAMUEL PERRY, MD, is an associate professor of psychiatry, Cornell University Medical College, New York, NY. Dr. Perry is the primary investigator for a research project involving the treatment of pain in burn patients at New York Hospital-Cornell Medical Center.

The authors express their deep appreciation to Ada G. Rogers, RN; Raymond W. Houde, MD; and Stanley L. Wallenstein, MS; all of the Analgesic Study Section of the Memorial Sloan-Kettering Institute for Cancer Research, for their willingess to share clinical insights.

This work was supported in part by NIH Grant P50 GM26145.

the subjects did not grimace, moan, clench their eyelids, or give other behavioral cues associated with pain. When questioned, however, the subjects stated that the injection was painful(2).

How, then, can pain be accurately evaluated? The answer was well stated over a hundred years ago by Peter Latham, a British physician and author: "Not only degrees of pain, but its existence, in any degree, must be taken upon the testimony of the patients"(3). Over the last 20 years, numerous analgesic studies have determined that asking the patient is the most reliable method of assessing pain and pain relief. The success of these studies has been in the ability of the researcher to develop questions that have answers that are quantifiable and meaningful to patients(4).

A commonly used set of questions for analgesic testing involves the use of categorical scales. Before the patient is medicated, his level of pain is assessed by asking, "How much pain do you have right *now*?" He then chooses one of four answers: no pain—0, slight pain—1, moderate pain—2, or severe pain—3. The reply is recorded by the researcher, and if the pain is moderate or severe, the drug is then administered. At hourly intervals the patient is asked again about his level of pain, but he is also asked, "How much pain *relief* is the medication giving you right now?" The patient replies no relief—0, slight relief—1, moderate relief—2, a lot of relief—3, or complete relief of pain—4.

This questioning and recording of the patient's responses continues until the patient reports that he is experiencing "complete pain relief" from the analgesic. This method provides information about the onset of action, the duration of analgesic effect, the hourly level of pain, and hourly pain relief afforded the patient(5). The method is neither difficult nor time-consuming. In a clinical situation, a nurse can use the categorical scales to document a patient's pain and how effective the pain medication has been. Based on the patient's responses, she can plan how much and how often to give an analgesic. The responses elicited by scales can be easily transferred to a permanent pain record, which can be placed in the patient's chart. Such a record is a dramatic representation of the patient's pain and response to the analgesic medication. A pain site diagram can also be used (see chart on p. 1831) and can be particularly helpful in keeping track of multiple pain sites in the patient with metastatic disease. When a new pain site is identified, the health care team can move quickly to evaluate the appropriateness of radiation therapy, surgical intervention, or another analgesic therapy.

The scales have additional value beyond reliably recording a patient's pain. Their use establishes an alliance between the patient and nurse. A patient may begin to take a more active role in dealing with his pain. Some patients choose to complete the scales themselves in order to gain some control over the emotion-laden issue.

Some individuals may fear that a patient will abuse the scales by overestimating his pain and understating its relief. Experience has shown, however, that the vast majority of patients are not eager to receive excessive medication and only want to make sure that their pain is fully appreciated.

When the analgesic does not work and the patient continues to complain, those providing care understandably become frustrated. If it is understood how a prescribed pain medication can be given most effectively, a therapeutic alliance between the staff and patient can be established. Effective administration includes knowing when to give an analgesic, whether to give the drug intramuscularly or orally, whether a placebo or psychotropic drug is indicated, and how to recognize signs of physical dependence, tolerance, and withdrawal.

How long should a patient wait?

At times a patient may be advised to "wait a little longer if you can," but such advice is usually given because a caretaker is not aware that analgesics are most effective if they are given *before* a patient's pain becomes severe. Thus, patients should be advised to *intercept* pain and not endure it. They will thereby suffer less, require lower dosages of analgesics, and be less anxious and more in control of their discomfort(6).

When should the analgesic be given IM and when PO?

The answer to this question is more complicated than one might think. First, consider that, in general, an injection offers quicker pain relief than does a pill taken by mouth. Parenterally administered narcotics usually achieve maximum effect within one hour, whereas it may take two hours for the oral form to peak(7). As the patient waits for pain relief, his pain becomes more severe and the medication is then less effective when it does take effect.

Second, in deciding whether to use the intramuscular or oral route, consider the nature of pain. If the pain is acute and intermittent, the parenteral route will rapidly curb the pain when it occurs; but if the pain is chronic and unfluctuating, the oral route may offer a more sustained relief and prevent a "roller-coaster effect." This effect is normally seen when the amount, frequency, and route of administration of the analgesic are varied within a 24-hour period.

A third consideration in choosing the route of administration relates to the comparative potencies of analgesic drugs in parenteral or oral form. A chart comparing the two routes is shown on page 1832. Using this table, consider a typical postoperative prescription: "Demerol 50-100 mg IM/PO every 3-4 hours prn." This prescription offers the nurse a wide range of analgesic options. The maximum dosage—100 mg meperidine (Demerol) IM—has approximately the same analgesic potential as 13 mg morphine IM. The minimum dosage—50 mg meperidine PO—has the equivalent analgesic effect of 2 aspirin. This prescription, therefore, gives the nurse a choice between 2 aspirin or 13 mg morphine IM. Furthermore, if the nurse on the next shift chooses to use the oral rather than the intramuscular route for the same dosage, the patient will receive far less analgesia than before and the "roller-coaster effect" will be produced. For the patient to have the same analgesic effect with an oral dose as he would with 75 mg of meperidine IM, the patient needs 300 mg meperidine PO.

Thus, on the basis of a nurse's discretion, the patient can receive a wide range of narcotic potencies over a 24-hour period. If he receives the maximum amount—100 mg meperidine IM every 3 hours for 24 hours, the total milligram dosage would be 800 mg IM, or the analgesic equivalent of 106 mg of morphine. If he receives the minimum amount—50 mg meperidine by mouth every 4 hours—his 24-hour total would be 300 mg PO or the analgesic equivalent of 10 mg of morphine IM. The range between 10 mg and 106 mg of morphine IM offers the nurse a number of options that are often needed when dealing with the fluctuations in pain. Care must be exercised, however, so that the patient is not experiencing highs and then lows in the relief of the pain.

Finally, patients with chronic pain who have been taking intramuscular narcotics over a long period may be reluctant to switch to the oral route. For example, a cancer patient being readied for discharge may be inadequately prepared for this transition. Instead of abruptly switching a newly discharged patient to the oral equivalent dosage (such as from 4 mg of levorphanol [Levo-Dromoran] IM to 8 mg of levorphanol PO), the patient can be given one-half the dosage by injection (2 mg) and the other half by mouth (4 mg). This way the patient will receive the quick onset of the intramuscular dosage and the longer-acting effect of the oral route. After a few days, when the patient is comfortable with this regimen, the intramuscular dosage can be reduced to 1 mg and the oral dosage increased to 6 mg. Over the course of a week or so, the patient can be gradually converted to oral analgesics alone.

How can you tell if a patient is becoming addicted?

This question reflects a concern of nurses and physicians who observe a patient requesting larger dosages of pain medication, asking for the drugs more frequently, or both. First a difference between addiction and tolerance must be understood.

Tolerance simply means that *increasingly larger dosages of narcotics are necessary to provide the effect produced by the original dose*. Tolerance has been compared to inflation: when the cost of a bus ride is raised from 35 cents to 50 cents, the reason for taking the bus remains unchanged. What *has* changed is that the 35-cent fare will no longer pay for the same ride to the same place. More money—or analgesic—is necessary.

Addiction, on the other hand, is "*a behavioral pattern of drug use, characterized by overwhelming involvements with the use of a drug (compulsive use), the securing of its supply, and high tendency to relapse after withdrawal*"(8). Once it is acknowledged that tolerance is the inevitable pharmacological effect of using narcotics continuously over time and that the development of tolerance should not be confused with drug abuse, it is easier to accept the early signs of tolerance and alert the patient's physician to make the necessary adjustments.

One of the first indications of tolerance is that the period of analgesic effect of the drug is shortened. Because the narcotic is not working for as long a period of time, the patient will request medication more frequently and will begin "watching the clock" in anticipation of the next dose. This preoccupation with receiving the analgesic on time may lead the staff to believe that the patient is beginning to crave the drug and is on his way to becoming an addict. Actually, the development of tolerance and the unrelieved pain are dictating the patient's request.

For patients who have had acute pain, such as those recovering from surgery, tolerance is not usually an issue, because the pain will diminish sufficiently before tolerance to the drug develops. Tolerance is more commonly a problem in patients whose pain is more chronic, such as those who have metastatic bone cancer. When tolerance is developing and narcotics remain the pain treatment of choice, the dose of the drug ought to be increased or the time interval between doses shortened. Increasing the dosage does not increase the risk of respiratory depression. Tolerance to the respiratory depressant or sedative, and other CNS effects develop at essentially the same rate as tolerance to the analgesic effect(9).

Along with being alert to the early signs of tolerance, one also ought to be aware of the possible development of physiological dependence, which can occur over time. For example, if 10 mg morphine IM are given a few times a day, physical dependence will become evident after about 10 days(10). Like tolerance, physiological dependence does not mean that the patient has become addicted; it only means that a withdrawal syndrome will occur if the narcotic is stopped abruptly. In most clinical situations, pain seldom stops all at once. Usually, as healing takes place, pain gradually subsides. With less pain, the patient makes fewer requests for analgesics and thereby slowly withdraws himself without ever realizing physiological dependence has occurred. In those rare situations in which pain stops abruptly, as with a nerve block or surgical intervention, the patient may become inexplicably anxious and report abdominal cramps and rhinorrhea. These symptoms, which signal withdrawal, can be managed by tapering the narcotics on a fixed schedule over the course of 7 to 10 days, using one-fourth of the original dose of a long-acting oral narcotic (methadone) every six hours for the first few days, then increasing the time interval every two to three days until the patient is gradually taken off the drug(11).

When should you give a placebo?

Placebos are sometimes administered when a patient is given an analgesic and continues to complain of pain. This issue is complicated both from an ethical and pharmacological point of view(12). Before giving a placebo, it must be understood that a response to a placebo does not mean that pain is not real or severe. Many patients with documented physical pain respond to a placebo the first few times but then request a "stronger" medication(13). As a general rule, rather than threatening to break the necessary trust between patient and staff, the nurse and physician ought to work out a treatment plan.

When should you give a tranquilizer?

Along with the standing analgesic orders, a physician will often prescribe a psychotropic drug, such as promethazine (Phenergan), to be given as necessary. It is often tempting to use these drugs to calm the patient who is in pain. Although some psychotropic agents have been shown to have analgesic properties, most tranquilizers do *not* help relieve the pain and only potentiate

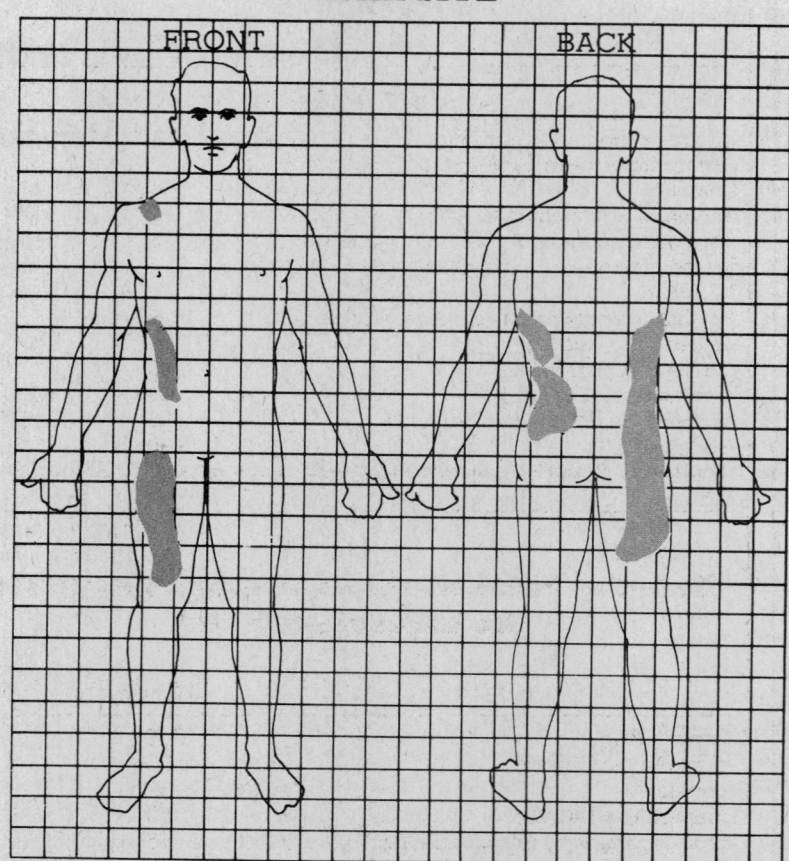

the sedative effect of the analgesic(14-16). Sedation can lead to confusion, disorientation, and agitation. The result, then, is a drowsy patient who is more frightened about pain and has less capacity to cope with it. Therefore, as a general principle, when patients become anxious, distraught, and hypersensitive because of unrelieved pain, treat these secondary psychological phenomena by treating the pain itself with more effective analgesia. If the pain is relieved, often the associated anxiety and depression are relieved as well.

The idea of combining analgesics with other types of medication, such as psychotropics, has recently become more popular because of the numerous articles, particularly in the lay press, about Brompton's cocktail. Though the ingredients of this combination vary at each institution, a typical solution includes an analgesic (morphine, methadone, or heroin), an antiemetic (chlorpromazine), a stimulant (cocaine, amphetamine), a bacteriocidal base (ethyl alcohol), and a sugared syrup. It is usually given on an around-the-clock schedule every 3 to 6 hours for patients suffering with chronic pain from advanced cancer.

Because patients in pain are often desperately looking for the "magic bullet" and may ask about this acclaimed combination, the nurse ought to be aware that numerous clinical problems are beginning to emerge as more institutions use these cocktails. One problem has been caused by the stimulant additive. Cocaine or an amphetamine is used to overcome sedative effects from the narcotic, but in elderly or debilitated patients such stimulants can cause agitation and disorientation. This confusion is not easily distinguished from the CNS effects of the disease itself. The opposite kind of problem has been caused by the antiemetic, which is usually a tranquilizer such as chlorpromazine (Thorazine). These drugs produce a depressant effect and the resulting lethargy can limit the amount of narcotics used. A third problem has been attributed to the ethyl alcohol or vodka. Although the amount is small and probably not an additional depressant, many patients find that the alcohol irritates mucous membranes already sensitized by the disease and chemotherapy.

Those who originally advocated the use of Brompton's cocktail have recently simplified its list of ingredients(17-20). Some made this change because they found oral morphine was as good for pain relief as the heroin in the cocktail. Twycross, for example, gives his patients a pain cocktail consisting only of morphine and water(21). In defense of Brompton's cocktail, its use helped clinicians realize the importance of medicating terminally ill patients before their pain became severe, using a fixed time schedule and a carefully titrated dosage.

What other methods can be used?

The experience with Brompton's cocktail is a reminder that no one analgesic method is perfect for treating all types and severities of pain. Nonpharmacological methods must be used as well. Such strategies as hypnosis, biofeedback, acupuncture, and autosuggestion, however, require training and experience in using them. Some patients may be too physically ill or skeptical to accept these techniques.

All pain has a psychological

Relative Potencies of Analgesics Commonly Used for Severe Pain*

	IM (mg)	PO (mg)
morphine	10	60
oxymorphone (Numorphan)	1	6
hydromorphone (Dilaudid)	1.5	7.5
levorphanol (Levo-Dromoran)	2	4
heroin	4	—
methadone (Dolophine)	10	20
oxycodone (Percocet—5, oxycodone and acetaminophen; Percodan, oxycodone and APC)	15	30
methotrimeprazine (Levoprome, Nozinan)	20	
anileridine (Leritine)	30	50
alphaprodine (Nisentil)	45	
pentazocine (Talwin)	60	180
meperidine (Pethidine, Demerol)	75	300
codeine	130	200

*Expressed in IM and PO doses approximately equivalent in total effect to a morphine 10 mg IM.

Relative Potencies of Analgesics Used Orally for Less Severe Pain*

	PO (mg)
aspirin (ASA)	650
pentazocine (Talwin)	30
codeine	32
meperidine (Demerol)	50
propoxyphene hydrochloride (Darvon)	65
propoxyphene napsylate (Darvon-N)	100
phenacetin (acetophenetidin)	650
acetaminophen (Tylenol)	650
sodium salicylate	1,000

*Expressed in doses approximately equivalent in total effect of ASA 650 mg.

Adapted with permission from Rogers, A. G. Pharmacology of analgesics, J. Neurosurgical Nsg., 10:182, 1978.

component; that is, pain is not something that is just felt; pain also means something to the patient. Moreover, this meaning is not usually vague or general; pain has a specific meaning for this particular patient at this particular time in his or her life. The nurse has an opportunity to determine specifically what that meaning is. For the most part, this determination is not difficult. The majority of patients will answer directly if asked directly: "What do you think is causing this pain and what are you worried will happen?" Some patients may have distortions and exaggerated fears: a baseball-sized lump must be pressing on the nerves in my back; I'm going to bleed to death; because this pain is not getting better, it means that the doctors don't know what's the matter with me, or that I will be crippled, or that I have cancer, and so on.

The nurse should not avoid discussing specific disease-related questions with the patient. In fact, the patient's misconceptions can usually be quickly relieved by providing information that offers some hope and insight, such as, "The pain is caused by an irritation of your nerves. We are aware of your pain and know that its presence is not a sign that you will fail to improve." A more detailed explanation about the disease process and the prognosis is rarely necessary as long as the patient's specific fear has been addressed. Statements with a focus on the patient's personal concerns are far better than blanket reassurances.

A study done by Beecher points out how any assessment of pain must take into account the meaning of the pain to the patient(22). During World War II, Beecher cared for soldiers who were wounded on the beaches of Anzio. He was surprised to find that these soldiers complained little about their pain and took morphine very infrequently. When he questioned them, he learned that they were indeed experiencing pain but their wounds meant that they would be freed from an extremely dangerous situation and they would be sent home to recuperate.

In the same way, patients with postoperative pain, having undergone a successful surgical procedure, may view their pain as a sign of the healing process and can look forward to discharge and resumption of normal activities. In contrast, patients with unrelenting chronic pain may view their discomfort not as a sign of recovery but as a reminder of their disease. Many times it can quite honestly be pointed out to patients that the presence of pain does not in itself mean a poor prognosis or that because of the pain, the patient is going to be crippled or die. When a patient begins to view his pain not as a death knell, but as a signal that he is ill, he is less likely to expect the staff to relieve the pain totally and may be more tolerant of the inevitable mild discomfort.

Even after the steps suggested have been taken, the patient may still be experiencing sufficient pain to warrant a change in the route, dose, frequency, or kind of analgesic medication he is receiving. A discussion with the prescribing physician then becomes necessary. To make a comment such as "Ms. Jones is still complaining about pain" is of little service in communicating significant information. Instead, a more effective statement would be "Ms. Jones's pain continues to be severe. The analgesics are only effective for two hours. Her surgical wound is draining well; she is alert and has no respiratory compromise or fever. How would you like to increase her analgesic regimen?" If the physician fails to respond, perhaps because of an unsubstantiated fear of iatrogenic addiction, the placement in the chart of the categorical pain assessment scales may prove to be of assistance(23,24). Hourly, documented recordings of severe, unrelieved pain are difficult to ignore. Like laboratory values, the categorical scales can be seen as "numbers" that require an adjustment.

Managing a patient's pain can be an intriguing and gratifying process. If the nurse is knowledgeable about the pain experience and the use of analgesics, a potentially frustrating clinical problem can be transformed into a mutually rewarding situation.

References

1. Bellville, J. W., and others. Influence of age on pain relief from analgesics. *JAMA* 217:1835-1841, Sept. 27, 1971.
2. Lim, K. S., and Guzman, F. Manifestations of pain in analgesic evaluation in animals and man. In *Pain Proceedings of the International Symposium on Pain*, ed. by A. Soulairac and others. New York, Academic Press, 1968, pp. 119-152.
3. Latham, P. M. *Lectures on subjects connected with clinical medicine*, 2nd ed. Philadelphia, Barrington and Haskell, 1847, pp. 108-117.
4. Wallenstein, S. L., and Houde, R. W. The clinical evaluation of analgesic effectiveness. In *Methods in Narcotic Research*, ed. by M. S. Ehrenpreis and A. Neidel. New York, Marcel Dekker, 1975, pp. 127-145.
5. _____, and others. Clinical evaluation of mild analgesics: the measurement of clinical pain. *Br.J.Clin.Pharmacol.*10(Suppl.):319S-327S, Oct. 1980.
6. Saunders, Cicely. Control of pain in terminal cancer. *Nurs.Times* 72:1133-1135, July 22, 1976.
7. Rogers, A. G. Pain and the cancer patient. *Nurs.Clin.North. Am.* 2:671-682, Dec. 1967.
8. Jaffe, J. H. Drug addiction and drug abuse. IN *Goodman and Gilman's The Pharmacological Basis of Therapeutics*, 6th edition edited by L. S. Goodman and others. New York, Macmillan Publishing Co., 1980, p. 536.
9. Houde, R. W. The management of pain. IN *Oncology 1970 Vol. 3. Diagnosis and Management of Cancer*, ed. by R. L. Clar and others. Chicago Year Book Medical Publishers, 1971, pp. 489-496.
10. Jaffe, *op.cit.*, pp. 535-584.
11. Rogers, A. G. Pharmacology of analgesics. *J.Neurosurg.Nurs.* 10:180-184, Dec. 1978.
12. Perry, S. W., and Heidrich, George. Placebo response: myth and matter. *Am.J.Nurs.* 81:720-722, Apr. 1981.
13. Mosteller, F., and others. Study of the placebo response. *Am.J.Med.* 16:770-779, June 1954.
14. Beaver, W. T., and Feise, G. Comparison of the analgesic effects of morphine hydroxyzine, and their combination in patients with postoperative pain. IN *Advances in Pain Research and Therapy*, ed. by J. J. Bonica and others. New York, Raven Press, 1976, Vol. 1. pp. 553-557.
15. Houde, R. W., and Wallenstein, S. L. Analgesic power of chlorpromazine alone and in combination with morphine. (abs) *Pharmacol.Exp.Ther.* 14:353, March 1955.
16. Keats, A. S., and others. "Potentiation" of meperidine by promethazine. *Anesthesiology* 22:34-41, Jan-Feb. 1961.
17. Mount, B. M., and others. Use of the Brompton mixture in treating the chronic pain of malignant disease. *Can.Med.Assoc.J.* 115:122-124. July 17, 1976.
18. Twycross, R. G. Diamorphine and cocaine elixer BPC 1973. *Pharm.J.*:153, 159, Feb. 1974.
19. Mount, B. M., and others. The Brompton mixture: a comparison of the standard mixture and orally administered morphine. (abs) *Pain* 1:201, Aug. 27-Sept. 1, 1978.
20. Twycross, R. G. The relief of cocaine in the Brompton cocktail. (abs) *Pain* 1:78, Aug. 27-Sept 1, 1978.
21. _____. The relief of pain in far advanced cancer. *Regional. Anesth.* 5:2-11, July-Sept. 1, 1980.
22. Beecher, H. K. Pain in men wounded in battle. *Ann.Surg.* 123:96-105, Jan. 1946.
23. Marks, R. M., and Sacher, E. J. Undertreatment of medical inpatients with narcotic analgesics. *Ann.Intern.Med.* 78:173-181, Feb. 1973.
24. Porter, J., and Jick, H. Addiction rare in patients treated with narcotics. (letter) *N.Engl.J.Med.* 302:123, Jan. 10, 1980.

HYPERTENSION

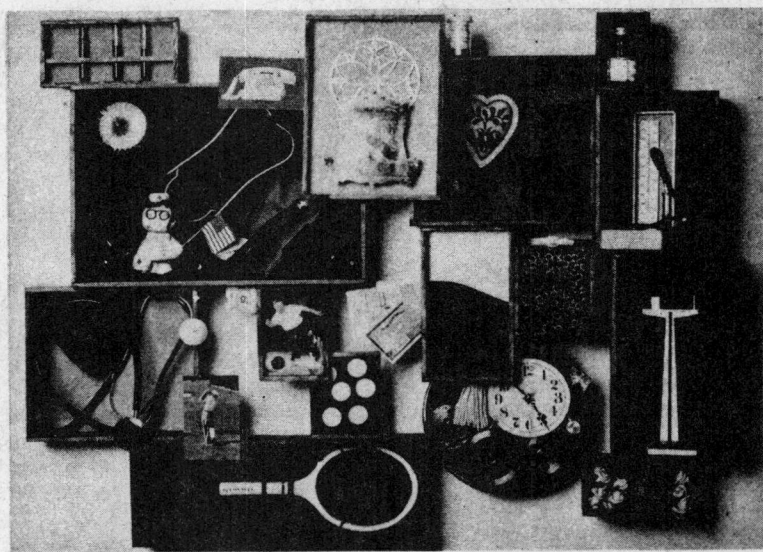

What Patients Need to Know

MADELEINE L. LONG / ELIZABETH H. WINSLOW / MARY ANN SCHEUHING / JULE A. CALLAHAN

Reprinted from American Journal of Nursing, May 1976.

Hypertension menaces 20 to 25 million Americans producing premature sickness, disability, and death. Its prevalence rises steadily with age and is twice as great in blacks as in whites.

Disability and death are directly related to the level of blood pressure elevation; the higher a pressure is, the worse the prognosis becomes. For example, mortality in men ages 35 to 45 with a blood pressure of 160/100 mm. Hg is five times higher than in those with a blood pressure below 140/90 mm. Hg. Patients with even a slight elevation in blood pressure risk heart attack, stroke, or heart failure with two to six times greater frequency than normotensive individuals[1].

Reducing elevated pressure reduces the sickness, disability, and death that prolonged hypertension causes. Reports of the Veterans Administration Cooperative Study Group on Antihypertensive Agents dramatically demonstrated the efficacy of 18 months' of drug therapy for men with severe hypertension: only 2 of 73 treated men died or had serious complications, but 27 of 70 untreated men died or experienced major complications of hypertension[2,3].

In spite of such evidence, hypertension remains a massive health threat. One half of all persons with hypertension probably have not been identified. One half of known hypertensives are untreated, and one half of treated hypertensives are inadequately treated[4].

The major determinants of blood pressure are cardiac output and total peripheral resistance. Any factor that increases these will increase mean blood pressure. Most cases of hyper-

MADELEINE L. LONG, R.N., M.S., is a staff nurse in the Intensive Care Unit, Philadelphia General Hospital.

ELIZABETH H. WINSLOW, R.N., was a cardiovascular clinical specialist, Hospital of the University of Pennsylvania, Phila., when this article was written. She is now a cardiovascular clinical specialist, St. Paul Hospital, Dallas, Texas.

MARY ANN SCHEUHING, R.N., PH.D., is an assistant professor of anatomy and physiology at Peirce Jr. College in Philadelphia.

JULE A. CALLAHAN, R.N., MPH., is coordinator of ambulatory care at the Hospital of the University of Pennsylvania.

tension, however, are caused by increased peripheral resistance, with cardiac output remaining normal[5].

Most of the peripheral resistance to systemic circulation occurs in the arterioles. The marked narrowing in the radius of the arteriolar lumen that accompanies sustained high blood pressure exerts particularly deleterious effects on four target organs: the brain, retina, heart, and kidneys.

High pressure in vessels leading to the brain increases the incidence of strokes due to hemorrhage and thrombosis. The principal retinal changes include vascular sclerosis, exudation, and hemorrhage. Elevated pressure increases cardiac work, resulting in left ventricular hypertrophy, congestive heart failure, angina pectoris, and myocardial infarction. Vascular damage to the kidneys causes diminution of function and eventual renal failure. Adequate therapy usually can mitigate or prevent these complications.

A precise definition of high blood pressure is needed to identify persons

HYPERTENSION

requiring evaluation and therapy. The American Heart Association recommends an age-related definition of hypertension:

    under 40 .... 140/90 or greater
    over 40 .... 160/95 or greater

Either systolic or diastolic elevation necessitates secondary screening or referral for evaluation and therapy(6).

A single high blood pressure reading does not establish a diagnosis of hypertension because stress, anxiety, discomfort, and physical activity may cause sharp but transient blood pressure elevations. The following guidelines are helpful to document sustained hypertension:
- take blood pressure with the patient in the upright position on three occasions at least one week apart;
- reevaluate as an outpatient any normotensive hospitalized patient suspected of having elevated pressure because bedrest reduces blood pressure;
- consider any hospitalized patient hypertensive if three out of four diastolic pressures are greater than 100 mm. Hg on two consecutive days;
- reevaluate pregnant women six weeks after delivery;
- reevaluate women suspected of hypertension while taking birth control pills after they have used some other form of contraception for four to six months, because oral contraceptives may elevate pressure(7).

Hypertension is classified as primary or secondary. Approximately 90 percent of all patients with elevated pressure have primary hypertension (without known cause). Primary hypertension also may be referred to as idiopathic, essential, or benign hypertension. The nurse should make sure that the patient does not think "essential" means "necessary." "Benign" should not be used, because it is misleading and may hinder understanding of the seriousness of the disease. Multiple factors are involved in the etiology of primary hypertension, including nervous, vascular, and endocrine mechanisms.

Recent evidence suggests that the renin-angiotensin-aldosterone system is a factor in the pathogenesis of primary hypertension.* Primary hypertension may be subdivided into low, normal, or high renin categories, and treated accordingly. Malignant hypertension, an accelerated phase associated with extremely high blood pressure levels, occurs in one to five percent of persons with primary hypertension. If therapy is not effective, death occurs rapidly from uremia or intracranial vascular accident.

Secondary hypertension includes

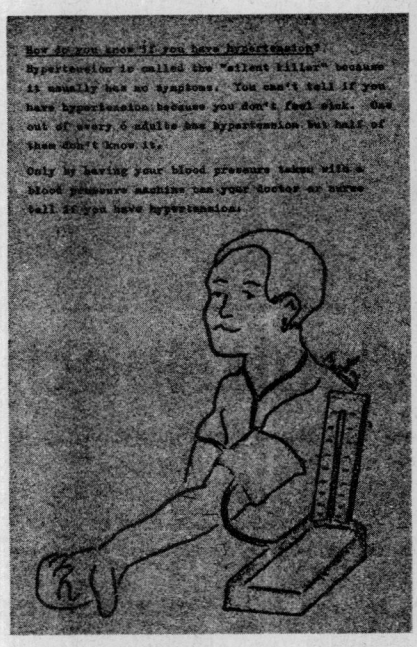

Sample page from booklet prepared by authors for use with patients.

only 5 to 10 percent of all hypertensive disease and is caused by specific conditions, many of them curable. Consequently, the diagnosis of primary hypertension is reached by excluding secondary forms. Usually, causes of secondary hypertension can be ruled out by physical examination and routine laboratory studies. Only in selected cases are complicated and expensive diagnostic workups necessary.

General measures for treating primary hypertension are patient education, weight control, sodium restriction, and reduction of cardiac risk factors.

Obesity and hypertension are interrelated. Sometimes, weight reduction

*See "Renin and Blood Pressure," September 1975 *AJN*.

is the only measure needed to lower the blood pressure. There is also evidence that hypertension is related to high sodium levels; moderation in the use of salt is necessary, especially if diuretics are not prescribed.

The presence of cardiac risk factors significantly increases morbidity and mortality in the hypertensive person. Smoking should be discontinued, hyperlipidemia and diabetes mellitus controlled, regular exercise encouraged, and anxious, restless individuals should be helped to find ways to relax. If these measures do not lower blood pressure to acceptable levels, drug therapy is considered.

The indications for drug treatment of mild hypertension are not as definitive as those for moderate and severe hypertension. The VA cooperative study group suggested that patients with diastolic blood pressures averaging 105 mm. Hg or higher receive drug treatment(2,3,8).

For people whose diastolic pressures average 90-104 mm. Hg, the benefits of treatment must be weighed against the possible untoward effects, expense, and inconvenience of lifelong drug therapy.

The decision to medicate borderline hypertensives is influenced by the following risk factors: target organ damage, male sex, age under 50, black race, smoking, and a family history of diabetes or hypercholesterolemia.

The goal of drug therapy is to reduce pressure to the lowest level the patient will tolerate. Usually a diastolic pressure of 90 mm. Hg or lower in the standing position can be achieved without serious medication side effects. Frequently, treatment is initiated with a thiazide diuretic; dosage is titrated and other drugs added or deleted until optimal effects are attained. Potent diuretics are reserved for patients with impaired renal function. If hypokalemia becomes a problem, the potassium-conserving diuretics are used.

If the blood pressure is not controlled by diuretic therapy alone, antihypertensive agents that affect the sympathetic nervous system or vascular smooth muscle are added. Hydralazine (apresoline) is rarely given alone because it is better tolerated and more effective when used with other agents. It is often the third or fourth agent in a drug combination, and its many side effects are minimized by methyldopa (Aldomet) or propranolol (Inderal). Reserpine (Serpasil) is used infrequently because of its recent association with breast cancer and past association with depressive reactions.

The use of propranolol for hypertension is still under investigation in the United States. It seems to be the drug of choice for hypertensive patients with tachycardia, high cardiac output, or angina.

If drug treatment is kept as simple as possible and clearly explained to patients, compliance can be expected.

Because most people with hypertension are symptomless, they do not seek medical advice. To identify victims of this "silent killer," well-publicized mass screening programs with *systematic follow-up* are a critical need. Every time a patient sees a health provider—at school, office, community agency, or hospital—his blood pressure should be checked and he should be referred for evaluation of any abnormal finding. Hypertension tends to be hereditary, so hypertensives are encouraged to have their family members evaluated.

Merely identifying hypertensive individuals and initiating therapy does not solve the problem, because many patients arbitrarily stop treatment, particularly if therapy produces unpleasant side effects. Patient education is important in all illnesses, but especially in asymptomatic hypertension. Patients' cooperation with treatment increases as they learn about the disease and the rationale behind the therapeutic methods and goals.

A nurse is often the best person to teach the patient. An assessment of his knowledge about his condition is fundamental. What additional information he would like and what he is ready to learn must be determined. Family members should be included in teaching sessions whenever feasible.

Myths about hypertension often undermine treatment efforts. Patients may refer to hypertension as "high blood," the opposite of "low blood" (anemia); or attribute hypertension to eating too many spices, or believe that

---

LIVING WITH HYPERTENSION

When Mr. R.'s blood pressure, taken routinely in a dental clinic, was 160/120 mm. Hg, he was referred for medical follow-up. Although he "felt fine" Mr. R. went to a medical clinic, where a physician diagnosed essential hypertension and started treatment. A year later he was referred for nursing conferences to help him better understand and control his hypertension.

A 42-year-old high school graduate who was married and had three children, Mr. R., worked as a machine operator in a printing plant. He was an interested, cooperative patient who was capable of following his treatment program, but several problems interfered with his adjustment to his illness and his compliance with therapy. The following problems and approaches emerged during several months of nursing conferences.

PROBLEM	APPROACH
Reluctance to express concerns about disease. "No, I don't have any questions. I know all about 'high blood.'"	Encouraged Mr. R. to voice feelings, suggested questions he might have, assured him that they were normal and expected.
Misconceptions about disease. "I almost have it licked. I've been taking my medicine and I feel good."	Repeatedly explained nature of disease, stressing chronicity and control versus cure.
Incorrect medication administration. "I don't always take the water pill because I'm not swollen or bloated. Besides, it keeps me up at night. When I'm on evening or night shift, I sometimes forget the blood pressure pills. Now I'm trying to get them all in by taking them every couple hours."	Reviewed action of drugs, expected side effects, and times to best take them. Helped patient devise medication time schedule for each shift.
Unwillingness to have wife accompany him to clinic. "She gets upset and nervous too easy."	Phoned Mrs. R., briefly discussed hypertension and its treatment, invited her to phone whenever she had concerns or questions about her husband.
Denial of symptoms. "I feel great. No problems." Wife said Mr. R. was having symptoms but "he's afraid to report them because they mean he's getting worse."	Stressed that reporting even minor symptoms would enable us to regulate treatment and gain better control.
Twenty pounds overweight and unable to reduce. "I don't look good thin."	Discussed effect of excess weight on hypertension and general health, gave diet instruction to patient and wife.
Extremely anxious and tense. "I worry a lot, then my nerves get tight. I snap at my wife and kids."	Encouraged patient to talk about things that were worrying him, suggested participating in activities he liked (walking, reading, listening to music). Recommended counseling at Mental Health Center, but Mr. R. refused. "I can talk better to you."
Minimal physical activity. "I like to just sit around after work. I don't play sports and I can't afford to do a lot of things."	Discussed value of regular exercise, explored interests, encouraged walking since it was most appealing and practical exercise for Mr. R.

After Mr. R. understood his disease and its treatment better, his blood pressure usually was well controlled. However, if his pressure was high, he would still say, "It's the beer" or "I've been eating spicy foods." He did accept the chronicity of hypertension and "having to take medicine for the rest of my life." Although Ms. R. never came to clinic, her interest and support, encouraged through phone conversations, were important in maintaining blood pressure control and in helping Mr. R. adjust to the changes in life-style that hypertension treatment demanded.

DRUGS USED TO TREAT HYPERTENSION

Name	Usual Daily Oral Dose	Action	Common Side Effects
THIAZIDE DIURETICS benzthiazide (Exna) chlorothiazide (Diuril) hydrochlorothiazide (Oretic, Hydrodiuril, Esidrix)	50-150 mg. 500-1000 mg. 25-100 mg.	increases sodium and chloride excretion by inhibiting renal reabsorption enhances potassium excretion relaxes peripheral arteriolar smooth muscles	*hypokalemia*—weakness, paresthesias, muscle cramps, nausea, paralytic ileus, cardiac disturbances *hyponatremia*—thirst, diminished sweating, fever, weakness, confusion
POTENT, RAPID ACTING DIURETICS ethacrynic acid (Edecrin) furosemide (Lasix)	50-200 mg. 40-240 mg.	increases sodium and chloride excretion by inhibiting renal reabsorption enhances potassium excretion	*hyperuricemia*—usually asymptomatic; can cause gouty arthritis *hyperglycemia*—usually asymptomatic; can cause nausea, vomiting, polydipsia, polyphagia, weight loss, dehydration sensitivity reactions gastrointestinal disturbances
POTASSIUM CONSERVING DIURETICS spironolactone (Aldactone)	50-100 mg.	blocks aldosterone, a mineralocorticoid secreted by the adrenal cortex which causes sodium and chloride reabsorption and potassium excretion; aldosterone blockage increases sodium and chloride excretion and decreases potassium excretion—effectiveness depends on the degree of aldosterone activity	*hyperkalemia*—weakness, paresthesias, cardiac disturbances *hyponatremia* gastrointestinal disturbances sensitivity reactions
triamterene (Dyrenium)	100-200 mg.	blocks reabsorption of sodium and chloride and causes no or minimal increase in potassium excretion	
SYMPATHETIC INHIBITING AGENTS reserpine (Serpasil, Reserpoid, Sandril, Rau-sed)	0.1-0.5 mg.	act by various complex mechanisms to inhibit synthesis, storage, and/or transport of norepinephrine, thereby depressing sympathetic nerve activity—as a result, cardiac output and/or peripheral vascular resistance are decreased reserpine and methyldopa also have central depressant effects	depression, nightmares, suicidal ideas drowsiness bradycardia G.I. disturbances increased appetite excessive gastric secretion nasal congestion
methyldopa (Aldomet)	500-2000 mg.		depression—less than reserpine drowsiness—tends to subside with continued use decreased mental acuity G.I. disturbances sodium and water retention loss of libido and sexual impotence postural hypotension— less than guanethidine
guanethidine (Ismelin)	25-150 mg.		postural hypotension generalized muscle weakness especially on arising diarrhea and other G.I. disturbances sodium and fluid retention failure to ejaculate sensitivity to sympathomimetics found in some cold remedies—can result in hypertensive crisis
propranolol (Inderal)	20-180 mg.	inhibits sympathetic action of beta receptors by competing with catecholamines for effector sites; causes a decrease in cardiac rate and force, thus reducing cardiac output decreases renal renin secretion	gastrointestinal disturbances bradycardia congestive heart failure bronchospasm sodium and fluid retention
VASODILATING AGENT hydralazine (Apresoline)	100-300 mg.	acts directly on vascular smooth muscle to decrease peripheral resistance—relaxant effect more marked on arterioles than veins increases cardiac output, renal blood flow, and plasma renin activity	headache, flushing, tachycardia, palpitation, angina gastrointestinal disturbances lupus-like syndrome—especially long-term administration with high doses sodium and fluid retention

FOODS HIGH IN POTASSIUM

Food	Portion	Calories	Potassium mEq.
Milk, whole	1 cup	166	9.0
Meat, broiled	3 ounces	220	9.6
Apricots, canned	4 halves	97	7.9
Banana	1 small	60	9.5
Honeydew	⅛ medium	50	9.6
Orange, fresh	1 medium	70	9.5
Plums, fresh	2 medium	60	7.7
Prunes, stewed, with sugar	4 medium	120	8.4
Prunes, dried	4 large	94	12.0
Raisins	4 tbsp.	104	7.8
Watermelon	½ slice 1 inch thick	156	15.3
Beet greens	½ cup	20	8.4
Carrot, raw	1 large	21	8.7
Cow peas	½ cup, cooked	75	8.6
Spinach	½ cup	23	7.4
Potato, baked	1 medium	100	12.9
Potato, boiled	1 medium	100	8.7
Potato, sweet, baked	1 medium	141	7.7
Lima beans	½ cup	76	8.3
Lima beans, dried	½ cup, cooked	127	14.5
Red kidney beans, canned	½ cup	90	8.4
Red kidney beans, dried	½ cup, cooked	118	10.9
Soybeans	½ cup, cooked	130	13.8
White beans, dried	½ cup, cooked	118	10.6
Winter squash	½ cup	45	10.0

blood pressure elevation is unimportant unless they have headaches and dizziness. These and other misconceptions must be elicited and corrected.

It is essential for every patient to perceive hypertension as a controllable but not a curable disease, one that will probably require life-long treatment. In presenting the potential crippling complications of untreated hypertension, care is taken to emphasize the necessity for compliance with ongoing medical management without causing undue alarm.

Stopping smoking is one of the most difficult therapeutic measures for some people. Many groups, the American Cancer Society's Smokers' Clinics, for example, provide counseling and support. Personnel and visitors should not smoke in front of these patients, and hospitalized hypertensives should have nonsmokers as roommates.

The harmful influence of stress on the blood pressure should be discussed, and the patient helped to identify his sources of stress and means to cope with them.

Patients requiring special diets need written and oral instructions that consider their cultural backgrounds and eating habits, and offer advice about substitute foods and seasonings. Patients on diets with no added salt may avoid table salt carefully but use celery, onion, or garlic salt liberally; avoid pork but eat ham; or eat unsalted French fries but douse them with catsup.

With all good intensions, a patient may use salt substitutes. This is hazardous because salt substitutes contain potassium and may cause hyperkalemia if taken in conjunction with potassium supplements or potassium-conserving diuretics.

It is important for patients to know the appearance, name, dosage, action, and possible side effects of their medicine(s). Some patients benefit from having this information written on a take-home card, as well as the instruction to take the medication even when they are feeling well, and to notify their doctor or nurse when they are not well. Patients should be told that alternate drugs or combinations of drugs can be prescribed if side effects become troublesome.

When a patient is taking a medication which can cause orthostatic hypotension, he is advised to sit down immediately if he feels faint or dizzy, not to rise quickly from a sitting or lying position, and not to stoop to pick up objects. Also, he should be aware that alcoholic intake, hot weather, exercise, and other causes of vasodilatation, as well as the fluid depletion following vomiting and diarrhea, will accentuate symptoms of orthostatic hypotension.

It is not always wise to warn patients about the sexual dysfunction sometimes associated with methyldopa and guanethidine, because the prophecy may fulfill itself. Sexual dysfunction may develop gradually, quickly, or not at all. Patients' responses to this problem vary. Some suspect the medication and discontinue it; others immediately question a doctor or nurse; many are too shy or distraught to broach the subject.

One patient did not notice any sexual dysfunction until he took a "vacation" from his medications as well as his job! Because of his suddenly revitalized sexual function, he later asked his nurse if the medications "affected his nature." It is extremely important, therefore, to seek specific information about recent sexual problems. Alternate drugs or a dosage adjustment can be tried to minimize this side effect.

Measures to prevent diuretic-induced hypokalemia include the use of dietary potassium, potassium supplement, intermittent diuretic therapy, or a potassium-conserving diuretic. Patients receiving long-term diuretic therapy are often encouraged to increase their intake of high potassium foods, and this may be adequate. However, some patients require 40 to 100 mEq. of potassium daily in addition to the 50 to 100 mEq. in the normal diet. If 60 mEq. of potassium were required it would be necessary to eat seven small bananas or drink four cups of orange juice. This additional caloric intake is unacceptable for a patient on a caloric restriction, and cost might also limit the usefulness of a dietary approach.

Despite dietary supplements, some patients require additional potassium, especially those who eat capriciously or take digitalis. Several salts are available but potassium chloride is

HYPERTENSION

preferred. If there is an associated alkalosis, the chloride is required to correct both hypokalemia and alkalosis.

The unpleasant taste of any potassium solution, the gastrointestinal distress it sometimes causes, and the feeling that powdered and liquid medications are not as important as pills all contribute to patients' tendency to discontinue potassium without informing a nurse or doctor. Explaining the importance of potassium and suggesting ways to make it more palatable, such as mixing it in chilled fruit juice or taking it after meals, encourages proper potassium intake.

The chance of developing hypokalemia may be lessened by using intermittent diuretic therapy or by joint administration of potassium-conserving and potassium-depleting diuretics. But since these measures involve more complicated medication schedules, they may confuse patients and decrease compliance.

A medication schedule based on a person's meal or work routine minimizes error and forgetfulness. Commercial aids for organizing daily or weekly medications can be recommended.

Selected patients benefit from taking their own blood pressures, unless the stress of doing so causes a transient elevation. Seeing his pressure rise when he does not follow treatment suggestions may persuade a patient to comply. The technique for taking blood pressure and the implications of readings are thoroughly explained; inaccurate findings and unreported high or low readings are of no value.

Most people grasp a concept better when they read it or see it graphically illustrated. Audiovisual aids and written take-home information supplement teaching. A list of teaching aids can be obtained by writing to the National High Blood Pressure Information Center, National Heart and Lung Institute, 120/80 Bethesda, Maryland.

Because most of these are geared to the college-educated person they are inappropriate for many patients. Therefore we have developed a new teaching aid and a take-home booklet, which have proved helpful in instructing patients about hypertension.

References

1. AMERICAN MEDICAL ASSOCIATION, COMMITTEE ON HYPERTENSION. Drug treatment of ambulatory patients with hypertension. *JAMA* 225:1647-1653, Sept. 24, 1973.
2. VETERANS ADMINISTRATION COOPERATIVE STUDY GROUP ON ANTIHYPERTENSIVE AGENTS. Effects of treatment on morbidity in hypertension; Part 1. *JAMA* 202:1028-1034, Dec. 11, 1967.
3. ———. Effects of treatment on morbidity in hypertension; Part 3. *Circulation* 45:991-1004, May 1972.
4. AMERICAN HEART ASSOCIATION. *Heart Facts 1976.* Dallas, The Association, 1975, p. 4.
5. KOCH-WESER, J. Correlation of pathophysiology and pharmacotherapy in primary hypertension. *Am.J.Cardiol.* 32:502, Sept. 20, 1973.
6. AMERICAN HEART ASSOCIATION, SUB-COMMITTEE ON REDUCTION OF RISK OF HEART ATTACK AND STROKE. *High Blood Pressure Control; a Guide for Community Programs.* New York, The Association, 1974, p. 3.
7. AYERS, C. R., AND OTHERS. Standards for quality care of hypertensive patients in office and hospital practice. *Am.J.Cardiol.* 32:534, Sept. 20, 1973.
8. VETERANS ADMINISTRATION COOPERATIVE STUDY GROUP ON ANTIHYPERTENSIVE AGENTS. Effects of treatment on morbidity in hypertension; Part 2. *JAMA* 213:1143-1152, Aug. 17, 1970.

Hyperalimentation

Definition: Infusion of hypertonic solutions of dextrose, nitrogen, and additives (vitamins, minerals, electrolytes) into a central vein, preferably the superior vena cava.

LONG TERM GOAL: To fulfill the body's energy needs, to achieve a positive nitrogen balance, and to maintain immuno-competence.

General Considerations:
- **Hyperalimentation is frequently given to patients with severe malnutrition or protein loss,** as in gastrointestinal illness (such as malabsorption syndrome, ulcerative colitis), major body burns, large wound infections, carcinoma (especially when the patient is being treated with radiation or chemotherapy), acute renal failure, and central nervous system dysfunction.
- **The procedure** involves three aspects:
  1) **Preparing the solution:** this is done by a registered pharmacist using strict aseptic technique under a laminar flow hood, since the hyperalimentation solution is a fine medium for bacterial and fungal growth. Each bottle is labeled identifying the patient's name, components of solution, and solution's expiration date (not to exceed 24 hours). The standard liter provides 250 gm dextrose (25%), six gm nitrogen, plus electrolytes, vitamins, and minerals according to individual needs as determined by lab tests. The solution is kept refrigerated and brought to room temperature before administering it to the patient.
  2) **Placing the catheter:** a large (#14) intracatheter is inserted infraclavicularly by an MD into the subclavian vein. During insertion, the patient is in Trendelenburg position (makes subclavian easier to reach, increases venous pressure, dilates vessels, and assists in preventing air emboli) and is performing the Valsalva maneuver (bearing down with mouth closed assists in preventing air emboli by increasing intrathoracic pressure and thus the central venous pressure). Have the patient practice the Valsalva maneuver before insertion. Reassure the patient that s/he will experience some pressure in chest during insertion. X-ray confirms location before solutions are administered. A dry, air-occlusive aseptic dressing is placed on the site and changed Q48 hours.
  3) **Giving the solution:** inspect the bottle carefully for cracks and solution clarity. Start infusion slowly (usually one liter QD) and gradually increase to amount needed (two to four liter QD). Administer solution continuously: replace one bottle by another at a steady drip. If delivery is ahead of schedule, add 20% D/W to keep system open.
- **Nursing responsibilities** include emotional and physical preparation of the patient, strict sepsis control, maintenance of the IV system, observation of patient for common complications of catheterization (pneumothorax, artery laceration, phrenic or brachial plexis nerve injury, mediastinal hematoma), and charting pertinent information.

Specific Considerations, Potential Patient Outcomes and Nursing Actions:

1) **Prevention of Infection** — The patient will be monitored for early signs of infection; strict aseptic technique will be carried out to prevent contamination of the puncture site, catheter, tubing, and/or solution:
   - change dressing Q48H, using strict aseptic no-touch technique, sterile gloves & supplies; follow hospital protocol for procedure; apply an air-occlusive dressing;
   - assign same nurse to do dressing change in order to decrease chance of contamination & to allow for continuing observations of insertion site by same person for signs of inflammation, swelling, &/or drainage (in many hospitals, dressings are done by the IV nurse);
   - change tubing Q24H (should coincide with expiration of current day's supply to eliminate added break in system);
   - notify MD & terminate the solution immediately if unexplained temperature spike occurs (add 20% D/W to keep vein open);
   - never use infusion line for piggy-back infusion, CVP monitoring, blood withdrawal, or other procedures;
   - never irrigate IV catheter.

2) **Maintenance of System** — The catheter will be maintained in correct position; the infusion will proceed safely and accurately at the prescribed rate; the patient will be monitored for early signs of impending complications:
   - caution pt. against scratching or pulling back the tape (hyperalimentation solution & dressing are irritating to skin);
   - check IV Q1-2H to prevent & control alterations in infusion; maintain solutions at constant uniform rate; *do not catch up*;
   - check tubing for kinks or loose connections;
   - observe the following *at least Q4H & PRN* & report any untoward signs to MD:
     - check solution for *turbidity &/or sediment* (notify pharmacist if any found)
     - check vital signs & report any *temperature elevation, dyspnea, or shortness of breath*
     - check urine for S&A to determine *sugar overload* (greater than 3 requires a blood sugar determination)
     - observe *complaints of pain or swelling in shoulder and neck* (may indicate infiltration or thrombosis)
     - observe pt. for signs of *circulatory overload* (prominence of neck veins, shortness of breath, edema, moist rales) or *peptide sensitivity* (headache, myalgia, fever, nausea, rash, abdominal pain);
   - maintain I&O record; check weight daily to maintain proper fluid balance.

3) **Comfort and Exercise** — The patient will verbalize an understanding of the procedure; the patient will exercise within capabilities and limitations in order to promote weight gain of lean muscle rather than fatty tissue:
   - explain rationale for hyperal & give proper explanations for every step of the procedure; answer all the pt.'s questions; allow pt. to verbalize any comments & fears;
   - encourage pt. to exercise within his capabilities & restrictions; provide passive ROM exercises PRN ambulate when not contraindicated.

© 1983 by Margo Creighton Neal. © 1985 by Williams & Wilkins. Guide No. 3:50 from *Nursing Care Planning Guides, Set 3*, 2nd Ed. Baltimore: Williams & Wilkins, 1983. Used by permission.

Bowel Management In Dialysis Patients

Reprinted from American Journal of Nursing, July 1983.

By Jeanette K. Chambers

Yes, dialysis sustains life by removing metabolic wastes and restoring fluid and electrolyte balance. But most people who have end-stage renal failure also learn to live with a number of other treatment measures. These measures include using phosphate-binding agents to counteract hyperphosphatemia, controlling fluid intake, and restricting the diet. All of these measures lead to constipation, a common problem experienced by most patients requiring dialysis. At the same time, the usual guidelines for teaching normal bowel management do not apply to these patients.

For instance, health teaching for regular bowel elimination in most people typically includes such suggestions as getting plenty of rest and exercise, drinking large amounts of fluid, and eating a diet high in fiber. And if constipation occurs at times, laxatives or enemas can be used. But these measures may all be specifically harmful for the chronic renal failure patient.

Since end-stage renal disease patients develop hyperphosphatemia, elevated serum levels of phosphorus are treated by phosphate-binding agents, which are aluminum hydroxide compounds, such as ALternaGEL, Amphojel, or Alu-Caps. These agents must be taken regularly to achieve a normal phosphorus level, but the primary side effect is constipation. Phosphorus is a chemical element distributed so widely in food that restriction of these foods is impractical.

JEANETTE K. CHAMBERS, MDN, RN, CS, is a renal clinical nurse specialist, Riverside Methodist Hospital, Columbus, Ohio.

If untreated, hyperphosphatemia has serious consequences. Normally calcium and phosphorus exist in a 2:1 ratio; that is, the calcium level is twice that of the phosphorus level. If this 2:1 balance is disturbed, the body will attempt to restore the normal balance.

When the phosphorus level becomes elevated, calcium binds with the phosphorus to form calcium phosphate. Calcium phosphate precipitates and may produce renal calculi and soft tissue calcifications. But in such binding, only the serum calcium level is lowered; the phosphorus level is too high to be reduced significantly. The parathyroid glands monitor the serum calcium level and are sensitive to lowered levels of calcium. Thus, when the serum becomes hypocalcemic, the parathyroid glands produce parathormone in an attempt to raise the low calcium level. Parathormone mobilizes calcium from bone cells. However, the all-too-available phosphorus also overwhelms this newer mobilized supply of calcium.

Failure to control hyperphosphatemia and the resultant hypocalcemia can lead to long-term problems for the chronic dialysis patient. Constant stimulation of the parathyroid glands results in secondary hyperparathyroidism. Calcium depletion leads to bony deformities and pathological fractures in a condition known as renal osteodystrophy.*

Calcium phosphate is also deposited in the arteriolar smooth muscle and in the conduction system of the heart. The resultant arteriolar rigidity heightens vascular resistance, thus making blood

*Binkley, Lowanna F., ed., Renal Osteodystrophy, J.Nephr.Nurs, Sept./Oct. 1979, p. 45.

pressure even more difficult to control. Deposits in the cardiac conduction system cause arrhythmias. Soft tissue deposits in the hips, thighs, and conjunctiva produce painful irritated areas that can become potential sites for infection. Therefore, management of the initial problem, high serum phosphorus, is important in preventing this sequence of pathology, but the remedy—the phosphate binders—also causes constipation.

Modifying the Rules

Getting plenty of fluids, particularly water, is probably the most common advice given for managing constipation. Fluids, however, are restricted for those dialysis patients who are oliguric or anuric—and most are. By definition, oliguria refers to the production of less than 400cc urine in 24 hours and anuria refers to the production of less than 100cc in 24 hours. In general, end stage renal failure patients are restricted to a 24-hour fluid intake equal to the amount of their urine output for 24 hours plus 600cc. The goal is to control the patient's water weight gain to 0.45 to 0.68 kg (1 to 1½ lb.) per day between dialyses. Fluid overload will all too quickly result in peripheral edema, hypertension, heart failure, and pulmonary edema. Frequent volume overload will make dialysis treatment uncomfortable because of muscle cramping associated with shifts in fluids and electrolytes. Consequently, dialysis patients do not have the option of increasing fluid intake to combat constipation.

The second most common advice is to eat foods high in fiber. Sources of fiber are generally fresh fruits and vegetables and bran products. But these foods are also high in potassium and phosphorus. Because it is not excreted by the kidneys, serum potassium increases between dialysis treatments. The rate of increase is directly related to the patient's dietary intake. Foods high in potassium must be limited. Depending on the patient, however, bran may be used as a cereal additive or mixed in applesauce, if necessary. Although patients with chronic renal failure tolerate slightly higher serum potassium levels—6.0mEq/L or perhaps even 6.5mEq/L—than the normal 3.5-5.0 mEq/L, they run the risk of arrhythmias when the serum potassium approaches 7mEq/L or higher, and cardiac arrest may result. In addition, such higher levels allow little safety margin and do not represent ideal management.

Finally, the third recommendation is to get plenty of exercise, balanced by rest. End-stage renal disease results in chronic anemia that is both normocytic and normochronic. The anemia is mainly caused by the lack of erythropoietin production that is needed in turn to stimulate the bone marrow to produce red blood cells. Some blood is also lost through hemodialysis and frequent lab work. Obviously, then, fatigue is one of the most noticeable symptoms in patients requiring dialysis. Although the fatigue may be influenced by the patient's psychological adjustment to his illness and by the quality of his support system, it is real and must be addressed in counseling the patient. Therefore, advising exercise as a method of managing constipation is not likely to be realistic. Encouraging the patient to make some effort in physical activity should be offered, however, since the adage "If I think I can, I can" is often true.

Management is most effective when a plan of aggressive prevention is used. Contrary to usual bowel management that suggests minimal reliance on stool softeners, people on dialysis often require such softeners. However, careful consideration must be given to the types of available agents, their mode of action and their potential side effects. Random selection of over-the-counter products and reliance upon recommendations of family and friends will probably yield less satisfactory results and may cause electrolyte imbalance.

Stool softeners are classified as emollients; they alter the surface tension of the feces and promote entry of water and fats into the fecal contents. Since these agents require 24 to 48 hours to act, their use is to prevent constipation, not to treat hardened stool.

Two common examples of emollient/stool softeners are docusate calcium (Surfak) and docusate sodium (Colace). The sodium and calcium in these products are not sufficient to warrant concern.

The usual advice for constipation— fluids, exercise, high fiber foods— may create new problems for the dialysis patient.

Bulk laxatives, such as psyllium hydrophilic mucilloid (Metamucil) may also be used regularly for management of chronic constipation. Such laxatives act by increasing the water content and, thus, the bulk of the stool. In turn, peristalsis is stimulated by mechanical distension of the bowel. Bulk laxatives are mild in the gastrointestinal tract; however, their effectiveness depends on fluid intake. Generally, the person is advised to take the laxative with a full glass of water. For renal patients who are restricted to 1000-1200cc of fluids per day, the glass of water, 240cc, would have to be included in their fluid allotment. Although bulk laxatives contain sodium, the amounts are minimal.

Stimulant laxatives should generally be reserved for acute constipation. If emollients and bulk agents become temporarily ineffective, a stimulant laxative may be indicated. Examples include castor oil, senna preparations (Senokot), danthron (Doxidan, Modane), and bisacodyl (Dulcolax). They act by stimulating sensory nerves, which in turn stimulate parasympathetic reflexes via Auerbach's plexus, which controls peristaltic activity in the large colon. Stimulant laxatives are site specific and do not alter motility in the stomach or small intestine.

Lubricant laxatives such as mineral oil alter the consistency of the feces, but do not influence peristalsis. The coating on the stool prevents the absorption of water by the intestinal mucosa; thus, feces do not become dry and hardened. Mineral oil is best used occasionally, since long term use is believed to interfere with absorption of the fat soluble vitamins. For this reason, mineral oil should be taken at bedtime, not immediately before or after meals. Some patients might also run the risk of aspirating the oil, which could cause pulmonary problems.

Laxatives and/or cathartics should be carefully selected. Compounds containing magnesium (milk of magnesia, Maalox) or phosphorus (Fleet's Phospho-Soda) can cause electrolyte toxicities. Serum magnesium levels can become elevated with repeated use of magnesium compounds. Attaining normal phosphorus levels will be further compromised by the ingestion of phosphorus compounds. Occasional use of these products may be necessary because of their stonger laxative properties. In such case, electrolyte levels must be monitored. Chronic use should be discouraged.

Caution is also needed regarding enemas. The usual rule of avoiding regular use also applies to the patient with renal failure. Generally small volume, gentle stimulant enemas, such as a Fleet or oil retention enema, are acceptable if used sparingly. They provide minimal fluid and interfer least with the electrolyte balance. Large volume saline or water enemas must be avoided; the fluid and saline may be absorbed through the intestines causing volume overload and sodium imbalance.

Patients and their families can learn effective bowel management and ways to alleviate constipation problems. The key is recognizing that the usual guidelines must be modified when the patient has renal disease.

ND
The Person with a Spinal Cord Injury

After you have studied the information presented here you will be able to:

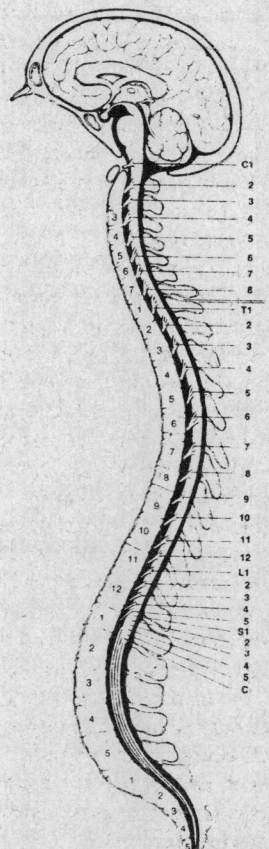

1. Identify the major cause of spinal cord injury (SCI) and discuss the implications of this for the patient's immediate care.
2. Describe the steps to prevent further neurological deficit when transporting a person with a suspected SCI.
3. Describe the spinal shock that all SCI patients develop, its average duration, and the probable underlying mechanism.
4. Identify two reasons why SCI patients may develop vascular shock.
5. Discuss the rationale for using tongs, body casts, or internal devices.
6. Explain why the patient may have some return of neurological function in the weeks (months) following SCI.
7. Describe the mechanisms by which SCI patients might develop pneumonia.
8. List specific nursing measures that help prevent pneumonia.
9. Describe three nursing mesures to prevent urinary tract infection in the SCI patient.
10. List three nursing measures that help to prevent the formation of decubitus ulcers in the SCI patient.
11. Given the level of a complete spinal cord lesion, list the organ systems that might (a) lack all innervation, (b) have reflex functioning.
12. List two metabolic disturbances common to paralyzed patients and the nursing measures to prevent these.
13. Explain the mechanism involved in autonomic dysreflexia, its symptoms and treatment, both immediate and long-term.
14. Explain when and why (a) emotional regression, (b) aggression, and (c) compulsive-obsessive behavior may be expected psychological reactions following catastrophic injury.
15. Name the patient's main psychological task in each of the three phases of adjustment after a catastrophic injury.
16. Describe the nursing approaches that will support the patient in accomplishing these tasks.
17. Define the meaning of the word "success" in relation to the rehabilitation of the patient who has sustained a spinal cord injury.
18. Discuss the average cost of the patient's initial hospitalization and rehabilitation following cord injury.

Reprinted from American Journal of Nursing, August 1977

The Person with a Spinal Cord Injury

Physical Care During Early Recovery

Whether the nurse works in an emergency room, intensive care unit, or on a general unit, she helps the patient to survive initially and to be ready eventually for the extensive rehabilitation that follows the intermediate stage of spinal cord injury. The complications that can delay rehabilitation are time-consuming and costly, and may be fatal. Good nursing in the general hospital can prevent or relieve most of them.

JUNE HANSEN LARRABEE

John's mind was on the party as he drove away from the fraternity house that May night. The road was a bit hazy to the 20-year-old, due to all the beer he'd drunk. He did not notice the embankment looming ahead until it was too late. When he regained consciousness, he had severe pain in his neck and some tingling in his arms. Rescue workers carefully secured him on a rigid stretcher and rushed him by ambulance to the nearest emergency room. The neurosurgeon who examined John in the ER thought he might have a spinal column fracture even though he had the full use of his fingers and toes.

John was taken to the x-ray department and transferred from the rigid stretcher to an x-ray table. After several exposures were taken, he was put back on the stretcher, returned to the ER, and transferred to a bed in the holding area. When room was available in the intensive care unit, he was transferred to a regular hospital bed and taken to the ICU.

The neurosurgeon reexamined John on arrival in the ICU and found that he had lost all sensation and movement in his arms, trunk, and legs. What had gone wrong? Why did he now have a neurological deficit when he had not on reaching the ER? Did everyone handling John know how to prevent neurological damage in a person with a suspected spinal fracture?

Knowledge about spinal cord injury (SCI) and its management, especially during the acute phase, is a growing need. Before the advent of antibiotics, most people who sustained an SCI died from urinary tract or respiratory infections, or from septicemia generated by decubitus ulcers. Over the past 30 years, specific antibiotic therapy and rapid advances in rehabilitation medicine have greatly increased the long-term survival rate of people with SCI(1).

The impact of SCI on the individual is immeasurable. It can only be worsened by an increase in neurological deficit or by urinary, respiratory, or skin infections. To enhance the patient's well-being, both physical and psychological, and to prevent unnecessary complications, the nurse must intervene knowledgeably.

The goal of care during the acute and intermediate phases following SCI is twofold: first, to resolve any life-threatening situation caused by or occurring with the injury; second, to provide care that prevents complications and moves the patient toward readiness for rehabilitation.

Transfer After Injury

When a patient is brought to an ER with a suspected SCI, the neurological deficit may or may not be the primary concern. Massive hemorrhage from other wounds; head injury, often associated with spinal cord trauma; and other problems may demand immediate attention if the patient is to survive.

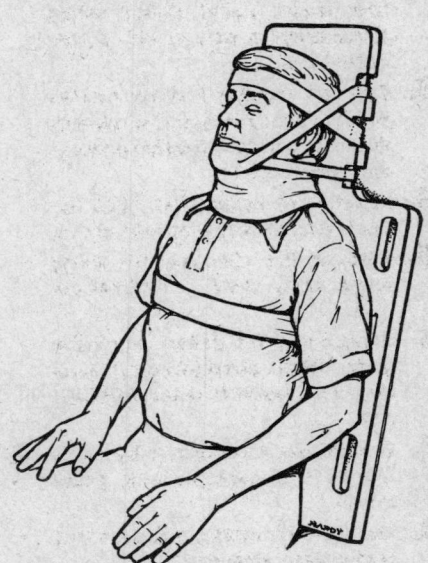

Before removing person with suspected back injury from car, (1) stabilize cervical spine with improvised collar (heavy towel, scarf); (2) slide rigid support (door, board, table leaf) behind him; (3) secure him to board with broad straps (wide belts, ties).

JUNE LARRABEE, R.N., M.S.N., was a surgical clinical nurse specialist at St. Vincent's Medical Center, Jacksonville, Fla., when she wrote this article. Now she is medical-surgical clinical nurse specialist at Kennestone Hospital in Marietta, Georgia.

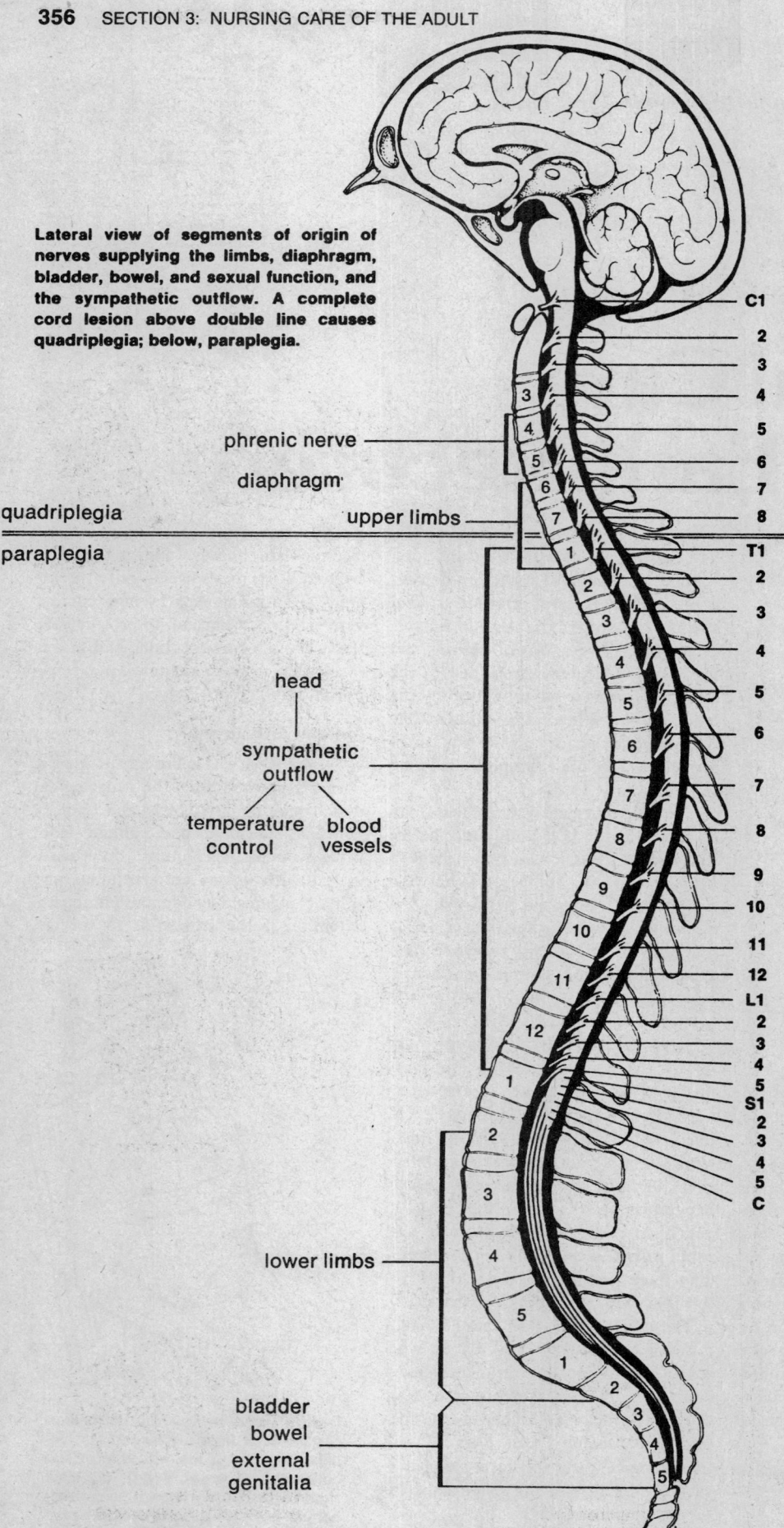

Lateral view of segments of origin of nerves supplying the limbs, diaphragm, bladder, bowel, and sexual function, and the sympathetic outflow. A complete cord lesion above double line causes quadriplegia; below, paraplegia.

However, efforts to prevent further neurological damage must be started along with the management of life-threatening injuries.

From the time of injury until the patient's spine has been immobilized, all transfers must avoid any movement, particularly flexion, of the spinal column.

Any person with a possible spinal injury, including all patients with head injuries, should be placed immediately on a rigid surface—a board, door, or table leaf. Transfer to this surface must be accomplished without flexing the spine. The patient should remain on the board until he arrives at the hospital unit where he will be cared for.

The only truly effective way to ensure that the patient's cervical spine is kept immobile is for a nurse or other responsible person to accompany him during all transfers, supporting his head to prevent flexion or extension, which might further traumatize the cord. Because the patient may have difficulty managing secretions in this position, suction equipment must be at hand to clear his airway and to prevent aspiration if he vomits.

If the person has sustained a cervical cord injury, a primary concern is the possible interruption of automatic respiration, secondary to lost or depressed innervation of the intercostal muscles, the diaphragm, or both. Weak or labored respirations or diaphragmatic breathing usually indicate the need for a tracheostomy. Endotracheal intubation is contraindicated as the need to hyperextend the neck while placing the tube could damage the cord further.

Because most spinal cord injuries are caused by accidents, the presence of severe wounds elsewhere in the body is a distinct possibility and should be investigated. Any hemorrhaging must be controlled immediately. If a frank bleed is not obvious and the patient does not have hemothorax, an abdominal tap usually is done to rule out that site. Intracranial hemorrhage is not sufficient to cause hypovolemic shock.

The management of fluid replacement is a difficult medical problem because the patient's shock with low blood pressure may be due to a frank bleed ((hypovolemic shock), to massive vasodilation secondary to the loss of

SCI-Physical Care

sympathetic tone caused by the cord injury (vasomotor shock), or to both bleeding and vasodilation(2).

Because the hypotension due to vasodilation usually is not severe enough to require support and because it is self-correcting over time, many physicians treat with fluid replacement, supplementing with steroid therapy.

Fluids extravasate from the microvasculature of the spinal cord within 30 minutes after it is injured. This edema, if allowed to run its full course, will cause local damage to the cord, called traumatic necrosis. Overhydration tends to exacerbate this condition. To prevent the edema responsible for traumatic necrosis, large doses of steroids may be administered.

A still-experimental method for reducing traumatic necrosis is to perfuse cold normal saline into the subarachnoid or epidural space. This produces local hypothermia of the cord(3,4).

Stabilization of Injury

After any life-threatening disorders have been controlled, the specific vertebral and cord injury is attended to. X-rays will help in determining the type of fracture. Basically, there are four types of spinal column injuries:

- *wedge or compression fracture*—the anterior portion of the vertebral body is compressed between the upper and lower vertebral bodies; posterior portion is intact and stable
- *burst fracture*—one or more intervertebral discs are forced through the end plate of the vertebrae by a vertical force on the whole spine
- *dislocation and rotational fracture dislocation*—one or more vertebrae are displaced or displaced and fractured by flexion and rotation of the spine or by a severe, direct, shearing force.

Dislocation and fracture dislocation are grossly unstable injuries because the ligament complex, which gives stability to the spine, is severed. They are the injuries that most often damage the

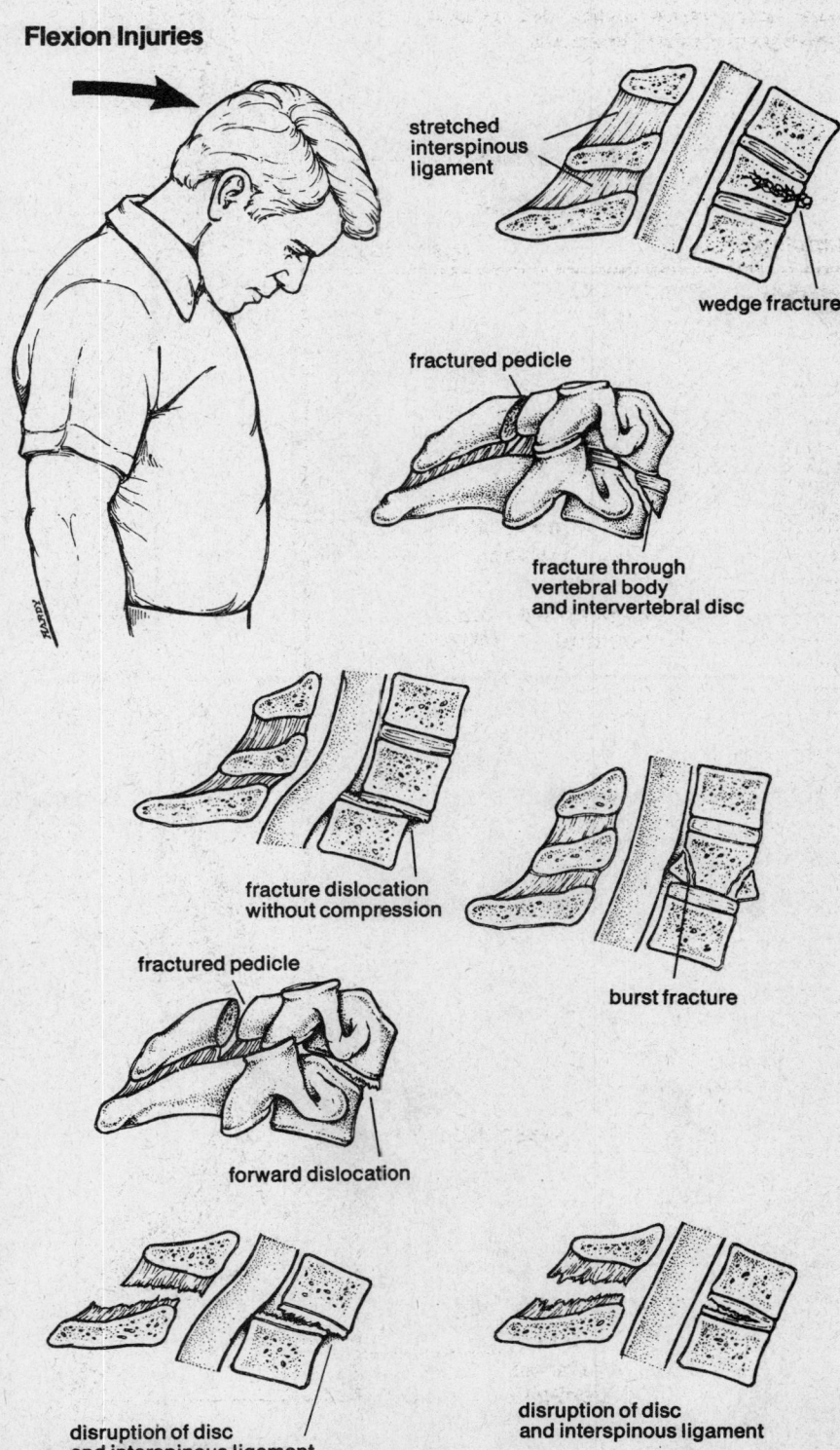

Flexion Injuries

Rotation with Flexion Injury

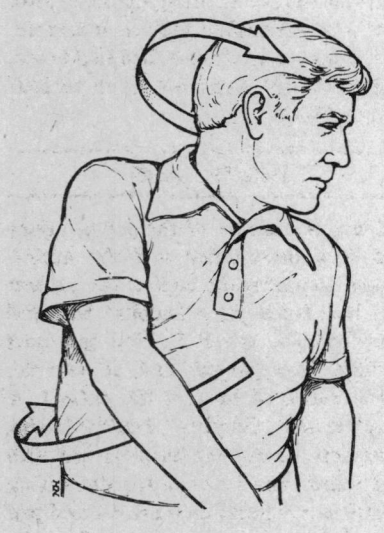
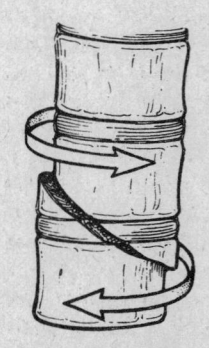

displacement of vertebrae with fracture of 2 vertebral bodies and 1 disc

Lateral Flexion Injury

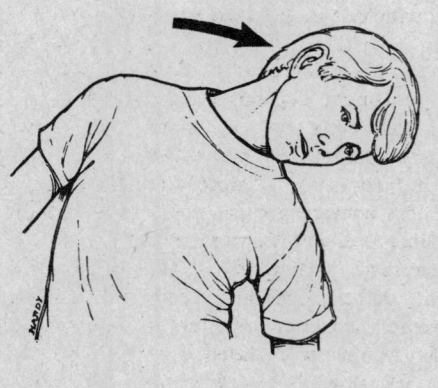
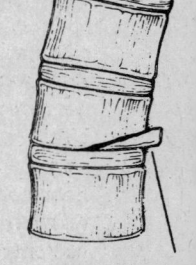

wedge fracture of vertebral body

Vertical Compression Injury

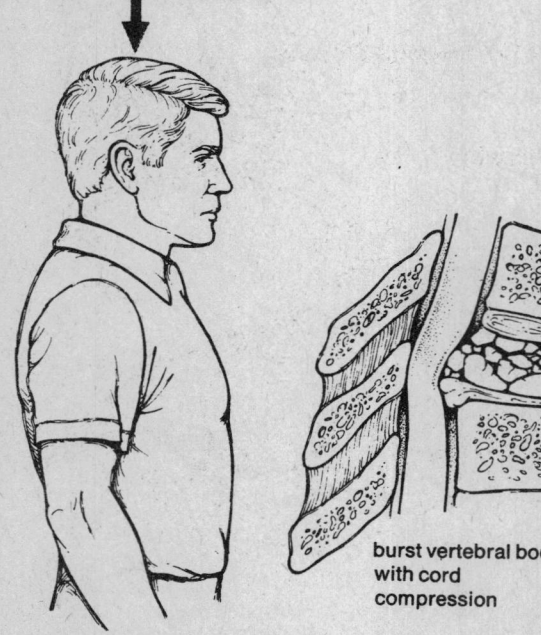

burst vertebral body with cord compression

Hyperextension Injury

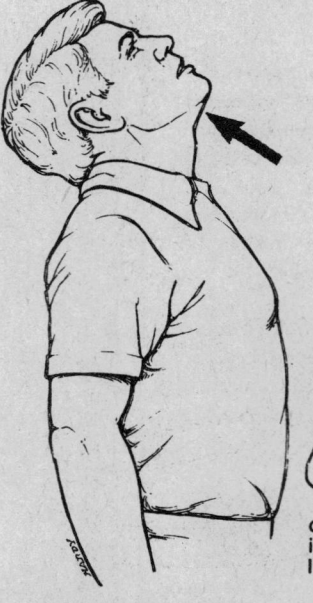
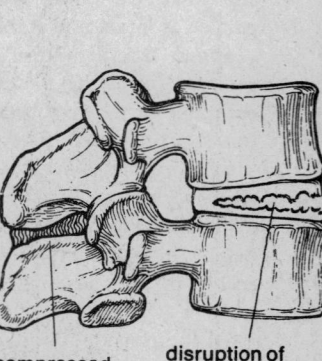

compressed interspinous ligament

disruption of intervertebral disc

SCI - Physical Care

spinal cord and nerve roots, with resulting neurological deficit. Injudicious movement of the patient can increase the pressure of the vertebral body or bony fragments on the spinal cord and change an incomplete lesion, which damages part of the cord, into a complete lesion, which damages most or all of the cord.

Whether the physician uses medical or surgical treatment depends on the stability or instability of the spinal column injury and on the possibility that bone fragments are compressing the cord. If cord compression is a possibility, a decompression laminectomy may be necessary, particularly if the neurological deficit becomes progressively worse. Decompression laminectomy also would be indicated if an increase in neurological loss was accompanied by evidence of blockage of the cerebrospinal fluid, such as a positive Queckenstedt sign.

To test for this sign, a lumbar puncture may be done and the CSF pressure determined. The patient's internal jugular veins are then compressed manually and changes in CSF pressure observed. Normally, pressure rises with jugular compression and returns to normal when it is released. Absence of this response indicates a block in the circulation of CSF.

The Queckenstedt test would be omitted if the patient had a concomitant head injury and a possibly elevated CSF pressure, because of the risk that brain tissue might herniate into the foramen magnum.

If the fracture is stable, the patient can be treated medically by stabilization of the spine with Crutchfield tongs or a halo body cast. The patient with Crutchfield tongs has to remain in bed for six to eight weeks, or until a stabilizing callus forms at the fracture site. A person wearing a halo body cast can be out of bed much sooner.

For an unstable fracture, surgical stabilization is required, by the placement of Harrington rods, by laminectomy and fusion, or by anterior fusion, in which the lamina are not encountered. The bone to be grafted is taken from the iliac crest, tibia, fibula, or ribs. About a week after such a procedure, the patient can be out of bed in a brace, which he will wear for three to four months(5-7).

ACUTE CARE

Once the nature of the spinal injury has been determined and the appropriate management begun, the patient can be placed on a hospital bed and transferred to the ICU. The bed must provide firm support and, if possible, some means of turning the patient. A CircOlectric, Stryker, Foster frame, Roto-rest, or regular hospital bed with bed boards may be used. An alternating pressure or a flotation mattress and pad should be put on the bed before the patient is placed on it.

The most obvious disability following SCI is paralysis of the extremities,

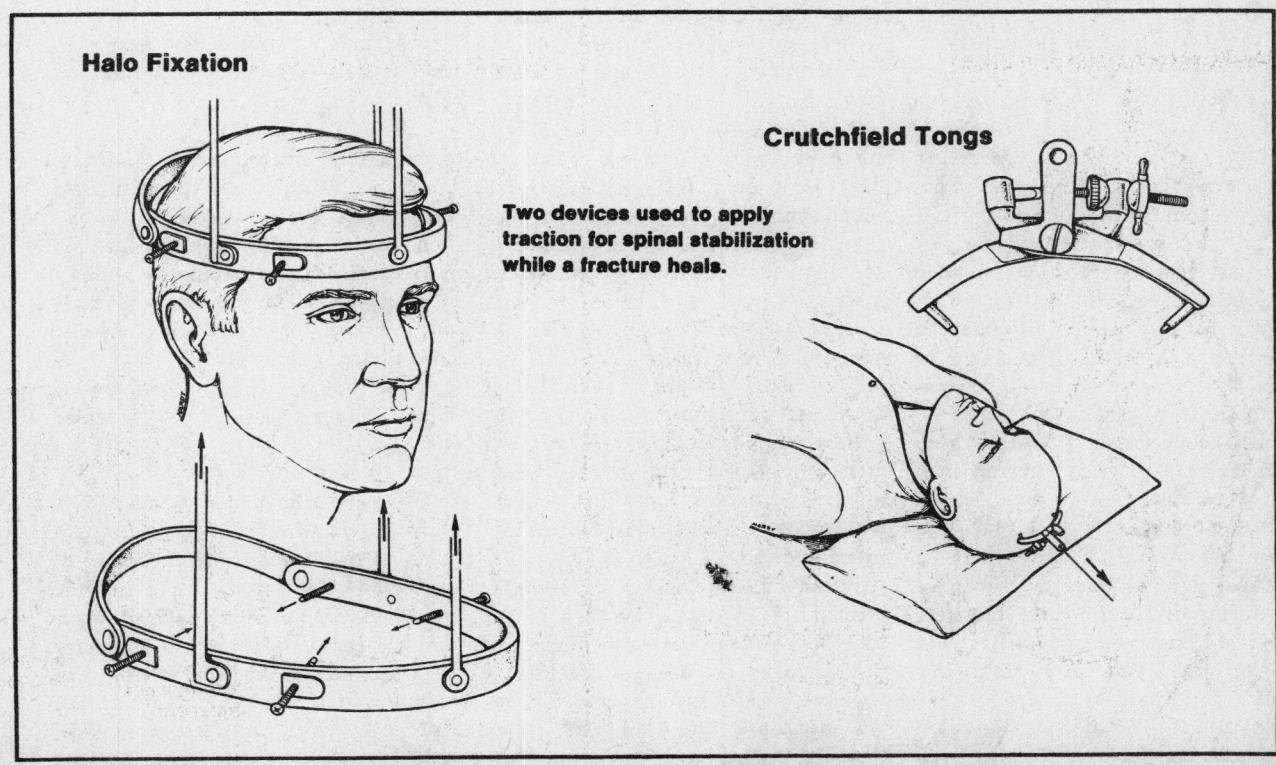

Halo Fixation

Crutchfield Tongs

Two devices used to apply traction for spinal stabilization while a fracture heals.

but this is only one manifestation of the injury and not necessarily the chief threat to survival. Other disorders occur as direct or indirect results of neurological trauma. Some of these problems reflect disturbances of nervous system function; others are secondary to the trauma and are manifested by symptoms related to other body systems. Each disorder must be managed if the person is to survive.

Many problems during the acute phase are due to spinal shock and to edema surrounding the site of injury. Although they may be serious and even life-threatening at this time, the deficits caused by spinal shock are transient. Edema can cause permanent damage.

Spinal shock involves the complete or nearly complete suppression of all reflexes at all spinal segments below the level of injury. The suppression is caused by "jamming" of neurological mechanisms. It results in the loss of temperature control, vasomotor tone, and sweating, as well as in the retention of feces and urine. Jamming is caused by the sudden cessation of efferent impulses and by inadequate microcirculation to the cord.

Spinal shock and edema develop within 30 to 60 minutes postinjury. Therefore, a person who *gradually* loses neurological function after an accident has some chance of recovering at least partial function when spinal shock dissipates. Return of function is not due to regeneration. Any patient who eventually demonstrates an improvement in level of function had an incomplete or partial lesion that appeared to be complete because of spinal shock.

Spinal shock wears off any time from two weeks to two years after an accident; three months is average. Edema resolves more quickly if steroids and proper alignment are used. Because some patients do have a chance of regaining some neurological function, the nurse must ensure maintenance of straight spinal alignment until this occurs.

The antacid Maalox (magnesium and aluminum hydroxide) may be given by nasogastric tube or orally to prevent the development of stress ulcers secondary to high-dose steroid therapy and to the emotional impact of the injury.

Maintaining Respiratory Function The nature and extent of respiratory involvement depend on the level of the spinal cord lesion. The diaphragm and the intercostals are the major muscles of respiration. Impulses are delivered to the intercostals by spinal nerves in the thoracic segments of the cord. The diaphragm receives its motor impulses via the phrenic nerve, which arises from the cervical plexus (C1-C4). If a person has a cervical injury, intercostal muscle function is lost, along with the ability to cough and take a deep breath.

If the injury is at the level of the cord involving the phrenic nerve, or if post-traumatic edema extends involvement to that level, the person loses involuntary control of respiration. To maintain life, artificial respiration must be provided. Some patients require respirator assistance for the rest of their lives; others recover involuntary respiratory control, particularly if their loss of respiration was gradual and caused by cord edema.

Another consequence of SCI is a susceptibility to pneumonia. Some patients arrive on a nursing unit without a reliable history about possible aspiration after the SCI. The breath sounds of such patients should be auscultated at least every eight hours, more frequently if the nurse detects changes. The tendency to develop pneumonia continues and is related to the impairment of intercostal muscle function and to the patient's supine position while at bed rest. Paraplegics may develop pneumonia, but quadriplegics and patients with higher thoracic injuries are more prone to do so.

Pneumonia develops by the following mechanisms. When a person is in the upright position, the bronchioles are held open by the outward traction of negative intrapleural pressure. The supine position, on the other hand, causes the diaphragm to rise because of greater pressure from abdominal contents. The great vessels of the chest fill with blood and the negative pressure falls. This reduces the diameter of the bronchioles, increasing their tendency to be obstructed by mucus.

When the person is upright, mucus coats the walls of the bronchioles evenly; when the person is supine, gravity pulls the mucus to the dependent side of the bronchioles. The upper surface of the bronchiole dries out and may crack, providing a site for infection. The lower surface is covered with a pool of mucus, increasing the chances of a mucous obstruction.

Coupled with the narrowing of the bronchioles and the pooling of mucous secretions is the patient's inability to cough effectively, due to neurological deficit. These events predispose him to develop hypostatic pneumonia.

For these reasons, it is essential to prevent excessive drying or pooling of secretions. If the patient must be maintained on bed rest, it is crucial to turn him every two hours around the clock. He also should receive chest physiotherapy as soon as possible and be mobilized as soon as spinal stabilization has been accomplished.

Maintaining Hydration and Nutrition Adequate hydration and nutrition must be provided parenterally until the patient can eat and drink. Overhydration is avoided because it promotes traumatic necrosis of the cord in the early postinjury period. Not uncommonly, cord-injured patients have paralytic ileus, so they should be tolerating clear liquids before progressing to a regular diet.

Maintaining Elimination A major risk immediately after injury is the possibility of overdistention and rupture of the bladder. Spinal shock prevents the involuntary reflex emptying of the bladder in a person who has lost voluntary control. Catheterization to prevent overdistention must be done in the emergency room, then repeated until reflex functioning has returned and

SCI-Physical Care

bladder retraining has been accomplished. An indwelling catheter or intermittent catheterization are used to prevent overdistention.

INTERMEDIATE CARE

After the acute phase of SCI has passed and life-threatening disorders are controlled, attention is turned to preparing the patient for rehabilitation while preventing complications that might result from the neurological deficits and from prolonged bed rest.

Neurogenic Bowel and Bladder Despite specific antibiotic therapy, recurrent bladder infections and their sequelae are still the leading threat to the long-term survival of spinal-cord-injured persons. Intermittent (every eight hour) straight catheterization with aseptic technique is recommended. Research has shown that this method is far superior to indwelling catheter drainage in lowering the incidence of urinary tract infections(8-10).

Intermittent catheterization prevents the hazards of reflux of the urine accumulated in a drainage bag or tube, and the inevitable trauma at the meatus produced by indwelling catheters. Then, too, because an indwelling catheter keeps the bladder constantly empty rather than alternately stretched and contracted as in normal function, prolonged use of an indwelling catheter can lead to a contracted, atonic bladder that is not easily retrained. If the patient must wear an indwelling catheter, bladder atony can be prevented by instituting a regular clamping-unclamping routine.

Measures are taken to discourage bladder infection in persons with indwelling catheters. For example, the catheter and collection system should be changed every two weeks, and a closed system of drainage used, with no break, ever, in its connections.

Urine specimens are obtained through sampling ports or by needle-and-syringe aspiration if special ports are not available. Collection systems with a drip chamber are preferable, as these prevent backflow of urine from the bag into the tubing and, possibly, the bladder. The tubing is positioned to allow drainage by gravity and taped securely to prevent the trauma of traction on the urethra and bladder. The urinary meatus is cleaned at least twice daily with a povidone-iodine (Betadine) solution, and Betadine ointment is applied lightly.

To help prevent bladder infection and renal calculi, the patient is encouraged to drink at least 3,000 ml. of fluids daily. Drinking cranberry juice several times a day helps keep the urine acidic, which discourages bacterial growth and bladder stone formation. The consumption of such alkaline ash foods as orange juice and grapefruit juice should be avoided or at least limited.

During the period of spinal shock, bowel function is affected in much the same way as bladder function. There is no voluntary or involuntary elimination, so impactions can occur. Soap suds enemas or saline enemas must be given about every three days during this period, simply to wash out the bowel. As spinal shock dissipates, the patient begins to have reflex emptying of the bowel following a stimulus, such as a meal, abdominal effleurage, or light tugging on the pubic hair.

After spinal shock has dissipated, bowel function is stimulated by using stool softeners, abdominal massage, and glycerin or bisacodyl (Dulcolax) suppositories. If evacuation does not occur with this regimen, a small enema—sodium biphosphate and sodium phosphate (Fleet, Phospho-Soda)—may be required. Some SCI centers prefer that staff remove the fecal mass digitally. At this stage, soap suds enemas should be given only as a last resort, not routinely(11).

A record is kept to document evacuations and the aids used to accomplish them. At this time a bowel retraining program can be started, taking into consideration the person's preinjury bowel habits(11-13).

Bladder and bowel as well as sexual function are innervated through S 2-4 (the sacral micturition center). During the period of spinal shock, there is no voluntary or reflex activity because both the upper and lower motor neurons are affected.

The upper motor neuron consists of the motor cell body in the cerebral cortex and its axon in the descending motor pathway (the pyramidal tract or corticospinal tract) to its synapse with the anterior horn cell in the spinal cord. Interruption of this neuron disrupts regulation by higher nervous system centers and leads to reflex activity.

The lower motor neuron consists of the anterior horn cell in the spinal cord and its efferent motor axon to its synapse with peripheral cells. Interruption of the lower motor neuron disrupts reflex activity *at the level of the lesion*. If the spinal cord lesion is above the sacral micturition center (S 2-4), reflex activity of bowel, bladder, and sex organs may occur after spinal shock resolves. For example, if the lesion is cervical, thoracic, or high lumbar, a man may have reflex penile erection after spinal shock has passed. Some may even attain reflex ejaculation.

A lesion above the sacral micturition center results in reflex urination, and the bladder is called an "upper motor neuron" or "automatic" bladder. If the lesion is at the level of the sacral micturition center, the reflex arc is disrupted, no reflex activity can occur, and the results are a "lower motor neuron" or "autonomous" bladder and bowel. Any functioning is merely the organ's response to filling, and consists of weak, asynchronous, incomplete contraction.

The lower motor neuron, or asynchronous, bladder or bowel cannot be retrained. A person with automatic bowel, bladder, and sexual function, on the other hand, is more likely to experience some success with retraining.

Skin and Musculoskeletal Complications Septicemia secondary to decubitus ulcers is another threat to the patient's long-term survival. These ulcers can be prevented through conscien-

SCI - Physical Care

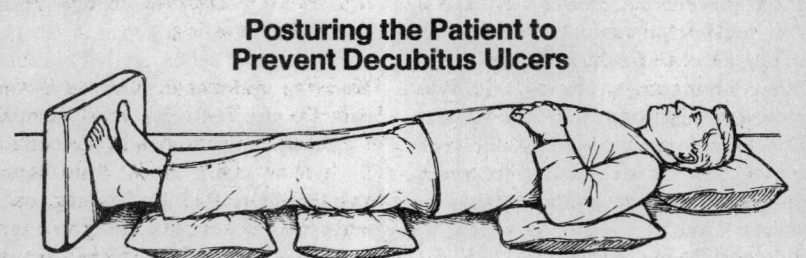

SUPINE Distribute body weight evenly, align correctly, and prevent pressure on bony prominences and genitalia (males) by placing patient on firm pillows or foam cushions (2"-4" thick depending on body weight). Support feet in dorsiflexion with padded footboard, bolster, or sandbags, with heels off mattress.

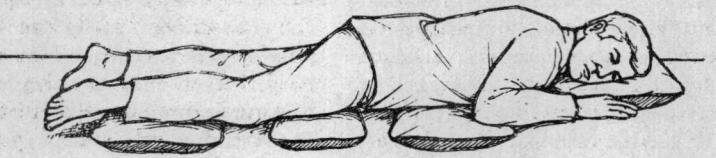

PRONE Arrange cushions to prevent or decrease pressure on insteps, toes, knees, genitalia, iliac crests, ribs, and the female breasts. Encourage face lying as patient's condition permits.

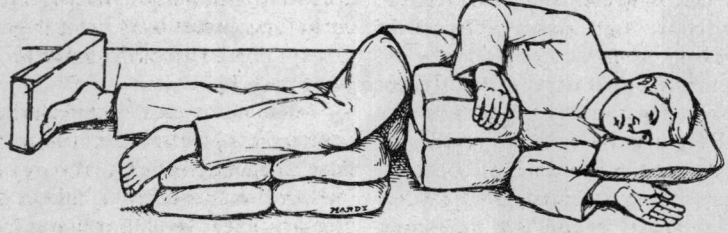

SIDE LYING Support upper extremities on firm, double pillows to prevent overstretching shoulder and hip muscles. Place lower leg in slight hyperextension, flat on bed, with foot supported at right angle to leg, and malleolus protected. Usually, no back support is needed if the patient has been correctly postured.

Suggested by Nicholas F. Saverine, L.P.N., New Jersey

tious nursing care. The greatest contributor to decubitus ulcers in any patient is prolonged pressure, especially over bony prominences.

For the spinal-cord-injured patient, who cannot move in bed, pressure is a special problem. His paresthesias or sensory losses prevent him from feeling the discomfort that prolonged pressure causes, so he does not recognize the need to be turned. Also, circulation to all areas below the level of the spinal lesion, including the skin, is decreased by the depressed autonomic nervous system function and decreased muscle tone.

Bedfast patients are in a metabolic state of catabolism, in which body cells break down faster than they can be built. This means that the nitrogen balance is negative rather than positive. Consequently, if the SCI patient develops a decubitus ulcer, it is difficult to heal. Prevention is imperative.

The best way to prevent prolonged pressure is to turn the patient frequently and mobilize him as soon as possible. The *maximum* time any paralyzed person should stay in the same position is two hours. Beyond that time, irreversible changes may take place in the integrity of the dependent tissues. If the patient in Crutchfield tongs and traction is on a turning bed or frame, the nurse's task is simplified. If the patient is on a regular hospital bed with bed boards and an alternating pressure mattress, turning him is more difficult but no less important.

Before changing the patient's position for the *first* time, the nurse must verify with the physician the amount and extent of turning that are safe. These limits are communicated to all personnel involved in changing the patient's position. If he cannot be turned at all, even more diligence is required to prevent skin breakdown. Skin care can be given by depressing the mattress with one hand and applying massage with the other. Particular care is taken to keep the back relatively dry, because excessive moisture will macerate the skin.

Turning also helps maintain adequate respiration, facilitates drainage of urine from the kidneys into the ureters, and provides an opportunity to carry the patient's limbs through their range of motion. When positioning the patient, the nurse aligns the extremities carefully.

A footboard is used to prevent footdrop; splints to prevent wristdrop, and the feet positioned so that the heels do not rest on the mattress. While the patient is on his side, his upper arm and leg are supported on pillows to prevent overstretching of muscles. If the patient receives adequate attention to joint mobility during the intermediate phase of care, he can progress more rapidly into the rehabilitation phase.

Muscle spasms that may be strong enough to cause violent contracture of the limbs and trunk often develop after spinal shock dissipates. Spasticity occurs only when lower motor neurons are intact. The higher the cord injury, the more lower motor neurons remain intact and the greater the body area involved in spasms. In one study, all patients with cervical-cord injury had spasms; 75-80 percent with thoracic cord lesions had spasms, and 44 percent with lumbar lesions had spasms(15).

Spasm occurs spontaneously or in response to such external or internal stimuli as pressure of bed clothing, a decubitus ulcer, tight shoes or clothing, ill-fitting braces, renal calculi, and range of motion exercises. Whatever the stimulus, it causes the lower motor neuron to fire impulses that result in contraction of skeletal muscles. The normal dampening control from the cerebellum and brainstem structures has no influence over these lower motor neurons below the level of the spinal cord lesion, so impulses for muscle contraction continue to be fired for a prolonged period, often until the stimulus is identified and removed.

Mild spasticity can benefit the patient. It helps prevent disuse atrophy of muscles and osteoporosis, and may aid in maintaining trunk posture. Extensor spasticity of the legs allows for weight bearing. If the spasticity is severe, however, its detrimental effects far exceed its benefits. Severe spasticity can make it difficult to stay in a wheelchair or even in bed. Reflex resistance to passive ROM exercises causes stiffness of the extremities and trunk, and interferes with proper positioning and, later, with vocational rehabilitation.

Although strong spasms often subside when the offending stimulus is removed, in many patients spasticity increases, and may prevent participation in their rehabilitation programs. No antispasmodic drug controls spasticity without impairing mental functions, so other medical or surgical means must be employed. These include rhizotomy, cordectomy, and subarachnoid alcohol or phenol blocks.

Such procedures obliterate or sharply decrease lower motor neuron function. Therefore they are used only after the patient has considered the alternatives. If he decides to keep the spasticity, his activities will be hindered greatly. If he eliminates spasticity, he will sacrifice those activities that the intact lower motor neurons allowed him to have. Among those activities are reflex bowel, bladder, and sexual function(16).

Metabolic Disturbances Research has demonstrated that the stress of trauma and surgical procedures stimulates an overproduction of adrenocortical hormones(14). One result is the conservation of fat and glucose while protein stores are used for energy. The breakdown of large amounts of amino acids for energy produces a negative nitrogen balance. This leads to anemia, loss of muscle mass, decreased healing power, and lowered resistance to infection. Routine analysis of blood-nitrogen and urine-nitrogen levels will indicate whether nitrogen intake and depletion are balanced. If nitrogen balance becomes negative, the patient should be placed on a high protein diet with protein supplements.

Experts disagree on the desirability of encouraging milk as a protein supplement. Some believe milk should be urged during the intermediate phase of recovery, to combat nitrogen depletion. Others restrict or prohibit milk and milk products, because their high calcium content may contribute to renal calculus formation. After the SCI patient is eating a regular diet and has progressed to a specialized rehabilitation program (beyond the acute and intermediate phases of recovery), milk consumption usually is sharply restricted(17).

Another major metabolic change related to immobility is the absorption of calcium from the bones into the circulatory system, which occurs in the absence of weight bearing. Decalcification causes two complications: (a) pathological fracture or increased susceptibility to fracture under minimal trauma, and (b) the formation of renal calculi(18). As soon as the patient's spine is stabilized, physical therapy should be started with tilt-table exercises to provide for some weight bearing.

Managing Autonomic Nervous System Disturbances These are most common in patients with injuries in the cervical or thoracic cord. Such disturbances may be manifested by flushing, occasional mild headaches, and goose pimples. All are caused by marked sympathetic stimulation. Sweating may constitute a major problem, by its presence or its absence.

Excessive sweating, besides being uncomfortable, can endanger the patient's health, especially if he is exposed to drafts. Sweating usually can be controlled by various drugs of the atropine group, but extreme sweating may require sympathectomy. Excessive sweating may diminish over a period of years.

Absence of sweating disturbs the patient's thermoregulatory mechanism, particularly in extremely hot weather. Because patients who cannot sweat cannot release excess body heat, they need closely regulated environmental temperatures(19).

The most serious manifestation of autonomic dysfunction is the alternations in blood pressure that may occur. *Postural hypotension*—a fall in blood pressure when the patient moves from a horizontal to a vertical position—results from depressed sympathetic control over blood-vessel contractility.

When light-headedness or syncope occurs, the patient must be returned to the horizontal position immediately. Vasopressor drugs may be required to support the blood pressure following such an episode. Postural hypotension and syncope can be prevented by using support hose and by raising the patient very gradually on a tilt table to a vertical position.

Autonomic dysreflexia (hyperreflexia or pressor reflex) is a rise in blood pressure to uncomfortable, sometimes fatal, levels. It is a medical emergency. Hyperreflexia is a reflex response to stimulation of the sympathetic nervous system. If the stimulus is not removed, the blood pressure continues to rise. The normal dampening control over such reflex activity is located in higher centers of the central nervous system, which cannot influence areas below the level of the spinal cord lesion.

Most often, the stimulus responsible for autonomic dysreflexia is a distended bladder or rectum, but it can be spasticity, decubitus ulcers, infection of the bladder, chilling, or even pressure on the skin. Symptoms include extremely severe headache, paroxysmal hypertension, bradycardia, profuse sweating, flushing, pilo-erection, and nasal congestion. Immediate intervention is necessary to avert a cerebrovascular accident[19].

The cycle of stimulus-response must be broken by removing the stimulus, administering a ganglionic-blocking agent, or both. The nurse's first intervention is to check the patient's bladder for distention; second, to catheterize the bladder if it is distended or to irrigate the indwelling catheter, if present, to clear it and allow the bladder to empty[20]. If symptoms are not alleviated promptly by such measures, the intravenous administration of a ganglionic-blocking agent like hexamethonium chloride may be necessary. Once the stimulus has been identified, efforts are made to prevent future episodes. If the stimuli are too numerous to eliminate, the patient may require daily maintenance with hexamethonium chloride, or surgical intervention as described for the elimination of spasms.

Autonomic hyperreflexia rarely occurs until after spinal shock has subsided and usually is first seen when the patient enters an active rehabilitation program. Unlike postural hypotension, autonomic hyperreflexia does not tend to correct itself over time. It is such a constant problem for some patients that the reflex arc must be interrupted surgically.

Emotional Support The nursing care to aid the patient's emotional adjustment is discussed in detail in the following article. Briefly, the emotional adjustment faced by a spinal-cord-injured person parallels the grief experience of those who have lost a loved one.

The injured person needs to recognize and come to accept the loss or "death" of portions of his previous self-image before he can begin to establish a new self-image. Lindemann has described the grieving process as consisting of stages, including initial realization, denial, realization, anger and dismay, and acceptance[21]. The literature indicates that denial is the stage of grief at which many SCI patients become fixed during the acute and intermediate care periods[22]. A healthy emotional adjustment cannot occur unless the person goes through all stages of the grieving process. The nurse supports the patient as he adjusts—a process that may take months to years—and is careful not to "push" him faster than he can progress.

Immediately following injury, the patient is overwhelmed by the personal and social implications of the lost body functions. Often, the patient copes by denying that the injury happened or that it is permanent.

Denial, the second step the paralyzed person must go through in the grieving process, is a normal reaction. Most patients believe that they eventually will recover completely. They tend to think that their early rehabilitation efforts are not very important —that time will work miracles. Because denial is a defense mechanism, health personnel must be careful not to strip the patient of this means of coping until he is able to deal with reality.

When the patient moves from denial in the grieving process, he faces, once again, all the implications of his loss. The normal emotional reaction is anger, then despair. The person may send out "SOS" signals to relatives, friends, or hospital personnel. It is essential, during this time, that the staff and family help the patient recognize that they consider him worthwhile and "good" despite his loss. Over time, these efforts can help the patient reassess his values, changing some, adding or dropping others, as he develops a self-image that reflects and emphasizes his essential worth rather than his status as a disabled person.

References

1. ABRAMSON, A. S. Modern concepts of management of the patient with spinal cord injury. *Arch.Phys.Med.Rehabil.* 48:113-121, Mar. 1967.
2. MCKIBBEN, B., AND BROTHERTON, B. J. The early management of cervical spine injuries. *Resuscitation* 2:245, Dec. 1973.
3. OSTERHOLM, J. L. The pathophysiological response to spinal cord injury. *J.Neurosurg.* 40:7-9,23-25, Jan 1974.
4. NEGRIN, JUAN, JR. Spinal cord hypothermia in the acute and chronic post-traumatic paraplegic patient. *Paraplegia* 10:336-343, Feb. 1973.
5. BEDBROOK, G. M. Pathological principles in the management of spinal cord trauma. *Paraplegia* 4:43-56, May 1966 .
6. LUSSKIN, RALPH, AND PENA, ARTURO. Orthopedic management of transverse myelopathies. *NY J.Med.* 68:2046-2049, Aug. 1, 1968.
7. ALPERS, B. J. *Clinical Neurology.* 5th ed. Philadelphia, F. A. Davis Co., 1963, p. 359.
8. GUTTMANN, L. Statistical survey of one thousand paraplegics. *Proc.R.Soc.Med.* 47:1,101, June 19, 1954.
9. BORS, E. Intermittent catheterization in paraplegic patients. *Urologia Internationalis* 22:236-249, 1967.
10. TALBOT, H. S. Pathogenesis of renal infection in spinal cord injury. *Paraplegia* 7:101-110, Aug. 1969.
11. ROSSIER, A. B. Rehabilitation of the spinal cord injury patient. *Documenta Geigy:Acta Clinica.* No. 3, North American Series, 1963.
12. CORNELL, S. A., AND OTHERS. Comparison of three bowel management programs. *Nurs.Res.* 22:321-328, July-Aug. 1973.
13. TALBOT, H. S. Adjunctive care of the spinal cord injury. *Surg.Clin.North Am.* 48:754-755, Aug. 1968.
14. GUYTON, A. C. *Textbook of Medical Physiology.* 3d ed., Phila., Pa., W.B. Saunders, 1967, pp. 1055-1056.
15. RUGE, DANIEL. *Spinal Cord Injuries.* Springfield, Ill., Charles C Thomas, Publisher, 1969, pp. 148-152.
16. HIRSCHBERG, G. G., AND OTHERS. *Rehabilitation.* 2nd ed., Phila., Pa., J. B. Lippincott Co., 1976, pp. 286-288.
17. KRAUSE, M. V., AND HUNSCHER, M. A. *Food, Nutrition and Diet Therapy.* 5th ed., Phila., Pa., W.B. Saunders, 1972, pp. 324-325.
18. BROWSE, N. L. *The Physiology and Pathology of Bedrest.* Springfield- Ill., Charles C Thomas, Publisher, 1965, pp. 95-96.
19. RUGE, DANIEL. op.cit. pp. 110-113, 133.
20. FEUSTEL, DELYCIA. Autonomic hyperreflexia. *Am.J.Nurs.* 76:228, Feb. 1976.
21. LINDEMANN, ERICH. Symptomatology and management of acute grief. *Am.J. Psychiatry* 101:143, Sept. 1944.
22. NAGLER, BENEDICT. Psychiatric aspects of cord injury. *Am.J.Psychiatry* 107: 49-56, July 1950.

The Person with a Spinal Cord Injury

Psychological Care

Correlating the emotional adjustments of the severely injured person with the developmental tasks of the infant, child, and adolescent may help nurses understand the disabled person's often perplexing behavior.

GINETTE A. PEPPER

Persons who become physically disabled from a sudden catastrophe, such as paralysis or loss of a limb after an accident, experience intense psychological reactions. The abrupt, overwhelming onset of the disability prevents the gradual development of awareness and acceptance that disorders with a slower onset may allow.

The variety and intensity of the patient's emotional reactions, coupled with the nurse's personal and culturally determined attitudes toward the deformed and disabled, may challenge the nurse's perceptions of her professional competence, and lead to frustration, anger, or avoidance.

"I feel terrible after I take care of him," a nurse said of a quadriplegic patient. "I can't even begin to meet his needs."

Nurses in rehabilitation centers can rely on an established approach to care that emphasizes patient independence,

GINETTE PEPPER, R.N., M.S., a senior instructor at the University of Colorado School of Nursing, Denver, has practiced as staff and head nurse in several orthopedic/neurologic units. She coauthored "Geriatric Nurse Practitioner in Nursing Homes," *AJN*, Jan., 1976.

an approach that usually succeeds. However, in acute-care hospitals as well as in rehabilitation centers, several important questions arise: What are the ranges of normal behavior following sudden catastrophic injury? Is the emphasis on independence appropriate at all times during the postinjury course? If not, how does the nurse determine when to alter her approach?

The theoretical model presented here proposes that a similarity exists between the psychosocial developmental stages postulated by Erikson and the adjustment phases experienced by patients who suddenly become paralyzed or severely disfigured. The model is based on the assumption that there is a natural regression and an obligatory reworking of some previously surmounted developmental tasks, namely, the first three stages described by Erikson.

Although the assumption that regression is normal or even requisite is far from universally accepted, much evidence supports the assumption. The dependent position into which the necessarily intense medical and nursing care places a severely injured person, as well as the devastating impact of the injury, demand a realignment of self-concept and body image.

Regression may allow the person time to reintegrate his ego in light of his new body image and curtailed abilities, then to align with a new social identity as a member of the disabled minority, and, finally, to form new expectations for himself.

Correlating this process with the psychosocial development process described by Erikson and others(1,2) accounts for many of the behaviors

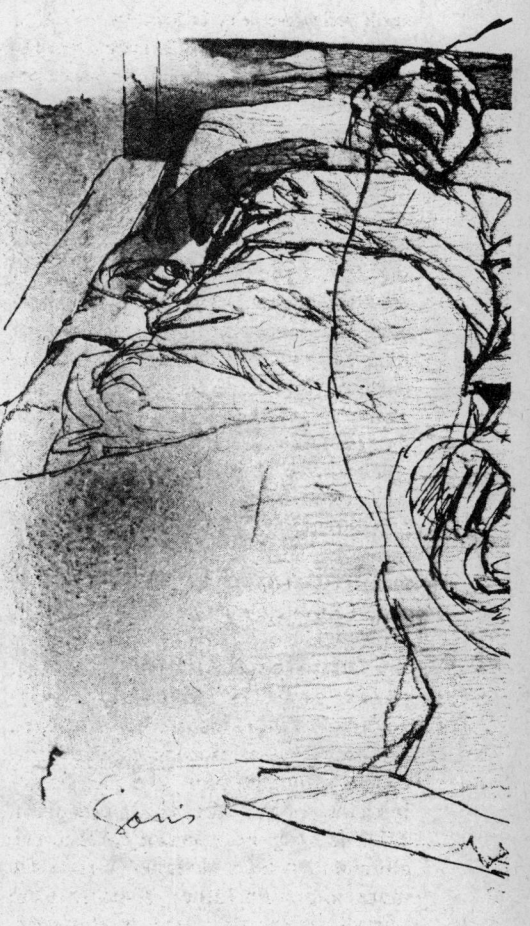

nurses see as they care for disabled patients, and begins to answer many questions about dependence and independence. Also, a valid theoretical model may aid in reducing the nurse's uncertainty about her ability to help a patient who is adjusting to severe disability, thereby reinforcing rather than threatening her feelings of competence.

Erikson's psychosocial stages are based on the psychosexual phases identified by Freud. The stages follow the epigenetic principle which maintains that psychosocial progress re-

SCI - Psychological Care

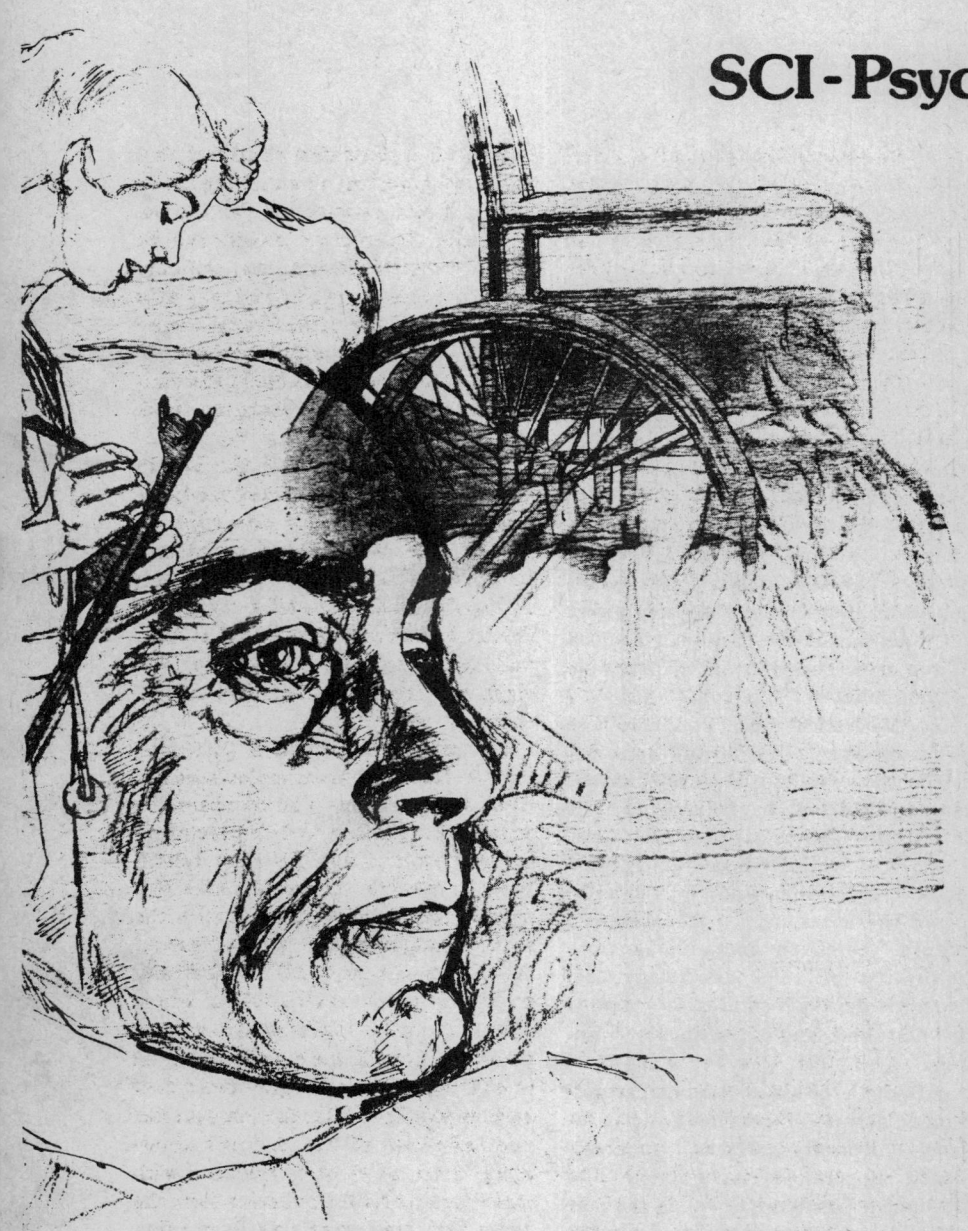

quires a person to surmount the critical task of each developmental phase at the proper time and in the proper sequence.

For each of eight phases, Erikson postulated a psychosocial task, expressed as a dichotomy (for example, a sense of basic trust or a sense of mistrust in the oral stage). The overall personality is determined by a favorable ratio of one to the other; but in each person the negative sense continues to exist as a dynamic counterpart of the positive sense.

Erikson related each "crisis," or dichotomy, to an ego strength, an organ mode, and a psychopathology (see table). The "eight ages of man," from birth to old age, are basic trust versus mistrust; autonomy vs. shame and doubt; initiative vs. guilt; industry vs. inferiority; identity vs. role confusion; intimacy vs. isolation; generativity vs. stagnation; and ego integrity vs. despair.

This discussion is limited to the first three crises, for several reasons. First, the person who sustains a catastrophic injury usually is an adolescent or young adult. Consequently, he may not have surmounted more than the third or fourth task at the onset of the disability. Second, more is known about early adjustment to such injuries, as indicated by the relative emphasis on this period in the literature. Finally, except for occasional encounters with community-based nurses, these people seldom interact with nurses after mastering the first three developmental stages following injury. As a result, there is little case material to draw on in explaining these persons' progress through later stages.

Trust: The First Task. The infant's need and ability to take in by mouth become the focus of the first approach to life, the *incorporative* approach. Initially, the pattern is receptive incorporation, not only of food but of other stimuli, through the senses. Later, the child becomes more assertive in seeking stimuli. To gain a sense of trust, the infant must have his needs met fairly readily and consistently, and must have an expectation that they will continue to be met. When this occurs, he gains a sense of outer predictability and a recognition that there is a corresponding inner certainty of remembered and anticipated sensations and images. These result in a basic sense of his own trustworthiness.

If an infant's needs are sporadically met, he may never experience the necessary consistency and constancy, and therefore may grow to mistrust others and himself. Temporal organization and willingness to let the mother out of his sight are important achievements of this stage.

Mahler postulates a period of *normal autism* in the newborn infant, when the primary task is maintaining inner homeostasis and he is shielded naturally against the bombardment of external stimuli. During the next period, which Mahler calls *normal symbiosis,* the child becomes aware that nurture comes from outside himself, and regards himself and his mother as one. It is the mother who screens the external stimuli at this stage.

Immediately following the sudden onset of disability, the patient is acutely ill and in a situation analogous to the infant's. He receives all therapy from others, including medication, intravenous infusion, oxygen, respiratory assistance, and frequent position changes. His relationship to his environment becomes literally incorporative. The physical limitations, the restrictions imposed by therapy, and the overwhelming psychological assault combine to enforce dependence. Camille Cayler, a psychiatrist who became paraplegic following an accident, stated:

The first phase is dominated by severe bodily discomfort, shock, confusion, excitement. The patient suddenly becomes the center of worried attention of doctors, family and friends. This may provide him with some narcissistic gratification and draw his attention away from the outside world, the tragic consequences of his disability, and the difficult future. . . . Because of psychological traumata, and dependency on others . . . the patient's ego has, as a rule, been weakened. Because he cannot take care of himself physically he regresses to the position of a child not only physically but also psychologically. His dependency on the hospital, where he literally has to repeat the training procedures of his childhood, fosters much emotional regression. (3)

During this initial shock period, the patient is protected from external stimuli much as an infant is protected. Each has the major task of establishing or reestablishing homeostasis. Several researchers have documented a dissociation from self and the development of infantile thought patterns. Studies of persons with spinal cord injury and poliomyelitis have revealed that patients have a tendency toward immature emotional behavior, including impulsive, egocentric explosiveness; ambivalence; and a tendency to think autistically about future problems(4,5).

A patient implied this in describing her reactions during the acute phase: "I had a peculiar inability to identify myself with my name; we didn't come together, my name and I." Noreen Linduska wrote of her experience in the acute stage of polio, "Something happened and I became a stranger. I was a greater stranger to myself than to anyone"(6). This absence of ego boundaries, comparable to the situation of the infant who has not yet defined his, may allow the patient to form a symbiotic relationship with the nurse until he is again able to cope.

After the initial shock, the patient becomes more aware of his environment. This contributes multiple stimuli that are meaningless to anyone unfamiliar with hospital equipment and routines, and the patient must begin to organize them. In an intensive care unit, where there often are no windows and the activity level is always high, it is difficult for the patient to gain temporal organization(7). The incorporative relationship becomes less receptive and the patient begins to indicate his needs more aggressively as he becomes less acutely ill.

Nursing Implications

Independence is *not* a realistic goal during this stage, but neither should the goal of nursing care be to maintain dependence. Rather, the primary goal is to establish the *dependability* and *consistency* of nursing care. Dependence is caused and maintained by the physical and psychological assault. Purposefully consistent nursing care helps the patient acquire a sense of trust in the nurse and in himself—the foundation for successful rehabilitation.

In responding to the patient's serious and often labile condition, the nurse constantly and regularly meets his physical needs through observation, hygiene and nutrition measures, and the alleviation of discomfort. These very actions also help to satisfy his psychological needs.

During this early period, the patient rarely initiates futuristic discussion of sexual and vocational adjustment, and it is rarely appropriate for the nurse to begin such a discussion or to feel that she is not providing an accepting atmosphere if the patient does not do so. Similarly, the patient should not be forced to perform all the self-care which he appears to be physically able to perform. As the patient gains a sense of trust, he will assume these responsibilities. The nurse offers him opportunities to perform these tasks as he is ready.

Mathews demonstrated the importance of consistency in care of the quadriplegic(8). Designating one nurse to provide care helps ensure a constant approach. However, the approach must be consistent among shifts and when the designated nurse has a day off. This underlines the need for written care plans and intra- and intershift conferences.

The professional nurse is best qualified to deal with the complex needs of these patients and to plan care based on accurate assessment of their psychological adjustment, but this may not always be feasible outside the ICU. Regardless of the setting, it remains the nurse's responsibility to understand thoroughly the patient's physical and emotional status, to ascertain if care is effective, and to reinforce and support those who provide the care. Although it is best that the nurse give the actual care, especially during the early period, one indication of the patient's developing sense of trust is the ease with which he accepts less attention from the nurse and more attention from other members of the staff.

As the shock wears off and the patient becomes aware of the environment, screening and interpreting the many stimuli which bombard him become important nursing functions. Clocks, calendars, and familiar personal items encourage temporal perspective and reality orientation. Family members, too, need to be included in the care, and their part in each phase of adjustment must be explained. The experience of C.M. demonstrates the importance of the development of trust and temporal organization.

C.M., a 17-year-old female, sustained a head injury in a motorcycle accident. Ultimately this resulted in left hemiparesis with severe spasticity and motor aphasia. Tests revealed that her intelligence level was essentially unchanged despite a long period of unconsciousness during her stay in a neurological ICU. On transfer to the rehabilitation unit shortly after she regained consciousness, C.M. showed extreme regression. A nurse began to work with C.M. and her family.

Initially, C.M. covered her head with a blanket when anyone approached. She confused day and night, and responded to questions or discomfort with a piercing wail. The nurse began by telling C.M. how long the visit would last, and sat quietly beside the bed. On leaving, she said when she would return. Family members did the same.

After several days, C.M. came out from under the blanket and grasped the nurse's hand. The staff then began to interpret and explain daily routines and expectations to her. Her eating and sleeping patterns became normal after two weeks, but she continued to be easily frustrated and lacked restraint in expression. At first she ignored her disability, but did permit therapy. After C.M. noted her deformed hand, she tried to persuade everyone to exercise it, often refusing therapy to her other extremities. Ultimate rehabilitation was considered very successful because C.M. was employed one year later.

When the patient begins to express his needs more assertively, staff may be annoyed that this person, in whom they have invested so much care, has become difficult to satisfy. The staff's response is often negativism and avoidance or a demand that the patient assume more independence in self-care.

Unfortunately, just at this time, when aggressiveness corresponds with improved physical condition, the patient often is transferred to a different unit. Here, he meets a new staff whom he is uncertain about, and the staff meets a demanding and testing patient whom they do not understand and tend to avoid.

This avoidance further threatens the patient. Nursing care should continue to emphasize consistency, which not only reaffirms the patient's sense of trust in others and himself but also sets limits that provide predictability in the new environment. Until trust and predictability have been established, emphasis on independence is still premature.

The patient whose needs are met consistently develops a hope for successful rehabilitation. If he finds that he must often wait for care, he develops behaviors indicating a lack of trust and he may be unable to move on from dependence. He may despair or express unrealistic hope, such as the expectation of complete recovery. L.H. was a patient who maintained extreme overdependence, based on a lack of trust.

A leader in family, church, and community, L.H., aged 46 and father of five, sustained a spinal cord injury at work. On admission, he had no motion or sensation below C-6 (quadriplegia). Because the census was low in the ICU, he received much attention from staff.

On transfer to a busy orthopedic ward, L.H. became demanding, required many hours to be bathed or fed, and was uncomfortable if not turned at least every hour—a difficult task due to his large size.

No staff member could care for anyone in the room without constant interruption, and most staff began to avoid L.H. Finally, he demanded the total attention of a nurse, refusing care from

ERIKSON'S PSYCHOSOCIAL STAGES*

Psychosexual Stage	Organ Mode	Psychosocial Stage	Rudimentary Ego Strength	Relation to Psychopathology
oral sensory cutaneous	incorporative	basic trust vs. basic mistrust	hope	addictive psychotic
muscular anal urethral	retentive-eliminative	autonomy vs. shame and doubt	will	compulsive impulsive
phallic-locomotor	intrusive	initiative vs. guilt	purpose	hysterical phobic

*Adapted from Erikson, E. Insight and Responsibility, W. W. Norton, 1964, p. 186.

The phases of a patient's emotional adjustment following sudden catastrophic injury resemble the psychosocial developmental stages described by Erikson.

SCI - Psychological Care

aides and orderlies. Because of his generally apprehensive behavior, episodes of dyspnea were discounted until he became so ill that he was transferred back to the ICU. There, multiple pulmonary emboli were diagnosed.

When L.H. returned to the orthopedic ward, the staff was defensive and rejecting. L.H. expressed his mistrust of staff and continued to demand and manipulate. His commitment to physical therapy was minimal as he waited passively for return of function. Although much function actually did return, he left the hospital almost completely dependent on others for care.

Autonomy: The Second Task. Erikson says that muscular maturation establishes holding on (*retentive*) and letting go (*eliminative*) as the social modalities of the second psychosocial stage (Freud's anal stage). In this stage the child discovers conflict between his desires and his mother's. The dichotomy of this stage is autonomy—the lasting sense of pride, goodwill, and self-control without loss of self-esteem— versus the shame and doubt that result from a loss of self-control and from foreign overcontrol. For the child, the focus of conflict and control often is bowel and bladder training. Mahler describes this phase as *separation-individuation*, a time of moving away but constantly checking to gain reassurance from the mother's presence. It is a time of negativism.

Following transfer to a general unit or rehabilitation center, the disabled person usually is placed on a fairly rigid therapy schedule, and bowel and bladder retraining is begun. Therefore, progress in bowel and bladder training and in physical mobility represents progress in self-control and influences the patient's self-esteem and ego reformation.

Cayley stressed the significance of this phase: ". . . specific areas of the body and bodily functions assume tremendous psychological importance. These are the excretions. . . . Some patients overcome gradually the exaggerated value of their excretory functions, while the lives of others continue to revolve around their urination and defecation"(9).

Another important factor during this stage of recovery is control by hospital staff as opposed to self-control. "Most patients want to be 'good patients'," Cayley said, "to accept the routine of the hospital blindly, in order to please the paternalistic hospital authorities. They do it at the expense of their spontaneity" (9). Too strong control by the staff may become internalized, creating a compulsive patient who is unable to adapt to change.

While many patients exhibit a certain compulsiveness which may actually benefit rehabilitation at this point, too much compulsiveness may halt progress by limiting the desire to take the gambles necessary to improve.

Patients may react to a strongly controlling staff by becoming negative and rejecting therapy or by demonstrating overt anger or prolonged depression. On the other hand, too little guidance and control, infrequent though this may be in the average institution, forces the patient to flounder in a sea of uncertainty.

If there is adequate—not excessive—control, the patient gains a sense of pride in his ability to cope and in his self-control, and a goodwill toward others. When control is rigid, he becomes compulsive, angry, and anxious from a sense of doubt in his ability to cope and in others' ability to help him. R. S. typifies this stage:

A 30-year-old man with two children, R. S. became paraplegic following a car accident. His relationship with the nursing staff was warm and trusting. Because he was in a private room and unable to compare himself with other patients, he questioned staff on all shifts to learn whether he was a "good patient." He established strict routines for eating, bathing, and transfer to a wheelchair; he seemed lost if this routine was broken. One night he was unable to sleep because a small sore on his foot, which previously had been open to air at night, had been rebandaged by a new nurse.

When the indwelling catheter was removed, R. S. achieved bladder control readily, an accomplishment he had been worried about. Now his pride was evident and for two weeks he quoted his intake-output total to anyone who would listen. Within a month, however, he began to adjust and the topic of excretion no longer occupied his attention.

Nursing Implications

To gain a sense of mastery, the patient must experience success. Hence, the nurse helps him establish reasonable early goals so that he does not learn failure. She does not expect him to assume too many or too complex tasks rapidly. At this point, the patient begins to be a full member of the health care team.

He makes decisions, an important component of independent functioning that is often overlooked. While the decisions should be small in scope initially, they should not be confined for too long to inconsequential matters. After the patient has resolved dependency needs, the nurse does not foster dependence in order to meet her needs. As he becomes increasingly autonomous, she remains available, reassuring him and coordinating his widening experiences.

The importance of bowel and bladder control to the patient's growing sense of autonomy dictates that nursing staff never show revulsion or foster shame by word or action. Responsibility for helping him regain bowel and bladder control rests primarily with the nurse. Control of elimination is a strong determinant of rehabilitation outcomes, so the nurse continually updates her knowledge about techniques of training, to afford patients the maximum opportunity for success. When the patient soils himself, this may threaten his developing sense of control; inappropriate emphasis by nursing staff on control of elimination can foster a life that revolves around elimination.

Extreme, persistent, obsessive-compulsive behavior is abnormal. But in relation to physical therapy, the transient compulsiveness of many patients may be beneficial. If a patient is learning one method of transfer in the physical therapy department, nursing staff should use the same method on the unit because learning a second method is confusing and potentially dangerous.

Reinforcement and practice of activities learned in the various therapy departments are included in the patient's nursing care. This requires open communication among all disciplines. The nurse does not challenge the patient's compulsions. Necessary changes in therapy or routine are explained thoroughly before they are implemented. Again, a limited number of staff who know the patient well should provide his nursing care.

Many disabled persons say that at one time they felt overwhelmingly ashamed, as though they had committed a terrible crime against society. Rigid expectations, rules, and a prison-like atmosphere foster this feeling. Nurses must evaluate the rules governing patients' lives, then work to eliminate all but those that are essential for people who must live for months in an environment where eating, sleeping, and even social contact are controlled.

Part of the patient's adjustment entails a change in value system. Therefore, nurses provide a value system that serves as a reference point; other patients may serve as models (see "Eddie—A Successful Quad"). Wright suggests that the disabled must subordinate physique, enlarge the scope of values to include those still available, and contain the disability effects(10). A sense of autonomy and containment of disability effects—that is, belief that the whole self is not worthless because a part does not function—developed simultaneously in M. D., a 19-year-old soldier wounded in Vietnam.

On return to a stateside hospital, M. D. had an above-knee amputation. On the stump sock he drew the cartoon figure Snoopy. Soon everyone called him Snoopy, and he introduced himself that way.

On this orthopedic unit, the patients, mostly veterans, were given weekend passes. Those who lived far from home went out in groups—usually with patients who had been around longer—to parties, discotheques, and the beach.

"Snoopy" had gone with the group on several weekends before the time he became separated and walked several miles back to the hospital on a temporary prosthesis. Shortly thereafter, he asked that he not be called Snoopy, but by his legal name. This request suggested that he no longer considered himself and the disability as synonymous.

Initiative: the Third Task. Mahler and Erikson believe that the child becomes a more distinct individual during the next period. The organ mode for this stage is *intrusive*: the male "making" and the female "on the make." Freudian theory calls this the oedipal stage, in which the child loves the opposite-sexed parent but, fearing retaliation by castration, represses the love for the opposite-sexed parent and identifies with the same-sexed parent.

The oedipal stage has been called the "self-centered sexual stage," because many advantages of loving augment personal worth rather than the desire to give. Erikson identified the danger of this stage as guilt—guilt over the goals contemplated or the inability to achieve them. The child gains a basic sense of initiative through awareness of moral responsibility, roles, and institutions. He finds accomplishment in manipulating tools and weapons.

By the time the disabled person has resolved dependence and gained some measure of self-control, he has begun to question the effect of the disability on his sexual functioning and desirability. Confusion and conflict in this area may complicate the interpersonal situation. To prove or test their sexual desirability, patients often express romantic or sexual desire for a staff member.

The loss of sexual function or fear of its loss may reawaken the guilt of the oedipal phase; the patient may believe that his injury is punishment for wrongdoing. This can impede rehabilitation, for it limits initiative. Cayley says that patients who lose sexual function "are then inclined to consider themselves as failures, and feel inadequate not only sexually, but in every respect"(11).

Some patients become obsessed with sexuality while others sublimate it completely. Comarr and Gunderson described a paraplegic who invested his total energy in job, church, and school, a behavior that caused severe marital stress(12). Other patients identify with a staff member of the same sex, and the desire to become a nurse or therapist often is voiced.

C. M., for instance, had a crush on an intern for some time and carried his picture with her. Shortly after the crush terminated, she spoke of becoming a nurse. Eventually she was employed in the hospital in a clerical position.

The re-alignment of the value system continues. The patient begins to sever ties with the staff, for soon he will leave the hospital. This may cause some ambivalence. He may revert temporarily to dependence, but will recover his initiative after a period of reassurance. This is the time he will begin to consider his societal role and to prepare for a job.

Nursing Implications

If the patient is ambivalent and retreats to dependence, the nurse offers the support he needs, recognizing that this is not an unusual reaction. If a sexual counselor and vocational counselor are available, the nurse may only need to coordinate and augment their contributions. If such counselors are not available, she will need to work closely with other health care professionals and may need to assume these functions herself to ensure that total rehabilitation is achieved.

Role definition by patients is more than merely vocational; it requires a

SCI - Psychological Care

total interaction with family and community, and always entails anticipatory guidance. Some institutions use role playing successfully to help patients and families identify future problems.

Because sexuality is an emotion-laden topic for patient and nurse, sex counseling is difficult, but it should not be avoided. Ideally, counseling is based on a physiological and humanistic approach. Rather than leave sex counseling to physicians by default, Smith and Bullough recommend a system that uses a primary sex counselor, who can be a specially prepared nurse, with secondary support by other team members[13]. These authors state that a generally hopeful attitude characterized by interest and concern is the best approach to the topic of sexuality, and they stress the need to include the patient's partner, if possible.

When a patient attempts to form a romantic relationship with the nurse, she recognizes the need this demonstrates and maintains her acceptance while assisting him to channel these energies elsewhere. A patient's identification with the nursing role can be used as a positive force in rehabilitation if the goal is not unrealistic. Referral to a psychiatrist is appropriate for any patient with severe, prolonged guilt feelings.

The astute nurse can use the theoretical framework presented here to identify the patient's progress and needs, and to determine what approaches best foster his ultimate independence. The limitations of using any model include the tendency to fit patient to model by ignoring important individual variations. This particular developmental model could introduce the risk of treating patients like children rather than adults with established personalities who have suffered overwhelming physical and psychological assault.

The nurse's day-by-day sensitivity to the patient's feelings and unique pace in adjusting are the best assurance that the patient gradually will again become a "whole" human being, no matter how devastating the injury.

References

1. ERIKSON, E. H. *Identity: Youth and Crisis.* New York, W. W. Norton, 1968.
2. MAHLER, M. S., AND FURER, MANUEL. *On Human Symbiosis and the Vicissitudes of Individuation.* New York, International Universities Press, 1968.
3. CAYLEY, C. K. Psychiatric aspects of rehabilitation of the physically handicapped. *Am.J.Psychotherapy* 8:518-529, July 1954.
4. MUELLER, A. D. Personality problems of the spinal cord injured. *J.Consult. Psychiatry* 14:189-192, 1950.
5. ARNOLD, N. Adjustment of adolescents to poliomyelitis; A study of six patients. *J.Pediatr.* 45:347-361, Sept. 1954.
6. LINDUSKA, NOREEN. *My Polio Past.* New York, Pellegrini and Cudahy Co., 1947.
7. SORENSEN, K. M., AND AMIS, D. B. Understanding the world of the chronically ill. *Am.J.Nurs.* 67:811-817, Apr. 1967.
8. MATHEWS, N.C. Helping a quadriplegic veteran decide to live. *Am.J.Nurs.* 76:441-443, Mar. 1976.
9. CAYLEY, *op.cit.,* p. 519.
10. WRIGHT, B. A. *Physical Disability, a Psychological Approach.* New York, Harper & Row, 1960.
11. CAYLEY, *op.cit.,* p. 520.
12. COMARR, A. E., AND GUNDERSON, B. B. Sexual function in traumatic paraplegia and quadriplegia. *Am.J.Nurs.* 75:250-253, Feb. 1975.
13. SMITH, JIM, AND BULLOUGH, BONNIE. Sexuality and the severely disabled person. *Am.J.Nurs.* 75:2194-2197, Dec. 1975.

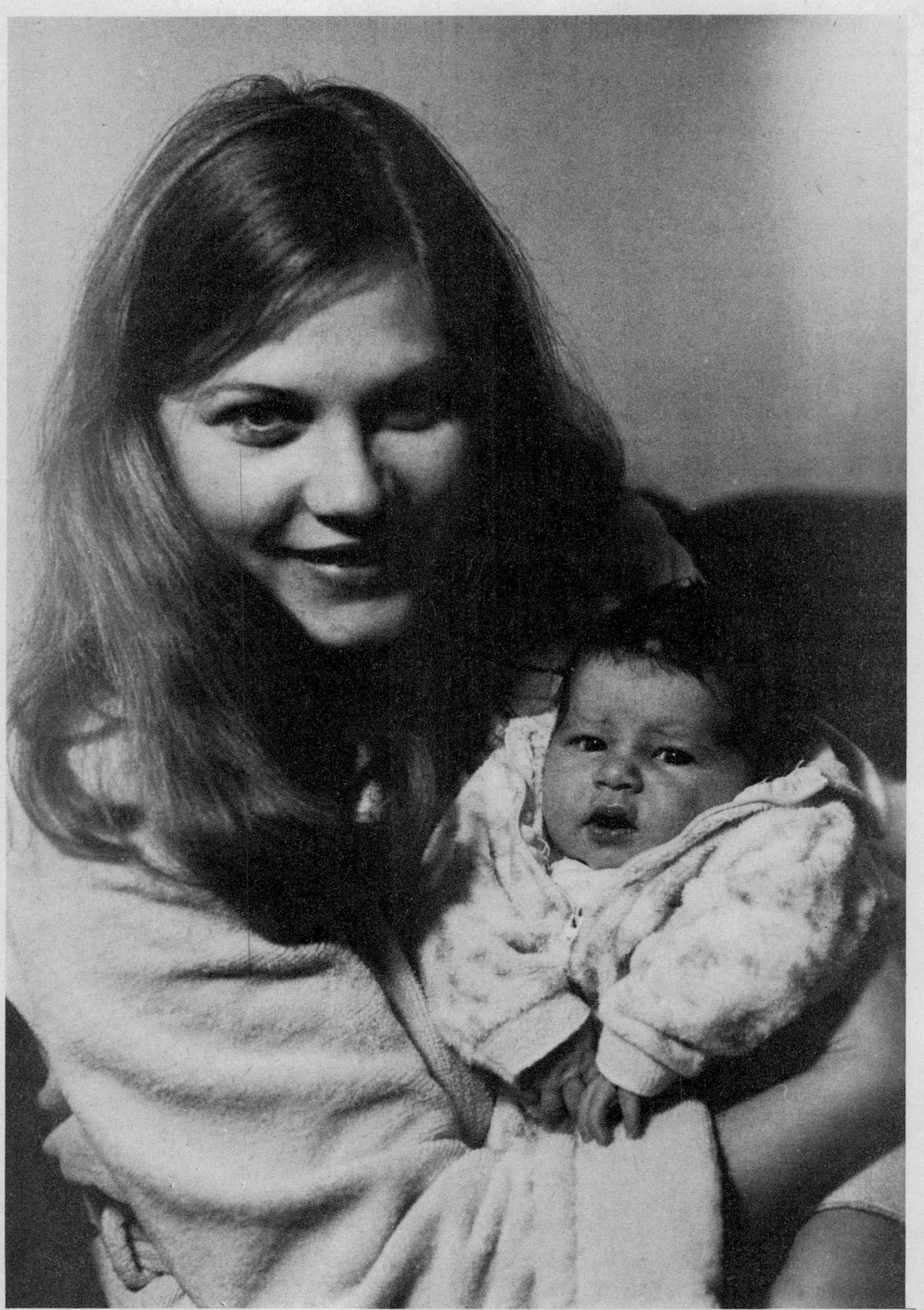

Section 4
Nursing Care of the Childbearing Family

Marybeth Young, RN, MSN, Coordinator

Gita Dhillon, RN, MEd
Cynthia Dunsmore, RN, MSN
Michele M. Kamradt, RN, EdD
Deborah Koniak, RN, EdD
B. Patricia Nix, RN, MSN
Karen Stefaniak, RN, MSN
Quilla D. B. Turner, RN, PhD
Deborah L. Ulrich, RN, MA
Francene Weatherby, RNC, MSN

Section 4: Nursing Care of the Childbearing Family

FEMALE REPRODUCTIVE ANATOMY AND PHYSIOLOGY 375

ANTEPARTAL CARE 381
General Concepts 381
   Normal Childbearing 381
   Overview of Management 385
   Application of the Nursing Process to Normal Childbearing, Antepartal Care 386
   High-Risk Childbearing 389
   Application of the Nursing Process to High-Risk Childbearing 394
Selected Health Problems 394
   A. *Abortion* 394
   B. *Incompetent Cervical Os* 395
   C. *Ectopic Pregnancy* 395
   D. *Hydatidiform Mole* 396
   E. *Placenta Previa* 397
   F. *Abruptio Placentae* 398
   G. *Pregnancy-Induced Hypertension* 399
   H. *Diabetes* 401
   I. *Cardiac Disorders* 402
   J. *Anemia* 404
   K. *Infections* 404
   L. *Multiple Gestation* 405
   M. *Adolescent Pregnancy* 407

INTRAPARTAL CARE 408
General Concepts 408
   Normal Childbearing 408
   Ongoing Management and Nursing Care 411
   Application of the Nursing Process to Normal Childbearing, Intrapartal Care 416
Selected Health Problems 420
   A. *Dystocia* 421
   B. *Premature Labor* 423
   C. *Emergency Birth* 425
   D. *Induction* 425
   E. *Episiotomy* 426
   F. *Forceps* 427
   G. *Vacuum Extraction* 428
   H. *Cesarean Birth* 428
   I. *Rupture of the Uterus* 430
   J. *Amniotic Fluid Embolism* 430

POSTPARTAL CARE 432
General Concepts 432
   Normal Childbearing 432
   Application of the Nursing Process to Normal Childbearing, Postpartal Care 434
Selected Health Problems 437
   A. *Postpartum Hemorrhage* 437
   B. *Hematoma* 438
   C. *Puerperal Infection* 439
   D. *Mastitis* 440
   E. *Postpartum Cystitis* 441
   F. *Uterine Prolapse With or Without Cystocele or Rectocele* 441
   G. *Uterine Fibroids* 442
   H. *Pulmonary Embolus* 443
   I. *Psychologic Maladaptations* 443

THE NORMAL NEONATE 444
Definition 444
General Characteristics 444
Specific Body Parts 445
Systems Adaptations 448
Gestational Age Variations 450
Application of the Nursing Process to the Normal Neonate 452

THE HIGH-RISK NEONATE 457
General Concepts 457
   Definition 457
   Antepartum Risk Factors 457
Selected Health Problems 457
   A. *Hypothermia* 457
   B. *Neonatal Jaundice* 457
   C. *Respiratory Distress* 459
   D. *Hypoglycemia* 461
   E. *Neonatal Infection* 462
   F. *Neonatal Narcotic Drug Addiction* 463
   G. *Fetal Alcohol Syndrome* 463
   H. *Intracranial Hemorrhage* 464
   I. *Brain Injuries* 464
   J. *Neonatal Necrotizing Enterocolitis* 465
   K. *Congenital Anomalies* 465
   L. *Parental Reaction to a Sick, Disabled, or Malformed Infant* 466

REPRINTS 469

Female Reproductive Anatomy and Physiology

General Concepts

(*NOTE:* The concept development in the sections on the Adult, Child, and the Client with Psychosocial Problems also applies to the mother and her newborn. However, this section has been organized according to the normal childbearing cycle, from conception to postpartum.)

A. Overview

1. The Structure of the Female Pelvis
   a. Pelvic Structure (four united bones): two hip bones (right and left innominate), the sacrum, and the coccyx
   b. Pelvic Divisions: two parts divided by the inlet or brim
      1) false pelvis: upper portion above brim; supports uterus during late pregnancy
      2) true pelvis: located below brim; composed of three parts: the pelvic inlet, the mid-cavity, and the pelvic outlet; forms birth canal through which fetus passes during parturition
   c. Pelvic Variations: pelvic structures differ in shape and size
      1) android: normal male type; heart-shaped inlet, narrow pubic arch; influence on labor is not favorable
      2) gynecoid: true female type; slightly ovoid or rounded inlet; influence on labor *most favorable*
      3) platypelloid: flattened antero-posteriorly, oval-shaped inlet; influence on labor not favorable
      4) anthropoid: apelike type; inlet oval shaped; influence on labor favorable
   d. Pelvic Measurements
      1) diagonal conjugate (DC): distance between sacral promontory and lower margin (inferior border) of symphysis pubis; adequate size for childbirth is 12.5 cm or more; *estimated on pelvic exam*
      2) true conjugate or conjugate vera (CV): distance between upper margin, superior border of symphysis pubis to sacral promontory; adequate size for childbirth 11 cm or more (1.5–2 cm less than diagonal conjugate); *measured accurately by x-ray*
      3) obstetric conjugate: the shortest distance between the inner surface of the symphysis and the sacral promontory; *measured by x-ray*
      4) tuber-ischial diameter: transverse diameter of the outlet, the distance between the ischial tuberosities; adequate size for childbirth 9–11 cm or more; *estimated on pelvic exam*

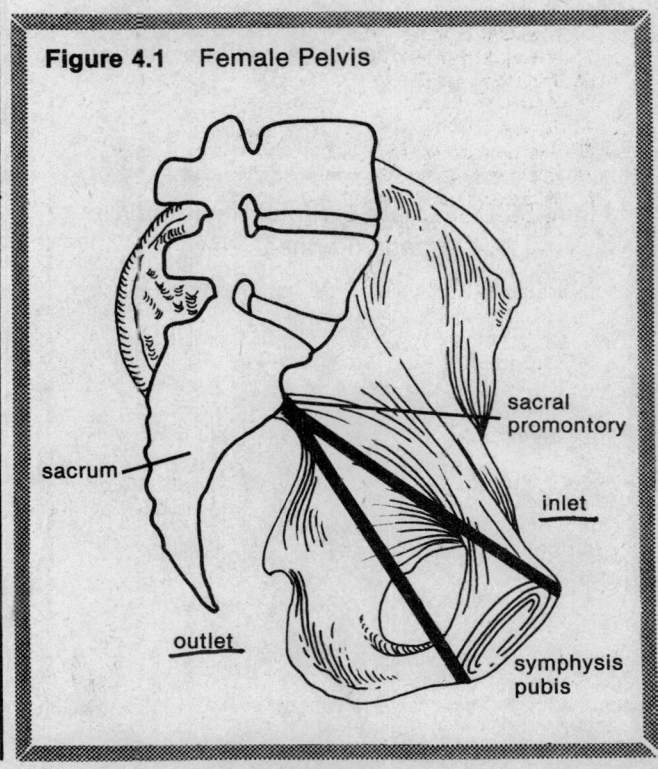

Figure 4.1 Female Pelvis

5) assessment of size
   a) estimate of pelvic dimensions: diagonal conjugate and tuber-ischial diameter
   b) x-ray or internal pelvimetry: use is limited to suspected pelvic bony contractions and suspected cephalopelvic disproportion (most accurate measurement of pelvic size)
   c) ultrasonography: employs use of high-frequency sound waves for determination of gestational age
2. The Female External Organs
   a. Mons Veneris or Pubis: rounded, soft, fatty pad over symphysis pubis, covered by coarse hair in adult
   b. Labia Majora: two folds of skin containing fat and covered with hair; located on either side of the vaginal opening
   c. Labia Minora: two thin folds of delicate tissue without hair; located within labia majora
   d. Glans Clitoris: a small body of erectile tissue partially hidden between the anterior ends of the labia minora; highly sensitive to touch, temperature, and pressure
   e. Hymen: thin mucous membrane; located at the opening of the vagina, can be stretched or torn during intercourse, physical activity, tampon insertion, or vaginal examination
   f. Urinary Meatus: external opening of the urethra
   g. Openings of Vulvovaginal or Bartholin's Glands: two small glands situated between the vestibula on either side of the vaginal orifice; secrete alkaline mucus during coitus
   h. Openings of Skene's Ducts: two paraurethral glands open onto posterior urethral wall
   i. Perineum: area between vagina and rectum consisting of fibromuscular tissue
3. The Female Internal Organs
   a. Ovaries: two oval-shaped organs located on either side of the uterus in the upper pelvic cavity; responsible for producing the ovum and the female hormones, estrogen and progesterone
   b. Fallopian or Uterine Tubes: two thin muscular canals extending from the cornua of the uterus to the ovaries; responsible for transport of the ovum from the ovaries to the uterus; fertilization occurs in middle 3rd (ampulla) of either fallopian tube
   c. Uterus: a hollow muscular organ that is the site of implantation, retainment, and nourishment of the products of conception. It is also the organ of menstruation in the nonpregnant female. The upper segment of the uterus is known as the *fundus* and the lower segment is called the *cervix*. In the nonpregnant female, the uterus is located in the pelvic cavity between the bladder and rectum and weighs approximately 60 gm. The uterus is composed of smooth muscle (myometrium) and an inner mucoid lining (the endometrium), which responds to estrogen and progesterone during the menstrual cycle.
   d. Vagina: a thin-walled dilatable canal located between the bladder and rectum that serves as the passageway for menstrual discharge, copulation, and the fetus
   e. Accessory Structures (breasts): two mammary glands composed of glandular tissue and fat, which are capable of producing and secreting milk for nourishment of the infant
4. The Menstrual Cycle
   a. Hormones
      1) follicle-stimulating hormone (FSH): secreted by anterior pituitary gland during the first half of the menstrual

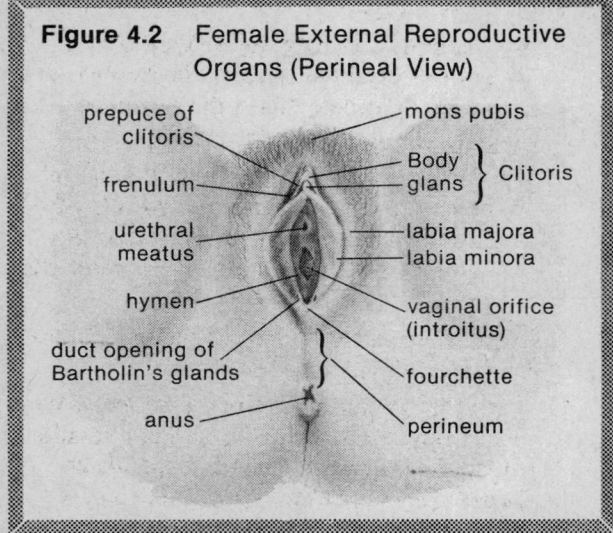

Figure 4.2 Female External Reproductive Organs (Perineal View)

Figure 4.3 Female Internal Reproductive Organs (Side View)

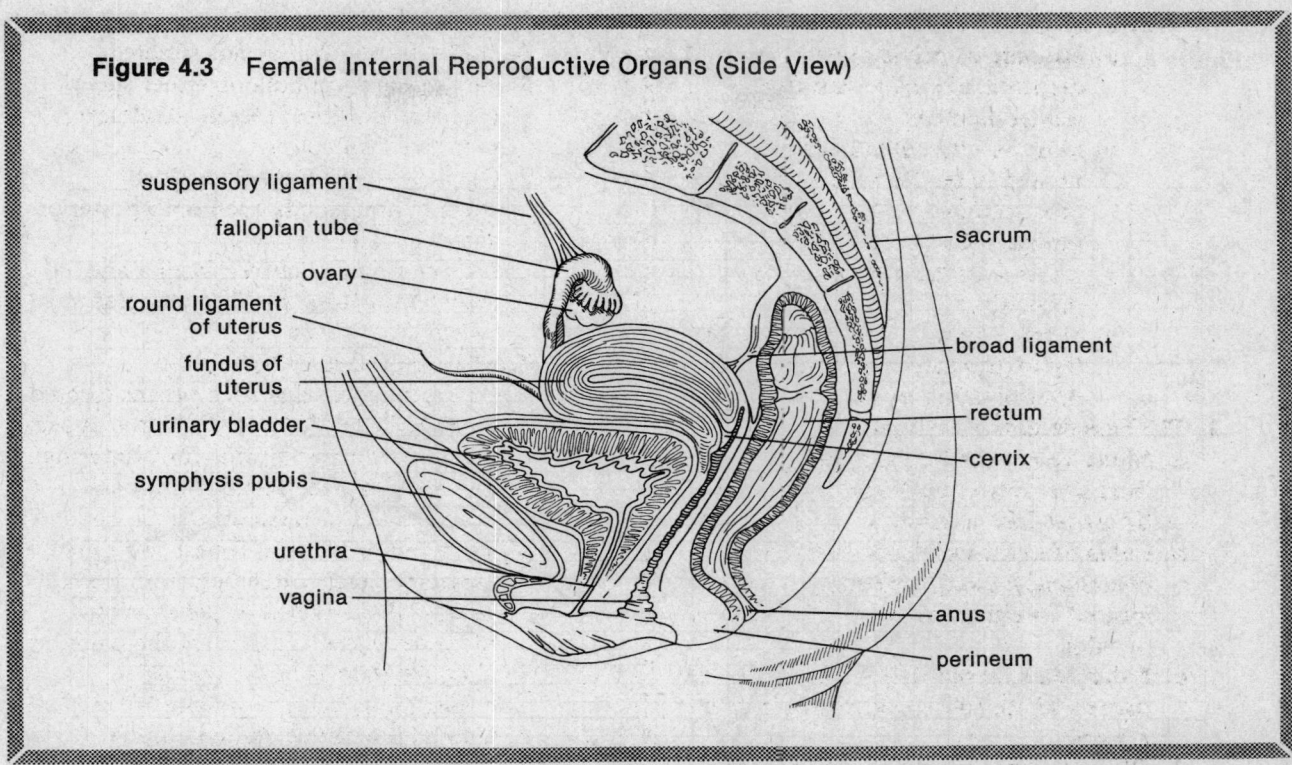

cycle; stimulates development of graafian follicles and thins the endometrium

2) interstitial-cell stimulating hormone (ICSH) or luteinizing hormone (LH): secreted by the pituitary; stimulates ovulation and development of the corpus luteum; causes the endometrium to thicken

3) estrogen: secreted primarily by the ovaries and by the adrenal cortex (in small amounts), and by the placenta in pregnancy; assists in maturation of ovarian follicles, stimulates thickening of the endometrium, causes suppression of FSH secretion, and is responsible for development of secondary sex characteristics; in pregnancy, it maintains the endometrium, causes fatigue, and stimulates contraction of smooth muscle

4) progesterone: secreted by corpus luteum and by the placenta during pregnancy; supplements estrogen effect on endometrium by facilitating secretory changes; relaxes smooth muscle; decreases uterine motility; has thermogenic effect (i.e., increases temperature); causes cervical secretion of thick viscous mucus; allows pregnancy to be maintained

5) prostaglandins: fatty acids categorized as hormones, produced by many organs of the body, including the endometrium; affect the menstrual cycle and may influence the onset and maintenance of labor. *NOTE*: Thyroid function affects production of reproductive hormones

b. Ovulation: growth and release of a nonfertilized ovum from the ovary; generally occurs 13–15 days prior to next menses in regular cycle

c. Menstruation: cyclic vaginal discharge of blood and superficial fragments of endometrium and other secretions in response to falling levels of estrogen and progesterone

d. Menopause: cessation of menses at the end of fertility cycle

5. Fertilization: impregnation of an ovum by a spermatozoon, occurring in the ampulla of the fallopian tube; egg life span is 24 hours after ovulation; sperm life span is 48–72 hours after ejaculation

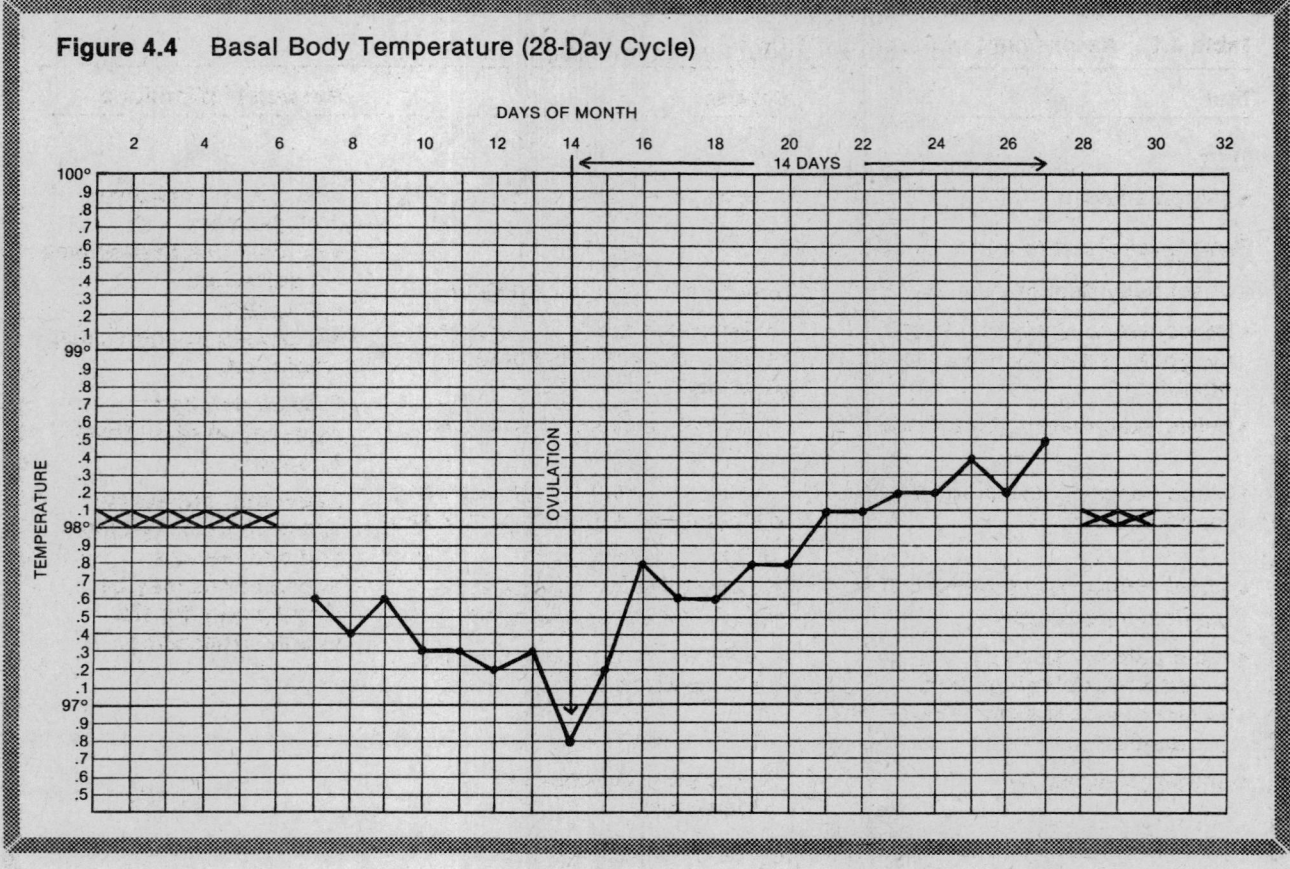

Figure 4.4 Basal Body Temperature (28-Day Cycle)

6. Implantation: the imbedding of the fertilized ovum into the uterine mucosa (usually in the upper segment); occurs approximately 7–10 days after ovulation (also known as nidation)
7. Menopause: cessation of menses at end of fertility cycle
   a. A normal developmental process that occurs naturally between the ages of 35 and 60 (average age: 53)
   b. Early menopause may be stimulated by
      1) multiple, frequent pregnancies or abortions
      2) hypothyroidism with obesity
      3) surgical removal of the ovaries
      4) hard physical work or exercise
      5) overexposure to radiation
   c. Medical Treatment: for symptom relief
      1) estrogen replacement therapy: often controversial
      2) increased vitamin B complex and vitamin E for hot flashes
      3) vaginal creams and lubricants for painful intercourse (dyspareunia)
      4) increased calcium and decreased phosphorus intake for osteoporosis
      5) positive emotional support during this developmental change/crisis

B. Application of the Nursing Process to Female Reproductive Anatomy
   1. Assessment
      a. Health History: onset of menarche, duration of menstrual periods, menstrual problems (e.g., amenorrhea: absence of menses as a result of hormonal problems or surgery; dysmenorrhea: painful menses), use of family planning, past and current pregnancies, infertility problems, hot flashes, dizzy spells, palpitations, osteoporosis (decrease in skeletal bone mass)
      b. Physical examination of external reproductive organs; breast palpation for masses; mammography, thermography in at-risk clients; bimanual internal examination; and

Table 4.1 Assessment of Fertility/Infertility

Test	Purpose	Nursing Implications
Male		Take careful history of both partners
• semen analysis	To determine sperm count, mobility	• chronic health problems
Female *(simplest to more complex)*		• medications
• basal body temperature	To determine time of ovulation	• drug use
• cervical-mucus examination (self-done, basis for natural family planning)	To determine elasticity for sperm mobility and time of ovulation (*Spinnbarkheit*)	• exposure to chemicals, radiation.
• pelvic examination (bimanual)	To identify obvious reproductive problems	Provide detailed explanation of all tests to couple.
• blood hormone levels and thyroid function tests	To measure levels of estrogen and progesterone, and influence of the thyroid	Know that process of assessment of fertility and subsequent interventions may be lengthy and, for the couple, frustrating.
• Sims-Huhner test (postcoital cervical mucus test)	To determine pH of cervical mucus, effects of hormones	
• tubal patency tests — hysterosalpingogram (x-ray) — laporoscopic exam (direct visualization)	To determine condition, patency of Fallopian tubes	
• endometrial biopsy	To determine condition of endometrium	
• culdoscopy (examination through cul-de-sac with dye injection)	To determine function of Fallopian tubes	

observation of cervical-vaginal discharge (by physician or nurse)

2. **General Nursing Goals, Plans/Implementation, and Evaluation**

   <u>Goal 1:</u> Client will understand her reproductive system and capabilities; will report gynecologic problems to the physician. *Report abnorm + aware of body*

   Plan/Implementation
   - discuss anatomy and physiology of female reproductive system
   - review menstrual cycle, ovulation, and fertilization
   - teach client reportable problems

   Evaluation: Client can give a basic explanation of reproductive anatomy and physiology; can explain relationship of menstrual cycle, ovulation, and fertilization.

   <u>Goal 2:</u> Client will be knowledgeable about various methods of birth control.

   Plan/Implementation
   - assess client's learning needs
   - provide information as needed; refer to "Birth Control: Permanent, Temporary Measures" in reprint section

   Evaluation: Client is aware of birth control measures; asks questions about them; uses chosen method consistently according to directions.

   <u>Goal 3:</u> Client understands the importance of <u>periodic examinations</u> in maintaining reproductive health.

   Plan/Implementation
   - explain the need for periodic Papanicolaou (<u>Pap</u>) smears (cells taken from cells of squamo-columnar junction) to detect cancer of the uterus and abnormalities of cervical, vaginal cells
   - explain importance of regular self-breast examination after cessation of menstrual period (days 5–7 of menstrual cycle)

- demonstrate self-breast examination; ask client for return demonstration
- discuss meaning, purposes, and interpretation of various test results with client
- provide supplemental reading materials to increase client's knowledge

Evaluation: Client performs self-breast examination regularly and states she will do it at end of each menstrual cycle; understands need for periodic checkups and Pap smears.

<u>Goal</u> **4:** Client will be physically and psychologically prepared for menopause and will be able to make informed choices for treatment.

Plan/Implementation

- allow client to <u>voice feelings</u> about menopause
- teach client how to maintain good health and nutritional status
- discuss normal changes that occur with menopause
- dispel "myths" concerning menopause
- discuss implications of estrogen therapy
- discuss sexuality needs

Evaluation: Client can list the signs and symptoms of menopause; participates in decisions about treatment as an informed consumer.

Antepartal Care

General Concepts
A. Normal Childbearing
1. Definition: care provided to a woman and her family during pregnancy
2. Normal Adaptations: changes that occur in body systems of childbearing women due to the influence of hormones and growth on the embryo/fetus
   a. Integumentary System
      1) chloasma (mask of pregnancy): brown blotches that appear on face and neck, often visible in 2nd trimester; usually fade after delivery
      2) linea nigra: a dark line that extends from umbilicus to mons veneris; will lighten after delivery
      3) striae gravidarum: pink or slightly reddish streaks on abdomen, thighs, or breasts, resulting from stretching of underlying connective tissue due to adrenal cortex hypertrophy; grow lighter after delivery but never disappear completely
   b. Reproductive System
      1) changes in the uterus
         a) size: increases in length (6–32 cm), width (4–24 cm), and depth (2.5–22 cm)
         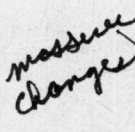
         b) weight increase: 60–1,000 gm
         c) shape: from globular to oval; wall thickens and then becomes thin at term
         d) location: rises out of pelvis at 12th week; near xiphoid process at term
         e) structure
            - body of uterus
              - three distinct uterine segments in pregnancy
              - vascularity increases
              - muscle fiber changes, mainly enlargement of preexisting fibers
              - new fibroelastic tissue develops and strengthens uterine wall
            - softening of the lower uterine segment (Hegar's sign)
            - cervix: softens (Goodell's sign) and increases in vascularity
            - formation of mucus plug (prevents bacterial contamination)
         f) contractility: Braxton Hicks' contractions occur intermittently throughout pregnancy
      2) changes in the vagina
         a) increased vascularization, which results in purplish discoloration (Chadwick's sign) beginning 6th week of pregnancy
         b) thickening of mucosa
         c) loosening of connective tissue
         d) increased vaginal discharge (thick, whitish) without signs of itching or burning
      3) changes in the breasts
         a) enlargement and prominence of superficial veins
         b) increase in size and firmness
         c) Montgomery's glands in areola enlarge
         d) nipples become more prominent, areolae darken and increase in diameter
         e) colostrum may be expressed by 4th or 5th month
         f) alveoli and duct system enlarge
      4) changes in joints and ligaments
         a) relaxation of pelvic joints and ligaments
         b) hypertrophy and elongation of
            - broad, round ligaments (stabilize uterus)
            - uterosacral ligaments (support cervix)

5) changes in abdomen: occur to accommodate progressive growth in uterine size
   a) at end of 3rd month, uterus is at level of symphysis pubis
   b) at end of 5th month, uterus is at level of umbilicus
   c) at end of 9th month, uterus is at level of xiphoid process
   d) decrease in fundal height after lightening in primiparous women

c. Endocrine System (Placenta)
   1) function of placenta
      a) secretes estrogen, progesterone, human chorionic gonadotropin (HCG), and human placental lactogen (HPL)
      b) acts as a barrier to some substances and organisms
      c) transports nourishment to fetus and removes wastes
      d) exchanges
         - diffusion, e.g., O_2 and CO_2 (low molecular weight)
         - facilitated and active transport, e.g., glucose, amino acids, calcium (high molecular weight)
         - leakage: *slight* mixing of fetal and maternal circulation
         - pinocytosis, e.g., gamma globulin, albumin
   2) dimensions
      a) 15 x 3 cm
      b) discoid
      c) 400–600 gm at term
      d) covers ¼ of uterine wall
      e) fetal-placental weight ratio at term is 6:1
   3) structure and development
      a) developed by 3rd month from the decidua basalis and chorion of the embryo
      b) normally develops in the posterior surface of the upper uterine segment
      c) two surfaces
         - fetal (amniotic) surface: chorionic villi and their circulation; membranes: amnion (inner), chorion (outer) fused
         - maternal surface: decidua basalis (hypertrophied endometrium of pregnancy) and its circulation; cotyledons present
      d) umbilical cord: 55 cm at term; most commonly is centrally inserted into fetal surface of placenta
   4) hormones
      a) estrogen and progesterone: after 1st 2 months of gestation, placenta is major source of production; responsible for growth of uterus and development of breasts
      b) human chorionic gonadotropin (HCG): secreted by 3rd week after fertilization, detected in urine 10 days after missed period (basis for pregnancy tests); HCG prolongs life of corpus luteum; radio-immunoassay (RIA) for HCG will be positive the 2nd day after implantation
      c) human chorionic somato-mammotropin (human placental lactogen): secreted by 3rd week after ovulation; prepares breasts for lactation, influences somatic cell growth of fetus

d. Musculoskeletal System
   1) waddling gait common
   2) increase in normal lumbosacral curve
   3) stress on ligaments and muscles of mid and lower spine
   4) backache and leg cramps may occur
   5) relaxation and increased mobility of pelvic joints

e. Cardiovascular System
   1) heart and vessels
      a) heart rate increases 10–15 beats/minute in 2nd trimester; persists to term
      b) blood pressure should remain constant during pregnancy
      c) increase in vasculature: dilation of pelvic veins, varicose veins, varicosities of the vulva, hemorrhoids
   2) blood volume altered in pregnancy
      a) total volume of blood increases approximately 25%–40%
      b) physiologic anemia of pregnancy: plasma volume increase that is not proportional to the cell increase results in hemodilution; this makes the woman appear to be anemic

c) hemoglobin range 10–14 gm/100 ml
d) hematocrit range 32%–42%; may decrease approximately 10% in 2nd and 3rd trimesters
e) average white count
3) cardiac output increases 20%–30%
4) palpitations: common in early and later pregnancy because of sympathetic nervous system disturbance and increased intra-abdominal pressure

f. Renal System
1) dilation of ureters, especially on the right, leading to possible urinary stasis
2) decreased bladder tone, caused by progesterone effect
3) increased pressure on bladder by enlarging uterus (1st and 3rd trimesters), therefore decreased capacity and frequency
4) glomerular filtration rate increases 50%
5) increased amount of urine; decreased specific gravity
6) reduced renal threshold for sugar

g. Respiratory System
1) diaphragm rises as much as 1 inch; dyspnea may occur until lightening (60% of pregnant women)
2) thoracic cage is pushed upward and widens
3) increased vital capacity, tidal volume, respiratory minute volume
4) increased vascularization due to elevated estrogen can cause nasal stuffiness; nosebleed, voice changes, eustachian-tube blockage [Avoid nasal sprays.]

h. Digestive System
1) gastrointestinal motility and digestion slowed, because of progesterone effects
2) delayed emptying time of stomach; reflux of food
3) upward displacement and compression of stomach
4) displacement of intestines
5) common problems
a) nausea and vomiting (morning sickness, 50%–75% of pregnant women)
b) pica or food cravings
c) acid indigestion or heartburn
d) constipation
e) hemorrhoids

i. Psychosocial Changes
1) factors influencing a woman's response to pregnancy
a) memories of her own childhood
b) cultural background
c) existing support systems
d) socioeconomic conditions
e) perceptions of maternal role
f) impact of mass media
2) maternal adaptations to pregnancy
a) 1st trimester: initial ambivalence about pregnancy; pregnant woman places main focus upon self, i.e., physical changes associated with pregnancy and emotional reactions to pregnancy
b) 2nd trimester: increased awareness and interest in fetus, acceptance of reality of pregnancy, feeling of well-being, and preoccupation with self
c) 3rd trimester: anticipation of labor and delivery and assuming mothering role, heightened introversion, viewing infant as reality vs fantasy; fears and fantasies about pregnancy common; "nesting" behaviors
3) psychologic tasks of pregnancy (Rubin, 1961)
a) acceptance of pregnancy as a reality and incorporation of fetus into body image
b) preparation for physical separation from fetus (birth)
c) attainment of maternal role
4) paternal reactions to pregnancy
a) 1st trimester: ambivalance and anxiety about role change
b) 2nd trimester: increased confidence and interest in mother's care; difficulty relating to fetus; "jealousy"
c) 3rd trimester: changing self-concept; fears about mutilation/death of fetus [for wife also]
5) sibling reactions to pregnancy
a) normal rivalry dependent on developmental stage
b) may need increased affection and attention
c) regressions in behavior (may appear in bed-wetting and thumb sucking)

3. Signs and Symptoms of Pregnancy
   a. Presumptive Symptoms (Subjective)
      1) amenorrhea
      2) breast sensitivity and fullness
      3) nausea and vomiting
      4) urinary frequency
      5) fatigue
      6) quickening: maternal perception of fetal movement 18–20 weeks in primipara, 16 weeks in multipara
      7) constipation
   b. Presumptive Signs (Objective)
      1) dark blue discoloration of the vaginal mucosa (Chadwick's sign)
      2) skin pigmentation and striae
   c. Probable Signs (Objective)
      1) enlargement of abdomen
      2) changes in the uterus: size, shape, and consistency (Hegar's sign)
      3) softening of the cervical tip (Goodell's sign)
      4) ballottement: movement of the fetus in the pregnant uterus by the examiner
      5) Braxton Hicks' contractions
      6) positive pregnancy test: biologic and immunologic tests based on secretion of HCG in maternal urine or in serum
   d. Positive Signs (Objective)
      1) fetal movements felt by examiner
      2) presence of fetal heart sounds detected by fetoscope at 16 weeks (Doppler, 10 weeks)
      3) x-ray outline of fetal skeleton (rarely used)
      4) delineation of pregnancy by ultrasonography
4. Fetal Development
   a. During 1st Lunar Month
      1) following fertilization, the ovum (zygote) begins a process of rapid cell division (mitosis or cleavage) leading to formation of *blastomeres*, which eventually become a ball-like structure called the morula
      2) the *morula* changes into a *blastocyst* after entering the uterus
      3) implantation occurs within 1–2 days, when the exposed cells of the trophoblast (cellular walls of the blastocyst) implant in the anterior or posterior fundal portion of the uterus
      4) the cells of the embryo will differentiate into three main groups: an outer covering (ectoderm), a middle layer (mesoderm), and an internal layer (entoderm)
         a) ectoderm: later differentiates into epithelium of skin, hair, nails, nasal and oral passages, sebaceous and sweat glands, mucous membranes of mouth and nose, salivary glands, the nervous system
         b) mesoderm: later differentiates into muscles; bones; circulatory, renal, and reproductive organs; connective tissue
         c) entoderm: differentiates into epithelium of gastrointestinal and respiratory tracts, the bladder, thyroid
   b. Subsequent Lunar Months
      1) end of 1st lunar month: heart functions; beginning formation of eyes, nose, digestive tract; arm and leg buds
      2) end of 2nd lunar month: recognizable human face, rapid brain development, appearance of external genitalia

Table 4.2 Signs and Symptoms of Pregnancy

Symptoms	Signs
Presumptive	
Amenorrhea	Chadwick's sign
Breast sensitivity	Breast enlargement
Nausea, vomiting	Skin pigmentation, striae
Fatigue	
Quickening	
Probable	
Enlarged abdomen	Ballottement
Hegar's sign	Braxton Hicks' contractions
Goodell's sign	Positive pregnancy tests
Positive	
	Fetal movements
	Fetal outline
	Fetal heart tones

3) end of 3rd lunar month: placenta fully formed and functioning; sex determination apparent; bones begin to ossify; length—3 in, weight—1 oz
4) end of 4th lunar month: external genitalia obvious; meconium present in intestinal tract; eye, ear, and nose formed; fetal heartbeat heard with fetoscope; length—6½ in, weight—4 oz
5) end of 5th lunar month: lanugo present; fetus sucks and swallows amniotic fluid; quickening (mother can feel movement); length—10 in, weight—8 oz
6) end of 6th lunar month: vernix present; skin reddish and wrinkled; considered viable, but usually doesn't survive if born now; length—12 in, weight—1 lb 5 oz
7) end of 7th lunar month: surfactant production begins; nails appear; better chance of survival if delivered; length—15 in, weight—2 lb 8 oz
8) end of 8th lunar month: more reflexes present; good chance of survival
9) end of 9th lunar month: well padded with subcutaneous fat; survival same as term
10) end of 10th lunar month: lanugo mostly gone, nails firm, full term
c. Fetal Circulation
1) fetus receives oxygen via placenta (refer to *Nursing Care of the Child* reprints page 620)
2) oxygenated blood enters fetal circulation through umbilical vein of cord to the ductus venosus and liver; ductus venosus attaches to inferior vena cava and allows blood to bypass liver
3) from inferior vena cava, blood flows into right atrium and goes directly on to the left atrium through the foramen ovale
4) blood enters right atrium through superior vena cava, flows to right ventricle, to pulmonary artery (small amount enters lungs for nourishment); the ductus arteriosus shunts blood from pulmonary artery into the aorta, allows bypass of fetal lungs
5) two umbilical arteries return deoxygenated blood from fetus to placenta
d. Amniotic Fluid
1) multiple origins; composition changes in pregnancy (mostly fetal urine at term)
2) appearance: clear, pale, straw colored, with faint characteristic odor; neutral to slightly alkaline (pH 7.0–7.25)
3) approximately 1,000 ml at term; oligohydramnios is less than 500 ml of fluid; polyhydramnios is greater than 1,500 ml of fluid
4) contains albumin, urea, uric acid, creatinine, lecithin, sphingomyelin, bilirubin, epithelial cells, fat, fructose, leukocytes, enzymes, lanugo
5) functions
a) protects fetus from injury
b) separates fetus from fetal membrane
c) serves as excretion-collection system
d) allows fetus freedom of movement
e) helps control fetus's body temperature
f) exchanges at rate of 500 ml/hour (at term)

B. **Overview of Management**
1. Interdisciplinary Health Team: nurses, nurse practitioners, midwives, physicians, social workers, dietitians, and other specialists
2. Schedule of Visits
a. Routine
1) every 4 weeks, up to 32 weeks
2) every 2 weeks from 32–36 weeks
3) every week from 36–40 weeks
b. Initial Visit
1) obtain complete family and obstetric history
a) personal/social characteristics of childbearing family, including cultural patterns, education, economic level, support systems
b) maternal factors affecting course of pregnancy: smoking, use of alcohol and/or drugs, past and current medical problems, activities of daily living, sleep patterns, nutrition, bowel habits

Table 4.3 Naegele's Rule

If first day of last menstrual period was
June 17, 1986
subtract 3 months
+
add 7 days
Estimated date of delivery is March 24, 1987

---

    c) use of family planning measures and health history during pregnancies; history of infertility
    d) attitudes toward present pregnancy
    e) history of preceding pregnancies and perinatal outcomes (TPAL)
- T: number of term births
- P: number of premature births
- A: number of abortions (spontaneous or induced)
- L: number of living children
- *gravida*: all pregnancies regardless of duration or outcome, including present pregnancy
- *parity*: past pregnancies resulting in viable fetus, whether born dead or alive (twins considered as one)

    f) past personal and family medical history

2) calculate expected date of delivery (confinement) (EDC) using Naegele's rule: count back three calendar months from the 1st day of the last menstrual period (LMP) and add seven days (see table 4.3)

c. Initial and Subsequent Visits
  1) assess vital signs and blood pressure
    a) BP: BP 90–140/60–90; upper limits of increase: 10/15 mm Hg systolic/diastolic above normal baseline
    b) pulse: 60–90/minute
    c) respiration: 16–24/minute
    d) temperature: 36.2°–37.6°C (97°–100°F)
  2) check urine for albumin and glucose: ideally negative and not more than 1+ sugar

3) monitor weight gain: a total gain of 20–30 lb is recommended
    a) 2–4 lb in the 1st trimester
    b) 11–14 lb in the 2nd trimester
    c) 8–11 lb in the 3rd trimester
4) assess changes in fetal development over duration of pregnancy (40 weeks or 280 days)
    a) fetal heart rate
    b) abdominal palpation
    c) fundal height
5) allow time for client to express perceived problems or complaints

C. **Application of the Nursing Process to Normal Childbearing, Antepartal Care**
1. **Assessment**
  a. Refer to "Initial Visit," this page
  b. Refer to "Initial and Subsequent Visits," this page
2. **Goals, Plans/Implementation, and Evaluation**

Goal 1: The pregnant woman and fetus will maintain optimal well-being through preventive health measures and regular antepartal/prenatal care.
Plan/Implementation
- measure vital signs, including temperature, blood pressure, pulse, respiration, height and weight
- assist with physical examination and bimanual pelvic examination
  - prepare and arrange necessary equipment (gloves, lubricant, vaginal speculum, pelvimeter, materials for Pap smear, light)
  - prepare client for procedure by providing explanation, instructing her to empty bladder, and placing her in lithotomy position
  - provide emotional support and maintain comfort of client during examination

---

Table 4.4 McDonald's Rule

Height of fundus (in cm)
- × 2/7 = duration of pregnancy in *lunar months*
- × 8/7 = duration of pregnancy in *weeks*

- measure fundal height using McDonald's rule (in 2nd and 3rd trimesters): place tape measure at notch of the symphysis pubis and measure up over fundus
  - height of fundus (cm) x 2/7 = duration of pregnancy in lunar months
    height of fundus (cm) x 8/7 = duration of pregnancy in weeks
- estimate fetal weight (EFW): rump-to-crown length in utero in cm x 100 = EFW in gm
- check for fetal heart beat, detectable as early as 16th week with fetoscope, and by 10-12 weeks with Doppler device
- assist in obtaining samples for laboratory studies
  - clean catch urine for urinalysis, albumin, and glucose
  - blood for hemoglobin, hematocrit, type, Rh, rubella titer (greater than 1:8 of immunity present)
  - standard tests for sexually transmitted diseases (syphilis, gonorrhea, herpes)
- encourage regular antepartal care
  - explain need for continuity
  - describe "danger signals" (e.g., vaginal bleeding, dizziness or visual spots, swelling of face or fingers, epigastric pain, physical trauma) and need for immediate medical care
- provide anticipatory guidance re rest and exercise, personal hygiene, sexual activity, dental care, substance abuse
  - tell client to expect an increased need for sleep during entire pregnancy; exact sleep needs vary among individuals (average 8 hours/day); plan rest times during day
  - teach relaxation methods in preparing for sleep
  - advise to continue usual exercise regimen; avoid introduction of strenuous sports
  - client may continue to work except if exposed to toxic chemicals, radiation, biologic or safety hazards (if job requires sitting for long period of time, encourage frequent movement)
  - maintain skin care; daily baths if desired (caution re transfer into and out of bathtub); avoid soap on nipples; towel-dry breasts
  - be aware that changes in sexual desire and response may occur, related to discomforts or anxieties of pregnancy; encourage couple to verbalize their concerns about sexual activity
  - counsel couple on alternative coital positions and other methods of satisfying sexual needs; coitus may be continued unless premature labor, rupture of membranes, or bleeding occur
  - know that hypertrophy and tenderness of gums is a common problem; encourage dental checkup early in pregnancy and delay extensive dental work and x-ray examinations when possible
  - recommend wearing comfortable, nonrestricting maternity clothing and low-heeled, supportive shoes
  - advise client to stop or reduce cigarette consumption; maternal smoking is associated with a decrease in birth weight of infants
  - know that alcohol, even in minimal-to-moderate amounts, may be harmful to fetus; advise client to avoid alcohol consumption during pregnancy
  - advise client to avoid medication, particularly in the 1st trimester (over-the-counter and prescription drugs may cross placental barrier); physicians must weigh advantages versus risks of medications for individual clients
  - know that attenuated, live vaccines are contraindicated for immunization

Evaluation: The pregnant woman receives initial and regular follow-up antepartal care to prevent/detect any early complications; avoids substances that may potentially harm the fetus. The fetus maintains a growth and development pattern appropriate for gestational age as evidenced by maternal weight gain, fundal height, activity level, and other antenatal screening techniques; is protected from environmental hazards and stresses (e.g., alcohol, nicotine).

Goal 2: The pregnant woman will be advised of common discomforts of pregnancy and how to relieve them.

Plan/Implementation
- *morning sickness*: eat dry crackers or toast before slowly arising; eat small frequent meals; avoid greasy, highly seasoned food
- *breast tenderness*: wear a well-fitted, supportive bra with wide, adjustable straps
- *heartburn and indigestion*: avoid overeating, ingesting fatty or fried food; take small, frequent meals; avoid taking sodium bicarbonate
- *backache*: maintain proper body alignment (pelvic tilt) and use good body mechanics; use maternity girdle in selected situations; wear comfortable shoes; use proper mattress; rest frequently; do pelvic-rock exercise
- *leg cramps*: stretch involved muscles (extension of leg with dorsiflexion of the foot); may be related to alterations in calcium, phosphorus
- *varicose veins*: elevate legs frequently when sitting or lying down in bed; avoid sitting or standing for prolonged periods of time or crossing legs at the knees; do not wear tight or constricting hosiery or garters; physician may suggest wearing supportive hose from morning to night
- *hemorrhoids*: apply warm compresses; upon recommendation of physician, reinsert hemorrhoids (place client in a side-lying or knee-chest position; use gentle pressure and a lubricant), avoid constipation; take sitz baths
- *constipation*: increase fluid intake (to 6–8 glasses/day), roughage; develop good daily bowel movement habits, exercise
- *urinary frequency*: regular emptying of bladder; report any burning, cloudiness, blood in urine, or dysuria
- *ankle edema*: change position, lie on left side; report any edema in face and in hands; rest with legs and hips elevated
- *uterine contractions* (Braxton Hicks'): normal during pregnancy; report if they progressively increase and are accompanied by signs of labor
- *faintness*: avoid staying in one position over a long period of time; get out of bed from a lateral position, rising on elbow and hand (supine hypotension)
- *shortness of breath*: use proper posture when erect; sleep with head elevated by several pillows

Evaluation: The pregnant woman identifies own basic discomforts of pregnancy and appropriately relieves them.

Goal 3: The pregnant woman will have adequate knowledge of nutrition to meet her own developmental needs, the physical requirements of pregnancy and lactation, and fetal growth and development.

Plan/Implementation
- obtain complete dietary history
  - prepregnant nutritional intake and status (i.e., over/underweight, anemic)
  - dietary habits: pica, use of junk foods, regularity of meals, peer pressure
  - knowledge of nutritional needs, basic four food groups
  - socioeconomic status: lack of finances for a balanced diet; customs and special beliefs
  - physical symptoms possibly indicative of poor nutrition (e.g., dry scaly skin, lack of skin turgor, fatigue)
- consider mother's age, present weight, routine activity, developmental needs, and cultural dietary patterns as basis for teaching
- assess client's knowledge of basic four food groups and recommended dietary allowances for pregnant women; teach good nutritional practices; see tables 4.5 and 4.6
  - discuss well-balanced diet including basic four groups as adapted during pregnancy
  - additional calories, protein, and calcium will be recommended for pregnant adolescents
  - a minimum fluid intake of 6–8 glasses of water/day is recommended
  - discuss possible vitamin and mineral supplements (e.g., iron, folic acid)
  - monitor weight gain each antepartal visit; a total weight gain of 20–30 lb is usually recommended
  - recognize when restrictions in calories and salt may be indicated (e.g., situation of high-risk childbearing)
  - refer to nutritionist for intensive teaching/counseling

Evaluation: The pregnant woman can identify the basic four food groups and their components; knows the number of calories needed each day; states she will

Table 4.5 Recommended Dietary Allowances for Females Aged 11-50*

Nutrients	Non-pregnant Girls and Women (Age in Years) (Mean Weight in Lbs.)				Pregnant Women	Lactating Women
	11-14 (101)	15-18 (120)	19-22 (120)	23-50 (120)		
Energy (kcal) (mean)	2,200	2,100	2,100	2,000	+300	+500
Protein (gm)	46	46	44	44	+ 30	+ 20
Vitamin A (mcg)	800	800	800	800	+200	+400
Vitamin D (mcg)	10	10	7.5	5	+ 5	+ 5
Vitamin E (mg)	8	8	8	8	+ 2	+ 3
Vitamin C (mg)	50	60	60	60	+ 20	+ 40
Thiamin (mg)	1.1	1.1	1.1	1.0	+ 0.4	+ 0.5
Riboflavin (mg)	1.3	1.3	1.3	1.2	+ 0.3	+ 0.5
Niacin (mg)	15	14	14	13	+ 2	+ 5
Vitamin B_6 (mg)	1.8	2.0	2.0	2.0	+ 0.6	+ 0.5
Folacin (mcg)	400	400	400	3	+400	+100
Vitamin B_{12} (mcg)	3	3	3	800	+ 1	+ 1
Calcium (mg)	1,200	1,200	800	800	+400	+400
Phosphorus (mg)	1,200	1,200	800	300	+400	+400
Magnesium (mg)	300	300	300	18	+150	+150
Iron (mg)	18	18	18	15	Suppl†	†
Zinc (mg)	15	15	15	150	+ 5	+ 10
Iodine (mg)	150	150	150		+ 25	+ 50

*From the Committee on Dietary Allowances, Food and Nutrition Board, Division of Biological Sciences. Assembly of Life Sciences, National Research Council, *Recommended Dietary Allowances*, 9th rev. ed. Washington, D.C.: National Academy of Sciences, 1980.
† Recommendation: Iron supplement of 30-60 mg during pregnancy and for 2-3 mc postpartum. Iron needs during lactation do not differ substantially from those of nonpregnant women. The supplement is to replenish stores depleted by pregnancy.

follow balanced diet; gradually and steadily gains between 20 and 30 lb during the pregnancy. Fetus maintains a growth and development pattern appropriate for gestational age.

Goal 4: The pregnant woman and her family will receive educational preparation for childbirth.

Plan/Implementation
- explain the purpose and scope of childbirth education (to decrease fear and anxiety through increasing knowledge and ability to effectively use coping mechanisms, i.e., relaxation techniques, concentration, breathing exercises)
- discuss various methods, e.g., Lamaze, Read, Bradley, Le Boyer (Lamaze differs from other methods in use of conditioned responses)
- offer direct instructions or referral to appropriate resources (e.g., International Childbirth Education Association)

Evaluation: Childbearing family expresses a positive attitude toward pregnancy and is adequately prepared for birth experience; members are able to openly express their needs and provide emotional support to each other; begin role transition to parenthood.

D. High-Risk Childbearing
1. Definition: any existing or developing condition or factor that prevents or impedes the normal progress of pregnancy to the delivery of a viable, healthy, term infant.
2. Assessment of Risk Factors (some that already exist cannot be altered)

Table 4.6   Pregnant Woman's Daily Food Intake

Food Group	Recommended Daily Amount
Dairy products	Three to four 8-oz cups
Meat group	Two 3-4 oz servings; 1 egg
Grain products, whole grain or enriched	4-5 servings
Fruits/fruit juices	3-4 servings; include 4 oz of orange or grapefruit juice
Vegetables/vegetable juices	3-4 servings (1 or 2 servings raw; 1 serving of dark green or deep yellow)
Fluids	4-6 glasses (8 oz) water plus other fluids to equal 8-10 cups/day

SOURCE: Olds, S. et al. *Obstetric Nursing.* Menlo Park, CA: Addison-Wesley, 1984

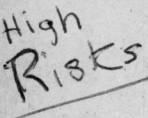
High Risks

a. <u>Age</u>: under 17 or over 35
   1) pregnant adolescents: have a higher incidence of prematurity, pregnancy-induced hypertension, cephalopelvic disproportion, poor nutrition, and poor antepartal care
   2) women over 35: have an increased risk of chromosomal disorders in infants (e.g., Down's syndrome), pregnancy-induced hypertension, and cesarean delivery
b. <u>Parity</u>
   1) multiparity: two or more pregnancies
   2) grand multiparity: six or more pregnancies
c. <u>Past Health History</u>
   1) diabetes
   2) heart disease
   3) renal conditions
   4) essential hypertension
   5) anemia
   6) thyroid disorder
d. <u>Past Obstetrical History</u>
   1) abortions: spontaneous or ruptured ectopic pregnancy
   2) premature deliveries or intrauterine-growth retardation
   3) congenital malformations: result of genetic disorders
   4) cesarean births
   5) <u>lack of antepartal care</u> ↑ infant mortality
   6) previous fetal death
   7) pregnancy-induced hypertension, gestational diabetes
   8) maternal vaginal bleeding
   9) isoimmunization
   10) multiple gestation
e. Current Obstetric History
   1) Rh incompatibility
   2) pregnancy-induced hypertension
   3) bleeding
   4) exposure to toxic agents or drugs
   5) infections
      a) sexually transmitted diseases
      b) TORCH syndrome (*T*oxoplasmosis, *O*ther, *R*ubella, *C*ytomegalovirus, *H*erpes)
      c) other viral or bacterial diseases
   6) multiple gestation
   7) abnormal presentation
   8) premature rupture of membranes
   9) diabetes or cardiac disease
   10) other medical problems
   11) abnormal antenatal test results (e.g., amniotic-fluid analysis)
f. Socioeconomic-Cultural Status
   1) low socioeconomic status: often associated with
      a) inadequate nutrition
      b) lack of general knowledge about health care needs
      c) inability to detect problems during pregnancy
   2) Asian and black women have higher incidence of small-for-gestational-age babies
g. Malnutrition or Deprivation: less than 4 kg weight gain by 30th week of gestation
h. Drug or Alcoholic Addiction: associated with congenital anomalies, intrauterine-growth retardation, and numerous other problems

i. Smoking: associated with low-birth-weight infants
j. Frequent, Repeated Pregnancies: with spacing 2-3 months between birth and conception

3. Diagnostic Tests
   a. Daily Fetal Movement Count (DFMC)
      1) definition: periodic recording of fetal movements to assess active and passive fetal states in normal pregnancies, as well as in those with complications
      2) procedure: a noninvasive test that may be done directly by pregnant woman
      3) interpretation
         a) normally 3 or more movements felt in an hour when lying down, although fetal states normally vary (cyclic periods of rest and activity)
         b) marked decrease in fetal activity (unrelated to sleep) of 2 or less movements/hour should be reported and NST may be scheduled
   b. Nonstress Testing (NST)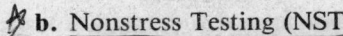
      1) definition: observation of fetal heart rate (FHR) associated with fetal movement; accelerations are a predictor of fetal well-being
      2) procedure
         a) requires external electronic monitoring (indirect) using ultrasound transducer to measure FHR and tokodynamometer to trace fetal activity and/or spontaneous uterine activity
         b) pregnant woman placed in semi-Fowler's position, may be turned slightly to the left
         c) maternal BP recorded initially
         d) requires 30-50 minutes to administer test (10- to 12-minute tracing obtained)
         e) performed in an ambulatory setting or in the hospital obstetrical unit by nurse trained in test administration
      3) interpretation
         a) reactive (normal): 2 FHR accelerations (greater than 15 bpm) above baseline—lasting 15 seconds or more—occur with fetal movement in a 10- to 20-minute period
         b) nonreactive (abnormal): none or one FHR acceleration (greater than 15 bpm) above baseline—

Table 4.7 Laboratory Studies of Fetal Well-Being

Study	Purpose/Indication	Interpretation
Urinary/serum estriol	Assess placental functioning	Sudden drop = fetal hypoxia
		Continuous low levels = fetal compromise
Amniotic fluid analysis	Chromosomal studies	Detection of genetic disorders
	Determination of sex chromatin	Detection of sex-linked disorders
	Biochemical analysis of fetal cell enzymes	Detection of inborn errors of metabolism
	Fetal lung maturity (lecithin/sphingomyelin ratios)	L/S ratio of 2:1 or greater = fetal lung maturity
	Alpha-fetoprotein (AFP) levels	High levels = neural-tube defects
	Creatinine levels	2.0 mg = fetal age greater than 36 weeks
	Identification and evaluation of Rh incompatibility	Increased bilirubin = evaluate for intrauterine transfusion and/or delivery
	Lipid cells (Nile blue stain)	20% cells stained orange = fetal weight at least 2,500 gm
	Meconium presence	Fetal hypoxia (except with breech presentation)

lasting 15 seconds or more—occurs with fetal movement in a 10-minute period, or accelerations less than 15 bpm or lasting less than 15 seconds; a nonreactive test indicates the need for additional evaluation using OCT (Oxytocin Challenge Test)
- c) unsatisfactory result: uninterpretable FHR or fetal activity recording; test repeated in 24 hours or OCT done

c. Oxytocin Challenge Test (OCT) or Contraction Stress Test:
1) definition: the response of the fetus (i.e., FHR pattern) to induced uterine contractions is observed as an indicator of uteroplacental and fetal physiologic integrity
2) indications: pregnancies at risk for placental insufficiency or fetal compromise
3) procedure
   a) requires external electronic monitoring (indirect) using ultrasound transducer to measure FHR and tokodynamometer to trace uterine activity
   b) pregnant woman placed in position for NST (see above)
   c) maternal blood pressure recorded initially and at intervals during test
   d) requires 60 minutes to 3 hours to administer
   e) performed on an outpatient basis in or near the labor and delivery unit
   f) increasing doses of oxytocin are administered as a dilute intravenous infusion according to hospital protocol or physician's orders until uterine contractions occur
4) interpretation
   a) negative (normal): the absence of late decelerations of FHR with each of three contractions during a 10-minute interval; known as "negative window"
   b) positive (abnormal): the presence of late decelerations of FHR with three contractions during a 10-minute interval; known as "positive window"
   c) equivocal or suspicious: the absence of a positive or negative window, i.e., criterion of three contractions in a 10-minute interval is not achieved
   d) unsatisfactory tests occur when interpretable tracings are not obtained or adequate uterine contractions are not achieved
   e) high-risk pregnancies are usually allowed to continue if a negative OCT is obtained; test is repeated weekly for these clients

d. Ultrasonography
1) definition: a noninvasive procedure involving the passage of high-frequency sound waves through the uterus in order to obtain an outline of the fetus, placenta, uterine cavity, or any other area under examination
2) purposes
   a) early diagnosis of pregnancy
   b) determination of fetal viability
   c) placental localization
   d) confirmation of fetal death
   e) estimation of fetal age through measurement of the biparietal diameter of the fetal head; most accurate at 16-18 weeks
   f) detection of fetal abnormalities
   g) monitoring fetal growth
   h) identification of multiple gestation
3) procedure
   a) advise pregnant woman to consume one quart of water 2 hours prior to procedure and avoid emptying bladder; scanning is done when the bladder is full (exception: prior to amniocentesis)
   b) transmission gel spread over maternal abdomen
   c) sonographer scans vertically and horizontally in sections across abdomen
4) possible risk: none known *Not sure*

e. Amniocentesis
1) definition: an invasive procedure for amniotic fluid analysis to assess fetal health and maturity; done from the 14th week of gestation
2) procedure
   a) pregnant woman must empty bladder before procedure, if greater than 20 weeks gestation

b) ultrasonography is first performed to locate the placenta
  c) baseline vital signs and FHR are assessed; monitor every 15 minutes
  d) pregnant woman is placed in supine position and given an abdominal prep
  e) a needle is passed through the abdominal and uterine walls into the amniotic sac and a small amount of amniotic fluid is withdrawn
 3) possible risks: overall less than 1%
  a) maternal: hemorrhage, infection, Rh isoimmunization, abruptio placentae, labor
  b) fetal: death, infection, hemorrhage, abortion, premature labor, injury from needle
 4) instruct client to report any side effects (e.g., unusual fetal activity, vaginal discharge, uterine contractions, fever, or chills)
f. Fetal Blood Sampling
 1) definition: a small volume of fetal blood is taken (from a small puncture into the fetal scalp) to assess fetal hypoxia during labor
 2) procedure
  a) an invasive technique requiring rupture of the fetal membranes and cervical dilation (3–4 cm); performed when fetus is in jeopardy
  b) pregnant woman generally placed in a lithotomy position
  c) an amnioscope (plastic or metal truncated cone) is employed for visualization of presenting part of fetus during the procedure
  d) electronic fetal monitoring is desirable during the procedure
  e) after procedure, observe for vaginal bleeding (of fetal origin) and fetal tachycardia
 3) laboratory analysis of fetal pH, Po_2, and Pco_2 is done from blood sample (normal pH: 7.25–7.35; pH of 7.20 is associated with hypoxia)
g. Laboratory Studies
 1) urinary or serum estriol determination: to assess placental functioning
  a) steroid precursor produced by the adrenals of the fetus is synthesized into estriols in the placenta and is excreted by the maternal kidneys; mother's levels normally rise during pregnancy
  b) serial estriol determinations are obtained with repeat blood samples or 24-hour urine collections after 20th week of gestation (preferably after 32 weeks)
  c) a sudden drop in estriol level is associated with fetal hypoxia; continuous low levels associated with compromise of fetus
 2) analysis of amniotic fluid: purposes include
  a) chromosomal studies to assess genetic disorders (e.g., Down's syndrome, cell culture for karyotype)
  b) determination of sex chromatin in fetal cells to assess sex-linked disorders
  c) biochemical analysis of fetal-cell enzymes to assess inborn errors of metabolism
  d) determination of lecithin to sphingomyelin ratios (L/S ratios) to assess fetal lung maturity
   • lecithin and sphingomyelin are important components of surfactant, a phosphoprotein that lowers surface tension in the fetal lungs and facilitates extrauterine expiration
   • an L/S ratio of 2:1 or greater is generally associated with fetal lung maturity except for selected high-risk neonates (e.g., infants of diabetic mothers)
  e) determination of alpha-fetoprotein (AFP) levels to assess neural-tube defects such as anencephaly and spina bifida; high levels also associated with congenital nephrosis, esophageal atresia, fetal demise
  f) determination of creatinine level: 2.0 mg or greater suggests fetal age greater than 36 weeks
  g) identification and evaluation of isoimmune disease; usually done

Post op – ABORT. emotional support

after 24th week to assess bilirubin levels and optical density
h) determination of lipid cells (Nile blue stain); if more than 20% of cells stain orange, fetus weighs at least 2,500 gm
i) identification of meconium (often indicative of fetal hypoxia)

E. **Application of the Nursing Process to High-Risk Childbearing**
1. Assessment
   a. Risk Factors
   b. Results of Diagnostic Tests
2. Goal, Plan/Implementation, and Evaluation
   Goal: The pregnant woman and partner will learn about symptoms (danger signals) of high-risk conditions to be reported immediately.
   Plan/Implementation
   - teach woman/partner to immediately report any of the following danger signals
     - vaginal bleeding
     - generalized edema
     - infection
     - trauma
     - leaking amniotic fluid
     - elevated temperature
     - headache
     - visual changes, i.e., spotting before eyes
     - abdominal, epigastric pain
     - projectile vomiting
     - decreased fetal activity
   - reinforce the importance of keeping appointments as scheduled and of complying with therapeutic regimen
   - at each visit, assess client for above danger signals
   Evaluation: The pregnant woman or partner reports danger signals immediately upon detection; she seeks regular care to minimize problems related to high-risk conditions.

Selected Health Problems in the Antepartal Period

A. Abortion
1. **General Information**
   a. Definition: one of the bleeding disorders of pregnancy, it is termination of pregnancy before viability (less than 20 weeks gestation or less than 500 gm fetus) as a result of elective procedures or reproductive failure. Approximately 75% of all spontaneous abortions occur during the 2nd or 3rd month of gestation.
   b. Types
      1) *therapeutic* (or induced): pregnancy that has been purposefully terminated
      2) *spontaneous:* natural termination of pregnancy without therapeutic intervention
      3) *threatened:* possible loss of the products of conception
      4) *inevitable:* threatened loss of the products of conception that cannot be prevented or stopped
      5) *incomplete:* the expulsion of part of the products of conception and the retention of other parts in utero *(D&C)*
      6) *complete:* the expulsion of all the products of conception
      7) *missed:* retention of the products of conception in utero after the fetus dies
      8) *habitual:* spontaneous abortion in 3 or more successive pregnancies
   c. Predisposing Factors (Spontaneous Abortion): often unknown (20%-25%), may be associated with
      1) embryonic/fetal problems (50%-60%): disorganization of germ plasma, ovular defects, chromosomal aberration, faulty placental development
      2) maternal problems (15%-20%): systemic infections, severe nutritional deprivation, abnormal pathologic conditions of the reproductive tract, endocrine dysfunction, trauma, medical diseases
2. **Nursing Process**
   a. Assessment
      1) identify symptoms (spontaneous vaginal bleeding, uterine cramping, contractions)
      2) evaluate blood loss: save pads; assess saturation, frequency of change
      3) recognize signs and symptoms of shock (e.g., rapid, thready pulse; pallor; decreased BP; restlessness; clammy skin)
   b. Goal, Plan/Implementation, and Evaluation

Nontherapeutic when saying can become preg. again

ANTEPARTAL CARE

Goal: The pregnant woman will be monitored and treated for signs of developing complications.

Plan/Implementation
- note and record blood and tissue loss
- institute nursing measures to treat shock if necessary
- monitor I&O
- replace fluids as ordered
- prepare for dilatation and curettage as necessary (incomplete abortion)
- provide emotional support of grieving process (refer to *The Client with Psychosocial Problems* page 28)

Evaluation: Client is free from preventable complications (e.g., excessive blood loss, fluid imbalance, infection).

B. Incompetent Cervical Os

1. **General Information**
   a. Definition: mechanical defect in the cervix, often a cause of habitual 2nd trimester abortions or preterm labor
   b. Predisposing Factors: anatomical deviation of the cervix
   c. Medical Treatment: surgical intervention such as suturing of cervix during the 14th–18th weeks of gestation
      1) permanent suture (Shirodkar procedure); subsequent delivery will be by cesarean section
      2) temporary purse string (McDonald procedure); delivery will be vaginal

2. **Nursing Process**
   a. Assessment
      1) history of miscarriages/abortions
      2) relaxed cervical os on pelvic examination
   b. Goal, Plan/Implementation, and Evaluation

Goal: The pregnant woman with an incompetent cervical os will be identified and treated; will maintain gestation to term.

Plan/Implementation (Post-op)
- suggest limited activity for 2 or more weeks following this procedure
- tell client to report signs of labor
- monitor fetal growth to term and continue routine prenatal assessment and care
- observe for signs of labor, infection, and premature rupture of the membranes

Evaluation: Client complies with activity restrictions; carries fetus to term.

C. Ectopic Pregnancy

1. **General Information**
   a. Definition: an extrauterine pregnancy, implantation occurring most often in ampulla of the fallopian tubes
   b. Incidence: 1 in 80 to 1 in 200 live births, 7th cause of maternal mortality (from rupture of tube leading to hemorrhage, infection, and shock)

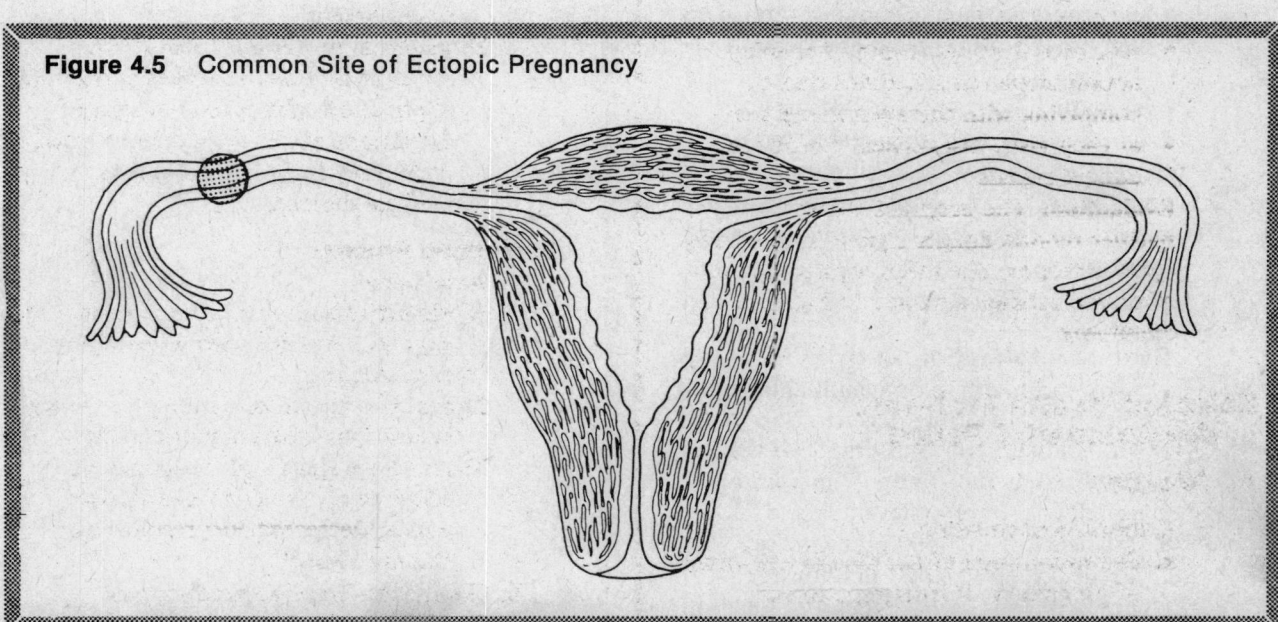

Figure 4.5 Common Site of Ectopic Pregnancy

c. Predisposing Factors: any condition that causes constriction of the fallopian tube (e.g., pelvic inflammatory disease, puerperal and postabortion sepsis, developmental defects, prolonged use of an IUD)
d. Medical Treatment: diagnosis, ultrasound, surgical intervention (laparoscopy, laparotomy with salpingectomy)

2. Nursing Process
    a. Assessment
        1) signs and symptoms
            a) lower abdominal pain related to stretching of the tube
            b) knifelike pain in lower quadrant (only when tube has ruptured)
            c) profound shock, if ruptured
            d) vaginal spotting
        2) history: last menstrual period
        3) prior history of infection, IUD use
    b. Goal, Plan/Implementation, and Evaluation

    Goal: Client will be monitored to detect early signs of complications; will return to a homeostatic state.
    Plan/Implementation
    - monitor vital signs; carry out an ongoing assessment for shock
    - maintain intravenous infusion for administration of plasma/blood, antibiotics, or other required medication
    - prepare client for surgery, physically and emotionally
    - post-op, continue to monitor vital signs, I&O; have client cough and deep breathe q2h

    Evaluation: The pregnant woman has diagnosis confirmed and treated before rupture of tube (or other site); post-operatively, regains homeostasis (vital signs stabilized, I&O adequate, no indication of infection).

D. Hydatidiform Mole
    1. General Information
        a. Definition: a developmental anomaly of the chorion causing degeneration of the villi and formation of grapelike vesicles; fertilized ovum is initially present but usually no embryo develops
        b. Incidence: 1 in 1,500 pregnancies
        c. Predisposing Factors: unknown; however, it is associated with induction of ovulation by clomiphene therapy and increased maternal age
        d. Medical Treatment
            1) surgical intervention (D&C or, if malignant, hysterectomy)
            2) medical intervention: chemotherapy, if indicated
            3) close supervision for one year

    2. Nursing Process
        a. Assessment
            1) signs and symptoms
                a) initially appears as a normal pregnancy
                b) uterus larger than expected for reported gestational age
                c) lower uterine segment soft and full upon palpation
                d) excessive nausea and vomiting (hyperemesis gravidarum)
                e) brownish discharge or vaginal spotting; onset around 12th week of gestation
                f) hypertension and other symptoms of preeclampsia (e.g., proteinuria)
            2) pregnancy test: HCG often very high
        b. Goal, Plan/Implementation, and Evaluation

    Goal: The pregnant woman will have hydatidiform mole removed without

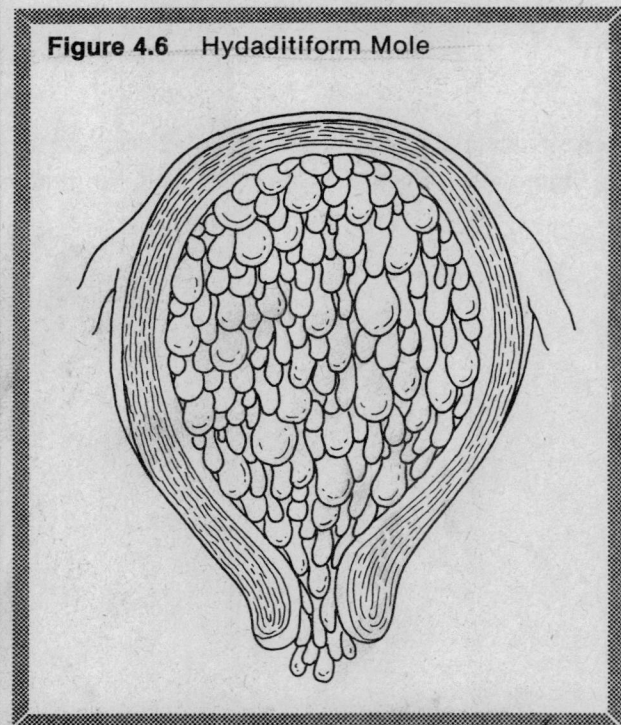

Figure 4.6 Hydaditiform Mole

complications and will obtain close supervision for one year to detect signs of choriocarcinoma; will delay pregnancy at least one year.

Plan/Implementation
- administer plasma/blood replacement as ordered
- maintain fluid and electrolyte balance through replacement
- follow-up supervision for 1 year includes HCG measurement, examination to detect choriocarcinoma, chemotherapy if indicated; emphasize importance of regular visits to physician
- provide emotional support

Evaluation: Client has had hydatidiform mole removed and complies with regular schedule of visits following therapy; knows to avoid pregnancy until cleared by physician.

E. Placenta Previa

1. **General Information**
   a. Definition: abnormal implantation of placenta in lower uterine segment
   b. Incidence: 1 in 170 pregnancies; most common cause of bleeding in late pregnancy
   c. Predisposing Factors: decreased vascularity of upper uterine segment; multiparity
   d. Degrees of Placenta Previa
      1) partial: placenta partially covers the internal os
      2) complete: placenta totally covers the cervical os (cesarian birth necessary)
      3) low-lying or marginal: placenta encroaches on margin of internal os
   e. Placental Abnormalities (in Formation or Implantation): associated with maternal bleeding during the 3rd trimester or intrapartum period; hemorrhage is the leading cause of maternal mortality
   f. Medical Intervention: diagnosis; blood and fluid replacement and cesarian birth if placental placement prevents vaginal birth of fetus

    ultrasound used to determine placement of and contents

2. **Nursing Process**
   a. Assessment
      1) signs and symptoms
         a) painless, bright red, vaginal bleeding; often begins in 7th month of pregnancy; usually early episodes have small amount of bleeding and are rarely fatal; several episodes of bleeding may occur
         b) soft uterus
         c) manifestations of hemorrhage, shock
      2) diagnosis is confirmed by ultrasound

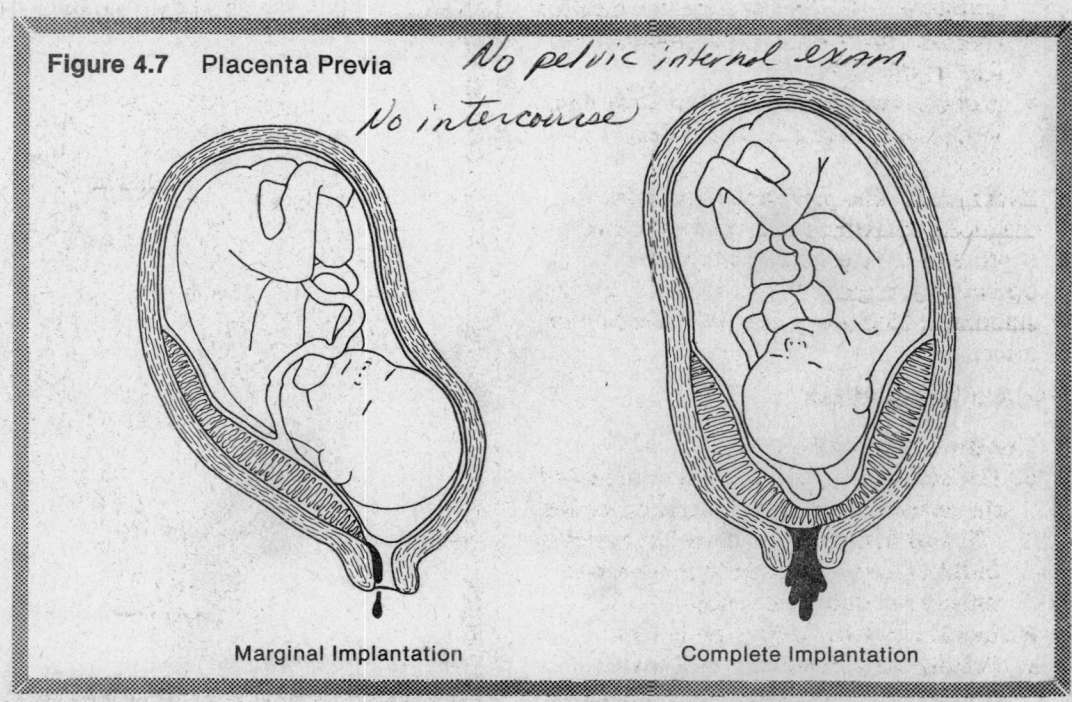

Figure 4.7 Placenta Previa

No pelvic internal exam
No intercourse

Marginal Implantation   Complete Implantation

b. Goal, Plan/Implementation, and Evaluation

Goal: The pregnant woman will be monitored for indications of abnormal placental implantation; will be prepared for surgery (if necessary).

Plan/Implementation
- maintain bed rest, avoid vaginal examinations, and observe carefully (conservative management)
- continuously assess quality and nature of blood loss
- monitor maternal vital signs
- evaluate FHR
- institute appropriate nursing measures if shock develops (i.e., administer fluids, transfusions)
- give physical and emotional preparation for possible cesarean birth; physician may perform "double setup"
- observe for associated problems (e.g., prematurity of newborn, DIC)

Evaluation: Client is free from frank hemorrhage; client and partner are adequately prepared for possible cesarean birth; a healthy newborn is delivered at or near term.

F. Abruptio Placentae

1. General Information
a. Definition: partial or complete separation of normally implanted placenta; also known as accidental hemorrhage or ablatio placentae
b. Incidence: 1 in 80 to 1 in 200 pregnancies
c. Predisposing Factors: pregnancy-induced hypertension, fibrin defects; associated with older multigravidas
d. Types
   1) marginal: evident external bleeding; placenta separates at margin
   2) concealed: bleeding not evident or inconsistent with extent of shock observed; placenta separates at the center
e. Medical Intervention: diagnosis; blood and fluids replacement; cesarean birth as necessary to save fetal or maternal lives

2. Nursing Process
a. **Assessment:** signs and symptoms
   1) bleeding: 3rd trimester, amount of bleeding is not an accurate indicator of degree of separation
   2) severe abdominal pain
   3) rigid distended uterus
   4) enlarged uterus
   5) shock
   6) associated problems, e.g., renal failure, hypofibrinogenemia
b. Goal, Plan/Implementation, and Evaluation

Goal: The pregnant woman will be monitored for increasing signs of placental

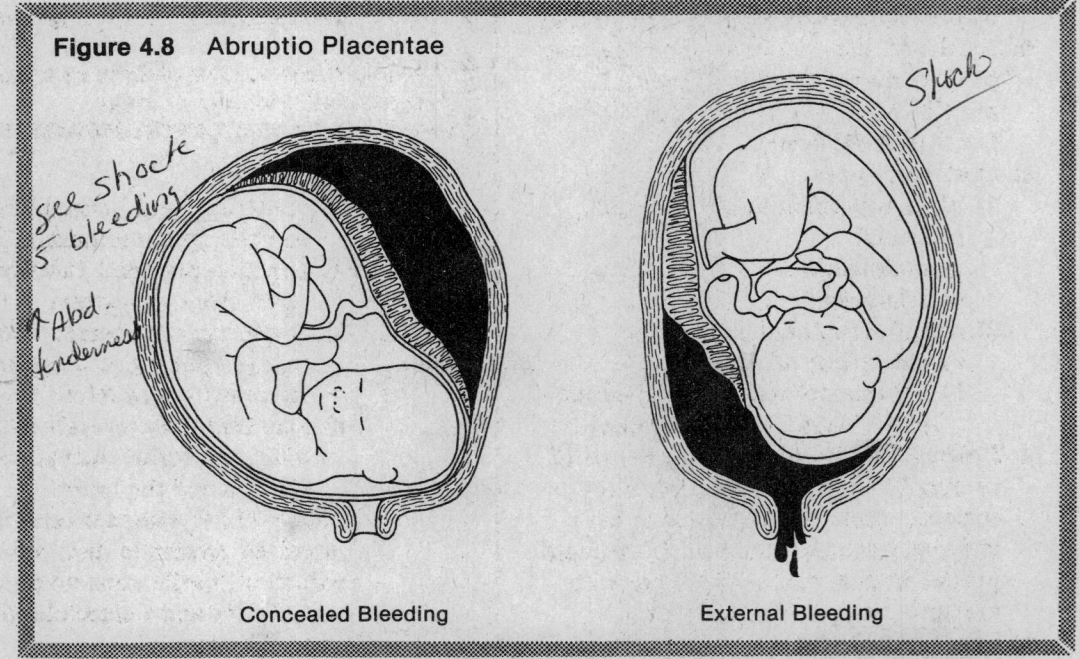

Figure 4.8 Abruptio Placentae

Concealed Bleeding   External Bleeding

separation; will be prepared for emergency surgery or vaginal delivery as indicated; fetal hypoxia will be prevented or minimized; a live infant will be delivered.
Plan/Implementation
- maintain bed rest
- monitor FHR and maternal vital signs
- assess blood loss and uterine pain
- administer blood replacement as ordered by physician
- if shock present, institute nursing measures (e.g., flat in bed, monitor vital signs frequently, keep warm, increase IV fluids)
- provide emotional support; explain what is happening and all procedures; encourage to express feelings, ask questions
- prepare for emergency cesarean birth or prompt delivery
- observe for associated problems after delivery, e.g., DIC, poorly contracted uterus, fetal neonatal hypoxia

Evaluation: The pregnant woman delivers a healthy infant; blood loss is controlled; receives blood and fluid replacement; receives preoperative preparation.

G. Pregnancy-Induced Hypertension (Hypertensive Disorders)

1. **General Information**
   a. Definition: a group of disorders characterized by presence of hypertension, with onset during last 10 weeks of pregnancy or in preceding pregnancy
   b. Incidence: 6%–7% of all gravidae; one of three major causes of maternal mortality and a significant cause of fetal/neonatal deaths
   c. Common Types
      1) pregnancy-induced hypertension (toxemia)
         a) preeclampsia
         b) eclampsia
      2) chronic essential hypertension
         a) antecedent to pregnancy
         b) with superimposed preeclampsia (coincidental with pregnancy)
   d. Predisposing Factors: age (less than 17 or over 35 years), primiparity, low socioeconomic class, absence of early and regular antepartal care, inadequate protein intake, diabetes, mother with previous history of hypertension
   e. Etiology: unknown

Table 4.8 Classification of Eclampsia

Preeclampsia

Mild

Elevated BP	An increase of 15-30 mm Hg or more above base × 2 at least 6 hr apart
Weight gain	1 lb per week in 3rd trimester
Edema	Generalized, slight
Proteinuria	1 gm/24 hr period (1+)

Severe

All changes associated with mild eclampsia, plus

Elevated BP	160/110 mm Hg or more with client on bed rest × 2, 6 hr apart
Edema	Massive weight gain, swelling, puffiness of face, hands, fingers
Proteinuria	5 gm/24 hr or more (4+)
Oliguria	400 cc or less/24 hr
Other	Severe headache, dizziness, blurred vision, retinal arteriolar spasm, spots before eyes, nausea and vomiting, epigastric pain, irritability

Eclampsia

All changes associated with preeclampsia, plus
Tonic and clonic convulsions or coma
Hypertensive shock or crisis

   1) vasospasm and ischemia believed to be underlying mechanism
   2) impaired placental function may result from vasospasm
   3) development of uteroplacental changes leading to decreased oxygen and nutrition to fetus
   4) may lead to degenerative changes in renal, endocrine, hematologic systems and the brain
   f. Medical Interventions: bed rest, (↓BP) increased protein in diet, possible salt reduction, medications to prevent convulsions and reduce blood pressure, early delivery

2. **Nursing Process**
   a. **Assessment:** symptoms include 3rd trimester onset of hypertension, edema, rapid weight gain, and proteinuria
      1) mild preeclampsia: symptoms generally appear after 24th week of pregnancy
         a) BP elevation: systolic increases 15–30 mm Hg and diastolic increases 10–15 mm Hg over baseline on 2 occasions 6 hours apart (or pressures are over 140/90 mm Hg and below 160/100 mm Hg)
         b) weight gain of more than 1 lb/week in 3rd trimester
         c) edema is present and generalized but not massive; no pulmonary edema
         d) urine protein is less than 1 gm in 24 hours (1+ proteinuria)
         e) urine output is greater than 500 ml in 24 hours
      2) severe preeclampsia
         a) BP rises above 160/110 or has risen 60/30 mm Hg or more above prepregnancy or early pregnancy level
         b) massive generalized or pulmonary edema
         c) urine protein is 5 gm or more per 24 hours
         d) urine output is 500 ml or less in 24 hours
         e) late symptoms include severe headache, dizziness, visual problems (blurred vision, retinal arteriolar spasm), nausea and vomiting; epigastric pain, irritability
         f) the only cure for preeclampsia is delivery of all of the products of conception
      3) eclampsia: diagnosed following the onset of clonic or toxic convulsions or coma in a woman with preeclampsia
   b. **Goals, Plans/Implementation, and Evaluation**

   Goal 1: The pregnant woman will maintain her fetus for as long as possible; blood pressure will be controlled; will be safely delivered of a healthy newborn.

   Plan/Implementation
   - prevent eclampsia by promoting early and regular antepartal care
   - monitor BP, weight, edema, urine, and reflexes (each antepartal visit)
   - provide dietary instruction; client may be asked to reduce sodium intake and maintain nutritional needs (ample protein)
   - instruct to take daily weight at home
   - bed rest, if signs of pregnancy-induced or pre-existing hypertension occur (at home for milder forms of preeclampsia; hospitalization for severe preeclampsia)
   - for the hospitalized client: monitor I&O, BP, weight, urine for protein, FHR
   - monitor administration of magnesium sulfate (anticonvulsant and sedative) if ordered and provide careful assessment for signs of toxicity
     - observe for symptoms of CNS depression (anxiety often first symptom preceding drowsiness, lethargy)
     - count respirations: do not administer drug if less than 12/minute
     - check BP
     - check deep tendon reflexes (1+ or higher)
     - check muscle tone for signs of paralysis
     - measure urinary output (greater than 30 cc/h)
     - keep calcium gluconate (10%) solution at bedside as an immediate antidote
   - administer sedatives, antihypertensives, and anticonvulsants, e.g., phenobarbital, diazepam (Valium), hydralazine (Apresoline), as ordered by physician to control symptoms and to prevent eclampsia and CVAs
   - monitor progress of labor
   - provide emotional support to couple

   Evaluation: The woman maintains her pregnancy as long as possible without compromising self or fetus; is safely delivered of a healthy infant; maternal blood pressure is controlled.

   Goal 2: The pregnant woman will be protected from physical injury, will receive care directed to regain homeostasis.

   Plan/Implementation (if convulsion occurs)
   - maintain patent airway
   - suction to prevent aspiration
   - protect mother from injury

ANTEPARTAL CARE **401**

Table 4.9	Magnesium Sulfate
Description	Anticonvulsant that decreases amount of acetylcholine liberated with nerve impulse, relaxes smooth muscle, reduces cerebral edema, depresses CNS, lowers BP
Uses	To lower seizure threshold in women with severe preeclampsia or eclampsia
Dose	1–4 gm (diluted) IV or 5–10 gm IM
Contraindications	Chronic renal disease
Side Effects	*Maternal:* severe CNS depression, hyporeflexia, flushing, confusion *Fetal:* tachycardia, hypoglycemia, hypocalcemia, hypermagnesemia
Nursing Implications	Monitor for seizures. Monitor for signs of severe CNS depression. Discontinue infusion if respirations fall below 12, if reflexes are severely diminished or hypotonic, if urine output falls below 20–30 ml/hour, or if client becomes lethargic or confused. Monitor FHR. Have calcium gluconate on hand (antagonist).

- note nature, onset, and progression of seizure
- monitor for signs of abruptio placentae
- administer O_2
- monitor FHR
- give medications as ordered

Evaluation: The pregnant woman recovers from convulsion(s) without physical injury; fetal heart rate is within normal limits.

H. Diabetes

1. **General Information**
   a. Definition: an inherited metabolic disorder characterized by a deficiency in insulin production from the beta cells of the islets of Langerhans in the pancreas
   b. Incidence: 1 in 300 pregnancies; the condition may be a concurrent disease in pregnancy or have its first onset during gestation
   c. Predisposing Factors
      1) family history of diabetes
      2) glucosuria
      3) obesity
      4) history of repeated spontaneous abortions or fetal loss (stillbirth)
      5) history of delivery of infants over 10 lb
   d. Classes (White's Classification): according to age at onset and pathologic changes
      1) Class A: gestational diabetes that is first diagnosed in pregnancy, can be controlled by diet, has no insulin requirement
      2) Class B: onset after age 20; duration 0–9 years; no vascular involvement
      3) Class C: onset age 10–19; duration 10–19 years; no vascular involvement
      4) Class D: onset before age 10; duration 20 or more years; calcification present in legs; retinitis
      5) Class E: presence of calcified pelvic vessels
      6) Class F: presence of nephritis
   e. Effects of Diabetes: maternal risk and fetal loss increase as classes change from A to E
      1) effects of maternal diabetes on the fetus/infant
         a) overall perinatal mortality increases when mother has diabetes
         b) as classes change from A to E, increased incidence of ketoacidosis for mother (high risk for fetus)
         c) greater risk (3–4 times) of congenital abnormalities that may result in neonatal death
         d) hypoxia and fetal death more common
         e) infants large-for-gestational-age (classes A, B, C)
         f) neonatal hypoglycemia common as a result of fetal response to hyperglycemia of mother
      2) effects of diabetes on the mother
         a) uteroplacental insufficiency often complicates pregnancy
         b) higher incidence of dystocia

f. Effects of Pregnancy on Diabetes
   1) insulin resistance progressively increases in most pregnant diabetics
   2) blood sugar less easily controlled
   3) insulin shock common
g. Medical Treatment
   1) diagnostic tests
      a) 2-hour postprandial blood sugar (screening test preferred for pregnant woman)
      b) oral glucose tolerance test very sensitive for pregnant diabetic *[late 2nd or early 3rd Trimester]*
         - normal fasting: less than 100 mg/100 ml
         - 1 hour: less than 200 mg/100 ml
         - 2 hours: less than 150 mg/100 ml
         - 3 hours: less than 120 mg/100 ml
      c) fasting blood sugar: normal 80–120 mg/100 ml
   2) surveillance of fetal well-being, i.e., serum or 24-hour estriol determinations, NST, OCT, ultrasound, and amniocentesis; refer to "Diagnostic Tests" in *High-Risk Childbearing* page 391.
   3) early delivery by cesarean birth or induction at 36-37 weeks if evidence of fetal compromise; otherwise, attempt to maintain pregnancy until fetal lungs are mature

2. **Nursing Process**
   a. Assessment
      1) signs and symptoms of hypoglycemia and hyperglycemia (see table 3.36, "Differentiating Hypoglycemia from Ketoacidosis" in *Nursing Care of the Adult*)
      2) indications of hydramnios, preeclampsia, infection
      3) history of large-for-gestational-age (LGA) babies
      4) insulin requirements
   b. Goal, Plan/Implementation, and Evaluation

   Goal: The pregnant woman will adhere to prescribed therapeutic regimen; will carry fetus as close to term as possible in optimal health.
   Plan/Implementation
   - stress importance of ongoing, regular antepartal care
   - assist in performance of diagnostic tests
   - demonstrate accurate urine-testing technique; have client return demonstration
   - educate client regarding nutritional needs: strict adherence to prescribed dietary regimen
   - teach to give own insulin; observe for accuracy and correct as necessary
   - know that insulin dose will be regulated by blood glucose levels, not by urine tests, due to lowered renal threshold
   - recognize and share with client changes in her diabetic state
     - as pregnancy develops, insulin need increases
     - insulin need will decrease postpartum
   - promote good personal hygiene to prevent infection
   - monitor for early signs of infection
   - assure mother that she will be able to breast-feed her infant, if she wishes
   - initiate ophthalmologic referral

   Evaluation: The pregnant woman complies with diet and insulin regimen during pregnancy; complications of diabetes are prevented during pregnancy and the puerperium; pregnancy is carried as close to term as possible; the infant of the diabetic woman is delivered with minimum problems and in satisfactory condition.

I. **Cardiac Disorders** *[More cardiac → more advanced tx of anomalies]*
1. **General Information**
   a. Definition: includes a number of heart diseases/defects, which include both congenital and acquired conditions. In the past, the majority of cardiac disorders during pregnancy were associated with rheumatic heart disease; today, pregnant women with heart disease are seen more frequently because of better care and screening. Refer to *Nursing Care of the Adult*, "Congestive Heart Failure" page 188.
   b. Effects of Pregnancy on Heart Disease: alters heart rate, blood pressure, and volume of cardiac output
   c. Incidence: 0.5%-2% of all pregnant women
   d. Predisposing Factors: syphilis, arteriosclerosis, renal and pulmonary disease, rheumatic fever, congenital defects of the heart, surgical repair of defects

e. Types: New York Heart Association's functional classification system for clients with heart disease (based on client history of past and present disability and uninfluenced by presence or absence of physical signs)
    1) Class 1: no limitation of physical activity; no symptoms of cardiac insufficiency
    2) Class 2: slight limitation of activity; asymptomatic at rest; ordinary activities cause fatigue, palpitations, dyspnea, or angina
    3) Class 3: marked limitation of activities; comfortable at rest; less than ordinary activities cause discomfort
    4) Class 4: unable to perform any physical activity without discomfort; may have symptoms even at rest
f. Prognosis: depends on
    1) functional capacity of heart
    2) likelihood of other complications that further increase cardiac load
    3) quality of health care provided
    4) maternal and fetal risk increases from Classes 1 to 4; risks include
        a) maternal heart failure
        b) spontaneous abortion or premature labor, caused by maternal hypoxia
        c) maternal dysrhythmias
        d) intrauterine-growth retardation
    5) Classes 1 and 2: may carry pregnancy without problems; Classes 3 and 4: physician may consider therapeutic abortion, dependent upon woman's health status and desire
g. Medical Treatment
    1) confirm diagnosis
        a) difficult to differentiate heart disease, because of normal cardiac changes that occur with pregnancy
            - functional systolic murmurs common
            - edema and some dyspnea frequently present in last trimester
            - changes in position of heart suggest cardiac enlargement
        b) criteria for establishment of diagnosis of heart disease
            - continuous diastolic or presystolic heart murmur
            - a loud, harsh systolic murmur, especially if associated with a thrill
            - unequivocal cardiac enlargement
            - severe dysrhythmia
    2) hospitalization: may be necessary 1-4 weeks before delivery
    3) prophylactic antibiotic treatment to prevent subacute bacterial endocarditis
    4) vaginal delivery (method of choice, using regional anesthesia and forceps) *less stressful*

2. **Nursing Process**
    a. Assessment
        1) fetal monitoring and maternal vital signs
        2) adherence to prescribed therapeutic regimen
        3) cardiac and respiratory status
    b. Goal, Plan/Implementation, and Evaluation

    Goal: The pregnant woman will comply with regimen and notify physician of changes; complications of cardiac disease during pregnancy will be prevented; pregnancy will progress to term.

    Plan/Implementation
    - encourage early and regular antepartal care; stress importance of keeping appointments and adhering to regimen
    - promote adequate nutrition; ensure adequate iron intake to prevent anemia
    - stress need for additional rest
        - Classes 1 and 2: some limits on strenuous activity
        - Classes 3 and 4: bed rest with expert medical supervision
        - semi-Fowler's position in bed *lateral side*
    - prevent exposure to persons with upper respiratory tract infections; provide early treatment of URIs
    - continuously observe for changes in condition indicative of congestive heart failure (e.g., rales with cough, decreased ability to carry out household tasks, increased dyspnea on exertion, hemoptysis, tachycardia, progressive edema)
    - administer medications as ordered by physician (e.g., diuretics, digitalis); explain actions, side effects to woman and significant other

- maintain continuous maternal and fetal monitoring during the intrapartum period; advise client to avoid pushing, position in semi-Fowler's
- postpartum, assess for signs of hemorrhage, puerperal infection, thromboembolism, congestive heart failure; avoid giving ergonovine and other oxytocics

Evaluation: The pregnant woman complies with regimen of rest, exercise, and care; complications of cardiac disease during pregnancy and puerperium are prevented; the woman delivers a healthy infant; mother and newborn are free from complications.

J. Anemia

1. General Information
a. Definition: decrease in the oxygen-carrying capacity of the blood
b. Cause: often because of low iron stores and reduced dietary intake
c. Incidence: 20% of all pregnant women; 90% of anemias are caused by iron deficiency; it is the most frequently encountered complication of pregnancy
d. Predisposing Factors: heredity, malnutrition
e. Prognosis: maternal and fetal mortality and morbidity rates are increased; specifically
   1) anemia aggravates existing problems such as cardiac disease during pregnancy
   2) anemic women have increased incidence of abortion, premature labor, infection, pregnancy-induced hypertension, and postpartum hemorrhage
   3) maternal anemia is associated with intrauterine-growth retardation
   4) severe anemia may cause heart failure
f. Types of Disorders
   1) iron deficiency: most common
   2) folic acid deficiency (megaloblastic anemia): less than 3% of all gravidae; caused by poor diet and malabsorption
   3) hemoglobinopathies: e.g., sickle cell anemia (refer to *Nursing Care of the Child* page 548), thalassemia

2. Nursing Process
a. Assessment
   1) signs and symptoms are usually absent in mild to moderate iron-deficiency anemia
   2) diagnosis based upon
      a) Hgb less than 11 gm/100 ml or HCT less than 37%
      b) Hgb less than 10.5 gm/100 ml or HCT less than 35% in 2nd trimester
      c) Hgb less than 10 gm/100 ml or HCT less than 33% in 3rd trimester
   3) nutritional intake
b. Goal, Plan/Implementation, and Evaluation

Goal: The pregnant woman is assessed for signs and symptoms of anemia; receives treatment for correction.

Plan/Implementation
- monitor hemoglobin or hematocrit levels at initial antepartal visit and in later pregnancy
- provide dietary counseling regarding importance of iron-rich diet
- instruct to take oral iron compounds (ferrous sulfate or gluconate) as daily supplement as ordered; teach regarding side effects
  - change in color of stools (become black)
  - take with food only if gastric distress occurs
- provide folic acid supplement of 5 mg/24h orally for folate deficiency, as ordered
- observe for symptoms of hemolytic crisis (e.g., chills, fever, pain in back and abdomen, prostration, shock) with hemoglobinopathies
- refer for genetic counseling (women with inherited disorders)

Evaluation: The pregnant woman eats a balanced, adequate, iron-rich diet during pregnancy; is free from iron-deficiency anemia.

K. Infections

1. General Information
a. Definition: a variety of infectious agents can affect maternal and fetal health, leading to increased morbidity and

mortality. Maternal disease that is mild or even asymptomatic can cause severe anomalies or death in the embryo/fetus/neonate.
  b. Types of Infectious Diseases
    1) the TORCH complex (*T*oxoplasmosis, *O*ther, *R*ubella, *C*ytomegalovirus infection, *H*erpes)
       a) *toxoplasmosis* (protozoa)
          - transmitted through ingestion of raw or undercooked meat; through improper hand washing after handling cat litter that has been contaminated with infected cat's feces
          - maternal symptoms may be absent or nonspecific
          - possible to detect virus by serologic screening
          - organism readily crosses placenta
          - may cause hydrocephaly, chorioretinitis, mental retardation in the neonate
       b) *other* most commonly refers to infection with group B beta-hemolytic streptococcus, syphilis, and gonorrhea
          - *streptococcal* infection: streptococci estimated to be present in genital tract of approximately 15% of women of childbearing age; associated with urinary tract infection, septic abortion, stillbirth, puerperal sepsis, neonatal sepsis
          - *syphilis:* prenatal serologic screening test is important for prevention of congenital syphilis; associated with abortion, stillbirth, prematurity, and congenital syphilis [*Systemic neurological*]
          - *gonorrhea*: may cause postpartum infection, pelvic inflammatory disease, sterility; danger to newborn is ophthalmia neonatorum; refer to "Sexually Transmitted Diseases" in *Nursing Care of the Child* page 582 [*localized eye sight*]
       c) *rubella*: extremely teratogenic in 1st trimester
          - transmitted transplacentally
          - congenital rubella syndrome in the neonate includes cataracts, hemolytic anemia, heart defects, mental retardation, deafness
          - infected infant can shed live viruses for many months after birth
          - women with low titers should receive vaccine in early postpartum period and avoid pregnancy for at least 2 months
       d) *cytomegalovirus* (CMV); also called cytomegalic inclusion disease (CMID): member of herpes virus group
          - adult usually asymptomatic or has mononucleosis-like symptoms
          - transmission in adults is respiratory, possibly venereal
          - transmission to fetus is transplacental; occasionally may be transmitted during passage through birth canal
          - no effective treatment
          - effects on neonate include mental retardation, intrauterine-growth retardation, congenital heart defects, deafness
       e) *herpes simplex virus type 2*
          - sexually transmitted, painful vesicles present on cervix, vaginal wall, vulva, and thighs; last 10 days to 2 weeks; remissions, exacerbations
          - usual mode of transmission to neonate is passage through birth canal; rarely occurs transplacentally
          - infection results in high infant mortality
          - cesarean birth, if pregnant woman has active herpes virus, type 2
    2) tuberculosis
       a) rarely transmitted to fetus
       b) disease must be arrested by usual methods of care for client with Tb
       c) if disease still active at birth, infant usually kept from close contact with mother, to protect from infection
    3) urinary tract infections

a) affect approximately 10% of gravidae, generally due to *E. coli*
b) increased urinary stasis, related to anatomic changes during pregnancy
c) increased incidence of pyelonephritis if bacteria present
d) associated with increased incidence of premature labor
4) nongonococcal urethritis (NGU)
   a) increasingly common
   b) organism: chlamydia
   c) both partners should be treated with tetracycline
   d) may cause ophthalmia neonatorum or pneumonia in newborn
5) condylomata (genital warts)
   a) viral transmission
   b) may be transmitted to fetus at birth
   c) should be treated with laser beam or cautery
   d) biopsy indicated for large warts

2. **Nursing Process**
   a. Assessment
      1) routine serologic studies for venereal disease and selected laboratory tests as indicated
      2) signs and symptoms of infectious diseases
   b. Goal, Plan/Implementation, and Evaluation

   Goal: Maternal exposure to infectious diseases during pregnancy will be minimized through careful management and client education; the pregnant woman who acquires an infectious disease will be diagnosed early and care will be appropriately managed to minimize maternal and fetal risk; the pregnant woman will comply with treatment for infectious disease.
   Plan/Implementation
   - review precautions to take in order to minimize exposure to infection
   - teach client to report any symptoms, i.e., vesicles, discharge, rash, elevated temperature
   - administer drugs as ordered (e.g., penicillin for syphilis)
   - instruct to take drugs as ordered (e.g., isoniazid [INH], streptomycin, PAS); explain expected actions, side effects; avoid self-medication

   Evaluation: The pregnant woman is free from controllable infectious disease; maternal or fetal risks have been minimized; mother complies with therapeutic regimen.

L. Multiple Gestation

1. **General Information**
   a. Definition: gestation of two or more fetuses. Twins may be produced from a single ovum (monozygotic or identical twins) or from separate ova (dizygotic or fraternal). Fraternal twinning is an inherited autosomal recessive trait and is more common (70%) than identical twins (30%). Triplets result from one, two, or three separate ova.
   b. Incidence: 2%–3% of all viable births
   c. Predisposing Factors
      1) blacks have higher incidence of multiple pregnancies, compared with whites
      2) family history of dizygotic twins
   d. Prognosis
      1) increased risk of premature labor, pregnancy-induced hypertension (25%), hemorrhage
      2) increased risk of delivery of low-birth-weight infants, often premature (50%)
      3) increased risk of maternal anemia (40%-50%)
      4) increased risk of uterine inertia (10%), hydramnios (5%-10%), intrauterine asphyxia (5%)
      5) increased risk of secondary cessation or weakening of effective uterine contractions
      6) monozygotic twins have higher mortality and morbidity rates than dizygotic twins, because of increased congenital anomalies, twin-to-twin transfusion syndrome, and intrauterine-growth retardation

2. **Nursing Process**
   a. Assessment
      1) early identification of multiple pregnancy based upon
         a) history
         b) weight gain
         c) abdominal palpation

d) asynchronous fetal heart beats
e) ultrasonography
2) maternal and fetal status: prenatal visits every 2 weeks
3) nutritional status

b. **Goal, Plan/Implementation, and Evaluation**

Goal: The woman with a multiple pregnancy will be monitored closely for early signs of maternal or fetal complications.

Plan/Implementation
- advise frequent rest periods; lateral recumbent position may be most comfortable and provides oxygenation for fetal/placental unit
- review diet, ensure it is adequate; give iron and vitamin supplements as ordered
- monitor FHR carefully for indication of fetal distress
- prepare for vaginal delivery unless complications arise (e.g., fetal distress, cephalopelvic disproportion); administer oxytocic agent as ordered immediately following birth to prevent postpartum hemorrhage (very important because of overdistention of the uterus)

Evaluation: The woman is free from complications (e.g., anemia); multiple pregnancy is carried to term (or close to term), resulting in delivery of healthy neonates.

M. Adolescent Pregnancy

1. **General Information**
   a. Definition: pregnancy in a female under 17 years of age
   b. Incidence: worldwide, 1/3 of all births are to girls under 17 years of age; one million teenage pregnancies per year (10% of all teenagers) (World Health Organization 1977)

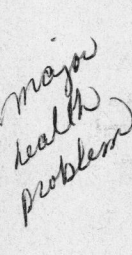
major health problem

   c. Predisposing Factors: teenage pregnancies are associated with
      1) earlier onset of menarche
      2) changing sexual behavior
      3) poor family relationships
      4) poverty
   d. Prognosis
      1) for pregnant girls under 15 years, a high risk of stillbirths, low-birth-weight infants, neonatal mortality, and cephalopelvic disproportion
      2) increased maternal risk of pregnancy-induced hypertension, prolonged labor, iron-deficiency anemia, gonorrhea, and urinary tract infections

2. **Nursing Process**
   a. Assessment
      1) nutrition status
      2) knowledge of physiology of pregnancy
      3) emotional status
      4) support systems
   b. **Goal, Plan/Implementation, and Evaluation**

Goal: The pregnant teen will maintain maternal-fetal well-being; will prepare for birth of the newborn; will achieve developmental tasks of adolesence.

Plan/Implementation
- assist pregnant teen to achieve developmental tasks
  - develop intimate, mature relations with peers (male and female)
  - accept changing body image
  - socialize into appropriate gender role
  - establish an independent and satisfying life-style
- provide dietary counseling regarding
  - importance of well-balanced meals
  - selection of nutritionally valuable, yet acceptable food
  - food preparation; increased protein, calcium, and iron intake
- refer to social service for
  - career and educational counseling
  - options regarding child care and adoption
  - support services in community
- prepare teen for childbirth; arrange for coaching assistance
- suggest follow-up classes on parenting
- teach family planning
- as indicated, instruct teen in child care

Evaluation: The pregnant adolescent is free from preventable complications (e.g., anemia, urinary tract infections); has a physically safe and emotionally satisfying childbirth experience; is delivered of a healthy neonate; achieves the appropriate developmental milestones for her age; is capable of safely caring for her newborn or has arranged for alternate, permanent, or temporary child care.

Intrapartal Care

General Concepts
A. Normal Childbearing
1. Definitions
   a. Labor: a series of processes by which the products of conception are expelled from the maternal body
   b. Delivery: the actual event of birth
2. Essential Factors in Labor: powers, passageway, passenger, person (four Ps)
   a. The Powers: uterine contractions, voluntary bearing down, abdominal muscle contractions, contractions of levator ani muscle
   b. The Passageway: bones, tissues, ligaments
      1) type of pelvis: gynecoid, android, anthropoid and platypelloid; refer to "The Structure of the Female Pelvis" page 375
      2) adequacy of planes of true pelvis
         a) true pelvis forms the birth canal through which fetus must pass
         b) three distinct levels
            - plane of inlet
            - midplane (plane of least dimensions)
            - plane of outlet
      3) condition of soft tissues (lower uterine segment, cervix, and vaginal canal)
   c. The Passenger: the fetus
      1) attitude (habitus or posture): the relation of the fetal parts to its own trunk; normal attitude of the fetus in utero is complete flexion
      2) engagement: the entrance of the greatest diameter of the presenting part through the plane of inlet and the beginning of the descent through the pelvic canal (biparietal diameter of head is fixed in pelvis)
      3) lie: the relation of the long axis of the fetus to the long axis of the mother; it is either transverse, longitudinal, or oblique
         a) transverse lie: long axis of fetus is at right angle to mother's long axis; it is a pathologic lie if present at term
         b) longitudinal lie: long axis of the fetus is parallel to mother's long axis; it has two alternatives
            - cephalic presentation (head first)
            - breech presentation (buttocks first)
      4) presentation and presenting part: that part of the fetal body that enters the true pelvis and presents itself at the internal os for delivery; the presentation is dependent upon the attitude of the fetal extremities to its body and the fetal lie
         a) in cephalic presentations (95% of term deliveries), the fetal head is the presenting part: the head may be
            - completely flexed upon the fetal chest (vertex presentation)
            - moderately flexed (sinciput presentation)
            - partially extended (brow presentation)
            - hyperextended with chin presenting (face presentation)
         b) in breech presentations (3% of term births)
            - the fetal knees and hips both may be flexed, positioning the thighs on the abdomen and calves on the posterior thighs (complete breech)

Figure 4.9 Six Possible Fetal Positions with Cephalic Presentation

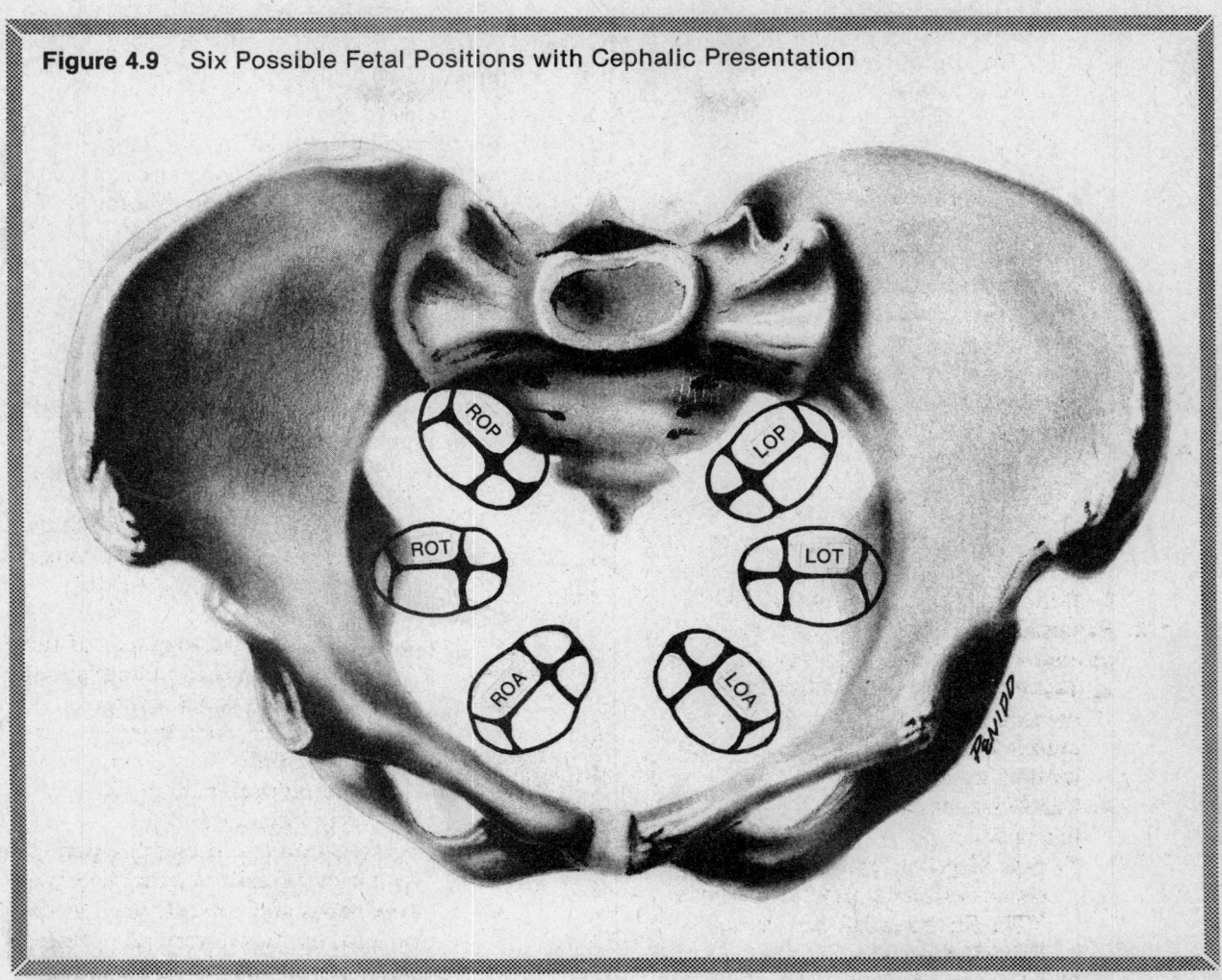

- the hips may be flexed and the knees extended (frank breech)
- extension of the knees and hips (footling breech)
- shoulder presentation is commonly known as a transverse lie

5) position: the situation of the fetus in utero is determined by the relation of the established point of direction of the presenting part to one of the quadrants of the mother's pelvis; established point of direction
   a) breech presentation: sacrum (S)
   b) cephalic presentation: occiput (O)
   c) shoulder presentation: scapula (Sc) (6 different positions are thus possible for each of the above by relating the established point of direction to the right or left side of the mother's pelvis)
6) station: the degree of engagement, measured in centimeters above or below the pelvic midplane from the presenting part to the ischial spines
   a) station 0 is at the ischial spines
   b) minus station is above the spines
   c) plus station is below the spines
d. The Person: pregnant woman's general behavior and influences upon her
   1) maternal response to uterine contractions
   2) cultural influences and perceptions about labor and delivery
   3) antepartal and/or childbirth education
   4) ability to communicate feelings to significant other(s) and staff
   5) support system

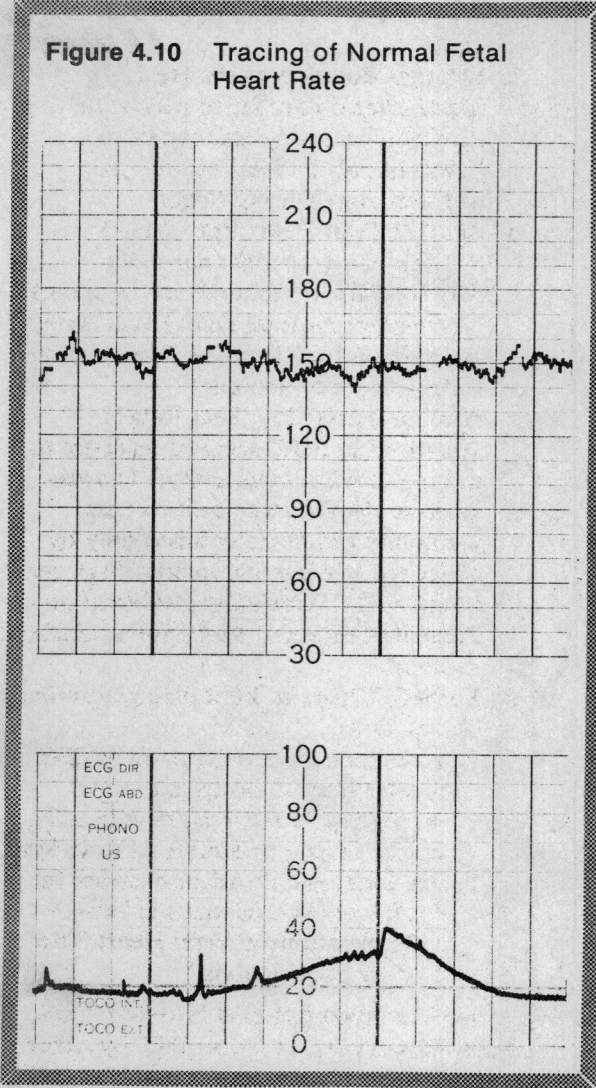

Figure 4.10 Tracing of Normal Fetal Heart Rate

3. Signs of Labor
    a. Premonitory Signs of Labor: changes indicative that labor will shortly be approaching
        1) increased Braxton Hicks' contractions: intermittent contractions of the uterus occurring throughout pregnancy; generally painless
        2) lightening or engagement: the descent of the fetus into the pelvic cavity; generally occurs 2-3 weeks before the onset of labor in primigravidas; causes increased bladder pressure and reduced diaphragm pressure
        3) show: blood-tinged mucus discharged from cervix shortly before or during labor
        4) sudden burst of energy: i.e., "nesting behaviors" exhibited
        5) weight loss resulting from fluid loss and electrolyte shifts
        6) increased backache and sacroiliac pressure due to fetal pressure
        7) spontaneous rupture of membranes may occur; woman will be advised to enter hospital immediately
    b. True Labor vs False Labor
        1) true labor
            a) contractions increase progressively in strength, duration, and frequency
            b) regular pattern, not relieved by walking (walking may increase the strength of the contractions)
            c) felt in back or radiating towards front
            d) effacement and dilation of the cervix
            e) fetal membranes
                • intact: generally in early labor, indicated by negative Nitrazine paper test (yellow to yellow-olive paper)
                • ruptured: generally in active labor, indicated by positive Nitrazine paper test (blue green to blue paper); meconium staining may indicate fetal distress, except in breech presentation
        2) false labor
            a) an exaggeration of the periodic uterine contractions normally occurring during pregnancy
            b) does not produce progressive dilation, effacement, or descent
            c) contractions are irregular and do not increase in frequency, duration, or intensity
            d) walking has no effect on contractions
            e) discomfort felt in lower abdomen and groin
            f) absence of bloody show
4. Labor Onset Theories *unsure*
    a. Oxytocin Stimulation: alone or in combination with other factors
    b. Progesterone Withdrawal: allowing uterine contractions to progress
    c. Estrogen Stimulation: causing hypertrophy of myometrium and

increased production of contractile proteins
- **d. Prostaglandin Secretion:** effect on uterine muscle (increased uterine irritability)
- **e. Fetal Endocrine Secretion of Cortical Steroids**
- **f. Distention of Uterus:** with subsequent pressure on nerve endings stimulating contractions and increased irritability of uterine musculature

5. **Physiologic Alterations Occurring During Labor**
   - **a. Dilation to 10 cm:** the process by which the cervix opens
   - **b. Effacement:** thinning and obliteration of cervix
   - **c. Physiologic Retraction Ring:** the separation of the upper (active, thicker) and lower (passive, thinner) uterine segments in labor

6. **Fetal Positional Response to Labor (Mechanisms of Labor)**
   - **a. Engagement:** descent of fetus into true pelvis
   - **b. Descent:** the passage of the presenting part through the pelvis
   - **c. Flexion:** further flexion of the fetal head when it meets resistance from the pelvic floor
   - **d. Internal Rotation:** the process by which the long axis of the fetal skull changes from the transverse diameter to an anteroposterior diameter at the outlet
   - **e. Extension of the head** as it leaves the outlet
   - **f. External Rotation of the Head (Restitution):** in order to rotate the shoulders and leave the outlet
   - **g. Expulsion of the total baby**

7. **Fetal Heart Rate During Labor**
   - **a. Baseline Fetal Heart Rate (FHR) Without Contractions:** normally between 120-160/minute; see figure 4.10 "Tracing of Normal Fetal Heart Rate," and table 4.10, "Baseline Fetal Heart Rate—No Contractions"
   - **b. Baseline Variability:** beat-to-beat variations in FHR occur in response to uterine activity, medications, hypoxia, acidosis (*NOTE:* true beat-to-beat variability can be determined only by direct fetal or internal monitoring); see figure 4.12, "Tracing of Acceleration of Fetal Heart Rate in Response to Uterine Activity"
   - **c. Periodic Changes:** FHR changes during contractions
     1) accelerations: transient rise in FHR greater than 15 beats/minute for more than 15 seconds; may or may not be related to uterine contractions
     2) decelerations: transient decrease in FHR; see classifications in table 4.11, "Decelerations in Fetal Heart Rate During Contractions"

B. Ongoing Management and Nursing Care
1. Fetal Monitoring: monitor FHR by either
   - **a. Periodic Auscultation:** count for 1 full minute, or

Table 4.10 Baseline Fetal Heart Rate—No Contractions
Normal Range: 120-160 beats/minute

	Tachycardia	Bradycardia
Mild	161-180 beats/minute	100-119 beats/minute
Marked	Greater than 180 beats/minute	Less than 100 beats/minute
Causes	Prematurity Maternal fever Mild fetal hypoxia Fetal infection Drugs	Fetal hypoxia Maternal hypothermia Drugs Congenital heart defects*

*A physiologic bradycardia may occur during contractions.

412 SECTION 4: NURSING CARE OF THE CHILDBEARING FAMILY

Figure 4.11 Types of Decelerations in Fetal Heart Rate

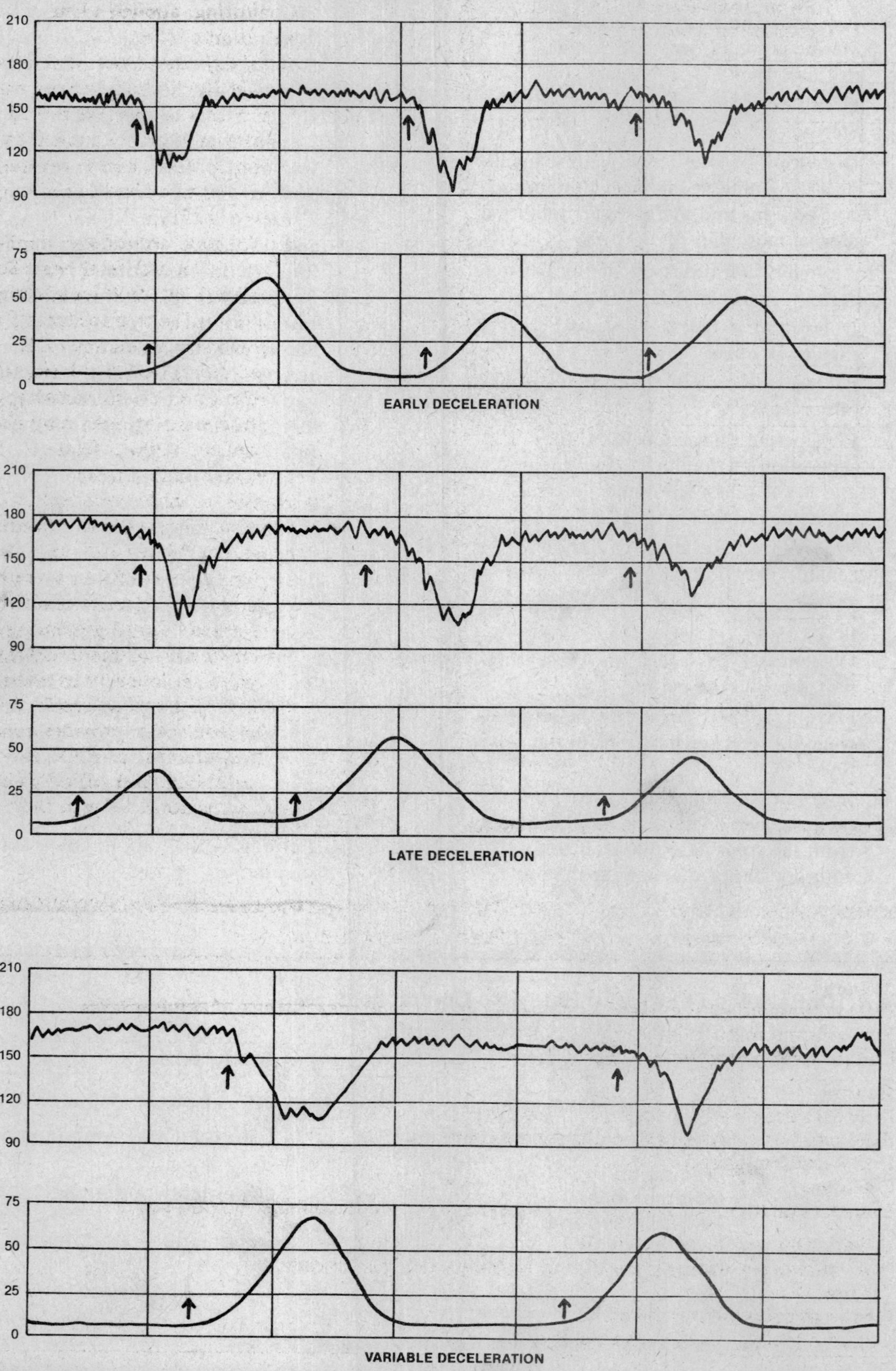

EARLY DECELERATION

LATE DECELERATION

VARIABLE DECELERATION

INTRAPARTAL CARE 413

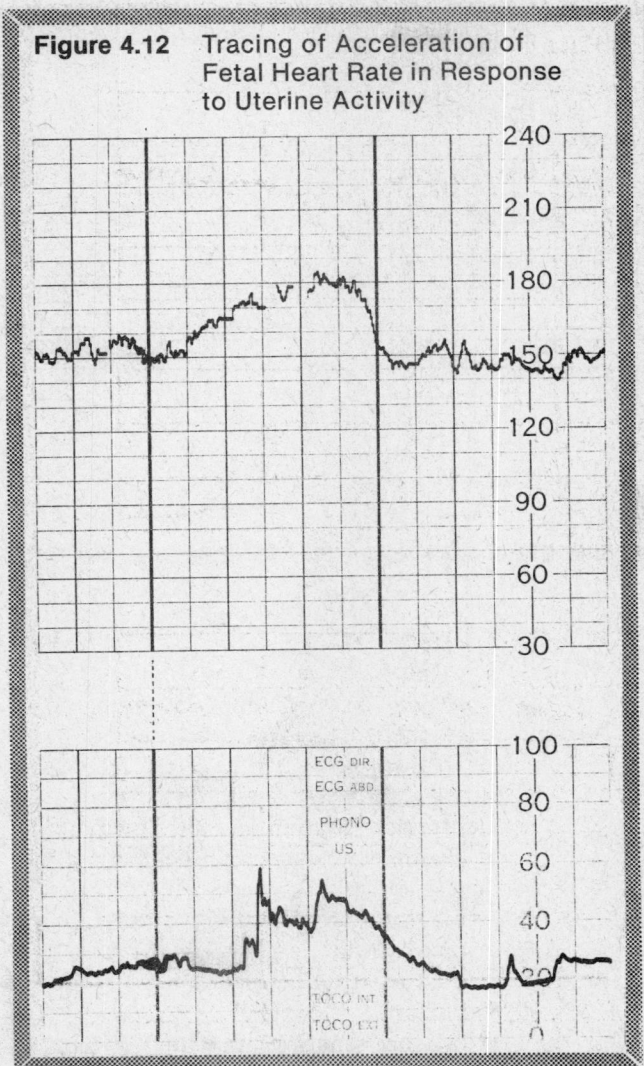

Figure 4.12 Tracing of Acceleration of Fetal Heart Rate in Response to Uterine Activity

b. Electronic Fetal Monitor
  1) external or indirect electronic monitoring: applied when membranes intact
    a) *tokodynamometer*: disk attached over fundus and secured with belt; provides continuous record of external pressure created by contractions, allows measurement of frequency and duration of contractions
    b) *ultrasonic transducer*: applied at site of loudest fetal heart beat, secured with belt (conducting gel is spread over transducer); provides continuous FHR recording, which is interpreted in relation to uterine activity; phonocardiography may also be used for indirect fetal electrocardiography
  2) internal or direct monitoring: applied when membranes have ruptured and cervix has dilated 2–3 cm
    a) *pressure transducer*: an intra-uterine catheter filled with water is inserted beyond presenting part; allows measurement of frequency, duration, intensity of contractions
    b) *internal spiral electrode*: applied to fetal scalp; provides continuous measurement of FHR, baseline variability, and periodic changes
2. Uterine Contractions: refer to table 4.12 and figure 4.13

Table 4.11 Decelerations in Fetal Heart Rate During Contractions

Type 1 (early)
- FHR decreased with onset of contraction and mirrors the pattern of contractions
- FHR returns to baseline as the contraction ends
- Cause: fetal head compression

Type 2 (late)
- FHR decreases *after* the onset of contraction
- FHR persists beyond completion of contractions
- Has a uniform shape
- Ominous
- Cause: fetal hypoxia, associated with a decrease in uteroplacental perfusion

Type 3 (variable)
- FHR decreases at any point *during or between* contractions
- Jagged V- or U-shape
- Range of drop in FHR is large
- Cause: umbilical cord compression

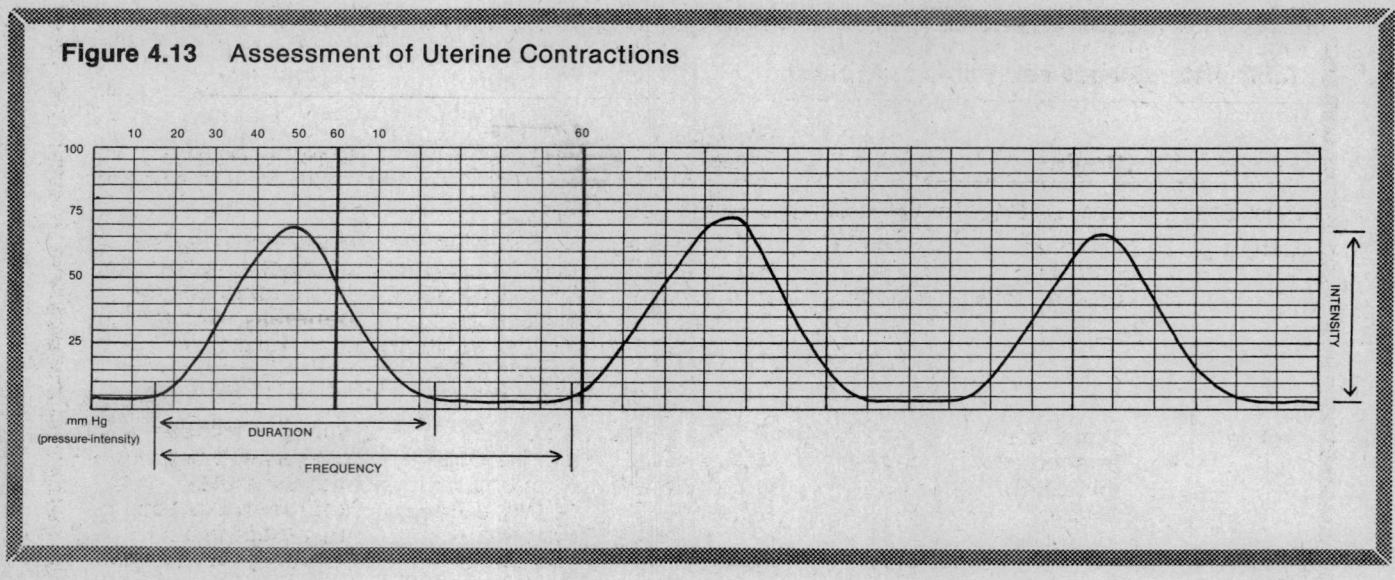

Figure 4.13 Assessment of Uterine Contractions

- a. Frequency: timed from beginning of one to beginning of next contraction
- b. Duration: timed from beginning to end of one contraction
- c. Intensity: degree of muscle contraction; may be mild, moderate, strong
- d. Tonus: pressure within the uterus in between contractions; only measurable with an intrauterine catheter
3. Analgesics: drugs that relieve pain or alter its perception may alter level of consciousness and reflex activity; administer as ordered and monitor effects; common obstetric analgesics include
    a. Narcotics
        1) may initially slow labor, have depressive effect on neonatal respirations
        2) examples: meperidine HCl (Demerol), alphaprodine (Nisentil)
        3) administered when client in active labor (4–5 cm); drug action may have long duration (Demerol) or short duration (Nisentil)
    b. Tranquilizers
        1) produce sedation and relaxation; often given with narcotics because of potentiating effects; when given alone, there may be little or no analgesia; may cause excitement and disorientation in presence of pain
        2) examples: promethazine HCl (Phenergan), hydroxyzine pamoate (Vistaril), promazine HCl (Sparine) and diazepam (Valium)
        3) effects
            a) peak action within 60 minutes
            b) may last 6–8 hours depending on stage of labor and activity of client
    c. Amnesics (rarely used today)
        1) produce sedation and alter memory
        2) example: scopolamine (belladonna alkaloid)
        3) may cause dysrhythmias and fetal tachycardia
        4) "cat reaction"
    d. Sedatives
        1) produce sedation; may depress fetus
        2) examples: secobarbital sodium (Seconal) and pentobarbital sodium (Nembutal) may be given in early labor
4. Anesthetics: produce a local or generalized loss of sensation
    a. General
        1) induce sleep
        2) examples: nitrous oxide, halothane (Fluothane), thiopental (Pentothal sodium), cyclopropane
        3) may depress fetus
        4) danger of pulmonary aspiration of gastric contents
        5) uterine atony
    b. Local
        1) used for pain relief during episiotomy and perineal repair
        2) example: lidocaine (Xylocaine)
        3) any agent may cause an allergic response

Table 4.12 Stages and Phases of Labor

Phase	Begins	Ends	Average Time	Uterine Activity	Manifestations
First Stage (Onset of Regular Contractions to Full Dilatation)					
Latent	Onset of regular contractions	Effacement complete; dilatation 0-3 cm	Primigravida: 8½ hours multigravida: 5½ hours	Mild uterine contractions, lasting 10-30 seconds; regular pattern every 15-20 minutes apart	Abdominal cramps, backache, rupture of membranes, client generally excited, alert, talkative, in control
Active	Complete effacement; dilatation 2-3 cm	Approximately 8 cm dilatation	Primigravida: 4 hours multigravida: 2 hours	Moderate uterine contractions, lasting 30-45 seconds; increased regularity in pattern; occur every 3-5 minutes	Show; moderately increased pain; client may be more apprehensive, fear losing control, focusing on self; skin warm and flushed
Transitional	Dilatation 8 cm	Cervix fully dilated	Primigravida: 1 hour multigravida: 10-15 minutes	Strong uterine contractions occur every 2-3 minutes, lasting 45-90 seconds	Client may be irritable and panicky, may lose control, be amnesic between contractions; perspiring, nausea and vomiting common; trembling of legs, pressure on bladder and rectum, backache, circumoral pallor
Second Stage (Full Dilatation and Effacement to Delivery of Infant)					
	Full dilatation and effacement	Delivery of infant	Primigravida: 30-50 minutes multigravida: 20 minutes	Strong uterine contractions every 2-3 minutes, lasting 45-90 seconds	Decrease in pain from transitional level; increase in bloody show, pressure on rectum, urge to bear down, bulging perineum; client excited and eager
Third Stage (Delivery of Fetus to Delivery of Placenta)					
	Delivery of fetus	Delivery of placenta	5-30 minutes	Strong uterine contractions; uterus changing to globular shape; gush of blood	Client focuses upon infant, excited about birth; feeling of relief
Fourth Stage (Placental Delivery to Homeostasis)					
	Delivery of placenta	Homeostasis	Usually defined as 1st hour postpartum	Uterus firm at level of two finger breadths above umbilicus	Exploration of newborn; parent-infant bonding begins; infant alert and responsive

c. Regional
   1) for relief of perineal and uterine pain
   2) usually safe for infant unless maternal hypotension occurs
   3) types
      a) paracervical block: given in 1st stage; rapid relief of uterine pain; relieves pain of contractions; no effect on perineal area; does not interfere with bearing-down reflex; fetal bradycardia may occur
      b) pudendal block: given in 2nd stage of labor; affects perineum for about ½ hour; safe for neonate; no effect on contractions
      c) peridural block: given in 1st or 2nd stage of labor; produces rapid relief of uterine and perineal pain; may be given in single doses or continuously
         • epidural: may cause maternal hypotension
         • caudal: same side effects as epidural
      d) intradural blocks
         • spinal block: rapid onset; relieves uterine and perineal pain; may cause maternal hypotension; client must remain flat for 8–12 hours
         • saddle block (low spinal): rapid onset of pain relief; used for forceps delivery; client must remain flat for 8–12 hours

C. **Application of the Nursing Process to Normal Childbearing, Intrapartal Care**
   1. Assessment
      a. Premonitory Signs of Labor
      b. Signs and Symptoms of True Labor
      c. Stage and Phase of Labor: refer to table 4.12
      d. Uterine Contractions
      e. Fetal Response to Labor
   2. **Goals, Plans/Implementation, and Evaluation**

   Goal 1: The pregnant woman will be admitted to the labor and delivery unit and will be appropriately monitored for intrapartal status.
   Plan/Implementation
   • orient client to physical setting and review basic procedures to be performed
   • determine onset, duration, and frequency of contractions
   • determine client's knowledge of the labor and delivery process
   • obtain baseline vital signs and BP
   • perform Leopold's maneuver; have client empty bladder and flex knees for abdominal relaxation; warm hands, then proceed with
     – fundus palpation: note breech or cephalic presentation
     – lateral palpation: note back and small parts of fetus
     – just above symphysis pubis, note position and mobility of fetal head
     – midline about 2 inches above Poupart's ligaments, note position and descent of head, location of back
   • observe FHR and pattern changes in relation to contractions (*NOTE:* The use of electronic fetal monitoring at this time is determined by hospital policy)
   • prepare and position client appropriately for initial vaginal exam and reinforce the rationale for exam; explain the results of exam
   • note color, consistency, amount, and gross appearance of amniotic fluid
   • obtain laboratory specimens: urine for protein (normally neg), glucose (normally neg), and ketones (normally neg); blood for Hgb (normal range 12–16 gm/100 ml), HCT (normal range 38%–45%), WBC (normal range 4,500–11,000 ml), VDRL
   • determine time of last food ingestion
   • review process of labor and provide emotional support
   • perform vulvar and/or perineal preparation as ordered
   • administer cleansing enema if ordered by physician; check FHR after procedure

   Evaluation: The pregnant woman is admitted to labor and delivery unit; receives appropriate monitoring and preparation for delivery.

   Goal 2: The health of the pregnant woman and fetus are maintained during the 1st stage of labor.
   Plan/Implementation
   • take maternal vital signs qh, if stable and within normal limits
   • take temperature q2h if membranes ruptured more than 24 hours previously

or if temperature is greater than 37.5°C (may indicate infection or dehydration)
- observe blood pressure between contractions q1–2h for supine-hypotensive syndrome caused by pressure of enlarged uterus on vena cava (decreased BP, pulse, pallor, clammy skin); condition may be prevented or corrected by placing client in left lateral position
- monitor fetal status
  - auscultate FHR using a stethoscope q30min (early labor) to q5min (transition); count rate for 1 full minute (normal is 120–160/minute) or observe FHR tracing from electronic monitor for baseline changes, variability, and periodic changes related to contractions
  - monitor uterine contractions through abdominal palpations q30min (in early labor) to q5min (in transition); note regularity, frequency, intensity, and duration or observe uterine tracings from electronic monitor for tonus, frequency, duration, and intensity of contractions
  - check FHR after rupture of membranes
  - check for prolapse of cord; if cord is prolapsed, place mother in Trendelenburg's or knee-chest position, give O₂, notify physician immediately; grave danger of fetal hypoxia because of cord compression
- assist with or perform periodic vaginal examination to assess dilatation and effacement of cervix, fetal descent, presentation, lie
- monitor fluid and electrolyte balance
  - record I&O
  - encourage voiding q2h; catheterize for bladder distention
  - observe for signs of dehydration
  - note diaphoresis
  - monitor parenteral therapy; specific use determined by medical regimen and duration of labor
- provide sufficient nourishment according to medical policy and client need
  - nothing PO routine in many hospitals, especially if client is receiving medication; observe for signs of hypoglycemia
  - ice chips or liquid diet may be given in some settings (*NOTE:* GI absorption and motility are decreased during labor)
  - observe for nausea and vomiting during transition (common)
- promote physical safety
  - client may ambulate in early labor if desired, unless there are contraindications (e.g., membranes ruptured, medications, IV infusion)
  - keep side rails up as necessary to prevent injury during active labor
  - advise to not smoke and no smoking in client's environment
- administer basic comfort measures: pillows to support body; frequent position change; bathe face and body as necessary; backrubs; effleurage for abdominal discomfort; change linen and pads frequently
- assist client with breathing techniques or provide direct coaching as necessary
  - utilize appropriate techniques taught in antepartal or childbirth classes or instruct as necessary (e.g., abdominal breathing, shallow chest breathing, panting)
  - advise client to rest between contractions but wake client and begin breathing techniques at onset of next contraction
  - observe for symptoms of hyperventilation (light-headedness, dizziness, tingling and numbness of lips); if it occurs, slow down breathing, breathe into paper bag or cupped hands
  - periodically relieve significant other of coaching role (give him a break and nourishment)
  - praise efforts and keep client and significant other informed about progress in labor
- assess ability to manage pain, desire for medications; administer analgesics (and assist with anesthetic administration) as ordered by physician, in accordance with client's preference
  - provide relaxing environment by maintaining calm manner and reducing external stimuli
  - administer medications as ordered; record administration of drug
  - note maternal and fetal response to medication; report any undesired side effects

- monitor maternal vital signs and FHR q5–15min, depending on drug given
- place client in appropriate position for administration of anesthetic
- if hypotension develops, place client in lateral position, increase IV fluids
- administer 6–8 liters of O_2/min for maternal hypotension or late decelerations in FHR

Evaluation: During the 1st stage of labor, the pregnant woman maintains normal vital signs, balanced fluid intake and output, is as comfortable as possible; is supported by an effective coach. The fetus maintains a normal heart rate in response to uterine contractions.

Goal 3: The health of the mother and fetus will be maintained during the 2nd stage of labor; a healthy newborn will be delivered with minimal trauma.

Plan/Implementation
- promote physical safety of childbearing family
  - if transfer to delivery room is required, do it between uterine contractions (transfer multiparas at 8–9 cm dilation, primiparas at full dilation with perineal bulging)
  - wear appropriate apparel and assist significant other in proper hand washing and obtaining appropriate attire (scrub dress/pants, cap, mask, and booties must be worn in delivery room; birthing room regulations may be less specific)
  - place client in optimal position on delivery table for birth of infant
- prep vulvar and perineal area, thighs, lower abdomen; wear sterile gloves and proceed from mons veneris to perineum
- continue to palpate fundus for uterine contractions, or assess via the electronic method
- continue monitoring FHR by either auscultation with a fetoscope or via the continuous electronic method
- continue to monitor BP
- encourage strong pushing with contractions
  - instruct client to begin by taking 2 short breaths, then hold and bear down; legs should be spread with knees slightly flexed
  - show the client which muscles are to be used by showing or touching those muscles in the pelvic floor
  - use blow-blow breathing pattern to prevent pushing between contractions
- assist physician/midwife as necessary
- promote emotional well-being of pregnant woman and significant other
  - inform them about progress and all procedures
  - position mirror so delivery may be viewed
  - encourage rest and relaxation between contractions
  - praise frequently for efforts

Evaluation: The pregnant woman is positioned appropriately and safely on delivery table; pushes and bears down effectively so as to enhance the power of uterine contractions; expels the fetus with minimal trauma; significant other appropriately supports pregnant woman.

Goal 4: The health of the mother and newborn is maintained during the 3rd stage; the placenta is safely expelled intact.

Plan/Implementation
- note time of delivery of infant
- provide immediate newborn care; refer to "Application of the Nursing Process to the Normal Newborn" page 452
- place newborn on mother's uncovered abdomen in delivery room, if possible
- allow mother to touch and explore infant
- after cord is cut, allow mother to hold and cuddle infant, to explore his or her body
- assess for signs that placenta has separated
  - uterus rises up in abdomen
  - uterus changes to globular shape
  - sudden trickle of blood appears
  - umbilical cord lengthens
- observe time and mechanism of placental delivery; chart on delivery record
  - Duncan mechanism: maternal surface of the placenta presents upon delivery; appears dark and rough; increased risk of retained placental fragments
  - Schultze mechanism: fetal surface of the placenta presents upon delivery; appears shiny, smooth

- inspect placenta for intactness
- palpate uterus to check for muscle tone at frequent intervals (firm and contracted)
- administer oxytocic agents as ordered
  - type and amount determined by individual need and physician's preference; may be given IM or added to existing IV
  - used to prevent/control postpartum hemorrhage by stimulating uterine contractility
  - very important with overdistention or poor muscle tone
    * ergonovine (Ergotrate): may also cause transient hypertension
    * Pitocin (synthetic): also has an antidiuretic effect
    * methylergonovine (Methergine): may cause tetanic contractions with little tendency toward uterine relaxation; less effect on BP; given IV or PO
- measure maternal BP at q5-15min intervals (decreases in BP are often associated with blood loss and administration of oxytocic drugs)
- antilactation agents may be given in delivery room or postpartal unit
  - Deladumone
  - bromocriptine (Parlodel) (nonestrogen)
- agents containing estrogen should be used judiciously and with client's consent
- send cord blood to lab if mother's blood is Rh negative or O positive (for direct Coombs' test)
- allow mother (and significant other if present) opportunity to see and directly touch infant (promotes bonding) after initial stabilization
- initiate breast-feeding (hospital policies may vary)

Evaluation: Mother and newborn safely complete the 3rd stage of labor; the placenta is delivered intact; parent-infant bonding is initiated.

Goal 5: Mother will be safely transferred to the recovery room and complications will be prevented during the 4th stage of labor; parent-infant bonding will be achieved.

1-2 hr after delivery – greatest adapt time & watch for complications.

Plan/Implementation
- take vital signs q15min until stable (obtain temperature only upon admission)
- check height of fundus
  - palpate q15min during 1st hour
  - note position in relation to umbilicus (at or just above umbilicus, 1–2 finger breadths)
  - note consistency: should be firm; if boggy, massage until firm (avoid overmassaging)
- observe lochia q15min during 1st hour; note amount (small, moderate, or heavy), color (rubra), consistency; presence of large clots may indicate retained placental fragments; flow is considered excessive if bleeding saturates pad within 15 minutes (flow may increase as oxytocics wear off)
- check perineum: note general appearance, any swelling, redness, bruising, drainage, condition of episiotomy
- palpate bladder for distention; measure initial voiding; catheterize if necessary (full bladder displaces the uterus)
- for afterpains and pain at episiotomy site, promote general comfort
  - cover client with warm blanket if chilling or shivering occur; may be caused by sudden release of pressure that has been on nerves, excitement, rapid decrease of hormone, fetal blood cells in maternal circulation
  - position for maximum comfort; encourage rest
  - give partial bath
- provide contact with newborn, if it was not done in delivery room
- perform peri care; apply pad from front to back and teach rationale
- maintain adequate fluid intake; state specific amounts of fluids to be taken in 8-hour period
- if transfer to recovery room required, ensure that both mother and baby are stabilized
  - monitor maternal vital signs q15min until stable
  - palpate position, firmness, and consistency of fundus
  - observe lochia for quantity, color, and consistency

- transfer to postpartum unit when condition stable (usually within 1-2 hours)
- if mother will breast-feed infant, help infant to breast

Evaluation: The mother is physiologically and psychologically stable (vital signs, fundus, lochia all within normal limits; asks questions about her own body functions); parents gaze at newborn; hold, touch, and cuddle infant; infant attempts to suck at breast; is transferred to postpartum unit.

Selected Health Problems in the Intrapartal Period

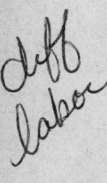

A. Dystocia

1. **General Information**
   a. Definition: difficult, painful labor and/or delivery characterized by abnormally slow progress as a result of abnormalities in the mechanics involved
   b. Incidence: approximately 5% of intrapartum women (largely primigravidae) experience some type of dystocia
   c. Types: fall into four categories, which may exist alone or in combination
      1) the *powers* (or forces): the main ones are
         a) hypertonic uterine dysfunction (primary inertia)
            - the uterine muscle is in a state of greater than normal muscle tension; contractions are of poor quality, and the force of the contraction is distorted
            - increased tonus
            - no cervical changes
            - is a problem in the latent phase of labor
            - treatment: sedation
         b) hypotonic uterine dysfunction (secondary inertia)
            - the tone or tension of the muscle is defective or inadequate, synchronous but not adequate
            - during active phase, uterine contractions reduce in intensity and get farther apart
            - treatment: stimulation of labor (e.g., rupture membranes, give oxytocin)
      2) the *passageway*: abnormalities in the size or character of the birth canal that form an obstacle to the descent of the fetus
         a) cephalopelvic disproportion (CPD): disproportion between the size of the infant's head and that of the birth canal
            - most frequently caused by a contracted pelvis: slight irregularities in the structure of the pelvis may delay the progress of labor; marked deformities often make delivery through the natural passages impossible
         b) types of pelvic contractions
            - contraction of the inlet
            - contraction of the midpelvis
            - contraction of the outlet
            - a combination
      3) the *passenger*: variations in position, presentation, or development of the fetus; includes a variety of conditions that are associated with prolonged labor, failure to progress, lack of engagement
         a) abnormal position: persistent occiput position (25% of pregnancies)
         b) faulty presentation
            - shoulders, face, or brow presentation
            - breech presentation
              - *frank breech*: buttocks present, the fetal legs are flexed and lie against the abdomen and the chest
              - *footling*: one or both feet present through the cervix

Table 4.13 Uterine Dysfunction in Labor

	Hypertonic	Hypotonic
Phase of labor	Latent	Active
Symptoms	Painful	Painless
Fetal distress	Early	Late
Treatment	Sedation	Oxytocin

SOURCE: Reeder, S. et al. *Maternity Nursing.* Philadelphia: Lippincott, 1983. Used with permission.

- *complete*: feet and legs are flexed on the abdomen, so that the buttocks and the feet present
    c) excessive size of fetus
      - a fetus over 4,000 gm (8 lb 13½ oz) may be too large to pass through the birth canal of some pregnant women; the fetal head also becomes less malleable when fetal weight increases
      - hydrocephalus (internus): excessive accumulation of cerebrospinal fluid in the ventricles of the brain with consequent enlargement of the cranium; incidence: 1 in 2,000 births
      - enlargement of the body of the fetus, e.g., abdominal distention, tumors
  4) the *person*: maternal factors (e.g., anxiety, lack of education, fear) can lengthen labor

2. **Nursing Process**
   a. Assessment
      1) vaginal exam, pelvimetry, or ultrasound to establish diagnosis
      2) false labor vs true labor
      3) fetal status
      4) trial labor period of 4-6 hours for
         a) effacement and dilation
         b) descent of fetal head
         c) fetal well-being
      5) cause of dystocia
      6) complications of uterine dysfunction
         a) maternal exhaustion
         b) intrapartum infection
         c) traumatic operative delivery
         d) fetal death and injury
      7) presentation of fetus by palpation (Leopold's maneuver)
      8) meconium staining of amniotic fluid (normal when associated with breech presentation)
      9) anxiety
   b. **Goals, Plans/Implementation, and Evaluation**

   Goal 1: The pregnant woman will be monitored for early signs and symptoms of dystocia; the woman with a dystocia will be safely managed during the intrapartum period; a healthy newborn will be delivered.

Plan/Implementation
- assess uterine contractions
- plot individual labor pattern, compare to Friedman curve (average labor curve of dilatation and time, figure 4.14)
- assist with ultrasonographic or radiographic studies for laboring woman with suspected CPD
- when physician artificially ruptures fetal membranes, immediately assess for prolapsed cord and FHR
  - if cord prolapsed, place mother in Trendelenburg's or knee-chest position (to minimize pressure of the presenting part on the cord); give O$_2$; notify physician; prepare for emergency cesarean birth
  - grave danger of fetal hypoxia
- monitor IV therapy and electrolyte replacement
- administer broad-spectrum antibiotics as ordered for treatment of intrauterine infection
- maximize rest for client
- support family

Evaluation: The pregnant woman receives prompt detection and treatment of signs of dystocia; potential dystocia due to abnormalities in the powers, passageway, or passenger is identified during the antenatal or early intrapartum period.

Goal 2: When indicated, the pregnant woman's hypotonic uterine contractions are corrected through safe oxytocin augmentation.

Plan/Implementation
- administer oxytocin (Pitocin) according to physician's order or hospital's protocol and pregnant woman's condition, see table 4.16; the physician must consider the following criteria before administration
  - there must be true hypotonic dysfunction; oxytocin ABSOLUTELY CONTRAINDICATED for *hypertonic* uterine dysfunction
  - the client must be in true labor (progressed to at least 3 cm)
  - there are no mechanical obstructions to safe delivery (e.g., cephalopelvic disproportion)
  - the condition of the fetus must be good: regular fetal heart rate, no meconium staining

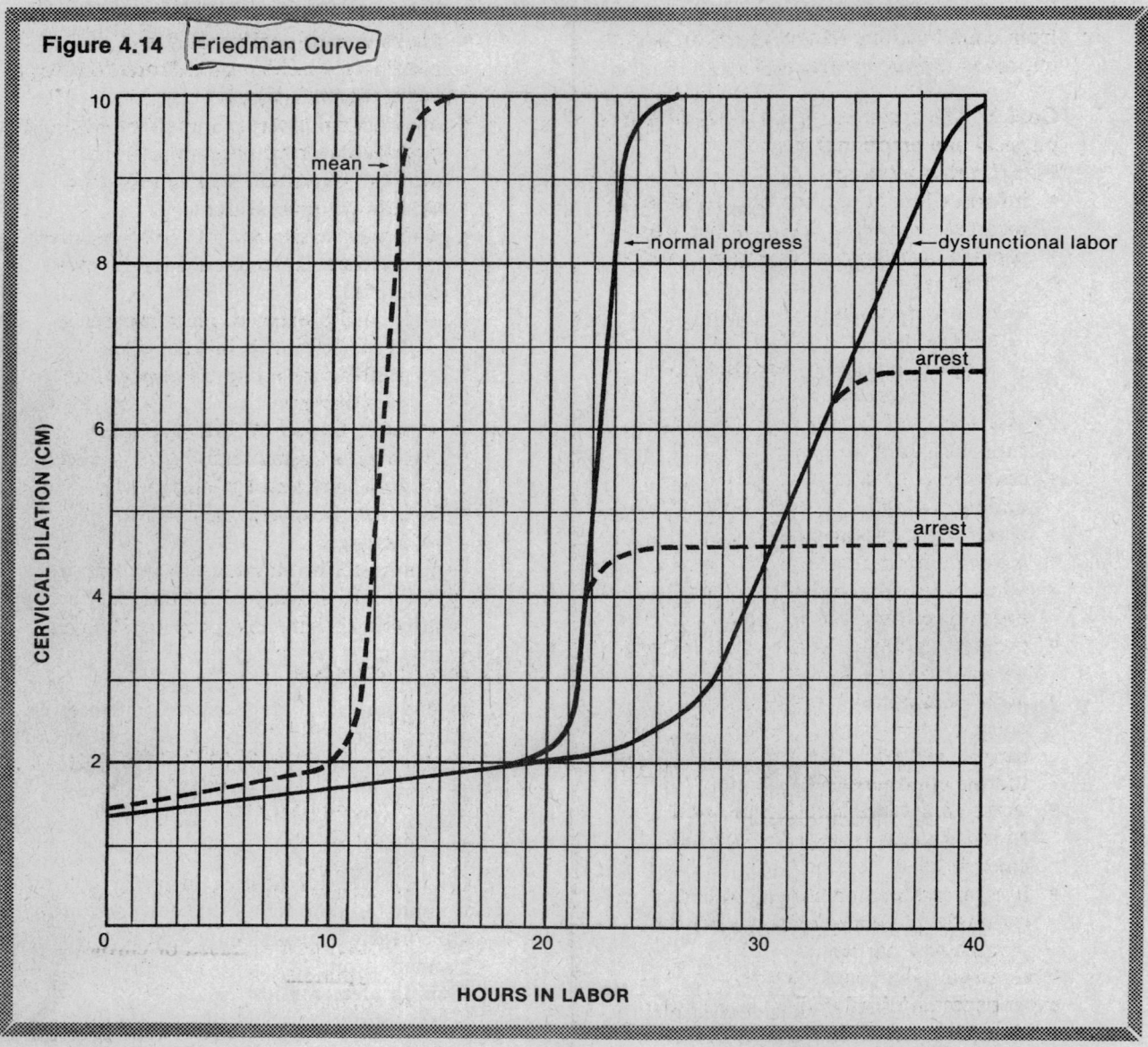

Figure 4.14 Friedman Curve

- the client usually must be less than 35 years old and less than a para 5 (greater age and parity increase the risk of uterine rupture)
- the uterus must not be overdistended because of a large infant (weighing 4,000 gm or more) or multiple gestation
- no previous cesarean births
• while administering oxytocin
  - use infusion pump
  - monitor maternal vital signs, drip rate, and infusion site with extreme caution and frequency
  - continue electronic fetal monitoring; observe fetal heart rate pattern and contractions (duration, intensity, tonus, and frequency)
  - place client in a left lateral position to maximize uterine blood flow by reducing pressure on vena cava and aorta
  - never leave client unattended (physician must be available)
  - assess for complications (e.g., rigid abdomen, water intoxication)
  - if uterine tetany occurs, or contractions exceeding 90 seconds duration, or if there is fetal distress (abnormal FHR pattern), discontinue oxytocin
  - give O_2 for signs of fetal distress

Evaluation: The pregnant woman is free from complications related to oxytocin; has improved uterine contractions.

Goal 3: The pregnant woman will receive physical and emotional support.
Plan/Implementation
- inform client about her status and what measures are being taken to help her
- provide basic comfort measures such as
  - back rubs
  - clean, dry linen
  - sponge bath
  - frequent change of position
  - quiet conversation
- assess level of fatigue and ability to cope with pain
- assess level of education and understanding (e.g., prenatal classes, breathing techniques learned)
- maintain hydration; monitor I&O
- administer sedatives and analgesics as ordered, to promote relaxation and rest
- provide emotional support to pregnant woman and significant other
- assist with administration of local anesthetic to interrupt peripheral neurohormonal mechanisms (hypertonic uterine contractions)
- assist with administration of anesthesia to relax uterus (hyperactive uterine contractions)
- if cesarean birth indicated, discuss rationale and expected outcomes with woman and partner

Evaluation: The pregnant woman experiences minimal anxiety; knows the status of labor and the fetus; rests comfortably between contractions, treatments.

Goal 4: The woman with an abnormal fetal position or presentation will be safely delivered of a neonate; will be free from preventable complications.
Plan/Implementation
- assist with vaginal or rectal exam to determine fetal presenting part
- explain and prepare pregnant woman for ultrasonic or radiographic studies to confirm previously unsuspected malpositions (anomalies often undetected before intrapartum period)
- continue electronic monitoring to assess effectiveness of labor and fetal well-being
- encourage lying on left side
- provide emotional support and childbirth coaching as indicated (labors are often prolonged)
- apply sacral pressure and offer frequent backrubs to keep pressure of fetal occiput off mother's sacrum (occiput posterior presentation)
- once membranes are ruptured, observe for cord prolapse (occurs in 1 in every 400 births)
  - if cord prolapsed, place mother in Trendelenburg's or knee-chest position; give O_2; notify physician immediately
  - grave danger of fetal hypoxia
- assist with vaginal delivery or cesarean birth as indicated by fetal presentation, labor progression, and maternal well-being

Evaluation: The woman receives care to enhance safe delivery of neonate (e.g., continuous monitoring, position change).

B. Premature Labor

1. **General Information**
   a. Definition: onset of labor before completion of 37 weeks gestation
   b. Predisposing Factors
      1) maternal
         a) diabetes
         b) cardiovascular and/or renal disease
         c) pregnancy-induced or chronic hypertension
         d) infection
         e) prematurely ruptured membranes
         f) incompetent cervix
         g) smoking
      2) fetal
         a) multiple pregnancy
         b) hydramnios
         c) infection
   c. Prognosis: fetal/neonatal mortality is less than 5% in pregnancies when gestation has lasted 35 or more weeks and the fetus is larger than 2,000 gm
   d. Maternal Complications Necessitating Delivery of Preterm Infant
      1) uncontrolled hemorrhage associated with placenta previa or abruptio placentae
      2) severe preeclampsia or eclampsia
      3) uncontrolled diabetes or cardiac disease

4) premature rupture of membranes (24–48 hours) prior to onset of labor (fetal maturity must be assessed)
5) chorioamnionitis
6) severe isoimmunization

2. **Nursing Process**
   a. **Assessment:** assess for true labor (contractions of increased frequency and duration, effacement and dilation of cervix)
   b. **Goal, Plan/Implementation, and Evaluation**

   Goal: The pregnant woman will progress to a safe delivery of neonate; or will experience a cessation of labor.
   Plan/Implementation
   - maintain bedrest in lateral recumbent position, a quiet environment
   - if fetus is immature, administer selected tokolytic agents to suppress labor as prescribed by physician (e.g., isoxuprine [Vasodilan], ritodrine, terbutaline, magnesium sulfate)
     - assess the effects of drugs upon the pattern of labor and fetal well-being via electronic monitoring system
     - assess for specific cardiovascular side effects, i.e., maternal tachycardia, hypertension, dysrhythmias, flushing if receiving ritodrine
     - have antidote available (propranolol)
     - do not administer these drugs for control of premature labor if contraindicated (e.g., client has a cardiac condition)
     - assess reflexes, respirations, and urinary output before and while giving magnesium sulfate
   - maintain adequate hydration through oral or parenteral intake
   - monitor I&O
   - take maternal vital signs
   - provide emotional support to mother and significant other
   - if indicated, administer glucocorticoid therapy (betamethasone) to prevent respiratory distress syndrome in neonate
     - drug is effective if delivery can be delayed 48 or more hours
     - do not administer if delivery is imminent or if maternal hypertensive or cardiovascular disorders exist
     - pulmonary edema has been reported in rare cases when ritodrine and corticosteroids are used together
   - administer minimal analgesics for pain during labor and delivery
   - prepare for delivery if maternal complications are present (e.g., diabetes, hemorrhage, eclampsia)

Table 4.14 Ritodrine Hydrochloride (Yutopar)

Description	Beta sympathetic agent that relaxes arterioles in uterine muscle
Uses	To stop uterine contractions in premature labor in pregnancy of at least 20 weeks gestation with intact membranes and absence of fetal distress
Dose	150 mg diluted in 500 ml fluid, administered up to 70 ml/hour; given IV initially; later may be given orally
Contraindications	History of cardiovascular disease, severe preeclampsia, hyperthyroidism, bronchial asthma
Side Effects	*Maternal:* tachycardia, tremors, palpitations, PVCs, hypertension or widening pulse pressure, headache, nervousness *Fetal:* tachycardia, hypoxia, acidosis
Nursing Implications	Monitor apical pulse, BP, FHR. Report pulse rate above 120 and FHR above 180. Check glucose and potassium levels. Keep I&O. Instruct client on expected cardiovascular responses and on value of additional maintenance of pregancy for fetal lung development. Anticipate that glucocorticoids (e.g., dexamethasone) may be administered to stimulate fetal surfactant production.

Evaluation: The pregnant woman is safely delivered of the neonate or retains her pregnancy.

C. Emergency Birth (Unassisted by Physician or Midwife)

1. **General Information**
   a. May occur in a hospital or community setting
   b. Predisposing Factors: precipitate labor, environmental problems, absence of physician/midwife
   c. Prognosis: increased maternal and fetal risk associated with possible
      1) intrauterine hypoxia (precipitate labor or delivery)
      2) laceration of the perineum
      3) infection

2. **Nursing Process**
   a. Assessment
      1) fetal status
      2) stage and phase of labor
   b. Goal, Plan/Implementation, and Evaluation

   Goal: The pregnant woman will be delivered of her neonate, free from complications.
   Plan/Implementation
   - do not leave woman alone; have another adult (if present) call for assistance
   - position pregnant woman comfortably
   - provide emotional support and remain calm
   - place clean towels or other protective material under buttocks
   - instruct mother to pant when head crowns
   - rupture amniotic sac (if intact) when fetal head crowns
   - apply gentle pressure on fetal head downward toward the vagina (this will prevent head from "popping out" and damaging fetal head, and prevent maternal lacerations)
   - deliver fetus between contractions
   - check for cord around neck; if wrapped around neck, slip cord over infant's head
   - allow restitution to deliver posterior shoulder
     - apply gentle downward pressure to bring anterior shoulder under symphysis
     - apply upward pressure to deliver posterior shoulder
   - place infant in head-down position to facilitate mucus drainage; do not hold upside down by feet or ankles
   - dry infant rapidly (maintain at level of uterus)
   - cover infant with blanket or towel to prevent heat loss
   - if equipment available, clamp cord in 2 places and cut between the 2 clamps; use sterile or clean (not contaminated) scissors or knife, or leave intact
   - do not milk the cord
   - wait for placental separation
     - do not pull on cord
     - instruct woman to gently push out placenta
   - put baby on mother's abdomen or to breast to stimulate uterine contractions
   - perform assessment of woman in 4th stage of labor and delivery

   Evaluation: The woman is delivered of a healthy newborn; is free from delivery complications.

D. Induction

1. **General Information**
   a. Definition: artificial stimulation of labor through a variety of mechanisms
   b. Predisposing Factors: induction is indicated for
      1) placental insufficiency
      2) prematurely ruptured membranes
      3) prolonged pregnancy (postmaturity)
      4) severe preeclampsia, eclampsia, or severe hypertension
      5) uncontrolled diabetes
   c. Prognosis
      1) increased risk of fetal and neonatal bradycardia
      2) increased risk of tetanic uterine contractions and premature separation of placenta

2. **Nursing Process**
   a. Assessment (see table 4.15): before beginning induction, assess that
      1) the cervix is thinning and dilating
      2) there is no cephalopelvic disproportion
      3) if oxytocin ordered, refer to "Dystocia" Goal 2 page 421
   b. Goal, Plan/Implementation, and Evaluation

   Goal: The pregnant woman will begin induced labor; will maintain a normal labor pattern without risk to the fetus.

Table 4.15 Bishop's Scale for Assessing Candidates for Induction of Labor

	Score 0	1	2	3	Subtotal Score
Dilatation (cm)	0	1–2	3–4	5–6	
Effacement (%)	0–30	40–50	60–70	80	
Station	–3	–2	–1	+1	
Cervical consistency	Firm	Medium	Soft		
Fetal position	Posterior	Midline	Anterior		
				Total Score*	

*Medical Guidelines: Parous woman: Induce at score 5
Nulliparous woman: Induce at score 7

Plan/Implementation
- administer oxytocin intravenously according to hospital protocol and physician's orders (see table 4.16)
- position pregnant woman on left side
- check fetal heart rate following amniotomy to evaluate for possible cord prolapse
- nipple stimulation may be used to stimulate contractions; research on safety/dangers not clear

Evaluation: The pregnant woman manifests positive signs of labor (e.g., contractions are strong and effective), leading to a safe and controlled labor and delivery; the fetus remains in good condition throughout course of labor and delivery.

(*NOTE:* The next four selected health problems [E through H] are classified as "Operative Obstetrics.")

E. Episiotomy

1. **General Information**
   a. Definition: an incision made into the perineum to facilitate delivery
   b. Indications: any condition that places the woman at risk for perineal tearing, e.g.,
      1) rapid labor
      2) large baby
      3) malposition of the fetus
   c. Prognosis: generally heals within 2–4 weeks following delivery; may cause mild to moderate discomfort in the postpartum period
   d. Types (see figure 4.15)
      1) median (midline)
         a) advantages: easily repaired; generally less painful; minimal blood loss
         b) disadvantages: increased risk of 3rd° or 4th° extension
      2) mediolateral (right or left)
         a) advantage: minimal risk of extension into rectum
         b) disadvantages: greater blood loss; repair more difficult; area more painful during healing; possible damage to pubococcygeal muscle

2. **Nursing Process**
   a. Assessment
      1) use Reeda method
         a) *R*edness
         b) *E*dema
         c) *E*cchymosis
         d) *D*ischarge
         e) *A*pproximation
      2) hematomas
   b. Goal, Plan/Implementation, and Evaluation

   Goal: The new mother will learn to do perineal care correctly; will be free from complications.

   Plan/Implementation
   - inspect site daily for normal healing (use Reeda method)
   - promote comfort and healing of the episiotomy site by
     – ice pack 1st 24 hours if ordered
     – sitz bath

Table 4.16 Oxytocin (Pitocin)

Description	Posterior pituitary hormone that stimulates smooth muscle of uterus and blood vessels.
Uses	To stimulate contractions and ensuing cervical effacement and dilatation in labor; to induce or augment labor in women with "ripe" cervix, full-term infant, and absence of cephalopelvic disproportion
Dose	Dilute 10 units in 1,000 ml IV solution; gradually increase rate to maximum 120 ml/hour
Side Effects	*Maternal:* overstimulation of uterus resulting in rapid labor, delivery; uterine rupture following tetany; abruptio placentae; water intoxication *Fetal:* hypoxia, fetal distress
Nursing Implications	Monitor FHR and vital signs. Monitor contractions. Record, report changes in contraction duration, frequency. Discontinue infusion if contractions exceed 70–90 seconds duration or occur more frequently than every 2 minutes, if tetany occurs, or if fetal distress is noted.

- heat lamp treatment for 20 minutes, 3 times/day, 10–20 inches from perineum if ordered
- analgesic spray or ointment applications as ordered
- use clean technique when giving peri care
- teach new mother techniques of perineal care: dry perineal area from front to back, blotting rather than wiping; apply perineal pad (do not touch inner surface of pad); cleanse area front to back in shower daily

Evaluation: The new mother experiences minimal discomfort from the episiotomy; the episiotomy site heals free from complications (no signs of redness, discharge) within 3 weeks.

F. Forceps

1. **General Information**
    a. Definition: obstetric instruments that are used to extract the fetal head during delivery. Each consists of a blade, shank, handle, and lock.
    b. Predisposing Factors
        1) maternal factors
            a) to shorten 2nd stage of labor in dystocia
            b) expulsive efforts that are ineffective or deficient
            c) if pushing is contraindicated because of a chronic disease or cardiac problem
        2) fetal factors
            a) premature labor (to protect fetal head)
            b) fetal distress
            c) arrested descent
            d) abnormal presentation

Figure 4.15 Types of Episiotomies

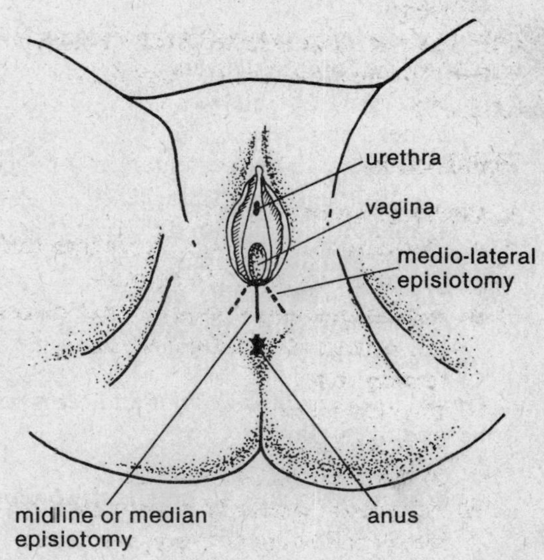

c. Prognosis
   1) perineal lacerations may occur with a difficult forceps delivery or may follow a precipitate delivery
      a) 1st degree laceration involves fourchette, perineal skin, and vaginal mucosa
      b) 2nd degree laceration involves skin, mucous membrane, muscles of perineal body
      c) 3rd degree laceration involves skin, mucous membranes, muscles of perineal body, and rectal sphincter
      d) 4th degree laceration involves all features of 3rd degree laceration plus tearing into the lumen of the rectum
   2) pressure by forceps on fetus's facial nerve may cause temporary paralysis of one side of the face
   3) perinatal morbidity and mortality increased, particularly with midforceps delivery
   4) increased risk of postpartum hemorrhage with midforceps delivery
   5) maternal implications following forceps or other traumatic delivery may include cystocele, rectocele, or uterine prolapse later in life
d. Types of Forceps Deliveries
   1) outlet or low forceps: fetal head on perineal floor
   2) midforceps: fetal head higher than level of ischial spines

2. **Nursing Process**
   a. Assessment: presence of prerequisites for low forceps delivery
      1) cervix fully dilated
      2) head engaged
      3) fetus in vertex presentation (or face with mentum anterior)
      4) membranes ruptured
      5) no cephalopelvic disproportion
      6) bowel and bladder empty
   b. **Goal, Plan/Implementation, and Evaluation**

   Goal: The pregnant woman and fetus will be free from trauma.
   Plan/Implementation
   - explain procedure to pregnant woman and significant other
   - provide physician with selected forceps
   - continuously monitor fetal heart rate during extraction procedure
   - assess neonate for forceps bruises

   Evaluation: The new mother is free from complications of forceps delivery; a healthy newborn is delivered with minimal trauma.

G. Vacuum Extraction
1. **General Information**
   a. Definition: the use of an obstetric instrument consisting of a suction cup attached to a suction pump for extraction of the fetal head; it employs negative pressure and traction
   b. Predisposing Factors
      1) prolonged labor
      2) fetal distress
      3) fetal malposition
      4) chronic maternal disease or complications that contraindicate pushing
   c. Prognosis
      1) increased risk of tissue necrosis of the fetal head, cephalhematoma, and cerebral trauma
      2) increased risk of trauma to vagina and cervix
      3) increased risk of postpartum hemorrhage

2. **Nursing Process**
   a. Assessment
      1) fetal status
      2) fetal position
   b. **Goal, Plan/Implementation, and Evaluation**

   Goal: The pregnant woman will understand procedure; the fetus will be delivered safely.
   Plan/Implementation
   - explain procedure to pregnant woman and significant other
   - assemble necessary equipment
   - provide continuous monitoring of fetal heart rate
   - pump the suction apparatus according to hospital protocol or physician's order
   - assess newborn for caput and cerebral swelling

   Evaluation: The newborn is delivered safely, using the vacuum extractor.

H. Cesarean Birth
1. **General Information**
   a. Definition: delivery of a newborn through abdominal wall and uterine incisions. The procedure may be prearranged and performed prior to the

onset of labor (elective) or unplanned and initiated after the onset of labor (emergency).
- b. Indications
  1) cephalopelvic disproportion
  2) weakened or defective uterine scar, caused by previous cesarean birth or other uterine surgery
  3) severe preeclampsia, eclampsia, or poorly controlled diabetes
  4) placenta previa or premature separation
  5) dystocia
  6) pelvic tumors
  7) maternal vaginal infection (e.g., herpes virus type 2 or gonorrhea)
  8) fetal distress
  9) prolapsed cord
  10) fetal abnormalities (e.g., hydrocephalus)
  11) abnormal presentations (e.g., breech)
  12) multiple birth
- c. Prognosis
  1) related to the reasons the cesarean delivery was performed, the type of procedure used, length of time membranes were ruptured, and the nature of complications occurring
  2) perinatal mortality increases with fetal immaturity and complications compromising uteroplacental blood exchange
- d. Types (see figure 4.16)
  1) classical: vertical incision is made through the visceral peritoneum and into the full body of the uterus above the bladder; performed infrequently
     a) advantages: simple and rapid to perform, useful when there is an anterior placenta previa
     b) disadvantages
        - potential for rupture of the scar with subsequent pregnancy
        - increased risk of small bowel adhesion to the suture line
  2) lower segment: incision made into the lower segment of the uterus
  3) extraperitoneal: incision is made into the lower uterine segment without entering the peritoneal cavity

2. Nursing Process
- a. Assessment
  1) indication
  2) maternal and fetal well-being
  3) pain and anxiety

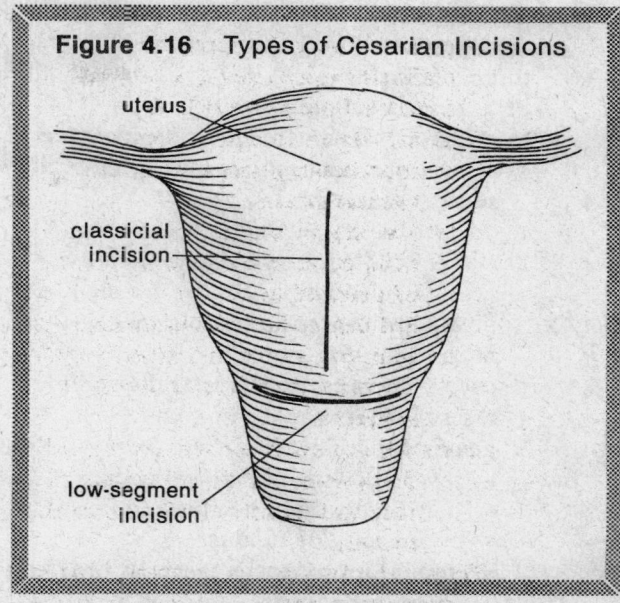

Figure 4.16 Types of Cesarian Incisions

- b. Goals, Plans/Implementation, and Evaluation

Goal 1: Preoperatively, the pregnant woman and fetus will be monitored for early signs of distress; will be physically and emotionally prepared for the cesarean birth.

Plan/Implementation
- pre-op care will vary with an elective versus an emergency cesarean birth
- explain procedures involved
- ensure that informed consent is obtained
- perform or request laboratory studies: type and crossmatch, CBC, Hgb, and Hct, Rh
- begin intravenous therapy as ordered
- shave abdomen from xiphoid cartilage down to the pubic area
- insert Foley catheter
- monitor maternal vital signs continuously
- monitor fetal heart rate
- assess for signs of labor
- teach post-op breathing exercises and coughing
- provide emotional support
- administer pre-op medications as ordered by physician
- have emergency equipment available for resuscitation of mother and newborn

Evaluation: The pregnant woman and fetus show no signs of distress.

Goal 2: The mother will tolerate surgery; postoperatively, will achieve homeostasis;

will initiate maternal-infant bonding. The neonate will be free from preventable complications.

Plan/Implementation
- assist physician with surgical procedure as necessary and monitor maternal-fetal status
- post-op, assess vital signs q15min until stabilized, then q2-4h as indicated by woman's condition; observe for signs of post-anesthetic recovery, e.g., leg movement after spinal
- encourage deep breathing and coughing
- assess for signs and symptoms of hemorrhage
  - inspect lochia on perineal pads
  - palpate position, height, and consistency of fundus
  - administer oxytocin agents as ordered by physician
- monitor I&O
- administer analgesics and sedatives as ordered by physician to promote comfort and relaxation
- provide assistance as necessary during mother-infant interactions
- know that Foley catheter and intravenous therapy may be continued until peristalsis returns and woman tolerates fluids (usually 24–48 hours)
- assess for signs of infection at wound site, perineum (e.g., redness, swelling, drainage)
- assess for respiratory problems
- ensure progressive ambulation
- instruct on techniques of perineal and breast care
- anticipate possible feelings of failure and provide emotional support to help mother and significant other integrate the experience

Evaluation: The mother is free from complications; maintains comfort during the postoperative period; maternal-infant bonding is initiated; mother and infant are discharged in satisfactory condition.

I. **Rupture of the Uterus**
  1. **General Information**
     a. Definition: the uterus ruptures from the stress of labor; rupture may be complete or partial
     b. Occurrence: rare, 1 in every 2,000 births
     c. Predisposing Factors
        1) previous surgery of myometrium or cesarean birth
        2) oxytocin (Pitocin) induction (2nd most common cause)
        3) nonprogressive labor
        4) very intense contractions
        5) faulty position or fetal abnormalities
        6) injudicious use of forceps
     d. Prognosis
        1) maternal mortality 5%–10%
        2) fetal mortality is high: 50%–75%
  2. **Nursing Process**
     a. **Assessment:** signs and symptoms (onset sudden)
        1) sharp abdominal pain (during contractions)
        2) tachypnea, tachycardia, anxiety, cool and clammy skin, confusion (shock)
        3) absence of uterine contractions (with complete rupture)
        4) uterus palpated as a hard mass adjacent to fetus
        5) hemorrhage into the abdominal cavity and/or vagina
        6) abdominal tenderness
     b. **Goal, Plan/Implementation, and Evaluation**

     Goal: The pregnant woman will have her condition diagnosed and treated before uterus ruptures; if rupture occurs, hemorrhage will be controlled.

     Plan/Implementation
     - take careful assessments during labor, reporting any signs of an impending rupture
     - implement appropriate measures with failure to progress
     - if surgery ordered in labor, rapidly prepare client for cesarean birth, possible hysterectomy
     - provide emotional support to couple

     Evaluation: Neonate is delivered safely; hemorrhage is controlled.

J. **Amniotic Fluid Embolism**
  1. **General Information**
     a. Definition: the entrance of amniotic fluid into the maternal circulation through the placental site and venous sinuses
     b. Occurrence: extremely rare complication that occurs in the intrapartum or early postpartum period
     c. Predisposing Factors: rapid, intense contractions from oxytocin infusion; multiparity with large fetus

d. Prognosis
   1) fetal death will result if delivery is not implemented immediately
   2) maternal death may occur within 1–2 hours if emergency interventions are ineffective
   3) presence of meconium and/or mucus in amniotic fluid is indicative of increased lethality, graver outlook

2. **Nursing Process**
   a. **Assessment:** signs and symptoms
   1) sudden dyspnea and cyanosis
   2) profound shock with uterine relaxation
   b. **Goal, Plan/Implementation, and Evaluation**

   Goal: The pregnant woman with an amniotic fluid embolism will be given the critical care necessary to sustain maternal-fetal well-being.

   Plan/Implementation
   - provide basic critical care
     - take vital signs q15min
     - assess level of consciousness
     - give fluid replacement as ordered, to prevent hypovolemia
   - administer oxygen under positive pressure
   - observe for complications such as disseminated intravascular coagulation (DIC) (the formation of multiple tiny blood clots, often due to the release of large amounts of thromboplastin into the maternal circulation as a result of damage to the uterus or placental site)
   - give fibrinogen IV as ordered
   - condition is characterized by hypofibrinogenemia

   Evaluation: The pregnant woman survives the critical period free from complications (e.g., pulmonary infarct).

Postpartal Care

General Concepts

A. Normal Childbearing

1. Definition: the postpartum period (puerperium) starts immediately after delivery and is completed when the reproductive tract has returned to the normal nonpregnant state (usually defined as 6 weeks)
2. Restoration to Pregravid Status
   a. Uterine Involution
      1) process of involution takes 4–6 weeks to complete
         a) weight of uterus decreases from 2 lb to 2 oz
         b) hormones decrease
         c) autolysis occurs (enzyme action)
         d) contractions increase muscle tone
         e) vasoconstriction occurs at placental site
         f) endometrium regenerates
         g) fundus steadily descends into true pelvis; fundal height decreases about 1 finger breadth (1 cm) per day; by 10 days postpartum, cannot be palpated abdominally
      2) factors delaying involution
         a) multiparity
         b) conditions causing overdistention of uterus
         c) infection
         d) retained placenta or membranes
         e) hormonal deficiencies
      3) cervical involution
         a) after one week, muscle begins to regenerate
         b) small lacerations may heal or need cauterization
         c) external os remains wider than in a nonparous woman
         d) internal os closed after one week
      4) lochia
         a) constituents: blood, mucus, particles of decidua, cellular debris, leukocytes, RBCs
         b) changes from rubra (delivery day to day 3: bright red) to serosa (days 4–10: brownish pink) to alba (days 10–14: white, due to increased leukocytes); normally has fleshy odor; decreases daily in amount; increases with ambulation
         c) signs of abnormal lochia
            • foul smell
            • excessive amount (any stage)
            • scant (during rubra stage)
            • return to rubra after serosa and/or alba
      5) after-birth pains due to contraction of uterus are reported primarily in multiparas as well as in mothers
         a) with a history of blood clots
         b) who were treated with oxytocic drugs
         c) who breast-feed their infant
         d) who had an overdistended uterus during pregnancy (large baby, multiple gestation, polyhydramnios)

Table 4.17 Lochia Changes

Time Postpartum	Characteristics
Delivery–day 3	Lochia rubra (red)
4–10 days	Lochia serosa (brownish to pink)
10–14 days	Lochia alba (white)

b. Perineal Healing
   1) vaginal distention decreases although muscle tone is never restored completely to its pregravid state
   2) vaginal rugae begin to reappear around 3rd week
   3) lacerations or episiotomy suture line gradually heal
   4) hemorrhoids common, generally subside
c. Bladder and Bowel Function: physiologic adaptations include
   1) increased urinary output due to normal diuresis
   2) increased bladder capacity; trauma to the bladder during delivery may diminish urge to void
   3) urine may show increased acetone, nitrogen, albumin, and lactose
   4) edema of the urethra and vulva
   5) GI tract motility sluggish because of
      a) relaxed abdominal and intestinal muscles
      b) decreased intra-abdominal pressure because of distention of the abdominal wall
d. Restoration of Abdominal Wall
   1) abdomen may be soft and flabby, usually returns to normal state by 6-8 weeks
   2) striae fade to silvery white; linea nigra fades
e. Breast Changes: condition of breasts during pregnancy maintained for 1st 2 days postpartum; physiologic adaptations include
   1) establishment of lactation
      a) colostrum secreted during 1st 2-3 days postpartum
      b) prolactin released from anterior pituitary gland
      c) oxytocin (released from posterior pituitary) causes let-down reflex
   2) engorgement
      a) onset usually day 3
      b) lasts 24-48 hours
      c) caused by venous and lymphatic stasis of the breasts
   3) mechanism of lactation: sucking activates nerve impulses from nipple to spinal cord to pituitary gland
      a) anterior pituitary gland produces prolactin only if breasts are emptied; seems to inhibit FSH and LH
      b) posterior pituitary gland secretes oxytocin, causing let-down reflex when milk is ejected from ducts
   4) effect on mother
      a) increased metabolic-system stress
      b) loss of large amounts of stored protein and fats
      c) increased need for calcium and phosphorus
      d) hastens involution of uterus, may decrease incidence of breast cancer
      e) enhances physical closeness with infant (usually pleasurable)
   5) infant's sucking stimulates milk production of 200–300 ml (6–10 oz) by day 4; by end of 6 weeks, about 600 ml/day
f. General Physiologic Status
   1) restoration of energy reserves
      a) immediate need for sleep
      b) subsequent need for sleep and rest increased
   2) blood
      a) decreased in volume
      b) moderate anemia if excessive blood loss at delivery
      c) leukocytosis immediately after delivery
      d) elevated fibrinogen levels during 1st week postpartum; may contribute to thrombophlebitis
   3) weight loss
      a) usually 1–12 lb immediately because of baby, placenta, amniotic fluid, and diuresis
      b) 5 lb in following week
   4) vital signs
      a) temperature: 1st day may be 38°C (100.4°F)
      b) pulse: initially decreases postpartum, range 50–70
      c) blood pressure: normal limits
3. Maternal Psychologic Adaptation
   a. Adaptive Responses to Parental Role (Rubin, 1961)
      1) taking-in phase: 1st 2–3 days postpartum
         a) passive and dependent behavior
         b) mother focuses upon own needs rather than baby's, i.e., sleeping and eating

434 SECTION 4: NURSING CARE OF THE CHILDBEARING FAMILY

- c) verbalizations center on reactions to delivery (help integrate experience)
- d) beginning to recognize child as an individual
2) taking-hold phase: 3rd to 10th day postpartum
   - a) mother strives for independence; wants to care for self and child
   - b) strong element of anxiety
     - unsure of mothering role (primipara)
     - unsure of own ability to physically care for child
   - c) stage of maximum readiness for learning
   - d) interested in learning baby care
   - e) may show mood swings
3) letting-go phase: 10 days to 6 weeks
   - a) achieves independent, realistic role transition
   - b) learns to accept baby as separate person and establishes new norms for self
  b. Parent-Infant Bonding and Attachment (Maternal and Paternal)
   1) parental behavior
     - a) holds infant in en face position
     - b) explores infant with fingertips/palms
     - c) addresses infant by name
     - d) verbalizes positively about baby
     - e) focuses on infant's eyes
   2) mastery of infant care skills (i.e., bathing, feeding, burping)
  c. Postpartum Blues: occur in some new mothers; timing and severity of symptoms vary and may occur in hospital but more likely to occur after discharge

1) manifestations
   - a) loss of energy and general fatigue
   - b) crying spells
   - c) anxiety and fear
   - d) insomnia
   - e) concerns focusing upon her body
2) theories of etiology
   - a) stress of labor
   - b) hormonal changes
   - c) immaturity
   - d) need for rest
   - e) family problems

B. **Application of the Nursing Process to Normal Childbearing, Postpartal Care**
  1. Assessment
     a. Degree of Homeostasis Achieved
     b. Vital Signs
     c. Fundus: height, consistency, and position
     d. Lochia: amount, color, consistency, and odor
     e. Perineum: swelling, redness, tenderness; episiotomy site: intactness, discharge, ecchymosis
     f. Bladder: distention and displacement
     g. Bowel: constipation
     h. Breasts/nipples: secretions, engorgement; nipple variations
     i. Psychologic Status
  2. Goals, Plans/Implementation, and Evaluation

  Goal 1: The mother will be monitored for increasing degree of homeostasis.
  Plan/Implementation
  - on admission to postpartum unit, take vital signs
    - bradycardia (50-70/minute) common 1st 6-10 days postpartum

---

Table 4.18 Maternal Psychologic Adaptation (Rubin)

Phase	Characteristics	Nursing Interventions
Taking in (1-2 days postpartum)	Mother passive, dependent, concerned with own needs; verbalizes delivery experience	Assist mother in meeting physical needs; structure day for her. Allow time for verbalization.
Taking hold (3rd-10th day postpartum)	Mother strives for independence; strong anxiety element; maximal stage of learning readiness	Teach infant care, stay with parents during care and activities. Provide positive reinforcement of parenting abilities.

- temperature may be elevated within 1st 24 hours because of dehydration
- temperature of 38°C (100.4°F) or above on any 2 consecutive postpartal days is considered febrile (excluding 1st 24 hours); possible causes: endometritis, urinary tract infection
- take BP; initially may drop after birth, then returns to normal
• orient to unit
• review antepartum and intrapartum records for
  - pertinent historic data
  - rubella titer (need for vaccination after postpartum checkup)
  - hemagglutination inhibition (HAI): less than 1:8 indicates susceptibility
• provide ongoing postpartal care
  - continue to monitor fundus, lochia, and perineal healing
  - check fundus a minimum of q8h for size, consistency, and position
  - take vital signs and BP q4–8h
  - increase fluid intake to avoid constipation; provide diet high in roughage
  - ambulate early
• promote perineal healing and relief of perineal and hemorrhoidal discomfort
  - inspect episiotomy daily for normal healing; observe for swelling, redness, lacerations, ecchymosis, and hematomas
  - ice pack during 1st 24 hours to prevent edema as ordered
  - sitz baths, cool astringent compresses, anesthetics
  - analgesics and/or topical medications as ordered
  - heat lamp treatments for 20 minutes, 3 times/day, 10–20 inches from perineum if ordered
  - use clean technique when giving peri care
  - teach self-peri care: dry perineal area from front to back, blotting rather than wiping; apply perineal pad (do not touch inner surface of pad when applying); cleanse area front to back in shower daily
• treat after-birth pains by
  - encouraging frequent voiding
  - advising mother to lie on her abdomen
  - giving analgesics as ordered
• give RhoGam if ordered; indication
  - unsensitized Rh negative women bearing Rh-positive children; given within 72 hours of delivery of Rh-positive infant
  - research is still in progress on antepartal use of RhoGam for selected clients
• check for tautness and pain in calf when foot is flexed and leg extended (Homans' sign of thrombophlebitis)
• observe abdomen for muscle tone, diastasis recti abdominis; measure degree of any diastasis
• assess bowel and bladder function
  - encourage usual voiding patterns; if mother is unable to urinate for 8 or more hours following delivery, catheterization may be necessary
  - recognize signs of bladder distention
  - measure initial voidings
  - check for signs of urinary infection (e.g., frequency, burning)
  - use stool softeners, cathartics, and enemas as ordered by physician
• observe lochia

Evaluation: The new mother has stabilized vital signs, adequate intake and output; experiences minimal pain and discomfort.

Goal 2: The new mother will be knowledgeable about breast changes, breast care, lactation, or suppression of lactation.

Plan/Implementation
• cleanse breasts daily; breast-feeding mother should wash nipples with clear water only (nipples are cleansed by natural antiseptic lysozyme)
• air dry nipples for 15–30 minutes after breast-feeding
• apply bland cream or ointment (e.g., lanolin) to sore nipples after feeding
• explain mechanisms of lactation
• help infant to breast as needed; explain and demonstrate proper positioning of infant to mother
• teach lactating mother to relieve breast engorgement (e.g., frequent emptying of breasts by nursing, manual expression, or breast pump)
• for discomfort, apply warm packs prior to feeding for 15 minutes; ice packs may be used in between feedings

- to prevent breakdown of breast musculature and provide comfort, advise to wear supportive nursing bra
- give analgesics as ordered
- observe breasts for
  - colostrum secretion
  - engorgement
  - nipple inversion or cracking
  - inflammation and/or pain
- for non-lactating client, provide supportive bra, ice packs, medications; do not express milk

Evaluation: The new mother demonstrates correct care of breasts, wears a supportive bra; lactating mother knows how to express milk (manually and via pump).

Goal 3: The new mother will have adequate nutritional knowledge to meet general nutrition needs and to supply additional calories/nutrients required for lactation.
Plan/Implementation
- review basic four food groups
- encourage nutritious snacks and increased fluids
- advise lactating mothers to increase amount of protein, calcium, iron, phosphorus, and vitamins (see table 4.5)

Evaluation: The new mother develops written menus for self and family for several days; can state amounts of daily requirements from each of the basic four food groups.

Goal 4: The new mother will learn requirements for immediate rest and appropriate exercises.
Plan/Implementation
- while in bed, elevate head to about 45° angle and elevate knees slightly (enhances circulation)
- avoid dangling feet when sitting on side of bed (constricts popliteal arteries and veins)
- ensure early ambulation to prevent thrombophlebitis and constipation. *NOTE:* If client had conduction anesthesia, have her maintain recumbent position for 10–12 hours
- encourage frequent rest periods during day and minimize interruptions
- teach client that postpartum exercises strengthen muscles of back, pelvic floor, and abdomen; Kegel or pelvic-floor exercises increase vaginal tone
- demonstrate exercises as needed; start mild exercises on 1st postpartum day and gradually increase

Evaluation: The new mother takes several rest periods during the day; performs postpartum exercises correctly.

Goal 5: Parents will continue to attach to the newborn.
Plan/Implementation
- encourage physical closeness between infant and parents; teach them to use eye-to-eye contact and en face position
- encourage physical examination of baby
- compare baby's likenesses to and differences from other family members
- explain how normal baby appears
- allow parents to verbalize their concerns and questions
- stay with parents during feeding and care activities as needed
- teach infant care and about infant behavior
- provide positive reinforcement of parenting abilities

Evaluation: Parents exhibit bonding behaviors (e.g., gaze at, cuddle, fondle, talk to infant), make positive statements about newborn.

Goal 6: The new mother will acquire knowledge regarding conflicts in maternal role.
Plan/Implementation
- explain the following
  - independency vs dependency
  - idealized vs realistic role
  - love and resentment of infant
  - self-fulfillment and motherhood
  - love for significant other and infant
- promote maternal psychologic adaptation
  - listen to and assist mother to interpret events of labor and delivery
  - clarify any misconceptions about the birth experience
  - encourage rooming-in or extended feeding periods with baby
  - obtain information for evaluating the future parent-child relationship, i.e., plans for newborn, naming
  - act as a role model in assisting the mother with her maternal tasks

Evaluation: The new mother states her own conflicts about maternal role, asks questions about own feelings, caring for baby.

Goal 7: Parents will receive adequate information for home care of selves, newborn, and siblings.
Plan/Implementation
- provide discharge planning and teaching information on
  - normal physiologic changes
  - expected weight loss
  - lochia: may last up to 3–6 weeks
  - changes in abdominal wall
  - perineal healing: episiotomy sutures dissolve in about 3 weeks
  - return of menses and ovulation (if mother not nursing, menses return within 6–12 weeks; in nursing mother, menses return within 4–18 months)
  - diaphoresis common in 1st 2–3 weeks ("night sweats")
  - maintaining lactation
- teach self-care needs: rest, sleep, balanced diet, increased fluids if nursing; proceed slowly with activities
- instruct to report any of the following
  - increased temperature
  - increased lochia or reverse in trend in lochia characteristics
  - signs of bladder infection (e.g., frequency, burning)
  - pain in calf
- demonstrate infant care skills as necessary (refer to General Nursing Goals 4 and 5 pages 455–456)
  - offer opportunity for mother to bathe infant in hospital, if possible
  - review feeding technique
  - answer questions about newborn care, behavior, and basic needs
- review approaches to manage sibling rivalry: extra attention and special times needed for other children
- discuss family planning
  - review of methods (pill, IUD, diaphragm, natural family planning) refer to reprints pages 471–477
  - use of previous methods
  - explain that breast-feeding is not a form of contraception
- discuss sexual adjustment
  - sexual intercourse may be resumed after cessation of lochia and when comfort permits (except if hematoma or infection)
  - fatigue and hormonal changes may influence desires
  - altered body image may affect satisfaction
  - if client plans to use birth control measures, instruct to begin as soon as she resumes coitus
  - consult physician before resuming use of birth control pills, diaphragm, IUD
- review need for follow-up medical care 4–6 weeks postpartum
  - to assess involution
  - to determine family planning needs
  - to provide early treatment of deviations (i.e., cauterize unhealed cervical lacerations)

Evaluation: Parents have knowledge and skills for self-care, infant care, and know what to expect in physiologic changes (e.g., decrease in lochia, perineal healing), when to resume sexual intercourse; plan to set aside separate and special times for newborn's siblings; have an appointment for follow-up care.

Selected Health Problems in the Postpartal Period

A. Postpartum Hemorrhage

1. **General Information**
   a. Definition: postpartum *bleeding of more than 500 ml* after delivery
   b. Predisposing Factors
      1) *uterine atony:* most common cause, often associated with
         a) conditions that overdistend the uterus
            - delivery of a large infant
            - multiple gestation
            - hydramnios
         b) multiparity
         c) use of deep general anesthesia
         d) premature separation of the placenta
         e) obstetrical trauma
         f) abnormal labor pattern (e.g., prolonged labor)
         g) oxytocin stimulation or augmentation during labor
         h) overmassage of an already contracted uterus
      2) *lacerations:* more common after operative obstetrics
         a) perineum
         b) vagina
         c) cervix

3) *retained placenta fragments*
c. Prognosis: leading cause of maternal mortality, 25% of all maternal deaths are from hemorrhagic complications
d. Types
   1) *early* postpartum hemorrhage occurs within the 1st 24 hours after birth; incidence is 1 in 200 births
   2) *late* postpartum hemorrhage occurs between the 2nd day and 6th week postpartum; incidence is 1 in 1,000 births; more common in women with history of abortions or uterine bleeding during pregnancy

2. **Nursing Process**
   a. **Assessment**
      1) inspection of placenta to determine intactness
      2) evaluation of vaginal bleeding postdelivery
         a) may be slow and continuous (most common) or rapid and profuse
         b) blood may escape from the vagina or accumulate in the uterus or maternal tissues
         c) bleeding from a laceration appears often as bright red vaginal bleeding in presence of a well-contracted uterus
      3) palpate fundus for firmness, height, and position
      4) signs of shock
      5) assess bladder distention
   b. **Goal, Plan/Implementation, and Evaluation**

   Goal: The woman will be monitored for signs of hemorrhage and shock; blood volume replacement will be safely administered as indicated.
   Plan/Implementation
   - remain with the client
   - massage boggy fundus gently but firmly, cupping uterus between 2 hands; avoid overmassage
   - administer oxytocic agents in 4th stage of labor as prescribed by physician
   - encourage frequent voiding
   - provide critical care during acute phase of hemorrhage
     - continually assess fundus (if hemorrhage due to atony); massage to firmness if boggy
     - give fluid replacement as ordered, to prevent hypovolemia
     - administer oxytocic drugs as ordered
     - O₂ per face mask at 4–7 liters
     - take vital signs q5–15min
     - assess level of consciousness
     - monitor I&O
     - monitor central venous pressure, if instituted
     - monitor blood replacement and observe for transfusion reaction
     - maintain asepsis, since hemorrhage predisposes to infection; give prophylactic antibiotics as ordered
   - assist with pre-op preparation if ordered (for surgical removal of retained placental fragments)
   - prior to discharge, teach mother signs and symptoms of possible late hemorrhage; this is especially important because of increasing number of early-discharge programs
   - counsel client to increase iron in diet; iron supplements and Imferon may be ordered Vit C.
   - arrange for follow-up care
   Evaluation: Mother is free from hemorrhage; has no signs of shock; knows signs and symptoms of late hemorrhage (e.g., vaginal bleeding, increased lochia) to watch for.

B. **Hematoma**
   1. **General Information**
      a. Definition: a collection of blood, often on the external genitalia, as a result of injury to a blood vessel during spontaneous or forceps delivery; occurs once in every 500–1,000 deliveries; most common site of a genital tract hematoma is the lateral wall in the area of the ischeal spines
      b. Predisposing Factors: prolonged pressure of fetal head on vaginal mucosa; forceps delivery
   2. **Nursing Process**
      a. **Assessment:** signs and symptoms
         1) complaints of *severe perineal pain or rectal pressure* (very important)
         2) visible large mass at the introitus or labia majora
         3) bruising
         4) pain upon palpation
         5) inability to void owing to pressure of hematoma on the urethra

6) signs and symptoms of shock in presence of well-contracted uterus and no visible vaginal bleeding
   b. Goal, Plan/Implementation, and Evaluation

   Goal: The new mother will experience no more than minimal discomfort while the hematoma is being absorbed.

   Plan/Implementation
   - carefully estimate size of hematoma and monitor to detect any enlargement
   - notify physician
   - promote general comfort
     - apply cold to site
     - administer analgesics as ordered
   - prepare woman for surgery, if indicated, to evacuate the hematoma
   - continuously assess for vaginal bleeding postpartum

   Evaluation: The new mother's hematoma does not enlarge; tolerates minimal discomfort well.

C. **Puerperal Infection**
   1. **General Information**
      a. Definition: any inflammatory process in the genital tract within 28 days following abortion or delivery of a newborn
      b. Criterion: an elevation in temperature of 38°C (100.4°F) for two consecutive days, with the onset after the 1st 24 hours postpartum
      c. Origin
         1) *endogenous*: infection from within or other preexisting infection
         2) *exogenous*: infection introduced by others and/or poor technique
      d. Predisposing Factors
         1) debilitating antepartal conditions
            a) anemia
            b) malnutrition
         2) debilitating conditions related to labor and delivery
            a) invasive procedures, e.g., multiple vaginal examinations
            b) operative obstetrical procedures, e.g., cesarean delivery, forceps delivery
            c) soft-tissue trauma and/or hemorrhage
            d) prolonged labor after membranes rupture
            e) prolonged labor resulting in weak, exhausted mother
         3) retention of placental fragments
      e. Prognosis
         1) one of three leading causes of maternal mortality
         2) outcome improved with early detection and appropriate medical and nursing management
      f. Types of Infection
         1) localized lesions of perineum, vulva, and vagina
         2) endometritis: localized infection of lining of uterus, usually beginning at placental site
         3) local infection may extend through venous circulation, resulting in
            a) infectious thrombophlebitis
            b) septicemia
         4) local infection may extend through lymphatics to cause
            a) peritonitis
            b) parametritis
            c) salpingitis
      g. Bacterial Causative Agents
         1) *Streptococcus hemolyticus*: very virulent, early onset and rapid progression; less common today
         2) *E. coli*
         3) mixed aerobic-anaerobic infection: low virulence, two or more species of bacteria present; tends to be contained locally (abscess)

   2. **Nursing Process**
      a. **Assessment:** clinical signs and symptoms of postpartum infection
         1) temperature greater than 38°C (100.4°F)
         2) lochia is abnormal
            a) remains rubra longer or becomes brown
            b) may have foul odor
            c) scant or profuse in amount
         3) tachycardia (may be 100–120/min)
         4) delayed involution
            a) fundal height does not descend as rapidly
            b) uterus may feel larger and softer
            c) woman may have pain and/or tenderness over the uterus
         5) pain, tenderness, or inflammation of perineum
         6) malaise
         7) fatigue

8) chills
9) abnormal lab results: leukocytosis, increased sedimentation rate
10) calf tenderness, positive Homans' sign

b. Goal, Plan/Implementation, and Evaluation

Goal: The new mother will be monitored for early signs and symptoms of a local or systemic infection; infection will be treated early, before complications arise.

Plan/Implementation
- determine source of infection and take measures to prevent a recurrence
- isolate woman, if indicated
- administer antibiotic therapy as prescribed by physician
- maintain adequate hydration with oral or intravenous fluids (2,000–4,000 ml/day)
- obtain specimens for culture and sensitivity as ordered
- take vital signs at least q4h
- administer oxytocic medications as prescribed by physcian
- encourage semi-Fowler's position to facilitate lochia drainage
- change peri pads frequently
- teach good perineal hygiene techniques and encourage hand washing
- use sitz baths and peri light to aid perineal healing
- maintain bed rest
- maintain increased high caloric fluids and high protein diet
- provide comfort measures; administer analgesics as ordered
- keep mother informed about condition of newborn
- if thrombophlebitis occurs
  - maintain bed rest with leg elevated
  - apply heat
  - administer anticoagulants if prescribed

Evaluation: The new mother shows evidence of response to treatment for infection (e.g., falling temperature, increasing energy).

D. Mastitis *rare*

1. General Information

a. Definition: an inflammation of the breast as a result of an infection, usually caused by *Staphylococcus aureus* or *Streptococcus hemolyticus*; mainly seen in breast-feeding mothers

b. Predisposing Factors: nipple fissure, erosion of the areola; overdistention, milk stasis

c. Prognosis: condition is generally preventable; prompt and appropriate treatment with antibiotic therapy significantly decreases maternal morbidity

2. Nursing Process

a. Assessment
1) blocked milk duct: hard, warm, reddened, and tender site; often in the outer, upper quadrant of the breast
2) mastitis
  a) fever
  b) breast may have red area, be warm to touch and tender; lump may be visible
  c) pain, chills
  d) engorgement
  e) axillary adenopathy
  f) tachycardia often present (usual time of occurrence is 2–4 weeks after delivery)
  g) headache

b. Goal, Plan/Implementation, and Evaluation

Goal: The new mother with mastitis will be treated to prevent further complications; will maintain lactation, if desired.

Plan/Implementation
- administer antibiotics as ordered by physician
- promote comfort of woman
  - support breasts (bra)
  - apply local heat or cold
  - administer analgesics as prescribed by physician
- maintain lactation in breast-feeding mothers
  - regular nursing of infant (controversial, will vary with physician) *[1–2 days don't breast feed]*
  - manual expression of breast milk
  - use of a breast pump
- encourage good handwashing and breast hygiene
- offer emotional support
- if necessary, prepare client for incision and drainage of abscess

Evaluation: The new mother does not develop a breast abscess; experiences only minimal discomfort; milk supply is maintained.

E. Postpartum Cystitis

1. **General Information**
   a. Definition: an infection of the bladder occurring in about 5% of postpartum women; usually caused by coliform bacteria
   b. Predisposing Factors: trauma to the bladder during vaginal delivery or cesarean birth; catheterization during and/or after labor

2. **Nursing Process**
   a. Assessment: clinical signs and symptoms
      1) frequency
      2) dysuria
      3) nocturia
      4) urgency
      5) hematuria
      6) slight elevation of temperature
   b. Goal, Plan/Implementation, and Evaluation

   Goal: The new mother will be free from signs and symptoms of cystitis; will maintain adequate fluid intake and output.
   Plan/Implementation
   - teach prevention
     - good perineal hygiene
     - frequent and complete emptying of bladder
   - increase fluid intake; monitor I&O
   - obtain specimen for culture and sensitivity
   - administer antibiotic therapy and analgesics as prescribed by physician
   - if woman unable to void within 6-8 hours of delivery and bladder distended, catheterization as indicated

   Evaluation: The new mother experiences decreasing signs and symptoms of cystitis (e.g., no burning on urination, no urgency); maintains adequate intake and output.

F. Uterine Prolapse With or Without Cystocele or Rectocele

1. **General Information**
   a. Definitions
      1) *prolapse*: downward displacement
      2) *cystocele*: relaxation of the anterior vaginal wall with prolapse of the bladder
      3) *rectocele*: relaxation of the posterior vaginal wall with prolapse of the rectum
   b. Predisposing Factors
      1) multiparity
      2) pelvic tearing during childbirth
      3) inappropriate bearing down during labor
      4) congenital weakness
      5) vaginal-muscle weakness associated with aging
   c. Medical Treatment
      1) preventive
         a) correctly performed episiotomy
         b) postpartum perineal exercises
         c) fewer pregnancies
      2) surgical intervention
         a) vaginal hysterectomy
         b) anterior and/or posterior vaginal repair (colporrhaphy)

2. **Nursing Process**
   a. assessment
      1) uterine prolapse
         a) dysmenorrhea
         b) cervical ulceration
         c) pelvic pain
         d) dragging sensation in pelvis and back
      2) cystocele
         a) incontinence or dribbling with cough, sneeze, or any activity that increases intra-abdominal pressure
         b) retention
         c) cystitis
      3) rectocele
         a) constipation
         b) hemorrhoids
   b. Goals, Plans/Implementation, and Evaluation

   Goal 1: Client will remain free from complications following vaginal hysterectomy and/or an anterior and posterior colporrhaphy.
   Plan/Implementation
   - general pre- and post-op care
   - administer cleansing douche and enema pre-op
   - instruct client to refrain from coughing
   - promote perineal healing as in postpartal care (page 435); note amount and character of vaginal drainage
   - avoid rectal temps or tubes

   Evaluation: Client's vaginal drainage is minimal, sutures are healing well.

   Goal 2: Client will regain normal urinary and bowel control and muscle tone.

Plan/Implementation
- monitor urinary drainage
- perform perineal (Kegel) exercises qh
- begin bladder training gradually
- gradually increase residue in diet
- administer stool softeners and mineral oil prior to 1st bowel movement

Evaluation: Client is voiding; passing soft, formed stool without difficulty.

G. Uterine Fibroids

1. **General Information**
   a. Definition: benign uterine tumors of connective tissue and muscle
   b. Incidence
      1) 20%–25% of women over 30 have myomas
      2) higher incidence in blacks
   c. Predisposing Factors
      1) infertility
      2) hormone usage
      3) age (often disappear with menopause)
   d. Medical Treatment: depends on symptoms such as bleeding, pressure, and client's age and reproductive status
      1) medical intervention
         a) close supervision
         b) no hormone administration
         c) reassess after menopause
      2) surgical intervention
         a) simple myomectomy
         b) hysterectomy
            - vaginal approach
            - abdominal approach

2. **Nursing Process**
   a. Assessment
      1) menorrhagia
      2) dysmenorrhea
      3) low back and pelvic pain
      4) constipation
      5) uterine enlargement
      6) history of infertility or miscarriage
      7) presence of predisposing factors
   b. Goals, Plans/Implementation, and Evaluation

Goal 1: Client will be maintained with conservative (medical) therapy until pregnancy and birth are achieved.

Plan/Implementation
- discourage hormone usage
- support client's decision for immediate pregnancy
- monitor for increased severity of symptoms

Evaluation: Client experiences no further increase in symptoms.

Goal 2: Client will remain free from respiratory, circulatory, or renal complications, or infections following abdominal hysterectomy with/without salpingo-oophorectomy.

Plan/Implementation
- collect baseline data pre-op and continue to assess post-op
- maintain fluid infusion; monitor I&O
- record blood loss: abdominal and vaginal
- turn, cough, and deep breathe q2h
- ambulate as soon as possible
- perform sterile abdominal dressing and perineal pad changes
- give Foley catheter or suprapubic catheter care as ordered

Evaluation: Client recovers from surgery free from infection; experiences relief of pain; is voiding well.

Goal 3: Client will experience minimal discomfort from abdominal distention.

Plan/Implementation
- know that this is a major complication of hysterectomy
- if NG tube in place, monitor patency
- give nothing PO for 24–48 hours
- be aware that post-op analgesics, particularly codeine, can cause constipation
- give enemas, rectal tube as ordered, if necessary
- ambulate as soon as possible
- give no carbonated beverages

Evaluation: Client remains free from abdominal distention; is passing flatus; has no nausea or vomiting.

Goal 4: Client will remain free from thrombophlebitis.

Plan/Implementation
- apply thrombo-antiembolic (TED) hose, thigh high
- give passive and active exercise to lower extremities qh
- ambulate as soon as possible and frequently thereafter
- put no pressure on popliteal space
- decrease pressure on femoral area
- evaluate calves for tenderness, positive Homans' sign

Evaluation: Client has adequate circulation in lower extremities.

H. Pulmonary Embolus

1. **General Information**
   a. Definition: the passage of a thrombus, often originating in one of the uterine or other pelvic veins, into a lung, where it obstructs the circulation of blood; usually occurs at end of 1st week postpartum
   b. Predisposing Factors
      1) infection
      2) hemorrhage
      3) thrombosis
   c. Prognosis: maternal mortality high with large and undetected clots

2. **Nursing Process**
   a. **Assessment**
      1) signs and symptoms
         a) sudden, intense chest pain
         b) severe dyspnea
         c) apprehension
         d) irregular, thready pulse
         e) pallor or cyanosis
         f) hemoptysis
         g) syncope
      2) shock
   b. **Goal, Plan/Implementation, and Evaluation**

   Goal: The new mother will receive early treatment of signs and symptoms of pulmonary embolus.
   Plan/Implementation
   - administer O$_2$
   - provide basic critical care to combat shock (flat in bed; monitor vital signs frequently; keep warm; increase IV fluids)
   - administer anticoagulants as prescribed by physician
   - know that streptokinase may be given to dissolve clots
   - continuously monitor vital signs
   - give emotional support to client and significant other

   Evaluation: The new mother receives prompt treatment for pulmonary embolus; is free from further complications (e.g., pulmonary infarct); shows signs of recovery (e.g., breathes easily, pulse regular and full).

I. Psychologic Maladaptations

1. **General Information**
   a. Definition: psychologic responses that reflect the new mother's distorted perceptions of self, infant, or family and which occur in the puerperal period
   b. Predisposing Factors
      1) separation because of maternal or neonatal problems
      2) physical health problems of mother
      3) social factors, e.g., family relationships, economics
      4) prior emotional problems

2. **Nursing Process**
   a. **Assessment**
      1) behavioral and psychologic responses, e.g., depression, anger, blues that persist
      2) maladaptations in attachment
      3) delusions, hallucinations
   b. **Goal, Plan/Implementation, and Evaluation**

   Goal: The new mother will receive early intervention for signs of psychologic maladaptation or psychosis.
   - refer client to resource: psychiatrist, nurse psychotherapist, pediatrician, support group, public health nurse
   - recognize early signs of problems
   - support positive parenting behaviors
   - refer client to obstetrician to evaluate physiologic status

   Evaluation: New mother receives prompt treatment and support for maladaptive responses or psychosis; shows signs of attachment to newborn, ability to care for baby, and feelings of self-worth.

The Normal Neonate

A. Definition: full-term neonate, appropriate-for-gestational age (AGA) (38-41 weeks; between 10th and 90th percentiles on growth curves)

B. General Characteristics
  1. Behavior
     a. Sleeping and Waking (Brazelton 1977)
        1) individuality from birth: each normal neonate has unique, *usually predictable* behavioral responses in the first days of life
        2) consciousness or state (reactivity)
           a) initial reactive period immediately after birth
           b) deep sleep state several hours after birth
           c) alternate periods of physiologic state and behavior
              - deep or light sleep
              - alertness (reactivity)
              - active alertness
              - crying
        3) unique ability to "comfort" self and to shut out stimuli (habituation or self-quieting)
     b. Sensory Responses to Environmental Stimuli
        1) *sight* (response to visual stimulation)
           a) pupillary and blink reflexes present
           b) vision present; can focus 8–12 inches
           c) some degree of color and pattern discrimination: prefers complex stimuli
           d) can fixate and track for short distance to midline
           e) focuses on human face
        2) *hearing* (response to auditory stimulation)
           a) *in utero*: responds to music and to sound of mother's voice
           b) *in neonate*: within hours of birth, responds to sound by generalized activity depending on reactive state
              - loud sounds elicit Moro's reflex
              - prefers appealing sounds
        3) *taste* (response to feeding)
           a) differentiates between sweet and bitter
           b) vigor of sucking may vary with arousal
        4) *smell* (response to olfactory stimulation)
           a) present as soon as nose is cleared of mucus and amniotic fluid
           b) sensitive, discriminates, e.g., odor of mother's breast milk
        5) *touch* (response to tactile stimulation)
           a) well developed
           b) reacts to painful and soothing stimuli
  2. Posture
     a. May assume prenatal position
     b. Assumes partially flexed position
     c. Resists having extremities extended
  3. Size (compared for length, weight, weeks of gestation on growth curves)
     a. Length
        1) normal range 45-55 cm (18–22 in)
        2) average: 49 cm (19.5 in)
        3) rapid growth in 1st 6 months
     b. Weight
        1) normal range 2,500–4,000 gm (5 lb 12 oz to 8 lb 13 oz)
        2) average weight 3,400 gm (7 lb 8 oz)
        3) 5%–15% of birth weight may be lost in 1st few days of life because of
           a) minimal intake of nutrients
           b) fluid shift
           c) loss of excess fluid (70% of neonate's body weight is fluid)
           d) passage of meconium

c. Head Circumference
   1) normal range 33–35 cm (13–14 inches)
   2) approximately 2 cm more than chest circumference
   3) essential assessment for suspected hydrocephalus
d. Chest Circumference
   1) normal range 30–33 cm (12–13 in)
   2) shape and measurements change as neonate grows
e. Symmetry
   1) face symmetrical
   2) ears symmetrical; placed opposite outer canthus of eyes
   3) bilateral asynchronous movements of extremities
4. Vital Signs
   a. Blood pressure: normal range 60–80/40–50 mm Hg
   b. Pulse: normal range 120–150/min (apical) if infant is quiet
   c. Respirations
      1) normal range 30–50/min
      2) irregular and shallow
      3) diaphragmatic and abdominal breathing normal
   d. Temperature
      1) normal axillary range 36.5°–37°C (97.6°–98.6°F)
      2) temperature should stabilize within several hours of birth

C. **Specific Body Parts:** usual findings and common variations
   1. Skin
      a. Texture: smooth, elastic
      b. Color
         1) pinkish or ruddy color over face and most of body
         2) color varies with ethnic background
      c. Erythema Toxicum (Newborn Rash)
         1) pink papular rash anywhere on the body, appearing within 24–48 hours of birth
         2) harmless and disappears within a few days
         3) must be differentiated from rashes found in infections
      d. Localized Cyanosis of Extremities (Acrocyanosis): peripheral circulation not well established
      e. Mottling (irregular discoloration of skin): due to vasoconstriction and lack of fat, hypoxia
      f. Birthmarks (e.g., port-wine stain, strawberry) may or may not disappear with age, depending on type and location
      g. Vernix Caseosa
         1) white, odorless, cheese-like substance on skin, usually found in folds of axillae, groin
         2) produced in utero; diminishes close to term
         3) gradually absorbed or washed off after birth
      h. Lanugo
         1) fine, downy hair on shoulders, back, upper arms, forehead, and cheeks
         2) gradually disappears close to term
      i. Desquamation
         1) dry peeling of the skin, particularly on palms and soles
         2) requires no treatment
         3) more pronounced in postmature infant
      j. Milia
         1) pinpoint white papules on cheeks, across bridge of nose, or on chin; caused by blocked sebaceous glands
         2) require no treatment
         3) disappear in a few weeks
      k. Nevi (stork bite): red spots found on back of neck and eyelids; usually disappear spontaneously before end of 1st year
      l. Mongolian Spots: areas of grayish-blue pigmentation most often found on buttocks and sacrum; increased frequency in specific racial groups; may disappear by school age
      m. Physiologic Jaundice
         1) yellowish discoloration of infant, skin, and/or sclera often appearing 48–72 hours after birth (physiologic jaundice or icterus neonatorum) (refer to "Neonatal Jaundice" page 457)
         2) is common and appears in 50%–70% of neonates
         3) disappears in 7–10 days
   2. Head
      a. Appears round and symmetrical; full movement to right and left, up and down; may be covered by silky hair in varying amounts
      b. Molding: the shaping of the fetal head to accommodate passage through the birth canal as a result of overriding of

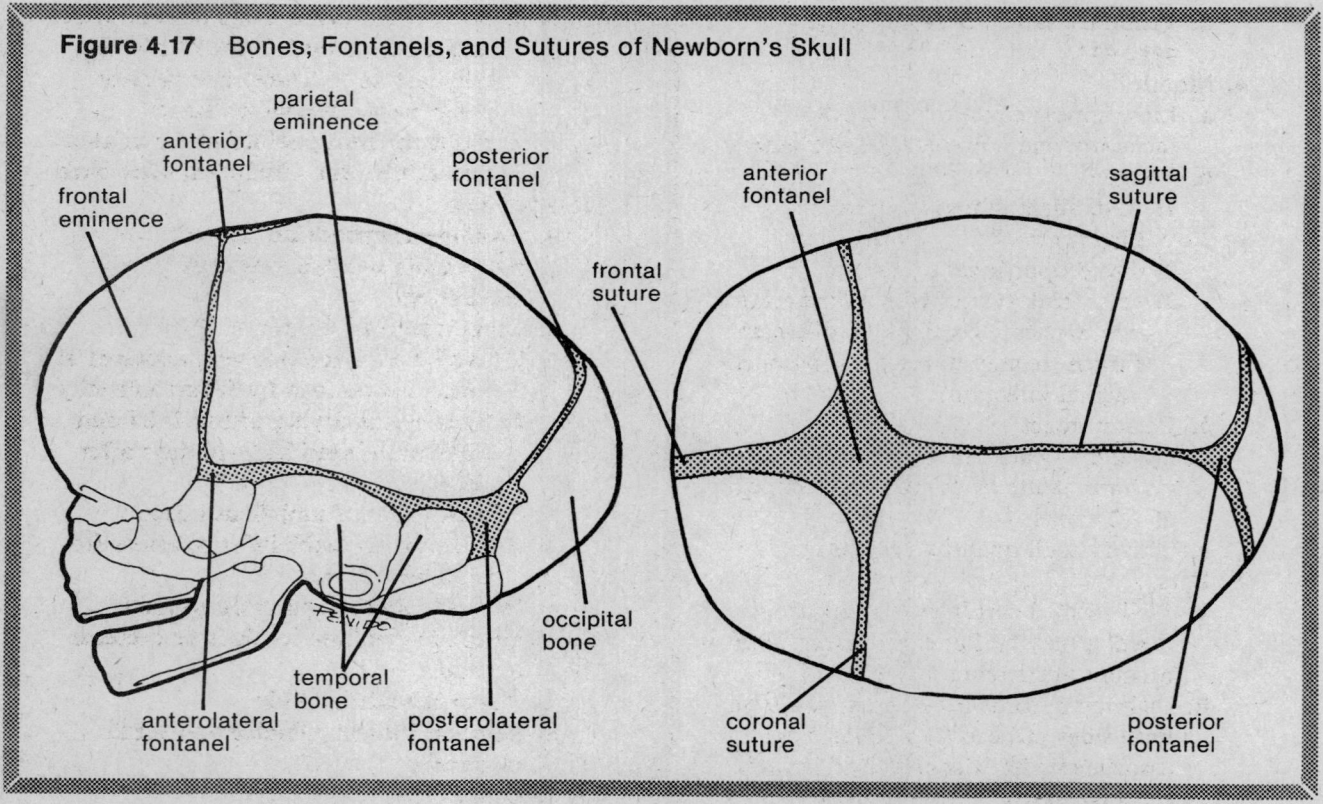

Figure 4.17 Bones, Fontanels, and Sutures of Newborn's Skull

the cranial bones; the head will return to its normal shape in about 2-3 days
  c. Cephalohematoma: a collection of blood between the periosteum and the bone of the skull
    1) caused by rupture of periosteum capillaries from pressure during the birth process
    2) swelling usually severe but does not cross suture lines
    3) spontaneously resolves in 3-6 weeks
  d. Caput Succedaneum
    1) edematous area under scalp, usually caused by birth process
    2) extends across suture lines
    3) is absorbed and disappears by 3rd-4th day of life
  e. Fontanels (soft spots)
    1) anterior
      a) diamond shaped, palpable
      b) 3-4 cm long, 2-3 cm wide
      c) found between frontal and parietal bones
      d) is closed within 18 months
    2) posterior
      a) triangular shaped, usually palpable
      b) 1-2 cm
      c) found between occipital and parietal bones
      d) is closed within 2 months
3. Eyes
  a. Appearance
    1) blue or grey-blue
    2) bright and clear
    3) pupils equal in size
    4) eyes evenly placed on face
    5) lacrimation in 50% of neonates not evident until 2-4 weeks old
  b. Movement
    1) to all directions
    2) poor neuromuscular control
  c. Common Variations
    1) subconjunctival hemorrhage: red spot on sclera, rupture of small capillaries during delivery; will be absorbed in about 2 weeks
    2) chemical conjunctivitis: inflammation with discharge, resulting from reaction of silver nitrate or other chemical agents (must be differentiated from infectious process)

d. Vision (refer to "Sensory Responses" page 444)
4. Mouth
   a. Lips: appear equal on both sides of facial midline; symmetry of movement
   b. Tongue
      1) in midline; moves freely in all directions
      2) size proportional to mouth
      3) color pink (varies with ethnic group); white, cheesy coating may indicate thrush (related to maternal monilial vaginal infection)
   c. Palate: intact
   d. Epstein's Pearls: small epithelial cysts on hard palate or gums; will disappear at 1-2 weeks
   e. Saliva: small quantity present
5. Ears
   a. Well-formed cartilage by term; recoil rapidly; may be flattened against skull because of pressure during birth
   b. Placement: same level and position on both sides of head (low set ears are associated with trisomy 13 or 18 and renal agenesis)
   c. Hearing (refer to sensory responses page 444)
6. Nose
   a. Shape: varies; may appear flattened because of delivery process
   b. Placement: evenly placed in relation to eyes and mouth
   c. Nares: bilateral patency; neonates are nose breathers
   d. Sneezing common
7. Neck
   a. Appears short; head moves freely
   b. Skin folds present
8. Chest
   a. Shoulders: sloping; width greater than length; bilateral expansion equal with respiration; no retractions
   b. Breath Sounds: loud and equal bilaterally; clear on crying
   c. Cough Reflex: absent; appears by 2nd or 3rd day of life
   d. Heart: rhythm regular, normal rate; usually heard to left of midclavicular space at 3rd or 4th interspace; may have functional murmurs (refer to page 445 for normal vital-sign values)
   e. Breasts
      1) flat; nipples symmetrical; breast-tissue diameter greater than 5 mm
      2) breast engorgement common in both sexes; occurs by 3rd day of life and may last up to 2 weeks; may have some nipple discharge due to maternal hormonal influence in utero and subsequent withdrawal after birth
9. Abdomen
   a. Prominent: cylindrical shaped; movements synchronous with respirations
   b. Umbilical Cord Stump
      1) two arteries and one vein apparent at birth, surrounded by Wharton's jelly
      2) cord begins drying within 1-2 hours after birth, shed by 7-10 days after birth
      3) protrusion of umbilicus often apparent in black infants; assess for umbilical hernia
   c. Diastasis Recti (separation of recti muscles): common in black or preterm neonates
   d. Bowel Sounds: audible
   e. Femoral Pulses: palpable and equal bilaterally
10. Genitalia
    a. Female
       1) labia majora cover labia minora; symmetrical, slightly edematous
       2) clitoris enlarged
       3) vaginal tag (hymen) may be evident
       4) a mucoid, vaginal discharge is common
       5) pseudomenstruation blood-tinged discharge is normal
       6) some vernix caseosa may be between labia
    b. Male
       1) urethral meatus evident at tip of penis
       2) foreskin covers glans; prepuce not easily retractable
       3) extensive rugae on scrotum
       4) testes descended in scrotal sac; if not, check inguinal, femoral, or abdominal areas for undescended testes
11. Buttocks and Anus
    a. Buttocks: symmetrical; anus patent
    b. Gluteal Folds: symmetrical
12. Extremities and Trunk
    a. Muscle Tone: good
    b. Position: extremities slightly flexed
    c. Arms and Legs: arms equal in length; legs equal in length; legs shorter than arms

d. Five digits on each hand and foot; freely movable, nails present
e. Normal palmar crease (simian line indicative of Down's syndrome)
f. Spine: straight and flat (prone position)
g. Fat pads and creases covering soles of infant's feet

D. Systems Adaptations

1. Neuromuscular: normal neonatal reflexes
   a. Sucking: neonate's tendency to suck any object that comes in contact with lips; essential for nutritional intake, oral satisfaction
   b. Rooting: neonate's tendency to turn head in direction of stimulus and open lips to suck when object touches cheek or mouth; disappears at 7 months
   c. Spontaneous Reflexes
      1) swallowing: usually follows sucking
      2) gagging: lifelong reflex
      3) yawning
      4) stretching
      5) sneezing
      6) hiccoughing
   d. Moro's: neonate's tendency to extend both extremities and then draw them up in normal flexed position in response to sudden movement or loud noise; most significant reflex indicative of CNS status; disappears at 1–4 months
   e. Grasp
      1) palmar grasp: neonate's tendency to grasp an examiner's finger when palm is stimulated; disappears at 4 months
      2) plantar grasp: neonate's tendency to curl toes downward when sole of foot is stimulated; lessens at 8 months
   f. Tonic Neck: neonate's tendency to assume a fencer's position when head is turned to 1 side; the extremities on the same side extend, while flexion occurs on opposite side; disappears at 3–4 months
   g. Stepping or Walking: neonate's tendency when held upright to take steps in response to feet touching a hard surface; disappears at 4 weeks
   h. Babinski's: neonate's tendency to hyperextend toes with dorsiflexion of big toe when one side of sole is stimulated from heel upward across ball of foot; disappears at 1 year
   i. Motor Function: head may be maintained erect for short periods of time; head lag less than 45°; movement of extremities may be jerky
2. Cardiorespiratory
   a. Circulatory Adaptations Occurring After Birth and Ligation of Umbilical Cord
      1) closure of ductus arteriosus, foramen ovale, and ductus venosus
         a) caused by changes in pressure in the 1st days of life
         b) allows oxygenation of all body systems
      2) closure of umbilical vessels after clamping of cord
   b. Pulses (reflect systemic circulation)
      1) femoral, brachial; easily palpable
      2) radial, temporal; more difficult to palpate
   c. Respirations
      1) initiation of respirations
         a) 1st breath: inflation of lungs in response to increased P_{CO_2} and lower pH
         b) reduction of pulmonary vascular resistance
         c) increased pulmonary blood flow
         d) recoil of chest causing replacement of fluids
         e) surfactant reduces alveolar surface tension
      2) respiratory secretions may be abundant
      3) may be irregular with short periods of apnea
   d. Blood Pressure
      1) may drop 1st hour of life
      2) crying and moving cause changes in systolic BP
3. Hematologic
   a. Blood Values (venous samples): average ranges for a normal, full-term neonate
      1) hemoglobin: 14–20 gm/100 ml (reflects oxygenation of tissues); broken down to bilirubin
      2) hematocrit: 42%–61%
      3) RBC: 5–7.5 million/mm^3
      4) WBC: approximately 20,000/mm^3 (10,000–30,000/mm^3)
      5) platelets: 100,000–280,000
      6) blood volume: 78–98 ml/kg depending on cord clamping
   b. Leukocytosis: normal; related to birth trauma

c. Fetal RBCs: have short life (100 days); hemolyzed RBCs deposit bilirubin in body tissues
d. Neonatal Jaundice (Physiologic Jaundice): common in 50% of neonates on 2nd or 3rd day of life because of deposits of bilirubin
e. Coagulation
 1) inability to synthesize vitamin K because of absence of intestinal flora normal in older people
 2) supplementary injection of vitamin K (AquaMEPHYTON) given prophylactically to promote normal clotting
4. Thermoregulation (temperature regulation)
 a. Adaptive Factors
  1) neonate responds to cold with increased motor activity and restlessness
  2) increased metabolism compensates for cold stress, since neonate does not shiver
  3) brown fat (or brown adipose tissue) is the neonate's major source of thermogenesis (2%-6% of body weight) (located between scapulae, around kidneys, sternum, adrenals, and in the axillae)
 b. Heat Loss: disproportionate to adult because of large skin surface to body mass; mechanisms of heat loss include
  1) *convection:* loss of heat from body surface to cooler surrounding air, e.g., infant placed in cool incubator
  2) *evaporation:* loss of heat from body occurring when fluid converts to vapor, e.g., wet infant loses heat immediately after birth in delivery room
  3) *conduction:* transfer of heat from warm object to a cooler surface, e.g., infant placed on a cold object
  4) *radiation:* indirect transfer of heat from a warmer object to a cooler one, e.g., infant loses heat to cool wall of incubator
5. Elimination (Gastrointestinal and Renal)
 a. Stools: change according to feeding
  1) meconium stool: viscous, dark green or black; formed of mucus, vernix, lanugo, hormones, carbohydrates; 1st one usually passed within 24–48 hours (if no stool passed, assess for imperforate anus, intestinal obstruction)
  2) 2nd–3rd day, transition stools begin: loose, slimy, green, and brown
  3) breast-fed neonates: golden yellow, mushy stools, often after each feeding
  4) bottle-fed neonates: soft, light-yellow stools; more formed
 b. Stomach Capacity: 50–60 ml; empties in about 3 hours
 c. Urination: neonate usually urinates in 1st 24 hours; if infant unable to void, assess for fluid intake and distention
  1) frequency: initially 6–10/day, then up to 20/day
  2) color: pale yellow (immature kidneys cannot concentrate); may appear cloudy if decreased fluid intake
  3) uric acid excretion is high; appears as red spots on diaper ("brick spots")
6. Immunologic
 a. In Utero: full-term fetus has had IgG (immunoglobulins) transferred; maternal antibodies may be present (depending on mother's immunity) for tetanus, diphtheria, pertussis, measles, mumps, rubella
 b. At Birth: immunologic system immature
  1) capable of some antibody response to immunizing agents
  2) phagocytosis ineffective
  3) cannot localize infection or respond with a well-defined recognizable inflammatory response, as can older child
  4) breast milk: contains IgA; gives immunologic protection from some infections
  5) elevated temperature may not reflect infection in neonate
7. Nutrition
 a. Sucks, swallows, and digests feedings; these reflexes may be weak in prematures
 b. Digestion
  1) unable to digest complete carbohydrates because of insufficient quantities of amylase
  2) can absorb simple CHO and protein
  3) fat absorption poor because of insufficient lipase
 c. Regurgitation is common
  1) cardiac sphincter is immature, nervous control of stomach incomplete

Table 4.19 Nutritional Comparison of Human and Cow's Milk

Nutrients	Human Milk (Breast)	Cow's Milk* (Whole)	Common Formulas†
Protein (gm)	10.12	32 §	15
CHO (gm)	67.82 ‡	45.4	72
Lipid	43.12	35.7	36
Calories	684.00	626.0	640

*Not given to newborns.
† Examples are Similac, Enfamil.
§ Because of the higher percentage of protein, cow's milk must be diluted to avoid kidney overload.
‡ Breast milk is higher in lactose, which limits pathogenic growth.

   2) neonates often spit up mucus in 1st 24 hours after birth
  d. Blood sugar normally 30–50 mg/100 ml (full term)
  e. Benefitted by immunoglobulins, enzymes, and lactobacilli in breast milk
  f. Psychologic Factors
   1) both bottle- and breast-feeding can be satisfying
   2) attachment facilitated by breast-feeding
   3) stress can inhibit successful breast-feeding
  g. Initial Feedings: breast milk or sterile water given 4–6 hours after birth to assess sucking reflex and absence of structural anomalies
  h. Subsequent Feedings
   1) bottle-fed neonates: q3–4h or on demand
   2) breast-fed neonates: q2–3h or on demand

E. **Gestational Age Variations Based on Neuromuscular Responses and External Physical Characteristics** (Dubowitz, Ballard)
 1. Premature Infant
  a. Definition: any infant born before 38 weeks gestation, regardless of birth weight
  b. Etiology: associated with chronic hypertensive disease, toxemia, placenta previa, abruptio placentae, incompetent cervix, infections, smoking, multiple gestation, inadequate maternal nutrition, maternal age under 20
  c. General Appearance: will vary with gestational age
   1) head large in proportion to body
   2) transparent appearance to skin
   3) lack of subcutaneous fat
   4) excessive lanugo
   5) immature neurologic system
   6) minimal flexion of extremities
   7) fontanels large; sutures prominent
  d. Associated Problems
   1) high mortality rate
   2) respiratory distress syndrome (RDS), related to immaturity of lungs and deficiency of surfactant (*NOTE:* L/S ratio determined by amniocentesis is helpful prior to delivery to determine lung maturity)
   3) infection: low WBC count, increased polymorphonuclear cells
   4) feeding problems
    a) regurgitates food easily
    b) may aspirate because of weak or absent suck-swallow reflexes
    c) may require gavage feedings
    d) breast milk or 24-calorie/ml formula advised
   5) hypoglycemia (glucose less than 20 mg/100 ml), caused by decreased glycogen and fat stores, decreased glyconeogenesis
   6) hypothermia and cold stress, owing to poor temperature control, increased surface area for cooling, extension of extremities, lack of brown fat
   7) jaundice because of impaired bilirubin conjugation in liver
   8) intracranial hemorrhage, related to birth trauma or hypoxia after birth

Table 4.20 High-Risk Conditions for Neonates by Gestational Age and Growth Classification

Growth Class	Gestational Age		
	Small for GA	Large for GA	Average for GA
Preterm	Apnea of prematurity Brain damage Congenital abnormalities Hyperbilirubinemia Hypoglycemia Infection Intracranial hemorrhage Meconium aspiration Neonatal asphyxia Polycythemia Pulmonary hemorrhage Respiratory distress syndrome Temperature instability	Apnea of prematurity Congenital abnormalities Hyperbilirubinemia Hypoglycemia Infection Intracranial hemorrhage Polycythemia Respiratory distress syndrome Temperature instability	Apnea of prematurity Congenital abnormalities Hyperbilirubinemia Hypoglycemia Infection Intracranial hemorrhage Respiratory distress syndrome Temperature instability
Postterm	Brain damage Congenital abnormalities Hypoglycemia Infection Meconium aspiration Neonatal asphyxia Polycythemia Pulmonary hemorrhage Temperature instability	Birth injuries Brain damage Congenital abnormalities Hypoglycemia Meconium aspiration Neonatal asphyxia Polycythemia	Birth injuries* Brain damage Meconium aspiration Neonatal asphyxia Polycythemia
Term	Brain damage Congenital abnormalities Hypoglycemia Infection Meconium aspiration Neonatal asphyxia Polycythemia Pulmonary hemorrhage Temperature instability	Birth injuries Congenital abnormalities Hypoglycemia Polycythemia	

*Large postterm infants
Source: Charles R. Drew Postgraduate Medical School, ©1978. Adapted from *Neonatal Postgraduate Program*. Reproduced by permission.

---

9) apnea, related to fatigue or immaturity of respiratory mechanism
10) oxygen therapy complications: retrolental fibroplasia, bronchopulmonary dysplasia (alveolar-bronchial necrosis)

2. Postmature Infant
   a. Definition: any infant born after 42 weeks of gestation (specific reference to potential intrauterine growth retardation)
   b. General Appearance: related to advanced gestational age and placental insufficiency
      1) thin, long infant
      2) dry, parchmentlike skin
      3) decreased or absent vernix
      4) little subcutaneous tissue; loose skin
      5) meconium staining of amniotic fluid (nails and skin stained yellow) related to hypoxia
      6) lanugo absent
      7) alert, wide-eyed (sign of hypoxia)
      8) nails lengthened
   c. Associated Problems: higher morbidity and mortality
      1) hypoxia: may be related to placental insufficiency
      2) hypoglycemia: caused by decreased glycogen stores

3) postmaturity syndrome with intrauterine asphyxia and fetal distress
4) polycythemia
5) seizure disorders: related to hypoxia (chronic)
6) cold stress related to minimal subcutaneous fat
3. Small-for-Gestational-Age (SGA) Infant
   a. Definition: any infant significantly underweight for gestational age (i.e., birth weight at or below the 10th percentile on intrauterine growth Denver curve); also known as intrauterine-growth-retardation or small-for-dates infant
   b. Etiology: associated with maternal malnutrition, pregnancy-induced hypertension, diabetes, drug addiction, alcoholism, smoking, maternal viral infections, prescribed or over-the-counter drugs, placental abnormalities or acute hypoxia, and other conditions affecting uteroplacental sufficiency
   c. General Appearance
      1) little subcutaneous tissue
      2) loose, dry skin
      3) loss of muscle mass in trunk and extremities
      4) desquamation
      5) length often normal yet weight decreased
      6) polycythemia: may be related to intrauterine hypoxia
      7) meconium staining of nails, skin
      8) appears alert because of hypoxia
   d. Associated Problems
      1) intrauterine infection if exposed to organisms while in utero
      2) asphyxia at birth: associated with intrauterine hypoxia
      3) hypoglycemia: caused by decreased glycogen stores and decreased glyconeogenesis
      4) hypothermia: related to decreased subcutaneous tissue and fat and poor thermal regulation
      5) congenital anomalies
      6) respiratory distress: often follows perinatal asphyxia
      7) hypocalcemia: may be related to asphyxia and respiratory diseases
      8) meconium aspiration; subsequent possible minimal brain dysfunction
4. Large-for-Gestational Age (LGA) Infant
   a. Definition: any infant significantly overweight for gestational age (birth weight at or above 90th percentile on intrauterine growth curve; usually over 9 lb 15 oz)
   b. Etiology: unclear; may be genetic predisposition associated with multiparity and maternal diabetes
   c. General Appearance
      1) fat and puffy
      2) may be edematous
      3) poor muscle tone
   d. Associated Problems
      1) birth trauma because of CPD
      2) hypoglycemia related to lack of maternal glucose
      3) hypocalcemia
      4) polycythemia
      5) congenital birth defects
F. **Application of the Nursing Process to the Normal Neonate**
   1. **Assessment**
      a. Immediate
         1) airway
            a) patency
            b) secretions: may contain mucus, blood, and amniotic fluid
         2) Apgar score: an assessment of heart rate, color, reflex irritability, muscle tone, and respiratory rate at 1 and 5 minutes after birth; provides index of infant's initial condition and baseline for subsequent assessments
            a) 0–2: severe asphyxia, extremely poor condition
            b) 3–6: mild to moderate asphyxia, fair condition
            c) 7–10: very mild or no distress, good condition
         3) gross appearance: appears to be free from obvious birth defects
         4) clamping of cord
            a) early: less possibility of placental transfusion
            b) late: expansion of neonate's blood volume, high systolic BP, higher Hgb
      b. Ongoing
         1) tracheoesophageal fistula or esophageal atresia, manifested by
            a) cyanosis during feeding
            b) immediate regurgitation
            c) inability to swallow feeding

Table 4.21 Apgar Scoring Chart

Sign	Score 0	1	2
Heart rate	Absent	Slow (below 100)	Over 100
Respiratory effort	Absent	Slow, irregular, weak cry	Good strong cry
Muscle tone	Flaccid	Some flexion of extremities	Well flexed
Reflex irritability			
• catheter in nostril	No response	Grimace	Cough or sneeze
• slap to sole of foot	No response	Grimace	Cry and withdrawal of foot
Color	Blue, pale	Body pink, extremities blue	Completely pink

d) fatigue
e) respiratory changes

2) body-temperature stability; heart rate, respirations
3) umbilical cord: check for 2 arteries and 1 vein; need cord blood sample if mother's blood is Rh negative or type O
4) eye care
5) parent-infant bonding

2. **Goals, Plans/Implementation, and Evaluation**

Goal 1: Neonate will adapt successfully to extrauterine life during the immediate period following birth.

Plan/Implementation

- immediately facilitate the establishment of respiration
  - clear air passages before onset of respirations (suction with DeLee or bulb syringe)
  - provide gentle tactile stimulation that aids breathing
  - assist physician with resuscitation as necessary (heart beat to respiratory ventilation rate is 3:1)
- prevent hypothermia: maintain neonate's body temperature and minimize heat loss
  - dry rapidly
  - wrap in receiving blanket
  - place on mother's skin, in warmed Isolette, or under radiant heater
  - LeBoyer method, bath may be given
- provide prophylactic treatment of eyes for protection against ophthalmia neonatorum with a 1% silver nitrate or other antibacterial agent such as penicillin (transient local redness and edema of neonate's eyes may follow instillation)
- when infant is stable, promote bonding/attachment
  - assist in positioning neonate
  - help initiate breast-feeding if mother plans to breast-feed infant
- place appropriate identification labels on neonate and mother; footprint may be taken
- weigh infant
- prevent hypoprothrombinemia by administering a single dose of vitamin K (AquaMEPHYTON) 1 mg IM, as ordered

Evaluation: Neonate maintains adequate oxygenation, breathes normally; maintains body temperature; is held by parent.

Goal 2: In the nursery, the neonate will be monitored closely for maintenance of homeostasis and early indications of difficulty (e.g., in breathing, feeding, eliminating).

Plan/Implementation

- check identification on admission to nursery, and re-weigh according to hospital protocol
- monitor neonate's condition (frequency of assessment determined by condition of baby and hospital policy)
  - assess apical pulse and respirations for 1 full minute
  - note periods of apnea
  - suction if mucus is excessive
  - position on side to promote drainage

Figure 4.18 Newborn Maturity Rating and Classification

Estimation of Gestational Age by Maturity Rating
Symbols: X – 1st Exam   O – 2nd Exam

Neuromuscular Maturity

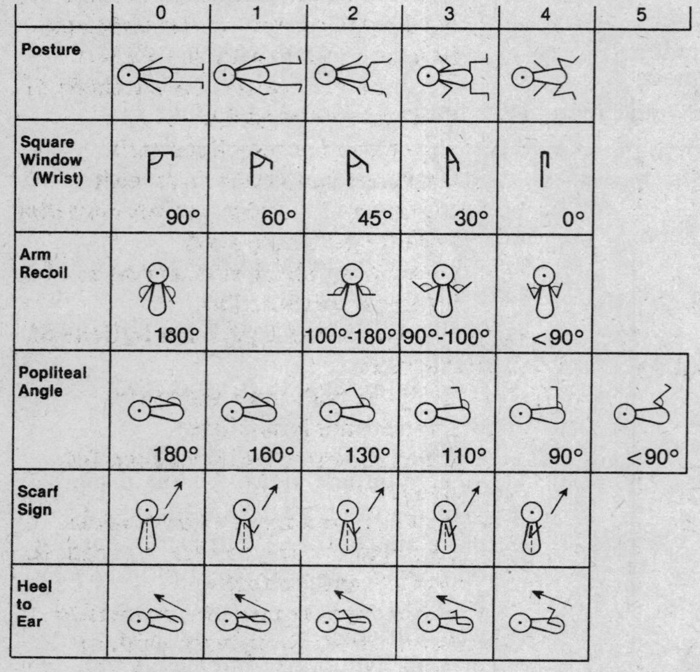

	0	1	2	3	4	5
Posture						
Square Window (Wrist)	90°	60°	45°	30°	0°	
Arm Recoil	180°		100°–180°	90°–100°	<90°	
Popliteal Angle	180°	160°	130°	110°	90°	<90°
Scarf Sign						
Heel to Ear						

Gestation by Dates _____ wks

Birth Date _____ Hour _____ am/pm

APGAR _____ 1 min _____ 5 min

Maturity Rating

Score	Wks
5	26
10	28
15	30
20	32
25	34
30	36
35	38
40	40
45	42
50	44

Physical Maturity

	0	1	2	3	4	5
Skin	gelatinous red, transparent	smooth pink, visible veins	superficial peeling &/or rash, few veins	cracking pale area, rare veins	parchment, deep cracking, no vessels	leathery, cracked, wrinkled
Lanugo	none	abundant	thinning	bald areas	mostly bald	
Plantar Creases	no crease	faint red marks	anterior transverse crease only	creases ant. 2/3	creases cover entire sole	
Breast	barely percept.	flat areola, no bud	stippled areola, 1–2 mm bud	raised areola, 3–4 mm bud	full areola 5–10 mm bud	
Ear	pinna flat, stays folded	sl. curved pinna, soft with slow recoil	well-curv. pinna, soft but ready recoil	formed & firm with instant recoil	thick cartilage, ear stiff	
Genitals Male	scrotum empty, no rugae		testes descending, few rugae	testes down, good rugae	testes pendulous, deep rugae	
Genitals Female	prominent clitoris & labia minora		majora & minora equally prominent	majora large, minora small	clitoris & minora completely covered	

Scoring Section

	1st Exam = X	2nd Exam = O
Estimating Gest. Age by Maturity Rating	_____ Weeks	_____ Weeks
Time of Exam	Date _____ Hour _____ am/pm	Date _____ Hour _____ am/pm
Age at Exam	_____ Hours	_____ Hours
Signature of Examiner	_____ M.D.	_____ M.D.

Scoring system: Ballard, J. et al. "A Simplified Assessment of Gestational Age." *Pediatric Research*. April 1977:374. Assessment of gestational age: Sweet, A. "Classification of the Low-Birth-Weight Infant" in *Care of the High Risk Neonate*, Klaus, M. and Fanaroff, A., Eds. Philadelphia: Saunders, 1979. Reprinted with permission.

- observe skin for color (jaundice or cyanosis)
- assess sclera and/or buccal mucosa (jaundice of these is a later symptom)
- observe for fatigue or respiratory changes during feedings
- after feeding, position on right side or prone to prevent aspiration
- maintain adequate nutrition by assisting new mother with bottle- or breast-feeding
  * fluid needs vary with age and size of infant
  * average intake of 17½ oz/day for 7-lb baby
  * calories: 80–120 cal/kg/day (birth to 5 months); most commercial formulas contain 20 calories/oz
- maintain a neutral thermal environment in which the neonate's metabolic rate and O_2 consumption are minimized, and body temperature is maintained within normal range
  - avoid unnecessary exposure of infant to cool air and environmental objects
  - neonate may need to be placed under radiant heater or in warmer–Isolette if axillary temperature is less than 36.6°C (97.8°F)
- note time of 1st urination and stool (passage of meconium); then monitor elimination
- weigh daily or every other day and record on chart; baby may take up to 10 days to regain birth weight
- prior to hospital discharge, obtain blood sample for phenylketonuria (PKU) (Guthrie test)
  - a disorder characterized by deficiency in the liver enzyme phenylalanine hydroxylase
  - leads to mental retardation if undetected
  - repeat PKU test will be needed if initial test was done prior to 48 hours of protein feeding

NOTE: in some states thyroid screening and other metabolic tests may be required

Evaluation: Neonate has vital signs within normal range; ingests nutritional fluids appropriate for size; has voided and passed meconium.

Goal 3: The neonate will remain infection free.

Plan/Implementation
- prevent infections from developing in neonate and spreading within nursery
  - use proper hand-washing/scrub technique to prevent staff-to-infant and infant-to-infant infection
  - exclude personnel with known infections from caring for neonates
  - instruct parents about importance of hand-washing and proper technique
  - isolate neonates with any signs of infection or neonates born outside of hospital delivery suite
  - assess skin for infectious rash
  - clean neonate's cord daily with alcohol and a designated antibacterial agent (e.g., Triple Dye)
  - periodically check cord for signs of infection and bleeding
- bathe and maintain personal hygiene of the neonate
  - delay 1st bath until neonate's temperature is stabilized
  - use plain water and mild soap for daily care
  - proceed from clean to dirty areas, i.e., eyes to face, to ears, to head, to genitals and buttocks
  - cleanse eyes from inner canthus to outer corner using wash cloth or cotton ball
- assess condition of circumcised male: keep area clean and observe for bleeding; a sterile dressing with petroleum jelly or antibiotic ointment may be applied to area during 1st 24 hours after circumcision

Evaluation: Neonate has normal temperature; no signs of an infection; is protected from exposure to infectious agents.

Goal 4: Parents will learn principles and techniques of infant care for home application.

Plan/Implementation
- assess parents' knowledge and past experience with child care (e.g., readings, care of other children)
- offer modified or complete rooming-in (provides an opportunity for mother to assume responsibility for her neonate's care before hospital discharge)
- encourage new parent's involvement in neonate care once condition is stabilized (fosters attachment)

- demonstrate techniques of bathing and daily care and safety
  - discuss need for bathing
  - emphasize safe handling of neonate
  - suggest timing of care (prior to feeding)
  - discuss environment and water temperature (room free from drafts; bath water warm to elbow 37°–38°C [98°–100°F])
  - teach correct cord care
    * use alcohol wipes to cleanse area
    * avoid tub bathing the neonate until the cord has fallen off (usually by 2nd week of life)
  - discuss diaper rash
    * emphasize frequent cleansing of diaper area to prevent rash
    * suggest exposure to room air several times per day
- allow mother to practice procedures in hospital
- assess and reinforce parent's handling of the neonate
  - emphasize support of head and back
  - discuss the importance of direct body contact and tactile stimulation
- assess parent's knowledge regarding feeding, and teach as necessary
  - schedule vs demand feedings
  - compare benefits of breast- vs bottle-feeding
  - burping of neonate
  - common feeding problems (e.g., regurgitation, constipation, hiccups)
  - position on side or abdomen after feeding

Evaluation: Parents demonstrate correct care of the neonate (e.g., feeding, bathing, holding).

Goal 5: Parents will know what to expect at home regarding neonate's sleep patterns, weight gain, and feeding.

Plan/Implementation

NOTE: criteria for discharge vary among hospitals; include variables of weight, gestational age, general health status of infant and mother, and status of home environment

- include a discussion of neonate behavior and development in discharge teaching
  - sleep needs: average 20 hours/day with wide variations among neonates; periods of intermittent alertness
  - crying: neonate's method of communicating basic needs (e.g., food, diaper change, affection)
  - nurturance: neonate needs to be held, loved, stimulated to develop a sense of trust
  - discuss plans for health care follow-up of neonate (clinic, physician, nurse practitioner)
  - refer to resource such as the public health nurse for assessment or assistance
  - teach reportable signs of problems, e.g., diarrhea, fever, vomiting, behavioral changes
- counsel on breast-feeding or formula preparation
  - frequency of nursing in home (every 2–3 hours on demand)
  - length of nursing time (infant obtains greatest quantity in 20–25 minutes)
  - importance of emptying breasts
  - positioning the baby for nursing (comfort of mother, infant to grasp nipple and areola)
  - discuss common concerns (sore nipples, supplementary feedings, expression of milk)
  - review methods of formula preparation, care of bottles and nipples (aseptic and terminal methods, dishwashing)
  - discuss bottle-fed infant's daily needs: intake approximately 3 oz, 6 times/day initially
  - introduction of solid food may be delayed up to 6 months
  - birth weight doubles by 5–6 months, triples by 1 year
  - average urination up to 20 times/day after first few days
  - average number of stools/day varies with feeding method (approximately 4–6/day)
- counsel regarding expected weight gain and elimination patterns (4–6 oz weight gain per week during 1st 5–6 months of life)
- discuss sibling adjustments to neonate

Evaluation: Parents demonstrate knowledge of correct infant care to provide at home; state home is equipped with adequate equipment; express confidence in ability to care for neonate.

The High-Risk Neonate

General Concepts

A. Definition: infant with higher than normal morbidity and mortality because of a situation or condition during the perinatal period.

B. Antepartum-Risk Factors: refer to "High-Risk Childbearing" in *Antepartal Care* page 389
   1. Previous History: abortions, premature deliveries, hypertensive disorders, diabetes, isoimmunizations
   2. Maternal Age: aged less than 17 years or more than 35 at time of conception
   3. Smoking, alcoholism, or drug abuse
   4. Infection
   5. Psychosocial Problems

Selected Health Problems (May Be Seen in Both Normal and High-Risk Neonates)

A. Hypothermia

1. **General Information**
   a. Definition: a drop in the newborn's body temperature below 36.5°C (97.7°F), produced by rapid heat loss to the environment. All newborns are at risk for heat loss because of their limited subcutaneous fat and large surface area in relation to body weight
   b. Predisposing Factors
      1) infants with reduced stores of subcutaneous fat, e.g., premature, postmature, SGA babies
      2) infants with reduced glycogen reserves, e.g., premature, nutritionally deprived, SGA babies

2. **Nursing Process**
   a. Assessment
      1) neonate's body temperature
      2) signs of cold stress
         a) increased activity level
         b) crying
         c) increased respiratory rate
         d) cyanosis
         e) mottling of skin
   b. Goal, Plan/Implementation, and Evaluation

   Goal: Neonate will expend a minimum amount of extra energy in the production of heat; periods of hypothermia will be avoided.

   Plan/Implementation
   - avoid heat loss in delivery room
   - refer to Goal 2 *The Normal Neonate* page 453
   - administer warmed air or O_2 to infant prn
   - monitor infant's temperature frequently; maintain axillary temp at 36.5°C (97.8°F), abdominal skin temperature at 36.1°-36.7°C (97°-98°F)
   - place crib or incubator away from draft and windows
   - keep portholes of incubator closed

   Evaluation: Neonate maintains a skin temperature of 36.1°-36.7° C.

B. Neonatal Jaundice

1. **General Information**
   a. Definition: excessive levels of bilirubin in the blood and tissues of the neonate (bilirubin is a product derived from the breakdown of erythrocytes and hemoglobin)
   b. Expected Levels of Serum Bilirubin
      (in mg per 100 ml)

	Full Term	Premature
1st 24 hrs	2-6	1-6
Day 2	6-7	6-8
Days 3-5	4-12	10-15

   c. Predisposing Factors
      1) prematurity
      2) isoimmunizations: maternal, red blood cell-destroying antibodies are

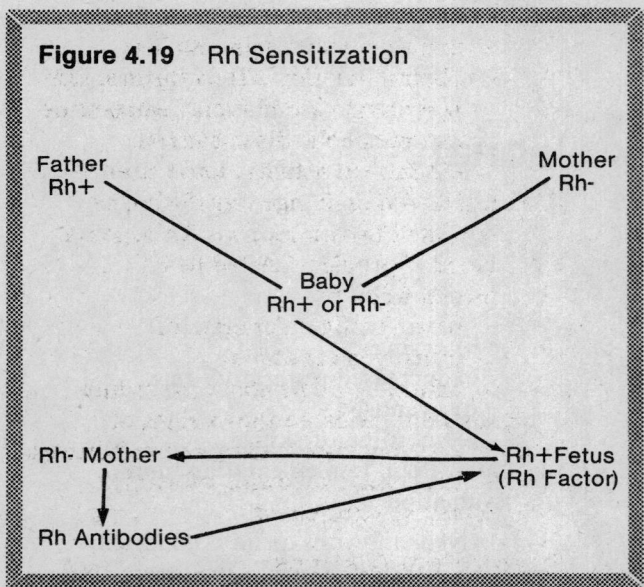

Figure 4.19 Rh Sensitization

transferred to the fetus, resulting in fetal erythrocyte destruction; after initial maternal sensitization occurs, the effects upon subsequent pregnancies with blood incompatibilities increase in severity
 a) Rh negative mother and Rh positive father may produce an Rh positive fetus; this leads to antigen-antibody response affecting subsequent fetus
 b) mother with type O blood and father with type A, B, or AB produce a fetus with type A, B, or AB (generally results in less severe disease than Rh incompatibility)
3) polycythemia
4) exposure to drugs in utero
5) sepsis
d. Common Forms
 1) neonatal (physiologic jaundice)
  a) onset
   • full-term infant: jaundice appears after 24 hours and disappears by end of 7th day
   • preterm infant: jaundice appears after 48 hours and disappears by 9th or 10th day
  b) bilirubin is unconjugated (indirect); below 6 mg/100 ml, and infant is without evidence of hemolytic disease or infection
  c) RBCs and WBCs are normal
 2) pathologic jaundice (hyperbilirubinemia)
  a) occurs within 1st 24 hours after birth
  b) characterized by rising bilirubin level in excess of normal
   • in full-term neonate: rises 6 mg/100 ml in 24 hours or value exceeds 12 mg/100 ml or persists beyond 7 days
   • in premature neonate: exceeds 15 mg/100 ml; persists beyond 10 days
  c) direct bilirubin greater than 1.5 mg/100 ml
  d) isoimmunization may lead to kernicterus (deposit of unconjugated bilirubin in basal ganglia of brain) when bilirubin levels rise over 20 mg/100 ml in full-term infants and over 9-10 mg/100 ml in preterm infants
   • signs and symptoms include problems such as
    – sluggish Moro's reflex with incomplete flexion of extremities
    – opisthotonic posturing
    – vomiting
    – bulging fontanels
    – twitching convulsions (late symptom)
 3) breast-milk jaundice: yellowing of newborn's skin caused by hormone pregnanediol, which inhibits glucuronyl transferase activity in conjugating bilirubin; bilirubin level begins to rise about 4th day, peaks at 10–15 days of age, returning to normal between 3rd and 12th weeks of age
e. Associated Problems
 1) hydrops fetalis (erythroblastosis fetalis) related to Rh or ABO incompatability: generalized edema, pleural and pericardial effusions, ascites
 2) hepatosplenomegaly
 3) progressive hemolytic anemia
2. Nursing Process
 a. Assessment
  1) prenatal history
   a) positive hemantigen test (maternal blood serum)
   b) positive indirect Coombs' (maternal blood serum)

2) early identification of infants at risk; includes those with
   a) predisposing factors
   b) delayed passage of meconium
   c) placental enlargement (may weigh ½–¾ of neonate's weight)
   d) visible jaundice of skin (bilirubin greater than 7 mg/100 ml)
   e) abnormal bleeding (e.g., extensive bruising or cephalohematoma)
   f) positive direct Coombs' test (neonatal cord blood)
   g) yellow-stained vernix on cord
3) signs and symptoms of polycythemia, especially in large-for-gestational-age infants
   a) decrease in peripheral pulses
   b) redness of hands and feet
   c) tachycardia
   d) respiratory distress
4) neonatal pallor with jaundice, appearing within 24–36 hours after birth
5) increased optical density of amniotic fluid

b. Goal, Plan/Implementation, and Evaluation

Goal: Neonate will be monitored closely for early signs and symptoms of neonatal jaundice; kernicterus (brain damage) will be prevented.

Plan/Implementation
- interpret laboratory values and recognize deviations from normal (i.e., rise in serum bilirubin, Hgb decrease, rapid decrease in hematocrit, positive Coombs')
- give appropriate dose of vitamin K as ordered (decreases prothrombin time)
- in case of antigen-antibody response due to Rh incompatibility (mother Rh negative, father Rh positive, infant Rh positive), phototherapy may promote absorption of bilirubin if neonate undergoes phototherapy
  - remove infant's clothing
  - protect eyes with eye patches (to prevent retinal damage)
  - turn frequently for maximum skin exposure
  - provide adequate fluids
  - feed q2–3h to prevent metabolic disorders
  - assess for signs of dehydration (e.g., sunken fontanels)
  - maintain lights 16″ from baby
  - monitor weight gain and loss
  - observe for side effects (bronze skin, peripheral vasodilation, temperature and metabolic disturbances, diminished activity, loose stools)
- assist with exchange transfusion as indicated (infant receives Rh negative blood if problem related to Rh incompatibility)
  - observe infant for signs of transfusion reaction
  - educate parents about procedure

Evaluation: Neonate shows signs of decreasing jaundice (falling serum bilirubin level, decreasing yellowing of skin); kernicterus is prevented.

C. Respiratory Distress

1. General Information
   a. Definition: difficulty in maintaining respiratory function adequate to meet oxygen needs; caused by a variety of complications in the newborn
   b. Predisposing Factors
   1) dysmaturity (SGA infants)
   2) prematurity (preterm infants)
   3) postmaturity (postterm infants)
   4) maternal diabetes
   5) maternal bleeding
   6) fetal asphyxia
   7) birth asphyxia
   8) pregnancy-induced hypertension
   9) prolonged labor after rupture of the amniotic membranes
   10) meconium-stained amniotic fluid
   11) low Apgar score
   12) cesarean birth
   c. Common Respiratory Disorders
   1) respiratory distress syndrome (RDS), also known as hyaline membrane disease
       a) definition: deficiency of surfactant activity leading to atelectasis, which prevents adequate gas exchange
       b) characterized by collapse of the alveoli
       c) most frequently affects preterm infants, especially those weighing between 1,000 and 1,500 gm; it is observed primarily in premature infants, infants of diabetic mothers, and infants of mothers whose pregnancies were

complicated by antepartum vaginal bleeding
2) meconium-aspiration syndrome
   a) aspiration of meconium-stained amniotic fluid into the lungs may occur with asphyxic or placental disturbances in utero
   b) associated with intrauterine-growth-retardation (SGA infants) and postmaturity (postterm infants)
d. Associated Problems
   1) hypoxia
   2) atelectasis
   3) bronchopulmonary dysplasia, retrolental fibroplasia (complications of O_2 administration)

2. **Nursing Process**
   a. **Assessment**
      1) using Silverman-Andersen scale: respiratory distress syndrome
         a) grunting: sound of air pushing past partially closed glottis, heard during expiration
         b) retractions: sternal and intercostal; due to use of accessory muscles to aid in breathing
         c) flaring nares: due to neonate's effort to lessen resistance in narrow nasal passages
         d) seesaw respirations: flattening of chest with inspiration and bulging of abdomen, caused by utilization of abdominal muscles during prolonged, forced respirations
      2) apnea: absence of breathing for more than 20 seconds
      3) cyanosis
      4) alterations in respiratory rate, rhythm, and depth
         a) tachypnea: respiratory rate greater than 60/minute or greater than 15/minute over baseline
         b) bradypnea: respiratory rate less than 30/minute
         c) apneic spells: absence of respiration for 20 seconds or more
   b. **Goal, Plan/Implementation, and Evaluation**

   Goal: Neonate will maintain adequate oxygen levels to meet physiologic demands.
   Plan/Implementation
   - collect blood gas samples and pH via umbilical line; interpret results of studies

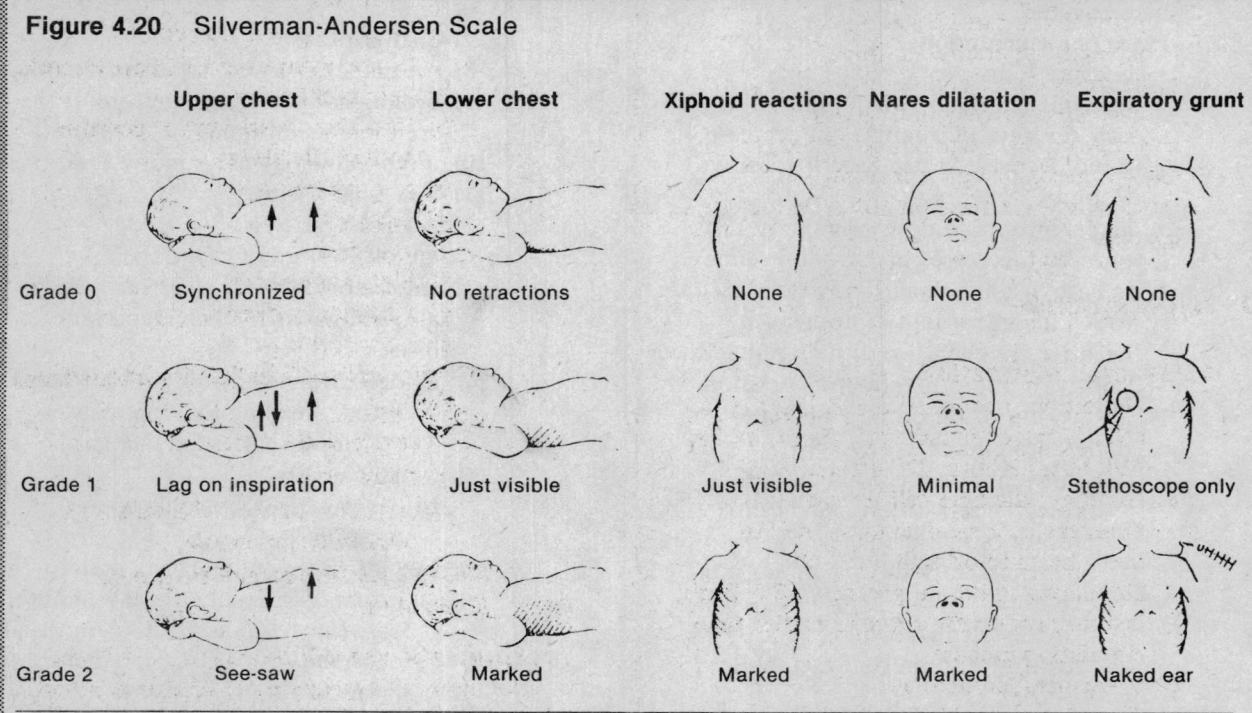

Figure 4.20 Silverman-Andersen Scale

SOURCE: Ross Laboratories, Nursing Inservice Aid #2, Columbus, OH; Reprinted with permission. W. Silverman and D. Andersen, *Pediatrics* 17:1, 1956, American Academy of Pediatrics.

- administer prescribed oxygen (dependent on results of blood-gas study)
  - give warmed and humidified oxygen
  - monitor concentration and pressure of oxygen
- monitor oxygen concentration through oximeter, blood gas and pH studies, and transcutaneous oxygen tension
- maintain infant in supine position, with head slightly extended to improve respiratory function
- evaluate skin color
  - pallor
  - plethora
  - cyanosis: circumoral, generalized, at rest or with activity
- maintain thermal environment
- minimize energy expenditure by keeping infant warm
- facilitate infant's respiratory efforts
  - continuous positive airway pressure (CPAP): controlled pressure exerted upon expiration to prevent collapse of alveoli
  - oxygen hood (to provide controlled oxygen and humidity)
- suction endotracheal tube q1–2h as needed; protect from extubation
- protect skin on nasal septum from breakdown and undue pressure from endotracheal tube
- provide for nutritional needs: IV, gavage, hyperalimentation
- prevent/detect complications
- give supportive care to parents

Evaluation: Neonate adequately meets oxygen needs of body; maintains respiratory rate between 30 and 60 without dyspnea.

D. Hypoglycemia

1. General Information
a. Definition: decreased blood glucose level (Dextrostix less than 30 mg/100 ml [full term] in first 72 hours of life)
b. Etiology: the beta cells in the fetal pancreas become overstimulated in utero because of high levels of circulating maternal glucose; after birth, insulin production remains higher than circulating glucose
c. Predisposing Factors
  1) malnourished infants
     a) premature infants
     b) SGA babies
     c) postmature infants
     d) smaller twin
  2) infants of diabetic mothers (usually LGA)
  3) large-for-gestational age (i.e., greater than 8.8 lb) and/or pregnancy-induced hypertension
  4) severe Rh incompatibility
  5) severely stressed infant, e.g., infants with cold stress, injections, RDS
d. Associated Problems
  1) jaundice
  2) hypocalcemia (serum calcium less than 7–7.5 mg/100 ml) especially in preterm infants

2. Nursing Process
a. Assessment
  1) signs and symptoms
     a) large-for-gestational age, usually over 8.8 lb
     b) poor muscle tone
     c) edema
     d) ruddiness
     e) lethargy
     f) irregular respiration
     g) feeding difficulties
     h) jitteriness
     i) twitching
     j) weak, high-pitched cry
  2) signs and symptoms of hypocalcemia
     a) neonatal tetany
     b) twitching from central nervous system irritability
     c) jerking tremors
     d) seizures
     e) cyanosis
     f) high-pitched cry
     g) respiratory distress
     h) poor feeding
  3) laboratory values for deviations from normal
  4) behavior and reflexes
     a) daily weight
     b) note frequency and amount of urination and stools
b. Goal, Plan/Implementation, and Evaluation

Goal: Neonate will be monitored closely for signs of hypoglycemic reactions before complications develop; will maintain adequate nutrition and fluid and electrolyte balance.

Plan/Implementation
- perform Dextrostix or laboratory blood glucose on admission to nursery, and for LGA babies, q30min 6 times, then qh 3 times, then q2h 6 times until stable; notify physician if Dextrostix result is less than 25 mg
- provide adequate calories for all neonates
- feed LGA babies sterile water within 1st hour of life, followed with formula (oral or tube feeding as indicated) or breast milk
- administer 10%-25% glucose, IV or orally, as ordered
- minimize handling of neonate
- observe carefully for signs of seizure related to low blood sugar
- at time of discharge, recommend regular pediatric care throughout childhood

Evaluation: Neonate maintains normal blood sugar level; hypoglycemic reactions are detected early; ingests calories appropriate for size; maintains fluid and electrolyte balance (moist mucous membranes, good skin turgor).

E. Neonatal Infection

1. **General Information**
   a. Definition: an invasion of the fetus or neonate by bacterial or viral microorganisms before, during, or following birth
   b. Predisposing Factors
   1) prematurity, especially gestational age less than 34 weeks
   2) prolonged labor after rupture of membranes
   3) intrauterine growth retardation (SGA)
   4) TORCH (toxoplasmosis, other, rubella, cytomegalo virus, herpes) syndrome
   5) poor maternal nutrition
   c. Modes of Transmission
   1) chronic transplacental infection, acquired in utero through the placenta
      a) usually due to viruses
      b) onset early in gestation
      c) may lead to growth retardation
   2) ascending intrauterine infection, acquired through the cervix after rupture of membranes
      a) onset late in gestation
      b) usually due to bacteria, often *E. coli*
      c) may lead to premature labor and subsequent premature birth
   3) neonatal infection, acquired after birth from organisms in the environment or via transmission from another person or infant (sepsis is most common infection seen in neonate)
      a) often due to staphylococcus, streptococcus, or *E. coli*
      b) preterm infants at greatest risk for this type of infection because of lower immunologic defenses
      c) more common in boys than girls
   d. Associated Problems
   1) generalized sepsis
   2) septic shock (evidenced by fall in BP and tachypnea)
   3) hyperbilirubinemia
   4) meningitis (evidenced by bulging anterior fontanel)
   5) increased mortality rate, especially in premature infants

2. **Nursing Process**
   a. Assessment
   1) antenatal and intrapartal history to identify infants at risk
   2) septic workup if infection suspected (blood culture, lumbar puncture, gastric aspiration, umbilical-stump culture, stool culture, amniotic-membrane culture)
   3) signs and symptoms
      a) lethargy
      b) infant doesn't "look right"
      c) poor feeding and sucking
      d) increased respiratory rate
      e) jaundice
      f) WBC increase
      g) loss of weight
      h) restlessness
      i) diarrhea and vomiting
      j) abdominal distention
      k) hypo- or hyperthermia
   b. Goal, Plan/Implementation, and Evaluation

Goal: Neonate will be monitored closely for signs of infection and will be treated promptly; generalized sepsis will be prevented.

Plan/Implementation
- treat immediately by administering antibiotics as ordered (e.g., penicillin, kanamycin, polymyxin); observe for side effects
- prevent spread of infection by isolating septic infants
- monitor thermal environment
- monitor body temperature (temperature rise is not an early sign of sepsis); in later stages, observe for severe hyper- or hypothermia
- take daily weight
- monitor I&O; observe for dehydration
- observe for central nervous system involvement (lethargy, apnea)

Evaluation: Neonate shows signs of decreasing infection (decreasing respirations, skin temperature between 36.1° and 36.7°C); generalized sepsis is prevented.

F. Neonatal Narcotic Drug Addiction

1. **General Information**
   a. Definition: drug dependence evident in the neonate as a result of maternal substance abuse
   b. Associated Problems
      1) convulsions
      2) hypothermia

2. **Nursing Process**
   a. Assessment
      1) signs and symptoms: onset according to time of last maternal use, type of drug taken, amount of drug taken, and length of addiction
         a) CNS signs
            - restlessness
            - jittery and hyperactive reflexes
            - high-pitched, shrill cry
            - convulsions
         b) GI system signs
            - feeds poorly
            - vomiting
            - diarrhea
            - dehydration
         c) respiratory system signs
            - nasal stuffiness
            - yawning and sneezing
            - apnea
      2) fluid-balance status
   b. Goal, Plan/Implementation, and Evaluation

Goal: Neonate will be protected from self-injury and severe symptoms associated with withdrawal; seizures will be prevented/controlled; the parent will receive a referral for follow-up care.

Plan/Implementation
- reduce stimuli in environment and minimize handling
- swaddle infant in snug-fitting blanket
- ensure infant receives required fluid and caloric intake; use pacifier between feedings
- use demand feeding schedule; give small amounts at frequent intervals
- give IV therapy as ordered
- position on side to avoid aspiration
- measure I&O; watch for signs of dehydration due to vomiting, loose stools, poor feeding
- weigh frequently
- give skin care with special attention to body folds; expose to air
- protect skin from injury (mittens on hands, sheepskin on crib, pads on sides of crib)
- give medications as ordered
   - phenobarbital (6 mg/kg/24h, IM, or 2 mg PO qid)
   - paregoric (2–4 gtts/kg orally q4–6h; dose may increase to 20–30 gtts/kg q4–6h)
- if seizure occurs, maintain patent airway

Evaluation: Neonate maintains comfort and safety; is free from seizures; receives adequate caloric intake; complications of withdrawal are prevented. Parent has an appointment with physician/clinic for follow-up care.

G. Fetal Alcohol Syndrome

1. **General Information**
   a. Definition: a group of disorders characterized by teratogenesis as a result of chronic maternal alcoholism during pregnancy; high incidence in female infants
   b. Associated Problems
      1) intrauterine-growth-retardation
      2) ocular structural defects
      3) limb anomalies
      4) cardiovascular disturbances and anomalies (e.g., atrial and ventricular septal defects)
      5) mental retardation
      6) fine-motor dysfunction

7) prematurity
8) convulsions

2. Nursing Process
a. **Assessment:** signs and symptoms
1) same as for "Neonatal Narcotic Drug Addiction", plus
2) onset generally within 1st 24 hours after birth
3) abdominal distention
4) tremors
5) sweating
6) irritability
7) seizures (late sign)

b. **Goal, Plan/Implementation, and Evaluation**

Goal: Neonate will be protected from self-injury during seizures; problems associated with fetal alcohol syndrome are detected and treated early before further complications arise.

Plan/Implementation
- protect from injury (swaddle infant in snug-fitting blanket)
- maintain adequate IV therapy if ordered
- maintain adequate warmth
- minimize environmental stimulation
- medicate (refer to "Neonatal Narcotic Drug Addiction" page 463)

Evaluation: Neonate is comfortable; seizures are prevented or controlled; parent has an appointment with physician/clinic for follow-up care.

H. Intracranial Hemorrhage

1. General Information
a. Definition: hemorrhage anywhere within the cranial cavity; in preterm infants, most often caused by hypoxia and hypovolemia
b. Predisposing Factors
1) prematurity
2) birth injury in full-term neonate
c. Associated Problem: hyperbilirubinemia

2. Nursing Process
a. **Assessment**
1) signs and symptoms (may be present immediately after birth or may be delayed)
a) respiratory irregularities
b) cyanosis
c) irritability
d) high-pitched cry
e) fullness or tenseness in fontanel
f) restlessness
g) convulsions
2) presence or absence of reflexes (e.g., Moro's sometimes disappears)

b. **Goal, Plan/Implementation, and Evaluation**

Goal: Neonate will be monitored for early recognition and immediate treatment of intracranial hemorrhage in order to minimize CNS sequelae.

Plan/Implementation
- position head higher than hips
- maintain warm environment
- administer O_2 (to treat cyanosis)
- promote rest
- maintain adequate nutrition by oral or IV therapy
- assist with lumbar puncture (to obtain sample cerebrospinal fluid)
- treatment will vary with nature of hemorrhage; may require evacuation of clot
- give medications as prescribed (vitamins C and K to control bleeding)

Evaluation: Neonate maintains adequate oxygenation; cerebral hemorrhage is detected and treated early before major CNS sequelae (e.g., convulsions, loss of consciousness).

I. Birth Injuries

1. General Information
a. Definition: trauma to the newborn resulting from the birth process
b. Predisposing Factors: large-for-gestational-age (LGA) infant; dystocia
c. Common Types of Injuries
1) brachial plexus injuries
2) cephalohematomas
3) fractures

2. Nursing Process
a. **Assessment:** signs and symptoms
1) decreased mobility of arm, abnormal positioning (brachial-plexus injuries)
2) swelling of head caused by rupture of the blood vessels between a cranial bone and the periosteum (cephalohematoma)
3) swelling, irritability associated with pain, decreased mobility of affected extremity, abnormal positioning at rest (fractures)

b. **Goal, Plan/Implementation, and Evaluation**

Goal: Neonate will be carefully assessed to detect any signs and symptoms of a birth injury; any injury will be treated promptly.

Plan/Implementation
- assess for asymmetrical movements by placing neonate on back and observing movements of arms and legs
- screen all LGA infants for birth injuries; listen for high-pitched, weak cry; observe muscle tone (poor), hypertonicity, hyperactivity, flaccidity
- palpate fontanels for bulging, tenseness
- observe pupillary response
- implement specific treatment, which varies with nature and extent of insult

Evaluation: Neonate receives early treatment of birth injury; is free from long-term sequelae, when possible (e.g., mental retardation).

J. Neonatal Necrotizing Enterocolitis (NEC)

1. **General Information**
   a. Definition: a disorder of vascular ischemia, affecting the gastrointestinal mucosa, often associated with perforation
   b. Incidence: approximately 5% of all newborns in intensive care nurseries; morbidity and mortality can be reduced by early detection and treatment of asphyxia (within 30 min of birth)
   c. Predisposing Factors
      1) neonatal asphyxia and hypoxia
      2) pregnancy-induced hypertension
      3) maternal vaginal bleeding
      4) excessive amounts of feeding
      5) immature immunologic system
      6) prematurity
   d. Associated Problem: sepsis

2. **Nursing Process**
   a. Assessment: signs and symptoms
      1) abdominal distention
      2) pallor
      3) poor feeding
      4) gastric residuals (2 ml or more) before feedings
   b. Goal, Plan/Implementation, and Evaluation

Goal: Neonate will be monitored for early recognition of signs and symptoms of necrotizing enterocolitis; will receive prompt treatment of any abnormalities before complications occur.

Plan/Implementation
- check bowel sounds
- monitor stools for blood (use guaiac test)
- discontinue oral or tube feedings and institute parenteral therapy or hyperalimentation as ordered
- monitor abdominal distention every shift
- record I&O, including nature and type of gastric secretion
- monitor for signs of dehydration (e.g., loss of skin turgor, sunken fontanels, dry skin, decreased urinary output)
- nasogastric suction to low, intermittent suction
- test all gastrointestinal secretions for blood; observe serum electrolytes
- test urine for glucose to monitor tolerance for hyperalimentation solution
- antibiotic therapy may be indicated
- provide appropriate pre- and post-op care when surgery is required (resection or colostomy)

Evaluation: Neonate receives prompt and appropriate treatment of any abnormalities (e.g., asphyxia, feeding problems); is free from sepsis and other complications.

K. Congenital Anomalies

1. **General Information**
   a. Definition: a variety of defects or disorders, which may be evident or concealed at birth. The physical and developmental consequences will vary with the selected problem(s).
   b. Incidence: 6 in 1,000 total births
   c. Predisposing Factors
      1) past personal or family history of congenital anomalies, genetic factors (e.g., chromosomal aberrations)
      2) exposure to toxic agents, viruses, or drugs during pregnancy
      3) genetic-environmental interaction

2. **Nursing Process**
   a. Assessment
      1) antepartum/intrapartum high-risk factors, including maternal history of
         a) chronic alcoholism or drug addiction
         b) family members born with congenital defects

- c) exposure to toxic agents in environment or viral disease (e.g., TORCH syndrome)
- d) living at high altitude
2) hydramnios: associated with
  - a) neurologic defects such as hydrocephalus, anencephalus, and spina bifida
  - b) gastrointestinal malformation such as esophageal atresia, cleft palate, pyloric stenosis
  - c) Down's syndrome
  - d) congenital heart disease
  - e) maternal diabetes
  - f) prematurity
3) oligohydramnios, associated with anomalies of the renal system

b. Goal, Plan/Implementation, and Evaluation

Goal: Neonate's anomalies will be recognized and treated early, before complications arise; will be supported to adapt physiologically to extrauterine life.

Plan/Implementation
- screen for apparent and hidden congenital anomalies (often done upon admission to nursery)
- implement appropriate therapeutic measures (will vary with type of disorder; some disorders require immediate intervention)
- provide pre- and post-op surgical care (if required) to promote physiologic adaptation, i.e., adequate nutrition, aeration
- refer family for genetic counseling

Evaluation: Neonate adapts successfully to extrauterine life; receives appropriate treatment for defect.

L. Parental Reaction to a Sick, Disabled, or Malformed Infant

1. General Information
a. The Grief and Mourning Process: initiated by birth (parents grieve over the loss of normality in their infant)
b. Stages of Grief and Mourning (refer to *Nursing Care of the Client with Psychosocial Problems* page 28)
  1) 1st stage
    - a) initial sadness
    - b) guilt feelings ("What did I do to cause this? What happened?")
    - c) shock over reality of situation
    - d) denial
    - e) general anger at situation; overprotectiveness of the infant
    - f) neglect of other family members
    - g) isolation/loneliness (increases after mother's discharge from hospital);
  2) 2nd stage: developing awareness of reality of situation
  3) restitution: coming to terms with situation)

2. Nursing Process
a. Assessment
  1) stage of grief and mourning
  2) parental behavior: adaptive or maladaptive

b. Goal, Plan/Implementation, and Evaluation

Goal: Parents will be supported in their adaptation to the ill, disabled, or malformed child.

Plan/Implementation
- allow parents to express grief (may be shown as anger, denial, depression, crying); be supportive
- modify hospital policies when possible to allow early contact with infant and frequent visitation; encourage parents to see infant, to touch and hold infant in neonatal intensive care unit
- point out normal characteristics of their infant to parents
- encourage parental participation in care (e.g., providing breast milk, bathing, feeding)
- recognize signs of maladaptive responses
  - possibility of abuse or neglect
  - overwhelming guilt
- expect repeated periods of sadness
- provide simple explanations for procedures
- refer parents to social worker for follow-up while infant is in hospital, according to family need
- encourage parents who are unable to visit to call nursery for progress reports
- refer to public health nurse (official agency or visiting nurse) for health supervision upon discharge of infant
- plan for follow-up or institutionalization as necessary

Evaluation: Parents grieve adaptively for their infant's condition; express feelings of sadness, anger; receive support from nursing staff.

References

*Blackburn, S. "The Neonatal ICU: A High-Risk Environment." *American Journal of Nursing.* November 1982:1708-1712.

Bobak, I. and Jensen, M. *Essentials of Maternity Nursing.* St. Louis: Mosby, 1984.

Brazelton, T. *Neonatal Behavioral Assessment Scale.* Philadelphia: Lippincott, 1973.

Brengman, S. and Burns, M. "Ritodrine HC1 and Preterm Labor." *American Journal of Nursing.* April 1983:537-540.

Clark, M. and Affonso, D. *Childbearing—A Nursing Perspective.* Philadelphia: Davis, 1979.

†Devore, N., Jackson, V., and Piening, S. "TORCH Infections." *American Journal of Nursing.* December 1983:1661-1665.

Friedman, B. "Infertility Workup." *American Journal of Nursing.* November 1981:2040.

*Floyd, C. "Pregnancy After Reproductive Failure." *American Journal of Nursing.* November 1981:2050-2053.

*Grad, R. and Woodside, F. "Obstetric Analgesics and Anesthesia: Methods of Relief for the Patient in Labor." *American Journal of Nursing.* February 1977:242-245.

Hammer, R., Bower, E., and Messina, L. "The Prenatal Use of Rh D Immune Globulin." *MCN: American Journal of Maternal-Child Health.* January/February 1984:29-31.

*Hoffmaster, F. "Detecting and Treating Pregnancy-Induced Hypertension." *MCN: American Journal of Maternal Child Health.* November/December 1983:398-405.

Ketter, D. and Shelton, B. "Pregnant and Physically Fit, Too." *MCN: American Journal of Maternal-Child Health.* March/April 1984:120-122.

Korones, S. *High Risk Newborn Infants.* St. Louis: Mosby, 1976.

McKay, S. "Squatting: An Alternate Position for the Second Stage of Labor." *MCN: American Journal of Maternal-Child Health.* May/June 1984:181-183.

*Neal, M. et. al. "Birth Control: Permanent Methods." *Nursing Care Planning Guides, Set 5.* Baltimore: Williams & Wilkins, 1981.

*_____. "Birth Control: Temporary Methods." *Nursing Care Planning Guides, Set 5.* Baltimore: Williams & Wilkins, 1981.

*_____. "Drugs: Birth Control Pills" *Nursing Care Planning Guides, Set 5.* Baltimore: Williams & Wilkins, 1981.

Olds, S., London, M., and Ladewig, P. *Maternal-Newborn Nursing.* Menlo Park, CA: Addison-Wesley, 1984.

*Pearson, L. "Climacteric." *American Journal of Nursing.* July 1982: 1098-1102.

*Perley, N. and Bills, B. "Herpes Genitalis and the Childbearing Cycle." *MCN: American Journal of Maternal-Child Health.* May/June 1983:213-217.

†Rancilio, N. "When a Pregnant Woman is Diabetic: Postpartal Care."*American Journal of Nursing.* March 1979:453-456.

Reeder, S., Mastroianni, L., and Leonide, M. *Maternity Nursing.* Philadelphia: Lippincott, 1983.

Rubin, R. "Basic Maternal Behavior." *Nursing Outlook*, November 1961:683-686.

†Schuler, K. "When a Pregnant Woman is Diabetic: Antepartal Care."*American Journal of Nursing.* March 1979:448-450.

†Schuler, K., Wimberly, D., Rancilio, N., and Vogel, M. "When a Pregnant Woman is Diabetic: A Case Study." *American Journal of Nursing.* March 1979:448-450.

Silverman, W. and Andersen, D. "A Controlled Clinical Trial of Effects of Water Mist on Obstructive Respiratory Signs, Death Rate and Necropsy Findings." *Pediatrics.* January 1956:1-10.

Whaley, L., and Wong, D. *Nursing Care of Infants and Children.* St. Louis: Mosby, 1983.

White, P. "Pregnancy and Diabetes, Medical Aspects." *Medical Clinics of North America.* July 1965:1015-1024.

†Wimberly, D. "When a Pregnant Woman is Diabetic: Intrapartal Care."*American Journal of Nursing.* March 1979:451-452.

†Vogel, M. "When a Pregnant Woman is Diabetic: Care of the Newborn."*American Journal of Nursing.* March 1979:458-460.

* See reprint section
† Highly recommended

Reprints
Nursing Care of the Childbearing Family

Neal, M. "Birth Control: Permanent Methods." 471
———. "Birth Control: Temporary Methods." 473
———. "Drugs: Birth Control Pills." 476
Floyd, C. "Pregnancy after Reproductive Failure." 478
Hoffmaster, J. "Detecting and Treating Pregnancy-Induced Hypertension: A Review." 482
Perley, N. et al. "Herpes Genitalis and the Childbearing Cycle." 490.
Grad, R. et al. "Obstetrical Analgesics and Anesthesia: Methods of Relief for the Patient in Labor." 495
Blackburn, S. "The Neonatal ICU: A High Risk Environment." 499
Pearson, L. "Climacteric." 504

Birth Control: Permanent Methods

Definition: Sterilization is an operation to remove the possibility of pregnancy or to render the person incapable of conception.

GOAL: The person will be able to virtually eliminate risk of pregnancy.

General Considerations:
- **Incidence:** voluntary sterilizations in the US exceed 1.1 million per year; about two-thirds are hysterectomies and nearly one-third are vasectomies; tubal ligation type operations are growing in popularity. Abortions, while not preventing pregnancy, are used as a major means of birth control by a growing number of women; there are over 1.6 million abortions per year in the US alone.
- **Advantages:** relief from worry and inconvenience of other birth control methods; relief from unwanted pregnancy and childbirth; a cessation of transmission of hereditary diseases.
- **Disadvantages:** nearly always permanent and irreversible consequences; with microsurgical and experienced surgical techniques, it is now possible sometimes to reconnect fallopian tubes or vas deferens in men, but surgery is difficult, expensive and successful in only a small percentage of cases.
- **Counseling** should be done with both sexual partners. There should be a complete exploration of feelings re: sexuality and sterility, possibilities of divorce and re-marriage, loss of child-bearing potential and psychological consequences, especially if there is a loss of an offspring, and any pressures or influences affecting decision. Postponement or cancellation of operation is advisable if there are any signs of emotional, economic or marital stress that signal doubt, distrust or absence of free, informed consent. After open and honest discussion, there should be complete understanding and acceptance of operation, its meaning and its effect on both partners.
- **Legal Consent:** Person must be over 21, fully aware and free of influences of drugs or coercion. While sterilization is now legal in all fifty states, policies and practices vary with local governments, doctors, hospitals, and insurance or Social Service Dept. guidelines. Written consent of marital partner is usually necessary.
- Literature is available from Association for Voluntary Sterilization, Inc., 708 Third Avenue, New York, NY 10017 and from local chapters of Planned Parenthood Federation of America. Teaching aids, counseling services, diagnostic tests for pregnancy and/or venereal disease, and physician referrals are also available from the latter as well as from local free clinic, Public Health Dept. or county clinic and student health clinic.

Methods:
1) **Hysterectomy**
   - Hysterectomy is removal of uterus: total (including tubes and ovaries) or sub-total (only the uterus), also known as a partial hysterectomy.
   - Refer to NCPG #1:12, "The Patient with a Hysterectomy."
2) **Laparoscopy and Cauterization or Clips for Tubes**
   - The insertion of a laparoscope through a small, one inch incision near the navel for purpose of viewing fallopian tubes that are then commonly cauterized (some doctors use clips).
   - Carbon dioxide gas is pumped into abdomen to facilitate lifting and viewing tubes. Frequently this remains in abdomen to be gradually absorbed. "Post insufflation syndrome" is the name for any resulting severe pain in chest, shoulder, and neck that patient experiences. Analgesic injections are often required to reduce discomfort and the normal 12 hour hospitalization may be prolonged. Some surgeons are now using a laparoscope "key" device to remove CO_2 before closing incision and this has been helpful.
   - Effectiveness: About 1 in 1,000 women can get pregnant after this type surgery. Cauterization makes this operation nearly always permanent, so clips are occasionally used for younger women.
   - Complications include: hemorrhage, infection, cardiopulmonary problems in about 1-5 per 100 cases.
   - Nursing care is similar to that of a patient with a mini-lap tubal ligation (see NCPG #5:19) although the surgery and hospitalization are often shorter. Most women recover in a few days from the sore throat (from general anesthetic tube), sore stomach, and mild to moderate cramps. Menstrual periods, hormone levels, and sexual abilities are unchanged.
3) **Tubal Ligation/Mini-Laparotomy**
   - A tubal ligation via mini-laparotomy is a small incision between the navel and the pubis for the purpose of cutting the fallopian tubes in half and tying them off.
   - Refer to NCPG #5:19, "The Patient with a Tubal Ligation (via Mini-Laparotomy)."
4) **Vasectomy**
   - Vasectomy is the resection bilaterally of the vas deferens or ducts that carry sperm from the testes to the penis.
   - Effectiveness: More than 99.5%; however, complete sterility may not be attained until several weeks or months after surgery. Other methods of birth control are necessary until follow-up sperm counts are negative. Operation is usually not reversible, and even if the tubes are re-connected, restored fertility is only 20% likely because sperm antibodies (which develop in many

men) lessen chances.
- Advantages: quick (10-20 minute operation under local anesthetic in an office or clinic), requires no hospitalization (only a couple of days rest with ice packs and elevation of scrotum), does not affect hormones, erections, climaxes, or ejaculations (except rarely — perhaps 5 per 1,000 men), sexual pleasure is same or increased.
- Complications are usually minor, self-limiting and arise in less than 10% of cases. These include: bleeding, hematoma inflammation, infection, ecchymosis (bruise), persistent swelling (due to epididymitis or spermatic granuloma). Aspirin, scrotal supports, ice or heat packs and occasionally, antibiotics, will be used PRN.

5) **Abortion**
- Abortion is the termination of pregnancy before the fetus is theoretically viable.
- Kinds: spontaneous, also called miscarriage, happens when natural body processes end pregnancy before birth — usually before the 20th week of pregnancy; induced abortion is a medical procedure used to end pregnancy.
- Legality: now legal in every state since the Supreme Court decision of 1973; abortions after the first trimester are subject to local state regulation and hospital policies.
- Induced abortion is currently used by many women as a substitute for other methods of contraception. Although a relatively safe procedure performed by a skilled doctor in the first trimester, it is not without some risk of hemorrhage, infection, and serious pyschological consequences. After the first trimester, abortions are much more dangerous, difficult, and expensive. Repeated abortions may increase the possibility of premature births in later, desired pregnancies.

© 1981 by Margo Creighton Neal. © 1985 by Williams & Wilkins. *Nursing Care Planning Guides, Set 5.*
Baltimore: Williams & Wilkins, 1983. Used by permission.

Birth Control: Temporary Methods

GOAL: The person(s) will be able to significantly reduce risk of pregnancy without harmful effects to self or partner.

General Considerations:
- Abstinence or continence is the only completely risk-free temporary method of birth control. Persons may choose either of these methods for various reasons: moral, religious, personal, physical, or psychosocial. In any case, the choice should be acceptable to both sexual partners and be respected by other persons, especially family and friends.
- Literature on the various methods of birth control and their relative effectiveness is available from local chapters of Planned Parenthood Federation of America. Teaching aids, counseling services, birth control aids and prescriptions, diagnostic tests for pregnancy and/or venereal disease, and physician referrals are also available from them as well as from the local "Free" clinic, the public health or county clinic, Right to Life Organizations, and student health clinics. *Hope Is Not A Method* is a recommended film (see references) which can be purchased or rented.
- Those who participate in counseling or providing birth control information and help are usually also responsible for detection of cancer, venereal disease, and for non-VD infection control activities (information, screening tests, referral for treatment, and required reports).
- Effectiveness rates are computed by subtracting failure rate from 100%; failure rates quoted are a combination of method and user failures per 100 women per year.
- **LESS RELIABLE** methods (than those listed later) include:
  - *Lactation:* breast feeding suppresses ovulation for some time, *for some women,* but the risk of pregnancy may be as high as 40%.
  - *Non-intercourse sex:* involves mutual masterbation, oral or anal copulation, interfemoral intercourse (between legs), "petting" to sexual climax (release of sperm), and/or astrological birth control. The latter involves avoiding sex each month during the sun/moon phase, corresponding to the time of one's birth. Astrologers believe, *without scientific basis,* that female eggs are released at this time.
  - *Intercourse mid-menstrual cycle:* although unlikely, it *is* possible for an egg to be in the fallopian tube at this time.
  - *Withdrawal:* involves removal of penis from vagina before ejaculation or leaking of any sperm occurs. Risk occurs if sperm is left on the woman's thighs or pubis, as they can still swim into vagina.
  - *Douching immediately after intercourse:* regardless of beliefs to the contrary, or the type of solution used (tea, vinegar, soapy water, cola, gingerale, etc.), this method is ineffective because of speed of sperm swimming into uterus before any douching can take place.
  - *Plastic food wrap used like a condom:* commonly breaks, slips off, or leaks.

Bona Fide Methods, Effectiveness, Advantages, and Disadvantages:
1) **Condoms** ("rubbers," "prophylactics")
   - A thin rubber sheath, slipped over an erect penis just before intercourse.
   - Effectiveness: 64-97%, depending on correct usage; effectiveness enhanced when used with other methods (see below).
   - Advantages: inexpensive, easily available without prescription, free from major side effects, no medical supervision needed, and provides some protection from venereal disease.
   - Disadvantages: for some they may inhibit sensation, enjoyment, spontaneity, and erection; they have been known to split, tear or spill during usage; sometimes allergies to rubber necessitate usage of other, more expensive types, such as lambskin.

2) **Diaphragms**
   - A thin, dome-shaped, shallow rubber cup surrounding a metal spring rim placed over the cervical os, between rear and side walls of the vagina and behind the symphysis pubis bone.
   - Concern over side effects of "The Pill" has caused an increase in the popularity for the diaphragm; other indications for use include: inability to use an IUD; non-allergy to spermicidal preparations; acceptability, motivation, and compliance readiness of both sexual partners; satifactorily meeting anatomical, medical, and other psychological criteria; and woman's informed choice over other less desirable methods. Contraindications include: a displaced or abnormal organ and surrounding structures (e.g., uterine prolapse, retroversion, anteflexion, cystocele, rectocele, inadequate muscular support, etc.) and a sexual pattern of behavior that includes a variety of partners and positions and/or multiple intercourse.
   - Effectiveness: 70-95%, depending on correct fit and usage.
   - Correct size should be carefully supervised. Size and fit should be re-checked at yearly intervals and after a pregnancy or a 10 pound weight gain or loss.
   - Wearer should be taught to check diaphragm once a month for holes or thin spots by holding up to light. Ordinary care includes washing with mild soap and warm water, thorough rinsing and completely air drying, and dusting with cornstarch (no scented talcs or vaseline to weaken rubber). One usually lasts two years with proper care. Newer, disposable models are now

available as is a type of polyurethane sponge impregnated and bonded with spermicide and designed for several days wear at a time.
- The standard diaphragm should be inserted less than six hours prior to intercourse, preferably a shorter time, and a teaspoonful of spermicidal jelly placed in the cup prior to insertion. The woman should leave it in place at least six hours after last sex act; if intercourse occurs within this six-hour period, additional spermicidal jelly or foam should be inserted into the vagina before each act. A tampon can be inserted to absorb contraceptive and/or sexual fluids if the diaphragm needs to remain in place for a longer time before it can be conveniently removed (no longer than 24 hours, however).
- Advantages: no ill effects such as other methods cause; high effectiveness when used correctly and with spermacide every time.
- Disadvantages: possible increased incidence of bladder infections; occasional allergic reactions to rubber or spermicide; sometimes wearer finds insertion to be distasteful, inconvenient or inhibiting; repeated fittings are needed for those who gain weight or lose weight readily; dislodgement problems due to vaginal wall expansion during state of sexual arousal related to frequent penile insertions, sexual position (woman on top), or both.

3) **Cervical Caps**
   - A small, rubber, thimble-like device that fits directly over cervix and needs only a small amount of spermicide.
   - Popular in Europe, not yet approved by FDA, but available here in US from physicians and clinics participating in FDA-approved studies of effectiveness.
   - Advantages and disadvantages thought to be same as those for diaphragms.

4) **Intrauterine Devices** (IUDs)
   - A small plastic device, some with copper, that is inserted into the uterus and remains there indefinitely; some release a synthetic hormone and these need replacing once a year; a nylon string hangs out of the cervical os into the vagina, making it possible for woman to check periodically to be sure IUD is still there.
   - Effectiveness rate: 90-99%, lower for those IUDs having copper or progesterone hormone in them.
   - If a menstrual period is more than a week late, or if woman thinks she is pregnant, she should contact her doctor or clinic right away. She should never try to remove IUD herself.
   - Because of increased susceptibility to pelvic infection, wearer should be warned to note and report to MD immediately signs of abdominal pain or tenderness, very heavy bleeding, fever, unusual vaginal discharge. Women who have a history of PID (pelvic inflammatory disease) or a variety of sexual partners should not use an IUD.
   - Advantages: convenient, frees wearer of concerns associated with other birth control methods, no daily routine or precautionary activity needed at time of intercourse; cannot be felt by partners.
   - Disadvantages: occasional displacement, expulsion, discomfort/pain, cramping, heavier than usual menstrual flow or irregular bleeding; increased risk of pelvic infection.

5) **Ovulation Method** (Fertility Awareness Method, Rhythm, Natural Method, Sympto-Thermal Method, Periodic Abstinence, Billings Method).
   - Currently gaining in popularity as a natural method without harmful effects of chemical usage, this method has evolved into a combination of the "calendar method" (based on menstrual history), the "temperature method," and the "vaginal mucus method." It is presently known as the Sympto-Thermal Method. It involves the total abstinence from sexual intercourse during the ovulation period, which is determined specifically for each woman. It was first described by Drs. Billings in 1952.
   - A chart or graph is made for each woman, noting the following on a *daily basis:*
     (a) cervical mucus secretions progressing from thick, sticky, and slightly yellow or cloudy to clear, slippery, and watery in nature;
     (b) signs of breast tenderness and/or "mittelschmerz" (lower abdominal tenderness on either side during mid-cycle); and
     (c) basal body temperatures to determine period when temperature rises and remains at consistently higher level for a few days. For most women, 96-98° (F.), orally is considered normal before ovulation and 97-99° typical after ovulation. Changes are fractional so a special *basal* thermometer that registers $1/10$ degrees is best to use.
   - The "Safe" period for intercourse is then determined to be a few "dry" days following menstruation prior to the onset of the above signs and again for a period of about ten days prior to the next menstruation.
   - Effectiveness: 75-98%, depending on regularity of woman's cycle, her correct observations of ovulation's signs, and the cooperation and discipline of both partners.
   - Advantages: no cost (except for thermometer), easily taught by professional, experienced instructors to well-motivated persons, acceptable to all religious groups, medical check-ups or supervision not required as part of method, no chemical or mechanical interference with body processes, easy to reverse when conception is desired, and some report 98% reliability in preventing conception.

- Disadvantages: requires consistent, persistent, accurate record-keeping and the mutual cooperation and self-control of sexual partners; inhibiting to spontaneous sex; no protection from impetuous contact, rape or incest; leukorrhea may interfere with women's observations of mucus character or chronic, frequent infections with normal temperature graphs.

6) **Spermicides** (Cream, Jelly, Foam, or Suppositories)
   - Contain an inert base that provide a physical barrier to sperm and a chemical that immobilizes and kills sperm.
   - Effectiveness: 70-98%, depending on whether they are correctly inserted into vagina with applicator provided (except for suppository form), and are inserted one hour prior to intercourse. Foam is considered to be more effective than cream or jelly types; effectiveness of spermicides is enhanced when used in combination with other methods (condom, diaphragm, etc.) Douching, after intercourse, should not be done for at least six hours to allow full spermicidal activity and protection.
   - Advantages: easy to obtain in drugstore without prescription, easy to use without major harmful side effects. Foam type is thought to provide a degree of protection from some venereal diseases.
   - Disadvantages: messy, inconvenient, interferes with spontaneity of mood; allergies can occur which may or may not be corrected by changing brands; more important, there is recent evidence to indicate that increased incidence of serious birth defects may occur in those who are or have recently used spermicides.

7) **Oral Contraceptives ("The Pill")**
   - Refer to NCPG #5:42, "Drugs: Birth Control Pills."

© 1981 by Margo Creighton Neal. © 1985 by Williams & Wilkins. *Nursing Care Planning Guides, Set 5.*
Baltimore: Williams & Wilkins, 1983. Used by permission.

Drugs: Birth Control Pills

GOAL: The woman will be able to minimize risk of pregnancy without seriously harmful side effects or complications.

General Considerations:
- "The Pill," as it is commonly called, usually contains two female synthetic hormones (estrogen and progestogen) that keep an egg from being released by the ovary. The estrogen suppresses secretion of Follicle Stimulating Hormones and Releasing Factors while the progestogen suppresses Luteinizing Hormones and Releasing Factors, thereby causing the cervical mucus to become more resistant to penetration and movement of sperm.
- Combination types are taken once a day for 21 days and then stopped for seven days, during which time menstrual flow occurs. The 21-day pill cycle is then repeated. Sometimes the doctor prescribes a different-colored, inert (inactive) pill to be taken during the 7-day period so that the daily pill taking habit is reinforced.
- The "Mini-Pill" is a progestogen only preparation that is taken daily on a continuous basis.
- **Effectiveness:** 99% when taken correctly *and consistently* according to directions.
- **Advantages:** most effective, temporary method of birth control; convenient, doesn't interfere with spontaneity or love-making activity; short-term (less than ten years' usage) risks of serious side effects are low in women under 35 who are healthy and non-smokers; more regular menstrual periods and less cramping than when a non-pill user; less iron deficiency anemia because menstrual flow is less in quantity and duration; some evidence that Pill may protect against endometrial or ovarian cancer and fibrocystic breast disease.
- **Disadvantages/Contraindications:** increased incidence of bladder and vaginal infections; increased incidence of blood clots (thrombophlebitis, emboli, strokes), cardiovascular and respiratory disease, especially among Pill users who smoke; at least twice the risk of MI as non-Pill users and risk is *greater* than twice as the age, amount of smoking, BP, and/or overweight increases; long-term risks of women who have used Pill more than ten years are still in question but are believed to include atrophy of ovaries, resulting in difficulty resuming normal menstrual periods and achieving normal fertility; higher incidence of cervicitis; higher incidence of breast cancer *when* there is a grandmother/aunt family history of breast cancer.

    The Pill should *not* be used by women who have had a stroke, heart attack, anginal chest pains, cancer, blood clots, renal or liver disease, high cholesterol levels, or high blood pressure. The Pill is contraindicated for those with a history of severe migraine headaches, depressions, or diabetes; for those who have a family history of breast cancer; for those who are overweight, over 35, or who are heavy smokers (more than 15 cigarettes per day). Lactating mothers should also avoid taking the Pill.
- Women new to the Pill should have a complete history and physical exam with screening and diagnostic tests (Pap smear, mammogram or Xerography, urine sugar and protein, prothrombin time, hemoglobin and hematocrit counts). Follow-up medical visits on a regular basis are necessary throughout the Pill-taking years to assess physical condition and untoward symptoms.
- **Side Effects:** Those that are relatively minor, transient and to be expected, although annoying, include for some: nausea, headaches, weight gain, sore or tender breasts, and "breakthrough bleeding" (pinkish spotting mid-cycle). These may disappear after a few months adjustment to the hormone level. Some women develop, after 1-2 years, melasma or chloasma (brown patches on face skin similar to "mask" of pregnancy). Use of sun screen lotions helps minimize this. Indications of serious problems should be reported to doctor immediately. These signs include: severe headache, loss of vision, shortness of breath, sudden chest, arm or leg pains and warmth, redness or swelling of calf, thigh, or forearm; persistent vaginal discharge or heavier than usual vaginal bleeding. After the initial adjustment period, if a woman misses a menstrual period, she should find out if she is pregnant before continuing to take Pill in order to reduce possibility of birth defects in the developing fetus.
- **Nursing responsibilities** include responsibility for or assistance with history, physical, and test on initial visit and preliminary patient teaching and counseling. Literature, complete explanations, and opportunities to answer all questions should be provided. Especially important are reminders to report immediately any serious side effects. Written information on what to do when one (or more) pill(s) is missed should be given to each woman to keep readily accessible. "If one Pill is missed, take it with the next day's Pill. If two are missed, take two Pills on each of the next two days and finish series as usual. Use another method of birth control until seven Pills are taken in succession, because disruption such as this can have a rebound effect so the chances of getting pregnant are greater. If three or more Pills are missed, all the remaining Pills in that series should be discarded and a new 21-day cycle should be started 7 days after taking the last Pill. If a period is missed, call your doctor or clinic and be tested for pregnancy."

Drug Trade Names	Ingredients	
Combination Types	**Estrogen**	**Progestin**
Brevicon 21 Day		
Brevicon 28 Day (with 7 inert tabs.)	Ethinyl estradiol 0.035 mg.	Norethindrone 0.5 mg.
Demulen -21		
Demulen -28 (with 7 inert tabs.)	Ethinyl estradiol 0.050 mg.	Ethnodiol diacetate 1 mg.
Enovid 5 mg. (20 day)	Mestranol 0.075 mg.	Norethnodrel 5 mg.
Enovid 10 mg.	Mestranol 0.150 mg.	Norethnodrel 10 mg.
Enovid-E (20 day or 21 day)	Mestranol 0.100 mg.	Norethnodrel 2.5 mg.
Loestrin -21 1/20		
Loestrin -Fe 1/20 (7 tabs. brown with ferrous fumarate)	Ethinyl estradiol 0.020 mg.	Norethindrone 1 mg.
Loestrin -21 1.5/30	Ethinyl estradiol 0.030 mg.	Norethindrone 1.5 mg
Lo/Ovral	Ethinyl estradiol 0.030 mg.	Norgestrel 0.3 mg.
Modicon (21 day or 28 day with 7 inert)	Ethinyl estradiol 0.030 mg.	Norethindrone 0.5 mg.
Norinyl 1+50 (21 or 28 day with 7 inert)	Mestranol 0.050 mg.	Norethindrone 1 mg.
Norinyl 1+80 (21 or 28 day with 7 inert)	Mestranol 0.080 mg.	Norethindrone 1 mg.
Norinyl 2 mg.	Mestranol 0.100 mg.	Norethindrone 2 mg.
Norlestrin 1 mg. (21 or 28 day, 7 inert) (or 28 day with 7 tabs. ferrous fumarate)	Ethinyl estradiol 0.050 mg.	Norethindrone 1 mg.
Ortho-Novum 1/50 (21 or 28 day, 7 inert)	Mestranol 0.050 mg.	Norethindrone 1 mg.
Ortho-Novum 1/80 (21 or 28 day, 7 inert)	Mestranol 0.080 mg.	Norethindrone 1 mg.
Ovcon -35	Ethinyl estradiol 0.035 mg.	Norethindrone 0.4 mg.
Ovcon -50	Ethinyl estradiol 0.050 mg.	Norethindrone 1 mg.
Ovral	Ethinyl estradiol 0.050 mg.	Norgestrel 0.5 mg.
Ovulen (20, 21, or 28 day with 7 inert)	Mestranol 0.100 mg.	Ethnodiol diacetate 1 mg.
Micronor		Norethindrone 0.35 mg.
Nor-Q.D.		Norethindrone 0.35 mg.
Ovrette		Norgestrel 0.075 mg.

© 1981 by Margo Creighton Neal. © 1985 by Williams & Wilkins. *Nursing Care Planning Guides*, Set 5. Baltimore: Williams & Wilkins 1983. Used by permission.

Pregnancy After Reproductive Failure

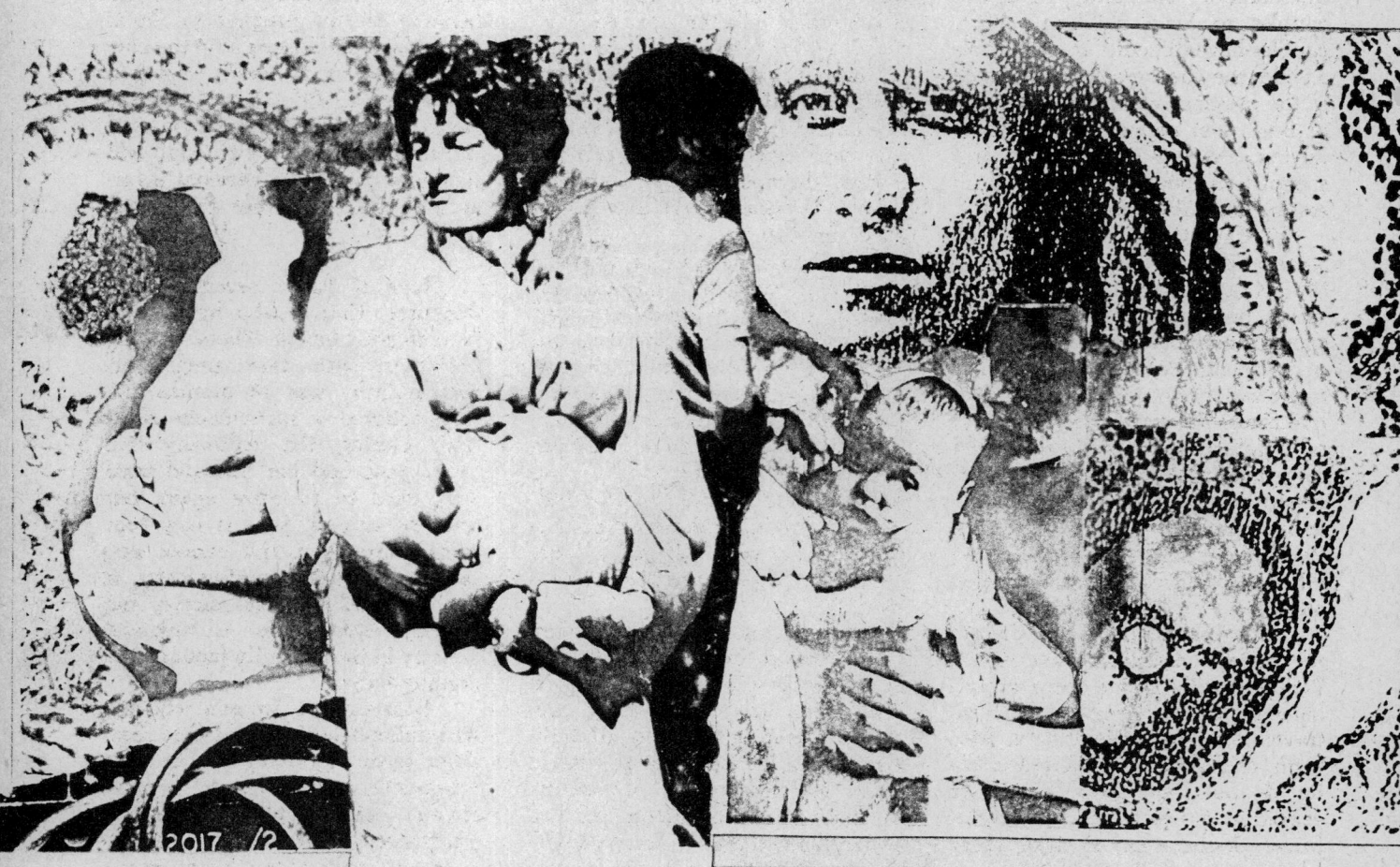

Reprinted from American Journal of Nursing, November 1981

By Cathy Cornwell Floyd

In families in which there has been previous reproductive disappointment—infertility, spontaneous abortion, prematurity, congenital anomaly, or stillbirth—there is usually a heightened anxiety level throughout a new pregnancy. The anxiety may persist into the early childhood period.

Previously disappointed women show great preoccupation with their diet and activity during pregnancy; phone calls to the obstetrician's office are more frequent; and women may experience disorganization at any usual occurrence, such as when Braxton Hicks contractions become noticeable, sometimes to the point of rushing to the hospital or imposing strict bed rest on themselves. Some women express a desire not to know anything during delivery, while others need to know everything.

This uptight behavior also extends to expectant fathers and grandparents. In some ways, the grandmother-to-be might be harder to deal with than the actual expectant parents. A grandmother tends to view a grandchild as a sacred trust—indeed, much too sacred to be completely entrusted to her own immature and irresponsible offspring and his or her mate!

Our society looks upon the production of a perfectly formed, healthy child as an indication of one's biological, sexual, and social worth. Men and women who have, in the past, failed to meet this expectation frequently feel com-

---

CATHY CORNWELL FLOYD, RN, MS, was an instructor in maternal-newborn nursing at the College of Nursing, Medical University of South Carolina, Charleston, when she wrote this article. She now is an assistant professor at Memphis State University, Tenn.

pelled to produce a healthy child in order to prove their fertility, virility, feminine adequacy, or human worth to themselves and to others.

Fears and Pressures

Family, friends, and mere acquaintances constantly pressure couples to have children. When couples have difficulty in producing a child, they become uncomfortable in the presence of pregnant women or find other people's children annoying. Pressure from others and speculation about "whose fault it is" can be very distressing.

Today, there is more public awareness about the causes of infertility. Couples who have had a previous pregnancy that ended in spontaneous abortion are aware that many spontaneous abortions are nature's way of getting rid of a defective fetus. They are also aware that such defects are sometimes related to genetic problems. This threat of genetic or biological inadequacy is a strong one. It is terrifying to think that there is something within oneself that could cause harm to one's offspring.

The public nurtures certain misconceptions of cause and effect. People readily blame the mother's behavior during pregnancy (work, travel, diet) for prematurity, stillbirth, or defects. Acquaintances often do not keep their theories of causation to themselves, which reinforces doubts that most of these families already have.

Then, there are those people whose scientific knowledge is unsound and who will say things like, "It's no surprise that Sally's baby has a heart defect. After all, her father had a massive heart attack last year"; or "They say that people who have syphilis have 'waterhead' babies." Such notions, even when the affected family knows that they are theoretically unsound, nevertheless awaken doubts in the couple that they are biologically inferior and could, therefore, never produce a healthy child.

While working with women who have given birth to defective children, I often hear them voice fears that the same thing will happen in future pregnancies. They are all hungry for knowledge about the causes of the defect so that they can reassure themselves that it will not happen again (1).

Similar fears are also present in families in which there has been a threatened abortion or other illnesses during pregnancy. If the pregnancy is salvaged, parents wonder if it should have been saved. What effect will the episode have on the child? DES, which was used to forestall miscarriages 15 to 20 years ago, has been linked to cancer in the offspring. This knowledge may lead families to be fearful of certain therapeutic regimens currently prescribed in cases of threatened abortion.

Reproductive failure and loss of an infant cause the couple a great deal of pain. One study revealed that half of the couples who lost infants planned never to try to have a child again. Two percent voluntarily chose sterilization. These actions may be due to an intense wish to avoid being hurt again or, more remotely, self-punishment for failure to reproduce (2). Some families who initially wish to avoid another pregnancy do change their minds later.

In working with these families, I have found that occasionally one of the couple will become subfertile. This subfertility, many times, cannot be traced to any organic problem, but is thought to be due to guilt, self-deprecation, avoidance, or other emotional factors that can suppress reproductive function. Often fertility returns as the person accomplishes resolution of the doubts and fears caused by the previous unhappy experience.

The following brief case studies describe behavior patterns that may be seen in such families.

Despite repeated admonitions from her mother-in-law, Carol C, a high school physical education teacher who was in good health, continued to work throughout her uneventful first pregnancy. During labor, the umbilical cord prolapsed and became strangulated. Her baby was born perfectly formed, but dead.

Last week, Carol was notified that her pregnancy test was positive. She immediately tendered her resignation; demanded full-time household help so that she would not have to lift or, worse still, reach for anything; and, she began making plans to shelter herself completely for the remainder of her pregnancy.

This patient, although well informed, is allowing superstition and old wives' tales to control her behavior during pregnancy. She is not taking any chances with the current pregnancy, nor is she willing to set herself up for further criticism from her mother-in-law. It is as if the rituals she is going through will somehow provide additional insurance in protecting her from mishaps.

Jane K has a seven-year-old daughter, Kathy, who has always been in good health. There were no problems with that pregnancy. When Kathy was 18 months old, Jane suffered a spontaneous abortion. During the following five years, Jane and her husband tried very hard to conceive again, but with no success. Jane is now four months pregnant and cannot stop talking about the coming baby. It has a name, and the nursery has already been set up. All talk and activity in the K family focus on the coming baby.

Sometimes a woman who has had difficulty conceiving is so reassured when she finally does become pregnant that she becomes very positive and confident that conception guarantees a beautiful, healthy baby. In other cases, this overpositive thinking may actually be an intense manifestation of the woman's anxiety or her denial of the possibility that this pregnancy might end in disappointment as well.

Two and a half years ago, Joe and Elizabeth T's son, born at 34 weeks' gestation, died when he was five days old. When Elizabeth realized that she was pregnant again, she changed physicians. In her search for a new obstetrician, she went to the other side of the city.

In planning for the new baby, Elizabeth got rid of everything she had before and bought an entirely new layette and new nursery furniture. She had a saddle block for her last delivery, but plans to try the Lamaze method for this delivery.

Does Elizabeth hope that by changing the props, setting, and even some of the principal characters, she can also change the outcome? It is not uncommon to find patients who have had experiences like this suffering from postpartum depression, even when they have healthy babies. The birth experience may be a painful reminder of the past.

Three years ago, Ellen and Rob S had a daughter who had multiple neurological and skeletal anomalies. Her condition was such that the child required institutionalization. Ellen is now pregnant, and her baby is due in the next three weeks. Her friends wanted to have a shower for her, but Ellen would not hear of it. When the nurse asked Ellen and Rob about the plans that they had made for the baby, she discovered that they had not set up the nursery and that the few baby clothes were still in a trunk in the attic. When the nurse pointed out that Ellen might deliver at any time and that she might find the event less hectic if provisions had already been made for the baby at home, Ellen replied that after the baby was born, her husband and her sister would go out and buy the necessary equipment and prepare the nursery.

In the light of Ellen's previous experience, we might find her behavior easy to understand. We also see this behavior sometimes in women who have a genetic or developmental anomaly in their family tree. It is not uncommon to see similar behavior even in nurses or other professionals who are aware of the hazards that can affect an infant.

Developmental Tasks

Clark describes four sequential developmental tasks that must be mastered during pregnancy and the intrapartum period in order to provide readiness for maternal roles and relationships. These tasks are pregnancy validation, fetal embodiment, fetal distinction, and role transition (3).

Pregnancy validation. Couples who have experienced repeated disappointment in their efforts to conceive or those who were deeply hurt by previous outcomes often have difficulty in accepting a pregnancy as a reality. Anxiety may be manifested in intensified physical symptoms, repeated requests for examinations by the obstetrician to prove that the pregnancy is real, or conversely, by failure to seek prenatal care. To help the patient achieve the task of validation, the nurse uses the individual's strengths and family resources for support. The patient who continues to need assistance in validating the pregnancy may need to be referred for additional professional counseling. During this period, feelings of ambivalence are common. These feelings may be especially disturbing to the woman who has tried very hard to become pregnant.

Fetal embodiment. Likewise, women who have had a long history of infertility or those who have lost a baby by spontaneous abortion may have difficulty in mastering the task of fetal embodiment: incorporating the fetus into the mother's body image. (4). The nurse can help the mother-to-be by allowing her to listen to the fetal heart tones, commenting positively on the progress of her pregnancy, and capitalizing on the significance of quickening.

Fetal distinction. When the mother starts to see the fetus as a separate entity, she begins to look for clues as to what her baby will be like and starts to make plans for him. At this point, dreams and fantasies may be heightened. The family who fears that a healthy baby will not become a reality may delay in making plans for him. They may not talk excitedly about the coming baby as other expectant parents do. The woman who fears premature labor will be particularly cautious. Here again, the nurse can observe for deviations from the expected behaviors and can assist the family in verbalizing their fears.

Role transition. At the very end of pregnancy, anxiety of couples who have doubts about the baby may increase due to the imminence of the delivery that will prove or disprove their biological and/or social worth. In such instances the woman who delivers prematurely may not have completed her psychological preparation for motherhood. The couple who has never been fully convinced that the pregnancy would result in a live normal baby may also be unprepared to take on their roles as parents and need nurses' help to adjust.

Counseling the Family

Sexual considerations. A "premium" pregnancy may strain the couple's sexual relationship. One member of the couple or both may fear that, once pregnancy is achieved, intercourse endangers the precious fetus. They will, therefore, avoid sexual expression of any kind. There may also be guilt feelings present in which intercourse was blamed for a previous fetal loss.

The nurse must help the couple express their fears and examine the validity of abstinence in protecting the fetus. Sexual relations usually involve closeness and provide for dependency needs, which are often more manifest during pregnancy for both partners. Many of the couples' fears are common and might be reduced by anticipatory guidance.

Discussion of sex in pregnancy should include the following information: although orgasm does cause uterine contraction, studies have not shown that orgasm leads to labor; some spotting may occur after intercourse, but this minimal spotting is not harmful; and the baby is usually well protected by the cervix, a mucous plug, and intact membranes(5). In situations in which vaginal intercourse is contraindicated, such as when the woman has an incompetent cervix, the nurse should assist the couple to explore alternate means of sexual expression.

Crisis intervention. Mild and moderate anxiety do not interfere with normal functioning. However, severe anxiety and panic do, and they have to be reduced. A severely anxious or panicky patient is limited in what he or she can take in. Therefore, interaction should be short, simple, and should set the stage for the patient to regain control. To prevent increasing anxiety, the nurse should be able to recognize lesser degrees of anxiety and help the woman talk about the origin of her fears and the circumstances surrounding it(6).

Four categories of anxiety responses may be applied to the obstetrical/setting:

1. *Somatization*, the symbolic expression of a problem through a bodily organ. It may show up as hyperemesis or various aches and pains that the woman might use to gain examination by the obstetrician and thereby gain reassurance that everything is all right.

2. *Acting out*, which involves outward behaviors, such as insomnia, restlessness, "taking it easy" to the point of excess, or keeping oneself so busy that one has no time to think frightening thoughts.

3. *Introspection*, withdrawal into private thought without verbal or outward concern shown to others.

4. *Investigation*, characterized by incessant reading and questions about pregnancy and/or the problem anticipated and talking about one's anxiety(7).

The investigation anxiety response provides the greatest growth potential. Investigation is useful if the patient takes time to study the anxiety-producing situation and its meaning to her, rather than quickly employing an anxiety relief behavior that makes her more comfortable but that also is an avoidance of resolving the anxiety(7). Sometimes our own anxiety as nurses makes this difficult; we may be more comfortable if patients engage in social chatter rather than questioning.

A couple of points should be kept in mind. Since these couples may see themselves as unlucky or as losers, the nurse might not succeed in reassuring them as much as she hoped to by supplying them with risk statistics, although this type of information should be provided to the family. Suppose the couple has had one child with a certain defect. Telling them that the chances of this particular problem repeating itself are one in 100 may not really encourage them. They may be unable to focus on their 99 percent chance for a normal child, but may instead be convinced that, with their luck, they will be the one couple who repeats this misfortune.

Even when the child is born and is healthy in every way, some of these parents constantly take their children to physicians because they are so fully convinced that they cannot produce completely normal children. Often they will not answer when professionals ask "What is it that you think is wrong with the baby?" We might be more successful if we ask, "What do you hope it is not?"(8). Such parents may actually be relieved if someone finds something wrong with the baby because whatever is found could not be as bad as what the parents had expected(9).

These parents may experience problems in developing relationships with their infants. "Couples appear to perceive their physiological inability to conceive as related to their psychological ability to parent children"(10). Often couples with long histories of infertility have dropped parental attitudes and abilities from their self-concepts. Later, if parenthood is achieved by conception or adoption, they may not be able to reintegrate parental roles successfully into their self-concepts. Their parent-infant attachment process proceeds slowly.

When parents take a new baby home from the hospital, there is often a difficult period of adjustment, which may lead to exhaustion and, finally, to some resentment of the baby. This can lead to guilt feelings.

In some cases, couples have tried to conceive immediately after the loss of a child, as a replacement scheme. It is usually difficult for parents to be successful at bonding with a new child if mourning for the lost child has not been completed. This is especially true when a new baby is conceived while parents are still grieving for a lost child or close family member(11).

Finally, getting the family members to verbalize their fears may not be easy. Some pregnant women verbalize their concerns freely—more freely even than if they were not pregnant. However, many mothers find thoughts of fetal deformity or loss too horrible to mention. They are afraid that if they verbalize their fears, they will come true.

One standard nursing approach to opening doors is to use knowledge of fears commonly held by expectant parents to initiate discussion of their individual fears. A lead, such as "You know, most of our patients report that they have had frightening dreams that something would be wrong with their babies. How is it with you?" might open the way for discussion. If the anxiety uncovered is great and the patient or her spouse express the fear that they don't know how they would cope if the outcome they fear materializes, the nurse might explore with the couple some of their strengths, resources, and support systems.

Using her knowledge of the individual patient and her family, the nurse might deem it appropriate to help them to formulate a plan for how they would meet the anticipated disaster. Anxiety of this level cannot be denied or eliminated, but it might be reduced by arming parents with a plan. This approach might at least calm the disorganization surrounding the feeling of "I-don't know what I'd do if____."

The far-reaching implications of the severity of the problem of reproductive disappointment appear even in pediatrics, where overanxious parents are often seen. In my own experience, I was struck by what seemed to be a high incidence of hospitalized psychiatric patients whose histories uncovered some guilt related to miscarriages, stillbirths, and birth defects. This guilt plagues relatives of the woman who lost a baby as well as the woman herself. The problems associated with reproductive failure extend to the whole family.

References

1. Floyd, C. C. *A Defective Child Is Born: A Study of Mothers*. (To be published)
2. Wolff, J. R., and others. The emotional reaction to a stillbirth. *Am.J.Obstet.Gynecol.* 108:73-77, Sept. 1, 1970.
3. Clark, A. L., and Affonso, Dyanne, eds. *Childbearing: A Nursing Perspective*. Philadelphia, F. A Davis Co., 1976, p. 255.
4. *Ibid.*, p. 256.
5. *Ibid.*, pp. 248-249.
6. Peplau, Hildegard. Anxiety. IN *Childbearing: A Nursing Perspective*, ed. by A. L. Clark and Dyanne Affonso. Philadelphia, F. A. Davis Co., 1976, p. 84.
7. *Ibid.*, pp. 83-84.
8. Clark and Affonso, *op. cit.*, p. 468.
9. Caplan, Gerald. *An Approach to Community Mental Health*. New York, Grune & Stratton, 1961, p. 84.
10. Wiehe, V. R. Psychological reactions to infertility: implications for nursing in resolving feelings of disappointment and inadequacy. *JOGN Nurs.* 5:29, July-Aug. 1976.
11. Klaus, M. H., and Kennell, J. H. *Maternal-Infant Bonding*. St. Louis, C. V. Mosby Co., 1976, p. 84.

Detecting And Treating Pregnancy-Induced Hypertension

Reprinted from American Journal of Maternal/Child Nursing, November/December 1983.

Although the etiology of pregnancy-induced hypertension remains unclear, women who are at risk of developing it can be identified and helped.

JOAN E. HOFFMASTER

Hypertensive disorders of pregnancy, variously called preeclampsia, eclampsia, eclamptogenic toxemia, gestational hypertension, and EPH (edema, proteinuria, hypertension) gestosis, are leading causes of maternal deaths. They contribute significantly to perinatal death rates also. Yet the causes of these disorders remain obscure.

Preeclampsia, which occurs primarily during first pregnancies, is characterized by the development of proteinuria and/or edema in conjunction with hypertension. It affects between 1.5 and 12 percent of expectant mothers. Women who are members of groups that have a high predisposition for hypertension, such as blacks, are at greater risk.

Generally, preeclampsia arises after 20 weeks' gestation and in the absence of preexisting hypertensive vascular or renal disease. With trophoblastic disease, signs of preeclampsia may develop prior to 20 weeks' gestation (1–3). When preeclampsia progresses to the occurrence of convulsions that are not caused by other cerebral conditions, it is called *eclampsia*. (For more information on the classification, definitions, and characteristics of pregnancy-induced hypertension, see "Pregnancy-Induced Hypertension: Prenatal

JOAN E. HOFFMASTER, R.N., M.S., is the coordinator of the Improved Pregnancy Outcome and Improved Child Health Projects, Public Health Region 2, Texas Department of Health. She helped establish a special program for adolescent pregnancy care at Texas Tech University Health Sciences Center/R. E. Thomason General Hospital in El Paso, Texas. She is a certified nurse midwife.

ASSOCIATIONS WITH PREGNANCY

Clinical Criteria	Early Indicators
Blood pressure	Persistent creeping-upward trend in diastolic blood pressure while still in normal range. Midtrimester blood pressure of 125/75 to 130/80 mmHg or greater; midtrimester arterial pressure of 82 mmHg or greater.

Proteinuria
  Quantitative (per liter)
  Qualitative/dipstick	

Edema	
Weight gain	2 pounds or more per week (no other signs).
Gastric/epigastric	
Central nervous system	
Extremities/reflexes	
Pulmonary	
Renal	
Placenta	
Fetus	

Laboratory findings:
  Plasma creatinine
  Hematocrit
  Blood viscosity
  Platelets
  Serum uric acid	

Prenatal, predictive blood pressure screening	Supine pressor test between 28 and 32 weeks' gestation; mean arterial pressure test (midtrimester).

A Review

...UCED HYPERTENSION

Mild to Moderate Preeclampsia	Severe Preeclampsia
...ersistent diastolic pressure ...f 90 mmHg. ...t least 140/90 mmHg but ...ss than 160/110 mmHg or ...0 mmHg or more rise in ...ystolic pressure over base-...ne or 15 mmHg or more ...se in diastolic pressure ...ver baseline.	160/110 mmHg or higher.
(Proteinuria may be absent.) ...3 gm to 2 gm per liter in ...4 hours. ...+ to 2+ qualitatively.	(Proteinuria may be absent.) 5 gm or more per liter in 24 hours 3+ to 4+ qualitatively.
...ossibly present.	Probably present; face edema.
...pounds or more per week ...r 6 pounds or more per ...onth.	2 pounds or more per week.
	Possible nausea and/or vomiting. Epigastric pain.
	Scotoma (blind spots). Photophobia, blurred vision. Headache.
...ossible hyperreflexia (not ...resent earlier).	Hyperreflexia; clonus.
	Pulmonary edema; cyanosis.
...ormal to decreased renal ...unction.	Decreased renal function. Oliguria (less than 500 ml/ 24 hours). Anuria possible.
	Decreased blood flow.
	Decreased fetal movement.
	Rising level. Rises. Elevated. Reduced. Level exceeding 7 mg/100 ml.

Potential Adverse Outcomes

Maternal death.
Fetal death.
Premature labor.
Fetal growth retardation.
Mental retardation.
Abruptio placentae.
Intravascular coagulation fibrinolysis (ICF) syndrome.
Massive intracranial hemorrhage.
Grand mal seizure (eclampsia).
Bilateral cortical necrosis of the kidney or tubular necrosis.

Factors Associated with Risk

First pregnancy.
Under age 20 or over age 35.
Malnutrition.
Chronic hypertension or other vascular disease.
Diabetes mellitus.
Multiple pregnancy.
Polyhydramnios.
Trophoblastic disease.
Chronic renal disease.
Hydrops fetalis.
Previous preeclampsia, eclampsia, or hypertension.
Poor health care.
Family history of preeclampsia, eclampsia, or hypertension.
Inadequate prenatal care.

Nursing Concerns" by Lois Sonstegard, MCN 4:90–95, March/April 1979.)

Dietary, endocrine, genetic, toxic, hemodynamic, stress, uterine stretch reflex, and immunologic mechanisms have all been cited as possible causes of pregnancy-induced hypertension. Researchers also have suggested that preeclampsia may involve a partial breakdown of mechanisms that ensure that the fetoplacental unit is not rejected as an allograft. The possible association of circulating antigen-antibody complexes with the development of pregnancy-induced hypertension continues to be investigated (2,3).

Judith Lueck and her colleagues more recently have observed multiple forms of a helminth-like organism, *Hydatoxi lualba*, in association with the trophoblast of hydatidiform mole and placentas from toxemic women (4). However, the exact mechanisms involved in the progressive development of toxemia remain to be determined (5). Uteroplacental ischemia is believed to play a key role in the genesis of pregnancy-induced hypertension, although it is not known whether it is a primary event or is secondary to hypertension-related vasospasm (6).

Associated Pathologic Changes

Various pathologic changes in many of the body's systems, particularly the vascular system, are associated with pregnancy-induced hypertension.(See table "Associations with Pregnancy-Induced Hypertension.") One of the most notable changes in the vascular system, vasospasm, causes arterial hypertension. Vasospasm and hypertension are in some way related to the presence of chorionic villi (with or without a fetus); these conditions are more likely to develop when there is an overabundance of trophoblastic tissue, which occurs in cases of multiple fetuses, hydatidiform mole, erythroblastosis fetalis, and maternal diabetes (2).

Other changes associated with pregnancy-induced hypertension include a lessening or absence of the normal rise in blood volume, resulting in hemoconcentration, coagulopathy, and hemolysis (7). Plasma levels of renin, angiotensin II, and aldosterone decrease, while vascular sensitivity to pressor hormones increases. Reduced maternal perfusion of the placenta, with increased uterine activity both spontaneously and in response to oxytocin, contributes to greater risk of uterine hyperstimulation with oxytocin. Decreased placental function, in turn, retards fetal growth. (See "Placental Function and Its Role in Toxemia" by Anna M. Tichy and Dianne Chong, MCN 4:84–89, March/April 1979.)

Renal blood flow and glomerular filtration are reduced as pregnancy-induced hypertension develops. The concentration of uric acid in blood plasma commonly is elevated because of decreased clearance by the kidney. Fluid changes often occur, with an accumulation of extracellular fluid above normal pregnancy levels. However, the presence of such edema by itself does not indicate a poor pregnancy outcome. Similarly, a lack of appreciable edema in instances of preeclampsia or eclampsia does not signal a more favorable pregnancy outcome (2).

Early Nursing Focus

Monitoring early for the potential or signs of preeclampsia helps to protect both mother and baby. Since the disease may be influenced by characteristics of the individual woman as well as the environment, the nurse must assess a number of variables, including the expectant mother's blood pressure, weight, and diet as well as the development of proteinuria and edema (8).

Blood pressure. Generally, hypertension is diagnosed when blood pressure is greater than 140/90 mmHg. It also is indicated if systolic pressure rises by at least 30 mmHg or diastolic pressure rises by at least 15 mmHg on at least two occasions six or more hours apart.

During pregnancy, however, certain variations in blood pressure are normal. For example, an older primigravida tends to have higher blood pressure than her younger counterpart, although blood pressure usually falls with succeeding pregnancies up to a parity of five. In addition, late in the first trimester until near term, systolic pressure often decreases by 20 to 30 mmHg and diastolic pressure by 10 to 15 mmHg. During this period, blood pressure greater than 120/80 mmHg may be considered elevated (6).

Of course, blood pressure measurements tend to vary according to the individuals recording them; the size of the arm cuff being used (narrow or short cuffs may cause readings to be 5 to 10 mmHg above their actual values); the position of the individual being examined; and the selection of the end point for recording diastolic pressure (9). Most American authorities use the fifth phase of Korotkoff, or disappearance of sound, to represent true diastolic pressure (3).

A persisting diastolic pressure of 90 mmHg or more is considered abnormal. Nearly 25 percent of all cases of eclampsia occur when blood pressure is considered to be borderline, while about 50 percent occur when blood pressure is less than 160/110 mmHg (10).

One study of blood pressure during and following the first pregnancies of adolescents suggests that gestational hypertension may simply be unmasking latent hypertension. When compared

RECORD OF FINDINGS AT PRENATAL VISITS

Neg− Pos+ Date	Headaches	Dizziness/Visual Problem	Nausea/Vomiting	Edema—Face or Hands	Bleeding/Discharge	Abdominal Pain/Cramping	Constipation	Urinary complaints	Fetal Movements Daily by History	Weeks of Gestation	Fundal Heights (cms)	Fetal Heart Rate Doppler (D) Fetoscope (F)	Presentation/Lie	Weight	Blood Pressure	Albumin	Sugar	Ketones	Remarks/Signed
Feb 11	−	Dizz +	−/−	−	−	−	−	−	−	10	−	(D)+ 156	−	133	116/64	−	−	−	urine pregnancy test Positive on Feb 5
Feb 20	−	−	+/+	−	−	−	+	−	−	11	−	(D)+ 152	−	132	102/60	+ Trace	−	−	Urinary complaints
Feb 28	Mild +	−	N+ V−	−/−	−	−	−	−	−	12	−	(D)+ 148	−	132½	100/60	−	−	−	Pregnancy classes recommended
Mar 15	+	−	N+ V−	−/−	−	−	−	−	14	6	(D)+ 156	−	134	100/58	−	−	−	Attending "early pregnancy" classes
Mar 29	Mild +	−	−	−/−	−	−	−	−	−	16	13	(D)+ 148	−	135½	98/56	−	−	−	Prenatal Vitamins
Apr 11	−	−	−	−/−	−	unsure	−	−	18	16	(D)+ 152	−	137½	98/58	−	−	−	Individual counseling c Social workers
Apr 22	−	−	−	−/−	−	−	−	+	20	18	(F)+ 144	−	139	100/58	−	−	−	FHT + c fetoscope Quickening 1 wk ago
May 6	−	−	−	−/−	−	+	−	+	22	20	(F)+ 152	−	141½	96/54	−	−	−	Attending "mid-pregnancy" classes
May 28	−	−	−	−/−	−	−	−	+	25	23	(F)+ 140	−	144	98/56	−	−	−	Low Hgb & Hct 11 gm 33.5%
Jun 18	−	−	−	−/−	−	Pain LLQ	−	+	28	27	(F)+ 156	Br	146½	96/54	−	−	−	Ⓛ Round Ligament pain Body mechanics Demonstrated
Jul 1	−	−	−	−/−	−	−	−	+	30	28	(F)+ 144	Ceph	148	98/56	−	Trace	−	Individual Counseling re: Plans Rollover test positive
Jul 15	−	−	−	−/−	−	−	−	+	32	30	(F)+ 136	Ceph	149¾	102/58	−	−	−	Attending "Childbirth prep" classes. Rollover ⊕
Jul 30	−	−	−	p.m. feet	−	−	−	+	34	32	(F)+ 152	Ceph	152	106/62	−	−	−	Low Back discomfort— exercises practiced
Aug 6	−	−	−	p.m. feet	−	−	−	+	35	33	(F)+ 138	Ceph	152½	112/66	−	−	−	Upward trend in B.P.— watch closely
Aug 9	−	−	−	p.m. feet	−	−	−	+	35½	33	(D)+ 150	Vtx	153	116/64	−	−	−	Hgb & Hct improved 12 gm 38%
Aug 12	−	−	−	Hands Face Feet	−	−	−	+	36	34	(F)+ 148	Vtx	159	124/82	Trace	−	−	Rapid wt & B.P. rise Admitted—high risk unit

Allergies:

with women in a matched control group six and nine years after giving birth, the women who had a history of hypertension during pregnancy still had higher blood pressure. Also, the blood pressure of these women correlated with the high blood pressure of their children and their own mothers (11).

Weight. Among primigravidas, the development of hypertension has been associated with obesity (12). After a woman's first pregnancy, obesity or increased weight gain above 30 pounds apparently does not predispose the expectant mother to hypertension. However, a pattern of weight gain of more than two pounds per week or six pounds per month should be suspect for impending pregnancy-induced hypertension (10). For some women, sudden and excessive weight gain is the first sign of preeclampsia.

Diet. Evidence suggests that diet has an influence on the etiology of preeclampsia. Thomas Brewer has shown that adequate nutrition reduces the incidence of hypovolemia and hypoperfusion during pregnancy (13). Expectant mothers need a sufficient amount of protein as well as adequate caloric intake, especially if they are predisposed to pregnancy-induced hypertension (14). (See "The Community Health Nurse's Nutrition Guidelines"

NURSING PROCESS RECORD

Date	Problem Identification	Nursing Diagnoses	Action/Intervention	Evaluation*
Feb. 11	Fifteen-year-old nullipara (Janet). Unplanned pregnancy. No continuing relationship or contact with father of baby; does not wish to see him. Requested prenatal care, expressing desire for provider staff assistance throughout pregnancy.	Health status altered; at risk in pregnancy (psychosocial and biophysical). Developmental adolescent tasks compromised by superimposed pregnancy developmental tasks. Relationship with significant other altered. Vulnerability in personal relationships and own self-concept. Sexuality development conflicts.	Ongoing assessment of family and other support units. Lend staff support as indicated. Encourage Janet to attend special adolescent group education and counseling (early-, mid-, and late-pregnancy groups) and to take responsibility for participating in her own health maintenance. Multidisciplinary team care by nurse, physician, midwife, social worker nutritionist, and others as indicated. Plan for postpartum follow-up counseling in regard to her feelings about sexual relationships and future decision making about her sexuality.	_Maintain frequent schedule of prenatal visits with close involvement of family._ (Janet and family kept all appointments; mother and father visited periodically to request information and to contribute to planning Janet's care.) _Everything that is done is to become part of the teaching process._ _Participates in group educational sessions with multidisciplinary team and in her own assessments at each visit._ (Checks her own weight and urine with supervision. Later in pregnancy, assists in measuring uterine growth and in palpating for fetal movements and position.) Assists in recording of these for her own health record.
Feb. 20	Occasional mild nausea and vomiting (morning only). Weight loss. Sometimes skips breakfast.	Alterations in hormonal and gastrointestinal functioning during first trimester. Nutritional sufficiency compromised for meeting pregnancy needs.	Suggestions given for diet changes to reduce nausea in morning, following assessment of present nutrition pattern. Encouraged to take along for morning snacks and eating en route to school: fruit, boiled eggs, raw vegetables, peanut butter, crackers, and so forth.	_Acceptance and use of information._ _Nausea decreased_ in one week, and weight gain resumed.
Feb. 20	"Burning" sensation while urinating and "hurting low" in abdomen. (Medical diagnosis: urinary tract infection.)	Urinary elimination altered by pregnancy; dysuria present. Health management: preventive self-care needed. Risk of urinary tract infection increased during pregnancy.	Instructed Janet about preventive care to follow throughout pregnancy to prevent bacteriuria and/or urinary symptoms; will recheck urinary status each visit. (Medical prescription of antibiotic for urinary tract infection.)	Janet reports increased intake of water (decreased soft drinks) and use of perineal washes after elimination. _Monthly urine cultures remained negative; no further urinary symptoms._
Feb. 20	Missing school and feels tired and nauseated; asks why she feels this way.	Lacks information about normal and abnormal pregnancy changes.	Encouraged to begin pregnancy classes; to write down questions to bring to each visit; and to go to school.	_Further questions stimulated and exploration of feelings and concerns precipitated_ as a result of classes. Continued school.
April 22	Concerned about getting heavier and hips and breasts becoming larger.	Altered body image because of pregnancy is intensified during adolescence.	Talked about body changes occurring, what they mean, and how she feels about them.	_Continued to gain weight_ appropriate for her.
April 22	Doesn't know what friends at school and others will think about her being pregnant; feels ashamed. Not going out with friends much anymore.	Fear of rejection or reaction by others. Self-esteem diminished; expressions of shame. Social isolation; less social contact with peers.	Special individual counseling, allowing Janet to explore her feelings and to help sort out her own decisions and their possible short-term and long-term consequences. Encouraged parents' involvement in Janet's pregnancy; learning and problem solving as	_Able to talk about concerns._ _Openly verbalized feelings and conflicts._ Maintained peer relationships throughout pregnancy and successfully completed the school year in which pregnancy and delivery occurred.

Date	Assessment	Intervention	Outcome*
May 6	Thinking about quitting school and getting a job; doesn't want parents' help.	Independence-dependence conflict; expresses anger and conflicting actions.	a family.	*Family support and consistency to facilitate growth in identity development and conflict resolution.* Both parents participated in counseling/planning sessions.
May 28	Constipation problem.	Altered bowel elimination because of pregnancy.	Suggested changes in diet: adding more fiber foods, fresh vegetables, fresh fruits, and fluids.	*Relief from constipation* after trial adjustments to diet and fluid intake.
June 18	Low hemoglobin (11 gm) and hematocrit (33.5%)	Altered nutritional-metabolic requirements during pregnancy. Fluid volume physiologic increase (hemodilutional effect).	Reassessment of nutritional pattern, counseling, and meal planning to supply identified deficiencies; emphasis on adequate protein and caloric content plus vitamin and mineral supplements.	*Appropriate weight gain pattern and rise in hemoglobin and hematocrit* indicated improved dietary pattern (goal for weight gain of about one pound per week during later half of pregnancy).
June 18	Wanted to talk about adoption for baby; tears in eyes. Father expressed concern about her feelings; mother put arm around her.	Family coping/stress tolerance alteration. Coping growth potential indicated by expressions and actions. Feelings of conflict and indecision expressed. Grieving/anticipatory sadness expressed about coming loss of baby.	Family came together with provider staff and Janet to evaluate and work out problems through family mechanisms. Special counseling provided to assist in decision making about adoption.	*Evidence of strength* of family shown by mutual support, and by taking responsibility. *Janet made decision* to have baby adopted. Anxious to return to school after delivery. Shows growth in making decisions and taking responsibility.
July 1	Supine pressor test is positive.	Indicator of risk for pregnancy-induced hypertension. High activity and low rest pattern.	Recommended daily rest periods in lateral recumbent position.	
Aug. 6	Complaints about not sleeping well; low backaches; and baby moving so much. Expressed fear of labor and delivery; wishes it was over.	Sleep pattern disturbance and discomforts of late pregnancy. Fears expressed (usual to late pregnancy). Vulnerable to embarrassment or being hurt physically or emotionally.	Normalcy of her fears explained; reassured her. Prepared in advance in as concrete terms as possible for what to expect and how to help; gentleness applied in all situations. Toured high-risk unit and labor and delivery area to familiarize Janet with setting.	*Able to express her concerns and verbalize fears.* Able to be dependent when needed. *Care administered by specially prepared staff* (antepartum, intrapartum, and later follow-up) and familiar persons throughout.
Aug. 8	Upward trend in blood pressure.	Indicator of risk for preeclampsia.	Bed rest at home; daily checks by community health nurse. On "homebound" school program.	*Close observation for early recognition of danger signs* for preeclampsia.
Aug. 12	Rapid increase of blood pressure and weight. (Medical diagnosis: preeclampsia.)	Potential alteration in fetal-placental circulation as well as compromise of fetal and/or maternal welfare.	Admitted to high-risk (limited ambulation) unit; accompanied to unit and introduced to the area by familiar staff persons. Family members were able to visit Janet daily. Main focus of care was ambulation as desired and a diet consisting of a minimum of 2,400 calories per day and one gram of protein per each kilogram of weight plus supplemental foods from home. Assessments of fetal and maternal well-being included laboratory tests (renal function, serial urinary protein and estriol levels), daily weight measurements, nonstress tests, frequent blood pressure measurements, and elicitation of symptoms.	*Delivered seven-pound girl spontaneously at 40 weeks without major problems.*

*Based on stated outcome criteria (underlined).

by Barbara B. Deskins and Mary Fucile Laska, MCN 7:202-205, May/June 1982.)

Proteinuria. An increase in perinatal mortality is associated with proteinuria during pregnancy, regardless of blood pressure levels. Proteinuria accompanied by hypertension further increases the chance of perinatal death. Studies indicate that the dipstick method of testing urine for the presence of protein is reliable when using clean midstream or catheter specimens of urine. A 2+ or more reading of proteinuria is considered significant, a 1+ reading is questionable, and a trace is negligible (9).

Proteinuria frequently develops later than excessive weight gain and nearly always later than hypertension (2). Although 41 percent of eclamptics do not manifest proteinuria, it may be the most ominous sign of preeclampsia when it does develop (3,10).

Edema. By itself, edema is a common physiologic occurrence of pregnancy. However, in association with hypertension and proteinuria, edema is linked to a poor pregnancy outcome (9). Eclampsia may occur in 60 percent of women with only slight to moderate edema and in about 20 percent of women without edema (10). Since only about 15 percent of women with generalized edema develop preeclampsia, it is a very rough clinical parameter (3).

Determining Who Is at Risk

Two clinical tests, mean arterial pressure and the supine pressor (rollover) test, are useful in predicting a woman's chances of developing pregnancy-induced hypertension. Mean arterial pressure reflects the resistance against which the heart works and thus is an indicator of cardiac work. It is calculated by adding the diastolic pressure to one-third of the pulse pressure. For example, a blood pressure of 140/90 mmHg would equal a mean arterial pressure of 107 mmHg. (Note that blood pressures of 134/68 mmHg, 110/80 mmHg, and 130/70 mmHg all yield a mean arterial pressure of 90 mmHg.)

An increase of 20 mmHg in mean arterial pressure is considered ominous, as is blood pressure as low as 125/75 mmHg if it occurs before the thirty-second week of pregnancy. Perinatal morbidity and mortality have been shown to increase when midpregnancy mean arterial pressure is greater than 95 mmHg or when blood pressure rises above 130/80 mmHg (3,6,8). Additionally, in the absence of proteinuria or edema, a trend toward increased perinatal deaths has been noted when mean arterial pressure exceeds 92 mmHg by the beginning of the third trimester (8).

The supine pressor test, developed by Norman Gant and his colleagues, is based on the supine hypertensive response (15). For this test, done between 28 and 32 weeks' gestation, blood pressure is measured in the superior arm in the lateral recumbent position until stable. The woman then rolls over to the supine position, and blood pressure is measured immediately and again five minutes later. An increase of 20 mmHg or more in diastolic blood pressure while in the supine position is considered a positive indicator of potential development of pregnancy-induced hypertension (6,15).

A negative supine pressor test generally is accepted as sound evidence that pregnancy-induced hypertension will not develop (6). A single positive supine pressor test is accurate in predicting the development of pregnancy-induced

> *Evidence suggests that diet can influence the etiology of preeclampsia. Thomas Brewer has shown that adequate nutrition reduces the incidence of hypovolemia and hyperfusion during pregnancy. Expectant mothers need both a sufficient amount of protein and calories.*

hypertension in about 25 to 75 percent of all cases. One study showed that women who had two positive supine pressor tests and an average mean arterial pressure during the second trimester greater than 85 mmHg had an 88 percent chance of developing pregnancy-induced hypertension (16).

Intervention Measures

When risk factors such as borderline elevations in blood pressure or rapid weight gain are present, prenatal assessments need to be made at weekly or biweekly intervals. Once the signs of preeclampsia are clearly recognized, hospitalization is indicated, with activities and care appropriate to the severity of the case. In instances of lesser severity, limited ambulation on a high-risk pregnancy unit may be appropriate. Bed rest in the lateral recumbent position is necessary for a large portion of the day, and a diet ample in protein and coloric content is essential.

Frequent surveillance for visual disturbance, epigastric pain, headaches, rapid weight gain, and proteinuria is required. Plasma creatinine is measured often. The precise age of the fetus is determined, and fetal growth, welfare, and size are evaluated regularly. The expectant mother can assess fetal movements by making a daily count (14).

The expectant mother's sodium and fluid intake is neither restricted nor encouraged. However, diuretics, especially thiazides, must be avoided. Diuretics are ineffective in deterring the course of preeclampsia/eclampsia, and they may further compromise intravascular volume as well as deplete sodium and potassium stores. For the infant, diuretics may cause decreased placental perfusion, thrombocytopenia, hyperbilirubinemia, and altered carbohydrate metabolism.

Antihypertensives also must be avoided unless diastolic pressure reaches 110 mmHg or more. Note that sodium restriction, antihypertensives, and diuretics have all been shown to decrease the placental clearance of dehydroepiandrosterone sulfate to estradiol and may thereby decrease uteroplacental perfusion (2,14,17).

A Case in Point

The following case example illustrates the kinds of basic care needed by women who are at risk of developing pregnancy-induced hypertension. It demonstrates how nursing care for an underlying medical problem is integrated with nursing care to meet other needs of the patient.

After a positive pregnancy test and early examination confirmed pregnancy, 15-year-old Janet received counseling and requested to continue being seen for prenatal care during her pregnancy. It was her first pregnancy. The health history for her family revealed that, for the previous two years, Janet's mother had regularly taken medication for high blood pressure. However, Janet had no previous health problems of significance.

Throughout her pregnancy, Janet was seen by a multidisciplinary team that worked closely with Janet's parents and a girl friend, her major support system. Because of her young age, the fact that she never had been pregnant before, a family history of hypertension, and positive supine pressor tests on two occasions, Janet was assessed at frequent intervals. When she experienced rapid weight gain and rising blood pressure, she was hospitalized.

Janet's care included limited ambulation, adequate diet, and close surveillance during the last weeks of pregnancy. (The findings for each prenatal visit are summarized in the accompanying charts.) As a result of this care, Janet's pregnancy culminated in an uncomplicated, vaginal birth.

A Better Chance

Expectant mothers who are at risk of developing pregnancy-induced hypertension need to be identified as early as possible. For the woman who has a hypertensive disorder, frequent monitoring of her condition throughout pregnancy and appropriate care measures can improve her chances of having a successful pregnancy outcome.

REFERENCES

1. BEER, A. E. Possible immunologic bases of preeclampsia/eclampsia. Semin.Perinatol. 2:39-56, Jan. 1978.
2. PRITCHARD, J. A. AND MACDONALD, P. C. Williams Obstetrics. 16th ed. New York, Appleton-Century-Crofts, 1980, pp. 665-697.
3. CAVANAGH, DENIS, AND KNUPPEL, R. A. Preeclampsia and eclampsia. In Principles and Practice of Obstetrics and Perinatology, ed. by Leslie Iffy and H. A. Kaminetzky. New York, John Wiley & Sons, 1981, pp 1271-1290.
4. LUECK, JUDITH, AND OTHERS. Observation of an organism found in patients with gestational trophoblastic disease and in patients with toxemia of pregnancy. Am.J.Obstet.Gynecol. 145:15-26, Jan. 1, 1983.
5. ALADJEM, SILVIO, AND OTHERS. Experimental induction of a toxemia-like syndrome in the pregnant beagle. Am.J.Obstet.Gynecol. 145:27-38, Jan. 1, 1983.
6. O'SHANUGHNESSY, RICHARD, AND ZUSPAN, F. P. Managing acute pregnancy hypertension. Contemp.OB/GYN 18:85-98, Nov. 1981.
7. CUNNINGHAM, F. G., AND PRITCHARD, J. A. Hematologic considerations of pregnancy-induced hypertension. Semin.Perinatol. 2:29-38, Jan. 1978.
8. WELT, S. I., AND CRENSHAW, M. C., JR. Concurrent hypertension and pregnancy. Clin.Obstet.Gynecol. 21:619-648, Sept. 1978.
9. DAVIES, A. M. Epidemiology of the hypertensive disorders of pregnancy. Bull.WHO 57(3):373-386, 1979.
10. HALVERSON, G. M. Toxemia in pregnancy. Wis.Med.J. 79:27-28, July 1979.
11. KOTCHEN, J. M., AND OTHERS. Blood pressure of young mothers and their children after hypertension in adolescent pregnancy: six-to-nine year follow-up. Am.J.Epidemiol. 115:861-867, June 1982.
12. FRIEDMAN, E. A., AND NEFF, R. K. Pregnancy Hypertension: A Systematic Evcluation of Clinical Diagnosis Critera. Littleton, Mass., John Wright—PSG, 1977, pp. 204-212.
13. BREWER, T. Role of malnutrition in pre-eclampsia and eclampsia. Am.J.Obstet.Gynecol. 125:281-282, May 15, 1976.
14. GILSTRAP, L. C., III, AND OTHERS. Management of pregnancy-induced hypertension in the nulliparous patient remote from term. Semin.Perinatol. 2:73-81, Jan. 1978.
15. GANT, N. F., AND OTHERS. A clinical test useful for predicting the development of acute hypertension in pregnancy. Am.J.Obstet.Gynecol. 120:1-7, Sept. 1, 1974.
16. PHELAN, J. P. Enhanced prediction of pregnancy-induced hypertension by combining supine pressor test with mean arterial pressure of middle trimester. Am.J.Obstet.Gynecol. 129:397-400, Oct. 15, 1977.
17. MATHEWS, D. D., AND OTHERS. A randomized controlled trial of complete bed rest versus ambulation in the management of proteinuric hypertension during pregnancy. Obstet.Gynecol.Surv. 38:94-95, Feb. 1983.

BIBLIOGRAPHY

GANT, N. F., AND OTHERS. Clinical management of pregnancy-induced hypertension. Clin.Obstet.Gynecol. 21:397-409, June 1978.
KELLEY, MAUREEN. Maternal position and blood pressure during pregnancy and delivery. Am.J.Nurs. 82:809, May 1982.
———., AND MONGIELLO, ROSANNE. Labor, delivery, and postpartum. Am.J.Nurs. 82:813, May 1982.
WILLIS, S. E. Hypertension in pregnancy, pathophysiology. Am.J.Nurs. 82:791-792, May 1982.
———., AND SHARP, E. S. Prenatal detection and management. Am.J.Nurs. 82:798, May 1982.

Herpes Genitalis And The Childbearing Cycle

Reprinted from American Journal of Maternal/Child Nursing, May/June 1983.

Nurses increasingly must contend with the fears and frustrations caused by this onerous disease and its effects on pregnancy and the newborn.

NANCY ZEWEN PERLEY/BARBARA J. BILLS

Statistics vary as to its incidence, but approximately 5 million to 20 million adults in the United States have already been infected with a herpes virus. The number of individuals contracting this ailment is increasing so rapidly that it may soon bypass gonorrhea as the most common sexually transmitted disease (STD).

Unfortunately, the growing incidence of herpes is not the only disturbing factor. Individuals can never rid themselves of this virus, and both symptomatic and asymptomatic pregnant women can transmit the disease to their newborns during delivery. The possible result is a serious, even fatal, infection.

The five herpes viruses that affect human beings are the varicella-zoster virus, the Epstein-Barr virus, the cytomegalovirus (CMV), the herpes simplex virus Type 1 (HSV-1), and the herpes simplex virus Type 2 (HSV-2). All share two important characteristics: *latency* (the ability to lie dormant within the body) and *reactivation* (the ability to cause symptoms without reinfection).

The two herpes simplex viruses (HSV-1 and HSV-2) have different chemical and biological properties as well as different clinical patterns. Most lesions that occur above the waist (mouth and eyes) are caused by HSV-1, while most lesions that occur below the waist (genital) are caused by HSV-2. However, approximately 10 to 15 percent of genital lesions are caused by HSV-1.

Genital herpes is thought to be sexually transmitted by vaginal intercourse, oral/genital and oral/anal contact, and anal intercourse. In addition, HSV-1 can be transmitted to the genital area by hand contact. Despite widespread popular belief that herpes can be transmitted to an individual via inanimate objects such as toilet seats, drinking glasses, or wash cloths, there is no documented evidence at this time to support the theory.

The incubation period of both HSV-1 and HSV-2 appears to range from two to ten days. After initial infection, the virus is thought to remain within the body by traveling along sensory nerve pathways and lying inside the sensory nerve ganglion (located in the spine). Approximately 14 percent of the individuals infected with HSV-1 and 60 percent of the individuals infected with HSV-2 will have a recurrence within the first year [1].

Women may experience four to six recurrences per year; the mean interval between infections varies from 40 to 60 days. The recurrence rate decreases one year after the primary infection. Researchers suggest that the inconsistency in recurrence rates may be related to the different specific strains of the herpes virus [1].

Although researchers have not been able to determine the cause of recurrent genital herpes, affected individuals have reported that the following may be provoking factors: ovulation, menses, heat, emotional stress, friction associated with intercourse, systemic infection, and pregnancy [2]. The role of immune responses such as antibody formation is unclear, but antibodies apparently do not form in every affected individual and do not protect against recurrences [3].

Clinical Course

Active primary genital herpes infections last an average of 21 days and can be caused by either HSV-1 or HSV-2. The clinical picture for both viruses is similar, although HSV-1 may cause a milder infection.

After the incubation period, the first stage of primary genital herpes is characterized by the formation of extremely tender and painful vesicles. In males, these thin-walled blisters usually are located on the glans or shaft of the penis or on the anus. In females, the lesions usually are located on the vulva,

---

MS. PERLEY, R.N.C., M.S.N., *is an instructor in women's health care for the nurse practitioner program at the Harbor U.C.L.A. Medical Center in Torrance, California.* MS. BILLS, C.N.M., M.S., *is a certified nurse midwife in private practice in Los Angeles, California.*

cervix, vagina, anus, or buttocks. The first stage lasts for approximately six days and may be accompanied by tender inguinal lymph nodes, fever, malaise, and dysuria.

After the vesicle breaks, a wet ulcer forms. Since the ulcer (a shallow crater with a yellow border) is an open area, exposure to other pathogens may result in a secondary infection. This second stage of primary genital herpes averages six days in length and is accompanied by severe pain.

The final stage of primary genital herpes (average length eight days) is characterized by the formation of dry crusts. The associated symptoms will disappear during this healing process. Also, viral shedding usually will cease when reepithelialization occurs. After the lesion has completely healed, the area may be free of any evidence that the lesion had existed.

Secondary (recurrent) genital herpes infections usually are shorter in duration and milder in intensity. About 70 percent of patients report that these infections begin with a recognizable prodromal period lasting one to two days. Symptoms include edema or itching in the previously affected area and posterior sacral neuralgia (4).

The progressive stages of secondary genital herpes lesions are similar to the stages of primary genital herpes lesions with the exception of the average length of each stage. The vesicular stage lasts about two days, the wet ulcer stage about three days, and the healing, dry crust stage about seven days. In addition, secondary infections usually have lower rates of complications and no systemic symptoms.

Available Laboratory Methods

Herpes usually can be diagnosed by taking a thorough patient history and having a skilled practitioner inspect the lesion. A number of laboratory tests are available to confirm the presence of the virus.

Tissue cultures are the most sensitive laboratory test for diagnosing the herpes simplex virus. They also can be used for differentiating HSV-1 from HSV-2. Since peak viral shedding occurs before the sixth day of the infection, the probability of false negative results will be decreased if the culture is obtained as early as possible.

To obtain a culture, first roll a sterile cotton-tipped applicator over the open lesion or, if possible, aspirate the fluid of the vesicle with a tuberculin syringe. Then, quickly inoculate (swab) the transfer media. Because of the heat liability of the virus, the media must be sent to the laboratory on ice or in a refrigerated compartment. Under optimal conditions, the culture can be positive within 24 to 48 hours. However, a culture cannot be assumed to be negative for at least 10 to 14 days.

The average cost of a herpes culture ranges from $36.00 to $100.00. Many state health departments

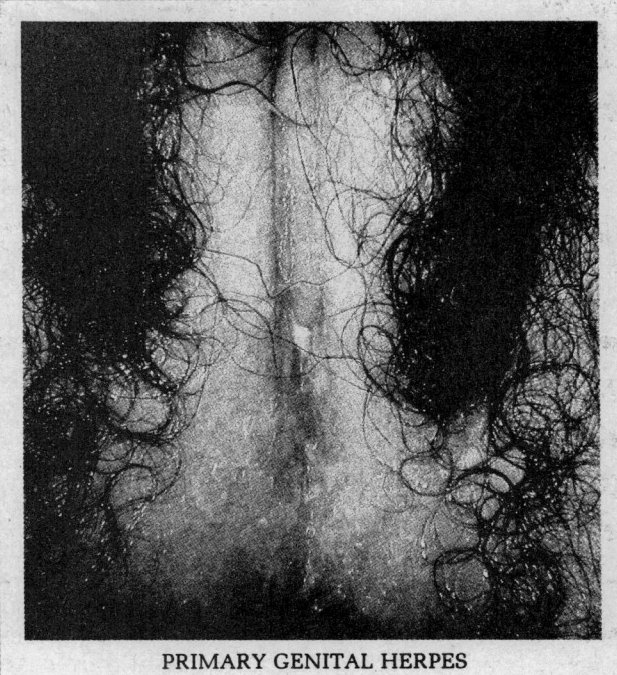

PRIMARY GENITAL HERPES

provide the service of culturing free of charge.

If a viral culture is not available or practical, a Papanicolaou (Pap) test or other cytological tests can be used to diagnose herpes simplex. However, they cannot be used to differentiate HSV-1 from HSV-2. The Pap test is positive in 50 percent of infections and is more accurate if done early.

To conduct a Pap test, first scrape an open active lesion with a Pap spatula. Then smear the virus on a slide and send it to the laboratory according to instructions. The test is diagnosed as positive if the multinucleated and inclusion-bearing cells indicative of herpes are seen microscopically. The cost is approximately $6.00.

Serum antibody titers have limited use in the diagnosis of herpes because they have a significant rate of false negative results and cannot be used to differentiate HSV-1 from HSV-2. Also, titers may not rise between primary and secondary infections (5).

Treatment Modalities

Presently, genital herpes infections cannot be prevented or cured. The current treatment modalities are either ineffective or limited or they provide only symptomatic relief.

Some of the ineffective agents are Betadine, ether, polio vaccine, iodine preparation, and Trimethopri-sulfa Methaxazole, all of which do not appear to have any long-term side effects. Agents such as photoactive dyes, neutral red, BCG, and smallpox vaccinations have been linked with adverse reactions. A few agents such as 2-deoxy-D-glucose and lysine have received considerable media attention, but they have been shown to be ineffective to date (2).

Another recent method of medical management that has received considerable press coverage is acyclovir (Zovirax Ointment 5%). This agent shows promise in the treatment of primary genital herpes infections by decreasing healing and viral shedding time, but it does not appear to significantly reduce herpetic pain.

According to the Food and Drug Administration (FDA), some research studies demonstrate that acyclovir significantly reduces the multiplication of the virus and decreases the duration of pain in immunodeficient patients. Further, the FDA recommends that acyclovir should be used during pregnancy only if the potential benefit to the mother justifies the potential risk to the fetus. The safety of this drug during lactation has not been established (6).

Since medical management of genital herpes still is limited, good hygiene is especially important in treating it. An affected individual can decrease the spread of infection that can occur by autoinoculation and help prevent secondary bacterial or yeast infections by washing hands thoroughly with mild soap and water and bathing daily. In addition, keeping the lesion dry helps decrease the period of viral shedding. Corn starch is effective for this purpose, as is drying the area carefully with a hair dryer or heat lamp and wearing only well-ventilated garments (cotton-crotched underpants, loose pants, and skirts). If a secondary infection develops, the area should be treated with an appropriate antibacterial or antifungal topical ointment.

Pain associated with herpetic lesions can be decreased by taking a mild analgesic such as A.S.A. or Tylenol, drying the infected area with a heat lamp for 20 minutes three times a day, taking sitz baths morning and evening for 15 to 20 minutes, applying wet compresses (Burow's solution) and gauze pads to the affected area for 20 minutes three times a day, and applying topical anesthetics (lidocaine jelly) to affected areas three times a day (7).

Potentially Greater Problems

The most common medical complication of genital herpes is urinary retention. Although primarily associated with the initial disease, this complication can occur with subsequent infections. Urinary retention develops in response to the dysuria, edema, and voiding hesitancy that accompanies genital herpes and may predispose the individual to a urinary tract infection (UTI).

Management and prevention of urinary retention includes drinking adequate fluids (6 to 8 glasses per day) and voiding frequently to decrease the incidence of UTI; pouring warm water over the vulva area and voiding while sitting in sitz baths to decrease the pain of dysuria; inserting an indwelling catheter if adequate elimination is not possible (an indwelling catheter may be contraindicated during advanced pregnancy because of the associated discomfort); and observing for signs and symptoms of UTI.

Viral encephalitis is a rare complication of herpes (the estimated frequency is several hundred to several thousand cases per year). Clinical assessment includes headaches, fever, behavioral disorders, speech difficulties, olfactory hallucinations, and facial seizures. The mortality rate of untreated cases ranges from 60 to 80 percent (3).

Research studies indicate that the incidence of cervical cancer may be higher among women who have a genital herpes infection. The risk of these women developing dysplasia or invasive cancer increases fourfold if they have antibodies to HSV-2. However, these findings remain inconclusive because the studies did not control for other factors that are associated with cervical cancer (early age of initial intercourse, multiple sexual partners, and other sexually transmitted diseases). Nevertheless, cervical Pap tests at six-month to one-year intervals are recommended for these women (1).

The Risks During Pregnancy

Some research studies indicate that spontaneous abortion and congenital anomalies may occur as the result of a primary herpes infection. Since these studies are not conclusive and the incidence probably is rare, the use of therapeutic abortion to avoid congenital anomalies is not recommended at the present time (8). The incidence of premature birth also may be higher among women who have genital herpes (9).

Transplacental exposure during pregnancy is documented but considered rare. The major problem associated with genital herpes and pregnancy is the possibility of transmitting the virus to the fetus during delivery. Studies demonstrate that approximately 25 to 60 percent of fetuses will develop serious neonatal herpes infections if delivered through an infected canal (10).

The incidence of genital herpes during pregnancy has been documented as being less than one percent, although 10 to 50 percent of pregnant women have been identified as asymptomatic carriers (characterized by viral shedding without the presence of symptoms). Yet, only an average of 121 cases of disseminated newborn herpes are reported annually in the United States. More research is needed to adequately assess the scope of the problem (11).

Despite the high percentage of pregnant women who appear to be asymptomatic carriers, screening all pregnant women for genital herpes is not indicated at the present time. However, all pregnant women should be questioned carefully. If a woman meets any of the following criteria, she is considered

to be at risk and should have viral cultures taken weekly after 34 to 36 weeks of gestation:
1. Any woman who has a suspicious lesion during pregnancy.
2. Any woman who has a known or suspected previous history of genital herpes.
3. Any woman who has had a sexual partner with a known or suspected previous history of genital herpes.

Tapping the amniotic fluid for herpes is not recommended since it has caused transplacental infection in a few cases (12).

Because of the increasing rate of cesarean deliveries and associated risk, much controversy surrounds the use of cesarean birth in the management of genital herpes during pregnancy. If a herpes lesion is suspected after 34 to 36 weeks gestation, the following generally accepted approach is recommended:
1. If all weekly herpes cultures are negative, allow a vaginal delivery.
2. If the initial culture is positive, reculture at weekly intervals.
3. If two consecutive cultures are negative (despite an initial postive culture) and there are no new lesions or positive cultures, allow a vaginal delivery.
4. If the culture is positive and labor begins, perform a cesarean delivery.
5. If the culture is positive and membranes have ruptured, perform a cesarean delivery within four hours since the fetus can become contaminated from an ascending herpes infection (12).

Postpartum Considerations

Minimal guidelines are available for controlling active herpes simplex in the postpartum women. Sidney Kibrick recommends that these mothers be given a private room in order to prevent cross-contamination. Nurses should use standard skin isolation techniques, including wearing a gown and gloves and double-bagging the mother's linen (13).

A mother with active herpes can handle and breast-feed her infant if she carefully washes her hands, uses a clean cover gown and possibly gloves, avoids hand contact with the lesion, and handles the infant away from her bed (12). Neonates born to mothers with herpes should be isolated from other neonates and carefully observed for the disease. Having the infant room with the mother may have the most advantages. Nurses who handle these infants need to wear a gown and gloves and follow the previously mentioned isolation techniques.

Newborns who have contracted herpes may have only a mild, localized infection, although they sometimes have a fatal, disseminated one. The incubation period is two to twelve days. Infants born to mothers with a primary herpes infection during pregnancy appear to be at a higher risk of developing a severe infection than infants born to mothers with a recurrent herpes infection (13).

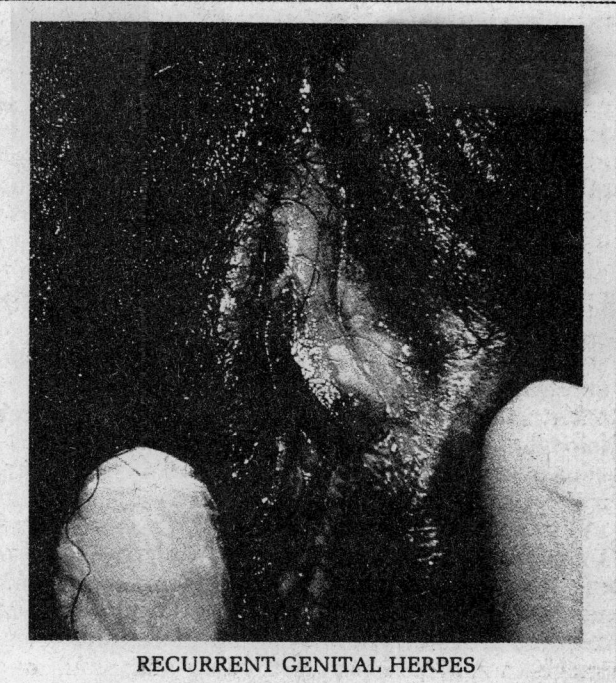
RECURRENT GENITAL HERPES

The mild form of herpes in the newborn may present itself as lesions involving the skin, eyes, or oral cavity. Severe, disseminated infections may cause sepsis, convulsions, jaundice, hepatosplenomegaly, central nervous system anomalies, chorioretinitis, encephalitis, D.I.C., irritability, and temperature instability (3).

In one study of 206 infants with herpes, the mortality rate was 65 percent. Of the survivors, 40 to 60 percent often had neurological or other organ sequelae (3). Vidarabine is available for treatment of neonatal hepatic infection, but for maximum efficacy it must be administered before signs and symptoms of illness develop. Further, this drug may have toxic systemic effect. Acyclovir also may be helpful in treating newborns (1).

Why Me?

Even in this age of more casual sexual mores, acquisition of a sexually transmitted disease can elicit many feelings of anxiety, guilt, and shame within the affected person. A recent study found that 35 percent of the people afflicted with herpes reported a sexual dysfunction related to the contraction of the disease (14).

The effect of the virus on sexuality probably is caused by fear that the disease may be transmitted to a present partner; fear that future transmission might prevent a sexual relationship with a new partner; rejection by present or future partners because of the disease; and/or decreased frequency of intercourse and sexual alternatives because of fear of transmission. These factors contribute to feelings of isolation, sexual inadequacy, and a lack of sexual fulfillment. Many individuals afflicted with herpes report that they approach sexual relationships with much more caution than they did before they contracted the virus.

Unfortunately, many meaningful relationships have dissolved over the acquisition of genital herpes. Partners may be wrongly blamed for a recent infection and often are accused of infidelity. The dormant characteristic of the virus makes it extremely difficult to accurately pinpoint the time of first exposure. Many people state they have no knowledge of recent exposure and do not recall a primary infection.

Genital herpes also can significantly affect an individual's body image and self-concept, resulting in feelings of anger, depression, guilt, anxiety, hopelessness, and despair. The intensity of emotions that are experienced depends on the strength of the individual's self-concept, the ability to cope with adversity, the frequency and intensity of infections, and the amount of support given by significant others.

The pregnant woman who has herpes experiences even greater psychosocial problems because the condition of pregnancy itself has a psychosocial impact on the woman and her partner. In addition, fear for the safety of the unborn baby may give rise to intense feelings of guilt and anger as well as inappropriate blaming. This can disrupt the couple's relationship and prevent them from adequately dealing with the psychological tasks of pregnancy. The couple also must face the possibility of a cesarean delivery, which of course increases risk, cost, and recovery time.

Teacher and Counselor

Patient education is extremely important in the management of genital herpes. The following areas need to be covered: characteristics and epidemiology of the virus, clinical manifestations, clinical course, methods of preventing transmission, comfort measures, need to have Pap tests every 6 to 12 months, diagnostic measures, new treatments, risk of transmitting herpes to fetus during delivery, need for viral cultures during the last month of pregnancy, cesarean versus vaginal delivery, postpartum precautions and precautions for controlling the spread of infection to the infant, clinical manifestations of herpes in newborns, and information about self-help groups.

Since all of the necessary patient education probably cannot be covered in one prenatal visit, several short sessions with printed handouts are suggested. The woman's partner should be encouraged to attend at least one prenatal visit so that his questions and concerns can be addressed. A dated checklist of all the teaching points covered helps ensure that areas are neither missed nor repeated.

Pregnancy complicated by a herpes infection magnifies the need for effective, empathetic counseling. In addition to having questions, the pregnant woman and her partner probably will feel varying degrees of fear, anxiety, shame, and anger. The nurse needs to encourage the expression of these emotions to promote understanding, give a feeling of control, and restore a sense of well-being within the couple.

Since sexuality may be disturbed by genital herpes, sexual issues need to be discussed with both the pregnant woman and her partner. A conservative but safe approach is to advise the couple to abstain from sexual intercourse and oral-genital contact from the time a lesion is suspected through complete healing of the lesion. Abstinence should be advised during both primary and recurrent infections, although transmission during recurrent infections is not clearly understood. Appropriate alternatives to sexual intercourse and oral-genital contact such as fondling and mutual masturbation can be suggested. If sexual problems appear to threaten the stability of the relationship, a referral to a sex counselor may be indicated.

Genital herpes during pregnancy can present many problems to the affected couple. Through medical management, patient education, and empathetic counseling, the nurse can help the couple achieve a positive outcome for the pregnancy and maintain the stable relationship necessary for the rewards and responsibilities of parenthood.

REFERENCES

1. BAKER, D. Prospects for treating herpes. Contemp. Ob/Gyn 19:179-187, Jan. 1982.
2. KELLUM, M., AND LOUCKS, A. Genital herpes infections: diagnosis and management. Nurse Pract. 7:14-18, 21, Feb. 1982.
3. DOUGLAS, G. DNA viruses. In Principles and Practice of Infectious Diseases, ed. by Mandell and others. New York, John Wiley & Sons, 1977, p. 1288.
4. DRY lesions may shorten periods of viral shedding: professionals urged to provide counseling. Sex.Transmitted Dis.Bull. 1:4, Dec. 1981.
5. ANTIBODY titer poor indicator for recurrent genital herpes: no difference found between infected and uninfected groups. Sex.Transmitted Dis.Bull. 2:9, Feb. 1981.
6. BETTOLI, E. Herpes: facts and fallacies. Am.J.Nurs. 82:924-929, June 1982.
7. GLOGAU, R. G. How I treat herpes simplex. Med.Times 108:66-68, Mar. 1980.
8. EDWARDS, M. S. Venereal herpes: a nursing overview. JOGN Nurs. 7:7-15, Sept-Oct. 1978.
9. WHITLEY, J., AND OTHERS. Natural history of herpes simplex virus infection of mother and newborn. Pediatrics 66:489-494, Oct. 1980.
10. BEHLMER, S. D., AND ANDERSON, P. C. Herpes simplex infections complicating parturition. Int.J.Dermatol. 20:242-248, May 1981.
11. ADAMS, S. K. Herpes simplex virus. In Protocols for Perinatal Nursing Practice, ed. by R. H. Perez. St. Louis, C.V. Mosby Co., 1981, pp. 149-155.
12. GROSSMAN, J. H., AND OTHERS. Management of genital herpes simplex virus infection during pregnancy. Obstet.Gynecol. 58:1-4, July 1981.
13. KIBRICK, S. Herpes simplex at term: what to do with mother, newborn, and nursery personnel. JAMA 243:157-160, Jan. 11, 1980.
14. SURVEY of patients finds high incidence of depression, sexual dysfunction; not related to severity of disease. Sex.Transmitted Dis.Bull. 2:3, Feb. 1982.

OBSTETRICAL ANALGESICS AND ANESTHESIA: Methods of Relief for the Patient in Labor

Reprinted from American Journal of Nursing, February 1977

RAE KROHN GRAD
JACK WOODSIDE

You are taking care of a woman in active labor who is complaining of severe pain. The physician orders 75 mg. of meperidine (Demerol) IM stat. Forty-five minutes later he tells you that the patient needs a cesarean section, and asks you to have the patient sign the consent form for the operation. Should you do it?

You are caring for a woman who delivered her baby by prepared childbirth 12 hours ago. Now she is trying unsuccessfully to breast-feed the baby, who is drowsy. You find out that the mother is upset because the resident physician insisted that she be given Demerol 50 mg. and hydroxyzine HCl (Vistaril) 50 mg. IM when her cervix was eight centimeters dilated, because she lost control during a few contractions. Now she feels that she failed and is sure the baby is too "doped up" to nurse. Is she right to be upset? How would you respond to her?

Information in textbooks and package inserts does not tell all you need to know about the nursing care of obstetric patients who are receiving medications. A pharmacology book may say that epidural anesthesia, if successful, blocks the pain of labor and delivery but also may cause maternal hypotension. Unfortunately, this is where much of the published information ends. Who describes the panic many mothers feel when they cannot move their legs or control their shaking after spinal anesthesia? Who talks about the temporary disorientation that may follow large doses of epidural medication?

The discomfort of labor and delivery is caused by traction on the adnexal, uterine, and cervical nerves. Pain also results from pressure on the uterus, bladder, urethra, and bowel, from dilatation of the cervix, from hypoxia and the accumulation of catabolites (waste products) in the myometrium, and not least of all from fear, tension, and anxiety.

The options for relieving these discomforts may be divided into six general types:

- positive conditioning, such as the Lamaze method of prepared childbirth
- sedatives/tranquilizers, which reduce anxiety and tension
- amnesics, which blot out the memory of pain
- general analgesia, which raises the threshhold of pain perception
- regional analgesia, which interrupts the afferent pathways of pain, and
- general anesthesia, which prevents central perception of pain.

We will discuss the nursing implications of the most common types of pain relief, excluding amnesics and general anesthesia, which now are rarely used.

Positive Conditioning

Prepared or natural childbirth is the major form of conditioning used to aid a mother in coping with anxiety, fear, tension, and discomfort by means of controlled breathing and relaxation during labor and delivery. Prepared childbirth and pain medication are not mutually exclusive, but the prepared woman usually needs less medication to overcome discomfort.

Your knowledge of how and when certain medications should and can be used may help the prepared mother to have a satisfying experience. Assure her that she has not "given up" if she asks for or needs medication. Keep in mind that medication must be given at the proper time to relieve discomfort.

The woman mentioned earlier who had maintained control until her cervix was eight to nine centimeters dilated and then had a few fleeting moments of doubt probably needed encouragement more than Demerol and Vistaril, because she would have been completely dilated and ready to push by the time the medication took effect. Because she did receive medication so close to delivery, however, this mother needed reassurance that her baby's drowsiness 12 hours after birth may have been a normal sleepiness rather than a drug-induced one, and that it would be temporary.

The management of labor and delivery is rarely a question of absolutes. Flexibility in the nurse's, physician's, and patient's attitudes about medication is extremely important.

Sedatives and Tranquilizers

These medications are used frequently, especially in the early stages of labor when some mothers are particularly tense. Such drugs as pentobarbital sodium (Nembutal), secobarbital sodium (Seconal), diazepam (Valium), and hydroxyzine HCl (Vistaril) lower the perception of stimuli and enhance mental and physical relaxation.

Given alone, sedatives and tranquilizers do not affect the pain threshhold, but they do reduce the amount of analgesic needed when given in combination with analgesics. Sedatives and tranquilizers can slow labor, and may lead to lethargy, sleep, or mood elevation; or to a lowering of inhibitions, restlessness, or delirium. These drugs may affect the attention span of the newborn for the first 24 to 48 hours, because the baby does not metabolize them as rapidly as an adult(1).

There are several implications for nursing of the sedated labor patient.

Remember the environment. Make it quieter by turning down the lights, lowering the shades, and minimizing

---

RAE KROHN GRAD, R.N., M.A., is an instructor in obstetrics at George Mason University, Fairfax, Va. She also works part time in labor and delivery at Alexandria Hospital, Alexandria, Va.

JACK WOODSIDE, M.D., is director of anesthesia at Alexandria Hospital, Alexandria, Va.

Effects of Agents Used for Pain Relief During Labor

Agent or Technique	Optimal Dose	Therapeutic Effect	Maternal Side Effect	Fetal/Newborn Side Effect	Miscellaneous Information
Sedatives secobarbital (Sconal) pentobarbital (Nembutal) phenobarbital (Luminal)	100 mg. IM, 50 mg. I.V. 100 mg. IM, PO, 50 mg. I.V. 100 mg. I.V., PO	sedation and sleep	vertigo, decreased perception of sensory stimuli, nausea and vomiting, decreased blood pressure	possible central nervous system depression or apnea	may cause restlessness when used alone; may slow labor
Tranquilizers diazepam (Valium) hydroxyzine (Vistaril) propiomazine (Largon) promethazine (Phenergan) promazine (Sparine)	2, 5, or 10 mg. I.V., IM, PO 5-15 mg. IM, PO 20-40 mg. IM, PO 25-50 mg. IM, PO 25 mg. IM, PO	lowered tension and apprehension levels	vertigo, drowsiness, decreased blood pressure	possible CNS depression	enhances analgesic drug action
Analgesics meperidine (Demerol) morphine sulfate alphaprodine (Nisentil)	50-100 mg. IM 8-15 mg. IM 20-40 mg. IM, I.V.	increased pain threshhold	nausea and vomiting, mild respiratory and circulatory depression	possible CNS depression	not given when delivery imminent; used in combination with tranquilizers
General Anesthetics trichloroethylene (Trilene) methoxyflurane (Penthrane) nitrous oxide cyclopropane diethyl ether halothane	0.5 percent 0.3-0.5 percent 40 percent 3-5 percent (inhalation) 2-5 percent 0.5-1 percent	analgesia during 1st stage of labor; loss of consciousness in 2nd stage	possible aspiration or cyanosis	possible CNS depression or hypoxia	Trilene volatile; Trilene and Penthrane can be self-administered by hand-held mask.
Local Anesthetics Procaine (Novocaine) Dibucaine (Nupercaine) Lidocaine (Xylocaine) Tetracaine (Pontocaine) Mepivacaine (Carbocaine) Chloroprocaine (Nesacaine) Bupivacaine (Marcaine)	concentration varies from 0.5-2 percent solutions	loss of sensation by blocking conduction of nerve impulses	effects depend on mode of administration	effects depend on mode of administration	
Types of Local Analgesia epidural block caudal block	5-15 ml. of 1, 1.5, or 2 percent sol.	high degree of pain relief	mild hypotension is frequent; loss of bearing down reflex in 2nd stage	none unless severe sustained maternal hypotension	may slow labor; epidural blocks pain at each stage of labor; caudal causes mild hypotension
paracervical block	5-10 ml. of 1 percent sol. bilaterally	temporary block of pain during labor	transient depression of contractions	occasional bradycardia	analgesia during labor, but no perineal anesthesia
pudendal block	5-10 ml. of 1 percent sol. bilaterally	nerve block for 2nd stage of labor	loss of bearing down reflex	rarely any	does not relieve contraction pain, anesthetizes perineum
saddle block	1-1.5 ml., concentration depends on agent used	high degree of pain relief	occasionally, post-spinal headache	rarely any	uncomfortable position while block administered; can be used only when delivery is imminent; excellent for delivery

OB ANALGESIA

interruptions, and by changing the linens and promptly clearing the room of any disagreeable odors or sights.

Use touch. When giving a mother medication, offer a backrub or abdominal effleurage. Sponge her face and hands with a cool cloth. Hold her hand and speak soothingly.

Use the power of positive thinking. Try a few encouraging words—"This medication will ease your contractions and let you sleep," or "This drug will help stop your nausea and shaking." Convincing reassurance and positive suggestion can do wonders in enhancing the drug's effectiveness.

Inform your patient. It helps a mother to know that after an injection of Vistaril she may feel lightheaded or have trouble being alert. If she is using special breathing techniques, reassure her that she will be awakened in time to breathe with each contraction.

Analgesics

Analgesics increase tolerance of pain by about 50 percent. When given intramuscularly, their peak action usually occurs within 60 to 90 minutes, and each dose has an effective duration of about two to three hours(1). The desired relaxation and easing of pain may be accompanied by such side effects as indifference, euphoria, apathy, lethargy, sleep, or nausea and vomiting. As with most other drugs, large doses of analgesics can slow labor, especially if given too early.

During the first stage of labor, Demerol is the most commonly used narcotic. This drug readily crosses the placenta, so the smallest effective amount should be used.

The effect of Demerol on the fetus is related to the amount of drug in the fetal circulation and to the time of administration. Such factors as gestational age, weight, length of labor, and birth trauma also affect the baby's reaction(1). Adverse effects, usually demonstrated by neonatal respiratory depression, probably are due to the drug's action on the fetal central nervous system(2). Respiratory depression occurs most commonly when large doses of the drug are given or when it is given two to three hours before delivery(3).

Inhalant analgesics are used less frequently but can be helpful when a patient needs quick relief without the full effect of I.V. or IM medications. The most widely used inhalants are methoxyflurane (Pentrane) or trichlorethylene (Trilene), self-administered by mask.

In giving analgesics consider the following:

Be realistic. Demerol will rarely alleviate all pain and does not become completely effective for about 60 to 90 minutes. The woman needs to know that relief will not be instantaneous, but that in a short while she will be able to relax more easily between contractions and that the edge will be taken off the peak of each one.

Inform your patient. All patients should be told that the medication may make them feel somewhat out of focus. Women using some method of prepared childbirth may become anxious and fear that the drug will cause them to lose control.

Know your responsibility. Medicated patients should not be left alone for long periods nor be allowed out of bed. If the couple is using prepared childbirth, you need to guide the coach and tell him not to help his medicated wife out of bed.

By state, hospital, or department policy, medicated patients usually are not allowed to sign a consent form for three to four hours after being medicated. The time to secure consent is before the medication is given, especially for planned procedures, such as circumcision or tubal ligation. In an emergency, the husband or guardian may sign a consent. Otherwise, consent can be obtained only after the effects of the drug have worn off.

Be cautious. Keep in mind all the safeguards about administering drugs: checking orders, dose, route, compatibility, allergies, and so forth. If the patient is receiving inhalants, never hold the mask for her because that might cause her to inhale too much medication and lead to general anesthesia. If she holds the mask herself, she will drop it when she begins to lose consciousness. Stay with this patient at all times since she is more likely to lose control or consciousness. Remember to aerate the room because the inhalant fumes leak out and begin to affect staff and visitors.

Regional Anesthesia-Analgesia

The commonest forms of regional pain relief are paracervical, pudendal, saddle, epidural, and caudal anesthesia. When properly given, regional analgesia has these effects:
- complete pain relief
- virtual elimination of pulmonary aspiration
- reduced risk of maternal or neonatal depression, provided no complications occur
- should not halt labor
- can be extended during delivery
- allows the mother to be awake during the birth of her child(4).

The first localized, or regional, analgesic is the **paracervical block.** The anesthetic agent is usually administered by the obstetrician when the woman's cervix is four or more centimeters dilated. The block takes effect within three to five minutes and lasts for an hour or two if the entire nerve plexus has been anesthetized.

A paracervical block may alleviate the pain of the contractions during the first stage of labor but may have to be repeated, depending on the duration of labor.

When the mother's cervix is more than eight centimeters dilated or the fetal head is at a +2 station, the administration of a paracervical block becomes more difficult(5). Side effects of the paracervical block may include a brief slowing of labor, maternal tachycardia, syncope, or convulsions, and transient fetal bradycardia(6).

The second regional nerve block is the **pudendal,** used when the patient's cervix is completely dilated and she is ready for delivery. It anesthetizes the pudendal and perineal nerves to permit the patient to deliver fully conscious but with a minimum of pain. The block takes effect in about five minutes, and does not affect the baby(7).

Some discomfort is felt during the

injection, depending on the speed of injection—the slower the injection, the less patient discomfort. Patients are frightened about injections that they cannot see or anticipate. It helps them relax when you tell them what will happen, the position used, and how the injection will feel. Fear—tension—pain is an unbreakable cycle unless you deal with it from the start. Other considerations for the patient with a local block:

Monitor vital signs. The physical signs of mother and fetus should be watched and measured. The mother's vital signs and the fetal heart rate should be taken every minute during the first 15 minutes after administration of the block and every 5 minutes thereafter until stable.

Give reassurance. Explain to the mother that the block will not deaden all sensation and that she will feel pressure and pulling during delivery.

The next series of regional anesthetics are spinal anesthetics. The **saddle block** is done only when delivery is imminent. It is a subarachnoid injection of an anesthetic agent, such as lidocaine (Xylocanine), dibucaine (Nupercaine), or others. The effects last about an hour. This block anesthetizes the mother's perineum, the area that would come in contact with a saddle during horseback riding. Thus a saddle block alleviates the pain of episiotomy, delivery, and repair(8).

A **caudal block** is achieved by the continuous or terminal administration of an extradural anesthetic into the caudal space, the area within the sacrum at the lower-most part of the bony spinal canal. A dural sac separates the caudal space from the spinal cord. One injection can be given at the caudal level to abolish pain sensation carried by the sacral nerves, or continuous doses can be given through a polyethylene catheter which is threaded into the caudal space(9). The physical and emotional aspects of nursing management are the same as with lumbar epidural anesthesia.

In the last 12 years or so, the **lumbar epidural block** has become the obstetric anesthetic of choice in most parts of the United States. It offers complete pain relief with less depression of mother and infant than do most of the other forms of medication.

There are several disadvantages to epidural anesthesia. It is not practical in a precipitate labor which requires immediate anesthesia. If started too early, the lumbar epidural may slow labor. If doses are excessive, oxytocin stimulation may become necessary.

An epidural anesthetic obliterates the bearing-down reflex, which means that forceps delivery may be necessary. Temporary paralysis or uncontrollable shaking of the legs may occur, and hypotension is common, especially if the mother is in the supine position. Fetal depression will occur if unusually large doses are needed or if maternal hypotension is not corrected promptly. Finally, the patient's ability to void is hampered, so careful bladder observation is required, and possibly catheterization(10). Nursing management of patients who have epidurals encompasses every aspect of good nursing care.

Prepare the patient. First, the patient should be prepared emotionally since her cooperation is imperative. She might be afraid of having a needle inserted in her back, as many people are.

The epidural tray must be set up under sterile conditions. Anticipate traffic patterns in the room before setting up the tray. Have the patient in the proper position on her side. Keep vital sign apparatus at your fingertips, so that vital signs can be taken immediately after the procedure and every 15 minutes thereafter, or more frequently if indicated. Be sure that an I.V. is in place so that therapeutic measures can be taken quickly if maternal hypotension develops.

Observe what is happening. Watch the patient's emotional as well as physical reactions. Toxic reactions, indicating possible injection of the agent into the epidural vessels, are manifested by complaints of ringing in the ears, vertigo, palpitation of the heart, metallic taste in the mouth; or by excitement or confusion.

Hypotension, signaled by nausea, lightheadedness, pallor, and abnormal vital signs, should be noted promptly because long, severe hypotension affects the fetus adversely(11). The immediate management of hypotension includes turning the patient on her left side to displace the uterus laterally and thereby relieve pressure on large abdominal vessels; initiating oxygen therapy; running I.V. fluids that contain no medications at a rapid rate; temporarily discontinuing any oxytocic; and placing the patient in Trendelenburg position. If all these measures fail, a vasopressor drug such as ephedrine may be required(11).

Know your medication. Besides knowing the different kinds of anesthetics, you should know the concentrations of each that are beneficial in specific situations. For instance, an epidural anesthetic should begin to work in 5 to 10 minutes and its effects should last 45 to 60 minutes, depending on the agent used. If this does not occur, the physician may have to restart the epidural. Epidural medication should not be instilled during a contraction, because pressure might force the anesthetic to a level that is higher than desired.

Keep communication open. Warn the mother that she may feel helpless over seeming paralysis or shaking of her legs, but that it is only temporary. An aware patient will be less inclined to panic, or if she does become upset, more easily calmed. The entire health team, including the patient and coach, must communicate with one another for a safe, successful delivery. Mutual trust can be earned by open, honest communication based on empathy, understanding, and knowledge.

References

1. BENSON, R.C. *Handbook of Obstetrics and Gynecology.* 5th ed. Los Altos, Calif., Lange Publishing Co., 1974, p. 148.
2. *Ibid.,* p. 148.
3. OXORN, H., AND FOOTE, W.R. *Human Labor and Birth.* 3rd ed. New York, Appleton-Century-Crofts, 1975, p. 376.
4. BONICA, JOHN. *Obstetric Analgesia and Anesthesia.* Seattle, Department of Anesthesiology, School of Medicine, University of Washington, 1972, p. 48.
5. ZIEGEL, ERNA, AND VAN BLARCOM, CAROLYN. *Obstetric Nursing.* 6th ed. New York, Macmillan, 1972, p. 322.
6. BENSON, *op.cit.,* p. 151.
7. ZIEGEL AND VAN BLARCOM, *op.cit.,* p. 320.
8. *Ibid.,* p. 323.
9. LERCH, CONSTANCE. *Maternity Nursing.* St. Louis, C.V. Mosby Co., 1974, p. 208.
10. BONICA, *op.cit.,* p. 62.
11. *Ibid.,* p. 70.

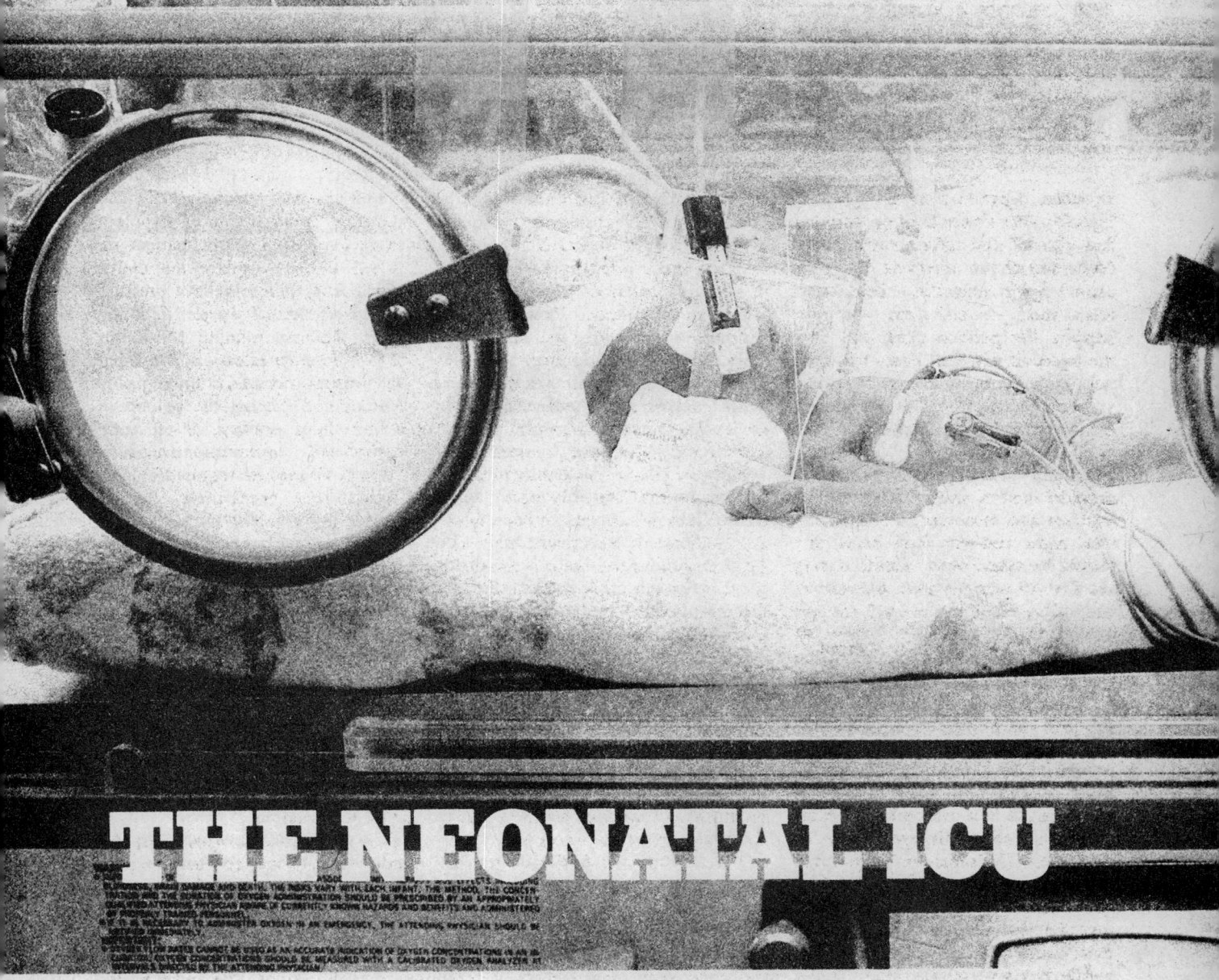

THE NEONATAL ICU
A High-Risk Environment

Reprinted from American Journal of Nursing, November 1982

By Susan Blackburn

The technological revolution has had a profound effect on perinatal health. Infants whose low birth weight and gestational age would have ruled out any chance of survival are now being saved, thanks to new knowledge about the nature of fetal and neonatal life and to our increased capability of applying the measures required to preserve such life. But these advances have had

SUSAN BLACKBURN, RN, PhD, is assistant professor and director, perinatal nurse specialist program, Department of Parent and Child Health, School of Nursing, University of Washington, Seattle.

some unexpected consequences that are raising troubling issues about the impact of the new technology on infants, their parents, health caretakers, and society.

Since it is estimated that 6 to 10 percent of the 3,600,000 births in this country each year are premature, infants born prematurely number in the hundreds of thousands. Most of them do well: 75 percent survive, and approximately 70 to 80 percent of those cared for in neonatal intensive care units (NICU) have minimal sequelae or none at all. These figures rise significantly, however, with decreasing **birth weight, especially for infants** who weigh less than 800 grams at birth(1-3).

At a conference on these issues at Hastings Center, experts from a number of disciplines identified three main concerns: resource allocation, appropriate intervention, and treatment decision(4).

Resource allocation. The application of the new technology has proved to be expensive. In 1976, Butterfield estimated that it cost $15,000 to equip one NICU bed, not including nursing staff or physician costs(5). Since then, the cost has probably doubled because of inflation. In addition, since smaller hospitals do not have NICUs, transport services must be available and the cost of such services is high. For example, a well-equipped vehicle to transport premature or infants-at-risk to an NICU has been estimated at nearly $100,000, not including personnel or other operating costs.(6).

Most infants needing intensive neonatal care require extended hospital stays, and NICU space is limited. As a result, the units often tend to be overfilled, resulting in less comprehensive and individualized care for the infants and their families. In turn, such crowding increases frustration and dissatisfaction for nursing staffs.

Perhaps more important, the allocation of funds to equip and staff expensive NICUs tends to divert health care funding away from preventive services. Steinfels reports that "so long as there is technology to handle prematurity, less attention will be given to prevention."(4)

Appropriate intervention. Babies weighing less than 1000 gm were once given little chance of survival, but the new technology has raised the survival rate of newborns weighing as little as 700 gm. Such infants require long hospitalization, however, and are at high risk of developing iatrogenic problems resulting from the intervention therapies necessary to ensure their survival(3). Iatrogenic problems, now endemic in perinatal care, include not only the physical side effects of treatment but possible psychological and behavioral consequences.

Treatment decisions. The third issue raised at the Hastings conference highlights the ethical dilemma posed for the professionals and families involved in making treatment decisions. Consideration must be given to the short- and long-term effects of treatment on the child, his development and his rearing, and the family's response to the use of technological intervention to save an infant who may have complex sequelae, yet who would otherwise die.

In sum, the application of advanced technology is costly in material as well as in human terms. In helping more infants survive, the cost of NICU care and prolonged periods of hospitalization after the immediate crisis are high for everyone involved. In human terms, the cost is almost impossible to gauge for the infant, his family, and the caretakers.

Cost to the Caretakers

The nursing staff—the main component of NICU care—must deal with the daily bombardment of stimuli from the equipment, numbers of people crowded into a relatively small place, parents in crisis, and the babies themselves. As nurses, we must also handle, on a regular basis, the ethical and moral issues that have accompanied the rapid advances in knowledge and adoption of extraordinary technology and the ability to keep smaller and smaller babies alive. The acute care nurse of the future will have to deal with being a "nurse-engineer." Biological instrumentation will frustrate, perplex, and challenge her. For nurses working in today's NICUs, however, it appears that tomorrow is already here.

Cost to the Consumer

For technology to be effective and efficient, there must be knowledgeable and skilled persons to use it. Nonetheless, individuals with minimal training are often assigned to operate expensive and potentially hazardous equipment. Equipment problems and failures can result from operator error as well as mechanical or electrical malfunction. Technology, therefore, requires training, education, problem-solving sessions, and regular updating.

Cost to the Families

Families have their own reactions to technology in the NICU. Such units certainly look, sound, and feel much different from the usual newborn nurseries, and the NICU may heighten parents' fear, anxiety, guilt, concern, and feelings of helplessness and hopelessness. Parents often describe the unit as looking like something in the realm of science fiction. They usually can't see their babies because of the tubes and equipment, and when they do, their babies may appear to them to be grotesque—like animals or little old men. Being separated from their infants, parents have to work harder to establish contact. While attempting to cope with their feelings and concerns about the infant himself, they are also trying to cope with other kinds of trauma—the financial costs of care and the disruption of their family lives. The costs can range from $10,000 to more than $100,000 for an infant with serious medical problems(2,7). Ultimately, parental perception of the infant as "different" or "abnormal" may cause problems later, when the child is being incorporated into the family.

Cost to the Infant

The costs to the infant are many. He is thrust from the intrauterine environment into one of constant bright lights, sudden loud noises, temperature changes, and cold hands; he is subjected to an environment without the containment and movement of the uterus, one in which people poke, prod, and stick things into him in a variable and unpredictable manner. The infant must constantly adapt to new faces, shapes, odors, touch, and voices.

Iatrogenic problems—consequences of treatment—occur even when the treatment is sound and used appropriately(8,9). Some specific treatment hazards follow:

Phototherapy—placing the infant under fluorescent lights—is used to reduce the need for exchange transfusions and the morbidity associated with high bilirubin levels in approximately 100,000 infants a year. Although no long-term detrimental effects have been documented, immediate negative effects include maculopapular rashes, diarrhea, increased insensible water loss, bronzing of the skin, and upper airway obstruction from slippage of the protective eye shields over the nose. The long-term subtle effect of coverage of the eyes is not yet well understood, but eye patches interfere with parent-infant interaction, unless nurses remove the patches at regular intervals to expose the infant's eyes to natural room light and during parent visiting. Another disadvantage of phototherapy is the tendency to use it without investigating for other causes of jaundice. Such infants need to be observed for signs of sepsis, hemolysis, and metabolic abnormalities.

Feeding tubes are a necessary adjunct to care because many premature infants have weak or absent sucking reflexes. Disadvantages of nasogastric tubes include injury to the stomach or intestine and possible association with enterocolitis as well as lack of opportunity for sucking.

Cardiorespiratory monitors, one of the earlier technological advances, provide information on the infant's cardiac and respiratory status. The most serious effect of these monitors is the false sense of security that they generate; they should supplement, not replace, close nursing observations. However, false alarms are frequent and often annoying. As a result, the alarms are sometimes ignored or disabled. These monitors require skill, time, and care in placement and adjustment. Sometimes when a monitor's alarm sounds, there is a tendency to attend to the monitor and only as an afterthought attend to the baby.

Radiant warmers not only help to stabilize an infant's temperature but also allow staff easy access to the infant. Such equipment, however, carries the risk of burns, over- or under-heating, electrical shock, and increased insensible water loss.

Umbilical catheters, which provide an access for fluids and medication, have potential hazards including trauma to the vessels, hemorrhage, blockage of circulation to the extremities, thromboemboli, and infection. Infusion pumps can also be a source of inaccurate fluid or drug administration if they are not monitored carefully, since the flow rates can vary from 10 to 40 percent(8).

Respiratory support methods have had a major impact on improving survival of high-risk infants, since respiratory problems are the major cause of premature infant mortality. However, oxygen therapy and mechanical ventilation are among the most invasive procedures commonly used in NICUs and can seriously affect respiratory, circulatory, renal, and metabolic systems.

Oxygen, for example, has known hazards for immature organisms, but it is physiologically necessary for treatment of respiratory insufficiency. Even though oxygen is currently given in carefully regulated and monitored quantities, there has been a recent resurgence of retrolental fibroplasia in many NICUs. In addition, the incidence of bronchopulmonary dysplasia may be as high as 15 to 20 percent among mechanically ventilated infants and occurs more often in the smallest, sickest infants(8,9). Many of these infants require hospital care for months—even years—with consequences for themselves, their families, and those who care for them.

Other complications are associated with endotracheal tubes and chest tubes. Continuous transcutaneous PO_2 monitoring, one of the more recent technological advances in caring for sick infants, records moment-to-moment changes in blood oxygen. One benefit of this technology has been insight into the effect of seemingly innocuous maneuvers such as handling the infant or changing the linen, or when infants cry. Although these drops in PO_2 were generally followed by satisfactory recovery, a prolonged series of hypoxigenic events could lead to a sustained lowering of PO_2, requiring assisted ventilation.

Starting or restarting an IV often causes one of the most serious diminutions of PO_2, leading to the recommendation that this be done as quickly as possible by the most skilled person, and if the first or second attempt fails, to let the baby rest and recover.(9)

Another procedure associated with potentially serious hypoxic consequences is chest physical therapy. Aggressive chest PT has been regarded as intrinsically good for *all* infants without much supporting physiologic data. The decision to do or not do chest PT, and how vigorously it should be done, should be a nursing decision based on the individual infant, not on routine orders.

Noise is another factor to consider. Bess recently reported on the potential additive noise effects from all the life-support apparatus within the incubator, from monitors, respirators, and pumps to noise caused by striking the side of the incubator or opening and closing its storage compartment(10). He found that these added as much as 20 decibels to the environmental noise levels already present. Most of this increase was in high-frequency range where most neonatal hearing loss has been demonstrated. Impulse noise from episodic striking or bumping of the incubator reached 140 db—a value above the adult criterion for risk of hearing damage. Bess suggests that when dealing with the incubated newborn one should walk and talk softly as well as handle the infant gently.

Caregiving Activities

How then can nurses modify some of the social and psychological consequences of advanced technology in NICUs? Studies by Sander and others suggest that early caretaker-

SECTION 4: NURSING CARE OF THE CHILDBEARING FAMILY

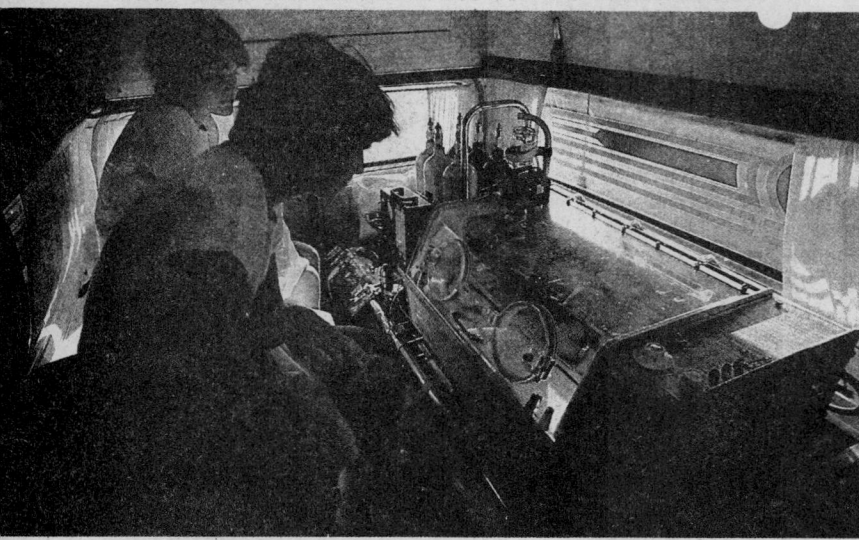
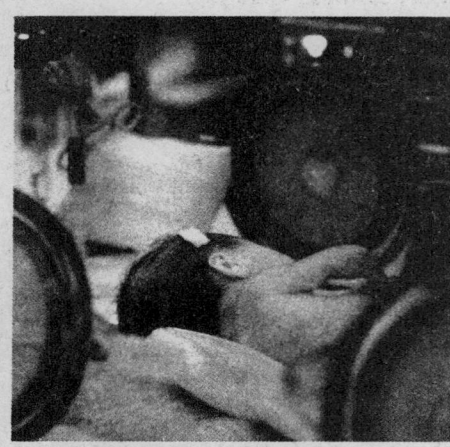
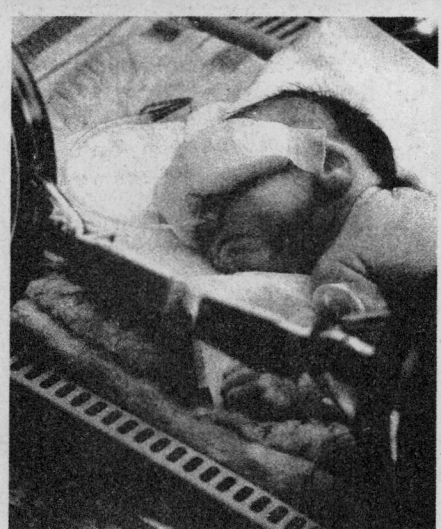
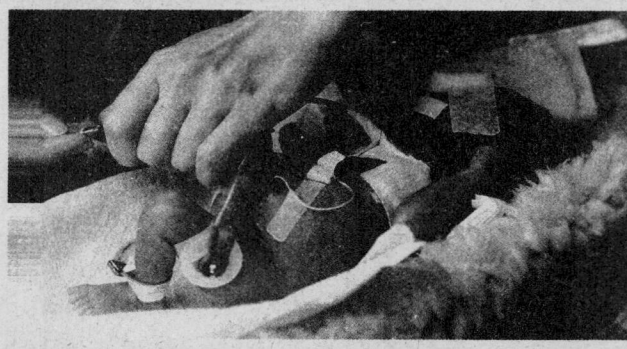
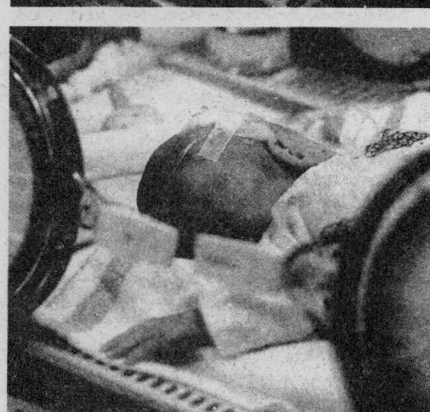
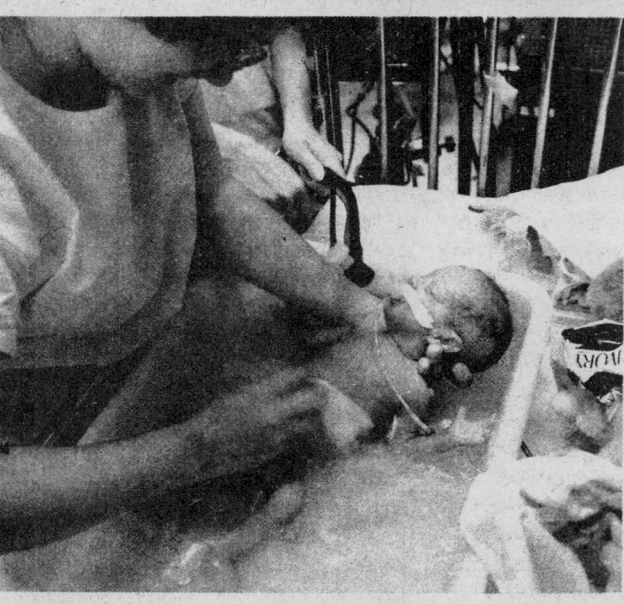

The high-risk infant who begins life in a neonatal intensive care unit has unprecedented chances of survival. But in this unnatural world of lights, noises, machinery, and invasive procedures, the danger of iatrogenic damage is always present.

infant interactions influence the infant's behavioral organization and development of diurnal rhythms. In other words, what happens in the intensive care unit can be critical and can either nurture or hinder the infant's early adaptations and interactions(11-12). The infant's ability to organize his behavioral and physiological rhythms after birth is crucial not only in his appropriate responses to environment but also in providing his caretakers—whether nurse or parent—with clearer and more consistent cues to understanding how to respond to his needs.

We have recently been studying the influence of the environment on premature infants by analyzing the types and amounts of handling that infants experience as part of regular caregiving activities in a NICU, and the infant's behavioral responses to these types of tactile contact. Data on caregiving activities were obtained from 24-hour time-lapse videotapes at three time points during the infants' hospital stay. Frequencies and durations of four types of caregiving activities—loving stroking, diapering/feeding, technical procedures such as injections, and holding the infant out of the crib or incubator—were examined on 102 premature infants born prior to 34 weeks' gestation. Caregiving activities were examined during the first two weeks after birth; when infants reached 34 weeks of gestational age; and again after transfer to crib prior to discharge.

At each time point, the most frequent caregiving involved handling related to miscellaneous technical activities. The least frequent was loving stroking (for some infants no episodes of loving stroking were recorded). While these premature infants were in incubators, they were handled during 14.8 percent of the 24-hour day. The amount of handling varied considerably from infant to infant, ranging from 5.4 to 38.1 percent of the day; when the infants were in cribs they were handled 19.1 percent of the 24-hour period. Variations in handling at different times of the day and of day versus night hours are currently being examined.

Thus, the majority of the caregiver-infant interactions in the NICU were related to technical procedures or involved relatively high levels of stimulus input, while few interactions were organized around soothing or attempts to decrease arousal. Since a primary function of the caregiver is to modulate levels of arousal in the infant, the lack of activities specifically designed to soothe the infant may contribute to impairment of the premature infant's ability to modulate his neurobehavioral state, resulting in an infant who presents fewer or less clear cues to his parents or caretakers.

Significant changes in infant motor activity were observed when infants were fed or held out of the crib or incubator. Before both types of caregiving activities began, infants showed significantly ($P=.01$) higher motor activity, and afterward distinct lowering of motor activity. It may be that certain caregiving activities facilitate an infant's ability to modulate his behavior from an aroused to a nonaroused state and provide a framework around which the infant can organize his behavior. Similar relationships were not observed between infant motor activity and loving stroking. It may be that such stroking occurs so infrequently and irregularly in the NICU that it does not provide the same stimulus input and have the same modulative effect as handling associated with other types of caregiving activities.

By attending to infants' physical and behavioral cues, nurses can provide care geared to promoting infants' neurobehavioral organization. Suggested actions are:

1. Feeding based on cues; that is, when the infant begins to become active and once a sleep-wakefulness cycle can be recognized.

2. Gentle handling and avoidance of sudden postural changes, and providing sensory experience and social interaction for the infant after feeding time. (During feeding time this may exhaust the infant.)

3. Offering visual and auditory feedback geared to the infant's own initiation; that is, when he reaches an alert state and is ready and organized to process such input.

4. Recognizing signs of stress and overload resulting in physiological deterioration, such as facial grimaces, increased jerky and startled movements, labile color changes, decreased muscle tone, paling, instability of respiration and heart rate, hiccupping, or spitting.

5. Responding appropriately to signs of stress and helping the infant to reorganize, such as helping him to disengage from a visual stimulus.

6. Teaching parents to recognize infant cues and respond to them appropriately.

In addition, Gorski describes instances in which nurses' observations of infant cues and needs influenced the outcome of nursing actions(13). For example, nurses who contained infant limbs while slowly positioning them to receive an IV observed that infants' heart rates, respirations, and skin color remained stable throughout the procedure. But if infants were abruptly positioned with their limbs uncontained, changes in color, heart rate, and respirations were observed. An increased number of severe apneic spells were noted in one infant, especially during morning and evening rounds when many staff members congregated at the infant's bedside. When rounds were moved away from the bedside, the apneic spells decreased. Nurses also noted that infants with chronic lung disease had more successful feedings when timed to coincide with the infants' alert periods, and also when the infants were fed where there was less noise, away from mainstream unit activity.

Although these are only observations and not controlled studies at this point, these nursing observations suggest ways to improve our understanding of infant behavior and how infants interact with their environments. In doing so, we can provide more personalized, humanistic care and send home an infant better able to cope with the world in which he lives.

References

1. Fitzhardinge, Pamela. Current outcome: ICU populations. IN *Neonatal Neurological Assessment and Outcome.* Report of the Seventy-Seventh Ross Confernce on Pediatric Research. Columbus, Ohio, Ross Laboratories, 1980, pp. 1-5.
2. Shannon, D. C., and others. Survival, cost of hospitalization, and prognosis in infants critically ill with respiratory distress syndrome requiring mechanical ventialtion. *Crit.Care Med.* 9:94-97, Feb. 1981.
3. Schechner, S. For the 1980s: how small is too small? *Clin.Perinatol.* 7:135-143, Mar. 1980.
4. Steinfels, M. O. New childbirth technology: a clash of values. *HastingsCent.Rep.* 8:9-12, Feb. 1978.
5. Richardson, C. J. Principles of organization of a neonatal intensive care unit from scratch. *Clin.Perinatol.* 3:331, Sept. 1976.
6. Greene, W. T. Organization of neonatal transport services in support of a regional referral center. *Clin. Perinatol.* 7:193, Mar. 1980.
7. Pomerance, J. J., and others. Cost of living for infants weighing 1000 grams or less at birth. *Pediatrics* 61:908, 1978.
8. Stavis, R. L., and Krauss, A. N., Complicastions of neonatal intensive care. *Clin.Perinatol.* 7:107-124, Mar. 1980.
9. Ross Conference on Pediatric Research. (69th) *Iatrogenic Problems In Neonatal Intensive Care.* Columbus, Ohio, Ross Laboratories, 1976.
10. Bess, F. H., and others. Further observations on noise levels in infant incubators. *Pediatrics* 63:100-106, Jan. 1979.
11. Sander, L., and others. *Changes in Infant and Caregiver Variables Over the First Two Months of Life.* Paper presented at conference on Origins of Infant Social Responsiveness, held at Nantucket, Mass., 1976.
12. Sander, L. Regulation and organization in the early infant-caretaker system. IN *Brain and Early Behavior* ed. by R. Robinson. New York, Academic Press, 1969, pp. 311-322.
13. Gorski, P. A., and others. Stages of behavioral organization in the high-risk neonate theoretical and clinical considerations. *Semin. Perinatol.* 3:61-72, Jan. 1979.

Climacteric

Reprinted from American Journal of Nursing, July 1982

By Linda Pearson

There are few clinical entities that the nurse who cares for adult female patients will encounter more frequently than the climacteric syndrome. For many women, the change of life signals the end of youth and the beginning of fast approaching old age. But in today's Western society, women at this stage still have an average of a third of their lives ahead of them.

LINDA PEARSON, RN, MSN, was assistant professor at the University of Colorado, School of Nursing, Denver, when she wrote this article. She is currently vice-president of the Colo. State Board of Nursing and clinical editor for the *Nurse Practitioner Journal*. She also works as a family nurse practitioner in a private family health care office.

The climacteric is the phase in the aging process that occurs during the woman's transition from fertility to a nonreproductive capacity. The mean age at which natural menopause, the final menstrual period, occurs is approximately 48. Premature menopause, which can have a familial tendency, may occur as early as 35 years of age, but an endocrine or emotional factor must first be ruled out before a diagnosis of menopause is made.

The variety of symptoms that each woman experiences in the climacteric syndrome result from an interplay of these three factors:

1. decreased ovarian activity with a resulting hormonal deficiency that produces such symptoms as hot flashes, perspiration, atrophic vaginitis, and later, end organ changes related to the altered metabolic state;

2. sociocultural factors within the female's environment; and,

3. psychological factors influenced by the female's inner and outer strengths and coping behavior.

Menstrual irregularity is usually the first symptom a woman notices. Her menstrual periods may alternate between scanty and profuse bleeding.

Hot flashes—brief periods of warmth confined to the chest, neck, and face—are frequently accompanied by diffuse or patchy flushing of the skin and/or sweating. Hot flashes may begin at any age but tend to become more frequent once menstruation ceases. About 85 percent of menopausal women experience this vasomotor instability; flashes occur most frequently when heat production is increased, such as with high humidity, heavy clothing, after meals, and after exercise. There seems to be an association between the rate of ovarian involution and the severity of menopausal symptoms. Complaints of dyspareunia and hot flashes are more frequent with a fast involution, whereas amenorrhea may be the only symptom with a slower ovarian involution.

The estrogen hormonal deficiency that follows decreased ovarian activity has a number of effects[1]. Atrophy of the vaginal skin is directly related to estrogen deficiency. The squamocolumnar junction usually retreats into the endocervical canal. The uterus becomes atrophied; fibroids frequently also atrophy and calcify. The ovaries diminish in size from age 30 on with a rapid decrease in size after age 60. The muscle tone of the pelvic floor diminishes and the ligaments lose their strength. The bladder mucosa and urethral tissue also lose their tone[2].

The effect of estrogen deficiency on nongenital body areas is less clear. The exact mechanism and effect of the deficiency and replacement estrogen on cholesterol, lipoproteins, triglycerides, skin, and thyroid function are still unknown.

Fatigue, insomnia, depression, and emotional instability are commonly blamed on the climacteric. Whether estrogens exert an influence upon mental functioning and emotions is still a disputed question[1,2]. Socioeconomic factors and the personal coping strategies of middle life may be more responsible for the stress in a person's life than the climacteric.

Other frequent presenting complaints of the climacteric include decreased libido, backache and body pains, faulty memory, irritability, and headaches. These symptoms are difficult to evaluate as results of estrogen deficiency, nor does the literature provide evidence of any well controlled studies that fully evaluate these complaints[1,2]. It is wise to maintain a high index of suspicion for causes other than the climacteric for such complaints.

Diagnosis

The diagnosis of menopause is fairly straightforward in a woman over 40 who experiences menstrual irregularity, whose periods have ceased for a year, or who has vasomotor instability or atrophic vaginitis. These symptoms are usually adequate for diagnosis, without the need for any hormonal assays.

The problem of confirming the diagnosis of menopause when presented with vague or less classic symptomatology becomes quite difficult. Experts disagree on the accuracy of laboratory confirmation of menopause. Some researchers have found that the level of estradiol-17B correlates excellently with the estrogenic state of the woman[3]. However, other researchers positively refute this claim. For example, one study found no correlation between the Maturation Index (the relation of parabasal to intermediate to superficial cells from the vaginal smear) or plasma estrogen levels to a women's symptomatology[4].

Laboratory tests can be inaccurate and costly. Cytological studies may show an estrogen-deficient smear, but they are not diagnostic unless they are read serially by the same expert cytologist and are correlated with a clinical picture which indicates the diagnosis clearly enough not to need laboratory confirmation in the first place[2]. Also plasma estradial assays may not be useful because of their cost and their inaccuracy due to diurnal variations within the ovarian cycle[2].

Confirmation of the diagnosis can be made with a careful history that elicits menstrual pattern, mood change, hot flashes, dry vagina, and so on. The nurse should also take a careful psychological history to determine the woman's individual strengths, weaknesses, and resources and her past coping behaviors and past mental health status.

The following criteria should be present before attributing the woman's various emotional complaints to a decrease in ovarian function:

• the first onset of symptoms occurs from age 40 to 55

• depression, fatigue, insomnia, have a periodicity that initially follows the menstrual cycle and gradually becomes more constant and severe as the menses cease

• the woman has experienced, in the past, other such psychological responses to hormonal changes as postpartum blues and premenstrual tension

• the woman is concurrently experiencing such vasomotor instability symptoms as hot flashes, sweating, and so on.

Pros and Cons of Estrogen Replacement Therapy

Experts do not agree on the use of replacement estrogen therapy in treating menopausal women. Estrogen compounds first became available for treatment of menopausal symptoms in the late 1930s and their use continued relatively unchecked until the early 1970s when studies began to link the use of estrogen with endometrial cancer. There has ensued a controversy over the justification for continued use of estrogen. Further evidence demonstrating the usefulness of estrogen replacement for treating such menopausal associated conditions as atrophic urethritis and postmenopausal osteoporosis have added additional fuel to this controversy(1,5,6).

Opinions on the proper treatment of menopause vary widely. At one end of the spectrum, the attitude prevails that menopause is a natural event and since the symptoms are relatively self-limiting, no therapy is required. Another view holds that the risk of endometrial cancer far outweighs the existence of benefits for estrogen replacement therapy(7). The other end of the spectrum is taken by those who advocate "femininity forever" or estrogen replacement from menopause to grave(8). By far the most predominate view in the medical literature today is that estrogens can be useful during the climacteric syndrome but that the therapy should be as brief and as low as possible while still alleviating symptoms(1,2,9-13).

The relative increased risks for women taking estrogen that have been reported include endometrial cancer, hypertension, gallbladder disease, carbohydrate intolerance, myocardial infarction, thromboembolic disease, cerebrovascular accident, and possibly, coronary disease(9-10). There is, however, considerable controversy and conflicting evidence about these reported associations. The most consistently reported association is between estrogen and endometrial cancer.

The accepted indications of estrogen replacement therapy include moderate to severe symptomatology of vasomotor instability, urogenital tract atrophy, early oophorectomy, and probably, the prevention of osteoporosis, especially if combined with adequate doses of calcium and exercise(1,9-14).

The exact dosage of the estrogen replacement varies with physicians, but cyclical low-dose estrogen replacement is most often recommended(1,9-14). The suggested length of replacement therapy ranges from one to three years to indefinitely(10,11). The addition of a progestrogen to the cyclical drug regime also is frequently suggested(1,9-12,14).

The woman who presents herself to her primary health care provider with menopausal symptoms has many needs. In addition to the history and physical exam, particular attention should be paid to weight, urine analysis, blood pressure, pelvic exam (especially an accurate Pap smear and checking the patency of the endocervical canal), breast exam, hemoglobin, and biochemical profile SMA 12. Any patient who reports a history of noncyclical spotting or bleeding should be referred to her physician for biopsy and/or curettage.

Care of the woman who is

Questions and Answers About the Menopause

By Laura Ryan Caldwell

During the four years I have conducted workshops for women on preparing for menopause, the same questions recur over and over. I suggest that women attending the workshop write down their questions and place them on my desk during the break so they can be anonymous if participants wish. Some of these questions with my answers follow:

How long are my hot flashes going to last? What causes them, and what can I do about them?

Unfortunately, no one can predict how long hot flashes will last. Some women have none; others have them for as long as 6 to 10 years. Although theories abound, the exact cause is not known. Instead of tightening your muscles and becoming upset when a hot flash begins, take a deep breath, relax your voluntary muscles, and visualize the hot flash passing over you in a calm, quiet way. Many women tell me they find that this helps alleviate the severity and frequency of hot flashes.

How long do I need to use birth control? What kind is the safest?

You should use birth control for at least one year after you have gone 12 *consecutive* months without a period. Some authorities even recommend that you use birth control for two years from this date. The diaphragm and foam plus condom are probably the best contraceptive methods for perimenopausal women. Your gynecologist may okay leaving your IUD in place or he may remove it. The "pill" is no longer advised for women over 40.

Will I lose my mind?

No. This fear is based on an old wives' tale about a mental illness once called "involutional melancholia," which was thought to be caused by menopause. As with any period of change or crisis in a woman's life, unresolved emotional issues can come into new focus at this time. A woman's sense of self-worth and her coping abilities play a large role in preventing psychological problems.

I find that women with a variety of interests or who have jobs they enjoy suffer least from the so-called "empty nest syndrome." However, a woman may suffer from a true depression that only coincidentally occurs at this time.

Anyone with serious sleep problems, a sense of helplessness including suicidal thoughts, or a cluster of such physical symptoms as loss of appetite, constipation, weight loss or gain should make an appointment with a health care provider. A referral for counseling or therapy may be advisable.

What is your opinion of "hormones?"

Estrogen replacement therapy (ERT) is a major concern for most middle-aged women today. Many women have taken or are still taking estrogens. Disturbing evidence in the last few

---

LAURA RYAN CALDWELL, RNC, BSN, FNP, is an assistant professor at Cuyahoga Community College, Cleveland, Ohio. She does menopause workshops and serves as a health consultant to a Displaced Homemakers Program. She is a mother of four and grandmother of seven.

going through the climacteric consists of two components. The first is information and support as she considers whether or not estrogen supplements are indicated. The second is adequate counseling and teaching concerning the expected physiological changes and problems.

The decision a woman must make concerning estrogen replacement is a difficult one, especially since the recognized authorities differ markedly in their advice. There are, however, certain guidelines to be followed in prescribing estrogen therapy.

• The use of estrogen in the following patient conditions is considered a much higher risk—obesity (extra ovarian conversion of adrenal androstenedione in body fat and muscle may be responsible for considerable amounts of extra estrogen); hypertension; diabetes; varicose veins; past or present estrogen-dependent tumors; history of thromboembolic disease; liver disease; heavy smoking; nulliparity; hyperlipidemia; or, immobilization. Under these circumstances, the physician will probably not prescribe the medication.

• Therapy should be *short-term* to aid the patient in accomplishing homeostatic adjustment to lowered estrogen level. It should be *cyclical* (20 to 25 days per month) to help avoid endometrial hyperplasia, and *low-dose* to prevent such complications and symptoms as breast pain, weight gain, cervical mucorrhea, edema, and atypical uterine bleeding.

• The addition of a progestagen should be given during the week off of estrogens and continued cyclically as long as bleeding follows (to lower the occurrence of adenocarcinoma of the endometrium) (1,2,15).

• All patients receiving estrogen replacement therapy should be seen every six months for a repeat Pap, breast examination, and blood pressure reading. All menopausal women should be taught by the nurse that any abnormal bleeding (if on estrogen-progestagen therapy) or spotting 12 months after cessation of the menses carries a 48 percent chance of carcinoma(16).

• Parenteral estrogen therapy is not advised(1,9,11). The use of injections does not allow for cyclical therapy, the absorption and length of action is unpredictable, and the cumulative effect frequently produces irregular bleeding.

Perhaps the most important role the nurse can play in menopause management is to teach the woman the expected physiologic changes and possible problems that may arise during this phase of life. The worst thing about the climacteric syndrome for most patients is not knowing what to expect. Women need to know what the change of life is and what its implications are. The nurse can, by counseling the patient, help her and her family understand her feelings and fears.

The psychological changes experienced by many women may result from a combination of a hormonal inbalance and adjustment to the aging process. Women need reassurance that some degree of emotional instability can be expected due to rapidly changing hor-

---

years indicates that women on ERT have three to eight times the risk of developing cancer of the lining of the uterus than do women who do not take such medication(1). The risk also seems to be related to the length of time and the dosage of the hormones taken.

ERT is not magic! It will not keep you young and "feminine forever." It will definitely help two major concerns of menopause: hot flashes and atrophic vaginitis. The decision is difficult and a risk/benefit ratio should be discussed. If ERT is undertaken, special health care and follow-up are necessary.

Are there particular danger signals that should make me seek health care at this time?

Yes. When periods have stopped, *any* spotting or bleeding should be immediately reported to and checked by a gynecologist. When periods are very irregular, it is difficult to determine intermenstrual spotting and an early period, but if the former is suspected, it should be reported. Postmenopausal spotting and/or perimenopausal intermenstrual bleeding may be the first signs of cancer of the uterus/cervix. Increasingly heavy periods also indicate the need for a careful pelvic exam and possible dilatation and curettage. These periods may be normal for you, but on the other hand, they may be symptomatic of what is known as atypical (adenomatous) hyperplasia, an overgrowth of the lining of the uterus. This is considered precancerous and normally requires a hysterectomy.

Intercourse is becoming very uncomfortable because my vagina seems so dry. What can I do?

Dryness can be a problem at any age if there is not enough clitoral stimulation to lubricate well. If adequate lubrication is a problem, a water-soluble KY jelly or baby oil can be used to help solve this problem. Vaginal estrogen creams can help severe vaginitis; however, recent studies show that a high percentage of these creams is absorbed systemically(2).

To quote Masters and Johnson, "Sex in middle age and beyond is a matter of use it or lose it!" An active sex life will keep both your vaginal membranes and your middle-aged male partner's prostate in better condition.

How can I have a healthy menopause?

PMZ (postmenopausal zest) depends on the development and continuation of a healthy life-style. Proper nutrition, aerobic exercise, maintenance of ideal weight, plus a personal relaxation/stress reduction program are more important to a woman at 50 than at 18. Smokers should try to stop and dependence on drugs, especially alcohol and tranquilizers should be avoided. Look for new friends and activities. Most of all, live life hour-by-hour and day-by-day—the recipe for a happy, healthy existence at any age.

References

1. Shoemaker, E. S., and others. Estrogen treatment of postmenopausal women: benefits and risks. *JAMA* 238:1524-1530, Oct. 3, 1977.
2. Martin, P. L., and others. Systemic absorption and sustained effects of vaginal estrogen creams. *JAMA* 242:2699-2700, Dec. 14, 1979.

mone levels. How a woman reacts depends a great deal on her feelings of self-esteem.

Many perceived losses can lead to depression. Four major areas include loss of femininity that may take the form of denial of adult achievements as a woman; loss of role as potential parent, even though many women desire no more children; loss of role of active mothering as the children leave home; loss of sexual desire and/or function.

Changes in themselves and their sexual partners can lead to pressure on sexual life. The devastating myth that "advancing age means the end of sex" needs to be destroyed. It is definitely not true. If sex is less dramatic as people age this should not be viewed as a decline; as bodies grow older, changes occur. Older persons cannot run as fast as they did when they were young, either.

Once the woman has passed through menopause, she may experience a sense of sexual freedom because she no longer has to worry about pregnancy or the anxieties and pressures of parenthood. So, sexual intercourse has the potential to become more enjoyable. What nurses have to keep in mind is that each woman will react differently to this stage in her life.

The climacteric syndrome is a clinical entity that represents for the woman a major change in her life. The nurse can ease the woman's adjustment by teaching and counseling her on what to expect and, if appropriate, advising her about drug management.

A Case Example

Ms. A, age 45, is a housewife and has three children, ages 17, 19, and 24. She came to the clinic with the chief complaint of menstrual spotting instead of her monthly period. She also complained of frequent episodes of a flushed feeling. Both symptoms had begun about four months previously.

Ms. A's health history was essentially negative. It included complaints of recent mild dyspareunia and insomnia. She told the nurse that she was worried that she might be going through the changes soon.

Ms. A felt that her marriage was a good one; she and her husband were able to share their feelings. Ms. A had experienced a moderate postpartum depression after the birth of her first-born. When her parents died 10 years earlier, she sought the aid of a counselor to help her overcome her grief. She felt somewhat lonesome at the thought of her youngest child leaving home. She considered her husband, children, and friends helpful to her in times of crisis.

The complete physical exam including breast and bimanual was entirely within normal limits. A Pap smear, SMA 12, and urinalysis were sent to the laboratory.

Analysis and Interactions

The timing of Ms. A's spotting was extremely important. If she had complained of midcycle spotting, she would have been immediately referred to gynecologist. Her menstrual irregularity, vasomotor instability, and age fell clearly into the classification of premenopausal symptoms signaling the onset of the climacteric. Since her physical exam showed no signs of vaginal atrophy, her mild dyspareunia probably reflected a decrease in natural lubrication.

It was important for the nurse to ascertain Ms. A's psychological history, so as to determine her coping abilities. The fact that she felt her family and friends were a support to her and that during a time of crisis she had sought counseling indicates that Ms. A has a positive history of present and past coping behaviors.

Ms. A's main needs center around her lack of information and support concerning the climacteric. The nurse began teaching her about premenopausal symptoms and the characteristics of the female climacteric. As part of the goal of treatment, Ms. A was reminded about her past history of psychological strength and her present support system. Increasing a person's self-esteem is vital in climacteric treatment.

At this first visit, the nurse also began an explanation of the risk/benefit ratio of estrogen replacement therapy. Ms. A's symptoms, at this time, were not severe enough to warrant the risk of estrogen replacement hazards. However, since her past family history, past medical history, and present physical were negative for increasing her risk on estrogen therapy and her present complaints could be relieved by short-term estrogen replacement, it could be an option for her. Her present mild dyspareunia could be approached initially by the use of a water-based lubricating jelly prior to intercourse.

Ms. A was asked to return in one week to review her lab results. During that visit, Ms. A needs to be encouraged to be proud of her accomplishments. Because her children are older, she may need to be encouraged to develop new interests and talents. The nurse also should be sure that Ms. A understands the need for regular follow-up, her options for additional support, and the warning signs that should prompt her to seek immediate medical attention.

References

1. vanKeep, P. A., and others. *Consensus on Menopause Research.* Baltimore, University Park Press, 1976.
2. Studd, John, and others. The climacteric. *Clin.Obstet.Gynecol.* 4:3-29, Apr. 1977.
3. Daw, E. Recent concepts in the treatment of menopausal symptoms. *Practitioner* 215:501-507, Oct. 1975.
4. Stone, S. C., and others. Postmenopausal symptomatology, maturation index, and plasma estrogen levels. *Obstet.Gynecol.* 45:625-627, June 1975.
5. Gordan, G. S. Postmenopausal osteoporosis: cause, prevention and treatment. *Clin.Obstet.Gynecol.* 4:169-177, Apr. 1977.
6. Horsman, A. Prospective trial of estrogen and calcium on postmenopausal women. *Br.Med.J.* 2:789-792, Sept. 24, 1977.
7. Oestrogen therapy and endometrial cancer. *Br.Med.J.* 2:209-210, July 23, 1977.
8. Mulvey, M. M. Management of the menopause. *Med.J.Aust.* 11:592-594, Dec. 1, 1979.
9. Kase, Nathan. Yes or no on estrogen replacement therapy?—a formulation for clinicians. *Clin.Obstet.Gynecol.* 19:825-836, Dec. 1976.
10. Shoemaker, E. S., and others. Estrogen treatment of postmenopausal women. *JAMA* 238:1524-1530, Oct. 3, 1977.
11. Kistner, R. W. Treatment of premenopausal and postmenopausal women. *J.Reprod.Med.* 19:103-110, Sept. 1977.
12. Campbell, Stuart, and Whitehead, M. Oestrogen therapy and the menopausal syndrome. *Clin.Obstet.Gynecol.* 4:31-47, Apr. 1977.
13. Proudfit, C. M. Estrogens and menopause. *JAMA* 236:939-940, Aug. 23, 1976.
14. Studd, John. Management of the menopause. *Practitioner* 216:546-549, May 1976.
15. Kaunitz, A. M. Estrogen use in postmenopausal women (Correspondence Department). *N.Engl.J.Med.* 303:1477-1478, Dec. 18, 1980.
16. Schindler, A. E. and Schmidt, G. Postmenopausal bleeding: a study of more than 1,000 cases. *Maturitas.* 2:269-274, 1980.

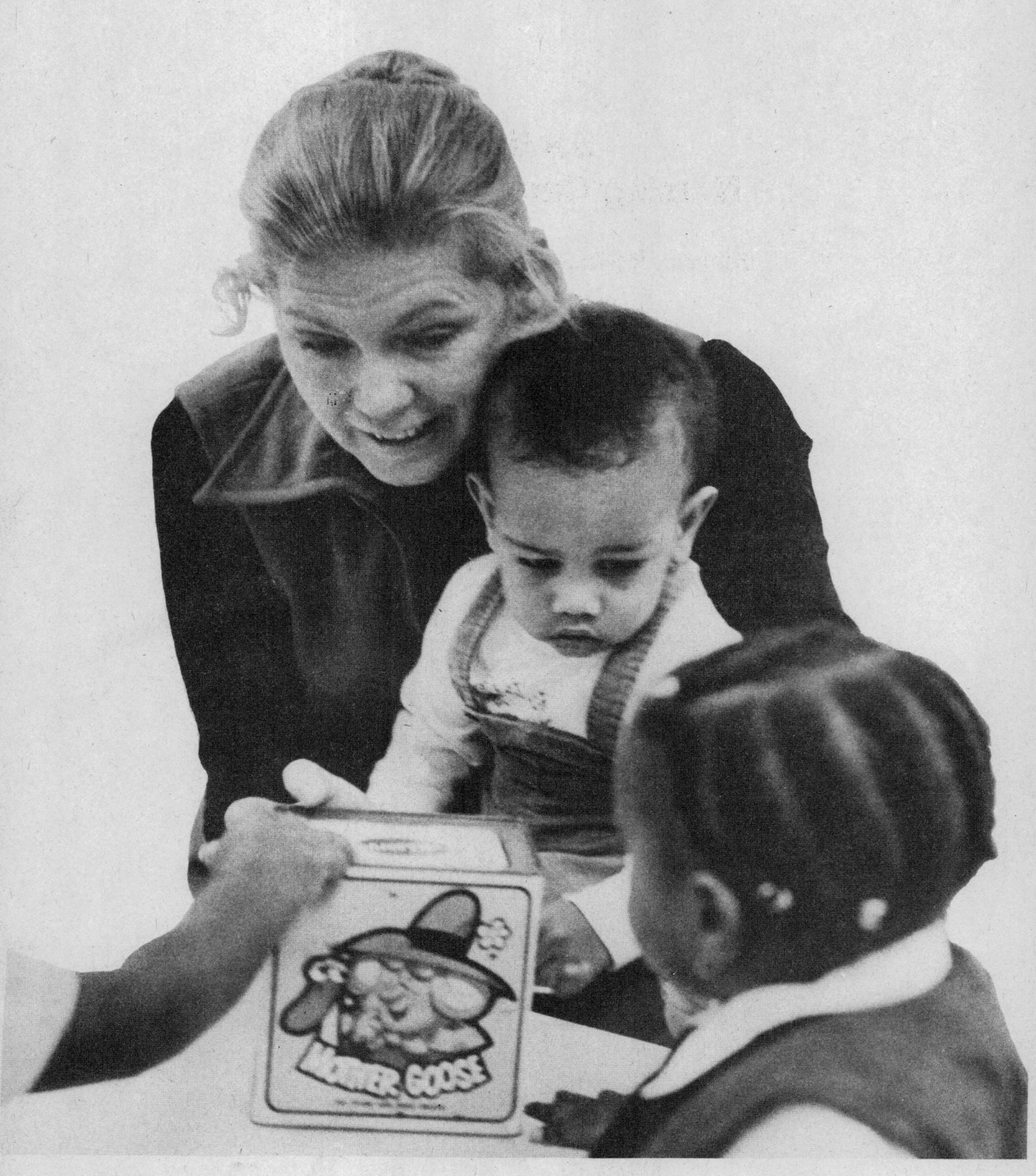

Section 5
Nursing Care of the Child

Janis P. Bellack, RN, MN, Coordinator

Cecily Lynn Betz, RN, PhD
Carolyn Vas Fore, RN, MSN
Elizabeth Anne Gomez, RN, MSN
Beverly Kopala, RN, MS
Judith K. Leavitt, RN, MEd
Mariann C. Lovell, RN, MS
Michele A. Michael, RN, PhD
Joan Reighley, RN, MN

Section 5: Nursing Care of the Child

THE HEALTHY CHILD 513

THE ILL AND HOSPITALIZED CHILD 525

OXYGENATION 532
General Concepts 532
   Overview 532
   Application of the Nursing Process to the Child with Respiratory Problems 532
Selected Health Problems Resulting in an Interference with Respiration 533
   A. *Sudden Infant Death Syndrome or "Crib Death"* 533
   B. *Acute Spasmodic Laryngitis (Spasmodic Croup)* 534
   C. *Acute Epiglottitis* 534
   D. *Laryngotracheobronchitis* 535
   E. *Bronchiolitis* 536
   F. *Bronchial Asthma* 536
   Application of the Nursing Process to the Child with Cardiac Problems 538
Selected Health Problems Resulting in an Interference with Cardiac Functioning 540
   Congenital Cardiac Disorders 540
   Rheumatic Fever 545
   Application of the Nursing Process to the Child with Hematologic Problems 546
Selected Health Problems Resulting in an Interference with Formed Elements of the Blood
   A. *Iron-Deficiency Anemia* 547
   B. *Sickle Cell Anemia* 548
   C. *Hemophilia* 550

NUTRITION AND METABOLISM 552
General Concepts 552
   Overview 552
   Application of Nursing Process to the Child with Problems of Nutrition and Metabolism 552
Selected Health Problems 553
   A. *Failure to Thrive Syndrome* 553
   B. *Vomiting and Diarrhea* 554
   C. *Pyloric Stenosis* 556
   D. *Cleft Lip and Palate* 556
   E. *Cystic Fibrosis* 558
   F. *Insulin-Dependent Diabetes Mellitus* 560

ELIMINATION 562
General Concepts 562
   Overview 562
   Application of the Nursing Process to the Child with Elimination Problems 562
Selected Health Problems 563
   A. *Hypospadias* 563
   B. *Urinary Tract Infection* 564
   C. *Nephrosis and Nephritis* 564
   D. *Lower GI Obstruction* 566

SAFETY AND SECURITY 568
General Concepts 568
   Overview 568
   Application of the Nursing Process to the Child with Neurologic or Sensory Problems 568
Selected Health Problems: Neurologic and Sensory Deficits 570
   A. *Mental Retardation* 570
   B. *Down's Syndrome (Mongolism)* 571
   C. *Cerebral Palsy* 572
   D. *Hydrocephalus* 573
   E. *Spina Bifida* 574
   F. *Seizure Disorders* 575
   G. *Bacterial Meningitis* 577
   H. *Otitis Media* 578
   I. *Tonsillitis, Tonsillectomy and Adenoidectomy* 579
   Application of the Nursing Process to the Child with a Communicable Disease 580
Selected Health Problems: Communicable Diseases, Skin Infections, Infestations 580
   A. *Communicable Diseases* 580
   B. *Sexually Transmitted Diseases* 582
   C. *Common Skin Infections and Infestations* 584
   D. *Pinworms* 584
   Application of the Nursing Process to the Child with an Interference with Safety 584
Selected Health Problems: Interference with Safety 584
   A. *Poisonous Ingestions* 584
   B. *Burns* 589

ACTIVITY AND REST 595
General Concepts 595
   Overview 595
   Application of the Nursing Process to the Child with Interferences with Activity and Rest 595
Selected Health Problems 599
   A. *Congenital Club Foot* 599
   B. *Congenital Hip Dysplasia* 599
   C. *Scoliosis* 600
   D. *Osteomyelitis* 601

CELLULAR ABERRATION (CHILDHOOD CANCER) 602
General Concepts 602
   Overview 602
   Application of the Nursing Process to the Child with Cancer 602
Selected Health Problems 606
   A. *Leukemia* 606
   B. *Hodgkin's Disease* 608
   C. *Brain Tumors* 609
   D. *Neuroblastoma* 611
   E. *Wilm's Tumor (Nephroblastoma)* 611

REPRINTS 615

The Healthy Child

General Concepts
A. Infant (1 Month to 1 Year)
1. Normal Growth and Development
   a. Psychosocial Development—Erikson: trust vs mistrust (see table 5.1)
      1) trust: infant's needs are met consistently resulting in feelings of physical comfort and emotional security
      2) depends on the quality of the primary care giver-infant relationship
   b. Physical Growth and Development
      1) length: 50% increase by 1 year (grows from average 20 inches at birth to 30 inches at 1 year)
      2) weight
         a) gains about 1½ lb/month during the first 6 months; ¾ lb/month the second 6 months
         b) doubles at 5–6 months (5½–8½ lb at birth)
         c) triples by 1 year (18–25 lb at 1 year)
      3) head circumference greater than chest circumference until age 2
      4) physical growth should follow standard growth curves
      5) vital signs (see table 5.2)
         a) pulse 80–150; average 100
         b) respirations 20–50
      6) developmental characteristics
         a) cephalocaudal (head to tail)
            - 2 months: lifts head and chest off bed
            - 5 months: turns over
            - 6 months: sits steadily without support
            - 8 months: pulls to a standing position
            - 1 year: stands upright, begins walking
         b) proximal to distal (central axis of body outward) and general to specific (differentiation)
            - 3–4 months: arm control; supports upper body weight; scoops objects with hands
            - 6 months: transfers objects from one hand to the other
            - 10 months: pincer (thumb-index finger) grasp
         c) fontanels
            - anterior: closes at 12–18 months
            - posterior: closes at 2 months (may be closed at birth)
         d) teeth
            - 4–8 months: central mandibular incisors
            - 1 year: 8 teeth (average)
   c. Cognitive Development—Piaget: sensorimotor stage (birth to 2 years)
      1) 1 month: reflexive
      2) 1–4 months
         a) visually follows objects 180°
         b) recognizes familiar faces and objects
         c) turns head to locate sounds
         d) discovers parts of own body (hands, feet)
      3) 4–8 months: beginning object permanence
         a) searches for objects that have fallen
         b) imitates expressions and gestures of others
         c) smiles at self in mirror (mirror-image play)
         d) begins development of depth and space
      4) 9–12 months: searches for hidden objects

Table 5.1 Erikson's First Five Stages of Psychosocial Development

Stage/Age Range	Core Conflict	Significant Persons	Description of Positive Resolution
Infancy (birth to 1 year)	Trust vs mistrust	Mother, father, primary caregiver	When infants' needs are met consistently and with a degree of predictability, they develop a sense of trust, a feeling that the world is a dependable and secure place.
Toddlerhood (1 to 3 years)	Autonomy vs shame and doubt	Parents	Children discover their world and their ability to explore and manipulate the environment. They assert independence (autonomy) in the face of parental control and develop a sense of will.
Preschool period (3 to 6 years)	Initiative vs guilt	Parents, siblings	Children move toward increasing independence from their parents and begin to assert themselves in the larger world outside the home. They involve themselves in mastering new tasks and acquiring new skills and capacities.
School-age period (6 to 12 years)	Industry vs inferiority	Peers, family, teachers	Children work hard to be successful at what they do. Belonging to and gaining the approval of the peer group is especially important.
Adolescence (12 to 18+ years)	Identity vs identity diffusion	Peers, significant adults other than parents (coach, teacher)	Children move toward becoming adults and achieving emancipation from parents. They struggle to find their place in society, establish career goals, deal with their sexuality, and give consideration to the problems of a complex world.

SOURCE: *Nursing Assessment: A Multidimensional Approach*, edited by J. Bellack and P. Bamford. Copyright © 1984 by Wadsworth, Inc. Reprinted by permission of Wadsworth Health Sciences Division, Monterey, CA 93940.

    d. Socialization
       1) 1 month: differentiates between face and object
       2) 2 months: social smile
       3) 4 months: recognizes primary care giver
       4) 7–8 months: shy with strangers
       5) 9–10 months: separation anxiety
    e. Vocalization (language development)
       1) 2 months: differentiated cry
       2) 3 months: squeals with pleasure
       3) 5 months: simple vocal sounds (ooh, aah), turns to voice
       4) 6 months: begins to imitate sounds
       5) 9 months: first word (da-da, ba-ba); says "dada," "mama" specifically
       6) 12 months: two words besides ma-ma and da-da
    f. Play (solitary)
       1) purposes: to practice motor skills and to learn to relate to objects and people
       2) toys
          a) washable
          b) easily handled
          c) bright colors
          d) safe, no sharp points or small removable parts
          e) nonlead paint
       3) types of toys
          a) mobiles
          b) large wooden beads, spools
          c) rattles

THE HEALTHY CHILD 515

Table 5.2 Vital Sign Ranges in Children

Pulse	1 month–1 year	80–150/bpm
	1 year–5 years	80–120/bpm
	5 years–10 years	70–110/bpm
	10 years–16 years	60–100/bpm
Respiration	1 month–1 year	20–50/min
	1 year–5 years	20–40/min
	5 years–10 years	18–30/min
	10 years–16 years	14–26/min
Blood Pressure	1 month–1 year	80/50 mm Hg
	1 year–5 years	90/60 mm Hg
	5 years–10 years	100–110/60–70 mm Hg
	10 years–16 years	110–120/70–80 mm Hg

Table 5.3 Average Daily Caloric Needs of Infants and Children*

Age	Calories
Birth–6 months	53 × weight in pounds = kcal/day
Example: 3-month-old who weighs 12 lb	12 × 53 = 636 kcal/day
6 months–1 year	48 × weight in pounds = kcal/day
Example: 10-month-old who weighs 19 lb	19 × 48 = 912 kcal/day
1–3 years	1,300 kcal/day
4–6 years	1,700 kcal/day
7–10 years	2,400 kcal/day
11–16 years	
Boys	2,700 kcal/day
Girls	2,200 kcal/day

* These daily averages may vary considerably for an individual child, depending on the child's activity level, length (height), and body build.

SOURCE: Food and Nutrition Board of the National Research Council, National Academy of Sciences

    d) musical boxes
    e) squeeze toys, sponge toys
    f) activity box for crib or playpen
    g) balls
    h) blocks
    i) pots and pans (9–10 months)
  4) games: peek-a-boo and patty-cake
2. Nutrition
  a. Caloric Needs: approximately 90–110 kcal/kg/day (see table 5.3 for recommended averages)
  b. Introduction of Solid Foods
    1) when to start solids: variety of opinions
    2) does not need solids first 5–6 months
      a) salivary enzymes and intestinal antibodies to aid digestion not present until 4–6 months
      b) extrusion reflex lasts until 3–4 months
    3) introduce foods one at a time; continue 3 or 4 days before introducing another
    4) give small quantities (start with 1 tsp)
  c. Types of Foods
    1) cooked cereal, e.g., rice (high iron content, easily digested, less likely to cause allergic reaction)

516 SECTION 5: NURSING CARE OF THE CHILD

- 2) strained fruits, vegetables, meats
- 3) egg yolks (delay egg whites until end of 1st year)
- 4) chewable and finger foods when teething (6–9 months): toast, crackers, zwieback, raw fruit, cheese
- 5) 9 months
  - a) chopped table foods
  - b) ground meat
  - c) bread
  - c) cooked vegetables (e.g., peas, carrots)
  - d) fruits (e.g., banana), desserts (e.g., gelatin pudding)
  - e) no nuts, raisins, popcorn (can be aspirated) *any sm. & firm*
- 6) 1 year: switch to whole or 2% milk *(No skim milk, not enough fat for CNS develop.)*
- d. Self-feeding: at 6 months infant begins handling spoon, finger foods; by 1 year, most infants are able to use a spoon well; ready for introduction of a cup at 6–8 months; drink independently from a cup at 1 year (may still want bottle or breast for security)
- e. Food Allergies
  1) common foods causing allergic responses include
     - a) milk
     - b) foods containing wheat, corn, or soy (protein gluten)
     - c) egg white (albumin)
     - d) chocolate
     - e) citrus foods *Not before 6 mo.*
  2) indications of hypersensitivity to food
     - a) urticaria
     - b) abdominal pain, vomiting, and diarrhea
     - c) respiratory symptoms
  3) diagnosis
     - a) singular addition of food
     - b) food diary or history *(listen to mom)*
     - c) skin testing not useful (because of immature immune system)
  4) treatment
     - a) removal of causative food
     - b) change to soy formula (if milk allergy)
     - c) elimination diet

3. Sleep
   a. Most infants have nocturnal sleep pattern by 3 months
   b. 6 months: sleep through night
   c. 8–9 months: two naps during day, sleep 10–12 hours at night
   d. Anticipatory guidance for parents
      1) each infant's sleep patterns are unique
      2) best indicators of adequate sleep are normal activity during waking hours and normal physical growth
      3) sleeping arrangements are influenced by family's cultural beliefs and customs

4. Health Care
   a. Immunizations

Table 5.4 American Academy of Pediatrics Recommended Immunization Schedule

Age	Immunization
2 months	DPT #1 (diphtheria/tetanus toxoid/pertussis) TOPV #1 (trivalent oral poliovirus)
4 months	DPT #2 TOPV #2
6 months	DPT #3 TOPV #3
12 months	tuberculin test
15 months 18 months	measles, mumps, rubella (MMR) DPT #4 TOPV #4
4 to 6 years	DPT #5 TOPV #5
14 to 16 years	tetanus and diphtheria toxoids (adult-type)—Td; repeat every 10 years

Primary Immunization for Children *Not* Immunized in Early Infancy

Age	Immunization
Under 6 years	
First visit	DTP, TOPV, Tb test
Interval after first visit:	
• 1 month	Measles, mumps, rubella (MMR)
• 2 months	
• 4 months	DTP, TOPV
10 to 18 months or preschool	DTP, TOPV
6 years and over	
First visit	Td, TOPV, Tb test
Interval after first visit:	
• 1 month	Measles, mumps, rubella
• 2 months	Td, TOPV
• 8 to 14 months	Td, TOPV
14 to 16 years	Td; repeat every 10 years

1) see table 5.4 for recommended schedule of the American Academy of Pediatrics
2) contraindications (see table 5.5)
   a) febrile illness
   b) previous severe reaction to toxoid
   c) presence of skin rash
   d) malignancy
   e) pregnancy
   f) poor immunologic response
   g) administration of gamma globulin, plasma, or blood in previous 6-8 weeks
   h) give measles vaccine only after Tb test has been found to be negative (Tb fulminates in presence of measles virus)
3) common side effects
   a) mild fever
   b) malaise
   c) soreness and swelling at injection site (DTP)
   d) mild rash (measles, rubella)
4) advise parents of possible side effects and use of antipyretics for fever

b. Accident Prevention: accidents are the second leading cause of death in this age group
1) aspiration/suffocation
   a) avoid propping bottles
   b) keep small objects out of reach
   c) check toys for small parts or sharp edges
   d) close pins when changing diaper
   e) keep plastic bags away
2) falls
   a) never leave on elevated surface unattended
   b) keep crib rails up
3) auto accidents: use infant car seats (crash-tested, rear-facing)
4) burns: check water temperature before immersing infant; keep hot substances away from infant (cigarette ashes, coffee, etc.)

B. **Toddler (1 Year to 3 Years) (Most Trying Time for Parents)**

1. Normal Growth and Development
   a. Psychosocial Development—Erikson: autonomy vs shame and doubt (see table 5.1)
      1) all activities move toward independence; expands independence

Table 5.5	Contraindications for Immunization
Febrile illness
Previous severe reaction to toxoid
Presence of skin rash
Malignancy
Inadequate immunologic response
Positive Tb test
Pregnancy
Administration of gamma globulin, plasma, or blood in previous 6-8 weeks

by exploring environment and extending its limits
      2) verbally negativistic ("No!") even when agreeable to request
   b. Physical Growth and Development
      1) vital signs: pulse and respirations decrease with increasing size and age (see table 5.2)
      2) teeth: all 20 deciduous present by 2½-3 years
      3) general appearance: potbellied, exaggerated lumbar curve, wide-based gait
      4) practices and increases muscle coordination and physical abilities
         a) climbs; goes up steps, cannot get down, and won't accept help
         b) jumps in place
         c) pushes and pulls toys
         d) scribbles spontaneously
         e) builds a tower of cubes
   c. Cognitive Development—Piaget: sensorimotor and preconceptual stages
      1) 13-18 months
         a) identifies geometric shapes
         b) opens doors and drawers
         c) points to body parts
         d) puts objects into holes, smaller objects into each other
      2) 19-24 months
         a) egocentric thinking and behavior
         b) beginning sense of time; waits in response to "just a minute"
      3) 24-36 months
         a) beginning magical thinking
         b) understands prepositions (e.g., over, under, behind, up, etc.)
         c) animism (attributes lifelike characteristics to inanimate objects)

518 SECTION 5: NURSING CARE OF THE CHILD

discipline @ time of act Not wait until other parent gets home

      d) understanding of cause and effect relationships is determined by proximity of two events
      e) increasing attention span
    d. Socialization
      1) 15 months
        a) resistant to sitting in laps
        b) wants to move independently
      2) 18 months to 2½ years: imitates parent behaviors (e.g., housework)
      3) dawdling and ritualistic behavior *← Promotes Security*
      4) temper tantrums may be used to assert independence and gain control, especially when desires are thwarted
      5) 18–24 months: learns to undress self
      6) 24–36 months: able to dress self with minimal help
      7) may be attached to transitional objects, such as a favorite blanket or stuffed animal *Security when mom gone*
      8) territorial: possessive of own toys and body
    e. Vocalization
      1) understands simple commands
      2) 18 months: 20 words
      3) 2 years: makes simple 2- or 3-word sentences; uses pronouns *me, mine*
      4) uses plurals
    f. Play (parallel)
      1) purpose: to help child make transition from solitary to cooperative play *learn how to share*
      2) types of toys
        a) cars and trucks
        b) push-pull toys
        c) blocks, building toys
        d) telephone
        e) stuffed toys and dolls
        f) large crayons, coloring books
        g) clay, finger paints *Don't like ears + mouth exam. Do last.*
        h) balls
      3) games: likes to throw and retrieve objects

2. **Nutrition and Dental Care**
    a. Growth slows, appetite smaller; "physiologic anorexia" (may eat a great deal one day and little the next); needs an average of 1,300 calories/day (see table 5.3)
      1) ritualistic food preferences
      2) likes finger foods (crackers, celery, carrot sticks)
      3) drinks from cup
      4) self-feeds by 18 months
      5) prone to iron-deficiency anemia, especially if milk intake is high

food items 1st.

    b. Anticipatory Guidance for Parents
      1) serve small portions
      2) do not give bottle as a substitute for solid foods
      (3) do not use food as a reward
      4) recognize ritualistic needs (same dishes, utensils, chair, etc.)
      5) do not force child to eat
    c. Dental Care Guidelines
      1) brush and floss twice daily with help from parents
      2) first visit to dentist as soon as all primary teeth have erupted (2½–3 years) *Caries — source infection*
      3) use fluoridated water or oral fluoride supplement (0.25–0.5 mg/day)
      4) limit concentrated sweets
      5) do not allow child to take a bottle containing juice or milk to bed since "bottle mouth caries" may result

3. **Elimination: toileting practices**
    a. Learning bowel and bladder control is one of the major tasks of toddlerhood
    b. Myelinization of nerve tracts occurs around 15–18 months of age (physiologic readiness)
    c. Toddler uses toileting activities to control self and others
    d. Independent toileting depends on
      1) physiologic readiness
      2) ability to verbally communicate need to defecate or urinate
      3) ability to get to toilet and manage clothing *Must be interested in.*
      4) psychologic readiness
    e. Ages
      1) 18 months: bowel control
      2) 2–3 years: daytime bladder control *Average*
      3) 3–4 years: nighttime bladder control

4. **Limit Setting and Discipline:** helps child learn self-control and socially appropriate behavior, promotes security
    a. Enforcement of limits should be consistent and firm
    b. Discipline should occur immediately after wrongdoing
    c. Positive approach is best
    d. Disapprove of the behavior, *not* the child
    e. Types of discipline
      1) redirecting child's attention
      2) reasoning and reprimanding, loss of privileges
      3) ignoring the behavior

THE HEALTHY CHILD 519

4) time-out
5) corporal punishment (controversial)
5. Accident Prevention: accidents are leading cause of death from 1–15 years of age. Safety is a problem because of move toward independence.
   a. Falls
      1) climbs over side rails; change to regular bed
      2) climbs stairs; use safety gates
      3) supervise at playgrounds
   b. Keep poisons and sharp objects out of reach; lock up
   c. Supervise when near cars; use car safety seats *also near water*
   d. Burns: cover electrical outlets; don't leave unattended in bathtub, near hot stove, fireplace, etc.; teach child what "hot" means

C. Preschooler (3–6 Years)
   1. Normal Growth and Development
      a. Psychosocial Development—Erikson: initiative vs guilt (see table 5.1)
         1) learns how to do things, derives satisfaction from activities
         2) needs exposure to variety of experiences and play materials
         3) imitates role models
         4) imaginative
            a) reality vs fantasy blurred
            b) may have imaginary friends
         5) exaggerated fears, e.g., fear of mutilation, monsters
      b. Physical Growth and Development
         1) body contours change: thinner and taller
         2) blood pressure 100/60 mg Hg
         3) motor skills: better control of fine and gross ones; posture more erect
            a) uses scissors and simple tools
            b) draws a person
               • 4 years: 3 parts
               • 5 years: 6 or 7 parts
            c) rides a tricycle or "big wheel"
            d) skips and hops
            e) throws and catches a ball well (5 years)
      c. Cognitive Development—Piaget: preconceptual and intuitive thought stages
         1) increased sense of time and space (tomorrow, afternoon, next week)
         2) less egocentric
         3) beginning social awareness

anticipate thing x-mas, meals.

         4) centration
            a) thinks of one idea at a time
            b) unable to think of all parts in terms of whole
            c) conclusions based on immediate visual perceptions
         5) increased ability to think without acting out
      d. Socialization
         1) capable of sharing *mostly*
         2) dresses self completely
         3) may be physically aggressive
         4) boasts and tattles
         5) learns appropriate social manners
         6) separates easily from mother
      e. Vocalization
         1) 3-year-old: constantly asks how-and-why questions; vocabulary 300–900 words
         2) 5-year-old: uses sentences of adult length
         3) knows colors, numbers, alphabet
         4) understands analogies ("If fire is hot, ice is [cold].")
      f. Play (cooperative)
         1) purpose: to learn to share and play in small groups, to learn simple games and rules *1st house play*
         2) play may be dramatic, imitative, or creative; expresses self through play
         3) types of toys
            a) housekeeping toys
            b) playground equipment
            c) wagons
            d) tricycles; big-wheel cycles
            e) water colors
            f) materials for cutting and pasting
            g) simple jigsaw puzzles
            h) picture books
            i) dolls
            j) TV (controversial, but a contemporary reality)

identify gender

   2. Nutrition: a slow-growth period; needs an average of 1,700 calories/day (see table 5.3)
      a. Appetite remains decreased; has definite food preferences *little less picky*
      b. Self-feeding: 4-year-old uses fork, can use knife to spread; able to get snacks for self
      c. Sets the table *Socially accept. table manners.*
      d. Able to pour from a pitcher
   3. Sleep *reg. pattern*
      a. Requires 9–12 hours/night
      b. May or may not take one nap during day

520 SECTION 5: NURSING CARE OF THE CHILD

    c. May have fears of the dark, or may awaken with nightmares
    d. Guidelines for care givers
       1) provide quiet time before bedtime
       2) use a nightlight
       3) adhere to a consistent bedtime pattern
  4. Sexuality
    a. Knows sex differences by 3 years
    b. Imitates masculine or feminine behaviors; gender identity well established by 6 years
    c. Sexual curiosity and exploration
       1) masturbation is normal
       2) curious about anatomical differences and seeks to "investigate" them
    d. Guidelines for care givers
       1) assess what child already knows when she asks a question
       2) answer questions simply, honestly, and matter-of-factly (avoid detailed explanations)
       3) use correct terminology
  5. Accident Prevention
    a. Motor Vehicle Accidents
       1) street safety: teach to wait at curb until told to cross
       2) wear seat belt
    b. Drownings: teach to swim; supervise near pools, lakes, etc.
    c. Burns: teach not to play with matches or lights; supervise near fireplace; teach how to escape from burning home
    d. General Safety: teach not to talk to strangers; child should know own name, address, telephone number, and how to seek help if lost

D. School Age (6–12 Years)
  1. Normal Growth and Development
    a. Psychosocial Development—Erikson: industry vs inferiority (see table 5.1)
       1) develops a sense of accomplishment academically, physically, and socially
       2) school phobias may occur as a result of increased competition, desire to succeed, fear of failure
       3) desire for accomplishment so strong that young school-age child may try to change rules of game to win
       4) gains competence in mastering new skills and tasks; assumes more responsibilities
       5) desires to get along socially; more responsive to peers
       6) still needs reassurance and support from family and trusted adults
    b. Physical Growth and Development
       1) growth is slow and regular (1–2 inches gain in height per year, 3–6 lb weight gain per year)
       2) motor skills: increases strength and physical ability, refines coordination
         a) 6 years: jumps, skips, hops well; ties shoelaces easily, prints
         b) 7 years: vision fully developed, can read regular-size print; can swim and ride a bicycle
         c) 8 years: writes rather than prints; increased smoothness and speed
         d) 9 years: fully developed hand-eye coordination; individual capabilities/talents emerge
         e) 10 years: increased strength, stamina, coordination
         f) 11 years: awkward; nervous energy (drumming fingers, etc.)
    c. Cognitive Development—Piaget: concrete operations stage (7–11 years)
       1) decentering: can consider more than one characteristic at a time
       2) reversibility: able to imagine a process in reverse
       3) conservation: able to conserve (mentally retain) physical properties of matter even when form is changed
       4) able to classify objects and verbalize concepts involved in doing so
       5) reasons logically
       6) able to think through a situation and anticipate the consequences; may then alter course of action
    d. Socialization
       1) prefers friends to family; life is centered around school and friends
       2) relationships with adults other than parents and peers of increasing importance
       3) increasing social sensitivity; learns to empathize and sympathize
       4) more cooperative; improved manners
    e. Vocalization
       1) curious about meaning of different words; rapidly expanding vocabulary
       2) likes name-calling, word games (e.g., rhymes)
       3) giggles and laughs a great deal; silly
       4) knows clock and calendar time
    f. Play (cooperative, team)

THE HEALTHY CHILD 521

↑ strenght + motor skills

1) purposes: to learn to bargain, cooperate, and compromise; to develop logical reasoning abilities; to increase social skills
2) types of toys, entertainment
   a) play figures, trains, model kits
   b) games, jigsaw puzzles, magic tricks
   c) books: joke and comic books, storybooks, adventure, mystery
   d) TV, video games, records, radio
   e) riding a bicycle
   f) organized activities (sports, Scouts, music and dancing lessons, camping, etc.)

2. Nutrition and Dental Health

   ↑ protein

   a. Appetite increases; needs an average of 2,400 calories/day (see table 5.3); breakfast is important for school performance
   b. More influenced by mass media; more likely to eat junk food because of increased time away from home
   c. Nutrition Education
      1) teach basic four food groups
      2) teach basic cooking skills, meal planning
      3) nutritious snacks
   d. Dental Health
      1) loss of deciduous teeth; eruption of permanent ones, including 1st and 2nd molars
      2) dental caries are a major health problem
         a) caused by poor nutrition, influence of TV advertising contributing to increased intake of carbohydrates and concentrated sweets, inadequate dental hygiene
         b) prevention: good brushing and flossing techniques, regular dental checkups, fluoridated water, good nutrition

3. Accident Prevention
   a. Motor Vehicle Accidents
      1) teach how to cross street
      2) bike safety
      3) use car safety belts
   b. Drowning
      1) learn to swim
      2) teach water safety
   c. Burns
      1) teach safety around fires (e.g., fireplaces, camp fires) *matches*

Test ↑ protein, No Na+ night before.

2) teach not to play with explosives or guns

E. Adolescence (12–19 Years)
1. Normal Growth and Development
   a. Psychosocial Development—Erikson: identity vs identity diffusion (see table 5.1)
      1) "Who am I?"
      2) "What do I want to do with my life?"
      3) accepts changes in body image
      4) experiences mood swings; vacillates between maturity and childlike behavior
      5) continually reassesses values and beliefs
      6) begins to consider career possibilities
      7) gains independence from parents
   b. Physical Growth and Development: puberty
      1) males: development of secondary sex characteristics *develop 2 yrs later than females*
         a) increase in size of genitalia
         b) swelling of breasts
         c) growth of pubic, axillary, facial, and chest hair
         d) voice changes
         e) increase in shoulder breadth
         f) production of spermatozoa; nocturnal emissions *norm*
      2) females: development of secondary sex characteristics
         a) increase in transverse diameter of pelvis
         b) development of breasts
         c) change in vaginal secretions
         d) growth of pubic and axillary hair
         e) menstruation: 12 years (average)
      3) both sexes
         a) acne
         b) perspiration
         c) blushing
         d) rapid increase in height and weight
         e) fatigue (since heart and lungs grow at slower rate)
   c. Cognitive Development—Piaget: formal operations (11 years and older); attained at different ages and depends on formal education, experience, cultural background
      1) abstract thinking
      2) forms hypotheses, analytical thinking
      3) can consider more than two categories at same time

↑ moral values unrealistic expect.

[Handwritten at top: Anorexia + Bulimia. Problem. Risk Taking Behaviors]

4) generalizes findings
5) thinks about thinking; philosophical
d. Socialization
  1) with adults
    a) may resent authority
    b) wishes to be different from parents: may ridicule them
    c) has need for parent figures
    d) develops crushes on adults outside the family
  2) with peers
    a) overidentifies with group: same dress, same ethical codes
    b) has close friendships with members of same sex
    c) develops heterosexual relationships, sexual experimentation (may be sexually active)
e. Recreation, Leisure Activity: expanding variety
  1) parties, dances
  2) movies, daydreaming
  3) video games, television, music (radio, records)
  4) telephone conversations
  5) sports, games
  6) jigsaw or crossword puzzles
  7) reading
  8) hobbies
2. Nutrition
  a. Appetite increases with rapid growth; needs basic four food groups
  b. Caloric needs vary with activity level, sex, body build (see table 5.3)
    1) girls need approximately 2,200 calories/day *[handwritten: c̄ ↑ Ca + Fe]*
    2) boys need an average of 2,700 calories/day
  c. Increased need for protein, calcium, iron, and zinc
  d. Sports activity may increase nutritional requirements
  e. Eating habits are easily influenced by peer group
    1) intake of junk food
    2) fad diets and dieting: can lead to health problems, including anorexia nervosa
    3) overeating or inactivity: may result in obesity
3. Accident Prevention
  a. Motor Vehicle Accidents: enroll in driver-training programs, wear seat belts
  b. Drownings: teach water safety, first aid, CPR
  c. Sports Injuries: educate for prevention
  d. Alcohol and Drug Abuse: education
  e. Suicide: be alert for signs of depression
F. Application of the Nursing Process to the Healthy Child *[handwritten: Review]*
  1. Assessment
    a. Health History
      1) general health status: incidence of illnesses in past year, visits to health provider, immunization history, current medications
      2) developmental history: parents' health status, mother's obstetric history with this child, child's neonatal history, achievement of developmental milestones, self-care abilities, behavior, and temperament
      3) parents' perceptions and concerns
      4) parents' knowledge of development, child care, safety, nutrition, etc.
      5) child's home and school environments: safety, appropriate stimulation, barriers to development
      6) nutrition: daily food and fluid intake, child's preferences and dislikes, self-feeding abilities, special needs (cultural/religious practices, allergies)
      7) dental care: number of teeth, tooth eruption (discomfort, management), daily oral hygiene, self-brushing and flossing, fluoride (water or daily supplement), dental visits
      8) elimination: daily routine, toilet trained or diapers, problems, e.g., diarrhea, constipation, enuresis, how managed
      9) activity/sleep: exercise and activity patterns; sleep habits: sleep environment, daily total, special needs, problems
      10) sexuality: gender knowledge and identity, sexual curiosity and exploration, sexual knowledge, primary and secondary sex characteristics; adolescent: knowledge, sexual activity, contraception, pregnancy, sexually transmitted disease
    b. Physical Examination
      1) development
        a) observation of age-appropriate developmental behavior and abilities

THE HEALTHY CHILD   523

   b) administration of developmental screening tools when indicated to screen for delays (e.g., Denver Developmental Screening Test)
   c) home environment: visit to appraise for support of or barriers to development
2) general physical appraisal
   a) growth: length, weight, head circumference; percentiles on standard growth curves
   b) vital signs: annual BP screening over age 3 (especially in high-risk children) (see table 5.2)
   c) general health: skin, activity, attention span, ability to communicate, etc.
   d) vision/hearing screening
- vision testing
  - binocularity tests for strabismus; if strabismus is not detected and corrected by age 6 years, amblyopia (dimness of vision, even blindness) may result [squinting]
    * corneal light reflex test
    * cover test
  - visual acuity tests; Snellen E (preschoolers or illiterate children) or Snellen alphabet chart
  - referral criteria
    * 3 years: vision in one or both eyes 20/50 or worse
    * 4-6 years: vision in one or both eyes 20/40 or worse
    * 7 years and older: vision in one or both eyes 20/30 or worse
    * children with one-line or more difference between both eyes (example: 20/30 in left eye, 20/40 in right)
    * abnormal findings from cover test or corneal light reflex test
- hearing testing
  - conduction tests
    * Rinne test (comparison of bone and air conduction)
    * Weber's test (bone conduction)
  - pure tone audiometry (audiogram) to test for conductive or sensorineural hearing impairments

2. **General Nursing Goals, Plans/Implementation, and Evaluation**

Goal 1: Child will achieve optimum development.
Plan/Implementation
- provide information to parents on normal growth and development
  - what to expect (skills, behavior)
  - age-appropriate play activities and materials
  - ways to stimulate development
- discuss child-rearing methods and styles, limit-setting, and ways to cope with child-rearing problems

Evaluation: Child grows and develops within expected range; is free from delays in development. Parents cope effectively with child-rearing concerns and problems.

Goal 2: Child will experience a safe environment and will be free from accidental injury.
Plan/Implementation
- provide anticipatory guidance to parents concerning age-related safety hazards, and ways to prevent accidental injury (safety-proofing the home, auto safety restraints, swimming and bicycling safety, safe toys, driver education)

Evaluation: Child is free from accidental injury.

Goal 3: Child will receive optimal nutrition and dental care.
Plan/Implementation
- provide teaching and counseling to parents concerning child's nutritional requirements, feeding techniques, dental hygiene, tooth eruption, food allergies, and feeding abilities

Evaluation: Child's physical growth follows growth curve; child receives daily nutritional requirements (calories, protein, CHO, fats, vitamins/minerals); feeds self in accordance with developmental abilities; receives appropriate dental hygiene and care and is free from dental caries; child's food allergies are detected and diet is adjusted as needed.

Goal 4: Child gets adequate rest and sleep.
Plan/Implementation
- provide anticipatory guidance to parents concerning child's sleep needs, patterns

of sleep in childhood, and ways to cope with sleep problems

Evaluation: Child gets amount of sleep required for optimal growth and development. Parents cope with child's sleep problems.

Goal 5: Child's sexuality and sexual development are fostered in healthy ways.

Plan/Implementation
- provide anticipatory guidance to parents concerning child's developing sexuality
  - what to expect (questions, behaviors)
  - answer child's questions matter-of-factly, honestly, accurately
- teach child about sex and sexuality appropriate to child's age and expressed interest

Evaluation: Child develops gender-appropriate sexual identity and healthy sexuality.

Goal 6: Child is free from preventable communicable diseases.

Plan/Implementation
- reinforce to parents the importance of childhood immunizations
- administer immunizations according to recommended schedule

Evaluation: Child receives immunizations according to recommended schedule; is free from preventable communicable diseases.

References

Bellack, J. and Bamford, P. *Nursing Assessment: A Multidimensional Approach*. Monterey, CA: Wadsworth, 1984

Chance, P. *Learning Through Play*. Skillman, NJ: Johnson and Johnson, 1979.

Euler, M. and McClellan, M. "Toilet Training: Ready or Not?" *Pediatric Nursing*. January 1981:15-20.

Malinowski, J. "Answering a Child's Questions About Sex and a New Baby." *American Journal of Nursing*. November 1979:1965-1968.

Nachem, B. and Bass, R. "Children Still Aren't Being Buckled Up." *MCN: American Journal of Maternal-Child Nursing*. September/October 1984:320-323.

Nelms, B. "What is a Normal Adolescent?" *MCN: American Journal of Maternal-Child Nursing*. November/December 1981:402-406.

O'Pray, M. "Developmental Screening Tools: Using Them Effectively." *MCN: American Journal of Maternal-Child Nursing*. March/April 1980:126-130.

Pipes, P. *Nutrition in Infancy and Childhood*, 2nd Ed. St. Louis: Mosby, 1981.

Pringle, S. and Ramsey, B. *Promoting the Health of Children*. St. Louis: Mosby, 1982.

Rybicki, L. "Preparing Parents to Teach Their Children About Sexuality." *MCN: American Journal of Maternal-Child Nursing*. May/June, 1976:182-185.

*Selekman, J. "Immunization: What's It All About?" *American Journal of Nursing*. August 1980: 1440-1443.

Slattery, J. "Dental Health in Children." *American Journal of Nursing*. July 1976:1159-1161.

Whaley, L. and Wong, D. *Nursing Care of Infants and Children*, 2nd Ed. St. Louis: Mosby, 1983.

Wieczorek, R. and Natapoff, J. *A Conceptual Approach to the Nursing of Children*. Philadelphia: Lippincott, 1981.

†Yoos, L. "A Developmental Approach to Physical Assessment." *MCN: American Journal of Maternal-Child Nursing*. May/June, 1981:168-170.

White, J. and Owsley, V. "Helping Families Cope with Milk, Wheat, and Soy Allergies." *MCN: American Journal of Maternal-Child Nursing*. November/December 1983:423-428.

* See Reprint section
† Highly recommended

The Ill and Hospitalized Child

General Concepts
A. Overview
1. Hospitalization and Illness are Stressful for Children
   a. Difficulty changing routines
   b. Limited coping mechanisms
   c. Reason for hospitalization is often less significant than consequences (e.g., separation from familiar persons and surroundings, painful procedures, restricted mobility)
2. Major Stressors for the Child
   a. Separation
   b. Loss of Control
   c. Body Injury *all age groups*
   d. Pain
   e. Immobility
3. Factors that Affect Responses to Illness and Hospitalization
   a. Developmental level (see below, "Developmental Responses to Hospitalization")
   b. Past experiences, especially with hospitalization and surgery
   c. Level of anxiety: child and parents
   d. Relationship between parents and child
   e. Nature and seriousness of illness or injury; circumstances of hospitalization
   f. Family background: education, culture, support systems
4. Developmental Responses to Hospitalization
   a. Infant
      1) separation: before attachment (under 4-6 months) not as significant; older infant's response is crying and rage, protest; stranger anxiety
      2) loss of control
         a) expects that crying will bring immediate response from care giver (changed, fed, held); may interfere with development of trust
         b) in hospital
            - immediate response may not occur
            - need may be met by unfamiliar person
            - doesn't understand explanations
      3) immobility: restrictions and restraints interfere with activity and sucking (see table 5.6)
      4) pain: procedures cause discomfort; responds by crying and withdrawal
   b. Toddler *3-6 yr.*
      1) separation
         a) fear of unknown and abandonment
         b) separation anxiety is similar to grief; so encourage protest behaviors as healthy response
            - protest: cries loudly, rejects attentions of nurses, wants parent
            - despair: cries in monotonous tone, state of mourning, "settling in"
            - denial: renewed interest in surroundings; seems adjusted to loss, but actually repressing feelings for parent
         c) disruption in routines (eating, sleep, toileting) decreases security and control
         d) regression: attempts to seek comfort by returning to earlier, dependent behaviors
            - clinging, whining
            - wetting
            - wanting bottle, pacifier
      2) loss of control: special concern because major task is to gain autonomy
      3) body injury: fears intrusive procedures (e.g., rectal temperature, injections) and reacts intensely

Table 5.6 Commonly Used Pediatric Restraints

Type	Indications	Precautions
Jacket	In crib (alternative to crib net) In high chair To maintain horizontal position in crib	Tie in back. Secure ties underneath crib or high chair.
Crib net	To prevent infant or toddler from climbing over side rails	Avoid nets with tears or large gaps. Tie to bedsprings, not to crib sides.
Crib cover	To prevent toddler from climbing out of crib	Ensure all latches are locked.
Mummy	For infant or small toddler needing short-term restraint • venipuncture • gavage feedings • eye, ear, nose, throat exams	Keep top of mummy sheet level with shoulder. Maintain arms and legs in anatomical position. Expose needed extremity only.
Clove hitch or commercial ties	For arm/leg restraints to limit motion for venipunctures	Observe for adequacy of circulation. Pad under restraint. Tie ends to crib springs. Remove q2h for ROM exercise.
Elbow	To prevent touching of head or face • scalp vein infusions • post-op, repair of cleft lip, palate	Pad stiff material. Use pins or ties to prevent slippage. Remove one at a time q2h for ROM exercise.

4) immobility: cannot freely explore environment; may interfere with motor, language development
5) pain: becomes emotionally distraught and physically resistant to painful procedures
  c. Preschooler
  1) separation
   a) may view as punishment for something thought or done
   b) more subtle responses than toddler (quiet crying, sleep problems, loss of appetite)
  2) loss of control: their active imagination may lead to exaggeration or misinterpretations of hospital experiences; fears and fantasies may get the best of them
  3) body injury/body integrity
   a) confusion between reality and fantasy
   b) casts and bandages are particular problems, since child is not assured that all body parts that were there before are there now; much worry over body integrity
  4) pain
   a) recognizes cues that signal an impending painful experience
   b) able to anticipate pain: may try to escape, may become physically combative
  5) immobility: prevents mastery of fears; preschooler often feels helpless
  d. School-Age Child
  1) separation
   a) from family and friends
   b) easier than other age groups because of cognitive level and better time concept
  2) fear of loss of control
   a) through immobility
   b) enforced dependence
   c) fear of injury and death; death anxiety peaks @ age 9
   d) doesn't want others to see loss of control (e.g., crying), tries to appear brave

3) pain: usually uses passive coping strategies (lies rigidly still, shuts eyes, clenches teeth and fists)
4) immobility: affects sense of physical achievement and need for competition
e. Adolescent: loss of control-enforced dependence when the need is to move toward identity and independence

loss of self esteem
Modesty, need time alone

B. **Application of the Nursing Process to the Ill and Hospitalized Child**
  1. Assessment
     a. Child's developmental level and major fear associated with age group
        1) infant: stranger anxiety
        2) toddler: separation anxiety, intrusive procedures
        3) preschooler: body mutilation
        4) school-age: loss of control
        5) adolescent: loss of control, change in body image and self-identity
     b. Child's perceptions/understanding of illness and hospitalization
     c. Family responses to child's hospitalization

Family's view impacts on child view of hosp.

        1) parents may react with denial, disbelief, guilt, fear, anxiety, frustration, and depression
        2) alterations in family routines and life-style
        3) parents' coping mechanisms
           a) support systems for parents, e.g., friends, extended family members
           b) financial resources
           c) family's ability to cope with the child's illness
           d) ability to express reaction to child's illness
     d. Child's responses to pain: unable to express verbally; often results in under utilization of pain-relief methods
        1) through observation
           a) verbally: younger child often uses incorrect words, e.g., "bad," "funny," "hot;" older child often reluctant to complain because of fear of "shots"
           b) behaviorally: pulling at area (ear), irritable, loss of appetite, lying or moving in unusual position
           c) physiologically: vomiting, change in vital signs, flushed skin, increased sleep time, sleep disruptions
        2) asking child to rate the pain, e.g., using happy/unhappy faces, or scale of 0–10
  2. **Goals, Plans/Implementation, and Evaluation**
     Goal 1: Child will be prepared psychologically for hospitalization.
     Plan/Implementation
     - encourage preadmission preparation
       - recommended time frame
         * before 2 years: explanation is ineffective; allow to take favorite toy and objects
         * 2–7 years: usually tell child ahead in days equal to years of age, e.g., 2 years = 2 days ahead, 6 years = 6 days ahead
         * over 7 years: tell child when parent knows
     - orient child and family to surroundings
     - anticipate and alleviate age-related needs and fears
       - to develop trust in infant
         * arrange for rooming-in
         * ensure consistency of care giver
         * provide security objects (e.g., toy, blanket)
         * make routine patterns as similar as possible to home
         * hold, cuddle, stroke
       - to help toddler maintain control
         * use familiar words (e.g., child's word for toileting)
         * ask parents to leave familiar objects with child (e.g., toy, blanket)
         * encourage rooming-in and parental participation in care
         * accept regressive needs but avoid promoting them (e.g., don't put toilet-trained child back in diapers)
         * provide explanations immediately prior to any procedure with use of simple, concrete words
         * use time orientation in relation to familiar activities (e.g., "after naptime")
         * prepare parents to recognize and accept regressive behavior following discharge
         * maintain limit setting to provide consistency for child
         * don't offer choices when there are none

- to help preschooler relieve body-mutilation anxiety
  * allow child to wear underwear
  * provide reassurance regarding invasive procedures
  * concept of time is related to routine activities (e.g., when you wake up, after lunch, etc.)
  * allow some choices to promote feelings of control and mastery (choice of fluids, play activities)
- to help school-age child maintain a degree of control
  * provide explanations of illness, treatment
    † pictures
    † simple anatomic diagrams
    † dolls: call them models or teaching models with older child
    † books
    † step-by-step illustrations
  * maintain educational level during long-term hospitalization to help meet need for accomplishment
    † homework; contact with own schoolteacher
    † in-hospital teacher
  * allow to participate in care planning
    † times for bath, treatments
    † food choices, etc.
- to help adolescent maintain some control
  * maintain peer contacts
    † visiting should be open to adolescents
    † place in adolescent unit or room
  * encourage participation in decision making regarding own body
- provide honest explanations, information, and support
  - determine level of understanding and preexisting knowledge
  - use age-appropriate language, terminology, and timing prior to instruction
- foster a sense of safety and security
  - encourage rooming-in, security objects for younger children
  - determine child's routine, rituals, nickname
  - implement age-appropriate safety measures, e.g., bubble top (covered) cribs, raised cribrails (see table 5.6)

Evaluation: Child maintains developmental level; expresses feelings/desires about hospital (e.g., wants to go home); maintains attachments (family, favorite objects, friends).

Goal 2: Parents will feel in control.
Plan/Implementation
- allow and encourage parents to participate in child's care; provide 24-hour open visiting and rooming-in facilities
- foster family relationships between ill child and family members; include siblings
- provide support; help family identify persons or community resources who can help
- provide information about child's illness, treatment, and care at rate that parents are able to accept and cope with

Evaluation: Parents express satisfaction with care givers and information provided; child and parents maintain/regain supportive relationships.

Goal 3: Child undergoing hospital procedures and surgery will be prepared.
Plan/Implementation
- refer to *Nursing Care of the Adult* "Perioperative Period" page 165
- additional concerns for children
  - measure child's height and weight (used for calculating medications and IV fluids)
  - explain procedure, recovery room, and post-op care to child (appropriate for age) and to parents
    * use concrete words and visual aids
    * use neutral words, e.g., "fixed" instead of "cut"
    * emphasize body part involved and any change in function
    * use drawings and storytelling to evaluate child's understanding
    * take child and parent to see equipment and rooms, if possible

Day of Surgery
- give nothing PO (shorter duration for a child compared with an adult)
- check for loose teeth
- allow favorite toy to accompany child to OR
- encourage parents to remain with child as long as possible
- clothe child for OR: diaper for non-toilet trained child; permit older child to wear underwear under hospital gown, if possible

- administer pre-op medications as ordered; oral or parenteral form is influenced by type, amount, age, accessibility; see table 5.7

Evaluation: Child takes nothing PO; is prepared correctly for surgery; child and family know what to expect postoperatively.

Goal 4: Postoperatively, child will maintain adequate pulmonary ventilation and circulation, fluid and electrolyte balance.
Plan/Implementation
- turn, position, and get child to cough at least q2h
- use inspirometer, straw games with older child to ensure deep breathing
- monitor IV closely
  - if microdrip (60 gtts/ml) used, gtts/min = ml/hour
  - check for fluid overload
- exercise restrained limbs q2h; fasten restraint ties to crib or bed

Evaluation: Child has adequate ventilation and circulation, normal color, no evidence of cyanosis, adequate fluid intake and output.

Goal 5: Child will be free from pain.
Plan/Implementation
- be alert to nonverbal messages in a very young child or child who may fear injections and not wish to communicate discomfort
- medicate for nausea and pain as ordered (often analgesics such as acetaminophen are used)
- assess for response to medications

Evaluation: Child experiences minimal pain.

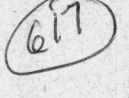

Goal 6: Child will use diversional activity and play to cope with the stress of hospitalization.
Plan/Implementation
- refer to "Healthy Child" page 513
- to help child participate in nursing activities, e.g., tea party for fluid intake, inspirometer for deep breathing, bean bags for range-of-motion
- use drawings, storytelling, puppets to help child express feelings about illness
- allow child to use syringes, needles with supervision

Evaluation: Child expresses fears and feelings during play; adapts to hospital routine with minimal distress.

Goal 7: Child and family will receive appropriate discharge teaching.
Plan/Implementation
- provide oral and written instructions regarding
  - activities and restrictions
  - diet
  - procedures
  - medications: schedule, administration, storage, side effects
- teach parents procedures that must be performed at home
- contact appropriate outside resources as needed, e.g., homebound teacher, Visiting Nurse Association

Evaluation: Child (as appropriate) and parent can state medical regimen that must be carried on at home (e.g., medications, diet, restrictions); can demonstrate how to do procedures or give medications, know how to obtain refills, arrange for follow-up appointments.

Table 5.7 Medication and Temperature Guide

Age Group	Usual Form of Oral Medication	Available Injection Sites	Usual Route for Temperature
Infant	L	VL	A R
Toddler	L P (crush)	VL	A R
Preschooler	L P (crush or chew)	VL VG GM D (immunizations)	A R O (older child)
School-Age Child	L P	VL VG GM D	O A
Adolescent	L P C	VL VG GM D	O A

P—pills
L—liquid
C—capsules

VL—vastus lateralis
GM—gluteus medius
VG—ventro gluteal
D—deltoid

O—oral
A—axillary
R—rectal

Table 5.8 Medication Administration for Young Children

Age	Developmental Considerations	Nursing Implications
1–3 months	Strong sucking reflex	Allow sucking for oral meds, e.g., nipples, syringes.
	Extrusion reflex	Give meds in small amounts to allow for swallowing.
		Keep head upright.
		Place liquid in center or side of mouth, toward back.
	Reaches randomly	Control child's hands when giving oral meds.
	Whole body reacts to painful stimuli	Use own body to control infant's arms and legs for parenteral meds.
3–12 months	Extrusion reflex disappears	Use medicine cup/syringe rather than spoon.
	Drinks from cup	Offer physical comforting more than verbal.
	Can finger feed	
	Can spit out medication	
12–30 months	Development of large motor skills	Never leave meds where child can reach or throw.
	Can spit out meds or clamp jaw shut	May need two adults to give injections (one to restrain).
	Can use medicine cup	Give ear drops by pulling pinna down and back.
	Auditory canal is not straight	Be honest about taste/pain, use distractions.
	Autonomy vs shame/doubt	Be firm, ignore resistive behavior.
	Ritualistic	Give choices when possible.
	Takes pride in tasks	
2½–3½ years	Has eating likes and dislikes	Disguise med taste.
	Little sense of time	Use chewable meds.
	Tries to coerce, manipulate	Use concrete and immediate rewards (stickers, badges).
	Has fantasies	
	Body boundaries are unclear	Give choices when possible, but do not offer if there are none.
		Be consistent.
		Give simple explanations; reassure child that medicine is not for punishment.
		Use Band-Aids for covering injection sites.
3½–6 years	Develops proficiency at tasks	Allow child to handle equipment (e.g., syringes).
	Refining senses	Unable to disguise tastes and smells.
	Has loose teeth	Consider teeth when deciding route.
	Can make decisions	Allow choice about route, if possible.
	Has a sense of time	Allow participation in choice of administration time when possible (e.g., before or after meals).
	Takes pride in accomplishment	Explain in simple terms reason for meds.
	Developing a conscience	Avoid prolonged reasoning.
	Fears mutilation, punishment	Use simple command by trusted adult that med is to be given.
	May master pill swallowing	Allow control when possible.
		Praise after med is given.

References

Birchfield, M. "Nursing Care for Hospitalized Children Based on Different Stages of Illness." *MCN: American Journal of Maternal-Child Nursing*. January/February 1981:46–52.

Evans, M. and Hansen, B. "Administering Injections to Different Aged Children." *MCN: American Journal of Maternal-Child Nursing*. May/June 1981:194–199.

Farrel, S. and Kiernan, B. "A Positive Approach to Nutrition for Hospitalized Children." *MCN: American Journal of Maternal-Child Nursing*. March/April 1977:113–117.

Hansen, B. and Evans, M. "Preparing a Child for Procedures." *MCN: American Journal of Maternal-Child Nursing*. November/December 1981:392–397.

Howry, L., Bindler, R. and Tso, Y. *Pediatric Medications*. Philadelphia: Lippincott, 1981.

Kline, J. "Recovery Room Care for the Child in Pain." *MCN: American Journal of Maternal-Child Nursing*. July/August 1984: 261–263.

Koss, T. and Teter, M. "Welcoming a Family When a Child is Hospitalized." *MCN: American Journal of Maternal-Child Nursing*. January/February 1980:51–54.

McCaffery, M. "Pain Relief for the Child: Problem Areas and Selected Nonpharmacological Methods." *Pediatric Nursing*. November/December 1977:31–55.

Nelson, M. "Identifying the Emotional Needs of the Hospitalized Child." *MCN: American Journal of Maternal-Child Nursing*. May/June 1981:181–183.

Ormond, E. and Caulfield, C. "A Practical Guide to Giving Oral Medications to Young Children." *MCN: American Journal of Maternal-Child Nursing*. September/October 1976:320–325.

*Sheredy, C. "Factors to Consider when Assessing Responses to Pain." *MCN: American Journal of Maternal-Child Nursing*. July/August 1984:250–252.

Weeks, H. "Administering Medications to Children." *MCN: American Journal of Maternal-Child Nursing*. January/February 1980:63.

Whaley, L. and Wong, D. *Nursing Care of Infants and Children*, 2nd Ed. St. Louis: Mosby, 1983.

Wieczorek, R. and Natapoff, J. *A Conceptual Approach to the Nursing of Children*. Philadelphia: Lippincott, 1981.

* See Reprint section

Oxygenation

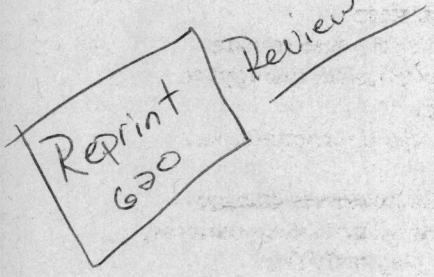

General Concepts

A. Overview
1. Respiratory System
   a. Chest configuration (AP diameter) changes from round to more flattened as child grows
   b. Steady increase in number and surface area of alveoli from birth to age 12
   c. Cricoid cartilage is at the level of the 4th cervical vertebra in infants, 5th cervical vertebra in children (important when positioning children for resuscitation, intubation, or tracheostomy)
   d. More susceptible to respiratory obstruction and atelectasis because of narrow tracheal and bronchiolar pathways
   e. More susceptible to infections because of immature immune system and frequent contacts with infectious organisms
   f. Respiratory infections are the most common cause of illness in infants and children
2. Cardiovascular System
   a. Heart is larger in proportion to total body size and lies at transverse angle during infancy
   b. Several changes take place during transition from fetal to postnatal circulation
      1) lungs inflate, resulting in increased pressure in left side of heart
      2) foramen ovale closes
      3) ductus arteriosus closes
      4) obliteration of ductus venosus and umbilical vessels
   c. Blood pressure gradually increases, and pulse and respiratory rates gradually decrease as child grows
   d. Cardiac problems are a major cause of illness and death in infancy
3. Hematologic System
   a. All components necessary for normal hematologic functioning are present at birth except vitamin K, which is administered intramuscularly to the neonate (refer to *Nursing Care of the Childbearing Family* page 449)
   b. *All* bones are engaged in blood cell production until growth ceases in late adolescence

B. Application of the Nursing Process to the Child with Respiratory Problems
1. Assessment
   a. Nursing History
      1) any known breathing problems, respiratory allergies, activity intolerance (does child have problems keeping up with other children during play?), incidence of respiratory illnesses, treatment, home management
      2) environmental factors: dust or pollen in home, play or school environments; do parents or client smoke?
   b. Physical Examination
      1) general appearance: color (pallor, cyanosis), respiratory effort (dyspnea, prolonged expirations), restlessness, irritability, fatigue, prostration
      2) respiratory rate, depth, character; presence of respiratory signs (cough: character, productive or nonproductive; rhinitis; retractions; nasal flaring)
      3) fever
      4) breath sounds: upper respiratory tract, all lobes of lungs; presence of wheezing, rales, rhonchi
   c. Diagnostic Tests (refer to *Nursing Care of the Adult* page 174)

2. **General Nursing Goals, Plans/Implementation, and Evaluation**

[Handwritten top notes: CPT - infected lobe 1st. give before eating - eat alot bottles - prevents vomiting]

[Handwritten top right: Acute resp distress → NPO & IV]

OXYGENATION

Goal 1: Child will maintain adequate oxygenation and a patent airway.
Plan/Implementation
- monitor respiratory status
  - vital signs (respirations, pulse, temperature) *↑ → resp distress*
  - skin and nail-bed color, dyspnea, cough, nasal flaring, retractions
  - lung sounds
  - use of sternal and thoracic muscles
  - behavioral changes (restlessness, irritability, disruptions in patterns)
- be alert for signs of airway obstruction
  - increased pulse and respiratory rates
  - restlessness, anxiety, agitation (indicate hypoxia)
  - increased stridor, retractions
  - pallor or cyanosis
- avoid sedatives that depress respirations and cough reflex (e.g., narcotics)
- keep endotracheal tubes, laryngoscope, and tracheostomy tray at bedside for emergency use

Evaluation: Child maintains a patent airway; exhibits signs of adequate oxygenation (normal skin color, quiet breathing, alert and oriented, clear lung sounds).

Goal 2: Child will be free from respiratory distress.
Plan/Implementation
- provide a humidified atmosphere (e.g., croup tent) and O₂ as ordered *cool mist*
- place child in semi-Fowler's position to facilitate lung expansion
- assist with chest percussion and postural drainage as needed

Evaluation: Child is free from respiratory distress.

Goal 3: Child will be adequately hydrated.
Plan/Implementation
- provide humidifed atmosphere to liquefy secretions
- ensure adequate fluid intake
  - withhold oral fluids until respiratory distress subsides
  - monitor IV fluids to prevent dehydration or fluid overload

[Handwritten left margin: Sp. gr. Norm 1.005-1.025 .025 → dehydration]

Evaluation: Child is adequately hydrated (elastic skin turgor, normal urine output, adequate fluid intake); is free from signs of dehydration or fluid overload.

Goal 4: Child will conserve energy.

Plan/Implementation
- schedule treatments and nursing activities to allow uninterrupted periods for maximum rest/sleep
- monitor child's response to care (feeding, chest physical therapy) to prevent tiring
- provide quiet age-appropriate play activities

Evaluation: Child conserves energy; approximates normal rest/sleep patterns; engages in quiet play activities.

Goal 5: Child will experience minimal anxiety.
Plan/Implementation
- administer sedatives (e.g., phenobarbital) as ordered
- encourage parent to stay with child or visit often
- allow child to keep favorite toy or attachment object
- assign staff familiar to the child
- reassure and comfort child following stressful procedures or separation from parents

[Handwritten margin: Is anything depress resp or cough - talk to Dr. about changing]

Evaluation: Child is calm and secure; cooperates with treatments and care.

Goal 6: Child will be physically comfortable.
Plan/Implementation
- keep child warm and dry
- administer antipyretics, tepid sponge bath for fever
- change child's position frequently
- encourage parents to participate in child's physical care

Evaluation: Child remains physically comfortable; rests quietly.

Selected Health Problems Resulting in an Interference with Respiration

A. Sudden Infant Death Syndrome (SIDS) or "Crib Death"

[Handwritten: 3RD leading cause]

1. **General Information**
   a. Definition: sudden unexpected death of an infant or young child, in which an adequate cause cannot be determined
   b. Incidence: 8,000–10,000 infants per year in the US; higher incidence in boys, infants who are premature or low birth weight, infants with CNS disturbances, nonwhites; five times greater incidence in siblings

[Handwritten bottom: Not preventive]

c. Etiology: unknown; evidence supports theory of relationship between periodic apnea and chronic hypoxia
d. Peak Occurrence: winter or early spring; between ages of 2 and 4 months

2. **Nursing Process**
   a. Assessment
      1) parents' knowledge of SIDS
      2) availability of support systems, i.e., family, friends, SIDS organization, mental health center
      3) apnea monitoring of high-risk infants (premies, subsequent siblings) or "near-miss" infants
         a) parents' knowledge of and adjustment to home apnea monitoring
         b) infant's apnea patterns
   b. Goals, Plans/Implementation, and Evaluation

   Goal 1: Parents will receive information and support to help them adjust to loss.
   Plan/Implementation
   - explain that they are not responsible for infant's death (parents feel guilty)
   - provide information about SIDS
   - allow expression of feelings; provide support as parents cope with loss, grief, and mourning
   - refer to local SIDS organization/support group: Foundation for Sudden Infant Death
   - refer to other community supports: church, community mental health centers, etc.
   - follow-up as indicated

   Evaluation: Parents ventilate feelings about loss of infant; have a referral for counseling.

   Goal 2: Parents will maintain and cope with home apnea monitoring.
   Plan/Implementation
   - teach parents mechanics of home monitoring equipment
   - teach parents infant CPR
   - provide emotional support to parents
   - help parents identify and utilize resources for relief (e.g., qualified sitters)

   Evaluation: Parents demonstrate ability to implement home monitoring, demonstrate correct infant CPR, adjust to home apnea monitoring.

B. Acute Spasmodic Laryngitis (Spasmodic Croup)

1. **General Information**
   a. Definition: acute spasm of larynx, resulting in partial airway obstruction
   b. Occurrence: occurs most frequently in 1- to 3-year-olds
   c. Cause: viral
   d. Medical Treatment
      1) differential diagnosis (from epiglottitis)
      2) emergency care: usually treated at home; may necessitate hospitalization, croup tent if severe
      3) medications
         a) single subemetic dose of syrup of ipecac (to help liquefy and expectorate secretions)
         b) mild sedation (phenobarbital 4–6 mg/kg body weight daily, divided into 3 doses)

2. **Nursing Process**
   a. Assessment: respiratory distress
      1) awakens with barklike, metallic cough
      2) hoarseness
      3) inspiratory stridor
   b. Goal, Plan/Implementation, and Evaluation

   Goal: Parents will implement specific home care of child.
   Plan/Implementation
   - teach emergency home care
     - run hot shower/water to create steam
     - remain with child in bathroom with door closed
     - give syrup of ipecac in subemetic doses: liquefies secretions; may also cause vomiting
     - contact physician if symptoms not relieved by home treatment
   - provide cool mist inhalation with humidifier at bedside
   - ensure adequate fluid intake (clear liquids)
   - prepare parents for the possibility of recurrence

   Evaluation: Child is free from severe respiratory distress; maintains adequate oxygenation; parents capably provide home care as taught.

C. Acute Epiglottitis

1. **General Information**
   a. Definition: severe inflammation of the epiglottis that progresses rapidly

b. Occurrence: primarily in 3- to 8-year-olds
c. Cause: bacterial, usually H influenza type B
d. Medical Treatment
   1) emergency hospitalization: <u>intubation or tracheotomy to maintain airway</u>
   2) medications
      a) IV antibiotics
      b) antipyretics
   3) supportive therapy: adequate oxygenation and high humidity (mist tent)

2. **Nursing Process**
   a. **Assessment:** respiratory distress
      1) sore throat: <u>inflamed, cherry-red epiglottis</u>
      2) <u>difficulty swallowing; drooling, retching</u>
      3) characteristic tripod posturing with mouth open and chin extended *(Tripod position)*
      4) <u>muffled voice</u>
      5) <u>froglike croaking on inspiration</u>
      6) substernal and suprasternal retractions
      7) <u>sits very still and quiet</u> *Don't lie down*
      8) fever
   b. **Goal, Plan/Implementation, and Evaluation**

   Goal: Child's airway will not become obstructed.
   Plan/Implementation
   - do not try to visualize child's throat <u>(may precipitate laryngospasm and sudden death)</u>
   - be alert for signs of airway obstruction
     - rapid increase in heart rate, respiratory rate
     - hypoxia
     - restlessness, anxiety, agitation
     - increased inspiratory stridor and retractions
     - pallor or cyanosis
   - have intubation and tracheotomy trays at bedside; assist with intubation or tracheotomy when indicated
   - <u>provide care for child with an endotracheal (ET) tube or tracheostomy</u>
     - perform ET tube/trach care and suctioning
     - restrain child as needed
     - provide reassurance to child and parents
     - change position q2h

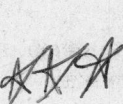 *loss of control*

- anticipate needs since child cannot verbalize
- inform child re inability to speak
- devise alternate means of communication

Evaluation: Child is free from obstructed airway; is adequately oxygenated (breathing via nasal passages, ET tube, or tracheotomy).

D. **Laryngotracheobronchitis (LTB)**
1. **General Information**
   a. Definition: primarily an inflammation of the larynx, to a lesser extent of the trachea and bronchi, resulting in spasm and partial airway obstruction; most common form of croup   *upper & lower affected esp.*
   b. Occurrence: predominantly infants and young toddlers
   c. Cause: viral; gradual onset
   d. Medical Treatment
      1) hospitalization; tracheotomy, if needed
      2) <u>medications: epinephrine, steroids</u> *relaxes smooth → severe cases only*
      3) supportive therapy
         a) adequate hydration (IV fluids)
         b) adequate oxygenation
            • high humidity (mist tent)
            • oxygen therapy

2. **Nursing Process**
   a. **Assessment:** respiratory distress
      1) preceded by URI
      2) <u>harsh brassy cough</u>
      3) <u>inspiratory stridor</u>
      4) substernal and suprasternal retractions, rales, and rhonchi
      5) <u>labored, prolonged expirations</u>
      6) fever
   b. **Goal, Plan/Implementation, and Evaluation**

   Goal: <u>Child will remain in croup tent until respiratory distress subsides.</u> *See as smothering*
   Plan/Implementation
   - maintain desired O_2 concentration (periodically analyze O_2 level)
   - plan care to minimize opening of tent
   - tuck sides of tent tightly to prevent loss of O_2 and mist
   - keep tent cooled
     - maintain ice chamber or cooling mechanism
     - monitor tent-chamber temperature
   - keep child as warm and dry as possible to prevent chilling (change clothing and bed linens frequently)

536 SECTION 5: NURSING CARE OF THE CHILD

- provide diversion and comfort measures to minimize child's fear and anxiety
- reassure child he won't be left alone
- provide favorite toy or object (no furry or mechanical toys) *due to mist*

Evaluation: Child cooperates with croup-tent treatment; is free from respiratory distress and does not chill; has adequate oxygenation.

E. Bronchiolitis *lower airway*

1. **General Information**
   a. Definition: inflammation of the bronchioles with resultant accumulation of mucus and exudate, impairing exhalation of air and resulting in lung hyperinflation, dyspnea, and cyanosis
   b. Occurrence: primarily 2- to 12-month-olds; third leading cause of illness in this age group
   c. Cause: viral
   d. Medical Treatment
      1) home care/possible hospitalization
      2) supportive therapy: adequate oxygenation (high humidity, mist tent, percussion and postural drainage)

2. **Nursing Process**
   a. Assessment
      1) paroxysmal cough
      2) flaring nares
      3) intercostal and subcostal retractions
      4) rales with prolonged expirations, wheezing
      5) decreased breath sounds, areas of consolidation
   b. Goals, Plans/Implementation, and Evaluation (refer to General Nursing Goals page 533)

F. Bronchial Asthma

1. **General Information**
   a. Definition: an obstructive reversible condition of the small bronchioles of the lower respiratory tract; a complex health problem that involves biochemical, immunologic, endocrine, and psychologic factors leading to
      1) edema of mucous membranes
      2) congestion of airways with tenacious mucus
      3) spasm of smooth muscle of bronchi and bronchioles
      4) trapping of air in alveoli

   b. Occurrence: a leading cause of childhood chronic illness; more common in boys (before age 12), equally common in boys and girls after age 12; onset usually occurs by early school-age years; attacks often begin suddenly at night, lasting several hours to 2–3 days
   c. Cause: believed to be an allergic hypersensitivity to foreign substances, such as plant pollens, mold, dust, smoke, animal hair, or foods; other contributing factors are changes in environmental temperatures (especially cold air), emotional distress, fatigue, physical exertion, and infections
   d. Medical Treatment: acute asthma is a medical emergency
      1) during acute episodes, treatment is directed toward relieving bronchial spasm, obstruction, and edema, and expectoration of secretions (see table 5.9)
         a) rapid-acting bronchodilators
         b) corticosteroids
         c) expectorants
         d) antibiotics (to treat any concurrent infection)
      2) supportive measures
         a) cool, humidified environment
         b) IV fluids to ensure adequate hydration
         c) sedatives to control anxiety
      3) status asthmaticus: continued severe respiratory distress in spite of medical intervention; child requires immediate hospitalization (to treat deyhdration and acidosis and improve ventilation)
         a) NPO or sips of clear liquids
         b) IV fluids for hydration and medication administration
         c) sodium bicarbonate (IV) to correct acidosis
         d) humified O₂
         e) mechanical ventilation in severe cases
         f) corticosteroids (hydrocortisone or methylprednisolone IV)
         g) aminophylline
         h) isoproterenol via intermittent positive pressure breathing
      4) long-term therapy includes removing the offending allergens, desensitization to allergens, normalization of respiratory function, and development of a personalized and effective therapeutic regimen

OXYGENATION 537

Table 5.9 Medications Used to Treat Bronchial Asthma*

Drug	Dose and Route	Nursing Considerations
Bronchodilators		
Epinephrine	0.01 ml/kg of body weight/dose (no more than 0.5 ml total) in 1:1,000 aqueous solution SC	Short acting; dose may be repeated in 20 minutes x 3-4 doses. Do not use solution if discolored. Observe for tachycardia, elevated BP, weakness, tremors, nausea, pallor. Metabolized more rapidly in children than adults.
Theophylline Aminophylline	5 mg/kg of body weight/q6h • IV during acute attacks • PO during home management	Observe for nausea, vomiting ("coffee grounds"), hypotension, restlessness, fever, convulsions.
Corticosteroids		
Hydrocortisone (Solu-Cortef) or methyl-prednisolone (Solu-Medrol)	20-240 mg/day depending on severity of attack IV during acute attack	Anti-inflammatory action relieves airway obstruction by reducing edema. *usually short term*
Expectorants		
SSKI (saturated solution of potassium iodide)	1 drop/year of age, tid, PO, in juice	These preparations liquefy secretions to aid expectoration.
Guaifenesin (Robitussin)	5 ml tid, PO	
Syrup of ipecac	Subemetic dose PO prn	

* Refer to *Nursing Care of the Adult* Tables 3.19-3.21 for additional drug information.

2. **Nursing Process**
   a. **Assessment**
      1) prolonged expiratory wheezing
      2) hacking, paroxysmal coughing, nonproductive at first, cough becomes rattling with thick, clear mucus
      3) deep red lips *resp acidosis*
      4) diaphoresis
      5) child sits in upright position
      6) intercostal and suprasternal retractions
      7) coarse breath sounds
      8) shallow irregular respirations with sudden increase in rate and ineffective coughing may signal impending asphyxia (status asthmaticus)
      9) barrel chest and hunched shoulders (chronic asthma)
   b. **Goals, Plans/Implementation, and Evaluation**

Detailed p4.

Goal 1: Child will resume normal breathing pattern, will maintain a patent airway, and will liquefy and raise secretions.
Plan/Implementation
- monitor frequency, amount, and appearance of expectorated mucus
- position in high-Fowler's or in a chair; administer O_2 to relieve cyanosis and anoxia (cyanosis appears in children with a Po_2 less than 55-65 mm Hg)
- teach child to use diaphragm rather than just lungs, to pull in and expel deep breaths of air when first feeling a tightening sensation in chest
- administer prescribed medications; know the action, dose ranges, side effects, and contraindications for all medications administered

Evaluation: Child resumes normal breathing pattern (no wheezing, rales, cyanosis), maintains patent airway, liquefies and raises secretions.

never leave child alone
anxiety + O_2 needs

Goal 2: Child will control anxiety during acute attacks.
Plan/Implementation
- *never* leave child alone during an acute attack; if parental anxiety is too high, it is better for child if someone who is calm and supportive stays with child; work with parent until parent can be a calming influence
- hold child in an upright position and rock (as effective as bed rest if a relaxed, confident approach is used)
- reduce the level of nonproductive stimuli by keeping room quiet, with dimmed lighting; use touch, soft music, and controlled noise levels to induce relaxation and rest
- teach child and parent panic control, i.e., to imagine how to stay calm (what works best) in stressful situations

[handwritten margin note: give child own element of control]

Evaluation: Child remains calm and copes with asthma attack.

Goal 3: Child will avoid and/or eliminate allergens or precipitating factors in environment.
Plan/Implementation
- identify possible precipitating factors with child and family; teach child and parent to avoid stressful experiences, extremes of temperature, unnecessary fatigue, and exposure to infections
- modify environment as indicated (no furry pets, damp dusting, nonallergic pillows and bedding, elimination of allergenic foods from diet, air filters)
- assist with immune therapy (hyposensitization for allergens such as dust, molds, and pollens)
- administer prophylactic antibiotics during periods of high susceptibility (e.g., winter, pollen or flu season)
- guide parents in planning a total program that promotes rest, moderate exercise, appropriate activities (swimming, baseball, skiing), balanced nutrition, controlled levels of emotional stress
- remind and urge child/parent to see physician regularly and at the first indication of a respiratory infection or attack
- refer family to psychologic/mental health services when indicated

Evaluation: Child/parent knows the importance of good nutrition and rest in preventing respiratory infections; can identify situations or agents that precipitate an asthmatic attack and conscientiously tries to modify or avoid these; recognizes signs of an impending attack (cough, wheezing, fever, N&V, increased anxiety or tension) and the steps to take to minimize distress (position, rest, medications, fluids).

C. Application of the Nursing Process to the Child with Cardiac Problems
1. Assessment
   a. Nursing History
      1) growth patterns
      2) past and recent infections
      3) activity tolerance, weakness, fatigue
      4) anorexia, weight loss
      5) chest pain, dyspnea, pallor or cyanosis
      6) medications: parent knowledge of; side effects
   b. Physical Examination
      1) general appearance: pallor, cyanosis, clubbing of fingers and toes, cold extremities, mottling, edema, distended neck veins
      2) delayed physical growth, motor skill development
      3) vital signs: apical pulse rate and character, presence of murmurs, gallops, friction rubs; blood pressure in upper and lower extremities; rate, depth, and character of respirations; rate, quality, and symmetry of peripheral pulses especially of lower extremities
   c. Diagnostic tests (refer to *Nursing Care of the Adult* page 174)
      1) cardiac catheterization in infants and children: aids in diagnosis of congenital anomalies, and abnormalities in oxygen saturation, pressure, and cardiac output; right-sided catheterization is usually done in children (see table 5.10)
      2) blood gas determination
         a) Po_2: 83–108 mm Hg (65–80 mm Hg newborn)
         b) Pco_2: 32–44 mm Hg (27–40 mm Hg newborn)
         c) pH: 7.33–7.43 (7.27–7.47 newborn)
2. General Nursing Goals, Plans/Implementation, and Evaluation
   Goal 1: Child will have decreased workload of heart.
   Plan/Implementation
   - monitor vital signs frequently

Table 5.10 Cardiac Catheterization in Children: Nursing Considerations

Preprocedural	Postprocedural
Psychologic preparation (see *Ill and Hospitalized Child* for developmental considerations) • explain in simple terms what child will experience and what it will feel like (e.g., skin prep: "cold"; catheter insertion: "pressure"; injection of contrast medium: "warm all over" [do not use the word "dye"]; darkness of room, and sounds of "picture-taking"); do not explain too far in advance of procedure. • allow child to play with and manipulate equipment, (e.g., gown and mask, syringes, sandbag). • arrange for child and parent to visit catheterization room the day before to see the equipment and meet staff. Physical preparation • NPO 4–6 hours before the procedure (give 5% DW orally as prescribed 2–3 hours before the procedure for infants with cyanotic heart disease and polycythemia); use pacifier for infants. • obtain baseline vital signs, including brachial and pedal pulses. • administer pre-op meds as ordered.	Maintain bed rest with frequent checks on vital signs until stable. Do not take blood pressure in affected extremity. Monitor skin color and warmth, especially distal to catheter-insertion site. *[handwritten: Distal to site, both sides]* Palpate brachial or pedal pulses distal to catheter insertion for presence, strength, symmetry. Observe operative site for bleeding, edema, hematoma formation. Maintain sandbag or pressure dressing on operative site as ordered. Notify physician of any signs of complications (e.g., poor circulation, unstable vital signs, fever, bleeding).

[handwritten: better measure how heart is doing]

- apical pulse while sleeping *[handwritten: 1 full min]*
- peripheral pulses
- BP
- respiratory status
- body temperature

• schedule treatments and nursing care to prevent tiring and promote adequate rest/sleep
• maintain bed rest as ordered
• provide age-appropriate diversional activities to prevent boredom and help child maintain bed rest
• avoid restrictive clothing and tight diapers
• minimize crying and emotional distress *[handwritten: suscept. to infect.]*
  - encourage parent to room-in or visit frequently
  - provide pacifier or favorite attachment object
  - hold and cuddle child
• relieve anoxic spells (congenital heart disease)
  - place child in knee-chest (squatting) position *[handwritten: ↓ peripheral blood flow]*
  - administer O₂ as ordered
  - administer sedatives, analgesics as ordered

Evaluation: Child is free from signs of respiratory or cardiac distress (e.g., no dyspnea, tachycardia); cooperates with bed rest, rests comfortably, plays quietly.

Goal 2: Child will be free from infections.

Plan/Implementation
• protect child from exposure to others with respiratory infections
• immunize child according to AAP recommended schedule (see Table 5.4)
• observe for signs of endocarditis (fever, malaise, anorexia) and pneumonitis (dyspnea, tachycardia, fever) *[handwritten: due to turbulence]*
• teach child and parents importance of antibiotic prophylaxis (long-term therapy or short-term course for dental work, surgery, childbirth)

Evaluation: Child remains free from upper respiratory infections; immunized on schedule; child and parents comply with antibiotic prophylaxis.

Selected Health Problems Resulting in an Interference with Cardiac Functioning

A. Congenital Cardiac Disorders

1. **General Information**
   a. Definition: a defect in the structure of the heart and/or great vessels that alters the flow of blood through the cardiorespiratory system. Two types of defects: acyanotic and cyanotic.
   b. Occurrence: 8–10/1,000 live births
   c. Cause: not known exactly; predisposing factors include
      1) certain chromosome disorders (e.g., Down's syndrome)
      2) maternal and fetal infections (e.g., rubella in first trimester)
      3) maternal alcoholism, maternal undernutrition
   d. Types of Defects
      1) acyanotic defects: those heart defects in which the blood flows from the arterial (left, oxygenated) side of the heart to the venous (right, deoxygenated) side; there is no mixing of unoxygenated blood with oxygenated blood in the systemic circulation (see figure 5.1)
         a) *atrial septal defect* (ASD)
            - flow of blood is from left atrium to right atrium
            - increased blood flow to right side of heart
            - treatment: surgical closure or patch graft of defect; 99% survival rate

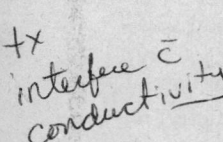

         b) *ventricular septal defect* (VSD)
            - most common cardiac defect
            - flow of blood is from left ventricle to right ventricle where oxygenated blood mixes with venous blood
            - may cause right ventricular hypertrophy and increased pulmonary vascular resistance
            - 50% close spontaneously within 1–3 years of age
            - often associated with other cardiac defects (tetralogy of Fallot, transposition of great vessels, patent ductus arteriosis [PDA], pulmonic stenosis)
            - infants with severe VSD may develop congestive heart failure
            - treatment: surgical closure or patch graft of defect
            - complications include conduction disturbances, CHF, or endocarditis
         c) *patent ductus arteriosus* (PDA)
            - ductus arteriosus (normal in fetus) fails to close; blood is shunted by higher pressure in aorta to pulmonary artery
            - pulse pressure is wide; left ventricular hypertrophy and congestive heart failure may develop
            - characteristic machinerylike murmur
            - treatment: surgical ligation (closed-heart surgery) at 1–2 years of age; 99% survival rate
            - in very ill newborns, medical closure of the ductus with the prostaglandin inhibitor, indomethacin, may be tried
         d) *coarctation of the aorta*
            - a narrowing of the aorta (usually on the arch after the first three branches and before the left subclavian artery [preductal])
            - because of obstruction, blood pressure is higher in upper extremities (BP may be unequal in arms)
            - bounding upper-extremity pulses, weak or absent femoral and popliteal pulses
            - lower extremities may be cool, pale, or dusky
            - headaches, dizziness, epistaxis
            - treatment: surgical resection and end-to-end anastomosis (or graft) at about age 4 (to allow for growth of aorta)
         e) *pulmonic/aortic stenosis*
            - pulmonic stenosis interferes with flow of blood from right ventricle to pulmonary artery
            - aortic stenosis interferes with blood flow from left ventricle to aorta
            - both pulmonic and aortic stenosis
              – may be asymptomatic
              – are usually of the valves
              – increased pressure can cause ventricular hypertrophy

OXYGENATION 541

Figure 5.1 Normal and Abnormal Hearts

a. Superior Vena Cava **b.** Aorta **c.** Pulmonary Artery **d.** Pulmonary Vein **e.** Right Atrium **f.** Right Ventricle
g. Inferior Vena Cava **h.** Left Ventricle **i.** Left Atrium

I. THE NORMAL HEART

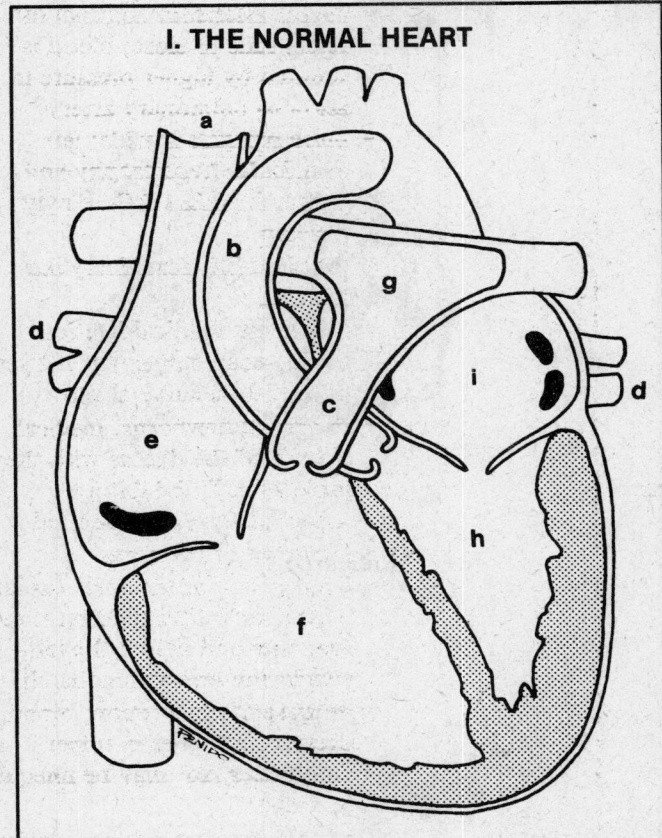

II. ACYANOTIC DEFECTS

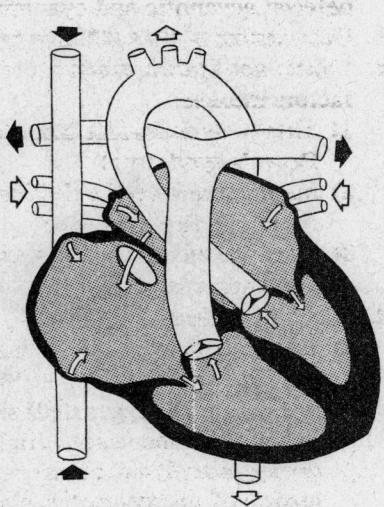

Atrial Septal Defect

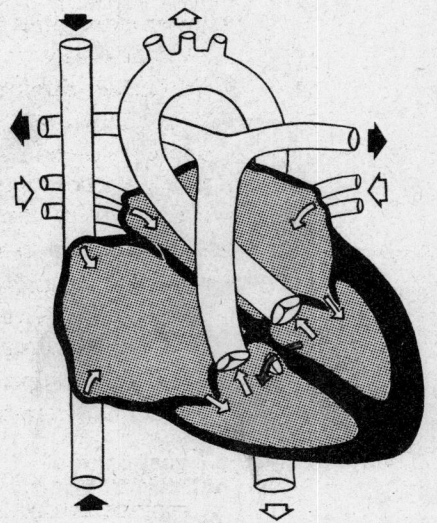

Ventricular Septal Defect

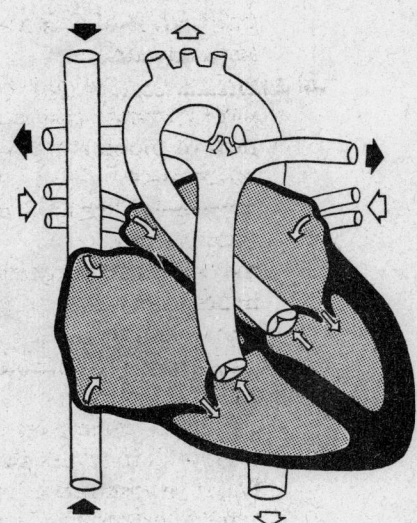

Patent Ductus Arteriosus

542 SECTION 5: NURSING CARE OF THE CHILD

Figure 5.1 Continued

(II. ACYANOTIC DEFECTS, Cont.)

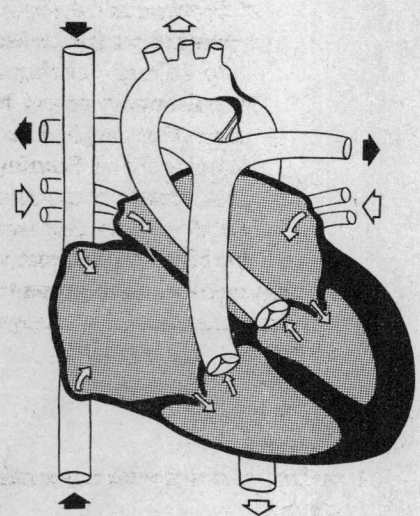
Coarctation of the Aorta

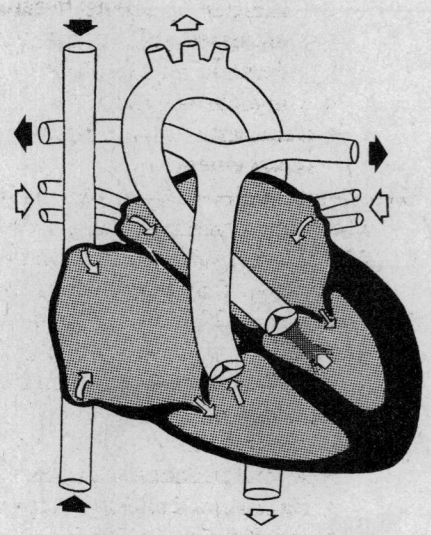
Subaortic Stenosis

III. CYANOTIC DEFECTS

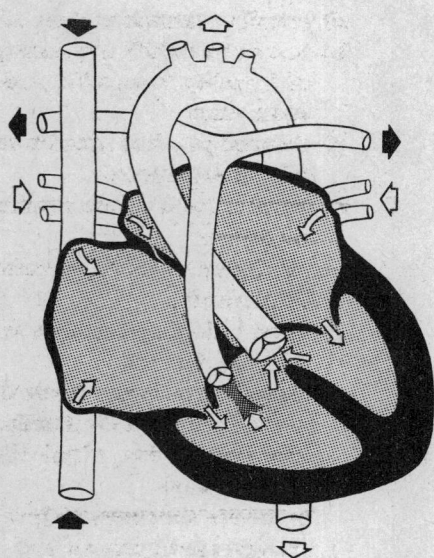
Tetralogy of Fallot

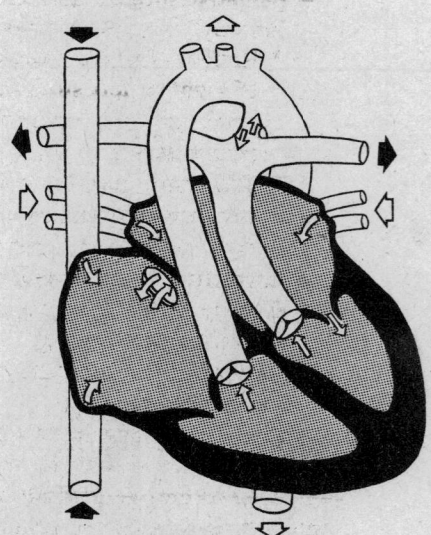
Transposition of Great Vessels

SOURCE: Nursing Inservice Aid #2, Congenital Heart Abnormalities Aid, Ross Laboratories, Columbus, OH 43216. Used with permission.

* in right ventricle with pulmonary stenosis
* in left ventricle with aortic stenosis
- aortic stenosis may result in sudden death after strenuous exercise or activity because of increased sudden oxygen demand and resultant myocardial ischemia
- treatment: valvulotomy or valve replacement

2) cyanotic defects: those defects in which unoxygenated blood from right side of heart mixes with blood on left side, so that a portion of the unoxygenated blood is circulated through the systemic circulation (right-to-left shunt); results in cyanosis

** a) *tetralogy of Fallot*
- severe VSD *congenital*
- severe pulmonic stenosis *congenital*
- right ventricular hypertrophy *acquired*
- overriding aorta: because the *congenital* aorta overrides the septal defect, much of the systemic flow is venous and, therefore, unoxygenated
- "boot-shaped" configuration of heart and great vessels
- treatment
  - palliative surgical correction: to increase pulmonary blood flow
    * Blalock-Taussig anastomosis of right or left subclavian artery and corresponding pulmonary artery
    * Waterston anastomosis between ascending aorta and right pulmonary artery
  - corrective surgical repair: closure of VSD (corrects overriding aorta) and pulmonary valvulotomy or valve replacement

b) *transposition of the great vessels:* the aorta arises out of the right ventricle so that venous blood enters directly into the systemic circulation, bypassing the lungs; the pulmonary artery arises out of the left ventricle and goes through the lungs; once the foramen ovale and ductus arteriosus close, the situation is incompatible with life

After complete repair watch for CHF.

- treatment
  - palliative surgical correction to prevent CHF and reduce pulmonary vascular resistance
    * surgical creation of an ASD (Blalock-Hanlen procedure)
    * balloon atrial septostomy during cardiac catheterization to enlarge existing ASD
    * pulmonary artery banding
  - corrective surgical repair (Mustard's or Senning procedure): creation of a new atrial septum that tunnels blood to the correct ventricle

e. additional medical management: digoxin, potassium, diuretics (if in congestive heart failure), antibiotics

2. **Nursing Process**
   a. Assessment
   1) infant or child with acyanotic heart defects
      a) poor weight gain, small stature
      b) increased incidence of respiratory infections
      c) exercise intolerance
      d) tachycardia, tachypnea, dyspnea
      e) *not* cyanotic
   2) infant or child with cyanotic heart defects
      a) usually cyanotic at time of birth
      b) babies have difficulty eating because of inability to breathe and suck at same time
      c) delayed physical growth because of chronic hypoxia
      d) frequent and severe respiratory infections
      e) moderate to severe exercise intolerance
      f) chest pain that becomes severe with O_2 demand
      g) hypoxic spell may occur during periods of high O_2 demand (feeding, crying, physical exertion during play)
         - severe shortness of breath
         - increased cyanosis and chest pain
         - squats with arms thrown over knees, and knees on chest to relieve respiratory distress
      h) chronic hypoxia causes erythropoietin to be released from kidneys

to stimulate bone marrow to produce more red blood cells; also causes clubbing of fingers and toes
- Hgb may rise 20–30 gm or more with a hematocrit as high as 60%–80%
- increased RBC results in increased blood viscosity (polycythemia)
i) polycythemia and sluggish circulation may cause cerebral thrombosis (stroke) and paralysis, sometimes occurring at a very young age

3) preoperative assessment
   a) baseline vital signs, including apical pulse; existence and quality of peripheral pulses, especially of lower extremities
   b) educational needs of child and parents for preoperative teaching and postoperative experience
4) postoperative assessment
   a) respiratory status, chest tubes, chest-tube drainage
   b) vital signs, including apical and femoral pulses
   c) hydration status and output
   d) signs and symptoms of congestive heart failure
   e) color of skin, mucous membranes, nail beds, and earlobes
   f) level of discomfort and anxiety
   g) surgical incisions (suture line)

b. Goals, Plans/Implementation, and Evaluation

Goal 1: Child will maintain adequate oxygenation and a patent airway.
Plan/Implementation
- pre-op and post-op
  - count respirations and apical pulse 1 full minute
  - pin diapers loosely, use loose-fitting pajamas
  - feed slowly with frequent rest periods; burp frequently
  - position at 45° after feeding
  - suction nose and throat if cough is inadequate
  - give O₂ as ordered and necessary
- administer prescribed medications
  - digoxin
    * give at regular intervals
    * do not mix with other foods or fluids
    * hold drug and notify physician if apical pulse rate is below 100 in infants, below 90 in toddlers, or below 70 in older children
    * give 1 hour before or 2 hours after meals/feedings
    * observe for signs of toxicity (bradycardia, nausea, anorexia, vomiting, disorientation)
  - diuretics
    * monitor I&O closely
    * ensure fluid intake within prescribed restrictions
    * encourage high potassium foods or administer prescribed potassium supplements
- post-op (palliative or corrective surgery)
  - monitor constantly
  - take precautions in care of closed chest drainage (bottles below level of bed, no kinks in tubing, do NOT empty bottles, monitor fluid level and fluctuation in tube, character of drainage)
  - avoid elevating foot of bed (causes intestines to put pressure on diaphragm)
  - administer O₂ as ordered
  - establish and follow coughing routine; allow crying post-op in infant and young child to facilitate lung expansion; use inspirometer (incentive spirometry)
  - when child has recovered from anesthesia, elevate head of bed to reduce pressure on diaphragm
  - use nasogastric suction to reduce gastric distention
  - be alert to signs of CHF, hypovolemic shock, pneumonia, hemothorax (dyspnea), atelectasis (dyspnea, increased pulse), cerebral thrombosis

Evaluation: Child has normal skin color, a patent airway, breathes freely; no signs of complications.

Goal 2: Child will maintain adequate hydration and electrolyte balance.
Plan/Implementation
- encourage fluid intake within fluid restrictions for child; monitor I&O *very* accurately (be especially alert to thoracotomy drainage, fluid used to administer IV medications or flush CVP or arterial lines)
- monitor daily weights

OXYGENATION 545

- check urine specific gravity and pH
- be alert to early signs and symptoms of pulmonary edema, cardiac overload, and congestive heart failure (e.g., tachycardia, dyspnea, tachypnea, moist respirations, rales, rhonchi, sweating [in infants], edema)
- be aware that dehydration with cyanotic heart disease increases blood viscosity, and therefore risk of thrombosis
- observe for signs of hypokalemia (altered lab values, cardiac dysrhythmias)

Evaluation: Child has adequate I&O; no signs or symptoms of fluid or electrolyte imbalance, stroke, or congestive heart failure.

Goal 3: Child and parents will experience no more than moderate anxiety.
Plan/Implementation
- encourage child and parents to disclose their feelings about the surgery, hospitalization, treatments (use projective techniques with child); answer their questions
- prepare child and parents for treatments, surgical routine, and discharge; consider developmental age, environment, culture and ethnicity, timing needs, ability to understand
- help parents and others understand the importance of treating child as normally as possible (to provide for optimal emotional-social development and to avoid overprotecting and sheltering)

Evaluation: Child and parents have realistic expectations about child's illness and hospitalization; age-appropriate limits are established and adhered to; parents and child demonstrate knowledge about procedures, medications, etc.

Goal 4: Child and parents will be adequately prepared for discharge and home care.
Plan/Implementation
- encourage and support parents in their attempts to allow child age-appropriate independence and responsibilities
- teach parents safe administration of medications, side effects, signs of complications, when to seek medical attention
- refer parents to community health nursing agency for home follow-up if indicated

Evaluation: Child gradually assumes self-care responsibilities and age-appropriate independence; parents are able to state signs of complications and when to seek attention; are able to administer medications correctly.

B. Rheumatic Fever and Rheumatic Heart Disease

1. **General Information**
   a. Definition: an inflammatory disease that affects collagen (connective) tissue such as heart, joints, central nervous system, and subcutaneous tissue
   b. Occurrence: primarily affects school-age children; higher incidence in cold or humid climates, crowded living environments, and with strong family history of rheumatic fever
   c. Medical Treatment
      1) antibiotics (penicillin or erythromycin)
         a) to eradicate any lingering infection
         b) for long-term prophylactic treatment
      2) salicylates to control joint inflammation, fever, pain

2. **Nursing Process**
   a. **Assessment:** revised Jones criteria (American Heart Association)
      1) major manifestations
         a) carditis: mitral and aortic valves most commonly affected with symptoms of tachycardia, cardiomegaly, pericarditis, murmurs, congestive heart failure; carditis is the only manifestation that may cause permanent damage
         b) painful migratory polyarthritis in large joints with manifestations of acute pain, warmth, redness, edema; permanent deformities do not follow
         c) chorea (Saint Vitus' dance or Sydenham's chorea): purposeless, irregular movements of the extremities, muscular weakness, emotional lability, facial grimacing
         d) erythema marginatum rheumaticum: macular rash with wavy, well-defined border on trunk
         e) subcutaneous nodules: small, nontender swellings in groups over bony prominences

546 SECTION 5: NURSING CARE OF THE CHILD

2) minor manifestations
  a) arthralgia
  b) fever
  c) elevated erythrocyte sedimentation rate (ESR)
  d) elevated C-reactive protein — indicate inflam process
  e) leukocytosis
  f) anemia
  g) prolonged PR and QT intervals on ECG
3) other
  a) positive throat culture
  b) elevated ASO titer — indicate recent strep infect.

b. Goals, Plans/Implementation, and Evaluation

Goal 1: Child will be free from pain and will rest comfortably.
Plan/Implementation
- administer salicylates as ordered
- use cradles to keep bed linen off painful joints
- position joints on pillows; handle gently

Evaluation: Child does not complain of pain, is able to rest and sleep comfortably.

Goal 2: Child with chorea will be protected from injury.
Plan/Implementation
- utilize side rails and pad sides of bed
- assist with ambulation
- use vest restraint in chair as necessary

Evaluation: Child ambulates without falling, does not sustain injury.

Goal 3: Child/family will be prepared for home care and long-term management.
Plan/Implementation
- emphasize importance of compliance with long-term antibiotic therapy for prevention of serious heart damage
  - prepare child for monthly injections of penicillin
  - stress seriousness of recurrence and possible consequences (death or severe disability from heart disease)
- plan for continuation of schoolwork, realistic career goals
- refer to community health nurse for follow-up as needed
- instruct parents to take vital signs, administer medications, ensure restrictions
- maintain child's contact with friends

Evaluation: Child returns to full activity with no residual cardiac involvement.

D. **Application of the Nursing Process to the Child with Hematologic Problems**

1. Assessment
  a. Nursing History
    1) dietary intake, especially dietary iron
    2) history of bleeding tendencies (easy bruising, gum bleeding, epistaxis), response to injury or trauma
    3) general symptoms: fatigue, irritability, anorexia, pain, edema
    4) recent stressful situations: exposure to temperature extremes, emotional stress
    5) family history of hematologic disorders
    6) current treatment, home management, general health
  b. Physical Examination
    1) general appearance: pallor, lethargy, bruising, physical growth (over or underweight for age)
    2) vital signs: tachycardia, tachypnea, hypotension
  c. Diagnostic Tests (refer to *Nursing Care of the Adult* page 174) 172

2. General Nursing Goals, Plans/Implementation, and Evaluation

Goal 1: Child will be free from pain.
Plan/Implementation
- administer prescribed analgesics (no aspirin!) ↓ bleeding time
- handle and move child gently
- provide bed rest with covers off affected areas
- provide age-appropriate diversional activities

Evaluation: Child is free from pain, rests comfortably.

Goal 2: Child will conserve energy.
Plan/Implementation
- schedule nursing care and treatment to prevent tiring and to provide uninterrupted periods of rest
- provide quiet age-appropriate play activities
- counsel parents concerning plan for activity and rest at home

Evaluation: Child engages in activities of daily living without tiring, has age-appropriate rest and sleep periods.

[margin notes: hemoglobin 11-16 Whites Asians; 10.5-16 Blacks; sore throat / have cultured; very painful; prolong care prophylactic antibiotics until 18 yrs]

OXYGENATION 547

Selected Health Problems Resulting in an Interference with Formed Elements of the Blood

A. Iron-Deficiency Anemia

1. **General Information**
   a. Definition: a decrease in the number of erythrocytes and/or a decreased hemoglobin (Hgb) level: less than 11 gm/dl for whites and Asians, less than 10.5 gm/dl for blacks; Hct less than 30% (normal Hgb levels 6 months to 12 years: 10.5–16 gm/100 dl); see table 5.11
   b. Occurrence: most common nutritional disorder in US resulting in reduced oxygen-carrying capacity of blood; most common childhood anemia
      1) primarily in children 6–24 months of age who have a diet low in iron
      2) in premature infants (inadequate iron stores)
      3) in adolescent girls, with increased growth and menstruation
      4) in adolescent boys, with androgen-related increase in hemoglobin concentration
   c. Cause: impaired production of red blood cells, resulting from deficient iron stores
      1) inadequate dietary intake
      2) impaired absorption
      3) blood loss
      4) excessive demand (prematurity, puberty, pregnancy)
   d. Medical Treatment
      1) oral iron supplements (ferrous iron), 10–15 mg/day for 3 months
      2) parenteral iron therapy (iron dextran [Imferon]) IM or IV
      3) blood transfusions with packed red cells (if Hgb is less than 4 gm/dl)

2. **Nursing Process**
   a. Assessment
      1) nutritional history (daily intake)
      2) pallor (porcelain-like skin)
      3) poor muscle development
      4) may be overweight ("milk baby")
      5) exercise intolerance, lethargy
      6) susceptible to infection
   b. Goals, Plans/Implementation, and Evaluation

   Goal: Child will ingest diet and medications to maintain adequate Hgb level.
   Plan/Implementation
   - explain the necessity for a proper diet to parents
     - provide adequate sources of iron and teach parent/child what they are
     - for infants: iron-fortified formula and cereal, iron supplements
     - for older children: foods high in iron, e.g., meat, vegetables, fruit
   - teach parents correct administration of oral iron preparations as ordered
     - usually ferrous sulfate (Fer-In-Sol), administered in 3 divided doses/day
     - * between meals
     - * with citrus juice
     - continue for 4–6 weeks after red blood cell count returns to normal
     - liquid iron temporarily stains teeth (use straw, or dropper to back of mouth, brush child's teeth)
     - oral iron causes stools to become dark green
   - administer parenteral iron as prescribed if oral preparations ineffective
     - use IM Z-track method: painful and stains subcutaneous tissue; do not use deltoid; no more than 1 ml/site; use air bubble, don't massage over injection site, avoid tight clothing over injection site
   - limit milk intake to 1 quart/day or less

   Evaluation: Child takes diet and medications as ordered; child's Hgb level returns to normal.

Table 5.11 Normal Blood Cells

Age	Hgb	WBCs
6 months to 6 years	10.5–14 gm/100 ml	6,000–15,000/mm
7 years to 12 years	11–16 gm/100 ml	4,500–13,500/mm

B. Sickle Cell Anemia

1. **General Information**
   a. Definition: autosomal recessive defect (see figure 5.2) found primarily in blacks, resulting in production of abnormal hemoglobin (hemoglobin S) and characterized by intermittent episodes of crisis
   b. Occurrence 1:400 black Americans, or 75,000 people in the US
      1) sickle cell trait: heterozygous form (carrier); 1 in 12 black persons is a carrier
      2) sickle cell disease: homozygous form (has the disease); may have vaso-occlusive crisis: painful, acute occurrence usually precipitated by decreased O_2 tension, which causes cells to become viscous and assume a sickle shape, obstruct blood vessels, and cause tissue ischemia, infarction, and necrosis
   c. Cause: defective form of hemoglobin (hemoglobin S), inherited by autosomal recessive genetic transmission
   d. Medical Treatment: symptomatic treatment of crisis
      1) bed rest to decrease O_2 expenditure
      2) adequate hydration: oral and IV fluids to increase blood volume and mobilize sickled cells
      3) electrolyte replacement (hypoxia causes metabolic acidosis)
      4) relief of pain
         a) acetaminophen
         b) codeine
         c) meperidine (Demerol)
      5) blood transfusions if Hgb falls below 4 gm/dl
      6) O_2 for severe hypoxia (on a short-term basis)
      7) antibiotics to treat concurrent infection

2. **Nursing Process**
   a. Assessment
      1) parents with sickle cell trait
      2) signs and symptoms (depend on organ involved)
         a) chronic hemolytic anemia
         b) frequent infections, related to decreased ability of spleen to filter bacteria
         c) organ deterioration (spleen, liver, kidney, heart, CNS)
         d) chronic pain: joints, abdomen, back
         e) bone deterioration (osteoporosis, skeletal deformities)
         f) leg ulcers
      3) manifestations of vaso-occlusive crisis
         a) severe abdominal pain: caused by organ hypoxia
         b) hand-foot syndrome: swelling of hands and feet
         c) fever: due to dehydration or possible concurrent infection
         d) arthralgia
   b. Goals, Plans/Implementation, and Evaluation

   Goal 1: Child's episodes of vaso-occlusive crisis will be prevented or minimized.
   Plan/Implementation
   - teach crisis-prevention methods to child/parent
     - avoid situations resulting in decreased O_2 concentration such as high altitudes, constrictive clothing, extreme physical exertion, exposure to cold
     - avoid emotional distress
     - maintain adequate hydration (child should receive at least *minimum* daily fluid requirement)
     - protect from infection
       * prevent exposure to persons with infections
       * promote adequate nutrition
       * obtain medical care at onset of infection (may need antibiotics)
       * keep immunizations current

   Evaluation: Parent/child adheres to plan for crisis prevention; child's crisis episodes are minimized.

   Goal 2: Child will receive appropriate supportive care during crisis.
   Plan/Implementation
   - relieve pain
     - administer analgesics
     - handle gently
     - use heating pad on painful areas
   - monitor hydration/electrolyte status
     - monitor I&O; offer liquids frequently
     - regulate IV fluids, blood transfusion
     - observe for fluid or electrolyte imbalance
   - assess for signs of infection; protect from exposure to infectious sources during crisis

   Evaluation: Child is relieved of pain during crisis; has no elevated temperature;

Figure 5.2 Common Modes of Genetic Transmission

A. Autosomal Dominant Diseases

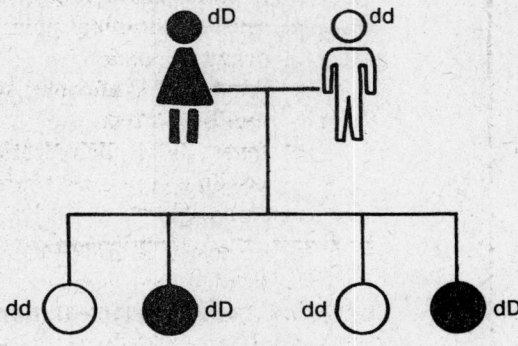

One parent affected
 50% offspring normal
 50% offspring affected

Key: d = normal gene; D = abnormal, *dominant* gene
Examples: Huntington's disease, osteogenesis imperfecta, polydactyly

B. Autosomal Recessive Diseases

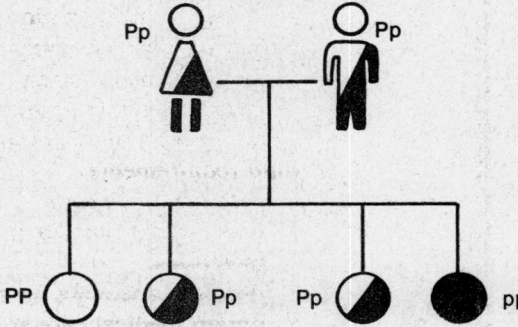

Both parents heterozygous (carriers)
 25% offspring normal
 25% offspring affected (homozygous)
 50% offspring carriers (heterozygous)

Key: P = normal gene; p = abnormal, *recessive* gene
Examples: phenylketonuria, cystic fibrosis, sickle cell disease, galactosemia, Tay-Sachs disease, thalassemia

C. Sex-Linked Recessive Diseases (X-Linked)

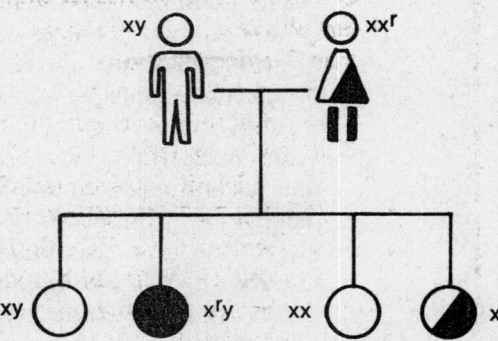

Female is carrier
 50% males normal
 50% males affected
 50% females normal
 50% females carriers

Key: xy = normal *male* sex chromosome pattern; xx = normal *female* sex chromosome pattern; r = sex-linked *recessive* gene
Examples: hemophilia, color blindness, agammaglobulinemia, G6PD deficiency, X-linked Duchenne's muscular dystrophy

OXYGENATION 549

has elastic skin turgor, moist mucous membranes, adequate fluid intake.

Goal 3: Parent/child will receive screening and genetic counseling.

Plan/Implementation
- teach parent about screening/diagnostic techniques
  - nonspecific screening tests for trait or disease
    * sickle cell slide preparation (sickling test)
    * Sickledex
  - specific identification of trait and disease: Hgb electrophoresis ("protein fingerprinting") used if screening tests are positive
- give information on available genetic counseling

Evaluation: Parents receive screening and genetic counseling as indicated; demonstrate knowledge of transmission and implications for subsequent pregnancies.

C. Hemophilia

1. **General Information**
   a. Definition, Occurrence, and Cause: hereditary coagulation defect, usually transmitted to affected male by female carrier through sex-linked recessive gene (see figure 5.2), resulting in prolonged clotting time; most common type is hemophilia A-factor VIII deficiency; severity of the deficiency varies from mild to severe
   b. Medical Treatment
      1) replacement of factor VIII: transfusion of plasma, factor VIII concentrate, or cryoprecipitate to prevent bleeding episodes
      2) additional treatment measures for more severe bleeding episodes
         a) immediate administration of factor VIII to control bleeding
         b) bed rest with covers off affected area to relieve pain; temporary immobilization of affected joints in a slightly flexed position with casts, splints, traction
         c) physical therapy to prevent contractures, beginning 48 hours after bleeding stops
         d) pain relief with sedatives/narcotics

2. **Nursing Process**
   a. Assessment
      1) infant
         a) umbilical-cord hemorrhage
         b) hemorrhage following circumcision
      2) any age
         a) hemarthrosis (bleeding into a joint space) is the most frequent site of bleeding; may result in crippling bony deformities
         b) epistaxis
         c) spontaneous hematuria
         d) hemorrhage following tooth extraction
   b. Goals, Plans/Implementation, and Evaluation

Goal 1: Parent/child will receive education to *prevent* bleeding, provide safety measures; will know how to treat minor bleeding episodes.

Plan/Implementation
- prepare parents and child for home care and administration of factor VIII (where available)
  - teach about the disease
  - teach venipuncture procedure and how to monitor the transfusion
  - provide regular follow-up (family must be sufficiently motivated and stable to maintain a home-care program)
- teach local treatment measures for minor bleeding episodes
  - apply direct pressure to site (10–15 minutes)
  - apply ice pack
  - immobilize and elevate affected part
- teach safe administration of medication
  - give orally if possible
  - avoid injections; if necessary, after injection, apply pressure until bleeding stops
  - avoid medications that increase bleeding time (aspirin, phenacetin, phenothiazines, indomethacin [Indocin])
- institute dental precautions: soft toothbrush, Water Pik, good dental hygiene to avoid extractions
- encourage appropriate toys/games/sports
  - soft toys for infants
  - quiet activities, e.g., reading, swimming
  - avoid body-contact sports

OXYGENATION

- careful handling of sharp objects
- use of electric shavers (not razors)
• use protective devices for young child: padded crib, playpen, side rails, protective padding and helmet for toddler
• teach to avoid overweight (causes strain on affected joints)
• teach to wear Medic Alert identification
• inform appropriate school personnel
• avoid stressful situations (they increase susceptibility to bleeding)
• seek emergency medical treatment in cases of uncontrolled bleeding

Evaluation: Parent/child demonstrate ability to correctly manage home administration of factor VIII; state medication precautions, activities to avoid, and those that are permitted; parent provides appropriate protective devices at home; adequately cares for minor bleeding episodes (e.g., local pressure, ice pack). School personnel/friends are informed about child's condition and necessary restrictions/appropriate action during a bleeding episode.

Goal 2: Child/parent will receive emotional support.

Plan/Implementation
• encourage realistic career goals
• allow child/family to discuss feelings and concerns about bleeding tendency and treatment, subsequent absences from school, reactions to peers, parental protectiveness
• encourage independence while maintaining safety
• refer to the local chapter of the National Hemophilia Foundation

Evaluation: Child seeks independence within reasonable limits; asks questions about reactions of school friends. Adolescent seeks out appropriate job opportunities.

References

Deal, A. and Bordeaux, B. "The Phenomenon of SIDS." *Pediatric Nursing*. January 1980:48–50.

Dressler, D. "Understanding and Treating Hemophilia." *Nursing 80*. October 1980:72–73.

Gottesfeld, I. "The Family of a Child with Congenital Heart Disease." *MCN: American Journal of Maternal-Child Nursing*. March/April 1979:101–104.

Graber, H. and Balas-Stevens, S. "A Discharge Tool for Teaching Parents to Monitor Infant Apnea at Home." *MCN: American Journal of Maternal-Child Nursing*. May/June 1984:178–180.

McFarlane, J. "Sickle Cell Disorders." *American Journal of Nursing*. December 1977:1948–1954.

Neal, M., Cohen, P., and Reighley, J. *Nursing Care Planning Guides, Set 3*, 2nd Ed. Baltimore: Williams & Wilkins, 1983.

†Sacksteder, S., Gildea, J., and Dassy, C. "Common Congenital Cardiac Defects." *American Journal of Nursing*. February 1978:266–277.

*Sacksteder, S. "Embryology and Fetal Circulation." *American Journal of Nursing*, February 1978:262–265.

†Shor, V. "Congenital Cardiac Defects." *American Journal of Nursing*. February 1978:256–261.

Whaley, L. and Wong, D. *Nursing Care of Infants and Children*, 2nd Ed. St. Louis: Mosby, 1983.

Wieczorek, R. and Natapoff, J. *A Conceptual Approach to the Nursing of Children*. Philadelphia: Lippincott, 1981.

* See Reprint section
† Highly recommended

Nutrition and Metabolism

General Concepts

A. Overview
1. Physiologic differences in infants and small children as compared with adults
   a. Greater proportion of body water, especially in extracellular space, until about 2 years of age
   b. Water-turnover rate per unit of body weight is three times greater in infants
      1) higher metabolic rate
      2) functional immaturity of kidneys which impairs ability to conserve water
   c. Greater skin surface area in proportion to body weight; more susceptible to insensible water loss
   d. Greater gastrointestinal surface area; proportionately greater fluid loss from diarrhea
   e. Average daily water requirements
      1) newborn: 250–500 ml
      2) infant: 750–1,300 ml
      3) 1–4 years: 1,200–1,800 ml
      4) 5–10 years: 1,800–2,500 ml
      5) adolescents: 2,000–2,600 ml
2. Digestive System
   a. High rate of peristalsis (increases susceptibility to diarrhea)
   b. Immature cardiac sphincter that relaxes easily *vomiting common*
   c. Immature liver
   d. Low production of intestinal antibodies until 6–7 months of age
   e. Development of digestive processes is complete by toddlerhood
3. Endocrine System
   a. Functionally immature
   b. Blood sugar levels fluctuate
   c. Hormonal feedback mechanisms are not fully operational; infant is less able to tolerate stresses and metabolic demands of illness

B. Application of the Nursing Process to the Child with Problems of Nutrition and Metabolism
1. Assessment
   a. Nursing History
      1) dietary-intake history: type, amount, frequency, how tolerated
      2) vomiting or diarrhea: onset, severity, duration, description, precipitating factors, how managed at home
      3) infant/child behavior: irritability, lethargy
      4) family history of hereditary disorders: cystic fibrosis, PKU, diabetes mellitus, cleft lip and palate
   b. Physical Examination
      1) general appearance: color, cry, behavior
      2) physical growth (refer to "Healthy Child" page 513)
      3) vital signs, presence of fever
      4) nutrition and hydration status, including signs of dehydration
         a) dry mucous membranes
         b) absence of tears
         c) poor skin turgor (folds, tenting)
         d) sunken fontanel and eyes
         e) pallor
         f) oliguria
         g) increased urine specific gravity
         h) tachycardia
         i) tetany, convulsions
         j) lab findings: elevated Hct and BUN
   c. Diagnostic Tests (refer to *Nursing Care of the Adult* page 211)
2. General Nursing Goal, Plan/Implementation, and Evaluation

   Goal: Child will maintain fluid and electrolyte balance.

Plan/Implementation
- administer fluids (PO, IV) as prescribed; usually includes sodium chloride and potassium replacement
  - use infusion pump to maintain accurate rate
  - restrain child as necessary to protect infusion site
  - observe infusion site for infiltration or redness, and report promptly
- provide pacifier if infant is NPO
- administer electrolytes as prescribed (give potassium only when urinary output is adequate)
- carefully monitor and record I&O (weigh diapers, indicate urine and stool output separately if possible)
- monitor response to therapy (improved skin color and turgor, moist mucous membranes, stable vital signs, urine output within normal limits, urine specific gravity within normal limits, i.e., 1.005–1.025)
- weigh child daily or every shift
- administer antiemetics as ordered
- gradually return to diet-for-age as tolerated

Evaluation: Child regains and maintains fluid and electrolyte balance; shows no signs of dehydration, electrolyte, or acid-base imbalance; returns to usual diet without recurrence of vomiting or diarrhea.

Selected Health Problems Resulting in an Interference with Nutrition and Metabolism

A. Failure to Thrive (FTT) Syndrome

1. General Information
a. Definition: psychosocial failure to thrive (attachment deprivation syndrome) resulting from sensorimotor deprivation due to some disruption in parent-child attachment; includes infants or children whose weight and sometimes height are below the 5th percentile in the absence of organic disease

b. Medical Treatment: rule out organic disease

2. Nursing Process
a. Assessment
  1) *infant*
     a) growth retardation: weight and height below 5th percentile
     b) developmental delays: social, motor, language, cognitive
     c) flat affect, withdrawn
     d) feeding or eating disorders (vomiting, anorexia, rumination)
     e) absence of stranger anxiety
     f) avoids eye-to-eye contact
     g) irregular sleeping, eating, elimination patterns
     h) posture stiff or floppy
     i) poor hygiene
  2) *parent*
     a) handles infant only when necessary
     b) does not talk to, play with, or cuddle infant
     c) bothered by infant's sounds and smells
     d) holds infant away from body, no eye contact with baby
     e) responds inappropriately and inconsistently to infant's cues, cannot discriminate among infant's signals of different needs
     f) refers to infant as "bad" and "unloving"

b. Goals, Plans/Implementation, and Evaluation

Goal 1: Infant will receive adequate nutrition and nurturing while hospitalized.
Plan/Implementation
- plan diet in accordance with needs of age and condition
- create a positive, structured feeding routine
- accurately record intake; weigh infant daily to monitor weight gain
- provide continuity with care givers, e.g., primary nurse
- hold, cuddle, talk to infant lovingly, reassuringly
- provide positive feeding environment and a structured routine
- give age-appropriate sensory stimulation

Evaluation: Infant shows a steady weight gain, shows improved feeding behaviors, has regular elimination pattern, coos and babbles, has eye contact with staff, allows being held closely.

Goal 2: Parents' self-esteem will be promoted, parental anxiety will be reduced, and parent-child attachment will be supported.
Plan/Implementation
- welcome parents when visiting

- encourage parent participation, teaching infant-care techniques through example and demonstration; praise parents' involvement with child
- provide anticipatory guidance concerning infant's capabilities, physical care, emotional needs
- urge parents to talk to infant; point out positive responses
- encourage parents to express feelings about infant and how parenting has affected their lives
- identify stressors in family; refer to social services and family counseling as appropriate
- maintain a nonjudgmental, caring attitude

Evaluation: Parents provide appropriate care to infant; hold, cuddle, and talk to infant; express feelings about infant and self.

Goal 3: Parent will participate in follow-up care after discharge.

Plan/Implementation
- review infant's regimen with parent: diet, elimination, sleep patterns, developmental stimulation
- assess home environment and family relationships
- arrange for follow-up visit for infant to physician or pediatric nurse practitioner
- refer to community resources (e.g., community health nurse, parent support group) as needed
- refer to agencies that can provide family counseling, financial assistance, babysitting and respite services

Evaluation: Parent keeps all appointments, including those with community resources, groups; infant shows age-appropriate developmental progress.

B. Vomiting and Diarrhea

1. General Information
a. Although vomiting and diarrhea are symptoms of other underlying problems or diseases, they are often the primary diagnosis in infants, because fluid and electrolyte imbalance can develop rapidly and become critical in a few short hours.
b. Occurrence: these are very common health problems in infancy; younger infants and children who are debilitated, and those who are exposed to unsanitary environmental conditions are at greater risk of developing diarrhea
c. Causes
  1) vomiting
     a) infection
     b) allergy to formula, food, medications
     c) emotional upsets
     d) GI obstruction
     e) toxin ingestion
     f) increased intracranial pressure
  2) diarrhea (may be acute or chronic)
     a) infection
        - viral (self-limiting)
        - parasites
        - enteropathic organisms such as shigella, salmonella, *E. coli*
     b) diet: formula or food allergy, high sugar or fat content, high bulk, overfeeding
     c) emotional upsets
     d) prolonged use of antibiotics (may destroy normal flora)
     e) intestinal malabsorption
     f) inflammatory bowel disease
d. Medical Treatment: depends on severity of symptoms
  1) medical intervention
     a) bowel rest; IV and/or oral fluid and electrolyte replacement therapy; type and amount determined on basis of child's age, hydration status as determined by weight loss and lab values
     b) switch to soy formula for 1–3 weeks after symptoms subside
     c) antibiotic therapy for bacterial diarrhea
     d) antiemetics, usually by rectal suppository
     e) gradual reintroduction of solid foods
  2) surgical intervention for GI obstruction

2. Nursing Process
a. Assessment
  1) feeding technique and formula preparation (amount, type, formula reconstitution, position of infant, burping)
  2) type of vomiting and/or diarrhea
     a) vomiting
        - *forceful* vomiting: evacuation of stomach contents; usually caused

NUTRITION AND METABOLISM

by overdistention from formula or air
- *projectile* vomiting: stomach contents propelled 2–3 feet from infant; indicates GI obstruction or CNS lesion
- *regurgitation:* "spitting up" milk after feeding; smells sour; usually associated with rumination or gastroesophageal reflux

b) diarrhea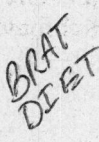
- *mild:* weight loss of 5% or less; stools are loose, runny, usually brown or brownish yellow
- *severe:* explosive, green watery stools, 10–12/day; weight loss 10% or more

3) character of vomitus or stool (ACCT)
  a) *A*mount: measure or estimate
  b) *C*olor/*C*onsistency
    - vomitus
      - undigested food, uncurdled milk
      - sour milk curds
      - bile stained
      - blood tinged or coffee ground
    - diarrhea
      - brown
      - green
      - yellow
      - bulky
      - watery
      - loose
      - mucoid
      - formed
      - seedy
      - pasty
  c) *T*ime
    - frequency of vomiting
    - number of stools/shift
    - precedents (feeding, stimulants, emotional upsets)

4) diagnostic tests
  a) stool pH and stool sugar with Clinitest
  b) stool culture for bacteria, ova, and parasites

5) associated symptoms: anorexia, nausea, cramping, abdominal pain, fever, association of vomiting with diarrhea

6) signs of dehydration

7) change in acid-base balance
  a) vomiting → loss of HCl → metabolic alkalosis
    - compensation: kidneys conserve Na^+ and K^+, excrete H^+
    - lab findings: urine pH greater than 7; serum pH greater than 7.43
  b) diarrhea → metabolic acidosis
    - compensation: respiratory hyperventilation (deep, rapid respirations)
    - lab findings: urine pH less than 6; serum pH less than 7.33

b. **Goals, Plans/Implementation, and Evaluation**

Goal 1: Others will be free from spread of infection.
Plan/Implementation — strict isolation
- obtain stool culture to determine infecting organism
- isolate infant; use good hand-washing technique; dispose of excreta and contaminated laundry appropriately
- teach parents protective measures
- administer antibiotics as ordered, observe for side effects

Evaluation: Individuals involved with care of child show no signs of spread of infection.

Goal 2: Child (with diarrhea) will maintain skin integrity.
Plan/Implementation
- cleanse perineum and buttocks well after each stool
- apply ointment
- expose to heat lamp or air
- take axillary temps to prevent stimulating peristalsis

Evaluation: Child is free from skin breakdown; previously excoriated areas are healed. — meticulous skin care

Goal 3: Child will maintain comfort and safety.
Plan/Implementation
- position to prevent aspiration (on side or abdomen, or in infant seat)
- give mouth care after vomiting and while NPO
- if child is NPO, offer pacifier to meet sucking needs
- change soiled clothing and linen immediately
- exercise restrained limbs

reinforce (+) parenting behaviors

Evaluation: Child does not aspirate vomitus; rests and sleeps comfortably.

C. Pyloric Stenosis

1. **General Information**
   a. Definition and Occurrence: narrowing of the pylorus due to hypertrophy of circular muscle fibers; more commonly affects firstborn white males, 2 weeks to 3 months of age
   b. Medical Treatment
      1) medical intervention
         a) barium swallow to confirm diagnosis
         b) IV fluids to hydrate and correct metabolic alkalosis
         c) nasogastric tube to decompress stomach
      2) surgical intervention: Fredet-Ramstedt procedure (pylorotomy); hypertrophied muscle is *split down to but not through* submucosa, permitting pylorus to expand (if mucosa is cut, gastric contents will leak into peritoneum)

2. **Nursing Process**
   a. Assessment
      1) vomiting: amount, color, consistency, time
      2) classic signs
         a) projectile vomiting (not bile stained since obstruction is above the duodenum)
         b) palpable, olive-size mass in RUQ
         c) observable left-to-right gastric peristaltic waves
      3) metabolic alkalosis, caused by loss of HCl and K+
      4) signs and symptoms of food and fluid loss
         a) hunger after feeding
         b) weight loss, or failure to gain weight
         c) dehydration
         d) scanty, concentrated urine
         e) decrease in size and number of stools
   b. Goals, Plans/Implementation, and Evaluation

   Goal 1: Postoperatively, child will be free from vomiting and will ingest adequate nutrition.

   Plan/Implementation
   - initiate glucose water or electrolyte solutions 4–6 hours post-op and gradually advance to full strength formula during 2nd post-op day
   - give small frequent feedings; feed slowly
   - burp every ½ oz; position on right side or in semi-Fowler's position after feeding
   - handle gently and minimally after feeding
   - keep accurate I&O

   Evaluation: Child ingests adequate caloric and fluid intake; has no vomiting, no signs of dehydration; gains or maintains present weight.

   Goal 2: Parent will be prepared for child's discharge.

   Plan/Implementation:
   - instruct parents on care of surgical incision
   - teach parent how to feed child; supervise as needed
   - allow parent to express feelings and concerns about care

   Evaluation: Parent demonstrates correct feeding of child; burps and positions child properly.

D. Cleft Lip and Palate

look for other anomalies

1. **General Information**
   a. Definition
      1) *cleft lip*: incomplete fusion of facial process; may be small notch in the upper lip (incomplete) or extend to nasal septum and dental ridge (complete); may be unilateral or bilateral — *boys*
      2) *cleft palate:* fissures in soft and/or hard palate and alveolar (dental) ridge; may be midline, unilateral, or bilateral — *more girls*
   b. Occurrence
      1) cleft lip (with or without cleft palate): 1:1,000 live births, higher in males, whites, and Asians
      2) cleft palate: 1:2,500, higher in females
   c. Cause: often unknown, multifactorial inheritance, chromosomal abnormalities
   d. Medical Treatment: lip defect is surgically repaired between ages of 2 weeks–3 months so infant can suck properly and for cosmetic effect; repair of palate usually delayed until about 12–18

months of age to allow for bone growth and changes in contour of palate

2. **Nursing Process**
   a. **Assessment**
      1) infant's ability to suck
      2) parents' reactions to birth of an infant with a facial defect
   b. **Goals, Plans/Implementation, and Evaluation**

   Goal 1: Preoperatively, child will maintain adequate nutrition and will not aspirate fluids.
   Plan/Implementation
   - feed slowly in upright position; use
     - soft nipple
     - special nipple
     - Brecht feeder
     - cup for older infant with cleft palate
   - burp frequently
   - rinse mouth with water after feedings to keep lip/palate cleansed
   - teach parents how to feed and burp infant
   - teach parents use and care of palate prosthesis

   Evaluation: Child ingests adequate fluids and caloric intake, does not aspirate; is free from infections of lip or palate; parents feed infant correctly.

   Goal 2: Postoperatively, child will maintain a patent airway.
   Plan/Implementation
   - observe for respiratory distress; assist in respiratory effort by repositioning child to facilitate breathing, aspirate oral secretions *gently*
   - cleft palate: place in mist tent
   - position infant to provide for drainage of mucus and to prevent trauma to suture lines
     - cleft lip repair: on side or in infant seat
     - cleft palate repair: on side or abdomen

   Evaluation: Child has patent airway and adequate oxygenation; has no signs of respiratory distress.

   Goal 3: Postoperatively, child will be free from trauma and infection of suture lines.
   Plan/Implementation
   - minimize crying by holding and soothing infant as needed
   - put elbow restraints on child; remove *one at a time* q2h for ROM exercises
   - position as stated above
   - maintain Logan bar on upper lip to decrease tension on suture line
   - cleanse suture lines after feeding with sterile swabs and solution as ordered
     - for cleft lip repair: *roll* applicator without rubbing
     - for cleft palate repair: rinse mouth with sterile water after feeding
   - encourage parents to stay with infant and participate in care

   Evaluation: Child's suture lines heal with no trauma and minimal scarring; no signs of infection present.

   Goal 4: Postoperatively, child will ingest adequate nutrition.
   Plan/Implementation
   - keep NPO initially, then introduce fluids in small amounts
   - feed with medicine dropper, Brecht feeder (cleft lip), or cup (cleft palate); no sucking, straws, or spoons
   - while suture line heals, give soft diet; avoid hard food items, e.g., toast, cookies, potato chips

   Evaluation: Child takes food and fluids (appropriate for age); is free from choking or aspiration.

   Goal 5: Child/parent will be referred for on-going, long-term intervention and promotion of habilitation.
   Plan/Implementation
   - teach parents signs of otitis media (fever, turning head to side, pulling at ear, discharge from ear, pain, crying); encourage parents to seek medical treatment for upper respiratory infections
   - refer for regular evaluation of child's hearing, speech, and dental development
   - assist parents to express feelings and concerns about defect and surgery
   - refer parents to community resources
     - parent groups; local and state cleft palate associations
     - Crippled Children's Services, social services

   Evaluation: Parent's can state early signs of ear infections and when to seek treatment. Child has no permanent hearing loss; has age-appropriate language development, intelligible speech; has normal tooth alignment. Parent/child receive community support (emotional, financial, social).

E. Cystic Fibrosis

[handwritten: some genetic trans as sickle cell disease]
[handwritten: muco viscidosis]
[handwritten: Know PATH.]

1. General Information

a. Definition
  1) hereditary condition (autosomal recessive disorder) involving the mucous secreting glands of the lungs, pancreas, and other exocrine glands whose secretions reach an epithelial surface, either directly or through a duct. The secretions are thickened and tenacious; they plug the gland ducts and cause obstruction of flow, fibrosis of the gland, and ultimately loss of function. Because of the wide distribution of affected glands and varying levels of involvement, a wide variety of symptoms may develop.
  2) pathophysiology
     a) *pulmonary effects:* depressed respiratory-cilia cells result in increased infection, bronchiole obstruction, and eventually pulmonary fibrosis; child ultimately develops chronic obstructive pulmonary disease; may progress to cor pulmonale; death can occur from respiratory infection or heart failure
     b) *pancreas effects:* pancreatic fibrosis and eventual decrease of digestive enzymes (lipase, amylase, trypsin) resulting in severe malnutrition; steatorrhea: fatty, bulky, foul-smelling stools that float because of undigested fat cells; also can affect pancreatic endocrine functions resulting in hyperglycemia, glucosuria, and ultimately requiring insulin replacement
     c) *salivary effects:* fibrosis and enlargement of glands caused by thickened secretions; elevated sodium and chloride in saliva
     d) *sweat gland effects:* elevated sodium and chloride in sweat
     e) *reproductive effects*
        • males: inability to produce sperm; the semen is thickened and tenacious; it plugs the duct in the testes, resulting in fibrosis; males are generally sterile but not impotent
        • females: difficult to conceive because cervical plug cannot be penetrated by normal sperm
     f) *hepatic effects:* since the liver secretes bile to emulsify fat in the duodenum, biliary cirrhosis and jaundice may occur; bile is thickened (inspissated) and may plug liver ductules; later can lead to esophageal varices; in newborn and infant, condition may be misdiagnosed as biliary atresia

b. Cause and Occurrence: believed to be autosomal recessive disorder (see figure 5.2); occurs predominantly in whites; 1 in 20 persons is estimated to be a carrier; incidence of children born with CF is approximately 1 in 1,600 live births; average life expectancy is currently late adolescence/early adulthood

c. Medical Treatment
  1) confirm diagnosis: pilocarpine electrophoresis (sweat chloride test) *[handwritten: ★ after 4 mo]*
     a) normal sweat chloride values: less than 40 mEq/liter
     b) suggestive of CF: 40–60 mEq/liter
     c) diagnostic: greater than 60 mEq/liter
  2) medication
     a) "high dose" antibiotics for respiratory infections: penicillins and aminoglycosides (Ticarcillin, Colistin, Piperacillin, Tobramycin); *NOTE:* with aminoglycoside therapy, toxic effects include renal and ototoxicity
     b) pancreatic enzymes by mouth (Pancrease, Cotazym)
     c) fat soluble vitamins A, D, E, K in water-miscible form *[handwritten: CAN'T Absorb vitamins.]*
     d) stool softeners, when necessary, for constipation
     e) in severe malnutrition in late stages of pancreatic insufficiency, may give Adroyd to increase protein metabolism (side effect: onset of male secondary sex characteristics)
     f) NaCl tablets added to diet in hot weather, during febrile illness, or strenuous activity
  3) oxygen therapy, aerosols, nebulizers, bronchodilators
  4) percussion, postural drainage, and breathing exercises

[handwritten: No screening test avail for carriers]

5) sweat chloride testing and genetic counseling for parents and other family members

2. **Nursing Process**
   a. Assessment
      1) effects of mucous gland involvement
         a) dry, paroxysmal cough
         b) wheezing
         c) barrel-shaped chest as child grows older
         d) cyanosis and clubbing of fingers and toes after repeated episodes of pneumonia and bronchitis
         e) thick, mucoid, tenacious pulmonary secretions expectorated following chest physical therapy
         f) since GI tract has a mucoid lining, newborn is at risk of meconium ileus (failure to pass meconium; impacted meconium causes bowel obstruction); older children are also at risk of bowel obstruction caused by fecal impactions
      2) effects of pancreatic involvement
         a) abdominal distention
         b) ravenous appetite
         c) small stature
         d) delayed puberty
         e) decreased subcutaneous tissue
         f) pale, transparent skin
         g) easy fatigability
         h) malaise
         i) fatty, bulky, foul-smelling stools
         j) rectal prolapse
      3) child tastes "salty" when kissed
   b. Goals, Plans/Implementation, and Evaluation

Goal 1: Child and parents will carry out pulmonary therapies as needed or prescribed to maintain adequate ventilation and prevent or lessen pulmonary complications.
Plan/Implementation
- teach parents how to administer nebulizer treatment with prescribed solution and postural draining at least twice daily, including on arising and at bedtime
  - percussion and postural drainage are carried out before and after nebulizer treatment
  - nebulizer solution is usually 10% propylene glycol and 90% distilled water

- teach child and family correct administration of medications (antibiotics, bronchodilators, expectorants)
- teach child breathing exercises (done after postural drainage)
- encourage child to engage in physical activities (swimming, gymnastics, baseball)
- teach child and family general health measures to prevent respiratory infections (e.g., immunizations on time, avoid crowds and people with URIs, prevent chilling, no smoking in the home, provide proper nutrition)
- observe and record sputum amount, color, consistency
- review social implications of sputum by age
  - 2-year-olds and under cannot expectorate
  - socially unacceptable for older children to spit, especially for teenager with beginning sexual identity and relationships
  - review with older children how to take care of bad breath
  - if tetracycline given, warn that it stains teeth

Evaluation: Child and parents implement daily pulmonary therapies; child is free from respiratory infections or they are detected and treated early and vigorously; child maintains optimal ventilation.

Goal 2: Child will maintain adequate nutritional and electrolyte intake.
Plan/Implementation
- give pancreatic enzymes as ordered
  - just prior to meals, to assist digestion
  - mix with pureed fruit for infants; older children can swallow capsules
- encourage intake of balanced diet high in protein and carbohydrate; give snacks with high food value (preceded by appropriate amount of enzymes); these children have additional protein and caloric requirements; fats should be unsaturated
- administer water-miscible vitamins daily

Evaluation: Child's nutritional intake is adequate to meet growth needs.

Goal 3: Child and parents will learn to cope with the chronicity of cystic fibrosis.

560 SECTION 5: NURSING CARE OF THE CHILD

Plan/Implementation
- encourage and permit child/parents to express their feelings regarding diagnosis and its effects, and prognosis
- refer for genetic counseling: essential for persons with CF and all family members
- support family in decision to seek genetic counseling
- refer to community support groups; Cystic Fibrosis Foundation

Evaluation: Child/parents relate their feelings (sadness, anger) about disease; have a referral to and plan to attend genetic counseling and community support groups.

F. Insulin-Dependent Diabetes Mellitus (IDDM)

1. **General Information**
   a. Definition: metabolic disease of unknown inheritance mechanism that results in insulin deficiency because of reduction in pancreatic islet cell mass or destruction of islets and consequent alterations of carbohydrate, fat, and protein metabolism; also results in long-term alterations in vascular, nervous, renal, and ocular systems; damage to other organ systems may be related to degree of control of diabetes
   b. Medical Treatment
      1) medication: insulin therapy (oral hypoglycemics not used with children) see table 3.34
      2) diet: exchange or free (more flexible than with adults)

2. **Nursing Process**
   a. Assessment
      1) initial
         a) polydipsia, polyphagia, polyuria (bed-wetting): classic signs
         b) weight loss
         c) irritability, fatigue
         d) abdominal discomfort
         e) may be mistaken for influenza, gastroenteritis

Table 5.12 Insulin-Dependent Diabetes in the Child (Comparison with Adult-Onset Diabetes)

General	Insulin-Dependent (Child)	Adult-Onset
Characteristics		
Proportion	5%	95%
Age of onset	Peak age 8 to 14	Over 35
Type of onset	Usually sudden	Gradual
Nutritional status	Usually trim	Usually obese
Symptoms	Polydipsia, polyphagia, polyuria	Maybe none
Remission	Present	Absent
Plasma insulin	Absent	Not always absent
Treatment		
Medication	Insulin only	Oral hypoglycemics frequently used
Diet	Free or exchange	Exchange
Urine Tests	Clinitest preferred	Testape OK
Hypoglycemia	Glucagon and oral sugars	Oral sugars only
Foot care	Same as adult, except bare feet OK	Keep clean and dry. Apply oil to prevent dry, cracked skin. Wear socks with shoes. No tight shoes. Do not walk barefooted. Toenails should be trimmed straight across, preferably by podiatrist.

2) often characterized by a remission or honeymoon period
   a) decreased amounts of insulin required
   b) occurs once, but may last a few weeks up to a year
3) DKA (diabetic ketoacidosis): polydipsia, polyphagia, polyuria; dehydration; nausea and vomiting; acetone breath; Kussmaul's respirations
4) hypoglycemia: irritability, trembling; headache; hunger; blurred vision; sweating

b. Goal, Plan/Implementation, and Evaluation

Goal: Child/parent will be prepared for home management.

Plan/Implementation

- demonstrate urine testing; 2- to 5-drop Clinitest preferred; first-voided specimens used because of difficulty in obtaining second-voided specimens from children
- teach management of hyperglycemia
  - importance of good control
  - food, activity, and insulin adjustment to improve control
- teach management of hypoglycemia: ingest a rapidly absorbed glucose-containing food or liquid, such as 4 oz orange juice, 2 teaspoonfuls honey, 5–6 Life Savers (chewed), instant glucose, glucagon
- demonstrate foot care: same as adult except bare feet OK
- prepare parents for developmental concerns with respect to management
  - for toddler and preschooler, review special concerns appropriate for this age
    * injections (bodily integrity concerns)
    * finicky eating habits
    * how to recognize hypoglycemia
    * toilet training and urine tests
  - for school-age child
    * inform school, teacher, peers about symptoms/treatment
    * arrange to participate in gym and sports, adjusting medication as needed
    * problem solve to anticipate diet needs of lunches, parties, holidays
    * feelings of being different
  - for adolescent
    * discuss feelings/concerns about future: career, marriage, pregnancy
    * acting out behaviors (anticipate and prevent)
    * onset of puberty ↑ needs of insulin
    * drugs, alcohol, birth control pills   suicide
- teach self-management as appropriate
  - at 8 or 9 years: physical readiness; teach to do urine tests and injections
  - at 12 or 13 years and beyond: cognitive readiness; teach diet planning, how to maintain food, activity, insulin balance

Evaluation: Child/parent has adapted necessary skills to daily routine; child does not have recurrent episodes of ketoacidosis or hypoglycemia; growth and development continues within normal range.

References

Harrison, L. "Nursing Intervention with the Failure to Thrive Family." *MCN: American Journal of Maternal-Child Nursing*. March/April 1976:111–116.

Hoette, S. "The Adolescent with Diabetes Mellitus." *Nursing Clinics of North America*. December 1983:763–776.

Johnson, M. "Self-instruction for the Family of a Child with Cystic Fibrosis." *MCN: American Journal of Maternal-Child Nursing*. May/June 1980:345–348.

Krauser, K. and Madden, P. "The Child with Diabetes Mellitus." *Nursing Clinics of North America*. December 1983:749–761.

Loman, D. and Galgani, C. "Monitoring Diabetic Children's Blood-Glucose Levels at Home." *MCN: American Journal of Maternal-Child Nursing*. May/June 1984:192–196.

†McGrath, B. "Fluids, Electrolytes and Replacement Therapy in Pediatric Nursing." *MCN: American Journal of Maternal-Child Nursing*. January/February 1980:56–62.

Whaley, L. and Wong, D. *Nursing Care of Infants and Children*, 2nd Ed. St. Louis: Mosby, 1983.

Wieczoreck, R. and Natapoff, J. *A Conceptual Approach to the Nursing of Children*. Philadelphia: Lippincott, 1981.

†Yoos, L. "Taking Another Look at Failure to Thrive." *MCN: American Journal of Maternal-Child Nursing*. January/February 1984:32–36.

† Highly recommended

Elimination

General Concepts
A. Overview
1. Urinary Elimination
   a. Kidney development is not complete until approximately one year of age
   b. Immature functioning of nephrons; poor filtration and absorption during first year of life; ability to concentrate urine gradually increases during first year of life
   c. Urinary bladder is an abdominal organ during infancy; as pelvic shape changes, the bladder gradually settles and becomes a pelvic organ
   d. Average daily urine output
      1) newborn: 150–300 ml
      2) infant: 400–500 ml
      3) 1–6 years: 500–700 ml
      4) 6–15 years: 700–1,400 ml
2. Bowel Elimination
   a. Large and small intestines serve as the major organs for detoxification during infancy while the liver and kidneys are maturing
   b. Development of digestive processes is complete by the early toddler years
3. Voluntary Control of Elimination
   a. Myelination of the spinal cord is complete by 18–24 months of age resulting in capacity for voluntary control of urinary and anal sphincters
   b. Bladder capacity increases (greater in girls than boys) as voluntary control is achieved

B. Application of the Nursing Process to the Child with Elimination Problems
1. Assessment
   a. Nursing History
      1) voiding patterns: day and night; frequency; color, clarity, estimated amount of urine output; recent changes or problems (e.g., nocturia, urgency, dysuria, infections)
      2) bowel elimination patterns: frequency, consistency, and color; recent changes or problems (e.g., diarrhea, constipation, abdominal cramping)
      3) alterations in elimination: neurogenic bowel and bladder, ostomy, enuresis, encopresis; problem management; medications (e.g., urinary antiseptics, laxatives, antidiarrheal drugs)
   b. Physical Examination
      1) observation of urine and stool
      2) palpation and auscultation of abdomen and bladder (normally nonpalpable), including bowel sounds (all quadrants)
   c. Diagnostic Tests (refer to *Nursing Care of the Adult* page 252)

2. General Nursing Goals, Plans/Implementation and Evaluation
   Goal 1: Child will achieve and maintain normal urinary and bowel elimination.
   Plan/Implementation
   - measure, describe, and record I&O
   - promote fluid intake (within restrictions, if any)
   - provide diet appropriate to health problem and age
   - carry out procedures (as indicated) to promote optimal elimination, e.g., colostomy care, catheter care, Credé of bladder, administration of medications

   Evaluation: Child's urinary and bowel output is within normal limits for age; child is adequately hydrated; receives necessary interventions to assist with elimination.

   Goal 2: Child will remain free from infection and complications.
   Plan/Implementation
   - take axillary temps

- administer antibiotics or antiseptics as ordered
- protect child from exposure to infection
- use aseptic technique and protective isolation as indicated
- teach handwashing technique to personnel and family
- observe for and report signs of complications

Evaluation: Child is free from infection (no fever, signs of wound infection, or respiratory involvement); is free from complications or long-term sequelae of disease.

Goal 3: Child will be comfortable and free from pain.

Plan/Implementation
- observe child for verbal and nonverbal signs of pain or discomfort
- position child for maximum comfort
- use diversion techniques (e.g., play, singing, counting)
- administer prescribed analgesics or sedatives when indicated

Evaluation: Child remains comfortable and free from pain (no complaints or nonverbal indicators of pain); rests and sleeps comfortably; engages in age-appropriate play.

Goal 4: Child and parents will receive appropriate health teaching and emotional support.

Plan/Implementation
- teach child/parent
  - diet restrictions
  - medications (actions, side effects, administration)
  - home care (ostomy, urine testing, dressing changes)
  - prevention of recurrence or complications
  - importance of compliance with therapeutic regimen
- encourage parents to express feelings and concerns about child's illness and care
- provide follow-up and home care as needed
- refer to community resources as needed

Evaluation: Parents demonstrate ability to provide needed home care (diet, medications, procedures); parents and child verbalize feelings/concerns about child's illness and care; make use of community resources and follow-up care as needed.

Selected Health Problems Resulting in an Interference with Urinary Elimination

A. Hypospadias

1. **General Information**
   a. Definition: congenital abnormality in which urethral opening lies on ventral surface of penis; frequently associated with chordee, which results in a downward curve of penis
   b. Medical Treatment
      1) surgical intervention to provide normal function and appearance
         a) urethroplasty: skin grafting to extend urethra and surgically reconstruct a new urinary meatus
         b) surgical release of chordee
      2) circumcision is contraindicated, since foreskin may be needed for reconstructive surgery

2. **Nursing Process**
   a. Assessment
      1) abnormal placement of urethral meatus
      2) abnormal urine stream
      3) associated problems
         a) chordee
         b) undescended testes
   b. Goal, Plan/Implementation, and Evaluation

Goal: Child will maintain integrity of surgical repair.

Plan/Implementation
- check pressure dressing for evidence of bleeding and to ensure intact dressing
- monitor function of urinary diversion apparatus (permits urine to bypass the operative site)
  - Foley catheter
  - suprapubic tube
  - perineal urethrotomy
  - check for adequate circulation to tip of penis
- observe for difficulties following catheter removal
  - inability to void
  - painful voiding (dysuria)
  - urinary tract infection
  - hematuria
  - frequency

Evaluation: Child can void normally; surgical dressing and site are dry and intact.

B. Urinary Tract Infection

1. **General Information**
   a. Definition: bacteriuria with or without signs and symptoms of inflammation of the urinary bladder or kidneys, resulting in risk of renal damage
   b. Incidence: 1%–2% of the childhood population; girls have a 10–30 times greater risk than boys (5% of girls have a urinary tract infection by age 18); peak age is 2–6 years
   c. Predisposing factors
      1) poor hygiene, prolonged use of a single diaper (especially disposable diapers)
      2) tight-fitting clothing, e.g., blue jeans
      3) ureteral reflux caused by congenital malposition of ureters
      4) concurrent vaginitis or pinworms
      5) neurogenic bladder
   d. Medical Treatment
      1) antibiotic therapy: usually ampicillin, amoxicillin, or sulfonamides for short, intensive treatment
      2) longer-term urinary antiseptic therapy: nitrofurantoin (Furadantin) or methenamine mandelate (Mandelamine) to maintain sterility of urine
      3) surgical correction of congenital malposition of ureters (ureteral reimplantation) to correct reflux

2. **Nursing Process**
   a. Assessment
      1) frequency, urgency, dysuria, dribbling
      2) foul-smelling urine
      3) lower abdominal pain
      4) fever, chills, flank pain (all usually indicate an acute infection of the upper urinary tract)
   b. Goals, Plan/Implementation, and Evaluation

   Goal 1: Child's urinary tract infection will be detected and treated early.
   Plan/Implementation
   - ensure child receives annual routine urinalysis (especially girls, ages 2–6 years)
   - provide age-appropriate preparation of child for intrusive diagnostic tests (usually done under general anesthesia)
   - emphasize importance of full course of antibiotic therapy and continuing antiseptics even when child has no signs of infection

   Evaluation: Child is free from urinary tract infection; recurrence is prevented.

   Goal 2: Child and parents will be educated concerning prevention of urinary tract infection.
   Plan/Implementation
   - teach good hygiene measures
     - wipe front to back
     - avoid tub baths, especially with water softeners such as bubble bath
     - wear loose-fitting clothing and cotton panties
   - caution child not to "hold" urine, but to void as soon as urge is felt
   - teach child to empty bladder completely with each voiding
   - advise an increase in daily fluid intake, especially fluids that acidify urine (e.g., apple and cranberry juice)

   Evaluation: Child is free from urinary tract infection; uses appropriate hygiene measures; empties bladder with each voiding; child's daily fluid intake is adequate.

C. Nephrosis and Nephritis

1. **General Information: Nephrosis**
   a. Definition: nephrosis (nephrotic syndrome) is a chronic condition with variable pathologic conditions that results in increased permeability of glomerular membrane to plasma protein, resulting in protein loss; acute phase (exacerbation) lasts approximately 4 weeks
   b. Peak Age: 2–3 years; cause is unknown; 60% of affected children are boys
   c. Medical Treatment
      1) bed rest until edema subsides
      2) medication
         a) prednisone
            - drug of choice
            - 2 mg/kg of body weight/day
            - to reduce proteinuria and, therefore, edema; to induce remission
            - given every other day
            - continued until urine is free from protein for 2 weeks (urine generally returns to normal in 4 weeks or less)
            - stop gradually to prevent adrenal insufficiency
         b) antibiotics to decrease risk of infection

Table 5.13 Comparison of Nephrosis and Nephritis

	Nephrosis	Nephritis
General Information	Chronic Unknown cause	Acute Caused by antigen-antibody response to group A beta hemolytic strep
Peak Age	2–3 years (toddler)	6 years (school age)
Medications	Prednisone	Antibiotic therapy
Diet	High potassium	Low potassium until urine output normal
Assessment		
Edema	Massive	Moderate, usually facial and periorbital
Blood pressure	Normal	Elevated
Proteinuria	Massive	Moderate
Hematuria	Microscopic	Gross
Serum K+	Normal	Elevated
Hypoproteinemia	Marked	Mild
Hyperlipemia	Elevated	Normal
Long-term sequelae	5%–10% develop chronic renal failure	10%–25% develop chronic renal failure

    c) IV salt-poor albumin: provides only a temporary response; administered q2–3days during acute phase
  3) diet
    a) may restrict fluid intake if edema is severe
    b) moderate sodium restriction to slow increase of edema
    c) high protein, high potassium
2. **Nursing Process: Nephrosis**
  a. Assessment
    1) insidious weight gain
    2) massive proteinuria
    3) hypoproteinemia
    4) oliguria, increased urine specific gravity
    5) anorexia
    6) diarrhea
    7) edema (severe)
      a) periorbital and facial; subsides during the day
      b) generalized: feet, ascites, genitals (scrotal or labial)
    8) blood pressure normal
    9) dark, frothy urine
    10) irritability, lethargy
    11) increased susceptibility to infection
    12) respiratory difficulty owing to pleural effusion
    13) hyperlipemia
3. **General Information: Poststreptoccal Nephritis**
  a. Definition: acute glomerulonephritis (AGN) is an inflammation of the glomeruli caused by an antigen-antibody response to group A beta hemolytic streptococcus, resulting in reversible changes in permeability of glomerular capillaries; glomerular filtration rate is reduced; water and sodium are retained, causing circulatory congestion and edema; acute phase lasts 1–3 weeks
  b. Peak Age: 6 years (range is 2–12 years); history of URI, scarlet fever, or impetigo 1–3 weeks prior to symptoms; 2 times higher incidence in boys
  c. Medical Treatment
    1) bed rest until edema, hypertension, and hematuria subside
    2) medication
      a) antibiotic therapy to eradicate lingering strep infection (indicated by elevated antistreptolysin-O [ASO] titer)
      b) antihypertensives to control BP

c) anticonvulsants (with hypertensive encephalopathy)
d) digitalis (with congestive heart failure)
3) diet
a) may restrict fluid intake
b) moderate sodium restriction
c) normal protein
d) low potassium until urine output is normal

4. **Nursing Process: Poststreptococcal Nephritis**
   a. **Assessment**
      1) moderate proteinuria
      2) hypoproteinemia (decreased serum albumin)
      3) oliguria, increased urine specific gravity
      4) anorexia
      5) diarrhea (caused by bowel edema)
      6) edema (moderate)
         a) primarily periorbital and facial
         b) may extend to extremities and abdomen during the day
      7) moderate hypertension
      8) hematuria (tea or cola-colored)
      9) irritability, lethargy
   b. **Goals, Plans/Implementation, and Evaluation (for both conditions)**
   Goal 1: Child will regain normal urine output and maintain fluid and electrolyte balance.
   Plan/Implementation
   - administer medications as ordered: prednisone, antihypertensives
   - teach parents administration, action, and side effects of medications (prednisone: Cushing's syndrome, increased susceptibility to infection [prednisone masks infection], GI distress, growth retardation)
   - restrict fluid intake as ordered; child should take maximum allowable limit to prevent dehydration
   - monitor I&O carefully; weigh daily
   - check urine for specific gravity, albumin, blood
   - restrict Na intake as ordered
   - restrict high-potassium foods during oliguria (in AGN)
   - check vital signs for deviations from normal parameters
   - maintain adequate nutritional intake with diet as ordered; allow child to participate in selecting foods within allowed limits
   - serve small portions to encourage appetite

   Evaluation: Child's urine output returns to normal and reflects normal specific gravity, is free from blood or albumin; child is free from edema, has adequate I&O, eats balanced diet of allowed foods, has no signs of electrolyte imbalance.

   Goal 2: Child with nephrosis will be free from skin breakdown.
   Plan/Implementation
   - give meticulous skin care
     - bathe and powder skin folds several times a day; separate skin surfaces with soft padding
     - utilize scrotal support as needed
     - cleanse eyelids with warm saline
     - turn at least q2h; use special mattress
   - place child in semi-Fowler's position to facilitate breathing and minimize facial and periorbital edema
   - handle gently

   Evaluation: Child's skin is intact; has no complaints of pain or discomfort.

   Goal 3: Child will conserve energy.
   Plan/Implementation
   - maintain bed rest when child has edema, hypertension, hematuria
   - explain reasons for bed rest and isolation
   - offer quiet, age-appropriate play activities

   Evaluation: Child does not become overly tired; engages in age-appropriate quiet play.

D. **Lower GI Tract Obstruction**
   1. **General Information**
      a. **Definitions**
         1) *intussusception:* telescoping of one portion of intestine into another, resulting in obstruction of blood supply with ischemia and death of telescoped portion; one of the most common causes of intestinal obstruction in infancy; most cases occur in children under 2 years of age; 3 times more common in boys; higher incidence in children with cystic fibrosis and celiac disease
         2) *Hirschsprung's disease* (aganglionic megacolon): congenital absence of parasympathetic ganglia of distal colon and rectum, resulting in inadequate peristalsis; stool and

flatus accumulate in colon proximal to defect, causing dilation and hypertrophy of bowel; usually diagnosed in neonatal period or early infancy; 4 times more common in boys; higher incidence in children with Down's syndrome

b. Medical Treatment
  1) *intussusception*
    a) hydrostatic reduction with barium enema before bowel becomes necrotic
    b) if bowel necrosis has occurred, surgical intervention: resection and anastomosis
  2) *Hirschsprung's disease*
    a) barium enema
    b) rectal biopsy to confirm absence of ganglion cells
    c) resection of aganglionic portion of bowel, temporary colostomy of sigmoid or transverse colon to rest bowel and restore nutritional balance; abdominal-perineal pull-through anastomosis at approximately 1 year of age

2. Nursing Process
  a. Assessment
    1) *intussusception:* acute, recurrent, severe, colicky abdominal pain; "currant jelly" stools containing blood and mucus, caused by bowel gangrene (occurs about 12 hours after onset of abdominal pain); palpable sausage-shaped mass in right upper quadrant
    2) *Hirschsprung's disease*
      a) delayed passage of meconium in newborn; failure to thrive
      b) chronic constipation
      c) ribbonlike, foul-smelling stools
      d) breath has foul odor
      e) severe abdominal distention with shortness of breath
      f) at risk for enterocolitis, which increases risk of fatality
    3) both
      a) bile-stained vomiting (the obstruction is below ampulla of Vater which empties bile into duodenum)
      b) abdominal distention
  b. Goal, Plan/Implementation, and Evaluation

  Goal: Child will maintain adequate hydration and nutrition, and regain normal elimination.

  Plan/Implementation
  - give IV fluids as ordered; hyperalimentation may be ordered for infants with Hirschsprung's disease
  - usually keep NPO; give mouth care, pacifier
  - keep accurate I&O; measure and record drainage (NG, colostomy); irrigate NG tube as ordered
  - assess bowel sounds frequently
  - gradually reintroduce feedings and return to normal diet post-op after NG tube has been removed and bowel sounds have returned

  Evaluation: Child is adequately hydrated (elastic skin turgor, moist mucous membranes, etc.), has adequate caloric intake; returns to normal diet without complications (e.g., vomiting); is free from abdominal distention and establishes normal bowel elimination postoperatively.

References

Hetrick, A., Frauman, A., and Gilman, C. "Nutrition in Renal Disease: When the Patient is a Child." *American Journal of Nursing.* December 1979:2152–2154.

*Ruble, J. "Childhood Nocturnal Enuresis." *MCN: American Journal of Maternal-Child Nursing.* January/February 1981:26–31.

Sugar, E. "Hirschsprung's Disease." *American Journal of Nursing.* November 1981:2065–2067.

Whaley, L. and Wong, D. *Nursing Care of Infants and Children*, 2nd Ed. St. Louis: Mosby, 1983.

Wieczorek, R. and Natapoff, J. *A Conceptual Approach to the Nursing of Children.* Philadelphia: Lippincott, 1981.

* See Reprint section

Safety and Security

General Concepts
A. Overview
1. Neurologic Differences in Children
   a. The greatest neurologic changes occur during the first year of life
   b. The brain reaches 75% of adult size by age 2, 90% by age 6
   c. Cortical development is usually complete by age 4
   d. Primitive neonatal reflexes disappear as higher centers of the brain take over; most neonatal reflexes disappear or diminish by 3–4 months of age; their persistence may indicate a neurologic problem
2. Immunologic Differences in Children
   a. Newborn receives passive immunity from mother for most major childhood communicable diseases (assuming mother is immune)
   b. The young infant's immune system is not fully developed; therefore, the infant is more prone to infectious disease
   c. The eustachian tube in infants and young toddlers is shorter and straighter than in older children and adults, leading to increased risk of middle ear infections [↑otisis media]
   d. Peak growth of lymphatic tissue occurs during early school-age years [↑tonsilitis]
   e. Increasing exposure of preschoolers and school-age children to sources of infectious disease leads to increased incidence during these years
3. Integumentary (Skin) Differences in Children
   a. The skin is less thick during infancy
   b. The epidermis is fragile and more prone to irritation
   c. The infant's skin is more sensitive to changes in temperature (especially extremes of heat and cold) and is more susceptible to invasion by bacteria and other infectious organisms
4. Developmental Disabilities
   a. Definition: any serious, chronic disability caused by an impairment of physical or mental functioning, or both, that occurs in childhood, is likely to persist throughout life, and results in limitations in daily functioning; it may cause significant and permanent interruptions in the child's physical, emotional, and social growth and development
   b. Includes chronic illnesses, such as asthma, cystic fibrosis, and diabetes mellitus, as well as motor-activity disorders; sensory deficits; mental retardation; and speech, learning, and behavioral problems
   c. Incidence: approximately 10% of all children and adolescents have some type of developmental disability

B. Application of the Nursing Process to the Child with Neurologic or Sensory Problems
1. Assessment
   a. Nursing History
      1) achievement of developmental milestones; child's self-care abilities
      2) developmental delays: motor, language, social, cognitive [Assess. focus on → detect + prevent long term disabil.]
      3) perceptual problems: vision, hearing
      4) perinatal history (refer to "High-Risk Neonate" in *Nursing Care of the Childbearing Family* page 457)
      5) family history: congenital anomalies, hereditary factors, infections
      6) child's health history: illnesses, allergies, medications, immunizations
      7) communication, memory, attention problems, school performance

SAFETY AND SECURITY

8) current health problem(s): signs and symptoms, medical treatment, home management, concerns or problems
9) parents'/family's perception of health problem
   a) child's adaptation to disability
   b) family's ability to cope with loss of "perfect child" (refer to *Nursing Care of the Client with Psychosocial Problems* page 29)
   c) stressors: economic, marital, lack of time and energy
   d) threats to self-esteem and control
   e) overprotectiveness or rejection of child

b. Physical Examination
  1) general: level of consciousness, affect, attention span; head and chest circumferences, cranial sutures and fontanels; vital signs, including BP
  2) persistent or absent neonatal reflexes
  3) posture: persistent extension/flexion of extremities, scissoring, frog-leg position, opisthotonos
  4) motor function: muscle size and tone; symmetrical, spontaneous movements of all extremities; involuntary movements such as tremors, spasticity, athetosis
  5) developmental skills: assess for developmental progress (e.g., Denver Developmental Screening Test), gross and fine motor development, language, self-help skills (dressing, feeding, toileting)
  6) vision: infant's ability to focus on small objects; vision screening tests for older children (refer to "Healthy Child" page 523)
  7) hearing: startle reflex is a rough estimate of sound perception in infants; audiometry is unreliable with infants, toddlers, and mentally retarded children

c. Diagnostic tests (refer to *Nursing Care of the Adult* page 289)

2. **General Nursing Goals, Plans/Implementation, and Evaluation**

Goal 1: Child will achieve optimum level of growth and development.
Plan/Implementation
- screen children at risk for developmental disabilities so problems are detected and treated early to minimize developmental delays
- keep child's activities in the mainstream as much as possible to promote self-sufficiency, adjustment, and mental development
  - refer family to infant stimulation, developmental, and special education programs
  - maintain open communication between family and all members of interdisciplinary team
- treat child according to developmental (not chronologic) age
- provide guidance for learning acceptable social behaviors
- include activities that enhance child's self-esteem and self-worth
- provide a variety of stimuli; help child pay attention to distinct stimuli [*struc & play one toy @ a time*]
- break tasks into small components; use positive reinforcement (verbal praise, hugs, stickers) [*not food*]
- provide visual and auditory cues, and opportunities for practice (repetition enhances learning)
- teach self-care skills for activities of daily living (e.g., hygiene, feeding, dressing)
  - allow child as much independence as possible (even if activities take longer)
  - acknowledge and positively reinforce parents' care of child and child's progress
  - help parents provide a stimulating, healthful environment for the child

Evaluation: Child achieves and maintains optimum developmental potential; is able to perform ADL as independently as possible; is maintained in a community setting.

Goal 2: Parents/family members will express feelings about having a child with a developmental disability, and their ability to cope.

Plan/Implementation
- allow parents/family members opportunities to express their grief; be supportive and anticipate repeated periods of sadness, anger
- help parents identify and reinforce child's capabilities and normal characteristics (this is *first* a child, and then a child with a disability)

- encourage family discussion and coping with changes that may occur in the family system as a result of caring for the child
- refer the family to appropriate community resources

Evaluation: Parents/family express feelings/concerns regarding child's limitations; develop realistic plans to care for the child at home; include child as a member of the family constellation; involve all family members in child's care; utilize appropriate community resources, e.g., parent-support groups, available programs.

Goal 3: The family will remain cohesive and function at its optimal level.

Plan/Implementation
- identify families at risk for adapting poorly to disability and chronic illness
  - recognize that certain family types (e.g., single-parent families, teen parents) may require more support and guidance in care of child
  - consider the availability of extended-family members and their ability and willingness to participate in care of child
- determine the family's perception of the child's disability and encourage realistic discussion about the child's capabilities and limitations
- identify support systems within the family and community (e.g., home health care)
- encourage activities that enhance individual and family development for *all* family members
- provide respite care to family when necessary

Evaluation: Family discusses realistic perceptions about the child; utilizes available support systems; participates in activities outside the home. Families at risk for poor adaptation are identified and receive the necessary support or referral for counseling and assistance.

Selected Health Problems: Neurologic and Sensory Deficits

A. Mental Retardation (MR)

1. **General Information**
   a. Definition: below average intellectual functioning that becomes apparent during childhood development and is associated with impairment in adaptive behavior; manifestations include impaired learning, inadequate social adjustment, and delayed or lowered potential capacity for achievement; see table 5.14 for classification levels
   b. Causes
      1) *prenatal:* chromosomal/genetic variations (Down's syndrome, PKU, Tay-Sachs), German measles or infection in mother during pregnancy, incompatible blood between mother and child (Rh or ABO), glandular disorders, toxic chemicals, nutritional deficiencies, excessive maternal drug or alcohol use
      2) *perinatal:* birth injury such as anoxia or intracranial hemorrhage
      3) *postnatal:* encephalitis, head trauma, glandular disturbances, inadequate developmental stimulation in early childhood, post-cardiac arrest, poisoning
   c. Incidence: 3% of the US population; 1 in 10 American families has an MR member; 70%–80% are in the borderline or mild (EMR) category (see table 5.14); 20%–30% are moderately, severely, or profoundly retarded (the latter are most often cared for in residential institutions)

2. **Nursing Process**
   a. Assessment
      1) developmental lags in motor and adaptive behaviors
      2) persistence of neonatal reflexes
      3) perceptual deficits
      4) level of functioning (see table 5.14)
   b. Goal, Plan/Implementation, and Evaluation (see General Nursing Goals above)

Goal: When hospitalized, the mentally retarded child will adapt to hospitalization, will maintain independence in ADL, will ingest adequate food and fluids.

Plan/Implementation
- adapt hospital routines to child's as much as possible
- explain all procedures and treatments carefully, at level child can understand
- maintain consistency to promote security within child's environment
- encourage parent/family participation in care

SAFETY AND SECURITY

Table 5.14 Levels of Retardation (Classification System of American Association on Mental Deficiency)

Level	IQ Range	Potential Mental Age	Rehabilitation Potential
Level 0: Borderline	68–83	Close to normal	Usually capable of marriage, being self-supporting (probable low socioeconomic living standard).
Level 1: Mild or educable	52–67	8–12 years	Can usually be maintained in community. Can work but needs supervision in financial affairs; 4th- or 5th-grade academic possibilities (special classes for educable mentally retarded [EMR]) and vocational skills, but often has difficulty holding a job in a competitive market.
Level 2: Moderate	36–51	3–7 years	1st- to 3rd-grade academic potential (special classes for trainable mentally retarded [TMR]) or vocational training in sheltered workshop or neighborhood job.
Level 3: Severe	20–35	Toddler	Minimal independent behavior and self-help skills (toilet training, dressing self). School placement in handicapped or TMR program. Some are able to work in a sheltered workshop.
Level 4: Profound	Less than 20	Young infant	May require total care; may have CNS damage.

- assist with feeding as necessary; bring special cups, feeding utensils from home
- be sure to follow through on what you tell child (e.g., if you say you will return at a certain time, be sure to do it)
- use positive reinforcement

Evaluation: Child accepts staff members' explanations and cooperates in care; feeds and dresses self; takes prescribed diet and fluids.

B. Down's Syndrome (Mongolism)

1. **General Information**
   a. Definition: extra chromosome 21 (trisomy 21), due to a failure of the chromosome to split during gametogenesis; mental capacity varies from level 1 (educable) to level 3 (severely retarded); one of the most common causes of mental retardation
   b. Cause: associated with increased maternal or paternal age
   c. Incidence: 1 in 600–650 live births
   d. Medical Treatment: diagnosis is usually based on clinical manifestations; chromosome studies may be done in some cases

2. **Nursing Process**
   a. Assessment
   1) physical manifestations
      a) small round head, flat nose, protruding tongue, high arched palate
      b) slanted eyelids, Brushfield spots (speckles in iris)
      c) muscle hypotonia, hyperflexible joints
      d) simian crease, short fingers, clinodactyly
      e) congenital heart malformations in 40% of cases
      f) weak respiratory accessory muscles
      g) increased incidence of leukemia and GI anomalies
   2) mastery of developmental tasks

3) intellectual functioning
4) child's routine for ADL
b. Goals, Plans/Implementation, and Evaluation

Goal 1: Child will be free from respiratory infection.
Plan/Implementation
- teach parents (and child as appropriate) preventive health measures
  - prevent exposure to individuals with URIs
  - encourage optimal nutrition, adequate rest
  - keep immunizations up-to-date
- obtain medical care at onset of infection (may need antibiotics)

Evaluation: Child has no more than a minimal number of URIs.

Goal 2: Child will ingest adequate food and fluids and will experience minimal feeding difficulties
Plan/Implementation
- ☆ teach parents appropriate feeding techniques
  - use bulb syringe to clear nasal passages before feedings
  - use a long-handled, infant spoon (rubber-coated) to place food to side and back of mouth
- reassure parents that infant's tongue thrust does not mean dislike of food
- adjust caloric requirements based on child's size and activity level to prevent child from becoming overweight
- provide high roughage and liberal fluids to prevent constipation *due to poor muscle tone*

Evaluation: Child experiences minimal feeding difficulties (airway remains clear during feeding, child ingests food sufficient for growth); maintains weight within expected limits for height as child grows older; remains free from constipation.

C. Cerebral Palsy *most common*
1. General Information *↑ incidence of low wt. babies.*
a. Definition: nonprogressive muscular impairment resulting in abnormal muscle tone and incoordination; spastic type most common (upper motor neuron involvement), dyskinetic (athetoid) type second-most common; may be mild to severe
b. Associated Defects: mental retardation (may have normal or superior intelligence), seizures, minimal brain dysfunction; speech, hearing, oculomotor impairment
c. Incidence
   1) 25,000 babies with cerebral palsy born annually (5:1,000 live births)
   2) most common developmental disability of childhood
   3) higher incidence in low-birth-weight babies or from birth with other complications, especially during the perinatal period, that result in cerebral anoxia
d. Medical Treatment
   1) braces, ambulation devices (crutches, walker)
   2) surgical correction of extremity deformities (especially lengthening of heel cord to improve stability and function)
   3) medications: muscle relaxants, anticonvulsants, tranquilizers

2. Nursing Process
a. Assessment
   ☆ 1) spasticity
      a) hypertonicity of muscles (continuous reflexive contraction of muscles leading to tightening and shortening)
      b) persistence of neonatal reflexes *head lag*
      c) scissoring
      d) poor posturing
      e) delayed gross and fine motor development
      f) uneven muscle tone
      g) intellectual functioning may be impaired
   2) dyskinesis (athetosis)
      a) continuous uncontrollable, wormlike movements of arms, legs, torso, face, and tongue
         - intensified by stress
         - absent during sleep
      b) drooling
      c) poor speech articulation
b. Goals, Plans/Implementation, and Evaluation

Goal 1: Child will ingest adequate nutrition.
Plan/Implementation
- provide adequate calories to meet additional energy demands of constant muscle activity
- feed slowly

[Handwritten margin notes: "- support jaw while feeding - massage gums to limit hyperplasia"; "- abnorm roof & teeth struc."]

- modify feeding technique to deal with extrusion reflex
- ensure adequate fluid intake
- use special silverware and dishes as needed (e.g., padded spoon, nonskid dishes)
- teach importance of daily dental hygiene; routine dental care

Evaluation: Child ingests calories and other nutrients needed for adequate growth; chews and swallows food adequately; has optimal dental hygiene and care; is free from dental caries or gum problems.

Goal 2: Child will develop maximum mobility and self-help skills.

Plan/Implementation
- teach parents appropriate stretching and range-of-motion exercises *[handwritten: get child to relax]*
- teach use of braces or splints, special support chairs, or wheelchairs as needed
- encourage participation in programs of physical and occupational therapy, speech therapy as needed
- avoid movement that triggers abnormal reflexes
- teach self-help skills, beginning with simplest ones first; teach only 1 skill at a time until it is learned
- provide needed adaptive devices (special utensils, Velcro fastenings)

Evaluation: Child is free from contractures; demonstrates maximum mobility (with assistance as needed); is able to participate in self-care tasks (e.g., feed self, dress self).

Goal 3: Child will be free from skin breakdown.

Plan/Implementation
- reposition frequently and gently massage pressure points with lotion
- check braces, splints for tightness and pressure; adjust as needed
- utilize special equipment ("egg-crate" mattress, sheepskin)
- keep linens and clothes dry; if wet with urine/stool, change as soon as possible

Evaluation: Child's skin is intact, free from pressure sores.

D. Hydrocephalus

1. **General Information**
   a. Definition: excessive accumulation of cerebral spinal fluid (CSF) within the ventricles of the brain; three common types
   1) excess secretion of CSF
   2) obstructive (noncommunicating): results from an obstruction in the ventricular pathway
   3) communicating: results when the CSF is not absorbed from the subarachnoid space
   b. Causes: developmental malformation (congenital), tumors, infections, head injury
   c. Medical Treatment
   1) diagnosis: lumbar puncture, CAT scan (refer to *Nursing Care of the Adult* page 289)
   2) surgical insertion of shunt to bypass obstruction or drain excess fluid
      a) atrioventricular (AV) shunt: lateral ventricle to right atrium of heart
      b) ventriculoperitoneal (VP) shunt: lateral ventricle to peritoneal cavity (see reprint page 636)
      c) one-way valves are used in both cases to prevent backflow of blood or peritoneal secretions
   3) rehospitalization is common for blocked or infected shunt, or for lengthening of shunt as child grows

2. **Nursing Process**
   a. Assessment
   1) for signs and symptoms of increased intracranial pressure to prevent/minimize brain damage (see table 5.15)
   2) shiny scalp with dilated veins (congenital hydrocephalus)
   3) sunset eyes (congenital hydrocephalus)
   b. Goals, Plans/Implementation, and Evaluation

Goal 1: Preoperatively, child will maintain skin integrity of scalp.

Plan/Implementation
- change position q2h
- use sheepskin or water mattress

Evaluation: Child has intact skin on scalp; no decubitus ulcers of scalp.

Goal 2: Child will maintain adequate nutrition and hydration.

Plan/Implementation
- offer small frequent feedings; do not overfeed
- burp often
- after feeding, position on side with head elevated
- provide rest period after feedings
- assess for dehydration

Table 5.15 Signs and Symptoms of Increased Intracranial Pressure in Infants and Children

Causes	Hydrocephalus
	Intracranial tumors
	Cerebral trauma
	Meningitis, encephalitis
Manifestations	
Infants	Bulging fontanels
	High-pitched cry
	Vomiting, feeding difficulty (poor suck)
	Seizures
	Opisthotonos
	Rapid increase in head circumference (especially occipital-frontal diameter)
Older children	Headache
	Nausea, vomiting
	Change in level of consciousness
	Papilledema
	Diplopia
	Motor dysfunction (grasp, gait)
	Behavior changes, irritability
	Change in vital signs (elevated systolic BP, wide pulse pressure, decreased pulse and respirations)
	Seizures

Evaluation: Child ingests food and fluid given; has elastic skin turgor, moist mucous membranes.

Goal 3: Postoperatively, child will be free from complications.

Plan/Implementation
- measure head circumference daily
- position on unoperative side relative to appearance of fontanel: if fontanel normal, elevate head; if fontanel depressed, position child flat in bed
- turn at least q2h
- do frequent neuro checks (LOC, PERRLA)
- observe for signs of infection
- *pump shunt only with a physician's order,* to maintain patency (usually done when shunt valve is a bubble type)

Evaluation: Child's fontanels remain flat (no bulging or depression) with no further increase in head circumference; no signs of infection or pneumonia (e.g., elevated temperature, increased pulse rate, reddened area around operative site).

E. Spina Bifida
1. **General Information**
   a. Definition: congenital defect involving incomplete formation of vertebrae, often accompanied by herniation of parts of the central nervous system
      1) meningocele: herniation of sac containing spinal fluid and meninges
      2) meningomyelocele: herniated sac containing CSF, meninges and malformed portion of spinal cord and nerve roots (most serious type); sac may be covered by skin or a very thin, transparent tissue layer that tears easily and permits leakage of CSF
   b. Motor and Sensory Impairment: relative to level and extent of defect; usually involves sensorimotor deficits of lower extremities, bowel and bladder dysfunction, associated orthopedic anomalies, and often hydrocephalus
   c. Medical Treatment
      1) prenatal diagnosis: amniocentesis shows increased alpha-fetoprotein;

done when mother has a history of having a child with a neural tube defect
2) surgical intervention to close defect within 24–48 hours to decrease chance of infection and minimize nerve damage

2. Nursing Process

a. Assessment
1) condition of sac
2) motor and sensory impairment: flaccid or spastic paralysis, response to painful stimuli, lower-extremity movement
3) bladder and bowel function: dribbling of urine, leakage of stool
4) associated orthopedic anomalies: clubfoot, congenital dislocated hip
5) signs of infection (fever, irritability, lethargy)
6) signs of increased intracranial pressure (see table 5.15), increased head circumference (especially following surgery)

b. Goals, Plans/Implementation, and Evaluation

Goal 1: Child will be free from rupture of sac and infection.
Plan/Implementation
- position on side or prone
- use Bradford frame
- protect sac with sponge doughnut when holding infant
- apply moist sterile dressings as ordered
- observe for leakage of CSF from sac
- observe for signs of meningitis (e.g., fever, irritability, nuchal rigidity)
- meticulously cleanse diaper area to prevent contamination of sac or post-op wound site with urine/stool

Evaluation: Child shows no signs of local or systemic infection (e.g., reddened skin around site, elevated temperature); sac remains intact (preoperatively); wound is free from infection postoperatively; wound heals normally.

Goal 2: Child will maintain skin integrity (lifelong goal).
Plan/Implementation
- observe for reddened areas, breaks in skin
- change position frequently
- use sheepskin or water mattress
- massage pressure areas to promote circulation

Evaluation: Child's skin is intact, no reddened areas or pressure sores.

Goal 3: Child will experience love and physical contact.
Plan/Implementation
- talk to infant (use face to face position)
- touch, stroke child
- encourage parents to caress, stroke, and talk to infant (cannot be held pre-op or early post-op) to promote parent-infant attachment

Evaluation: Child receives physical and voice contact from staff and parents/family; parents caress and talk to infant.

Goal 4: Child will gain optimal bowel and bladder function (long-term goal).
Plan/Implementation
- empty bladder manually by applying gentle downward pressure (Credé method)
- provide diet with adequate fluids (those that acidify urine such as apple and cranberry juice) and fiber (as child grows older)
- teach parent (and child when older) to care for
  - intermittent catheterizations (self-catheterization)
  - indwelling Foley catheter
  - ileal conduit
- administer urinary antiseptics, stool softeners as prescribed

Evaluation: Child has adequate urinary output, has an established bowel routine; no signs of urinary tract infection.

Goal 5: Child will be free from lower extremity deformity.
Plan/Implementation
- provide passive ROM exercises
- keep hips abducted using blanket rolls
- provide physical therapy; fitting with braces (usually long leg braces) and crutches for ambulation as child grows older

Evaluation: Child has full ROM of joints, no contractures of hip or lower extremity.

F. Seizure Disorders

1. General Information
a. Definition: episode of uncontrolled, electrical activity in the brain; neuronal discharges become excessive and irregular

resulting in loss of consciousness, convulsive body movements, or disturbances in sensations or behavior
  b. Incidence: occur in 0.5% of all children; it has been estimated that 4%-6% of all children will experience one or more seizures by the time they reach adolescence
  c. Cause: possible causes include infection, tumors, trauma, acid/base imbalances, epilepsy, allergies, anoxia, and hypoglycemia
  d. Types of Seizures and Manifestations
     1) generalized seizures
        a) *grand mal:* sudden loss of consciousness followed by tonic phase (stiffening of body) and clonic phase (jerky movements of trunk and extremities); periods of depressed or apneic breathing may occur; child may fall asleep after the seizure or be confused and irritable
        b) *petit mal* (absence seizures): child appears to be daydreaming; all verbal and motor behavior stops; may occur 10 or more times/day; usually lasts 10–30 seconds; child usually alert after the seizures; no memory of episode
        c) *akinetic:* child experiences a sudden loss of body tone accompanied by loss of consciousness; lasts a few seconds; resumes ADL afterwards
        d) *infantile spasms:* similar to a startle reflex; involves jerking of the head and clonic movements of the extremities; usually disappear by 2–3 years of age; may develop into more generalized seizures; usually accompanied by other problems (e.g., mental retardation)
     2) partial seizures
        a) *Jacksonian:* twitching begins at distal end of extremity, eventually involving entire extremity and possibly entire side of the body; no loss of consciousness; not commonly seen in children
        b) *psychomotor:* characterized by altered state of consciousness (e.g., dreamlike); may chew, smack lips, mumble; lasts several minutes; child has no memory of behavior
     3) febrile seizures: transient disorder usually the result of an extracranial infection (e.g., otitis media); peak incidence between 6 months and 3 years of age; resemble grand mal seizures
     4) breathholding: usually benign; child begins to cry, holds his breath and experiences brief cyanosis with loss of consciousness; precipitating factors may be anger or frustration
  e. Diagnosis: complete and accurate history and physical; thorough description of the seizure including onset, time of day, type of seizure, precipitating factors; EEG necessary for evaluating the seizure disorder
  f. Medical Treatment: anticonvulsants to elevate the child's excitability threshold and prevent seizures (refer to reprint page 635 for commonly used anticonvulsant medications)

2. **Nursing Process**
   a. Assessment
      1) history of seizure activity, recent episodes, management
         a) preseizure behavior: aura, loss of consciousness
         b) seizure activity: tonic/clonic phase; inappropriate behavior; fecal or urinary incontinence during the seizure
         c) postseizure behavior: memory lapse, headache, instability, loss of consciousness, lethargy
      2) use of anticonvulsant medications, side effects
   b. Goals, Plans/Implementation and Evaluation

   Goal 1: Child will maintain adequate respiratory function and be free from injuries during the seizure.
   Plan/Implementation
   - gently lower the child to the floor (supine position) if he is standing or sitting
   - maintain a patent airway by hyperextending the neck and pulling the jaw slightly forward; turn the head to the side to facilitate drainage of mucus and saliva
   - have O₂ and suction available (if possible)
   - *do not place anything in the child's mouth;* in the past it was believed that a padded tongue blade prevented the

child from "swallowing" or biting his tongue; simply turning the child's head to the side accomplishes the same effect and diminishes trauma
- do not restrain child
- remove any toys or dangerous objects that might injure the child during a seizure; pad side rails if possible
- loosen tight or restrictive clothing
- observe the seizure carefully
  - preseizure activity: aura, incontinence
  - seizure activity: include onset and initial focus of seizure, duration, change in respirations, progression of movement through body, changes in neurologic status
  - postseizure activity: duration, status, behavior
- administer anticonvulsant medication as ordered

Evaluation: Child maintains adequate respiratory function; is free from injuries.

Goal 2: Child and family will learn how to cope with the long-term problems associated with seizure disorders.

Plan/Implementation
- encourage good health practices including adequate sleep, good nutritional habits, and exercise
- provide appropriate explanations concerning cause of seizure activity, actions of medications, importance of periodic reevaluation
- teach the importance of adhering to medication routine, common side effects, importance of periodic blood and urine studies, behavior changes that may occur as a result of anticonvulsant medication
- stress the importance of never discontinuing anticonvulsant medication abruptly
- instruct family concerning care of child during a seizure
- encourage child/family to discuss fears, anxieties concerning seizure disorder
- inform child/family about situations that might precipitate seizures
  - illness, fever, stress
  - occur more frequently during menses or as a result of alcohol ingestion
- insure child wears a Medic Alert bracelet
- provide information concerning vocational guidance and federal and state laws regarding limitations that might be imposed on the younger child or adolescent
- provide information concerning support groups in the community

Evaluation: Child functions independently regarding ADL; adheres to medical regimen; child and family discuss fears and anxieties concerning seizure disorder; become involved in support groups.

G. Bacterial Meningitis

1. **General Information**
   a. Definition and Cause: a syndrome caused by inflammation of the meninges of the brain and spinal cord
      1) two basic types: bacterial (*H-influenza, streptococcus pneumoniae*, or *Neisseria meningitidis* [meningococcus]); aseptic (viruses, parasites, fungi)
      2) may be preceded by otitis media, tonsillitis, or other URI
      3) characteristics
         a) initially presents with vomiting, fever, headache, and stiff neck
         b) cerebral edema (may be intensified by secretion of antidiuretic hormone [ADH])
         c) meningococcal form usually accompanied by petechial or purpura rash (extravasation of RBCs)
         d) long-term complications
            - blindness, deafness
            - mental retardation
            - hydrocephalus
            - cerebral palsy
            - seizure disorders
   b. Incidence: occurs more often in boys; age of peak incidence is late infancy and toddlerhood
   c. Medical Treatment
      1) diagnosis: lumbar puncture to examine CSF; usual findings
         a) elevated WBC
         b) decreased glucose
         c) elevated protein
         d) positive culture
      2) medications
         a) antibiotics (large doses given IV)
         b) anticonvulsants
         c) antipyretics
      3) IV fluids for adequate hydration

[Handwritten at top: Aspirin 1gr/yr. of life for children]

2. Nursing Process
a. Assessment
1) vital signs (for respiratory distress, fever, increased ICP [see table 5.15])
2) neurologic signs (LOC, pupil reaction, nuchal rigidity, signs of increased ICP)
3) Brudzinski's sign (pain on flexion of neck)
4) Kernig's sign (pain on knee extension while lifting knee from a supine position)
5) headache
6) vomiting
7) irritability, hyperesthesia
8) lethargy
9) altered behavior
10) seizure activity
11) opisthotonus *[handwritten: extension of neck]*

b. Goals, Plans/Implementation, and Evaluation

Goal 1: Child will be free from infecting organism; disease will not spread.
Plan/Implementation
- administer antibiotics as prescribed
- place in strict isolation (for at least 24 hours after initiation of antibiotic therapy)
- teach parents, others isolation procedures

Evaluation: Signs or symptoms of infecting organism abate (CSF returns to normal); disease does not spread to others.

Goal 2: Child will be free from complications and long-term sequelae.
Plan/Implementation
- minimize environmental stimuli (lights, noise) and movement to lessen possibility of seizures
- administer anticonvulsants as ordered
- elevate head of bed slightly (to decrease intracranial pressure)
- implement seizure and safety precautions, e.g., side rails up (padded)
- monitor for signs of complications (seizures, acute cerebral edema, cerebral herniation, subdural effusion)
- monitor for long-term sequelae: seizures, hydrocephalus, mental retardation, ataxia, hemiparesis, deafness

Evaluation: Child shows no signs of complications (e.g., seizure activity); resumes normal activities.

Goal 3: Child will maintain adequate hydration and nutrition.
Plan/Implementation
- maintain NPO during acute phase of illness
- administer IV fluids as ordered; restrain as needed to maintain infusion site
- carefully monitor I&O to prevent fluid overload (can increase intracranial pressure)
- advance diet as tolerated as child recovers

Evaluation: Child is adequately hydrated; is free from signs of fluid overload; receives adequate nourishment.

H. Otitis Media

1. General Information
a. Definition: middle ear infection; two types:
   1) *serous otitis media:* nonpurulent effusion of middle ear
   2) *suppurative otitis media (acute or chronic):* accumulation of viral or bacterial purulent exudate in middle ear
b. Incidence: one of the most common illnesses of infancy and early childhood
c. Medical Treatment
   1) diagnosis
      a) otoscopic exam
         - inflamed, bulging tympanic membrane (acute) or dull gray membrane (serous)
         - no visible landmarks or light reflex
      b) tympanometry (measures air pressure in auditory canal): decreased membrane mobility
   2) antibiotic therapy: ampicillin (may cause diarrhea; given q6h) or amoxicillin (more expensive but fewer side effects; given TID) 10–14 days
   3) surgical intervention: incision of membrane (myringotomy) and insertion of myringotomy tubes in cases of recurrent, chronic otitis media

2. Nursing Process
a. Assessment
1) *suppurative otitis*
   a) pain (infants may pull or hold ears)
   b) irritability
   c) high fever
   d) lymphadenopathy
   e) purulent discharge (indicates rupture of membrane)

- f) nasal congestion, cough
- g) anorexia, vomiting
- h) diarrhea
2) *serous otitis*
    - a) ear "fullness"
    - b) popping sensation when swallowing
    - c) conductive hearing loss

b. **Goals, Plans/Implementation, and Evaluation**

Goal 1: Child will be free from infecting organism and recurrence of infection.
Plan/Implementation
- teach parents to administer antibiotics as prescribed
- educate parents concerning importance of adhering to medication regimen for full course of therapy
- clean drainage from ear with cotton balls and water

Evaluation: Child shows no signs or symptoms of continuing infection (e.g., pulling at ears, fever); no discharge from ears; disease does not recur.

Goal 2: Child will receive comfort measures and be free from pain and fever.
Plan/Implementation
- monitor body temperature
- teach parents to administer antipyretic analgesics (acetaminophen or aspirin)
- control fever with tepid baths or sponging
- avoid foods that require chewing
- apply external heat (warm water bottle or heating pad)

Evaluation: Child is free from pain, able to play and sleep comfortably; child's temperature returns to normal.

Goal 3: Child will have no permanent hearing impairment.
Plan/Implementation
- monitor for signs of hearing loss (decreased attention and responsiveness)
- conduct audiometry screening at routine intervals
- refer child to appropriate resources if results are abnormal

Evaluation: Child has normal hearing.

I. Tonsillitis, Tonsillectomy and Adenoidectomy   T + A

1. General Information
a. Definition: the tonsils and adenoids are lymphoid tissue located in the nasopharynx; tonsils are larger in children than adults and serve as a filtering mechanism to protect the body from infection
1) *tonsillitis:* acute infection of the tonsils; may be viral or bacterial (beta hemolytic *Streptococcus* group A)
2) *tonsillectomy and adenoidectomy:* surgical excision of the tonsils and adenoids; preferably done after age 3 (because of danger of excessive bleeding and tonsillar regrowth)

b. Medical Treatment
1) acute tonsillitis: penicillin/erythromycin for beta hemolytic *Streptococcus* group A
    - a) oral form: 10 days
    - b) IM: long-acting penicillin such as long-acting Bicillin or Penicillin G Benzathine
2) chronic tonsillitis: tonsillectomy and adenoidectomy may be indicated

2. Nursing Process
a. Assessment
1) sore throat, difficulty swallowing
2) enlarged tonsils
    - a) erythema of pharynx associated with viral pharyngitis
    - b) white exudate on tonsils indicates bacterial pharyngitis
3) enlarged cervical lymph nodes
4) persistent cough
5) fever
6) impaired nasal breathing, adenitis
7) impaired taste and smell
8) possible otitis media caused by blocked eustachian tubes

b. **Goals, Plans/Implementation, and Evaluation**

Goal 1: Parents of child with tonsillitis will adhere to drug therapy; child will experience minimal discomfort.
Plan/Implementation
- teach parents to continue oral penicillin/erythromycin for 10 days
- observe for allergic response (e.g., rash, diarrhea)
- promote throat comfort with warm (not hot) saline gargles
- provide soft or liquid diet
- give analgesics, antipyretics prn as ordered

Evaluation: Parent gives child all medications as prescribed; child's throat discomfort diminishes; child is free from infected tonsils.

Goal 2: Postoperatively child will maintain a patent airway.
Plan/Implementation
- position child on side with knee on upper side flexed, or in prone position until alert and recovered from anesthetic
- observe for excessive swallowing, vomiting of fresh blood, restlessness
- check pharynx for visible signs of bleeding
- monitor BP, pulse, and respirations

Evaluation: Child breathes easily, maintains adequate oxygenation; early signs of hemorrhage are detected.

Goal 3: Child will maintain integrity of surgical site; will experience minimal pain/discomfort.
Plan/Implementation
- *pre-op*
  - obtain baseline blood values
  - bleeding time
  - clotting time
  - prothrombin time (PT)
  - partial thromboplastin time (PTT)
  - Hgb and Hct
  - report abnormalities to physician
- *post-op*
  - apply ice collar to neck to decrease pain
  - administer analgesics prn *[Tylenol drug of choice]*
  - provide nonirritating, cool liquids (e.g., ice chips, popsicles and, later, soft foods)
  - discourage crying and coughing (can irritate the surgical site)

Evaluation: Child's surgical site remains intact, child remains free from excessive bleeding or hemorrhage; child's throat discomfort stays at a tolerable level.

Goal 4: Parents can state specific home-care instructions.
Plan/Implementation
- limit child's activities for 1–2 weeks
- provide daily rest periods
- provide nonirritating foods to child for 1–2 weeks; no hot, citrus, spicy, or rough foods
- have child refrain from coughing, clearing throat, or gargling
- observe for delayed hemorrhage (5–10 days post-op) caused by infection or tissue sloughing during healing process

[more than 1 tsp bright red bleeding bring in to DR.]

Evaluation: Parents carry out (above) home care for child; child's surgical site heals with no complications; child resumes normal diet/activities 1–2 weeks postoperatively.

C. **Application of the Nursing Process to the Child with a Communicable Disease**
  1. **Assessment**
     a. Nursing History
        1) immunization history
        2) history of exposure to disease
        3) previous communicable diseases, how treated
        4) signs and symptoms of current illness
           a) alterations in skin sensation
           b) skin lesions
           c) pain or tenderness
           d) itching
           e) fever
     b. Physical Examination
        1) skin lesions: size, color, distribution (general, localized), configuration (single, clustered, diffuse, linear), type of lesion (macule, papule, vesicle, pustule, crust)
        2) description of infestation (lice, scabies, ringworm, pinworms)
     c. Diagnostic Tests
        1) microscopic exam of lesions
        2) culture of organism
  2. **General Nursing Goal, Plan/Implementation, and Evaluation**
     Goal: Child will be free from communicable disease (infection, infestation) and will not spread communicable diseases to others.
     Plan/Implementation
     - explain prescribed treatment to parents/child and encourage them to comply with therapy
     - prevent child's exposure to others during communicable period
     - identify contacts who may also require treatment

     Evaluation: Child is free from communicable disease; does not transmit disease to others.

Selected Health Problems: Communicable Diseases, Skin Infections, Infestations

A. **Communicable Diseases**
  1. **General Information**
     a. Definition: a disease caused by a specific agent or its toxic products, transmitted

by direct contact or indirectly through contaminated articles; the incidence of communicable disease has significantly decreased with availability and widespread use of immunizations
    b. Types of Immunity
        1) active: antibodies formed by the body as a result of having had the disease or through immunization
        2) passive: introduction of antibodies formed outside the body, such as by placental transfer, breast milk, or gamma globulin injection
    c. Medical Treatment
        1) prevent through immunization (refer to table 5.4)
        2) antibiotic therapy for scarlet fever
        3) rubella titer before pregnancy or during 1st trimester

2. **Nursing Process**
    a. Assessment
        1) prodromal period
            a) malaise
            b) anorexia
            c) coryza
            d) sore throat
            e) fever
            f) lymphadenopathy
            g) headache
        2) specific characteristics
            a) *chickenpox (varicella zoster)*: rash in four stages at one time (macules, papules, vesicles, crusts) predominantly on face, trunk, and proximal extremities; intense pruritus
            b) *mumps (parotitis)*: pain and swelling of parotid glands, opening of mouth and chewing painful; intolerance of rough or acidic foods and fluids; after puberty, sterility in males is major complication
            c) *German measles (rubella)*: blotchy papular rash covers entire body, lasting only a few days; greatest concern is teratogenic effect on fetus during 1st trimester of pregnancy
            d) *measles (rubeola)*: Koplik's spots (red spots with white centers) on buccal mucosa two days prior to maculopapular rash; conjunctivitis, laryngitis, and photophobia; exanthem appears first on head and then spreads to entire body
            e) *roseola (exanthema subitum)*: occurs primarily in children age 6 months to 2 years; high fever for 3-4 days; temperature returns to normal with onset of rosy-pink, macular rash; rash fades with pressure and lasts 1-2 days
            f) *scarlet fever*: caused by beta hemolytic *Streptococcus* group A; high fever, strawberry tongue, and red pinpoint rash, especially in skin folds; rheumatic fever or acute glomerulonephritis may follow
    b. Goals, Plans/Implementation, and Evaluation

    Goal 1: Child will ingest adequate food and fluids to meet nutritional needs.
    Plan/Implementation
    - avoid rough or acidic foods; offer bland foods
    - use colorful glasses, straws, liquids to enhance appetite
    - offer favorite foods and fluids (ice cream, pudding, gelatin)
    - advance from liquids to regular diet as tolerated

    Evaluation: Child has adequate daily intake; is free from dehydration; eats a soft diet of sufficient caloric content.

    Goal 2: Child will experience minimal discomfort.
    Plan/Implementation
    - give antipyretics for fever or discomfort (dose: 1 grain per year up to 10 years q4h prn)
    - bed rest until fever subsides
    - change bed linen and clothing daily
    - provide humidifier as needed
    - use tepid baths to relieve fever and itching; keep skin clean
    - apply calamine lotion for itching (wash off completely once a day to prevent maceration of skin)
    - keep fingernails short and clean; apply mittens if needed
    - dim lights if photophobia present
    - warm compresses/irrigations of saline to eyes (measles)
    - local applications of heat or cold to relieve parotid discomfort (mumps)

    Evaluation: Child is able to rest and sleep comfortably; fever and itching are kept at minimal levels.

    Goal 3: Child will be prepared for isolation, will not spread disease.

582 SECTION 5: NURSING CARE OF THE CHILD

Plan/Implementation
- explain reason for isolation to child and parents
- provide age-appropriate play
  - diversion
  - plan time to play with child
  - TV in room (except if photophobic)
- accept expressions of fear, anger, restlessness, boredom
- if child is hospitalized, use appropriate isolation procedures
  - strict isolation (diphtheria, congenital rubella)
  - respiratory isolation (chickenpox, measles, mumps, rubella, pertussis, scarlet fever)
- discontinue isolation as soon as period of communicability is over

Evaluation: Child accepts restrictions of isolation (stays in room); other cases of disease do not occur; engages in age-appropriate activities.

Goal 4: Child will be free from complications and long-term sequelae.

Plan/Implementation
- observe and report signs of encephalitis: headache, bizarre behavior changes, seizures, fever, muscle weakness
- observe and report signs of vision or hearing loss
- observe and report signs of respiratory or cardiac complications: pneumonia, laryngotracheitis, otitis media, rheumatic fever
- observe and report signs of orchitis (mumps)

Evaluation: Child is free from complications and long-term sequelae (e.g., neurologic disability, sensory impairment, sterility, cardiac damage).

B. Sexually Transmitted Diseases (STDs) — *INDICATE Sexual Abuse*

1. **General Information**
   a. Definition: a communicable disease transmitted by direct genital contact or sexual activity; STDs are the most prevalent communicable diseases in the US; majority of cases occur in adolescents and young adults; some STDs are contracted by newborn (*Candida* [thrush], herpes, gonorrheal conjunctivitis); STDs in infants and children usually indicate sexual abuse and should be investigated
   b. Cause (see table 5.16)
   c. Medical Treatment (see table 5.16)

Table 5.16 Sexually Transmitted Diseases

Causative Agent	Incidence	Assessment	Medical Treatment
Gonorrhea *Neisseria gonorrheae*	Most commonly reported communicable disease	Males: dysuria, frequency, purulent urethral discharge Females: purulent vaginal discharge; 60% asymptomatic Diagnosis: by gram stain or culture (Thayer-Martin medium) Complications if untreated: Males: prostatitis and epididymitis Females: pelvic inflammatory disease, infertility, arthritis	Penicillin or other antibiotics Probenicid may be given to delay excretion of penicillin. *↑ blood level + delay excretion*
Herpes *Herpesvirus hominus* type 2	300,000–500,000 new cases/year	Active lesions: painful vesicular lesions that ulcerate Signs and symptoms of systematic illness: fever, headache, and/or general adenopathy Diagnosis: isolation of virus in tissue culture; demonstration of multinucleated giant cells on microscopic exam	Viscous lidocaine to ease pain Keep lesions clean and dry • apply cornstarch • use warm air blower • wear loose clothing Females: dysuria may be eased by voiding in warm water. Acyclovir (Zovirax) may decrease duration of the initial or subsequent episodes, but doesn't prevent recurrences.

Table 5.16 Continued.

Causative Agent	Incidence	Assessment	Medical Treatment
Syphilis *Treponema pallidum*	Third most commonly reported communicable disease	Primary (3 weeks postexposure): classic chancre (painless, red, eroded lesions with indurated border at point of entry) Secondary (1–3 months postexposure): cutaneous, nonpruritic, diffuse lesions on face, trunk, and/or extremities Tertiary (10–30 years postexposure): cardiac and neurologic destruction Diagnosis: positive darkfield slide of organism; VDRL, RPR, or FTA	Penicillin
Nonspecific urethritis (nongonococcal urethritis) Over 50% caused by *Chlamydia trachomatis*	Accounts for more than half of the cases of urethritis	Frequency and mild pain on urination Diagnosis: identification of organism through culture	Tetracycline hydrochloride
Trichomoniasis *Trichomonas vaginalis*	May be the most frequently acquired sexually transmitted disease in the US	Symptoms range from none to frothy, greenish-grey vaginal discharge Diagnosis: microscopic identification of motile protozoan	Metronidazole (Flagyl)
Candidiasis *Candida albicans*	Overall incidence in US is unknown	Erythematous, edematous, pruritic vulva Thick, white, "cottage-cheese"-like discharge	Nystatin (Mycostatin) vaginal suppositories or cream; if this fails, clotrimazole 1% (Lotrimin)
Scabies *Sarcoptes scabiei*	Epidemic in US	Intense, nocturnal genital itching Diagnosis: microscopic examination of shave excision of lesion	1% gamma benzene hexachloride lotion (Kwell) *[handwritten: Neurotoxic; Apply when dry & cool]*

SOURCE: Adapted from McConnell, E. and Zimmerman, M. *Care of Patients with Urologic Problems*. Philadelphia: Lippincott, 1983:114–115. Used with permission.

2. **Nursing Process**
   a. Assessment (see table 5.16)
   b. Goals, Plan/Implementation, and Evaluation

   Goal 1: Client will participate in treatment of STD.
   Plan/Implementation
   - use a straightforward, nonjudgmental approach when taking nursing history
   - teach client signs, symptoms, and transmission mode of STD
   - teach prevention: avoid sexual contact with partner when infected; use of condom
   - reassure client of confidentiality of information and exam
   - provide clear, specific, written and oral explanations of medical treatment

   Evaluation: Client participates in treatment plan; is free from disease.

   Goal 2: Recurrence of client's infection will be prevented; client does not transmit disease to others.
   Plan/Implementation
   - counsel women of childbearing age concerning transmission of STD to newborn

- gonorrheal conjunctivitis (may cause blindness)
- neonatal herpes infection (may cause blindness, deafness, mental retardation, or may be fatal)
- congenital syphilis (passively transmitted through placenta)
- oral candidiasis (thrush)
- assist with identification and treatment of sexual contacts
- report cases of gonorrhea, syphilis to health department
- teach client how to reduce risk of reinfection

Evaluation: Client is free from disease recurrence; does not transmit disease to others.

Goal 3: Client will resolve feelings of embarrassment, shame, guilt, and negative self-worth resulting from diagnosis.

Plan/Implementation
- treat client with respect, dignity
- ensure confidentiality
- provide sexuality education to dispel myths and misinformation
- encourage client to express any feelings of shame, embarrassment, guilt, loss of esteem
- refer to self-help groups (herpes) in community as appropriate

Evaluation: Client resolves negative feelings about diagnosis; utilizes support group (when appropriate); client's confidentiality is protected.

C. Common Skin Infections and Infestations

1. **General Information**
   a. Definition: bacterial infections or insect infestation of the skin, hair, or scalp; common in preschoolers and school-age children whose close contact increases their susceptibility
   b. Cause (see table 5.17)
   c. Medical Treatment (see table 5.17)

2. **Nursing Process** (see table 5.17)

D. Pinworms (Helminths)

1. **General Information**
   a. Definition: parasitic infestation primarily of the intestinal tract; worms deposit eggs in anal area causing severe itching; eggs attach to child's fingers causing reinfection when fingers are put in mouth

   b. Medical Treatment
   1) stool for ova and parasites
   2) cellophane-tape test
   3) antihelminth
      a) pyrvinium pamoate (Povan), single dose 5 mg/kg; stools turn red
      b) piperazine citrate 65 mg/kg daily for 3 days
   4) visual examination of infestation in early A.M.

2. **Nursing Process**
   a. Assessment
   1) intense anal itching (worsens at night)
   2) vaginitis
   3) irritability/restlessness
   4) night waking
   b. Goal, Plan/Implementation, and Evaluation

Goal: Child will be free from infestation, will not reinfest self.

Plan/Implementation
- identify other family members and close contacts who may also need treatment
- teach good handwashing and personal hygiene (after toileting and before eating)
- wear tight-fitting diapers or panties
- change and launder underwear, pajamas, and bed linens daily
- have child sleep alone
- wear mitts or socks to prevent scratching
- carry out proper disposal of feces
- ensure parents understand importance of carrying out these measures

Evaluation: Child is free from infestation; does not reinfest self or transmit it to others; parent establishes adequate sanitation.

D. Application of the Nursing Process to the Child with an Interference with Safety
See Selected Health Problems Below

Selected Health Problems: Interference with Safety

A. Poisonous Ingestions

1. **General Information**
   a. Definition: the swallowing of common non-nutritive materials that can cause health problems and/or poisoning. Common ingested substances: lead, corrosives, hydrocarbons, aspirin, acetaminophen, sedatives/hypnotics
   b. Incidence: poisonous ingestions are the 5th leading cause of death between

Table 5.17 Common Skin Infections and Infestations

Cause	Assessment	Medical Treatment	Plan/Implementation
Impetigo contagiosa: superficial bacterial skin infection			
Staphylococcus, Streptococcus	Vesicles that rupture to form honey-colored crusts; erupt most often on face, axillae, and extremities; highly contagious	Removal of crusts with Burow's solution. Topical bacteriocidal ointment (Neosporin). Penicillin in severe cases.	Teach child/parent how to soften and remove crusts, apply antibiotic ointment. Teach administration of oral antibiotics (penicillin/erythromycin). Prevent scratching by keeping nails clipped, using mitts or elbow restraints as necessary. Teach child to use own towels, washcloths until lesions heal.
Lice (pediculosis): parasitic infestation of head (capitis), body (corporis), or pubic area (pubis)			
Pediculus humanus	Ova (nits) on hair shafts. Itching, skin excoriation. Enlarged lymph nodes	Kwell (gamma benzene) shampoo or lotion. A-200 Pyrinate. RID.	Teach parents how to apply prescribed shampoo or lotion; caution against overuse (neurotoxicity). May need to cut long hair. Use fine-tooth comb dipped in vinegar to remove nits. Discard contaminated combs and brushes. Teach children not to exchange such personal items as towels, combs and brushes, hats. Launder bed linens, towels. Use gamma benzene spray on upholstered furniture.
Ringworm (tinea): superficial fungal infection of head (capitis), body (corporis), "jock itch" (cruris), "athlete's foot" (pedis)			
Various fungi	Scaly, circumscribed patches. Areas of patchy hair loss. Itching. Green concentric ring under Wood's light (ultraviolet) illumination. Positive culture	Oral griseofulvin: 20 mg/kg/day for 7–14 days. Local antifungal preparations • Whitfield's ointment • tolnaftate (Tinactin).	*Capitis* Teach parents how to administer oral and local antifungal agents. Shampoo frequently, using clean towels, combs, brushes. Keep child's hair short. *Corporis and cruris* Avoid wearing nylon underwear and tight-fitting clothes. Keep affected areas clean and dry. Identify and treat source (often from household pets). *Pedis* Wear clean, light, cotton socks. Wear well-ventilated shoes. Apply topical antifungal powder containing tolnaftate. Avoid bare feet in public places (such as school gym) until infection has cleared.

586 SECTION 5: NURSING CARE OF THE CHILD

  1 and 4 years of age; peak incidence is toddler years

c. Cause: incorrect storage of potentially toxic substances

d. Aim of treatment is to remove ingested toxic substance from body or to neutralize its effects as quickly as possible

e. Vomiting, or use of an emetic, is contraindicated when
  1) child is comatose, convulsing, or in severe shock (increases risk of aspiration)
  2) substance is a hydrocarbon (aspiration may cause a chemical pneumonia) *[gasoline, kerosine]*
  3) substance is a corrosive (acid or alkali) (emesis may further damage or perforate esophageal mucosa); see table 5.18 for general information, treatment, and assessment of specific ingestions *[bathroom cleaner]*

2. Nursing Process
   a. Assessment (see table 5.18)
   b. Goals, Plans/Implementation, and Evaluation (for all ingestions)

Goal 1: Child will receive emergency treatment for acute poisonous ingestion.
Plan/Implementation
- instruct parent to contact poison control center (provide telephone number) or take child to nearest emergency facility
- instruct to induce vomiting (if appropriate) by stimulating gag reflex and giving syrup of ipecac
- position child to avoid aspiration when vomiting
- tell parent to keep original container label for determining antidote
- analyze ingested substance, child's output
  - bring in container and any remaining substance

Table 5.18 Commonly Ingested Poisonous Substances

General Information	Nursing Assessment	Medical Treatment
Aspirin (salicylate poisoning)		
Most common cause of childhood poisoning. Toxic dose: 2 grains/lb body weight. Lethal dose: 3–4 grains/lb. Effects: stimulates respiratory center → respiratory alkalosis; increases metabolism → fever, metabolic acidosis (from high level of ketones)	GI effects • vomiting • thirst CNS effects • hyperventilation • confusion, dizziness • staggered gait • coma Hematopoietic effects • bleeding tendencies Metabolic effects • sweating • hyponatremia • hypokalemia • dehydration • hypoglycemia	Induce vomiting with syrup of ipecac • 6–12 months of age: 10 ml (2 tsp) and as much water as possible • over 1 year: 15 ml (1 tbsp) and 2–3 glasses of water. Gastric lavage. IV fluids, sodium bicarbonate (enhances excretion), electrolytes. Vitamin K for hypoprothrombinemia. Glucose for hypoglycemia. Diuretics: acetazolamide (Diamox). Dialysis when potentially lethal doses have been ingested.
Acetaminophen (Tylenol)		
Toxic dose: uncertain, do not exceed recommended levels. Effects: cellular necrosis of the liver resulting in liver dysfunction and, in some cases, hepatic failure	First stage (first 24 hours) • nausea • vomiting • sweating • pallor or cyanosis • weakness Second stage (24–48 hours) • SGOT, SGPT elevated • liver tenderness (RUQ) • prolonged prothrombin time Third stage (1 week) • liver necrosis • hepatic failure • possible death	Induce vomiting or gastric lavage (see aspirin). Acetylcysteine (Mucomyst) as an antidote, given PO with fruit juice or Cola, or via NG tube (offensive odor). IV fluids. Sodium-restricted, high calorie, high protein diet.

Table 5.18 Continued.

General Information	Nursing Assessment	Medical Treatment
Corrosives (lye, bleach, ammonia)		
Extent of damage depends on the causticity of the substance and the amount ingested	Grossly visible whitish burns of mouth and pharynx; color darkens as ulcerations form Edema Respiratory distress Difficulty swallowing Excess drooling Severe pain Shock	DO NOT INDUCE VOMITING. Dilute with small amounts of water. Tracheostomy if respiratory distress is severe. IV fluids while child is NPO. Analgesics, steroids, antibiotics, antacids. Possible gastrostomy. Possible esophageal dilatations to prevent strictures (or maintain patency of esophagus). Colon transplant if esophageal damage is severe (done when child is older).
Hydrocarbons (gasoline, kerosene, turpentine, mineral seal oil)		
Immediate concern is aspiration, which can cause severe (or fatal) chemical pneumonitis. Systemic effects from GI absorption of hydrocarbons are relatively mild.	Burning sensation in mouth and throat Characteristic breath odor Nausea, anorexia, vomiting Lethargy Fever	DO NOT INDUCE VOMITING. Supportive measures for respiratory effects, pneumonitis (O$_2$, antibiotics, IV fluids).
Lead (chronic poisoning)		
Approximately 4% of children under age 6 years have excessive lead levels in their blood; peak age is 2–3 years; black children have 6 times greater risk.	Hematopoietic effects • anemia CNS effects • irritability • lethargy • hyperactivity • developmental delays • clumsiness • seizures • disorientation • coma, possible death GI effects • anorexia • nausea, vomiting • constipation • lead line along gums Skeletal effects • increased density of long bones • lead lines in long bones Renal effects • glycosuria • proteinuria • possible acute or chronic renal failure	Remove child from lead source, hospitalize. Chelating agents: EDTA usually used in combination with BAL; given IM q4h for 5 days (causes lead to be deposited in bone and excreted via kidneys). Calcium, phosphorus, vitamin D to aid lead excretion. Anticonvulsants for seizure control. Oral or IM iron for anemia. Follow-up lead levels to monitor progress (lead is excreted more slowly than it accumulates in the body).

- bring in any vomitus or urine output since ingestion
• make appropriate referrals, e.g., social service

Evaluation: Parent institutes correct emergency care of child; child receives indicated follow-up care.

Goal 2: Child will maintain adequate oxygenation; ingestion will be recognized and treated early to prevent complications.

Plan/Implementation
• report difficulty breathing or swallowing *STAT*; may require a tracheotomy; keep

laryngoscope, endotracheal tube, and tracheotomy tray at bedside
- assess color of skin, nail beds, and mucous membranes
- monitor vital and neuro signs at least q15min until stable and as indicated
- administer O₂ therapy as ordered
- observe for seizure activity
- if breathing is labored, stay with child until it eases, to reduce anxieties
- observe for response to medications

Evaluation: Child breathes easily; has adequate oxygenation; no respiratory distress; is oriented to time, place, person.

Goal 3: Child will be free from severe pain and shock.
Plan/Implementation
- administer analgesics as ordered
- soothe child with gentle touching and soft voice
- check vital signs frequently until stable
- offer clear liquids in small amounts (if child is able to swallow); observe for nausea, ability to swallow
- do not induce vomiting following ingestion of hydrocarbons or corrosives

Evaluation: Child experiences minimal or no pain; vital signs are stabilized.

Goal 4: Child will be free from injury and kept safe during acute phase following ingestion.
Plan/Implementation
- give physical support when the child is vomiting
- institute seizure precautions
- record I&O accurately
- monitor urine output (EDTA is potentially toxic to kidneys)
- prepare child for painful injections (EDTA and BAL); mix with local anesthetic (Procaine HCl); rotate injection sites IV avail.
- increase fluid intake to 1-2 times maintenance (aspirin)
- check vital signs frequently until stable
- if child confused, provide safety measures as appropriate

Evaluation: Child returns to normal activities with no residual effects; is free from acquired injuries; fluid intake is 1-2 times child's usual.

Goal 5: Child will maintain normal fluid-electrolyte and acid-base balance.

Plan/Implementation
- observe and report signs of respiratory alkalosis (deep and rapid breathing, light-headedness, tetany, convulsions, coma)
- observe and report signs of metabolic acidosis (deep breathing, short of breath, disorientation, coma)
- observe and report signs of metabolic alkalosis (depressed respirations, hypertonicity, tetany)
- observe and report signs of hypokalemia: malaise, thirst, polyuria, cardiac dysrhythmias, decreased BP, thready pulse, depressed reflexes
- observe and report signs of hypo/hyperglycemia

Evaluation: Child maintains normal fluid-electrolyte and acid-base balance.

Goal 6: Child will maintain normal body temperature. 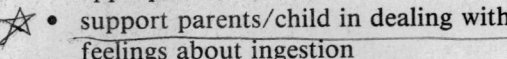 hyperthermia → hydrocarbons Aspirin
Plan/Implementation
- record temperature q2h and prn
- sponge bathe with tepid water
- use cooling blanket if sponging is insufficient to reduce fever

Evaluation: Child maintains body temperature within normal limits.

Goal 7: Parent will take steps to prevent recurrences.
Plan/Implementation
- teach the essentials of prevention
  - do not place substances in unmarked containers
  - keep harmful substances out of child's reach, in locked cabinets
  - teach child that medication is not candy
  - emphasize poisonous quality of abused over-the-counter drugs
- provide adequate supervision of the child
- provide love and attention to child
- observe child for pica
- obtain continued medical care as appropriate
- support parents/child in dealing with feelings about ingestion

Evaluation: Parent modifies home environment to prevent recurrence of ingestion.

B. Burns

1. **General Information**
   a. Definition: tissue damage that results from thermal, chemical, electrical, or radioactive agents (see table 5.19)
   b. Incidence
      1) third leading cause of accidental injury and death in children
      2) over 50% of burns occur in children 5 years of age and younger
      3) thermal burns are most common
   c. Classification
      1) percentage of body surface burned
         a) rule of nines (adults) (see figure 5.3)
         b) modified rule of nines (children) (see figure 5.3)
      2) degree of damage (depth of burn injury)
         a) 1st degree: superficial partial thickness; pain, redness, no tissue or nerve damage, superficial epidermis affected

Table 5.19 Systemic Responses to Burn Injury

Fluid and Electrolyte Changes	Increased capillary permeability results in shift of water, protein, and electrolytes from intravascular to interstitial spaces • severe edema of burned tissues with mild to moderate surrounding edema (greatest in first 48 hours) • sodium and potassium are exchanged (sodium enters cells; potassium enters intravascular [circulatory] compartment) • fluid is lost from burned surface, especially in first 3–4 days postburn • decreased renal blood flow leads to decreased urine output (impaired glomerular filtration); acute renal failure may develop if fluid replacement is not adequate
Circulatory Changes	• reduced blood flow to burned area caused by thrombosis of vessels • *burn shock:* decreased cardiac output, decreased circulating blood volume (in proportion to severity of burn injury) • capillary permeability returns to normal within 48 hours; fluid is reabsorbed primarily via lymphatic system • anemia results from RBC destruction, blood loss (initially and during debridement/excision)

Metabolic Changes	• increase in metabolic rate
	• stress of burn injury causes
	  – glycogen breakdown leading to depletion of energy stores within 24 hours postburn, followed by glyconeogenesis (breakdown of protein stores)
	  – negative nitrogen balance (elevated BUN and urine urea nitrogen)
	  – increased blood glucose levels
	• elevated aldosterone and antidiuretic hormone (ADH) levels
	• metabolic acidosis (often compensated for by respiratory alkalosis)

Complications of Burn Injury	• respiratory problems: inhalation injury, aspiration, bacterial pneumonia, pulmonary edema • wound infection (usually occurs within 3–5 days postburn; most often caused by gram-negative organisms, especially *Pseudomonas*) • Curling's ulcer (gastric or duodenal stress ulcer) • paralytic ileus (most common when burned surface is greater than 20%) • arterial hypertension • CNS disturbances: disorientation, personality changes, seizures (especially in burned children), coma

Figure 5.3 Estimation of Burn Surface Area

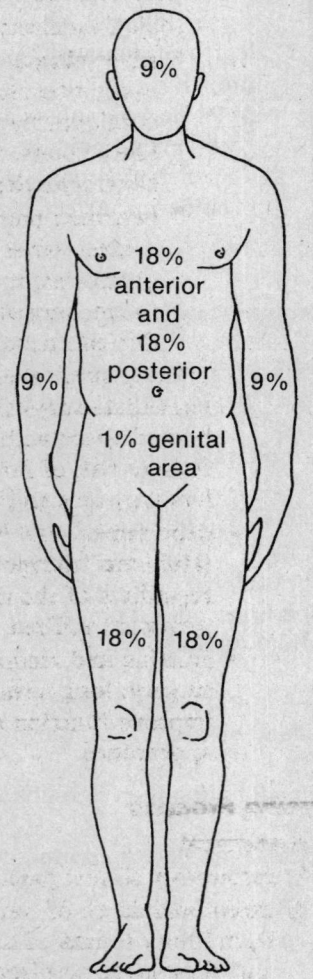

a) Over 12 years: Rule of Nines (see figure at left)

b) Under 12 years: Modified Rule of Nines

Head and neck	9% *plus* 1% for each year under age 12 years
Each arm	9%
Trunk	36%
Each leg	18% *minus* ½% for each year under age 12 years
Genital area	1%

Percentages include anterior and posterior aspects, except for genital area.

---

b) 2nd degree: deep-dermal partial thickness; pain, pale-to-red edematous skin, vesicles, entire affected area of epidermis and varying amounts of dermis affected
c) 3rd degree: full thickness; painless; skin white, red, or black; edematous; bullae; nerves, epidermis, dermis destroyed; subcutaneous adipose tissue, fascia, muscle and bone may also be destroyed or damaged

d. Medical Treatment (Moderate to Severe Burns)
  1) medical intervention
    a) immediate emergency care
      • extinguish burn
      • slowly immerse burn injury in cool water if possible (relieves pain, inhibits edema formation, slows tissue damage)
      • do *not* use ice water, ice packs, or topical ointments *[will macerate the tissue]*
      • cover burn with clean cloth

[handwritten at top: 1/2 1st 24° fluid replace given 1st 8° then rest given over 16°]

SAFETY AND SECURITY 591

- cover with blankets (uninvolved areas) if child is hypothermic
- remove constrictive clothing and jewelry before swelling occurs
- if child is alert and oriented, provide warm liquids
- transport to nearest medical facility if burn is extensive

b) admission care
- establish airway (O_2, intubation if laryngeal edema is a risk)
- *frequently* assess blood gases
- initiate fluid and electrolyte therapy
  - first 24 hours: crystalloid solutions, such as normal saline or Ringer's lactate
  - following diuresis, colloid solutions such as albumin or plasma
- assess other injuries
- insert urinary indwelling catheter for accurate assessment of urinary output
- insert NG tube to prevent vomiting, abdominal distention, or gastric aspiration
- administer IV pain medication as ordered
- administer antibiotics (penicillin or erythromycin) to prevent infection (broad-spectrum antibiotics are not used because of possibility of superimposed infections)
- immunize with tetanus toxoid (according to recommended schedule)

c) care of burn wounds
- open method: reverse isolation
  - burn exposed to air; crust or eschar forms a protective barrier
  - topical medication
    * mafenide acetate (Sulfamylon): penetrates wound rapidly, is painful, causes mild acidosis
    * silver sulfadiazine (Silvadene): penetrates wound slowly; is soothing, causes no acid-base complications, keeps eschar soft; debridement easier

- closed method
  - burn covered with nonadherent fine-mesh gauze and fluffed-gauze outer layer covered by stretch gauze bandages
  - topical medication
    * silver nitrate: reduces evaporative loss, must be continuously wet, causes black stains, may cause electrolyte depletion
    * betadine: painful, effective against variety of infectious organisms; may cause toughening of eschar and difficult debridement
- primary surgical excision: immediate surgical excision of burned tissue with grafting; reduces risk of infection; blood loss may be significant
- debridement and hydrotherapy (Hubbard whirlpool tank): done regardless of the method of treatment utilized
- grafting and reconstructive surgery: long-term treatment; to improve function and cosmetic appearance

2. Nursing Process
   a. Assessment
      1) respiratory status: patency of airway
      2) extent and depth of burn, location of burn injury (burns of head, neck, and chest areas predispose child to respiratory distress)
      3) pulse, blood pressure, urine output (for early signs of neurogenic, cardiogenic, or hypovolemic shock)
      4) presence of pain (often manifested in children by irritability, depression, hostility, or aggression)
      5) signs and symptoms of hemorrhage (decreased BP; rapid, thready pulse; diaphoresis; pallor; decreased body temperature)
      6) laboratory findings
         a) hematocrit, arterial blood gases *[handwritten: anemia]*
         b) sodium↓, chloride↓, potassium, CO_2
         c) BUN, creatinine↑
         d) serum protein↓
         e) urine pH, specific gravity↑

7) child's and parent's emotional responses to burn injury
b. **Goals, Plans/Implementation, and Evaluation**

Goal 1: Child will maintain adequate oxygenation.
Plan/Implementation
- observe for respiratory distress (wheezing, rales, dyspnea, increased rate, nasal flaring, stridor, air hunger)
- monitor arterial blood gases
- carefully monitor intubated child who is assisted by a respirator; humidified O_2 as ordered
- suction qh or prn
- prevent aspiration: maintain patency of nasogastric tube
- turn, cough, deep breathe; use inspirometer (to prevent hypostatic pneumonia)
- check eschar on neck and chest for constriction

Evaluation: Child is free from respiratory distress; maintains adequate oxygenation.

Goal 2: Child will be monitored for signs and symptoms of shock.
Plan/Implementation
- monitor vital signs qh and prn
- monitor I&O hourly (20–30 ml/hour) for child over 2 years; (10–20) ml/hour for child under 2 years
- observe for signs of hemorrhage (bleeding; decreased BP; decreased body temperature; rapid, thready pulse)

Evaluation: Child is free from shock, maintains adequate circulatory volume.

Goal 3: Child regains and maintains fluid and electrolyte balance.
Plan/Implementation
- observe for signs of dehydration (thirst, dry tongue, decreased urinary output, decreased BP, tachycardia, poor skin turgor)
- monitor urine output
- measure and record urine specific gravity and pH
- monitor IV therapy (*NOTE:* check for adequate renal function prior to adding potassium to IV)
- observe for signs of fluid overload (venous distention, increased BP, short of breath, rales)
- observe for signs of electrolyte imbalance (cardiac dysrhythmias, tingling of fingers, abdominal cramps, convulsions, spasms)

Evaluation: Child's fluid and electrolyte balance is restored (e.g., no signs of metabolic acidosis, hyperkalemia, hyponatremia).

Goal 4: Child will be free from pain or have it adequately controlled.
Plan/Implementation
- administer analgesics as ordered
- utilize comfort measures (e.g., pillows)
- teach child to change focus to music, TV, friends

Evaluation: Child experiences no more than minimal pain or discomfort; copes successfully with painful experiences (e.g., dressing changes).

Goal 5: Child will be free from infection.
Plan/Implementation
- maintain reverse isolation as ordered
- administer antibiotics and tetanus prophylaxis as ordered
- utilize sterile technique with wound care
- observe for and report signs of wound infection (temperature elevation, redness at wound edge, purulent or green-grey drainage, offensive odor)
- observe for and report signs of systemic infection (increased body temperature, chills, tachycardia, hyperemec)
- observe for and report signs of respiratory infection (increased body temperature, signs of respiratory distress)

Evaluation: Child is free from signs of infection (e.g., elevated temperature, offensive wound odor, etc.).

Goal 6: Child will maintain adequate nutritional intake to prevent nitrogen loss and GI complications.
Plan/Implementation
- provide a high protein, high calorie diet; determine special likes/dislikes
- offer small frequent meals
- assess bowel sounds for possible paralytic ileus (early postburn period)
- observe for signs of Curling's ulcer (coffee ground emesis, abdominal distention, anemia); usually occurs during the 3rd–4th week postburn in children (first week postburn in adults)
- give supplemental vitamins and minerals (vitamins A, B, and C; iron and zinc) antacids as ordered

Evaluation: Child ingests therapeutic diet as ordered; is free from gastrointestinal complications.

Goal 7: Child will have optimal wound healing.
Plan/Implementation
- handle wound carefully, to prevent damage to healing tissues
- keep child from picking at wound
- do not change donor site dressings (prevents tearing of underlying delicate epithelium)
- utilize sterile technique with wound care

Evaluation: Child does not scratch healing tissue; wounds heal without complications.

Goal 8: Child will regain/maintain maximal function of joints.
Plan/Implementation
- position to avoid contractures; use splints with involved joints
- assist with range-of-motion (ROM) exercises as ordered
- encourage ambulation when appropriate
- encourage child's participation in self-care and activities of daily living
- provide explanations to child and family for positioning requirements

Evaluation: Child has full (or increasing) ROM of affected/nonaffected joints; has no footdrop, contractures.

Goal 9: Child will verbalize concerns and feelings about altered body image.
Plan/Implementation
- assess child's/parent's adjustment to altered body image (child's verbalizations and nonverbal behavior)
- spend time listening to concerns and feelings
- utilize play therapy
- offer preprocedure preparation according to age
- utilize visual, auditory, and tactile stimulation
- problem solve with use of elastic bandages, camouflage clothes, and use of makeup to enhance appearance
- refer to support groups

Evaluation: Child talks about effect of burns on body; asks questions about what others will think of his body; participates in activities appropriate for age and personal interest.

References

Adams, J. et al. "Diagnosing and Treating Otitis Media with Effusion." *MCN: American Journal of Maternal-Child Nursing.* January/February 1984: 22–28.

*Coughlin, M. "Teaching Children About Their Seizures and Medications." *MCN: American Journal of Maternal-Child Nursing.* May/June 1979:161–162.

Fleming, J. "Common Dermatologic Conditions in Children." *MCN: American Journal of Maternal-Child Nursing.* September/October 1981:346–354.

Ford, P. "Management of Pediatric Poisoning." *Pediatric Nursing.* September/October 1980:35–36.

*Jackson, P. "Ventriculo-Peritoneal Shunts." *American Journal of Nursing.* June 1980:1104–1109.

Keim, K. "Preventing and Treating Plant Poisonings in Young Children." *MCN: American Journal of Maternal-Child Nursing.* July/August 1983: 280–286.

Killam, P. et al. "Behavioral Pediatric Weight Rehabilitation for Children with Myelomeningocele." *MCN: American Journal of Maternal-Child Nursing.* July/August 1983: 280–286.

*Meier, E. "Evaluating Head Trauma in Infants and Children." *MCN: American Journal of Maternal-Child Nursing.* January/February 1983:54–57.

†Muehl, J. "Seizure Disorders in Children: Prevention and Care." *MCN: American Journal of Maternal-Child Nursing.* May/June 1979:154–162.

Sataloff, R. and Colton, C. "Otitis Media: A Common Childhood Infection." *American Journal of Nursing.* August 1981:1480–1483.

Surveyer, J. and Halpern, J. "Age-related Burn Injuries and Their Prevention." *Pediatric Nursing.* September/October 1981:29–34.

Tudor, M. "Nursing Intervention with Developmentally Disabled Children." *MCN: American Journal of Maternal-Child Nursing.* January/February 1978: 25–31.

Vigliaroto, D. "Managing Bowel Incontinence in Children." *American Journal of Nursing.* January 1980:105–107.

Waechter, E., Phillips, J., Holoday, B. *Nursing Care of Children*, 10th Ed. Philadelphia: Lippincott, 1985.

Whaley, L. and Wong, D. *Nursing Care of Infants and Children*, 2nd Ed. St. Louis: Mosby, 1983.

†White, J. "Special Needs of Hospitalized Children with Learning Disabilities." *MCN: American Journal of Maternal-Child Nursing.* November/December 1983: 209–212.

Wieczorek, R. and Natapoff, J. *A Conceptual Approach to the Nursing of Children.* Philadelphia: Lippincott, 1981.

Young, R. "Chronic Sorrow: Parents' Response to the Birth of a Child with a Defect." *MCN: American Journal of Maternal–Child Nursing.* January/February 1977: 38–42.

* See Reprint section
† Highly recommended

Activity and Rest

General Concepts
A. Overview
1. Skeletal Maturation
   a. Accurate "bone age" is determined by x-ray of ossification centers
   b. Correlates closely with other measures of physiologic maturity (e.g., onset of menarche) rather than with height or chronologic age
   c. Complete when epiphysis fuses completely with diaphysis, usually 18–21 years of age (earlier in girls than boys)
2. Differences in Children's Skeletal System Compared with the Adults'
   a. Thick periosteum: stronger, more active osteogenic potential
   b. More plastic (pliable) bone: more porous, allows bending and buckling; this flexibility diffuses and absorbs a significant amount of the force of impact
   c. Rapid healing: decreases as child gets older (younger bones can be remolded more easily)
   d. Stiffness is unusual, even after lengthy immobilization

B. Application of the Nursing Process to the Child with Interferences with Activity and Rest
1. Assessment
   a. Nursing History
      1) development of motor skills: delays, recent changes or interferences
      2) signs and symptoms of current health problem: pain, altered structure or mobility
   b. Physical Examination
      1) muscle strength and symmetry
      2) balance, gait, and posture
      3) range-of-motion
      4) obvious structural deformities or functional deficits

2. General Nursing Goals, Plans/Implementation, and Evaluation

Goal 1: Child's deformity will be detected and treated early.
Plan/Implementation
- screen child for skeletal deformity
  - in newborn period for congenital clubfoot and congenital hip dysplasia
  - during preadolescence and adolescence for scoliosis
- refer child with possible deformity for immediate treatment
- teach child/parents the importance of adhering to prescribed treatment plan to minimize or prevent serious, permanent deformity
- stress importance of continued follow-up care to prevent recurrence

Evaluation: Child's deformity is detected and treated early; permanent deformity is prevented.

Goal 2: Child will maintain correct alignment of the affected body part during the period of treatment.
Plan/Implementation
- teach child/parents prescribed exercises, application of splints or brace, cast care
- provide care for child in traction (see table 5.20, figure 5.4)
  - maintain traction apparatus (elastic bandages, splints, rings, ropes, pulleys, weights)
  - do *NOT* allow weights to rest on floor
  - maintain correct body alignment
  - elevate head or foot of bed as needed to provide correct pull and countertraction
- provide care for child in cast
  - use palms of hands when handling wet cast

Table 5.20 Types of Traction

General

Skin traction	Direct pull to skin surface and indirect pull to skeletal structures by means of adhesive strips or elastic bandage
Skeletal traction	Direct pull to skeletal structures by means of pin, wire, or tongs inserted into bone distal to fracture

Specific

Bryant's traction	Unidirectional, lower extremity skin traction with child's hips flexed at 90° angle, knees extended, and legs and buttocks suspended
Buck's extension	Skin traction to lower extremity with hips and legs extended. Used mostly when short-term traction is needed
Russell traction	Two-directional, lower extremity skin traction with padded knee sling; immobilizes hip and knee in flexed position. One pull line is longitudinal; the other is perpendicular to leg. Traction pull is twice the amount of weight applied.
Balance suspension with Thomas ring splint and Pearson attachment	Two-directional, skin or skeletal traction that suspends leg with hip slightly flexed; Thomas ring circles uppermost portion of the thigh while Pearson attachment supports lower part of leg. Alignment is maintained even when child lifts off bed.
Halo-femoral traction	Metal rings (halo) are attached to the skull and pins are inserted into distal femur also. Progressive traction is applied upward to the halo and downward to the distal end of the femur, increasing weights twice daily until alignment is achieved.

- keep cast elevated and exposed to air to dry
- "petal" cast edges (protects cast and skin); use waterproof adhesive tape petals (see figure 5.5)
- protect cast from being soiled with urine or stool (position child with buttocks lower than shoulders during toileting)
- use Bradford frame for smaller children
- provide toys too large to fit down cast
- stay with child during mealtimes
- observe for signs of impaired circulation and infection (fever, lethargy, foul odor), do *NOT* rely on child to verbalize discomfort; change position frequently; do *NOT* use abduction-stabilizer bar on hip spica as a handle for turning child

Evaluation: Child maintains correct alignment of affected body part; permanent deformity is prevented; child/parents provide appropriate care of child in cast, splint, or brace; child has no infection or impairment of circulation.

Goal 3: Child's skin integrity will be maintained during period of immobilization.
Plan/Implementation
- assess for areas of skin breakdown
- change position frequently or encourage movement within limitations imposed by traction, cast, or brace to relieve pressure
- check pin sites (skeletal traction) for bleeding, redness, edema, infection
- provide pin care as needed
- monitor circulation of affected extremities (normal skin color, blanches easily, warm to touch, able to wiggle fingers and toes, peripheral pulses present)
- give meticulous skin care to areas near edges of cast or in contact with brace or traction apparatus

Evaluation: Child's skin integrity is maintained; circulation is maintained; child is free from skin breakdown.

Figure 5.4 Types of Traction

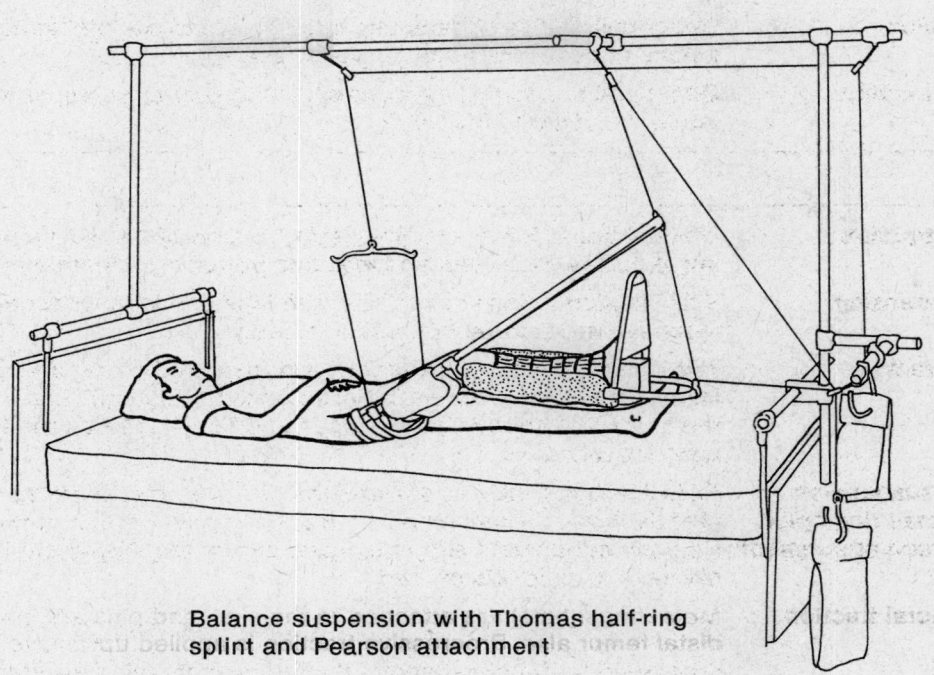

Balance suspension with Thomas half-ring splint and Pearson attachment

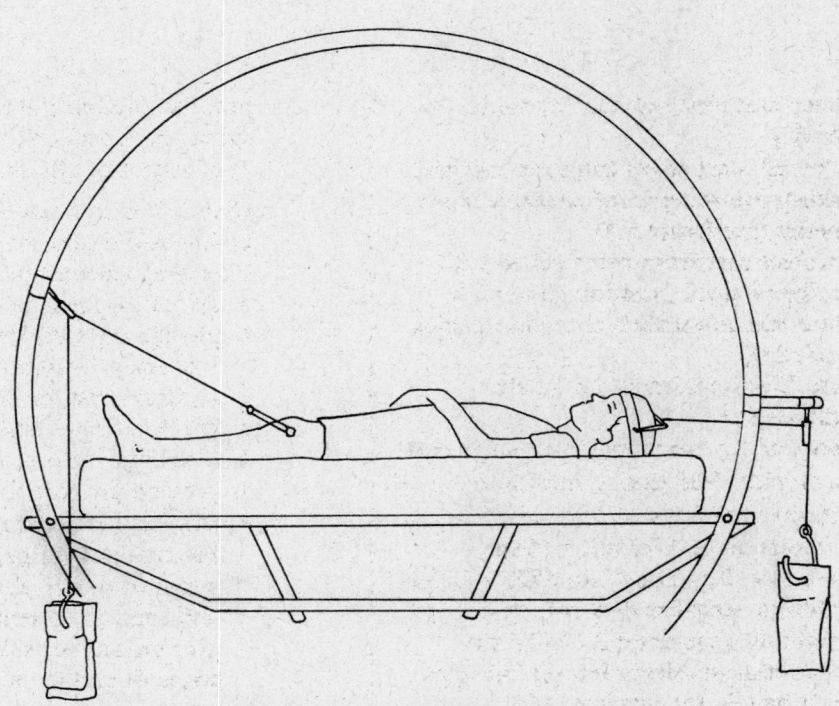

Halo-femoral traction

Figure 5.4 Continued

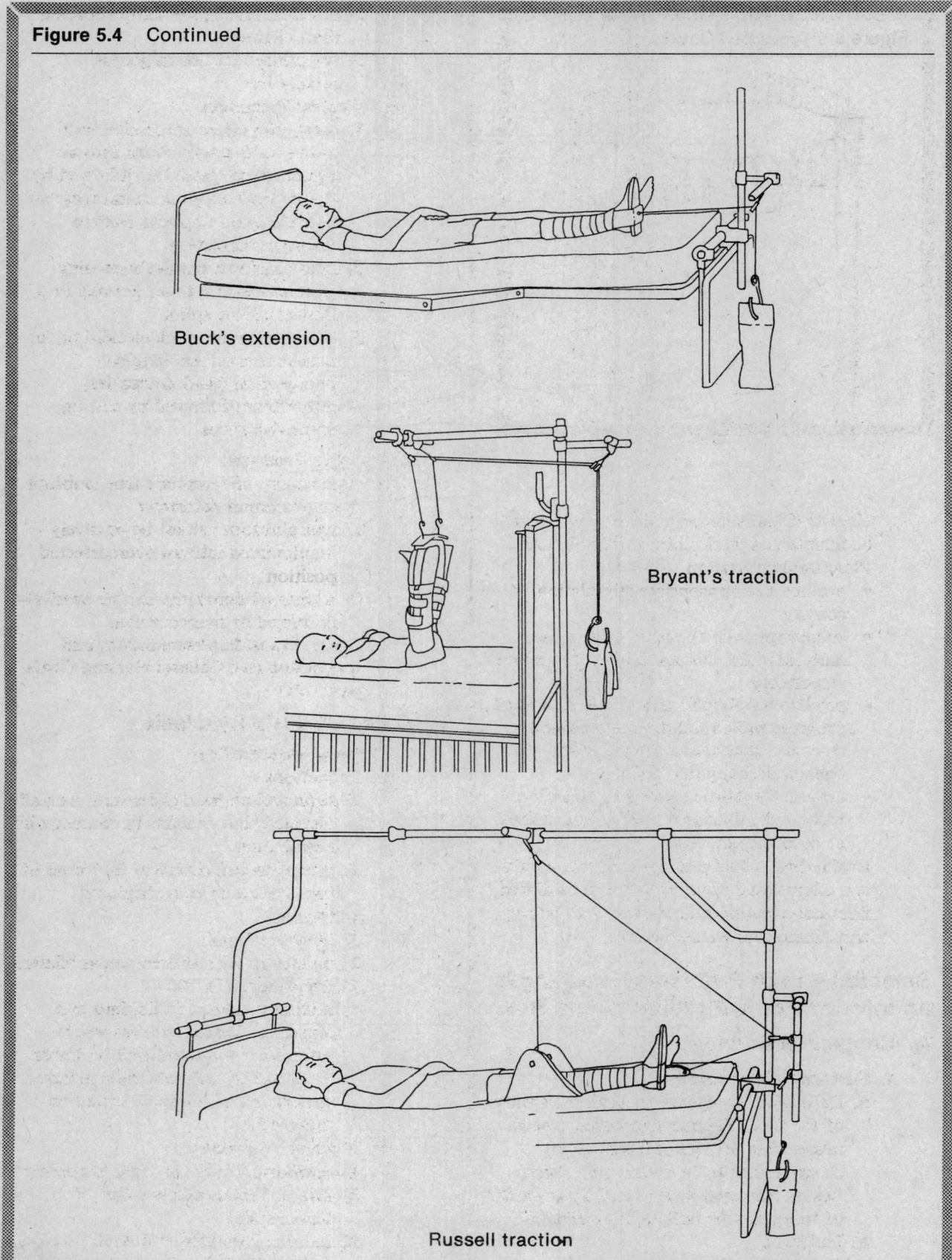

Buck's extension

Bryant's traction

Russell traction

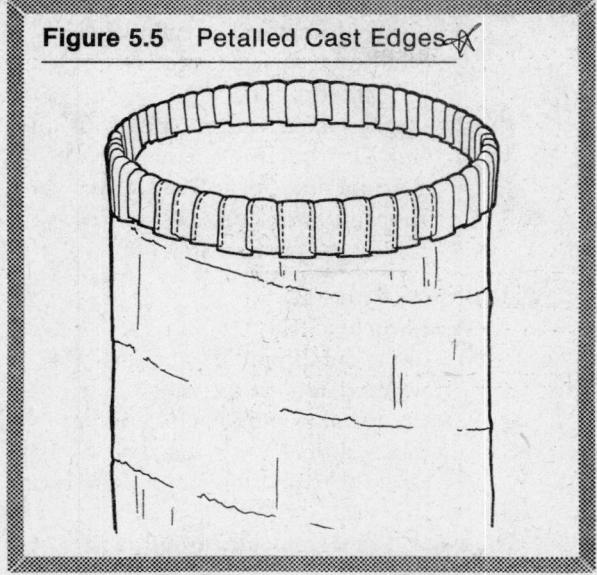

Figure 5.5 Petalled Cast Edges

Goal 4: Child's developmental progress will be maintained while child is immobilized.
Plan/Implementation
- provide age-appropriate stimulation, activity
- encourage child to participate in own daily care and maintain control as much as possible
- provide for child to maintain educational progress while immobilized (hospital teacher, homebound teacher, daily contact with regular teacher)
- arrange for and encourage interaction with peers, siblings if child is hospitalized or confined to home

Evaluation: Child maintains developmental and educational progress while immobilized; does not experience developmental delays; participates in own self-care.

Selected Health Problems Resulting in an Interference with Activity and Rest

A. Congenital Clubfoot

1. **General Information**
   a. Definition: congenital skeletal deformity of the foot. The most common type is talipes equinovarus (95% of cases), characterized by inversion and plantar flexion (directed inward and downward) of foot; may be unilateral or bilateral.
   b. Incidence
      1) boys are affected twice as often as girls
      2) unilateral is slightly more common than bilateral
      3) frequency: 1:1,000 in general population
   c. Medical Treatment
      1) early correction: successive casts until foot is manipulated into an overcorrected position, followed by Denis Browne splint (metal crossbar with shoes on opposite feet) to maintain correction
      2) mild clubfoot: passive stretching exercises several times per day or a Denis Browne splint
      3) later correction in older child or for recurrent clubfoot: surgical intervention (tendon transfer, arthrodesis) followed by casting, corrective shoes

2. **Nursing Process**
   a. Assessment: differentiate true clubfoot from positional deformity
      1) true clubfoot cannot be passively manipulated into an overcorrected position
      2) positional deformity can be passively corrected or overcorrected
   b. Goals, Plans/Implementation, and Evaluation (see General Nursing Goals page 595)

B. Congenital Hip Dysplasia

1. **General Information**
   a. Definitions
      1) *subluxation*: head of femur is partially displaced but remains in contact with acetabulum
      2) *complete dislocation of hip*: head of femur is completely displaced
   b. Incidence
      1) 70% are female
      2) unilateral twice as common as bilateral
      3) frequency: 1 in 500
      4) highest incidence in Eskimo and American Indian cultures where infants are swaddled tightly; lowest incidence in cultures where infants are carried with legs abducted on mother's hip
   c. Medical Treatment
      1) newborn: double or triple diapering
      2) infant: Frejka pillow splint, Von Rosen splint
      3) toddler: Bryant's or Russell traction, followed by hip spica cast or open reduction and casting

4) preschooler: combination of traction, open reduction, osteotomy, tendonotomy, casting; more difficult to treat because of secondary changes in hip joint
5) school age or older: total hip replacement when older; because of severe muscle shortening and bone deformity, may no longer be amenable to treatment

2. **Nursing Process**
   a. Assessment
      1) *infant*
         a) limited abduction of affected hip
         b) wide perineum
         c) shortening of leg on affected side
         d) asymmetry of thigh and gluteal folds
         e) positive Ortolani's sign: clicking when leg abducted, caused by femoral head slipping over acetabulum
      2) *older child*
         a) Trendelenburg's sign: when child stands on affected leg, pelvis tilts downward on unaffected side instead of upward
         b) limp on affected side
         c) flattening of buttock on affected side
   b. Goals, Plans/Implementation, and Evaluation (see General Nursing Goals page 595)

C. Scoliosis

1. **General Information**
   a. Definition: lateral curvature of the spine, which results in structural and functional alterations in spine, chest, and pelvis
   b. Incidence
      1) 15% of children between ages 10–21 are affected
      2) 7 times more common in adolescent females
      3) 70% of cases are idiopathic (i.e., without apparent cause)
   c. Medical Treatment
      1) medical intervention
         a) exercises (for curvatures less than 20°)
         b) braces, casts, traction (for curvatures 20°–40°)
            • Milwaukee brace (most common, most effective)
            • Risser plaster jacket/cast
            • halofemoral or halopelvic traction (continuous or intermittent)
      2) surgical intervention: spinal fusion with Harrington rods or Dwyer instrumentation, followed by application of body cast (for curvatures greater than 40°)

2. **Nursing Process**
   a. Assessment
      1) spinal curve may be obvious
      2) elevated shoulder or hip
      3) structural asymmetry (scapulae, waist, shoulders, breasts)
      4) rib hump apparent when child bends at waist
   b. Goal, Plan/Implementation, and Evaluation

   Goal: Adolescent and family will adjust to lengthy treatment regimen.
   Plan/Implementation
   - allow adolescent and parents to express feelings and concerns about long-term bracing or casting (6 months to 3 years)
   - help adolescent cope with altered body image
     - emphasize and enhance positive attributes (hair, makeup)
     - help with selection of attractive camouflage clothing
     - encourage involvement in appropriate activities (choir, school clubs, etc.)
   - demonstrate alternative ways of getting in and out of bed, dressing, etc.
   - advise standing at drafting table or easel for homework
   - teach application and removal of brace (must wear 23 hours/day; remove for 1 hour for hygiene or swimming)
   - teach adolescent to wear T-shirt under brace
   - check for loosening of brace; tighten as necessary
   - keep brace clean: wash plastic with soap and water, clean leather with saddle soap
   - provide for needs of adolescent following spinal fusion
     - keep bed flat; logroll q2h
     - assess circulatory and neurologic status in legs and feet
     - administer analgesics for pain
     - monitor incision sites for bleeding and signs of infection
     - monitor respiratory status

- cough and deep breathe; use inspirometer

Evaluation: Child with scoliosis copes with treatment regimen and altered body image; recovers from surgery free from complications; is free from permanent disability.

D. Osteomyelitis
1. **General Information**
   a. Definition: rapid-onset bacterial infection of the bone and its marrow; metaphyseal area of the long bones in the arms and legs is affected; causes bone destruction and formation of abscesses; staphylococcus aureus is causative organism in 80%–90% of cases
   b. Incidence
      1) most frequent in school-age children (5–14 years)
      2) boys affected 2–3 times more often than girls
      3) poor physical health, inadequate nutrition, and unsanitary environmental conditions are predisposing factors
   c. Medical Treatment
      1) medical intervention
         a) intravenous antibiotic therapy for 3–4 weeks; penicillin G (large doses) in conjunction with methicillin or oxacillin
         b) bed rest with immobilization of affected extremity *prevent spread in sec.*
         c) splint or bivalved cast to immobilize affected extremity
      2) surgical intervention: surgical drainage with insertion of polyethylene tubes in wound for antibiotic instillation
2. **Nursing Process**
   a. Assessment
      1) fever
      2) elevated pulse
      3) localized tenderness, warmth, redness, and swelling over affected area of bone
      4) limited, painful movement
      5) diagnostic tests
         a) elevated WBC count
         b) positive blood and wound cultures
         c) elevated ESR (erythrocyte sedimentation rate)
   b. Goals, Plans/Implementation, and Evaluation

Goal 1: Child's wound will heal; child will recover from illness free from complications.

Plan/Implementation
- carefully administer prescribed antibiotics (IV, wound) *ON TIME*
- provide wound care (irrigations, dressings, medications) as ordered
- encourage a nutritious diet (high calorie, high protein)
- maintain immobilization (positioning, cast, splint)

Evaluation: Child's wound heals; recovery is uneventful.

Goal 2: Child will experience minimal pain/discomfort.

Plan/Implementation
- assist child to achieve comfortable positions while immobilized
- check splint or cast for correct fit
- provide age-appropriate diversional activities
- administer prescribed analgesics as needed

Evaluation: Child experiences minimal discomfort during period of treatment.

References

Davis, S. and Lewis, S. "Managing Scoliosis: Fashions for the Body and Mind." *MCN: American Journal of Maternal-Child Nursing.* May/June 1984:186–187.

de Toledo, C. "The Patient with Scoliosis: The Defect-Classification and Detection." *American Journal of Nursing.* September 1979:1588–1591.

Hill, P. and Romm, L. "Screening for Scoliosis in Adolescents." *MCN: American Journal of Maternal-Child Nursing.* May/June 1977:156–159.

Meservey, P. "Congenital Musculo-Skeletal Abnormalities." *Issues in Comprehensive Pediatric Nursing.* October 1977:15–22.

Schatzinger, L., Brower, E., and Nash, C. "The Patient with Scoliosis, Spinal Fusion: Emotional Stress and Adjustment." *American Journal of Nursing.* September 1979:1608–1612.

Tacket, J. and Hunsberger, M. *Family-Centered Care of Children and Adolescents.* Philadelphia: Saunders, 1981.

Thorne, B. "A Nurse Helps Prevent Sports Injuries." *MCN: American Journal of Maternal-Child Nursing,* July/August 1982: 236–239.

Whaley, L. and Wong, D. *Nursing Care of Infants and Children*, 2nd Ed. St. Louis: Mosby, 1983.

Wieczorek, R. and Natapoff, J. *A Conceptual Approach to the Nursing of Children.* Philadelphia: Lippincott, 1981.

Cellular Aberration (Childhood Cancer)

General Concepts
A. Overview
1. Cancer is the leading cause of death from disease between the ages of 3 and 15
   a. Approximately 6,000 children receive a diagnosis of cancer each year
   b. Leukemias and lymphomas account for over 40% of childhood malignancies
   c. Brain tumors account for 20% of childhood cancers
   d. Embryonal tumors (e.g., Wilms' tumor and neuroblastoma) and sarcomas account for another 20% of childhood malignancies
   e. The survival rate for childhood cancer has dramatically increased in the last two decades 65%
2. Etiologic Factors
   a. No definitive etiologic agent has been identified
   b. Several causative agents have been linked with an increased incidence of cancer
      1) chemical carcinogens, such as DES (diethylstilbestrol) and asbestos
      2) physical carcinogens, such as radiation
      3) familiar and genetic factors
         a) higher incidence in children with Down's syndrome (leukemia)
         b) higher incidence in twin siblings of children with leukemia
      4) altered immune system (immune deficiencies or following organ transplantation and use of immunosuppressive therapy)
3. Malignant cells replicate in the same manner but not at the same rate as normal cells
4. All cancers are diseases of the cell; antineoplastic agents work in a variety of ways to interrupt the life cycle of malignant cells
5. Differences in childhood cancers as compared with adult cancers
   a. Higher incidence of embryonal tumors
   b. Occur more frequently in rapidly growing tissues, such as bone marrow
   c. Higher rate of metastasis
6. Medical Treatment
   a. Surgery: excision of all or part of solid tumors; may only be palliative if cancer has metastasized; most successful with localized and encapsulated tumors
   b. Chemotherapy: administration of antineoplastic agents, usually in a combination of two or more drugs (see table 5.21 for commonly used drugs)
   c. Irradiation: used as an adjunct to surgery and/or chemotherapy; may be curative or palliative
   d. Nonspecific immunotherapy:
      1) BCG (attenuated tuberculin bacillus): stimulates body's immune system to produce antitumor antibodies
      2) Interferon: is a newer immunotherapeutic agent that appears to also have antitumor effects (more often used with adults)
   e. Bone-marrow transplantation

B. Application of the Nursing Process to the Child with Cancer
1. Assessment
   a. Nursing history
      1) general health status, recent changes
      2) presence of any of the seven warning signals of cancer in children (American Cancer Society)
         a) marked change in bowel or bladder habits; nausea and vomiting for no apparent cause
         b) bloody discharge of any sort: blood in urine, spontaneous nosebleed or other type of hemorrhage, failure to stop bleeding in the usual time
         c) swellings, lumps, or masses anywhere in the body

Table 5.21 Commonly Used Chemotherapeutic Drugs

Drug/Route(s)	Types of Cancer	Side Effects	Nursing Implications
Antimetabolites			
Methotrexate IV, IT, PO	ALL, CNS leukemia, Osteogenic sarcoma, Non-Hodgkin's lymphoma, Brain tumors	Stomatitis, dermatitis, N&V, BMD (within 10 days), diarrhea, photosensitivity; may be highly toxic when given intrathecally	Do not give vitamins concurrently (folic acid antagonist); do not give aspirin or sulfonamides while child is receiving methotrexate (increase toxicity). Give leukovorin as an antidote for high doses of methotrexate.
Cytosine arabinoside (ara-C) IV, IM, IT	ALL, AML, Lymphomas, Brain tumors	N&V, anorexia, BMD, mucosal ulceration, hepatitis	Crosses blood-brain barrier. Monitor liver function.
Mercaptopurine (6-MP) PO	ALL	Abdominal pain, N&V, diarrhea, anorexia, BMD (in 4–6 weeks), stomatitis, dermatitis	Give allopurinol concurrently to inhibit uric acid production resulting from cell destruction, thereby increasing drug's potency.
Alkylating Agents			
Cyclophosphamide (Cytoxan) IV, PO, IM	Leukemia, Lymphomas, Neuroblastoma, Osteogenic sarcoma	N&V, BMD (except platelets), alopecia, stomatitis, hyperpigmentation, infertility	Push oral fluids to prevent chemical cystitis; report burning or hematuria to physician.
Mechlorethamine (nitrogen mustard, Mustargen) IV, IT	Hodgkin's disease, Neuroblastoma	N&V, BMD (in 2–3 weeks), alopecia, phlebitis	Use immediately after reconstitution. Avoid getting vapors in eyes; if solution comes in contact with skin, flush with liberal amounts of water. Ensure IV is in place to prevent tissue necrosis and sloughing.
Plant Alkaloids			
Vincristine (Oncovin) IV	ALL, Hodgkin's disease, Wilms' tumor, Neuroblastoma, Osteogenic sarcoma, Brain tumors	Alopecia, anemia, neurotoxicities (constipation, 1st weakness, ataxia, numbness, jaw pain, depression)	Ensure IV is in place while infusing to prevent cellulitis. Monitor for signs of toxicity.
Hormones			
Prednisone PO	ALL, Hodgkin's disease	Moon face, gastric irritation, mild BMD, hirsutism	Explain beneficial effects to family (increased appetite, elevated mood). Monitor weight gain (may need to restrict NA^+ intake); encourage high K^+ foods; administer with antacid. Monitor closely for infection (masks signs of infection). Screen stools for occult blood.

604 SECTION 5: NURSING CARE OF THE CHILD

Table 5.21 Continued.

Drug/Route(s)	Types of Cancer	Side Effects	Nursing Implications
Antibiotics			
Actinomycin D (Dactinomycin) IV	Wilms' tumor Neuroblastoma Osteogenic sarcoma	N&V, platelet depression, stomatitis, anorexia, alopecia, acne, desquamation of skin, abdominal cramps	Enhances effects of irradiation, but also increases its toxicity. Maintain IV in place to prevent tissue necrosis.
Doxorubicin (Adriamycin) IV	ALL Hodgkin's disease Osteogenic sarcoma Neuroblastoma	N&V, stomatitis, BMD, phlebitis, alopecia	Dilute with sterile water only. Maintain IV in place to prevent tissue necrosis. Monitor for cardiac dysrhythmias. Caution parents that child's urine will be red.
Enzymes			
L-Asparaginase IV, IM	ALL, AML Hodgkin's disease	N&V, anorexia, liver dysfunction, hyperglycemia, anaphylaxis	Monitor BUN and serum ammonia levels (causes elevation). Observe for allergic reaction (have epinephrine 1:1,000 at bedside). Monitor urine, glucose, liver functions.

Abbreviation key
ALL = acute lymphocytic leukemia
AML = acute myelocytic leukemia
BMD = bone-marrow depression
BUN = blood urea nitrogen
CNS = central nervous system
IT = intrathecal

    d) any change in the size or appearance of outward growth, such as moles or birthmarks
    e) unexplained stumbling in a child
    f) a generally run-down condition
    g) pains or the persistent crying of a baby or child, for which no reason can be found
  b. Physical Examination: physical findings will vary according to the type of cancer (see "Assessment" for each type of cancer)
  c. Diagnostic tests
    1) hematologic tests
      a) CBC, including blood cell characteristics (size, shape, maturation)
      b) chemistry: uric acid, electrolytes, glucose, and renal and liver function studies
    2) Bone-marrow aspiration: sterile procedure in which a needle is inserted into the anterior or posterior iliac crest to aspirate bone marrow for microscopic study
    3) lumbar puncture: to determine the presence of infiltration into the central nervous system
    4) radiologic examinations: to explore for sites of metastasis
      a) chest x-ray
      b) skeletal survey
      c) IVP
      d) ultrasonography
      e) computerized tomography (CAT scan)
      f) radioisotope scanning

2. **General Nursing Goals, Plans/Implementation, and Evaluation**

Goal 1: Child/family will be prepared for diagnostic tests.
Plan/Implementation
- provide age-appropriate explanation of procedure (what will happen, what it will feel like, what child is expected to do)
- give parents option of staying with child during procedure so they can provide needed emotional support to child

- hold child firmly during procedure to facilitate needle insertion (e.g., bone-marrow aspiration, LP)
- reassure child throughout procedure
- after the procedure, provide child opportunities to express feelings (verbally, through therapeutic play)
- provide positive feedback to child concerning child's cooperation during the procedure

Evaluation: Child copes with diagnostic procedures; cooperates with procedure; expresses feelings during and after procedure.

Goal 2: Child/family will be prepared for surgery (refer to "Ill and Hospitalized Child" page 525).

Goal 3: Child/family will be prepared for chemotherapy.
Plan/Implementation
- explain benefits of chemotherapy, using terms the child and family can understand
- reinforce physician's explanation of types of chemotherapy child will receive
- explain side effects that may occur and identify measures that will help lessen side effects
  - nausea and vomiting: administer antiemetics prior to chemotherapy
  - diarrhea: administer antispasmodics, adjust diet
  - anorexia: monitor weight; provide soft diet, small frequent feedings, favorite foods and liquids
  - stomatitis (see Goal 6)
  - alopecia: provide wig, scarf, hat as child desires
  - fatigue: provide frequent rest periods, encourage quiet activities

Evaluation: Child/family are able to state side effects; implement measures that minimize these effects and promote child's comfort.

Goal 4: Child/family will be prepared for radiation therapy.
Plan/Implementation
- reinforce reasons for and benefits of radiation
- prepare for and manage side effects of radiation therapy
  - nausea and vomiting: administer prescribed antiemetics as needed, bland diet, clear liquids
  - peeling skin: meticulous skin care; avoid direct exposure to sun; do not wash off skin markings (dark purple lines that define area to be irradiated)
  - risk of fracture: explain to child/family why child should avoid weight bearing; help plan to meet child's need for mobility through alternative means, such as crutches or stimulating activities while on bed rest
  - delays in physical development: discuss possible outcomes with parents and child (as appropriate) such as pathologic fractures, spinal deformities, growth retardation, sterility, delayed appearance of secondary sex characteristics, chromosomal damage

Evaluation: Child/family state reasons for radiation and knowledge of side effects that may occur.

Goal 5: Child will be free from infection.
Plan/Implementation
- maintain reverse isolation, or private room with strict hand washing if child is severely immunosuppressed
- prevent contact with anyone with infection
- rinse mouth regularly before meals, after meals, and q4h (removes debris as a source for growth of bacteria and fungi)
- administer antibiotics and observe for side effects
- take measures to prevent skin breakdown
- do not give immunizations until child's immune response is adequate
- permit return to school when WBCs approach normal level (2,000/mm³)

Evaluation: Child is free from infections, such as URIs, thrush, pneumonia; has intact skin.

Goal 6: Child will receive care for ulcerations of mouth and rectal area.
Plan/Implementation
- provide meticulous oral hygiene before/after meals
- offer mouthwash frequently; apply local anesthetic (viscous xylocaine) prn
- encourage fluids, nonirritating foods (soft foods, cool drinks)
- avoid rectal temperatures/suppositories
- encourage sitz baths; offer pericare after voiding or BM
- expose ulcerated anal area to air and heat

606 SECTION 5: NURSING CARE OF THE CHILD

Evaluation: Child is free from increased ulceration; lesions in mouth and rectum are healed.

Goal 7: Child will ingest foods and fluids to meet nutritional needs.
Plan/Implementation
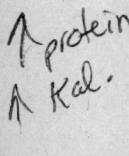
- rinse mouth before child eats
- offer small, frequent meals
- provide soft foods; permit favorite foods child tolerates
- use nutritional supplements

Evaluation: Child ingests fluid and diet as prescribed, including own preferences.

Goal 8: Child's pain will be relieved and comfort promoted.
Plan/Implementation
- administer nonnarcotic/narcotic analgesics as needed
- maintain comfortable body position, turning at least q2h and prn
- teach child to focus on TV, music, friend when having pain
- provide soothing skin care

Evaluation: Child experiences relief of pain; is positioned comfortably in bed or chair.

Goal 9: Child's growth and development will be fostered throughout the course of illness and treatment.
Plan/Implementation
- refer to "Healthy Child" page 513 for developmental needs appropriate to child's age
- encourage child to participate in self-care to the extent possible
- provide opportunities for child to exercise some control over daily routine (food choices, selection of play activities)
- maintain child's educational progress as much as possible
- maintain child's contact with siblings and friends (through visiting, telephone calls, letters)

Evaluation: Child is free from significant developmental or educational delays; demonstrates age-appropriate skills and behaviors.

Goal 10: Child and family cope with the stresses of living with cancer and its treatment.
Plan/Implementation
- encourage parents/family to continue to provide care of child as much as desired and possible
- encourage expressions of fears, feelings, concerns about cancer and its treatment
- refer to parent-support groups (Candlelighters, Compassionate Friends)
- help child express feelings through play and art
- encourage family to treat child as normally as possible (i.e., age-appropriate limit setting and enforcement, avoid excessive gifts or privileges)
- if child's condition becomes terminal, support family as they prepare for child's death; refer for home or hospice care, as appropriate and desired by family

Evaluation: Child and family cope with child's illness and treatment; parents participate in community support groups as desired, express their fears and feelings about child's illness and prognosis.

Selected Health Problems Resulting From Cellular Aberration

A. Leukemia

1. **General Information**
   a. Definition: malignant neoplasm of unknown etiology that involves all blood-forming organs and is characterized by abnormal overproduction of immature forms of any of the leukocytes. Interferes with normal blood cell production resulting in decreased erythrocytes, decreased platelets.
   1) types
      a) lymphocytic: predominance of stem cells, lymphoblasts, usually known as acute lymphocytic leukemia (ALL); 80% of childhood leukemias are of this type
      b) myelogenous: predominance of monocytes and immature granulocytes (more common in adults); 10%–20% of childhood leukemias are myelogenous
   2) pathophysiology: leukemic cells proliferate and deprive normal blood cells of nutrients needed for metabolism
      a) anemia results from decreased red blood cell production, blood loss
      b) immunosuppression occurs from large numbers of *immature* white blood cells or profound neutropenia
      c) hemorrhage results from thrombocytopenia

CELLULAR ABERRATION (CHILDHOOD CANCER) 607

d) leukemic invasion of other organ systems occurs (extramedullary disease)
- liver
- spleen
- lymph nodes
- CNS
- kidneys
- lungs
- gonads

e) hyperuricemia may result after the start of therapy when large numbers of cells are rapidly destroyed

b. Incidence
1) most common childhood cancer
2) peak age of onset is 2–5 years; more frequent in males
3) 50% of children with ALL who are treated in major research centers live 5 years or longer

c. Medical Treatment
1) diagnostic measures
a) bone-marrow aspiration
b) lumbar puncture
c) frequent blood counts
2) chemotherapy
a) induction course: to reduce leukemia-cell population
b) consolidation (sanctuary) course: after remission is achieved, different drugs are given to further reduce number of leukemia cells and prevent invasion of areas of body normally protected from cytoxic drugs, such as CNS
c) maintenance course: to maintain remission
3) additional therapies
a) radiation: irradiate cranium and spine as prophylaxis against CNS involvement *intrathecally*
b) bone-marrow transplantation

d. Prognosis: disease is characterized by remissions and exacerbations; outlook varies according to
1) type of cell involved
2) response to treatment
3) age at diagnosis
4) initial WBC
5) extent of involvement

2. **Nursing Process**
a. Assessment
1) bleeding tendencies
a) petechiae often the first sign, due to low platelet count

b) hemorrhage (nose bleeds, gingival bleeding; intracranial hemorrhage in advanced disease)
2) anemia: fatigue, pallor
3) neutropenia: immunosuppression leads to secondary infection and fever, since cells are not capable of normal phagocytosis
4) pain
a) abdomen: due to enlarged liver, spleen, lymph nodes, and other organs from cell infiltration
b) bones and joints
5) anorexia and weight loss; ulcers of mucous membranes of GI tract
6) vomiting and increased intracranial pressure from CNS involvement *(poor prognosis)*
7) impaired kidney function
8) emotional reaction, coping skills of parents, siblings, child, and significant extended-family members
9) developmental/educational needs of child

b. Goals, Plans/Implementation, and Evaluation

Goal 1: Child will be monitored for early signs of hemorrhage.
Plan/Implementation
- observe for epistaxis, gingival bleeding
- handle gently
- inspect skin and mucous membranes daily
- keep lips and nostrils clean and lubricated
- pad bed/crib to avoid trauma
- monitor blood work

Evaluation: Child is free from bruises/bleeding from traumatic handling; early signs of hemorrhage are detected and reported.

Goal 2: Child will receive transfusions properly and safely; will be monitored for early signs of reactions.
Plan/Implementation
- properly administer blood products
  - take baseline vital signs pretransfusion
  - check label with RN prior to transfusion for name, blood type, Rh, hospital number, and physician's name
  - flush tubing with isotonic saline solution (hemolysis can occur if dextrose in line)
  - administer blood at room temperature within 4 hours of refrigeration
  - administer transfusion slowly to determine possible transfusion

Stay c̄ child 1st 15 min

reaction, to prevent circulatory overload, and to protect small veins
- stay with child for 1st 15 minutes; have parent or other adult stay with young child throughout transfusion
- take vital signs q15min for 1st hour
- do not give IV medications while blood is infusing
- use blood filter
- monitor intravenous transfusions
  - whole blood/packed cells (cannot be continuously maintained on transfusions since preservative in whole blood functions as anticoagulant)
  - platelets last 1–3 days; do not need to crossmatch for blood group of type but doing so decreases chance of immunization to another platelet group; spontaneous hemorrhage can occur at platelet levels below 20,000/mm^3
  - leukocytes last 2–3 days; need compatible donors; febrile responses (with moderate to severe chills) are common; give antihistamines or antipyretics as ordered
- <u>observe for complications/reactions to blood transfusions</u>
  - chills
  - fever (give antipyretic prn)
  - headache
  - apprehension (give sedatives prn)
  - pain in back, legs, or chest
  - hypotension (give IV fluids, vasopressors)
  - dyspnea (give O$_2$, bronchodilator [epinephrine] as ordered)
  - urticaria (give antihistamines prn)
- promptly manage a transfusion reaction
  - <u>stop the transfusion of blood</u>
  - monitor vital signs
  - do not leave child alone
  - run IV fluids to maintain patency of the IV line
  - notify physician
  - return untransfused blood to blood bank

Evaluation: Child receives correct transfusion, is free from preventable complications (e.g., hemolysis); early signs of reaction (e.g., rash) are detected, and transfusion reaction is managed properly.

B. **Hodgkin's Disease**
  1. **General Information**
     a. Definition: malignancy of the lymphoid system characterized by a generalized painless lymphadenopathy; unknown etiology
     b. Incidence
        1) peak incidence between 15–30 years of age
        2) more common in males
        3) non-Hodgkin's lymphomas (lymphosarcoma, reticulum cell sarcoma) are more common in children under age 15
        4) 5-year survival rate is 90%; late recurrences (after 5–10 years) are not uncommon
     c. Medical Treatment
        1) diagnostic tests
           a) lymphangiography
           b) inferior venacavogram
           c) laboratory tests

Table 5.22 Staging of Hodgkin's Disease

Stage I:	Involvement of a single lymph node area or one additional extralymphatic organ (liver, kidney, lung, or intestine)
Stage II:	Involvement of two or more lymph node areas on the *same side* of the diaphragm or one additional extralymphatic organ on the same side of the diaphragm
Stage III:	Involvement of lymph node areas on *both sides* of the diaphragm; may be accompanied by involvement of one extralymphatic organ, the spleen, or both
Stage IV:	Diffuse involvement of one or more extralymphatic organs, with or without lymph node involvement.

Each Stage is also further categorized as subtype A or B:
Subtype A	Absence of generalized symptoms
Subtype B	Presence of generalized symptoms, such as fever, weight loss, night sweats

- erythrocyte sedimentation rate (ESR): elevated
- serum copper: elevated

2) clinical staging: surgical laparotomy to determine stage of the disease and best course of treatment; staging determines prognosis (see table 5.22)
   a) lymph node biopsy for characteristic cell (Reed-Sternberg)
   b) surgical clips are used to outline area for irradiation
   c) splenectomy
3) chemotherapy: combination drug MOPP (mechlorethamine [Mustargen], vincristine [Oncovin], prednisone, procarbazine) for 6–18 months
4) irradiation therapy

2. **Nursing Process**
   a. Assessment
   1) enlarged lymph nodes (most common sites: inguinal, mediastinal, axillary, retroperitoneal regions)
   2) anemia
   3) fever, infection (increased susceptibility to infection)
   4) anorexia, weight loss
   5) malaise
   6) night sweats
   b. **Goals, Plans/Implementation, and Evaluation**

Goal 1: Client will be prepared for lymphangiography and will be free from complications.

Plan/Implementation
- explain the procedure in terms of what the adolescent/family can expect
  - procedure lasts approximately 4 hours, may last longer
  - feet are anesthetized and immobilized for lymphatic vessel catheterization (initial injections of anesthetic are usually painful)
  - adolescent must lie still during procedure (this may be very tiring)
  - the dye may cause the following normal reactions
    * unusual taste sensations
    * fever
    * headache
    * insomnia
    * retrosternal burning sensation
    * bluish-green discoloration of urine
    * discoloration of skin, especially hands and feet, which may persist for weeks
- encourage family member to stay with adolescent to offer support and help time pass more quickly
- provide appropriate diversional activities such as reading or listening to music
- monitor for signs of complications
  - bleeding or infection from cutdown site
  - oil embolism (from oil-based dye)
    * fever, chills
    * dyspnea
    * cough
    * chest pain, soreness

Evaluation: Adolescent cooperates with and tolerates procedure; is free from complications.

Goal 2: Client/family are prepared for staging and splenectomy.

Plan/Implementation
- refer to "Ill and Hospitalized Child" page 528 for nursing care related to preparation for surgery
- inform adolescent/family of effects of splenectomy
  - increased susceptibility to infection
  - daily pencillin (or erythromycin) therapy for 1–3 years following splenectomy (especially in younger age clients because of less well-developed immune system)

Evaluation: Adolescent/family are able to state effects of splenectomy and implications for adolescent's life-style (daily medication, minimizing exposure to infection).

C. **Brain Tumors**

1. **General Information**
   a. Definition: neoplasms in the cranium; most brain tumors in children are *infratentorial* (below the tentorium cerebelli), thus affecting the cerebellum and brain stem, making them less operable than *supratentorial* tumors, which are more common in adults
   b. Common types
   1) infratentorial
      a) astrocytoma: located in cerebellum; most common childhood brain tumor; slow-growing tumor; if tumor is well defined, surgical excision may be accomplished
      b) medulloblastoma: most commonly invades cerebellum; fast-growing, highly malignant tumor; complete excision not usually possible; CNS

irradiation and aggressive chemotherapy prolong survival
- c) **brainstem glioma:** located in vital centers of brain; cannot be surgically removed; irradiation shrinks tumor and prolongs survival
- d) **ependymoma:** tumor of 4th ventricle, leading to signs of hydrocephalus; difficult to completely remove; irradiation and chemotherapy prolong survival
2) **supratentorial:** craniopharyngioma is a tumor located near pituitary gland and hypothalamus; interferes with pituitary function (may lead to growth impairment); usually cannot be completely excised, may involve repeated attempts at surgical removal; irradiation and hormone-replacement therapy are used as adjuncts to surgery
c. **Incidence:** 2nd leading cause of death from cancer in children; occurs most frequently in children under age 5
d. **Medical Treatment**
1) surgical excision (except brainstem gliomas) of as much of tumor as possible
2) irradiation of CNS
3) chemotherapy: vincristine, methotrexate, procarbazine in various combinations

2. Nursing Process
a. **Assessment:** manifestations of increased intracranial pressure (see table 5.15)
1) **infants:** usually not detected until tumor is quite large; manifestations do not become apparent until the tumor is large enough to obstruct CSF flow, leading to an increase in head circumference
2) **older children**
- a) early morning headache, aggravated by positions in which head is lower than rest of body, straining, and coughing
- b) nausea and vomiting: usually worse in morning; may become projectile
- c) gait disturbances and clumsiness: indicate cerebellar involvement
- d) visual disturbances
- e) behavior changes: irritability, lethargy, sleepiness, diminished interest in usual activities
- f) changes in vital signs: increased BP, wide pulse pressure, decreased pulse and respirations
- g) seizures

b. **Goals, Plans/Implementation, and Evaluation**

Goal 1: Child/family will be prepared for diagnostic procedures and craniotomy.
Plan/Implementation
- explain what child can expect to happen during CAT scan and that he must hold very still (younger children are often sedated to minimize fear)
- explain to child/family pre- and post-op care
  - prepare child for shaving hair
    * encourage parent to stay with child
    * allow child to watch in mirror, or to look at self as each section of head is shaved
    * save hair if child/family desire (long hair may be made into a wig)
    * suggest alternative head coverings, such as a wig, scarf, cap
  - explain that child will have a large head dressing post-op (demonstrate on doll for younger child)
  - prepare parents for child's post-op behavior (sleepiness)
  - explain to child he will be sleepy and may have a headache post-op
  - explain to child that he must lie still after surgery and can turn or move only with nurse's help

Evaluation: Child/family are prepared cognitively and emotionally for diagnostic procedures and craniotomy; cooperate with care (head shaving, positioning) pre- and post-op.

Goal 2: Child will be free from complications following craniotomy.
Plan/Implementation
- monitor vital signs frequently until stable
- use hypothermia blanket as ordered and as needed for temperature elevation
- assess LOC, pupils, grip, bilateral movement frequently
- observe cranial dressing for drainage; reinforce but DO NOT CHANGE dressing; record color, consistency of drainage (report clear fluid [i.e., CSF] immediately), lightly circle area of drainage on dressing with pen, noting time
- encourage deep breathing (no coughing)

- position child according to physician's orders
  - infratentorial tumors: flat in bed, on side (not back) with neck slightly extended (prevents tension on sutures)
  - supratentorial tumors: elevate head of bed slightly
- turn child very gently to prevent jarring movements
- monitor IV fluids carefully to prevent fluid overload
- provide sips of clear liquids once gag and swallowing reflexes are present (child is usually NPO first 24 hours post-op); stop fluids and notify physician if child vomits
- monitor urine output carefully, especially if child has received mannitol or dextrose (cause diuresis) to prevent cerebral edema
- minimize environmental stimulation (dim lights, no noise)
- avoid analgesics and sedatives post-op, especially those that cause CNS depression
- provide eye care
  - child's eyes are usually covered with eye patches to minimize stimulation
  - apply cold compresses at intervals to minimize edema
  - talk quietly to child, explaining exactly what is happening, what nurse is doing

Evaluation: Child is free from complications postcraniotomy.

D. Neuroblastoma

1. **General Information**
   a. Definition: malignant tumor of unknown etiology that originates from embryonic neural tissue; most develop from the adrenal gland or retroperitoneal sympathetic chain, thus they are usually abdominal tumors; known as the "silent tumor" because it is frequently not detected until metastasis has occurred; prognosis is best if detected in infancy, worst if detected after age 2 (survival is then less than 20%); child is considered cured if he is free from disease 2 years after treatment
   b. Incidence
      1) most common solid tumor in children (approximately 8% of all childhood malignancies)
      2) occurs primarily in children under age 4 (half of the cases occur under age 2); slightly more common in boys
   c. Medical Treatment
      1) diagnostic tests
         a) CAT scan to locate tumor mass
         b) urine catecholamines (VMA, HVA, dopamine, epinephrine, norepinephrine): elevated
         c) lung, bone, liver scans to detect areas of metastasis
         d) IVP if tumor is adrenal in origin
      2) staging: to determine extent of tumor, metastasis, and prognosis
         a) stage I or II: tumor confined, does not cross midline; tumor can be completely excised
         b) stage III: tumor extends beyond midline with regional lymph node involvement; excision of as much of tumor as possible, followed by post-op radiation (may be irradiated pre-op to reduce tumor size)
         c) stage IV: widespread disease; chemotherapy is treatment of choice (vincristine, cyclophosphamide, doxorubicin, nitrogen mustard in various combinations)

2. **Nursing Process**
   a. Assessment
      1) abdominal mass that may cross the midline (often used to differentiate neuroblastoma from Wilms' tumor)
      2) lymphadenopathy
      3) urinary frequency or retention caused by compression of kidneys, ureters, or bladder
      4) later signs
         a) bone pain
         b) pallor, weakness
         c) anorexia, weight loss
         d) periorbital ecchymosis
   b. **Goals, Plans/Implementation, and Evaluation** (see General Nursing Goals page 604)

E. Wilms' Tumor (Nephroblastoma)

1. **General Information**
   a. Definition: a malignant embryonal tumor of the kidney; a striking characteristic of this tumor is encapsulation for a fairly lengthy period of time; high rate of survival (90% survival stages I and II; 50% for other stages)
   b. Incidence: peak age of occurrence is 3 years; more common in boys; increased incidence among siblings and twins of child with Wilms' tumor; usually

unilateral with left kidney affected more often
- c. Medical Treatment
  1) radiographic studies, including IVP, to identify size and extent of tumor and presence of metastasis
  2) surgery and staging within 24–48 hours of detection of mass
     a) nephrectomy and adrenalectomy
     b) removal of adjacent affected organs
     c) staging
        - stage I: tumor limited to kidney, completely excised
        - stage II: tumor extends beyond kidney, but is still encapsulated, can be completely excised
        - stage III: tumor is confined to abdomen, as much as possible is removed
        - stage IV: tumor has metastasized to other sites (lung, liver, bone, CNS)
        - stage V: bilateral renal involvement; partial nephrectomy of less involved kidney, complete removal of other kidney
     d) radiation: all except stage I
     e) chemotherapy: all stages, for 6–15 months; actinomycin D and vincristine most commonly used

2. **Nursing Process**
   a. Assessment
      1) palpable abdominal mass
      2) abdominal distention (increased size of liver and spleen)
      3) anemia, weight loss
      4) may have hypertension (excess renin secretion)
      5) lymphadenopathy
   b. **Goals, Plans/Implementation, and Evaluation**

Goal 1: Child will have possibility of metastasis minimized preoperatively.
Plan/Implementation
- place sign on child's bed, "DO NOT PALPATE ABDOMEN"
- keep child on bed rest, engaged in quiet activities
- handle child very carefully to avoid pressure on abdomen or flank

Evaluation: Child's tumor is encapsulated at time of surgery; metastasis is prevented.

Goal 2: Child will maintain function of remaining kidney postoperatively.
Plan/Implementation
- carefully monitor I&O
- monitor BP; report hypertension
- protect child from exposure to infections
- emphasize importance of continued follow-up care to parents

Evaluation: Child's remaining kidney is free from disease; renal function continues normally.

References

Cleaveland, M. "Nursing Care in Childhood Cancer: Brain Tumors." *American Journal of Nursing.* March 1982:422–425.

Foley, G. and McCarthy, A. "The Child with Leukemia in a Special Hematology Clinic." *American Journal of Nursing.* July 1976:1115–1119.

†Gaddy, D. "Nursing Care in Childhood Cancer, Update." *American Journal of Nursing.* March 1982:416–421.

Green, P. "Acute Leukemia in Children." *American Journal of Nursing.* October 1975:1709–1714.

Green, P. "The Child with Leukemia in the Classroom." *American Journal of Nursing.* January 1975:86–87.

Hardin, K. "Solid Tumors in Children." *Issues in Comprehensive Pediatric Nursing.* February 1980:29–47.

Maul, S. "Childhood Brain Tumors: A Special Nursing Challenge." *MCN: American Journal of Maternal-Child Nursing.* July/August 1983:123–131.

Mills, G. "Preparing Children and Parents for Cerebral Computerized Tomography." *MCN: American Journal of Maternal-Child Nursing.* November/December 1980:403–407.

Sontesgard, L. et al. "A Way to Minimize Side Effects from Radiation Therapy." *MCN: American Journal of Maternal-Child Nursing.* January/February 1976:27–31.

Tealey, A. "Getting Children to Keep Still during Radiotherapy." *MCN: American Journal of Maternal-Child Nursing.* May/June 1977:178–181.

Waechter, E., Philips, J., and Holoday, B. *Nursing Care of Children*, 10th Ed. Philadelphia: Lippincott, 1985.

Whaley, L. and Wong, D. *Nursing Care of Infants and Children*, 2nd Ed. St. Louis: Mosby, 1983.

† Highly recommended

Notes

Reprints
Nursing Care of the Child

Sheredy, C. "Factors to Consider when Assessing Responses to Pain." 617
Sacksteder, S. "Congenital Cardiac Defects: Embryology and Fetal Circulation." 620
Ruble, I. "Childhood Nocturnal Enuresis." 624
Meier, E. "Evaluating Head Trauma in Infants and Children." 630
Coughlin, M. "Teaching Children about their Seizures and Medications." 634
Jackson, P. "Ventriculo-peritoneal Shunts." 636
Seleckman, J. "Immunization: What's It All About?" 642

Factors To Consider When Assessing Responses To Pain

Reprinted from American Journal of Maternal/Child Nursing, July/August 1984.

CAROLYN SHEREDY

To assess pain, the nurse must be familiar not only with the physiology of pain but also with the person's general physical condition as well as the person's cultural and historical factors that contribute to pain. (See box for a discussion of the physiology of pain.) Systematic observation skills are extremely important (especially when assessing children under five or six years old) since behavioral cues often are the primary source of data. Increased irritability, restlessness, and lack of appetite are important indicators of pain, as are pulling, rubbing, and guarding certain body parts. Young children may become so preoccupied with pain that they begin to limit involvement and interactions with others in the environment.

Since children often mimic parents' responses to pain, interactions between parents and children need to be assessed. If a child is told by parents that "big boys (girls) don't cry," the child may deny or minimize the degree of pain in order to please the parents. Thus a child soon learns what is an acceptable or unacceptable attitude and response to pain.

Vital signs also are considered. Heart rate and respirations increase when a person experiences pain and should improve after measures are taken to relieve pain (such as, repositioning, medicating, and/or distracting). The intensity of pain and whether it increases, decreases, or remains the same is determined after pain relief is provided. Individuals in the school-age years and older are able to rate the intensity of pain on a scale of one to ten.

A pain history is invaluable for assessing pain and evaluating pain-relief measures. Examples of variables affecting pain are listed in the table Variables Affecting Pain Responses. The nurse should consider not only physical, cultural, and historical factors that affect a person's response to pain but also the person's developmental level. The following discussion highlights the responses to pain of people at different developmental levels and some appropriate nursing interventions.

Infancy (birth to twelve months old). Infants usually indicate discomfort or pain through general body movements, changes in body state, stooling, hiccoughing, withdrawing the affected limb, and crying. Prolonged pain may lead to generalized body fatigue. Relief measures include removing the painful stimulus, if possible, as well as holding, touching, stroking, and providing a pacifier. Enabling the infant to assume a comfortable position also is helpful (see "The Neonate's Response to Pain" by Karen D'Apolito).

Toddler years (twelve months to three years old). Toddlers, like infants, may be unable to indicate the nature of pain in a meaningful manner. Language comprehension may be adequate, but the child may lack expressive language skills. Even if a toddler has mastered language skills, the unfamiliarity of the hospital may cause the child to be unusually silent or to regress in behavior. Often a toddler responds to pain through aggressive behavior such as biting, hitting, and temper tantrums or exhibits nonverbal cues such as clenching teeth, thumb sucking, or rocking.

A toddler's thinking basically is concrete and literal, and the toddler's concept of time is the

---

CAROLYN SHEREDY, R.N., B.S.N. is a clinical nurse at Group Health Association in Annandale, Virginia. At the time this article was written, she was a member of the p.r.n. staff at Children's Hospital National Medical Center in Washington, D.C.

present. Thus a toddler is unable to understand that "Mommy will come back" and needs to be familiarized with the hospital in order to reduce stress levels. Stress increases anxiety, which increases pain, which adds to the stress and anxiety that the toddler is experiencing. This cycle repeats itself unless the nurse intervenes.

Preschool years (three to five years old). The preschooler's greatest fear is of bodily injury. Placing a bandage over a cut or a scratch assures the child that his or her body will remain intact.

Because of increased maturity, the preschooler can verbalize fears and pains better than a toddler can. Also, the preschooler becomes adept at procrastination and believes that by saying "wait a minute" a painful procedure can be postponed or eliminated.

The preschooler's thinking is egocentric. All events and occurrences are believed to result from the child's own being. Consequently, hospitalizations may be viewed as a punishment. Parents may unknowingly reinforce this pattern of reasoning by saying, "If you aren't good, the nurse will give you a shot."

Prehospital visits familiarize the child with a new environment and reduce fearful misperceptions. Because fantasy and magical thinking are part of the preschooler's world, therapeutic play helps create a safe environment in which the child can work through feelings of fear, anger, or guilt about the trauma or pain.

Parents should be told how the child's developmental stage affects his or her response to pain and hospitalization. Often the child will cooperate with the nurse but exhibit aggressive behavior toward the parent. For example, a four year old may stoically receive an injection and then refuse a parent's comforting by turning over and hiding under a blanket.

School-aged children (five to twelve years old). Because the school-aged child has a greater awareness of the body and internal organs, fear of bodily harm increases, and fear of death develops. However, a five year old's thinking is still concrete and animistic. Objects are defined in terms of their use and effects upon the child. Thus the child may believe that a needle used for an injection caused the original pain. When another child is seen crying during an examination, the child may believe that the examination will hurt him, too.

Reasoning begins to occur by the time children become seven years old. The concept of time also develops. Past and future have meaning. Thus the pain experience is time-limited.

Whereas younger school-aged children describe pain mostly in terms of physical aspects, older school-aged children include psychological com-

---

VARIABLES AFFECTING PAIN RESPONSES

Variable	Example
Cultural background	An individual with an Oriental heritage may be stoic and not admit feeling pain.
Developmental level	Verbal communication in a toddler is inadequate.
Parents' attitudes	A parent may forewarn a child that an injection will or will not hurt.
Education (prehospital admission and preoperative teaching)	Fear of the unknown increases anxiety and pain.
Type of anesthesia	Local versus general.
Type of surgery performed	Cyst removal versus abdominal.
Nature of procedures	Intravenous insertion.
Frequency and duration of hospitalization	Repeated admission for renal dialysis.
Pain medication	Nurses may dispense medications conservatively because they fear addiction.
Parents' absence or presence	Pain increases in parents' absence because the child fears abandonment.
Nurses' attitudes	A nurse may draw conclusions about responses to pain on the basis of past experience or believe that an individual is "making a scene."

THE PHYSIOLOGY OF PAIN

The perception of and response to pain are dependent upon the maturation of the central nervous system. When a painful stimulus is felt by an older child or an adult, two types of nerve fibers (A delta and C) transmit pain signals to the brain. These afferent (ascending to the brain) pain fibers carry pain impulses from free, specialized nerve endings that serve as pain sensors in the skin, muscles, blood vessels, and organs.

The pain impulses travel to the dorsal horns of the spinal cord, where a synapse occurs. The axons of the activated neurons cross to the opposite side of the spinal cord and travel to the thalamus via the spinothalamic tract and finally to the cortex (see figure).

Because myelinated A delta fibers transmit impulses more rapidly than unmyelinated C fibers, two types of pain sensation are felt after the onset of a painful stimulus. Sharp, pricking sensations are caused by stimula-

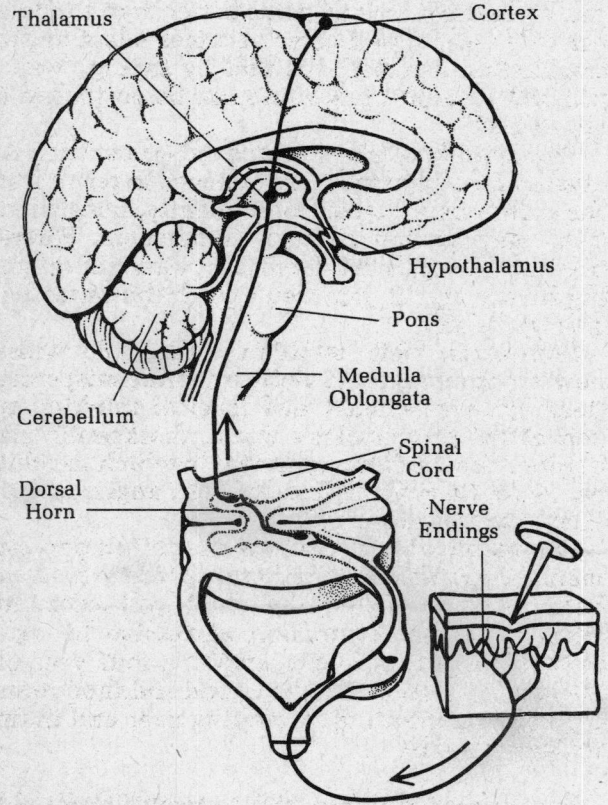

tion of A delta fibers, while prolonged, burning types of pain are caused by stimulation of unmyelinated C fibers. Activation of A delta fibers leads to a withdrawal response in the involved muscle or organ. The slow, burning sensation resulting from activation of C fibers tends to become more and more painful over time. This sensation causes the intolerable suffering of pain (2).

The sensation for chronic pain occurs in the medulla, reticular activating system, thalamus, hypothalamus, and other parts of the limbic system. As pain evolves from acute to chronic, different areas of the brain are involved in pain perception (3).

In addition to a sensory awareness of pain, visceral changes occur. They are caused by activation of the autonomic nervous system. Autonomic response fibers are located in the spinal cord, medulla, and midbrain. When a pain stimulus is received, blood pressure alterations, tachycardia, tachypnea, perspiration, or gastrointestinal disturbances may result. (For a detailed discussion of the infant's central nervous system, see "The Neonate's Response to Pain" by Karen D'Apolito.)

ponents (1). Both hospitalized and nonhospitalized children can describe interventions for pain such as pain medication, rest or relaxation, and the presence of a sensitive person or stuffed animal.

School-aged children between ten and twelve years old may deny pain because of a desire to be brave. They may pretend that they are not in pain by reading or by watching television. However, no child should be without some kind of pain relief. A simple explanation that refusing pain relief does not indicate that a person is brave or strong often helps children acknowledge that they feel pain and convinces them that their responses to pain are not signs of weakness. In addition, providing pain-relief measures other than injections may encourage children to describe their responses to pain.

Adolescence (twelve to twenty years old). Adolescents may find the threat of illness or alteration of the body physically or psychologically disturbing because they fear loss of control. They may be able to accept intellectually the reasons for hospitalizations or illnesses but unable to accept emotionally the separation from family or friends. Moreover, adolescents frequently experience mood changes and extremes of behavior. Consequently, an adolescent may refuse pain medication during one shift but request it repeatedly during the next shift even though pain has not increased.

Understanding this phase of development is vital. The nurse needs to establish a trusting relationship in order to encourage the adolescent to share and discuss any fears and concerns.

Young adult (twenty years old and older). Young adults are affected more by sociocultural forces and value changes than by physical or cognitive development. The young adult has new roles of responsibility at work, home, and in society. Coping with these new changes can be a source of physical and psychological stress.

In this special series, the young adult being discussed is the childbearing woman. Her response to pain or discomfort may be influenced by cultural and psychosocial attitudes about pregnancy and motherhood. These factors as well as various comfort measures will be discussed in Part III of this series.

Summary. Knowledge of growth and development as well as the other factors discussed is needed in order to make an accurate evaluation of a person's responses to pain. The assessment of pain is an ongoing and at times difficult undertaking. However, the long-range benefit is a reduction in the psychological hurt that often accompanies physical pain.

CONGENITAL CARDIAC DEFECTS

Embryology and Fetal Circulation

Reprinted from American Journal of Nursing, February 1978.

By Sara Sacksteder

Knowledge of the anatomical development of the fetal circulation and the changes that occur during the transition from intrauterine to extrauterine existence is helpful in understanding congenital cardiac defects.

From the time of fertilization, to implantation of the blastocyte in the uterine mucosa at the end of the first week of embryonic development, and into the third week of gestation, the developing embryo's nutritional needs are supplied by diffusion. After the third week of development, nutritional requirements of the embryo can no longer be met by diffusion alone; the heart and vascular systems develop rapidly. This developmental phase extends from the third to the eighth week of gestation.

Fetal lung tissue does not develop sufficiently to support extrauterine life until the twenty-sixth to twenty-eighth week of gestation. The fetal heart and vascular systems must therefore be structured in a fashion that will support intrauterine life but permit an instantaneous transition to extrauterine life at the time of birth.

By the third week of fetal development, a single tube composed of two layers of tissue (the endocardium, or inner layer lining the heart, and the epimyocardium, which will develop into the myocardium and epicardium) can be identified in the midline (figure A). The tube is fixed cephalically and caudally, leaving the midportion most capable of accommodating growth. Growth is rapid, and the midportion bends noticeably.

As the midportion of the tube grows and bends, future cardiac structures become indentifiable. These include the *sinus venosus*, formed by veins returning blood to the heart; a common *atrium*, connecting the atrium with the embryonic *ventricle*; the *conus cordis*, which will provide an outflow tract for the ventricles; and the *truncus arteriosus*, which will develop into the aorta and pulmonary artery (figures B, C). The heart remains relatively undeveloped, and blood flows through it in a continuous stream.

Transition to a four-chambered heart takes place between the fourth and eighth weeks of gestation. Tissue bundles, called *endocardial cushions*, arise on the dorsal and ventral walls of the atrioventricular canal. By the end of the sixth week, these cushions merge, dividing the canal into right and left channels. The tricuspid and mitral valves develop from proliferating tissues in the atrioventricular area.

The Atria

Atrial development begins with the incorporation of the sinus venosus into the wall of what will become the right atrium. Blood returning from the general circulation enters the right atrium through the superior and inferior vena cavae. Part of the wall of the left atrium is derived from the common pulmonary vein and two of its branches, leaving four pulmonary veins to return blood from the lungs to the left atrium.

Atrial septation begins with the development of the *septum primum*, formed by atrial wall fusion. The septum primum grows toward, but does not initially fuse with, the endocardial cushion. The communication remaining between the left and right atria is called the *foramen primum* (figure D). A second opening, the *foramen secundum*, now develops in the septum primum.

The author thanks Delores Danilowicz, M.D., associate professor of pediatrics and director of the Pediatric Cardiac Catheterization Lab., New York University Medical Center, New York, N.Y. for her advice in preparing this article.

The septum primum continues to develop, fusing with the endocardial cushion. The foramen primum is obliterated, but communication between the right and left atria continues through the foramen secundum (figure E).

A second septum begins to grow. This *septum secundum*, lying to the right of the septum primum, develops cephalically and caudally but does not fuse. Rather, an opening at about midpoint, known as the *foramen ovale*, remains and permits blood to flow between the atria (figure F). This flow is unidirectional, from right to left, because the septum acts as a one-way valve to prevent the flow of blood from left to right. The foramen ovale with its "valve" provides for flow of oxygenated blood from mother to fetal structures requiring highest oxygen saturation.

The Ventricles

Ventricular septation is completed about a week after atrial septation. The floor of the muscular ventricular tissue grows upward toward the endocardial cushion. Because the muscular tissue does not fuse with the endocardial cushion, an interventricular foramen exists for a time. This foramen will be obliterated by the end of the second month of fetal development. Closure is accomplished primarily with tissue derived from the endocardial cushion and the *conus ridges* of the truncus arteriosus.

The conus ridges in the ventricular septum are extensions of ridges present in the truncus arteriosus. These ridges fuse and divide the truncus in a spiral fashion, forming the aorta and pulmonary artery. Connective tissue grows from the endocardial tissue of the conus ridges to form the aortic and pulmonary valves.

The spiral fashion of fusion

DEVELOPMENT OF FETAL HEART

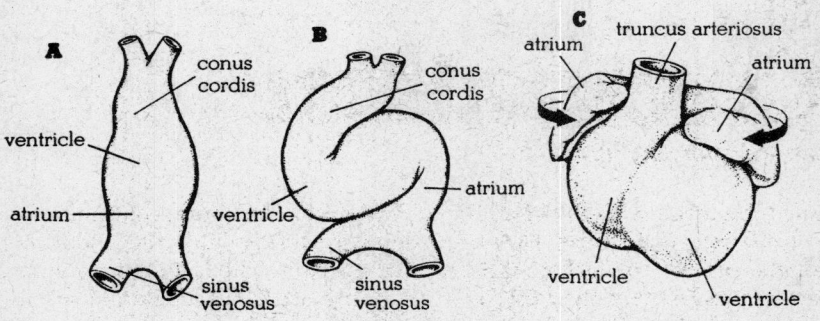

At about two and a half weeks (A), the embryo's heart consists of a tube at midline fixed cephalically and caudally. At about three weeks (B), structures are identifiable. Heart at 28 days (C). Atria have more dorso-cranial position; transverse dilatations of atria bulge on each side of truncus arteriosus.

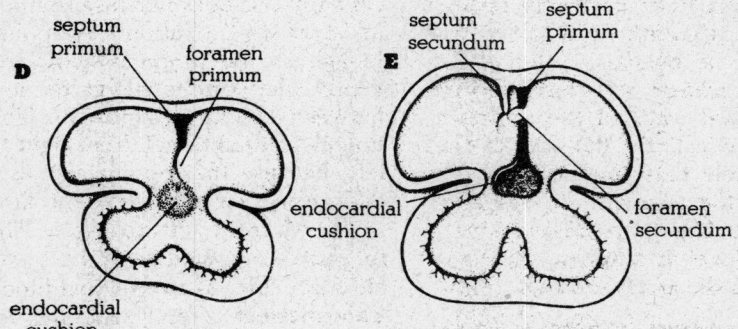

At 28 days (D) the foramen primum develops as septum primum extends toward endocardial cushion. At 33 days (E), septum secundum begins to grow, foramen primum closes, and a degenerative process divides upper portion of the septum primum, creating foramen secundum.

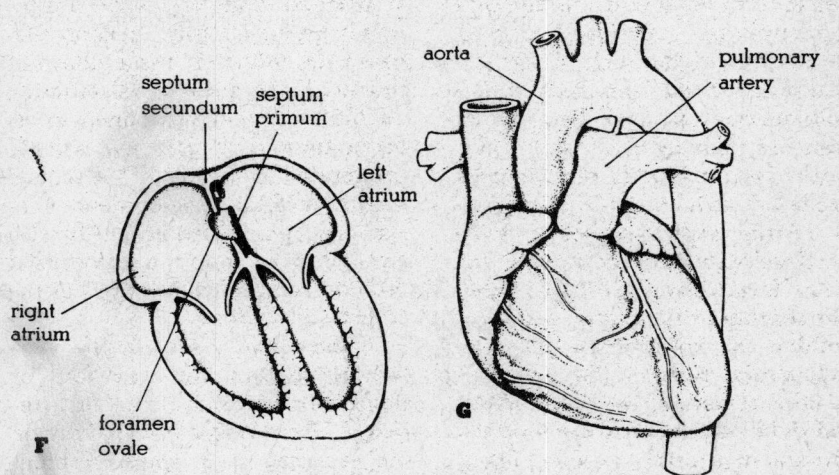

Septum secundum divides, creating foramen ovale. Septum primum act as a one-way valve preventing blood flow from left to right in fully developed heart (F). Conus ridges in the truncus arteriosus fuse, divide in a spiral fashion, and aorta and pulmonary artery twist around each other (G).

explains the position of the aorta and pulmonary artery as they emerge from the heart. Communication between the aorta and left pulmonary artery is maintained through the ductus arteriosus to shunt blood out of the pulmonary system before birth. The foramen ovale and ductus arteriosus direct flow away from the lungs, which remain collapsed in utero.

Fetal Circulation

Arteries are vessels that take blood away from the heart; veins bring blood to the heart. During fetal life, the placenta is the site of oxygenation. Oxygenated blood flows from the placenta via the umbilical vein to the liver. Here, the flow from the umbilical vein divides. Some blood is directed into the hepatic circulation, while the rest is shunted through the ductus venosus to the inferior vena cava.

Blood entering the heart from the inferior vena cava is a mixture of highly oxygenated blood received from the ductus venosus and blood with a lower oxygen saturation, returning from the alimentary canal, liver, and lower extremities of the fetus. On entering the right atrium, most of the blood returning through the inferior vena cava is directed through the foramen ovale into the left atrium, bypassing the right ventricle, and the lungs. Blood entering the left atrium through the foramen ovale is mixed with small amounts of blood entering via the pulmonary veins. This blood, high in oxygen content, passes from the left atrium into the left ventricle and out through the aorta to the most critical structures—the coronary arteries in the heart and the cerebral arteries in the brain.

Blood from the coronary arteries, head, and upper extremities then returns to the heart via the superior vena cava. This blood, low in oxygen content, as well as a portion of blood from the inferior vena cava flows into the right ventricle. It is ejected into the pulmonary artery where flow again divides. A small portion enters the lungs but most blood flows through the ductus arteriosus into the aorta. This blood is low in oxygen content and mixes with blood ejected from the left ventricle into the aorta.

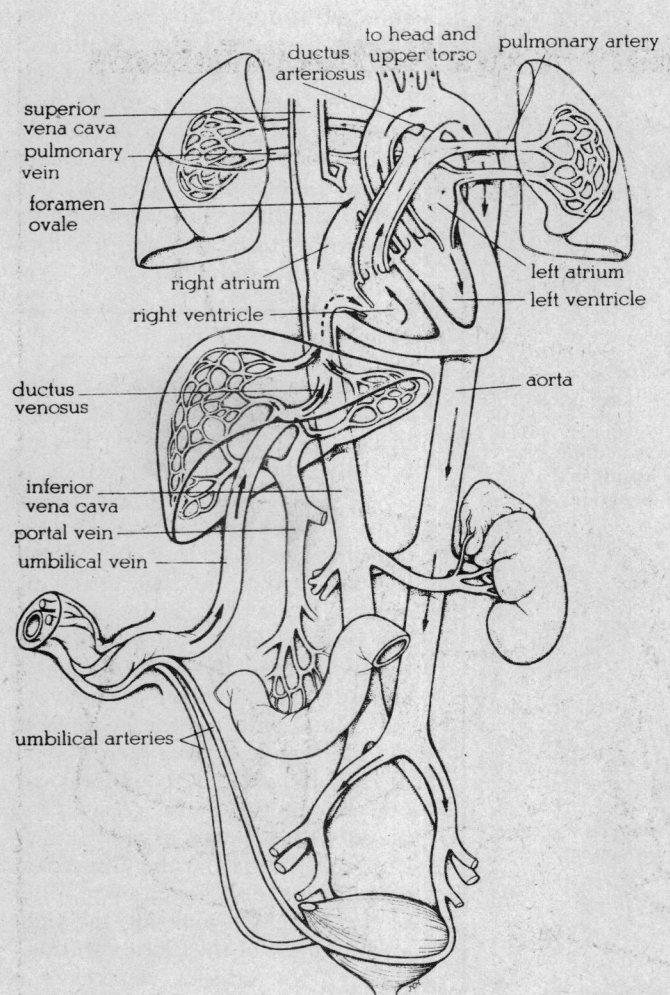
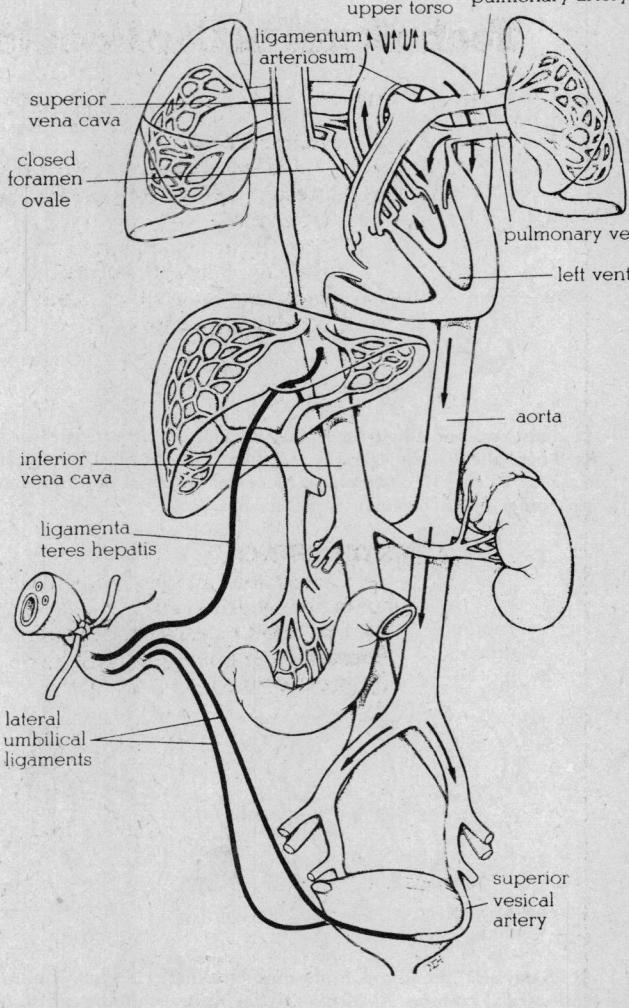

FETAL CIRCULATION (left). Oxygenated blood flows from placenta via umbilical vein to liver; into inferior vena cava, where it combines with some unoxygenated blood, and on to right atrium; through the foramen ovale to left atrium; left ventricle; and aorta. This blood perfuses the brain, coronary arteries, and upper torso. Venous blood returning to the right atrium from superior vena cava mixes with some oxygenated blood entering from inferior vena cava and flows into right ventricle and out through pulmonary artery. Some blood continues to lungs, but most is shunted through ductus arteriosus into decending aorta and eventually reaches placenta through umbilical arteries.
EXTRAUTERINE CIRCULATION (right). Ductus venosus, ductus arteriosus, and foramen ovale close as lungs take over function of oxygenation and carbon dioxide elimination.

This supplies the lower extremities and returns to the placenta via the umbilical arteries.

Circulatory Changes After Birth

At birth the lungs assume the function of oxygen and carbon dioxide exchange. The expansion of the lungs has profound effects on the neonate's circulatory system.

With the initiation of respiration, the alveoli expand and blood flow through the lungs increases. The increase in pulmonary blood flow and decrease in pulmonary vascular resistance cause left atrial pressure to rise while right atrial pressure falls. The foramen ovale, anatomically structured to permit flow only from right to left, closes. The increase in oxygen saturation following the changes in pulmonary vascular resistance stimulate constriction and closure of the ductus arteriosus.

With the ligation of the umbilical cord, the ductus venosus, umbilical vein, and umbilical arteries no longer transport blood. As blood flow through these structures ceases, they are obliterated except the proximal portions of the umbilical arteries, which remain open.

Unoxygenated blood now returns to the heart through the superior and inferior vena cavae to the right atrium, flows from the right atrium into the right ventricle and into the pulmonary arteries to the lung. Oxygenated blood returns to the left atrium via the pulmonary veins, flows from the left atrium to the left ventricle and out through the aorta. Extrauterine circulation is thus established.

Bibliography

Fink, B. W. *Congenital Heart Disease: A Deductive Approach to its Diagnosis.* Chicago, Year Book Medical Publishers, 1975.

Korones, S. B. *High Risk Newborn Infants: The Basis for Intensive Nursing Care.* 2d ed. St. Louis, C. V. Mosby Co., 1976.

Langman, Jan. *Medical Embryology.* 3d ed. Baltimore, Williams and Wilkins Co., 1975.

Patten, B. M. *Human Embryology.* 3d ed. New York, McGraw-Hill Book Co., 1968.

Techniques of Cardiopulmonary Resuscitation in Infants

AIRWAY
- Clear the airway of mucus, if present. Use your finger in a sweeping motion.
- Tilt the infant's head backward *slightly*. Forceful extension of the neck may obstruct the infant's pliable breathing passages.

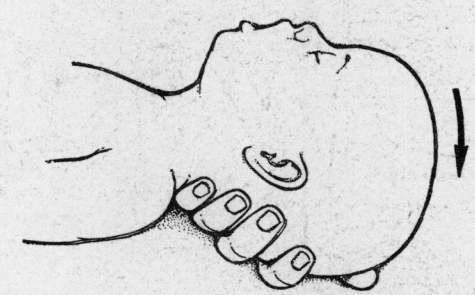

BREATHING
- Cover the infant's nose *and* mouth with your mouth.
- Use small breaths or puffs from cheeks to inflate the lungs once every three seconds.

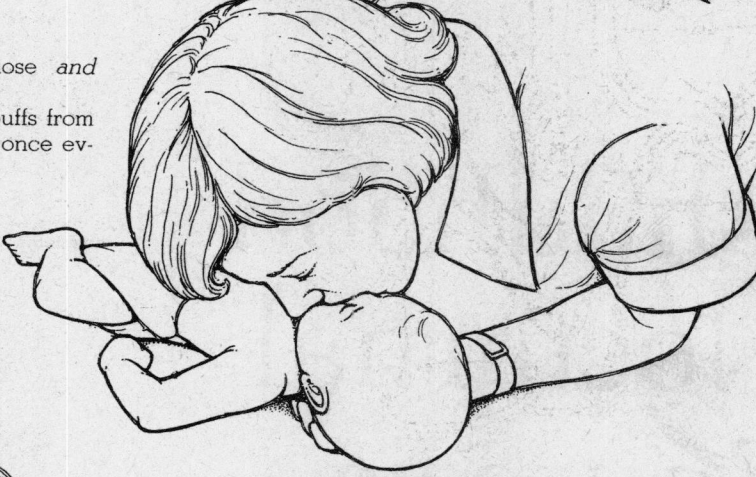

CIRCULATION
- Support the infant's back with your hand.
- Use the tips of your index and middle fingers to depress the midsternum about ½ to ¾ inches (left).
- Or, use alternate method (right). Circle chest with hands and compress sternum with both thumbs.
- Maintain a rate of 80 to 100 compressions per minute.
- Ventilate quickly, once after each five compressions.
- **Do not** interrupt compression during ventilation.

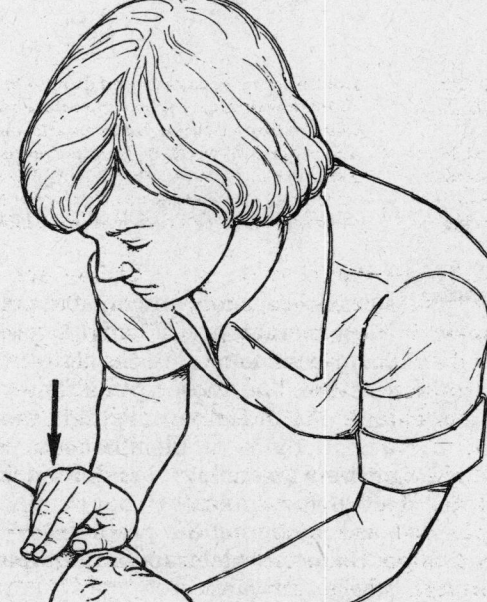
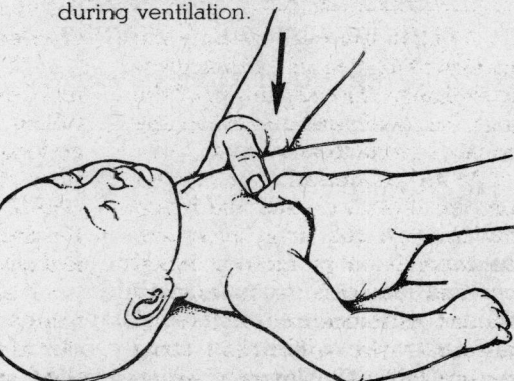

Childhood Nocturnal Enuresis

Reprinted from American Journal of Maternal/Child Nursing, January/February 1981.

Assuring the family that their child who bedwets will become dry, is not "bad," and they are not "to blame," are very important counseling messages.

JUDITH A. RUBLE

Childhood nocturnal enuresis, more commonly called bedwetting, occurs in children or adolescents usually between the ages of 5 and 18 years old. These children involuntarily urinate during sleep, one or more times a month. Moreover, the youngsters do not show any organic cause for the problem. Most commonly it affects children from lower socio-economic classes, males, children from large families, and those with a family history of enuresis (1-3). For the maternal child nurse, enuresis presents a challenging problem because confusion exists concerning its etiology; in addition there is a broad variety of and, typically, poor results from the treatments used to combat the problem.

Statistical data about childhood enuresis are not straightforward. Too many variables exist in the research that has been done, including differences in age among the children studied, varied frequency and history of the characteristics used to define the condition, and a reluctance among some groups of people to report enuresis. Moreover, some studies divide enuresis into two categories: "primary," where the child has never been dry, and "second-

REPRINTS: CHILDHOOD NOCTURNAL ENURESIS

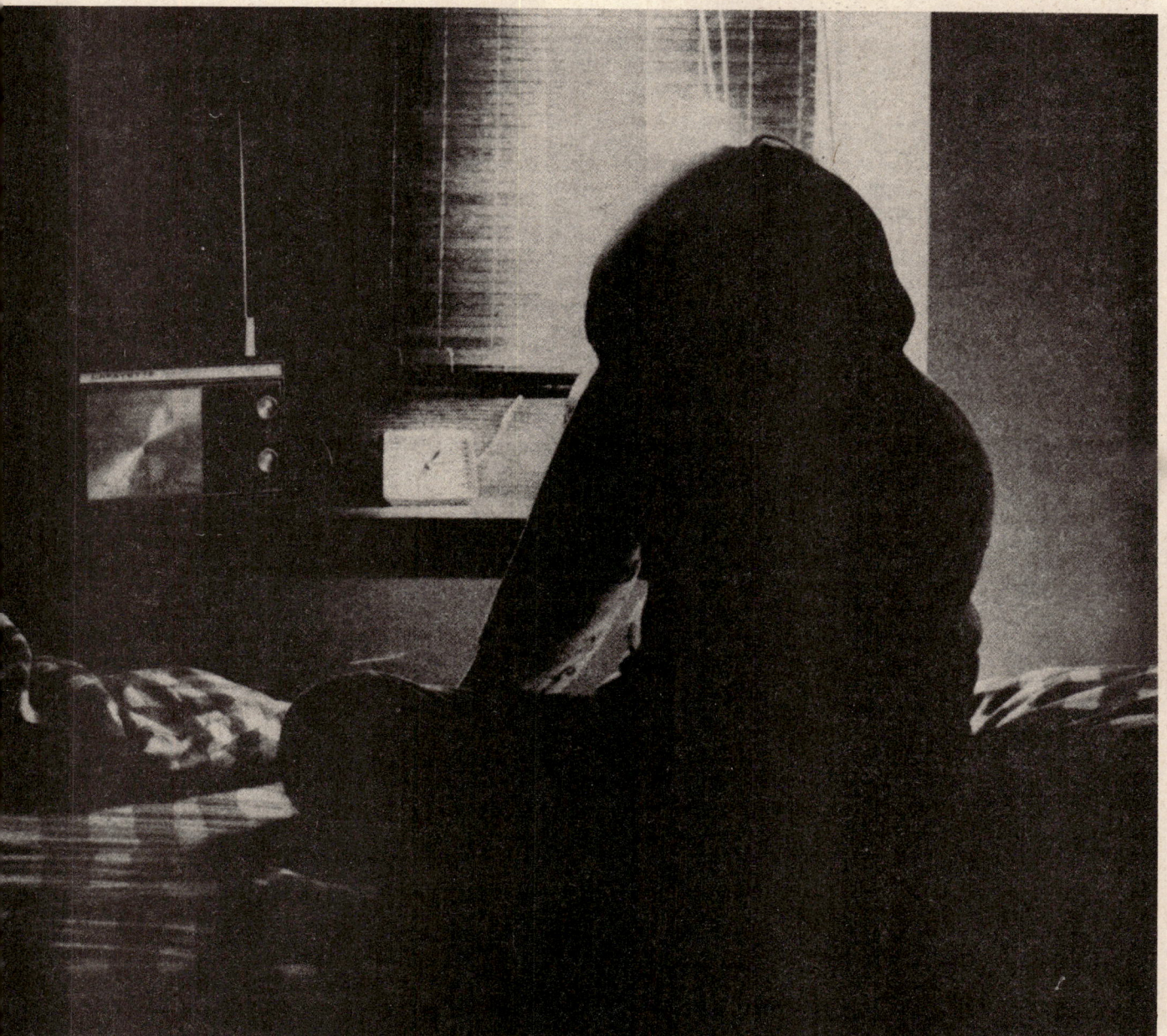

A child who suffers from enuresis faces many problems in our society. Often family rapport is negatively affected and relationships with other children his own age are severely limited.

ary," where the child has resumed wetting after having been dry for one month or more. Nonetheless, current management of these two groups does not differ significantly. To the affected child and his family, bedwetting causes manifold stresses, loss of self-confidence in the youngster, and troubled social and family relationships.

An enuretic child in our society faces considerable difficulties. Among these are that, usually, he is embarrassed to spend the night away from home and he is likely to be teased by schoolmates and siblings. Along with this, his family relationships are uneasy, irritated by the burden of constant bed-

MS. RUBLE, R.N., M.S., currently is associated with a physician in joint practice in Walnut Creek, California. Previously she was a maternal child nurse for the U.S. Public Health Service, assigned to three Appalachian counties. She was part of an improved pregnancy outcome program providing clinical and educational services to high risk mothers and infants.

changing and repeated punishments meted out by his parents. Enuretic children often suffer, as well, from low self-esteem, introversion, and psychological maladjustment (4,5).

Etiology of Childhood Enuresis

Although, as V.S. Werry writes, most of the research on the cause of enuresis "is remarkable for the absence of controls, for biased sampling and for lack of rigor in linking empirical fact with elegant theory", five popular etiologic theories exist (6). They are:

Emotional Disturbance. The concept of enuresis as a symptom of emotional disturbance is based on research done in the 1930s under the strong influence of Freudian psychology. These early studies involved small samples of children referred for psychiatric treatment. They had no controls and based their conclusions on highly subjective assessments of behavior (7,8). Later, longitudinal studies and studies of large populations of children in non-clinical settings refuted the 1930s research and found no significant differences in emotional adjustment ratings of enuretic and non-enuretic children (9,10). This evidence from clinical and non-clinical settings conflicts, suggesting the possibility that the enuretic children brought to the clinic formed a sample biased for signs of emotional disturbance. Therefore, the conclusion can be reached that while emotional disturbance may occur in enuretic children, it cannot be considered a necessary factor.

Deep Sleep. Parents commonly report that their child who has enuresis is an unusually deep sleeper. Therefore the belief that deep sleep is an etiologic factor in bedwetting persists—in spite of good evidence against it. Studies do not show any relationship between unusually deep sleep and enuresis, while EEG and bladder contraction tracings on enuretics do give convincing evidence that enuresis is associated with abnormal bladder contractions during transitions from deeper to lighter levels of sleep (11-13). It is possible that parents who awaken their enuretic child to void during the night inadvertently choose the deepest part of his sleep cycle when it is difficult to arouse him. They then wrongly assume he is an unusually deep sleeper.

Delayed Neurologic Development. This is another proposed etiology for enuresis. But the exact nature of the developmental delay is not known. It may result from slow myelinization of the neural pathways involved in inhibiting the bladder contraction reflex during sleep or by the child's slow response to a full bladder, so that he does not awaken in time to avoid bedwetting. Because studies show that approximately 14 to 16 percent of children who bedwet are "spontaneously" cured annually, it seems likely the cure is more closely related to increasing age than to treatment (14,15). These studies support the developmental delay theory, since enuretic children would be expected to outgrow the problem as they continue to develop and reach higher levels of neurologic maturity.

Small Functional Bladder Capacity. The theory that enuresis is due to a small functional bladder capacity is based on measurements of the volume the bladder can hold before a child feels an urgent need to void. This theory is supported by several studies using physiologic methods of bladder filling and volume measurements and show that enuretic children have a significantly smaller functional bladder capacity than non-enuretic children (16-18).

COMPARISON OF TREATMENTS FOR ENURESIS

	Bed Alarm	Bladder Stretching	Imipramine
Cure Rate	70 – 80%	Approximately 30%	25 – 50%
Speed of Effect	2 – 16 weeks	3 – 6 months	3 – 4 months
Advantages	Sound basis in psychological theory and research Most relapses quickly cured by re-treatment	No cost Non-invasive Child "cures" self Record-keeping may act as reinforcement Record-keeping shows compliance	Approximately 80% rapid improvement Easy to implement Little attention focused on enuresis by treatment
Disadvantages	Philosophical objections to conditioning Alarm may awaken family Cost of appliance ($25 – $100) Focuses attention on enuresis Cure achieved by "machine" Occasional reports of skin rash (with older devices) Relapse rate approximately 18%	Time-consuming procedures Focuses attention on enuresis	Lethal in overdose Common side effects (dry mouth, irritability, G.I. upset, wakefullness) Rare, reversible toxic effects (leukopenia, liver damage) Relapse rate approximately 20 – 80% Cure achieved by "pill"

The theory is further supported by the finding that as the enuretic child's functional bladder capacity is increased by bladder stretching exercises the enuresis improves (19).

Genetic Predisposition. There is good evidence for a genetic predisposition for enuresis. The tendency for bedwetting to occur in children with a family history of the condition is well documented, and the occurrence of enuresis in identical twins is nearly twice that for fraternal twins, which indicates a strong genetic influence (2,20). Yet there is no agreement among health professionals on the specific way in which genetic factors cause the delay in attaining nighttime bladder control.

Such conflicting evidence on the etiology of enuresis indicates that it has multiple causes. Possibly the underlying cause of enuresis is a genetic predisposition for developmental delay or abnormal bladder contraction during sleep. These factors in turn may result in a small functional bladder capacity, which is the immediate cause of bedwetting.

Managing the Problem

Current methods of treating childhood enuresis include drugs, conditioning devices, bladder stretching exercises, waking the child at regular intervals so he will void, fluid restriction, hypnosis, psychotherapy, behavior modification, and elimination diets. Reported cure rates for these methods range from no better than spontaneous cure rates to 100 percent. Each method has its benefits and drawbacks, and each has won only limited acceptance among clinicians and patients.

However, the first step in developing a management plan for children who bedwet is to take a complete medical and social history of the child and his family. This is essential so the problems produced by the enuresis can be assessed, possible causes and aggravating factors determined, and various treatment methods evaluated for that particular child and family.

Complaints of urinary frequency or urgency, dysuria, unexplained fevers, and abdominal or flank pain are investigated. Growth patterns are reviewed and a complete physical examination is performed. The health professional pays special attention to the child's general appearance, possible abdominal, suprapubic, or flank tenderness, and genito-urinary abnormalities, redness, or discharge. Laboratory studies are made and include urine culture, specific gravity, urinalysis including microscopic examination, and, for groups at risk, sickle cell screening (21). These procedures are carefully followed because it is necessary to rule out the possibility of any organic cause for the enuresis. Although only a small percent of childhood enuresis proves to have an organic cause, when such a cause is identified the child must be referred for further medical evaluation.

When functional enuresis is diagnosed it must be understood that it has no identified physical complications and has a 99 percent rate of cure, given time. Health professionals and parents should view it as a social problem, involving unmet expectations and reciprocal inappropriate behaviors of the child and family. In counseling the family, the health professional can impart the message that

- the child is not "bad"
- he will almost certainly become dry
- enuresis is very common
- it is not a conscious behavior
- no organic defect exists and no ill effects will result, and,
- the parents are not responsible for making the child enuretic

The nurse can discuss the child's enuresis as an involuntary delay in the development of the child's control of his bladder reflexes. This outlook relieves the parents of guilt and underlines the inappropriateness of punitive measures. Further, the nurse can assist the family as they deal with embarrassments and frustrations, by encouraging them to express and discuss their feelings during clinic visits.

Longitudinal studies of children found no significant differences in the emotional adjustment ratings of enuretic and non-enuretic children.

By praising the parents for their constructive efforts and discouraging critical comments about the enuretic child, a nurse helps to establish a supportive atmosphere within the family. For example, she can say to them, "You have already done several important things to help Mary. Asking her to avoid soft drinks in the evening, allowing her extra time in the morning to shower, and deciding to come here today are positive steps, and will be a part of the program we develop for Mary." This kind of positive approach is important and no critical remarks should be made to Mary about the enuresis.

The parents can be urged to give the child as much responsibility for changing his bed and doing laundry as he can handle. A five- or six-year-old can strip off the wet sheets or protective pads from his bed and a 10- or 12-year-old can do part or all of the laundering and bed-changing. By giving responsibility to the child in a non-punitive way, he is made to feel that he is participating in the management of his problem and that his parents begin to view their own role as primarily supportive.

Specific treatments used together with the counseling described above may quickly relieve some family stress by curing the enuresis. Although the use of "symptomatic" treatment has been criticized for ignoring possible underlying emotional disturbance and risking symptom substitution, there is no evidence to support this criticism.

Three such symptomatic treatments frequently used are:

Bed Alarm Condition Device. The bed alarm consists of a pad placed on the bed and an alarm device that is triggered by very small amounts of urine coming in contact with the pad. The cure is achieved as the child learns to inhibit urination in order to avoid the alarm. Cure is usually accomplished within three to four months, often within a few weeks. Relapse is common but is cured quickly with a second treatment (22).

Bladder Stretching Exercises. Bladder stretching exercises to increase functional bladder capacity employ a daily regimen of encouraging fluids and asking the child to hold his urine for as long as possible. When he does void, he's asked to stop and start several times to improve sphincter control. The amount voided is recorded on a calendar along with any dry nights. Significant increases in functional bladder capacity are found over the course of three to six months with a corresponding decrease in the frequency of enuresis (19).

Imipramine Drug Therapy. Drug therapy using anticholinergics, antihistamines, amphetamines, atropine, tranquilizers, or diuretics has been tried and not found effective in curing enuresis. At present the most promising drug for the treatment of enuresis is imipramine (Tofranil®), a tricyclic anti-depressant.

Imipramine acts in three ways that are considered useful in treating enuresis: (1) adrenergic action lightens sleep, (2) anti-cholinergic action allows increased bladder filling, and (3) anti-depressant action relieves underlying depression. This drug has proved highly effective in decreasing enuretic episodes within days and producing cures in approximately three to four months. Relapse is frequent, but the likelihood of this happening can be reduced by withdrawing the medication gradually after completing treatment (23).

All these treatments are acceptable currently, but each has a different set of implications for any given family. (See a Comparison of Treatments for Enuresis [22,19,23].) Since no clear cut research exists to guide the health professional's choice of treatment it is reasonable and desirable to involve the family in the decision-making process. I have adapted an outcome matrix from June T. Bailey and Karen Claus, which integrates patient participation in the evaluation of treatment alternatives while it provides an objective framework for the health professional and family for making a decision (24). (See Jones Family Outcome Matrix.)

Choosing a Treatment Method

In order to consider individual needs when using the outcome matrix, I have divided the criteria for choosing a treatment method into two categories:

1. General Criteria of Safety, Effectiveness, and Simplicity for Choosing Treatment. "Safety" refers to the absence of physical harm from treatment. (A high rating is ideal.) A high rating is given for no reports of physical harm, moderate for minor temporary effects, and low for permanent or serious harm.

"Effectiveness" refers to the documented probability of producing a cure. (A high rating is ideal.) A low rating is given for cure rates of 0 to 25 percent, moderate for 36 to 60 percent, and high for 61 to 100 percent.

"Simplicity" refers to the number of steps required to implement the treatment; a high rating is ideal. A high rating is given for one to three steps,

JONES FAMILY OUTCOME MATRIX

	General Criteria			Individual Criteria		
Alternatives	Safety	Effectiveness	Simplicity	Acceptability	Speed	Total
Bed Alarm	Mod/Low	(High)	Mod	(High)	(High)	3
Bladder Stretching	(High)	Mod	Low	Low	Low	1
Imipramine	Mod	Mod	(High)	Low/Mod	Mod	1
Ideal	High	High	High	High	High	5

*Alternative ratings which correspond with ideal ratings are circled.

moderate for three to four steps, and low for five and more steps.

2. Individual Criteria for Choosing Treatment Alternatives. "Acceptability" includes the feelings of the child and family toward the treatment and the suitability of the treatment for the family. (A high rating is ideal.) Special circumstances or needs are reflected in this criterion, for example, the risk of accidental poisoning with imipramine. Each treatment is rated by the family and clinician together.

"Speed in producing effect" refers to the expected length of treatment required for cure. (A high rating is ideal.) The value placed on the need for rapid results depends on the family situation; treatment ratings are assigned by the family.

Ideal ratings are assigned to each criterion as "high," "moderate," or "low," based on literature review, clinical judgment, and, for the individual factors, input from the child and his family. Each time an alternative corresponds with the ideal rating, it is given one point. Final choice of a treatment alternative is determined by the sum of the criteria scores.

For example, the Jones family is composed of Mr. and Mrs. Jones; John, age 13; and Mary, age 10. Mary has never been dry at night and presently wets from five to seven nights a week. She has no evidence of organic cause for the enuresis and no apparent emotional disturbance. Recently she has become increasingly withdrawn socially, refusing to go to camp or to slumber parties. Her brother teases her and calls her a "baby." Her mother has tried restricting fluids, awakening Mary during the night to void, offering rewards, and threatening punishment. All methods have been unsuccessful. As a last resort, the Jones family has come to the clinic for help. The mother is losing patience with Mary and Mary is close to tears when discussing the problem.

The family consults with the nurse about the different treatments available and their features. The nurse and family, together, assign the individual criteria ratings of "high" acceptability and speed for the bed alarm, "low" acceptability and speed for bladder stretching, and "low/moderate" and "moderate" acceptability and speed for imipramine (See Jones Family Outcome Matrix.) The bed alarm receives two points because its high ratings for acceptability and speed correspond with the high ideal ratings for these criteria. Therefore, two points for the bed alarm are added to the one point received for high effectiveness, giving a total of three. Bladder stretching has only one point (for high safety), as does imipramine (for high simplicity). The bed alarm, therefore, comes closest to the ideal total of five and is the treatment of choice. This choice is acceptable to the family and meets their desire for rapid results. The management plan is implemented with regular clinic visits to offer encouragement and support and to assess progress. If the nurse determines there is a need to measure the family's attitude changes during the treatment, suitable psychological tests can be administered at the first visit and again at the final treatment visit.

By gathering information about the effectiveness of different treatment alternatives from a number of families who have a child with enuresis, nurses will establish a basis upon which to make future recommendations about the treatment of bedwetting to parents of children with enuresis. Such data will influence the assigning of ratings to the criteria of the outcome matrix. In this way a feedback loop, which is essential to effective decision-making in the management of enuresis, will be established.

REFERENCES

1. LOVIBOND, S.H. Conditioning and Enuresis. New York, Macmillan Co., 1964.
2. HALLGREN, B. Enuresis: a clinical and genetic study. Acta Psychiat. Neur.Scand. 32(Suppl. 114):1-159, 1957.
3. BAKWIN, H. Enuresis in children. J.Pediatr. 58:806-819, June 1961.
4. SACKS, S., AND OTHERS. Psychological changes associated with conditioning functional enuresis. J.Clin. Psychol. 30:271-276, July 1974.
5. BAKER, B.L. Symptom treatment and symptom substitution in enuresis. J.Abnorm.Psychol. 74:42-49, Feb. 1969.
6. WERRY, J. S., AND COHRSSEN, J. Enuresis—an etiologic and therapeutic study. J.Pediatr. 67:423-431, Sept. 1965.
7. MICHAELS, J. J., AND GOODMAN, S. E. Incidence and intercorrelations of enuresis and other neuropathic traits in so-called normal children. Am.J.Orthopsychiatry 4:79, 1934.
8. GERARD, M. Enuresis: a study in etiology. Am.J.Orthopsychiatry 9:48-54, 1939.
9. MACFARLANE, J. W., AND OTHERS. Developmental Study of the Behavior Problems of Normal Children Between Twenty-One Months and Fourteen Years. (California University Publications in Child Development, vol. 2) Berkeley, University of California Press, 1954.
10. TAPIA, F., AND OTHERS. Enuresis: an emotional symptom? J.Nerv.Ment.Dis. 130:61-66, Jan. 1960
11. DITMAN, K. S., AND BLINN, K. A. Sleep levels in enuresis. Am.J. Psychiatry 11:913-920, June 1955.
12. BOYD, M. M. The depth of sleep in enuretic school-children and in non-enuretic controls. J.Sychosom.Res. 4:274-281, July 1960.
13. BROUGHTON, R. J. Sleep disorders: disorders of arousal? Science 159:1070-1078, Mar. 8, 1968.
14. FORSYTHE, W. I., AND REDMOND, A. Enuresis and spontaneous cure rate: study of 1129 enuretics. Arch.Dis.Children 49:259-263, Apr. 1974.
15. BARBOUR, R. F., AND OTHERS. Enuresis as a disorder of development. Br.Med.J. 2(5360):787-790, Sept. 28, 1963.
16 MUELLNER, S. R. Development of urinary control in children; some aspects of the cause and treatment of primary enuresis JAMA 172:1256-1261, Mar. 19, 1960.
7. STARFIELD, E. Functional bladder capacity in enuretic and nonenuretic children. J.Pediatr. 70:777-781, May 1967.
18. ESPERANCA, M., AND GERRARD, J. W. Nocturnal enuresis: studies in bladder function in normal children and enuretics. Can.Med.Assoc.J. 101:324-327, Sept. 20, 1969.
19. STARFIELD, B. Increase in functional bladder capacity and improvements in enuresis. J.Pediatr. 72:483-487, Apr.1968.
20. BAKWIN, H. Enuresis in twins. Am.J.Dis.Child. 121:222-225, Mar. 1971.
21. SUSTER, G., AND OSKI, F. A. Enuresis in sickle cell anemia. Am.J. Dis.Child. 113:311, Mar. 1967
22. LOVIBOND, S. H., AND COOTE, M. A. Enuresis. In Symptoms of Psychopathology, ed. by C. G. Costello. New York, John Wiley & Sons, 1970, pp. 373-396.
23. POUSSAINT, A.F., AND DITMAN, K. S. A controlled study of Imipramine (Tofranil) in the treatment of childhood enuresis. J.Pediatr. 67:283-290, Aug.1965.
24. BAILEY, J. T., AND CLAUS, K. E. Decision Making in Nursing: Tools for Change. St. Louis, C. V. Mosby Co., 1975, pp. 75-83.

Evaluating Head Trauma In Infants And Children

Reprinted from American Journal of Maternal/Child Nursing, January/February 1983

Nurses can play a significant role in screening, evaluating, and managing this common injury.

ELLEN M. MEIER

Acute head trauma is an extremely common problem among children, accounting for nearly 250,000 hospital admissions annually. Many more cases are evaluated and released through emergency departments and outpatient clinics or over the telephone. Because the nurse may be responsible for eliciting all or part of the injured child's history, she must know what screening questions to ask and what complications to caution parents to watch for.

The child's history is all-important in determining whether the child requires immediate medical attention or can be kept at home for observation by the parents. The specific information needed includes when the injury occurred; how the injury occurred (for example, how far the child fell and to what type of surface); and how the child behaved immediately after the injury.

In addition, the nurse must ascertain whether the child experienced loss of consciousness or memory, vomiting, disorientation, confusion, lethargy, bleeding or cerebrospinal (CSF) fluid drainage from the nose or ears, or any lacerations. She must also determine whether the child has any preexisting illnesses, such as a seizure disorder, gait disturbance, or physical handicap. Since head trauma among infants and young children may be the result of child abuse, the nurse also evaluates the history in terms of the child's developmental ability, the likelihood of the injury occurring as described, and the presence of limb fractures or other associated injuries.

If the child is alert and mature enough, the nurse can obtain the history directly from him. If not, any observer of the injury can provide the necessary information. Frequently, the nurse can obtain the history over the telephone, thereby eliminating the need for a clinic or emergency room visit.

If the head injury was minimal and there was no loss of consciousness, bleeding, or disorientation, the child can be safely observed at home. However, if parents are hesitant about observing the child, the child should be seen and evaluated by a health care provider.

Many children have headaches or vomit once or twice during the first 24 hours following minor head trauma. Unless these symptoms are progressive or accompanied by increasing lethargy, they usually are of little concern.

Loss of consciousness, severe or progressive vomiting or headaches, amnesia, disorientation, seizures or weakness, bleeding or CSF drainage from the ears or nose, and any unusual changes in behavior, however, warrant immediate medical evaluation and follow-up. Depending on their severity, open wounds or lacerations may also need attention. Even if a wound is not serious, the child's immunization status must be determined.

While eliciting the child's history, the nurse often will realize that the injury could have been avoided had safety measures such as car seats or restraints been used. Since the injured child's parents probably are already feeling anxious or guilty about the incident, the nurse must be careful not to increase their guilt feelings, although she can tactfully give appropriate guidance on safety procedures and precautions.

When a Physical Examination Is Needed

Positive or focal (pointing to a localized area of injury within the central nervous system) neurological findings are rare in cases of simple head trauma. However, any child who has sustained a significant blow to the head, has lost consciousness, or has any suspicious symptoms needs a thorough general physical examination and a neurological examination.

MS. MEIER, R.N., M.N., is the director of education and training for Kaiser Foundation Hospital in Panorama City, California. She is also a certified pediatric nurse practitioner.

Signs of shock (increased pulse and decreased blood pressure) or increased intracranial pressure are important to watch for. Any abnormalities found during the physical and neurological examinations require further evaluation by a neurologist or neurosurgeon and possibly hospitalization of the child.

The entire body, including the mouth, neck, chest, abdomen, and extremities, must be examined for evidence of injury. The scalp must be inspected for depression or areas of soft spongy hematoma over a depressed skull facture. For infants, the anterior fontanelle must be assessed for evidence of fullness or bulging.

Transillumination of the skull can be performed to detect intracranial or extracranial fluid. Other physical findings indicating possible basal skull fracture are periorbital hemorrhage with bilateral black eyes (raccoon eyes), blood behind the eardrum (hemotympanum), bruising behind the ear (Battle's sign), and bleeding or CSF drainage from the ears or nose.

A thorough neurological examination includes an evaluation of the child's level of consciousness, orientation, memory, and motor abilities. Level of consciousness can range from agitated to alert to lethargic, stuporous, or comatose. Orientation and memory can be evaluated by having the child identify himself and his surroundings and relate the incident of the injury.

The eyes are an important element in the neurological examination. Pupil size and reactivity as well as extraocular movements can be evaluated to determine cranial nerve function. The fundi can be examined for papilledema and retinal hemorrhage. Retinal hemorrhages often accompany subdural hematomas in small infants who are held by their shoulders and shaken vigorously, a relatively common form of child abuse. The child who is alert can be tested for visual acuity and peripheral vision.

To evaluate the motor system, the child's gait and symmetry of muscle strength can be observed. Parasthesias or numbness should be assessed. For the older child, cerebellar function can be evaluated with the Romberg test or by heel-walking and toe-walking. Eliciting deep tendon reflexes and attempting to elicit Babinski's reflex (dorsiflexion and fanning of the toes by stroking the lateral sole, an abnormal finding in infants and children over the age of one year) completes the motor system examination.

When Diagnostic Studies Are Necessary

Routine skull films for minor head trauma yield few findings or results. Further, skull fracture alone does not necessarily indicate serious brain injury

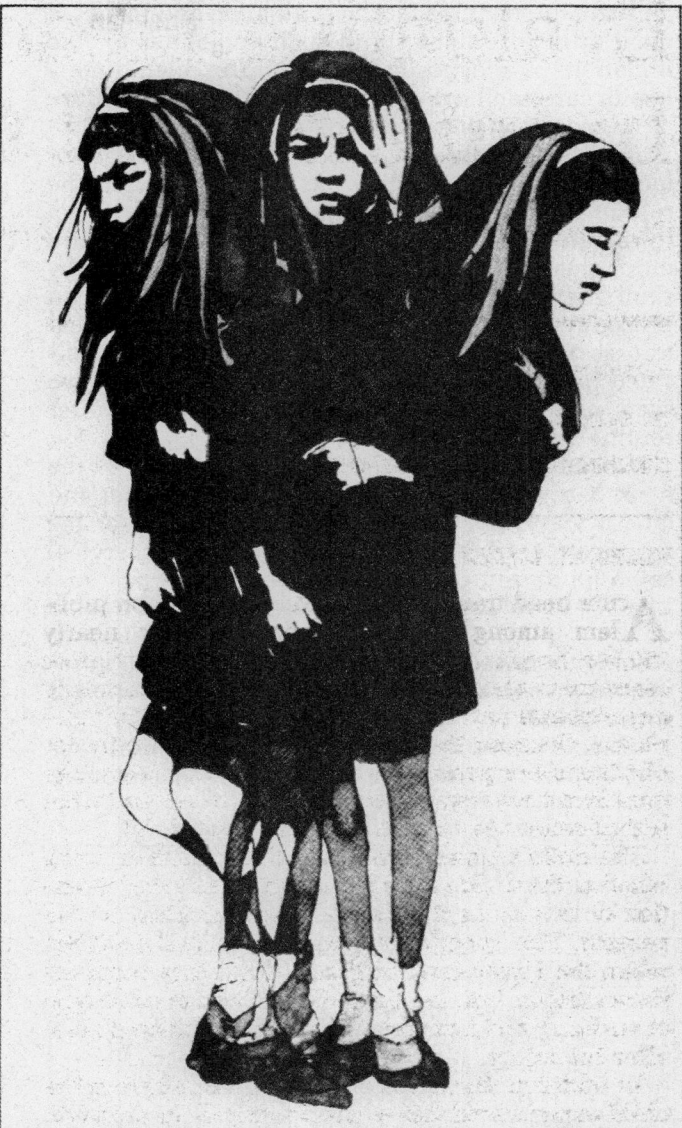

Evaluating all the symptoms accompanying head trauma is all-important in determining whether the child requires medical attention or can be kept at home for observation.

and does not change treatment plans, except for depressed and compound fractures, which require surgical correction. In a study of 354 infants and children who had skull roentgenography for head trauma, for example, only 4.2 percent had skull fracture and none had serious intracranial complications (1). Thus, unless there is significant reason to be suspicious of a pathological condition, routine skull films are unwise, especially in light of the ever-increasing concern about unnecessary exposure to radiation.

Criteria for determining when skull roentgenography is necessary were established in 1978 by Leon Phillips and modified in 1982 by John Leonidas and others (1,2). These criteria (listed in the table below) are useful to the nurse in the development of standardized procedures for the evaluation and management of head trauma. With such guidelines for the initiation of diagnostic studies, safe, high-quality health care can be provided without the expenditure of unnecessary time and money.

The availability of computerized transaxial tomography (CAT) scanning has greatly changed the role of radiology in the evaluation of head trauma. Intracranial hemorrhage and tissue structures are more clearly delineated by CAT scanning than by skull roentgenography. In addition, the CAT scan procedure is safe and painless and can be repeated to assess changing signs and symptoms. It is indicated for head trauma with localized or progressive signs or symptoms, although generally only after routine skull films have been obtained (3).

If head trauma is severe or there is injury to the neck, X-rays should also include anteroposterior and lateral views of the cervical spine. Because of the significance of spinal cord transection, cervical spine injury must be diagnosed as soon as possible. Lumbar puncture is not performed for head trauma unless central nervous system infection, such as meningitis, is suspected. It is contraindicated if intracranial pressure is increased or if a mass lesion is suspected (3).

Other diagnostic studies, such as subdural taps and ventricular drainage for subdural hematomas, may be necessary under selected and specific conditions. However, nurses usually are not involved in ordering or performing these studies.

Differentiating Diagnoses

Minor head injury without positive history or physical examination findings is simply called head trauma or uncomplicated head trauma. Frequently, the diagnosis of concussion is made incorrectly. Concussion is defined as head injury followed by a period of unconsciousness (loss of awareness and responsiveness). The period of unresponsiveness may last from several seconds to several hours. If the injury was unwitnessed, the diagnosis of concussion is sometimes made if the child experiences retrograde or posttraumatic amnesia (3).

The diagnosis of skull fracture is made on the basis of radiologic findings. About 75 percent of skull fractures in children are linear fractures; other types include depressed, compound, and basal skull fractures. Although skull fracture does not warrant any specific management, it indicates that a significant injury occurred. Often, children with skull fractures are hospitalized for observation.

In addition to radiographic evidence, racoon eyes, hemotympanum, and Battle's sign are indications of basal skull fracture. Characteristic features of an occipital fracture are tachycardia, hypotension, and irregular respirations caused by brainstem compression. CSF rhinorrhea may indicate a fracture of the cribriform plate, whereas CSF otorrhea may indicate fracture of the petrous temporal bone (3).

Actual epidural or subdural hematomas are diagnosed by the child's history and physical examination findings, specifically those findings associated with increased intracranial pressure. They are also diagnosed by skull films, CAT scans, and special studies such as subdural taps.

Contusion of the brain is a bruising or crushing injury to the brain. It usually results from blunt trauma to the head and may be accompanied by skull fracture (3). Diagnosis is based on the presence of focal neurological signs, such as seizures, and is frequently confirmed by a CAT scan.

Superficial injuries to the head include scalp lacerations and hematomas. Often, a significant amount of scalp swelling follows head trauma, but it does not require treatment. Aspiration is of no benefit and just increases the risk of infection.

Scalp lacerations must be evaluated to determine whether sutures are required, and the child's tetanus status must always be determined. A fully immunized child with a minor scalp laceration need not receive tetanus toxoid or antitoxin. However, if an open scalp wound has been unattended for more than 24 hours, the child must receive both passive and active tetanus immunization even if he was fully immunized previously (4).

PROPOSED CRITERIA FOR SKULL ROENTGENOGRAPHY FOR CHILDREN WITH HEAD TRAUMA*

Historical Criteria
- Age less than one year.
- Unconscious for more than five minutes.
- Gunshot wound or skull penetration.
- Previous craniotomy with shunting tube in place.

Physical Examination Criteria
- Palpable hematoma on scalp.
- Skull depression palpable or identified by probe in scalp laceration.
- Cerebrospinal fluid (CSF) discharge from ear or nose.
- Blood in middle ear.
- Battle's sign.
- Racoon eyes.
- Lethargy, coma, or stupor.
- Focal neurological signs.

*These criteria were established by John Leonidas and others and modified by Leon Phillips.

Most head injuries do not result in serious consequences. However, careful observation of the child during the first two days after a head injury is extremely important for recognizing complications. The following signs and symptoms must be reported and evaluated immediately:

- Persistent or progressive vomiting.
- Headache if it is long-lasting or increases in severity.
- Unusual drowsiness, confusion, irritability, or inability to awaken the child. (The child should be awakened every two hours for the first 24 hours following significant head trauma.)
- Convulsions or seizures.
- Dizziness, weakness, or numbness.
- Fever above 101°F.
- Visual disturbance or inequality of the pupil size.
- Clear fluid or blood coming from the nose or ears.

If you are uncertain or concerned about any of the above, call:

_____ at the following number _____

or return to _____

Head trauma may be complicated by meningitis, especially when a child has a basal skull fracture. Signs and symptoms include fever, irritability, and meningeal irritation such as nuchal rigidity.

Other syndromes following head injury include posttraumatic epilepsy and transient posttraumatic blindness. These syndromes are dramatic but poorly understood. Posttraumatic blindness generally lasts minutes to hours. Seizures can occur up to one week following head trauma; between 20 percent and 25 percent of the children who experience head trauma have seizure disorders (5).

The Role of the Nurse

In dealing with head trauma, the nurse is primarily responsible for observation, guidance, and deciding whether the injury is severe enough to refer the child for consultation with a physician and perhaps with a neurologist or neurosurgeon. If the child is sent home, the nurse must give the parents or caretaker specific instructions as to what signs and symptoms require further evaluation. These can be printed on a sheet for the parents to take with them (see example above).

Most signs of significant injury will appear during the first 48 hours following the trauma. Since it is unrealistic to expect a child who has sustained a head injury to remain awake during this period when observation is critical, the nurse must reassure parents that there is no inherent danger in allowing the child to fall asleep. Children often are drowsy after the physical and emotional upheaval of head trauma. Awakening them for evaluation at two-hour intervals is sufficient and safe. The important issue is the child's overall level of consciousness.

When counseling over the telephone, the nurse can refer to the head injury sheet as she instructs parents about the signs of possible complications and when to seek further medical attention for the child. If an open wound has been sustained, the nurse must also determine the need for suturing and the child's immunization status. At no time should the nurse discourage parents from bringing in a child for evaluation by a health care professional if they are uneasy about observing the child at home.

Generally Favorable Prognosis

Only 5 percent to 10 percent of children who are hospitalized for head trauma show neurological signs and symptoms (6). Most who are hospitalized because of loss of consciousness or skull fracture recover completely within 24 to 48 hours. A small percentage experience seizures, motor deficits, or intellectual impairment.

In contrast to adults, children who experience head trauma continue to show improvement for more than three years following a comparable injury (7). Children with signs of severe injury also have a more favorable outcome than do adults with similar signs (8). Because of this prognosis, the child or infant who experiences head trauma should be evaluated and treated quickly and aggressively.

Nurses can play a significant role in the screening, evaluation, and management of this common and frightening injury. At the same time, they can promote health and safety procedures as well as plans for follow-up for the injured infant or child.

REFERENCES

1. LEONIDAS, J.C., AND OTHERS. Mild head trauma in children: when is a roentgenogram necessary. *Pediatrics* 69:139-143, Feb. 1982.
2. PHILLIPS, L.A. *A Study of the Effect of High Yield Criteria for Emergency Room Skull Radiography.* (DHEW Publ. (FDA) 78-8089) Washington D.C., U.S. Government Printing Office, 1978.
3. ROSMAN, N.P., AND OTHERS. Acute head trauma in infancy and childhood. Clinical and radiologic aspects. *Pediatr.Clin.North Am.* 26:707-736, Nov. 1979.
4. AMERICAN ACADEMY OF PEDIATRICS, Committee on Infectious Diseases. *Report.* 18th ed. Evanston, Ill., The Academy, 1977.
5. JENNETT, B. Trauma as a cause of epilepsy in childhood. *Dev.Med. Child Neurol.* 15:56-62, Feb. 1973.
6. DEANGELIS, CATHERINE. *Pediatric Primary Care.* 2nd ed. Boston, Little Brown and Co., 1979.
7. RICHARDSON, F. Some effects of severe head injury. A follow-up study of children and adolescents after protracted coma. *Dev.Med.Child Neurol.* 5:471-482, Oct. 1963.
8. OVERGAARD, J., AND OTHERS. Prognosis after head injury based on early clinical examination. *Lancet* 2:631-635, Sept. 22, 1973.

The Child with Epilepsy
Teaching Children About Their Seizures and Medications

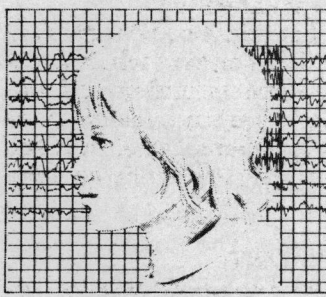

Reprinted from American Journal of Maternal/Child Nursing, May/June 1979.

Epilepsy remains a most misunderstood and feared disorder, a destructive tendency particularly among children who have seizures and their families.

MARY K. COUGHLIN

Children who have seizure disorders have many problems; it's the job of the health care team to make sure ignorance isn't one of them. To participate fully in their treatment programs, children and their parents need to understand what seizures are, how their medications work, what side effects to look for, and under what conditions their seizure frequency may increase. Too often this important teaching is overlooked.

To understand how her medication works, a child and her parents must first understand what happens when a seizure occurs. A simple explanation is often all that is necessary:

All living things are made of tiny parts called cells. Our brains are made of cells. The cells in our brains communicate with one another by sending electrical messages. These messages are what let us talk, see, walk, feel, and many other things. Sometimes a cell or group of cells gets too excited and sends messages when it shouldn't. When the other cells in the brain get these messages and obey, a seizure occurs.

MS. COUGHLIN, R.N., B.S.N., is a staff nurse in the Pediatric Neurology Clinic at the University of Illinois Medical Center, Chicago.

The nurse can then elaborate to say that the excitable cells may send messages without the other cells reacting to them and that these messages can be seen on an electroencephalogram. This will explain the purpose of these frequent tests.

Most anticonvulsants work in one of two ways: either they make the excitable cells less so or they make the other cells less responsive. Once the child and her parents understand this, it is a good time to stress the importance of always taking medication as prescribed. Too often patients and parents feel that if the child is no longer having seizures, she doesn't need the medicine. They must understand that absence of seizures only indicates that the medicine is working properly.

Side Effects and Toxic Signs

The best source of information about the side effects a child is experiencing is the child herself or her parents. Teaching them what to look for is critical. (See the list of common anticonvulsants and their side effects on the next page.) It should be pointed out that some side effects are more serious than others but that all such developments indicate a need to call their doctor to seek instructions.

The family must also be taught that some side effects are not obvious so that they will understand the need for periodic blood and urine tests. If a parent or child has difficulty understanding why a medication causes side effects, it can be explained that anticonvulsants are powerful drugs and sometimes affect areas of the body other than the brain.

The child and her parents must also be informed about when an increase in seizure activity may occur. This will help to alleviate fears that the medication is no longer effective or that the seizures are getting worse. Whenever the child is ill, especially with a fever; is overly tired; or is under unusual stress seizures may occur more frequently. As a young girl reaches puberty, she may also experience a greater number of seizures a few days prior to and during her menses. Some girls find that taking a diuretic during this time decreases the frequency of their seizures, but this should only be done under a doctor's supervision.

The adolescent also needs to know that drinking alcoholic beverages may increase the frequency of seizures. It may be beneficial to help the patient weigh the consequences of drinking against the stigma of being different in the eyes of peers. This decision is ultimately the individual's, but it helps if she has given some thought to the issue before she is in a situation where a decision is called for.

Teaching the child and her parents about medications is important in itself. Furthermore when someone spends time helping them to understand this aspect of care, the family will respond, feeling more at ease in expressing their questions, fears, and feelings and thus making it possible to provide comprehensive care.

BIBLIOGRAPHY

COOPER, C. R. Anticonvulsant drugs and the epileptic's dilemma? *Nursing* (Jenkintown) 6:45-50, Jan. 1976.
EPILEPSY FOUNDATION OF AMERICA. *Basic Statistics on the Epilepsies.* Philadelphia, F. A. Davis Co., 1975.
FORMAN, P. M. Therapy of seizures in children. *Am.Fam.Physician* 10:144, Sept. 1974.
SANDS, HARRY, AND MINTERS, F. C. *The Epilepsy Fact Book.* Philadelphia, F. A. Davis Co., 1977.

Common Anticonvulsants and Their Side Effects

Drug	Indication	Side Effects and Signs of Toxicity
Carbamazepine (Tegretol®)	Psychomotor	Nausea and vomiting, rash, vertigo, fever, aplastic anemia, liver damage, urinary frequency or retention
Clonazepam (Clonopin®)	Myoclonic Petit mal	Nausea and vomiting, rash, anemia, drowsiness, nystagmus, urinary retention
Ethosuximide (Zarontin®)	Petit mal	Nausea and vomiting, rash, drowsiness, headache, dizziness, albuminuria
Ethotoin (Peganone®)	Grand mal	Nausea and vomiting, rash, drowsiness, nystagmus, headache
Mephenytoin (Mesantoin®)	Grand mal Psychomotor	Nausea and vomiting, rash, aplastic anemia, ataxia
Mephobarbital (Mebaral®)	Grand mal Petit mal	Nausea and vomiting, drowsiness, hyperactivity, rash, gingival hypertrophy
Methsuximide (Celontin®)	Petit mal Psychomotor	Nausea and vomiting, rash, drowsiness, fever, ataxia, nervousness, headache, hiccoughs
Paramethadione (Paradione®)	Petit mal Grand mal Myoclonic	Nausea and vomiting, rash, leukopenia, photophobia
Phenacemide (Phenurone®)	Psychomotor Grand mal Petit mal	Nausea and vomiting, aplastic anemia, liver damage, personality changes
Phenobarbital	Grand mal Petit mal	Nausea and vomiting, drowsiness, hyperactivity, rash
Phenytoin Sodium (Dilantin®)	Grand mal Psychomotor	Gingival hypertrophy, anemia, nausea and vomiting, ataxia, nystagmus, rash, malaise
Primidone (Mysoline®)	Grand mal Psychomotor	Nausea and vomiting, drowsiness, ataxia, headache, gum pain
Trimethadione (Tridione®)	Petit mal	Nausea and vomiting, rash, photophobia
Valproic Acid (Depakene®)	Petit mal Complex absence Multiple other types	Nausea and vomiting, drowsiness, ataxia, nystagmus, rash, leukopenia, liver damage

Ventriculo-Peritoneal

Reprinted from American Journal of Nursing, June 1980

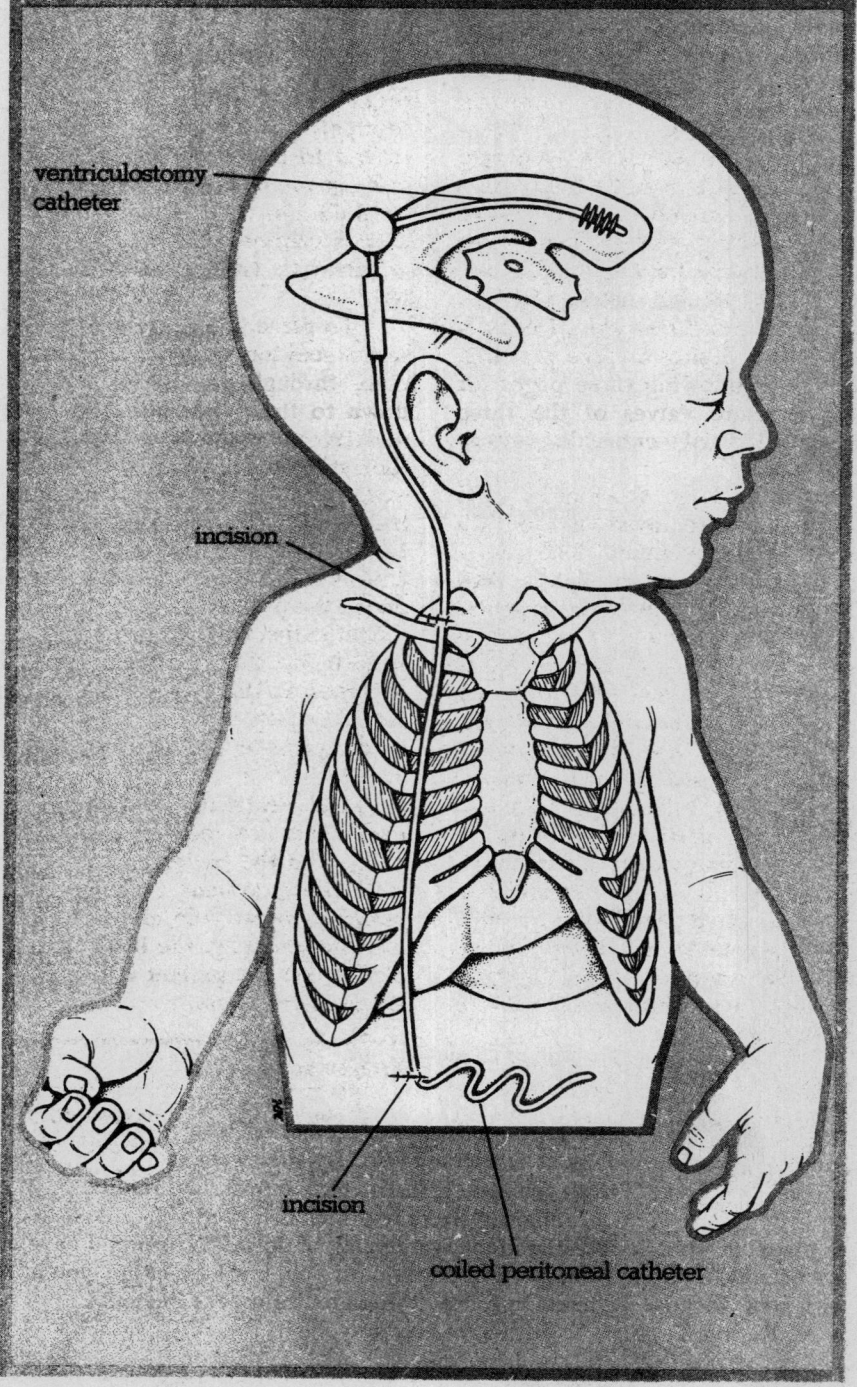

By Pat Ludder Jackson

Surgeons have been using the peritoneal cavity as a site for the drainage and absorption of cerebrospinal fluid in children with hydrocephalus since the late nineteenth century. These procedures, however, were not usually successful.

When polyethylene tubing was developed in the late 1940s, ventriculo-peritoneal shunting procedures were tried again. Unfortunately, the tubing frequently kinked, cracked, and clogged, and the polyethylene was thought to be responsible for omental reactions(1).

Because of these early problems with ventriculo-peritoneal shunts, ventriculo-atrial shunts gained favor. In the late 1950s, silicone rubber was developed and used for ventriculo-atrial shunting systems. As more shunts were inserted, however, the rate and significance of complications increased. Revisions were also frequently needed in children, owing to growth and subsequent displacement of the atrial catheter.

A new interest in ventriculo-peritoneal shunts with silicone catheters came about in the mid-1960s. Since that time, ventriculo-peritoneal shunting has become the more commonly performed and preferred shunting procedure because of the high incidence of serious complication from ventriculo-atrial shunts. Serious complications can still develop with peritoneal shunting, but in general, the problems tend to be less life-threatening

PAT LUDDER JACKSON, R.N., M.S., is a lecturer in the Department of Family Health Care Nursing at the University of California, San Francisco.

Shunts

and easier to correct than those associated with ventriculo-atrial shunts(2).

Peritoneal shunts are used in treating children and adults with hydrocephalus, which may be idiopathic or result from congenital malformation, neoplasms of the brain, infections of the central nervous system, brain cysts, or traumatic injury to the central nervous system by accident or operative procedure.

I will discuss the three major types of shunting systems. All three systems include a radiopaque ventricular catheter that is available in adult and pediatric sizes, and all are designed to permit only one directional flow of cerebrospinal fluid. In addition, all the systems described here provide a way of ensuring that the system is patent and thus functioning properly (see diagrams, on the following pages, for the details of the three systems).

Implantation of a ventriculoperitoneal shunt is a relatively easy neurological procedure. To insert the ventricular catheter, a small burrhold is made, usually in the right parieto-occipital region. This area is chosen because it offers the most direct approach to the third ventricle through brain tissue that is not highly specialized. Also, because the speech center is located on the left, there is no danger of damage to that area.

The catheter is passed, with the aid of specially designed surgical instruments, through a small slit in the dura and into the anterior portion of the lateral ventricles. Correct placement of the catheter is extremely important and should be verified by X-ray in the operating room. If the catheter is not placed in the anterior horn of the lateral ventricle, as the ventricle returns to normal size the ventricular walls may occlude the catheter tip and block the flow of cerebral spinal fluid. Once the catheter is in correct position, it is sutured in place at the dura.

Selection of the appropriate valve pressure is made before surgery. There are no absolute rules to guide selection, but past experience and an understanding of the patient's particular needs and the shunt's capabilities are all considered in choosing a valve pressure. (See the following three pages for the pressure valves of the three major kinds of ventriculo-peritoneal shunts.)

When large volumes of fluid have to be removed in order to achieve an acceptable intracranial pressure, such as in infants with rapidly progressing hydrocephalus or in draining postoperative meningeal cysts, large congenital subarachnoid cysts, and recurring subdural hygromas or hematomas, very low or low pressure valve settings are used. The low pressure permits easy drainage of the fluid.

When there is moderate or minimal enlargement of the ventricles, such as in individuals who have acquired hydrocephalus as a result of trauma or meningeal infection, or in a person needing shunt revision, a medium pressure valve setting is used.

In those situations where no further reduction in ventricular size is sought, such as in older adults with "normal pressure" syndrome, high pressure valve units are used.

All valves must be tested for accuracy prior to insertion. Each company supplies directions for testing its valve in the operating room.

After the valve unit is tested, it is placed subcutaneously down the occipital-parietal area toard the anterior portion of the neck. Cerebral spinal fluid is allowed to drain through the ventricular catheter to displace air. Then, the valve unit or reservoir and valve unit are attached to the ventricular catheter and also are filled with cerebral spinal fluid. The distal end of the valve unit is clamped until ready to be attached to the peritoneal catheter.

To place the peritoneal catheter, an incision is made in the abdomen, through the rectus muscle, down to the peritoneum. A small nick is made in the peritoneum, and the catheter is inserted. In a child, extra peritoneal catheter is coiled in the peritoneum to extend as the child grows. With the help of either a stainless steel or firm nylon introducer, the proximal end of the peritoneal catheter is slipped subcutaneously up the anterior abdomen and chest to the neck. A small incision is usually made at the clavicle to aid passage (see drawing, page 1104).

The ventricular catheter and valve unit are then attached and sutured to the peritoneal catheter. The entire system is filled with cerebral spinal fluid and tested. If all is functioning, the incisions are closed and the patient returned to the recovery room.

Preoperative Care

The preoperative care will depend greatly on the patient's diagnosis and reason for surgery. In the patient who has developed postmeningitis hydrocephalus, more extensive care will be required than for the person who has been admitted for an elective revision of a ventricular shunt.

However, regardless of the

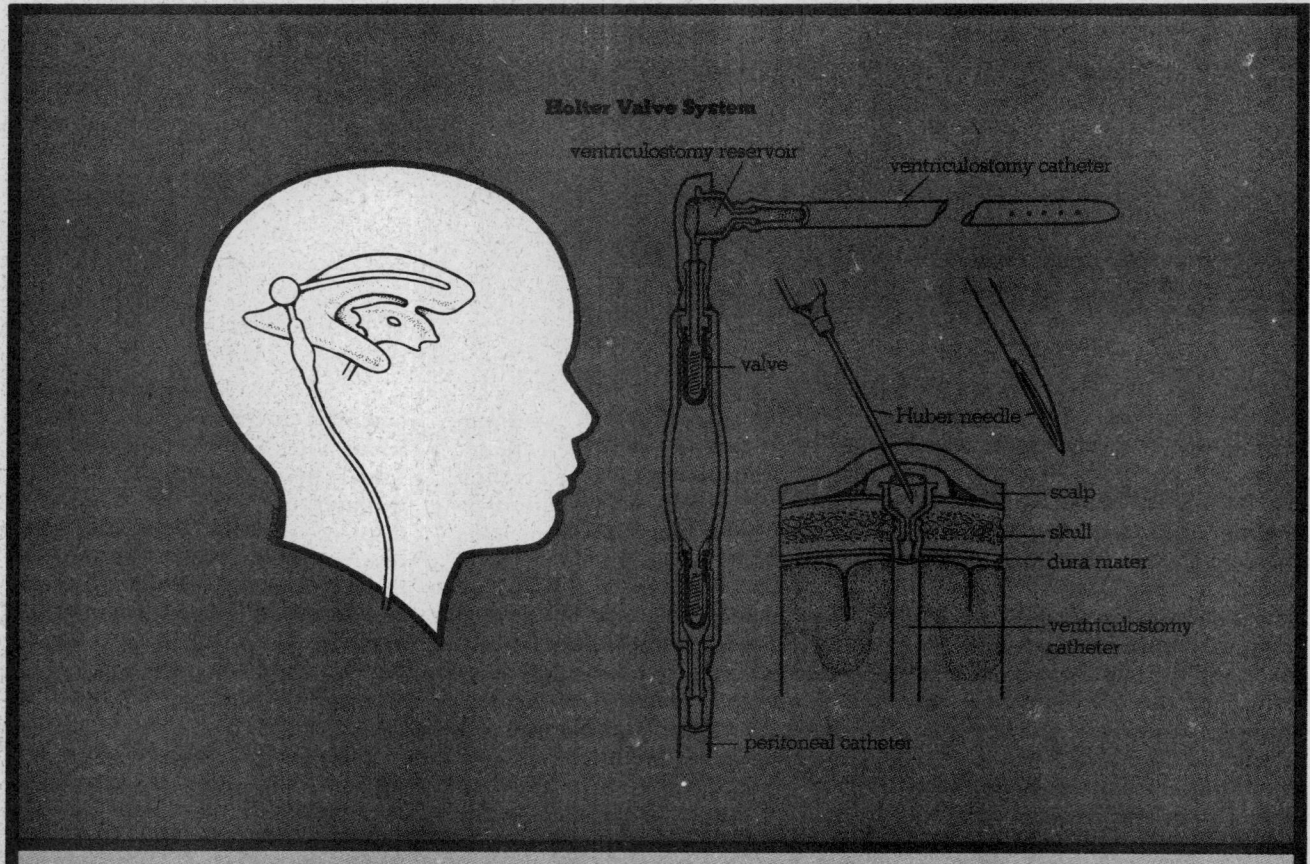

In the Holter Valve System, the ventriculostomy reservoir provides direct access to the ventricles and a means of irrigating the entire shunt system. A small-gauge Huber needle is recommended, rather than a conventional beveled needle. The Huber needle is slightly curved at the tip. The reservoir permits patency checks of both proximal and distal catheters radiographically and allows for injections of medications, aspiration of cerebral spinal fluid, and intraventricular pressure readings with a transducer.

The Holter dual valve comes after the reservoir. The valve is available in pediatric and adult sizes. The pressure and flow rate of cerebrospinal fluid are controlled by the length of slits in the valve and the hardness, tensile strength, and elasticity of the silicone.

The valves are available in four pressures: high (76-110 mm. H_2O), medium (41-75 mm.), low (11-40 mm.), and extra low (0-10 mm.). Normal cerebrospinal fluid pressure varies widely but is generally accepted to be between 70 and 200 mm. H_2O. The average is 125 mm. in adults, 50-100 mm. in children, and 30-80 mm. in newborns(3).

The peritoneal catheter is attached to the distal end of the valve. The company (Extracorporeal Medical Specialties, Inc.) makes two types of catheters: an "A" type that has an open end, and the "salmon" type that has a closed distal tip with multiple side slits. It is thought that the side slit design reduces the possibility of omentum occluding the distal end. It also manufactures an optional In-Line Shunt Filter that traps particles larger than 3.9 microns.

person's condition or developmental age, there are some important general principles of preoperative nursing. The primary indicator of changing intracranial pressure is a change in the person's level of consciousness and interaction with his environment. In order to identify a change, a baseline assessment must be made through observations and a detailed history of the patient's normal behavior, sleep patterns, eating habits, developmental capacities, and affect. This assessment must be charted in clear, objective terms that other staff members can easily interpret and use. This baseline assessment is important for evaluating the patient preoperatively for any change in condition, and the data become critical postoperatively, when evaluation of the shunt's function is a primary nursing responsibility.

As with all preoperative patients, maintenance of fluid and electrolyte balance and adequate nutrition are important. If the patient has increased intracranial pressure, nausea, vomiting, and anorexia may be a problem. Fluid balance must be observed for carefully so that cerebral edema as a result of overhydration does not compound the problem of increased intracranial pressure.

If the increase in cranial pressure is severe, the patient may be confused, become accident prone, or even develop seizures. The primary nursing responsibility is to protect the patient from injury. If seizures do occur, observe closely for duration; movement, whether tonic or clonic; focus and pro-

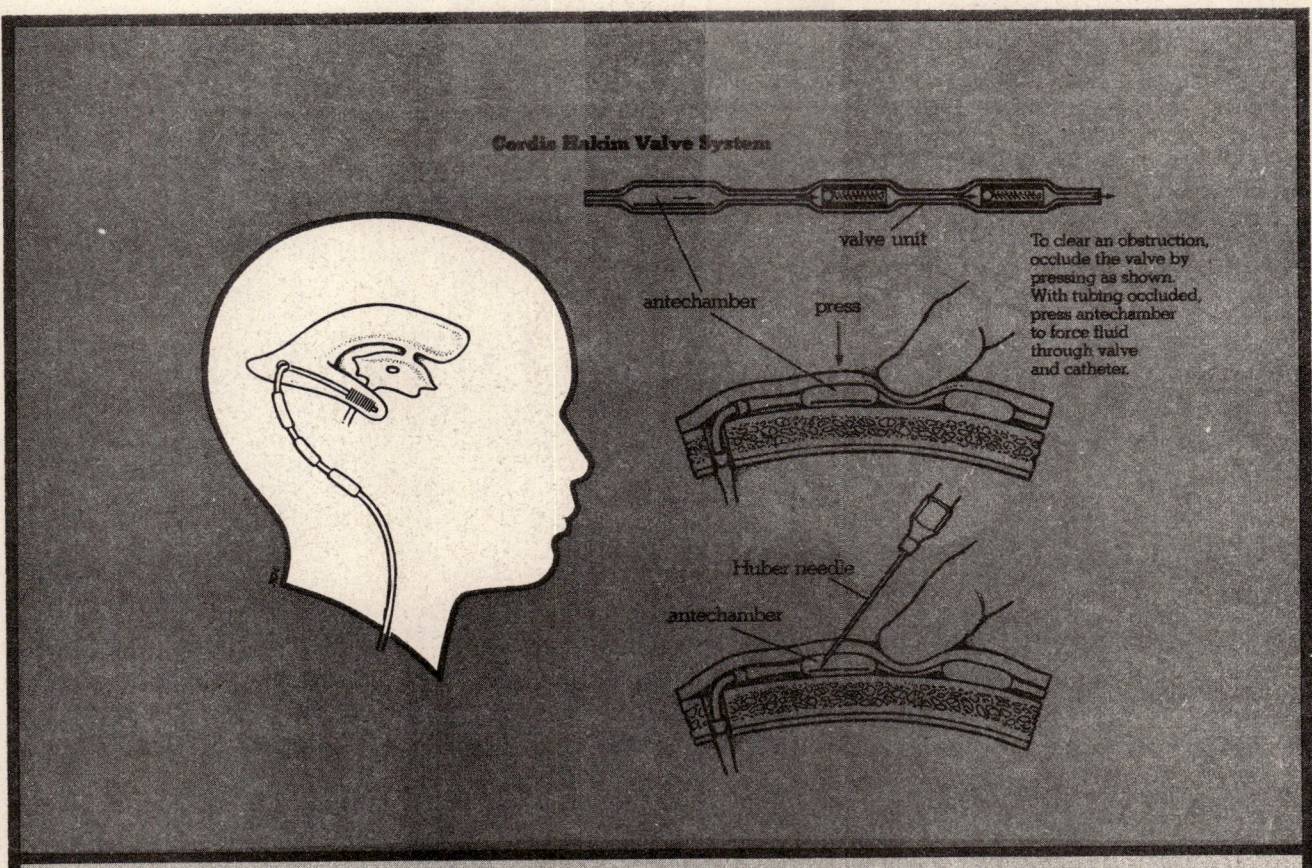

The Hakim Shunting Systems (Cordis Corporation) use a radiopaque silicone rubber ventricular catheter. With this system, cerebrospinal fluid enters the catheter through inlet holes that have overlying fins which protect the catheter from clogging.

The Hakim system does not have a separate reservoir but has an antechamber as part of the pressure valve unit. A small amount of cerebrospinal fluid collects in this antechamber. A stainless steel needle stop inside the antechamber allows Huber needles to be inserted to test the system without passing completely through the antechamber.

The antechamber can be used in much the same way for testing and treatment procedures as the reservoir that is part of the Holter Valve System. Cerebrospinal fluid from the ventricles can be aspirated by inserting a needle into the antechamber, compressing the tubing between the antechamber and the valve, and then aspirating the fluid.

The valve is designed to open when a specific pressure range is reached or exceeded by the cerebrospinal fluid. Each valve is contained in a stainless steel unit. The valves come in five different color coded sizes: green (140-165 mm. H_2O), brown (95-125 mm.), yellow (60-80 mm.), white (30-45 mm.), and blue (5-12 mm.).

The distal end of the peritoneal catheter has four rows of slits arranged in a staggered pattern for drainage of cerebrospinal fluid. The slits will open if the distal end of the catheter becomes obstructed.

gression of the seizure; and the patient's level of consciousness before, during, and after(4).

Preoperative preparation should include discussion of the details of the operation, the function of the shunt, the need for shaving the head, the number of incisions necessary, the types of dressings there will be, the normal postoperative course, and possible complications. Thorough preoperative education will reduce the anxiety, agitation, restlessness, and confusion often seen in people after surgery. Because these symptoms may also signify an early rise in intracranial pressure, their cause must be carefully analyzed.

Postoperative Care

When the patient returns from surgery, vital signs, level of consciousness, and pupillary reactions to light should be checked immediately. Check dressings for drainage, and note the amount of swelling and erythema along the peritoneal catheter tract. The peritoneal catheter can be palpated easily, and in young children and thin adults the outline of the catheter can often be seen. Some swelling, redness, and tenderness are normal for the first week after surgery.

The physician will indicate the desired position and activity of the patient. Elevating the head of the bed or allowing the person to sit up may increase drainage of the cerebral spinal fluid due to the effect of gravity on the fluid pressure. Depending on the amount of fluid drained during surgery, this may or

640 SECTION 5: NURSING CARE OF THE CHILD

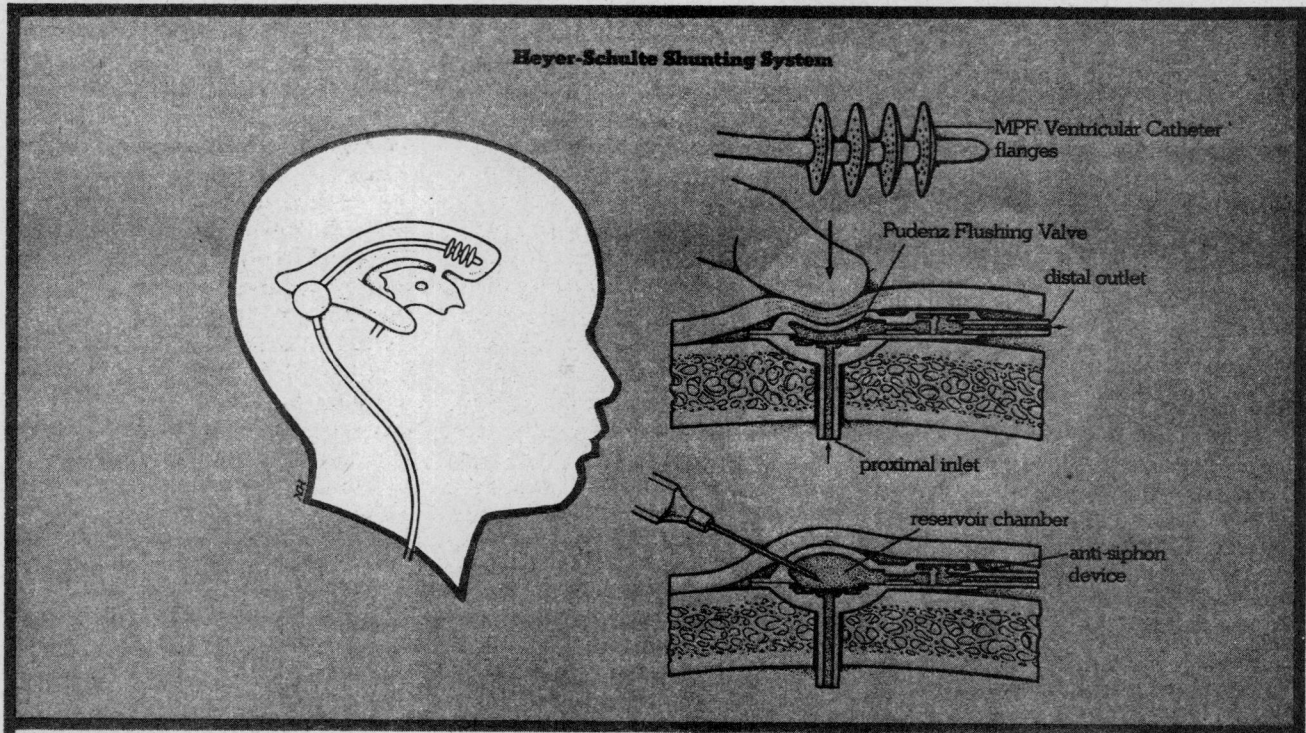

The Heyer-Schulte Corporation manufactures many different types of shunt components. The most commonly used components include the Heyer-Schulte Pudenz ventricular catheter that has many small perforations near the tip to facilitate drainage of cerebrospinal fluid. The extreme tip of the catheter is closed to prevent brain tissue from entering the tubing during placement.

Heyer-Schulte also makes the Multi-Perforated Flange (MPF) ventricular catheter that has silicone flanges encircling the tip of the catheter with the posterior side of each flange containing more than twenty small holes. During insertion the flanges fold back like an umbrella and then spring open when they enter the ventricle. The flanges help prevent the catheter tubing from resting against the ventricular wall or the choroid plexus.

The Heyer-Schulte Pudenz flushing valve combines the properties of a reservoir and a pressure valve. It is placed into a small burrhole and attached to the ventricular catheter. The valve controls the flow of cerebral spinal fluid by use of a diaphragm calibrated for low (5-75 mm. H_2O), medium (60-140 mm.), or high (120-200 mm.) pressure. The diaphragm also provides for one-way flow control. Because of the shape and size of the valve, it also acts as a reservoir. It can be injected with a small-gauge needle at an angle of not greater than 25 degrees. Because there is no metal stop in this valve, it must be entered carefully.

The Heyer-Schulte peritoneal catheter is different from the Holter and Hakim peritoneal catheters in that it has four slit valves at the distal end instead of plain perforated openings. These catheters come in three closing pressure ratings: low (1.5-5.4 cm. H_2O), medium (5.5-9.4 cm.), and high (9.5-14.4 cm.). These valves further aid the shunt valve in controlling the flow of cerebral spinal fluid and serve to resist retrograde flow of fluids into the catheter.

may not be desirable. Positioning the patient on his nonoperative side or his back, if postoperative vomiting is not a problem, will prevent pressure on the incisions.

Initially the patient's level of consciousness will be altered by anesthesia. Check with the anesthesiologist to determine how long the drowsiness caused by anesthesia will last, so that you can evaluate the patient's neurological status more accurately. The patient should show progressive awareness of his surroundings and be aroused from sleep easily. There is minimal pain involved with this surgery, and narcotics are rarely given because of their depressant effect on the central nervous system. Mild analgesics, such as aspirin or acetaminophen, are used.

For the first four to six hours after surgery, vital signs and neuro checks are done every 15 to 30 minutes. Compare each reading with previous readings to determine if there is any trend indicating an increase in the intracranial pressure. Pupils should be checked for progressive dilation. Increased intracranial pressure causes compression or stretching of the oculomotor (third cranial) nerve. This results in dilation of the pupil on the same side as the pressure.

Another sign of increased intracranial pressure is in blood pressure. The pulse will vary at first but then slow down as the blood pressure increases. Anoxia of the respiratory center in the medulla oblongata results in variable and intermittent respirations.

In the young child whose fontanels and sutures are not closed, the nurse has an additional way of observing for increased intracranial pressure. Evaluate the anterior fontanel for fullness and tension every hour. Because this is a subjective finding, continuity of nursing care is very important. The child's head circumference should also be measured carefully each day, preferably by the same nurse. Because the infant's skull is so malleable, an increase in cerebral spinal fluid pressure may cause enlargement of the head instead of the classic symptoms of increased intracranial pressure. Actual increases in circumference of 0.5 cm. are significant and must be reported.

If there is any indication of increased intracranial pressure, the shunt can be tested for patency by compressing the reservoir or antechamber (see diagrams). If cerebral spinal fluid is readily forced out of the reservoir, then the peritoneal catheter must be patent. If the reservoir fills readily, then you know that the ventricular catheter is also patent. Frequently, in the postoperative period, the shunt becomes partially occluded by cells or tissue dislodged during surgery. If this appears to be happening, the reservoir must be "pumped," or compressed, a specified number of times each shift.

Occasionally, too much fluid is drained from the cranial cavity, causing the cerebrum to pull away from the dura. This may result in formation of a subdural hematoma. Excessive drainage may be due to the insertion of a faulty valve, the use of too low a valve pressure unit, too frequent "pumping" of the shunt reservoir, other complications of surgery, or the patient's individual complex cranial hydrodynamics. In a young infant, sunken fontanels accompanied by agitation or restlessness are the primary symptoms of this complication. In an adult, a gradual depression in the level of consciousness is the primary symptom.

Shunt infections are another serious postoperative complication. Many physicians order pre- and post-operative antibiotics prophylactically. Observe incisions carefully for any signs of infection. Though it is quite normal for the patient to have a mild temperature two or three days after surgery, any temperature over 102°F, or lasting more than three days, is suspicious, and an infection workup including analysis of the patient's urine, sputum, and blood should be performed. If no source of infection can be found, a sterile sample of cerebral spinal fluid is obtained from the shunt reservoir for culture and sensitivity. Because of the inert properties of the shunt, infections of the shunt, or meningitis and ventriculitis, are extremely difficult to treat even with very large doses of intravenous and intrathecal (via the reservoir) antibiotics.

The most common organism cultured from ventricular peritoneal shunts postoperatively is *Staphylococcus epidermides*(5). If an infection is present, a one- to two-week course of antibiotics will be started in hopes of sterilizing the shunt. If the antibiotics fail, the shunt must be removed and replaced with a sterile shunt, followed by another course of antibiotics. Occasionally, it will be necessary to institute external drainage of cerebrospinal fluid via a ventriculostomy tube while an infection is being treated(6).

Long-Term Care

Most conditions that require ventricular shunting continue for the remainder of the person's life. Some children with congenital communicating or noncommunicating hydrocephalus do eventually have an arrest of their hydrocephalus and become shunt-independent, but the large majority of persons with hydrocephalus do not(7).

If there are no postoperative complications, the patient is usually discharged 7 to 10 days after surgery. Once the person has recovered from surgery and the wounds have healed, there are generally no restrictions on daily living, except exclusion from activities such as football, soccer, or ice hockey where there is a high incidence of head injury.

Long-term complications such as ascites, cerebral spinal fluid fistulas, hernias, hydroceles, ileus, migration of the peritoneal catheter, peritonitis, and perforation of the small bowel have all been reported, but blockage and infection of the shunt are by far the most common problems(1).

For this reason, it is important that the patient be followed closely by personnel who are well aware of the possible complications of ventriculo-peritoneal shunts. The patient and his family should also be taught the symptoms of increased intracranial pressure or infection and should be strongly encouraged to seek care for any unusual symptom. As patients learn to live with their shunts, they will learn what feelings or symptoms are danger signals.

Infants with shunts must continue their well-baby care and receive all their immunizations on time, if possible. A measurement of the baby's head circumference should be done on each visit. Once a child with hydrocephalus has had a shunt inserted, his head stops growing until his body and head are in approximately the same growth percentile. Therefore, continued growth of a baby's head after shunting, even in the absence of overt signs of increased intracranial pressure warrants further investigation(8).

The widespread use of EMI or CAT scanning has made evaluation of shunt function much easier. Tests are frequently ordered every six months to make sure no insidious enlargement of the ventricles is occurring, and the tests are repeated whenever symptoms warrant.

Even with the best possible care, shunt failures and other complications do occur and require surgical revision of part or all of the shunt. The average time between shunt revisions varies greatly. Young children appear to be more prone to complications and need shunt revisions more frequently than most adults.

References

1. Davidson, R. I. Peritoneal bypass in the treatment of hydrocephalus: historical review and abdominal complications. *J.Neurol.Neurosurg.Psychiatry* 39:640-646, July 1976.
2. Ignelzi, R. J., and Kirsch, W. M. Follow-up analysis of ventriculo-peritoneal and ventriculoatrial shunts for hydrocephalus. *J.Neurosurg.* 42:679-682, June 1975.
3. Krupp, M. A., and Chatton, M. J. *Current Medical Diagnosis and Treatment.* Los Altos, Calif., Lange Medical Publications, 1978, p. 1048.
4. Quesenbury, J. H., and Lembright, Pamela. Observation and care for patients with head injuries. *Nurs.Clin.North Am.* 4:237-247, June 1969.
5. Venes, J. L. Control of shunt infection. Report of 150 consecutive cases. *J.Neurosurg.* 45:311-314, Sept. 1976.
6. Bracke, Mary, and others. External drainage of cerebrospinal fluid. *Am.J.Nurs.* 78:1355-1358, Aug. 1978.
7. Holtzer, G. J., and DeLange, S. A. Shunt-independent arrest of hydrocephalus. *J.Neurosurg.* 39:698-701, Dec. 1973.
8. Becker, D. P., and others. Control of hydrocephalus by valve-regulated venous shunt: avoidance of complications in prolonged shunt maintenance. *J.Neurosurg.* 28:215-226, Mar. 1968.

Immunization: What's It All About?

Reprinted from American Journal of Nursing, August 1980.

By Janice Selekman

Many of today's parents have not experienced the impact of the contagious diseases of childhood. Many believe that immunizations are unnecessary now because the diseases are disappearing. However, except for smallpox, the antigens to most childhood diseases *cannot* be eliminated from the environment.

More than one-third of American children have not developed complete protection against measles, mumps, rubella, diptheria, pertussis, tetanus, and polio. This rises to almost 50 percent among the inner-city and disadvantaged populations. Not protecting children against these diseases is considered by some a form of child neglect.

Nineteen million Americans are not immunized against polio, and yet paralytic polio was reported in the U.S. in 1980. Twelve to fifteen million Americans are not immunized against DPT and rubella. Twelve million Americans are not immunized against measles, and many more probably don't have sufficient titers.

Americans have become lax in protecting their children from these communicable diseases, even though 48 states require immunization for entry into schools. Somehow, too many of our children are not being adequately immunized. We cannot afford this practice. Immunizations are vital to world health.

What is an immunization? How does it work? What diseases should we protect against and why?

The potential value of immunization was first recognized in 1796 by Edward Jenner when he developed an immunization against smallpox. This disease is the first one to be 100 percent eradicated.

The goal of immunization, to prevent or lessen the severity of an infectious disease process by the administration of an antigen (active immunity) or an antibody (passive immunity), has not changed since Jenner's day.

Immunity is defined as all those physiological mechanisms that endow the animal with the capacity to recognize materials as foreign to

---

A Problem: Immunization Records

One obstacle that nurses working on immunization projects encounter over and over again is lack of accurate documentation. Parents often cannot recall exactly what immunizations their children had or when and have great difficulty acquiring records from past care givers.

To help families maintain accurate records, the U.S. Public Health Service is developing a standardized national record. In the meantime, in California, the "California Kids" campaign urges care providers to supply clients with immunization records and encourages parents to take these records whenever they take their child for a health care visit.

Our county immunization unit decided to take an indepth look at this record-keeping problem. We wanted to find out how many families keep records; whether parental possession of records is related to the age of the child or to the source of care; and what records are kept.

We selected children served by the Child Health and Disability Prevention program, which provides preventive health care to Medicaid-eligible children. Fifty-nine children were randomly selected.

In a telephone survey, parents of these children were contacted and asked a series of questions. Fifty-seven percent of the parents had preschool age children (0-4 years) and 43 percent had school-age children (5-14 years).

In our sampling, 74 percent of the parents reported that they did have a record of the child's immunizations. Seventy-one percent of the parents of preschoolers reported having a record and 79 percent of the parents of school-age children said they did.

Seventy-one percent of the children had been immunized by a private physician and 29 percent at a public health immunization clinic. Children who received immunizations at clinics were more likely to have up-to-date records: 94 percent as opposed to 66 percent who had seen private physicians.

Results of this study imply that any attempt to improve immunization record-keeping must involve private physicians. Since nurses are in a key teaching position, we must teach families to *expect* to receive records from providers and *assure* them that they are valuable.—DIANE L. GOLD, R.N., M.S.N., and JOANNE MARTIN, R.N., M.S.N., *Santa Cruz, Calif.*

Types of Immunity

Natural—immunity that is permanent from birth, innate or genetic.
Naturally acquired active—protection obtained by having the disease.
Naturally acquired passive—obtained antibodies via placental transmission or by breast milk.
Artificially acquired active—development of protection by vaccination with a live, attenuated, or dead organism or its toxin (toxoid) so that the immune system produces antibodies—all immunizations.
Artificially acquired passive—prophylactic protection obtained by injecting antibodies directly into the individual. It produces no active involvement of the individual's immune system and, therefore, immunity steadily decreases—gamma globulin.

JANICE SELEKMAN, R.N., M.S.N., was an instructor of pediatric nursing at Bryn Mawr Hospital School of Nursing, Bryn Mawr, Pa., when she wrote this article. She now is a full-time doctoral student and a part-time teaching assistant at the University of Pennsylvania School of Nursing, Philadelphia.

itself and to neutralize, eliminate, or metabolize them with or without injury to its own tissue. The immune system includes the ability to defend the body against invasion, to perceive mutant cells, and to provide the homeostatic function of removing worn-out and damaged cells.

The vaccine's function is to stimulate the immune system to provide immunity in the individual as if the body were actually fighting the disease itself. The person should not suffer from the disease nor suffer more than a minimal reaction from the vaccine. The terms "immunization" and "vaccination" are now used synonymously, although the latter term was once used mainly in relation to smallpox.

Newborn infants are passively immunized by the placental transfer of maternal antibodies (via immunoglobulin G). IgG has a half-life of three to four weeks, so that as the months go by the infant's protection lessens. This passive protection virtually disappears by 15 months of age.

Maternal IgG suppresses the infant's own synthesis of IgG. This suppression, plus the decreasing maternal antibodies, makes the infant more susceptible to a variety of illnesses between two and six months of age. If an infant receives a vaccine while maternal antibodies are still present, the maternal antibodies may interfere with seroconversion, which will prevent active immunity, especially against viral agents. This may lead to the misconception that a child is immune when, in fact, the immunity is not at a protective level.

Children vaccinated earlier than recommended by current stan-

Recommended Immunization Schedule for Normal Infants and Children

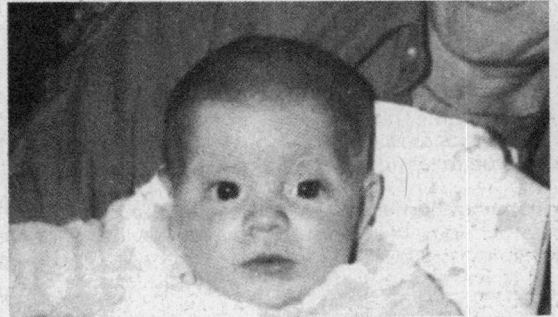

2, 4 & 6 mos. Diphtheria, Measles, Tetanus, Pertussis, Oral Polio*   *(6-month dose optional)

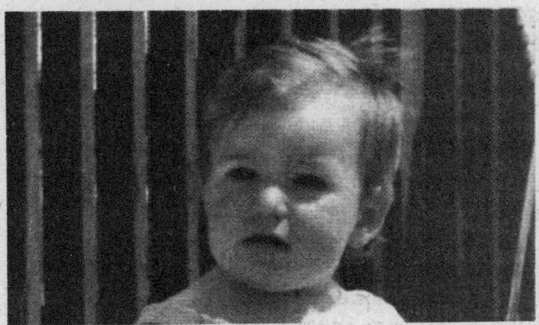

12 mos. Tuberculin test *(repeat every 1 or 2 years)*

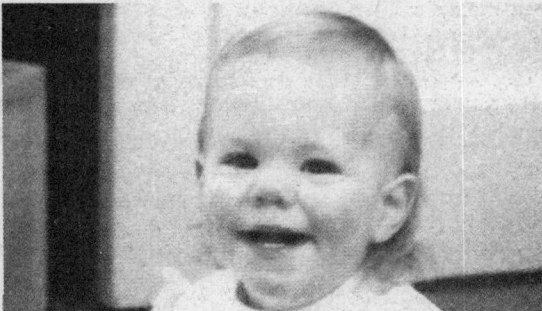

15 mos. Measles, Mumps, Rubella.

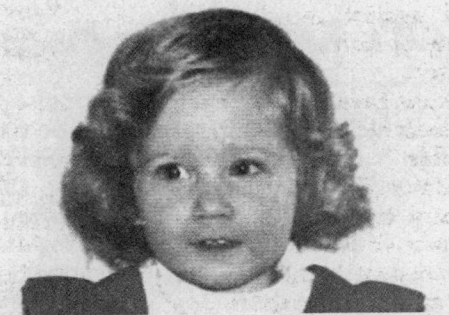

18 mos. Diphtheria, Tetanus, Pertussis, Oral Polio.

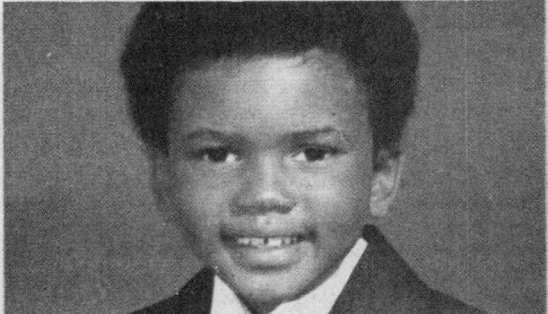

4–6 Yrs. Diphtheria, Tetanus, Pertussis, Oral Polio.

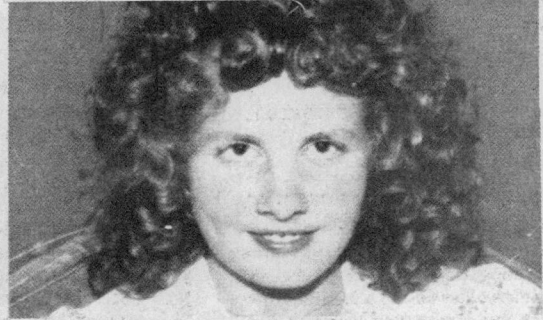

14–16 Yrs. Tetanus, Diphtheria *(repeat every 10 years)*

Schedule: American Academy of Pediatrics, 1977

> Before giving an immunization, the nurse should ask herself the following questions:
>
> 1. Does the child fall into the group for which the vaccine is indicated?
>
> 2. Do any contraindications exist?
>
> 3. By what route should the vaccine be given?
>
> 4. Has the parent given consent?
>
> 5. Has the parent been informed of the vaccine's benefits and risks?
>
> 6. Has the parent been told of what action to take if side effects develop?
>
> 7. Has the parent been informed that antigens to various diseases may be given separately?
>
> 8. Have accurate records been kept of the previous vaccines given and the reactions, if any, that occurred?
>
> 9. Is the child allergic to any of the consituents of the vaccine?
>
> 10. Has the vaccine been stored (usually refrigerated) according to the manufacturer's suggestions? (Failure to do so could cause vaccines to deteriorate and be entirely useless.)

dards, especially against measles, may be revaccinated. Breast-fed babies are vaccinated the same as bottle-fed infants. If there is no documentation that the child has been immunized or if there is any question, they should receive the full immunization series.

Even after a child has received all the immunizations, some diseases require a "booster shot," especially since maternal antibodies may have been present during some of the earlier doses. A "booster shot" restimulates the immune system. The need for booster shots is determined by the type of vaccine used, the desired length of protection, and the length of protection provided by the initial active immunization. Some physicians choose to give the initial immunization when the child is older, in order to get a better immunological response. This practice increases the risk of the child getting the disease first.

Immunizations come in many different forms. MMR and polio (Sabin) are live attenuated viral vaccines that multiply in the body and stimulate a strong antibody production. The original polio vaccine (Salk) as well as influenza antigens

An Adult's Reaction to Measles Vaccine

By Helen-Louise Boling

Sometimes health problems begin in unexpected ways. When I started a new job as a community health nurse, I had to have a physical examination in the Employee Health Clinic. Blood was drawn for what I assumed was the usual CBC and VDRL.

A few week later, I was called to go to the Employee Health Clinic for a rubella shot—my rubella titer at my physical was zero. When I received the immunization, the nurse informed me of the risks and possible side effects. I read the information on the consent form and in the *PDR*—frequent occur-

---

HELEN-LOUISE BOLING, R.N., BSN, is a community health nurse at the Bureau of Community Health Nursing, Health and Hospital Corp. of Marion County, Indianapolis, Ind.

rence of self-limited arthralgia and possible arthritis beginning two to four weeks after the vaccination.*

On December 27, 1979, I was immunized. On January 14, while working in our pediatric clinic, I squatted down to talk to a patient. When I stood up, my left knee locked. I have a history of mild joint instability in both knees, so I assumed that this locking sensation was part of that problem. However, during the day, the knee did not improve, and by 3:30 P.M., it was obviously swollen to one and one-half times its normal size.

I had the knee checked by our clinic physician. Crepitus was present, so he recommended that it be x-rayed. I did not have any pain, but did have difficulty flexing the

---

Physicians' Desk Reference. 34th ed. Oradell, N.J., Medical Economics Co., 1980, p. 1147.

knee. There was also a real feeling of instability at the joint—a feeling that it would not bear weight.

The x-rays were normal. I was told to wrap the leg with an Ace bandage and rest it as much as possible. The next morning, the left knee was virtually normal, but the right knee was beginning to swell. By that night, I had only 20° to 30° movement in the right knee.

By January 16, the right knee was swollen to twice it· normal size, my right index finger was swollen, and my right wrist had decreased flexion.

I went to the Employee Health Clinic where, as good fortune would have it, the physician on call was a rheumatology resident. He took a thorough history, examined all my joints, and concluded that this was, indeed, some kind of arthritis-connected problem. He sent me to the

are killed or inactivated. These vaccines do not multiply in the body, have a limited ability to stimulate the body to build a sufficient defense against the disease, and require revaccination.

Active immunizations work by mimicking the actual disease antigen and stimulating the body to produce its own antibodies. Passive immunization involves the administration of human immunoglobulin or human serum globulin. This provides temporary protection from a potential or imminent disease antigen by giving sufficient serum antibody levels quickly. It does not stimulate the body to make more antibodies, and the passive protection fades in a few weeks.

Some of the factors to consider before receiving (or giving) a vaccine include the composition of the antigen, the route, the dose, the side effects, when it should be given, and whether the vaccine prevents the disease or just decreases the severity of it. For example, doses of DPT may be given no closer than four weeks apart. Meanwhile viral antigens such as MMR and polio may be given either at the same time but no closer than six to eight weeks apart if they are administered separately.

Prolonging the interval between injections does not interfere with the final immunity. Interruption in immunizations during the first few years of life does not require that extra doses be given, nor does it mean that the individual must begin receiving vaccinations from the beginning. If vaccinations are not done during the first year of life, at least three doses of DPT, three doses of TOPV, and one dose of MMR should be given at the appropriate intervals.

Some reasons for delaying or postponing immunizations are:
- acute febrile illness
- an immunological deficiency or malignancy
- immunosuppressive therapy being given
- pregnancy
- skin irritation or dermatitis, which would delay the smallpox vaccine
- administration of gamma globulin, plasma, or a blood transfusion in the previous six to eight weeks, which postpones the immunization until passively received antibodies decrease.

The big fear for most parents is possible reactions from the vaccine, especially from pertussis. The link between the vaccine and brain damage or Sudden Infant Death Syndrome has not yet been established, although some parents blame the pertussis vaccine. The fear of the side effects of the pertussis vaccine and pending lawsuits may make the general public hesitant about immunizations.

Certainly, if a child should have a minor reaction to the vaccine, the remaining doses may be cut in half or in thirds to decrease the possibility of systemic reaction. DPT reactions occur within hours of the administration and subside within two days. Viral antigens may not cause symptoms for 10 to 28 days, but these may linger. Aspirin or Tylenol can help minimize a child's discomfort.

The nurse and pediatrician are the main sources of information for parents about immunizing their children. To give this information and administer the immunizations, nurses need to understand why immunizations are necessary, complications of the vaccines, how the vaccine works, and what are the contraindications to giving it.

Rheumatology Clinic for a workup and possible tapping of the right knee.

At the clinic, the rheumatology fellow and the attending physician went over my history. When the rubella shot was mentioned, the attending physician immediately commented that about a quarter of adult women who are immunized against rubella have reactions involving their joints. That probably was the reason for my trouble.

They decided to tap my knee, and 40 ml. of slightly cloudy, light straw-colored fluid was removed. The knee immediately felt better, and flexion markedly improved. The plan of care was discussed with me: blood work would be done—CBC and sedimentation rate, rheumatoid factor, and serum protein electrophoresis; the synovial fluid would be tested for glucose and cultures done, including a viral culture for rubella. I was to stay off my feet as much as possible and return to the clinic in three to four weeks.

In the next two weeks, the following joints were affected: right index finger, which remained swollen the longest of any joint (about 10 days), right wrist, right metatarsal area, and left ankle. I had some stiffness of the neck and shoulders that may have been related.

On February 4, I returned to the clinic for follow-up. All the laboratory results were normal. The physician reconfirmed that what I had experienced was probably a reaction to the rubella immunization. He could not predict how long I would continue to feel the effects. He recommended that I begin taking aspirin every four hours as a prophylactic measure. Gradually, the symptoms decreased, and I stopped the aspirin. I returned to the clinic in early April for my last visit.

After a very dramatic and frightening beginning, this reaction settled back into a low-key annoying problem—not serious enough to warrant bed rest. I still have intermittent aching in the joints of my right knee and right index finger. My physicians cannot predict how long this will last.

Looking back, I don't see that I had any choice about being immunized if I was to continue to work in community health nursing. However, this was not a pleasant experience. Since the risk of reaction for adult women is greater than for children, it is an additional reason for parents to insure that their children receive their rubella immunization in childhood.

Childhood Diseases, Immunization, and Nursing Care

Disease	Causative Agent	Incubation Period	Main Symptoms	Complications
diphtheria	*Corynebacterium diphtheriae*	2-7 days	pseudomembrane on pharynx, tonsils, and larynx nasal discharge swallowing and respiratory difficulty	bronchopneumonia respiratory and circulatory failure myocarditis nephritis
pertussis (whooping cough)	*Bordetella pertussis* *Hemophilus pertussis*	5-21 days	begins with nighttime cough three stages: catarrhal, spasmodic, convalescent paroxysmal cough with inspiratory whoop sticky phlegm	mental retardation convulsions hemorrhage pneumonia otitis media
tetanus (lockjaw)	*Clostridium tetani*	5-21 days	trismus muscular rigidity clonic convulsions difficulty swallowing irritability intramuscular hemorrhage cyanosis asphyxia	hemorrhage asphyxia malnutrition fluid & electrolyte imbalance
measles (rubeola)	rubeola virus (droplet infection)	7-21 days	Koplik spots photophobia conjunctivitis cough temperature elevation pruritic maculopapular rash that spreads down the body	encephalitis otitis media pneumonia cardiac damage neurological damage
rubella (*German* measles)	rubella virus	14-21 days	enlarged lymph glands of the head and neck rash—maculopapular begins on face and spreads downward rash disappears usually in three days	none in children birth deformities in the developing fetus
mumps (parotitis)	*Myxovirus mumps*	14-24 days	enlarged parotid glands sensitive to sour foods prodromal—fever, headache, pain on chewing, malaise	orchitis epididymitis deafness encephalitis myocarditis arthritis hepatitis
chicken pox (varicella)	varicella zoster	7-21 days	clear, oval vesicles in crops → crusts on trunk—all stages at same time pruritis lymphadenopathy irritability elevated temperature	viral pneumonia in adults shingles in adults encephalitis 2° infection from scratching
poliomyelitis (infantile paralysis)	poliovirus (3 types) (droplets from nose or throat, and in feces)	5-14 days	flaccid paralysis stiff neck and back nerve involvement	paralysis respiratory difficulty

Period of Contagion	Peak Incidence	Treatment and Nursing Measures	Immunization Available	Route	Possible Reactions
infectious for weeks if untreated 1-2 days in patients who have received treatment	2-5 years of age (passive protection 3-6 months)	antitoxin ice collars analgesics bed rest soft or liquid diet high humidity possible tracheostomy	diphtheria toxoid diphtheria antitoxin	IM	no major ones
at least 4 weeks	0-3 months of age most severe in young infants (no passive protection)	maintain patent airway humidified oxygen quiet environment antibiotic therapy (ampicillin and erythromycin)	pertussis vaccine human pertussis immune serum globulin (minimal value)	IM	CNS involvement sterile abscess fever irritability anorexia
not transmitted man to man spores usually enter body during injury—puncture wound or burns	all ages having the disease does not provide immunity	decrease external stimulation seizure precautions sedation possible tracheostomy antibiotic therapy	tetanus toxoid absorbed (aluminum phosphate absorbed) tetanus immune globulin (Hypertet)	IM	sterile abscess— (if both types are given at same time, use different syringes and different sites) erythema stiffness tenderness
from 5th day of incubation to 1 week following symptoms	highest in school-age increase in adolescents (passive protection 15 months)	antipyretics dimly lit room tepid baths keep skin dry cool mist vaporizer	live measles attenuated measles immune globulin	sc	fever (rare) slight rash
1-7 days before rash and until rash has faded	older school-age children adolescents (passive protection first six months)	keep pregnant woman away from child symptomatic relief	live rubella attenuated	sc	rash peripheral neuritis arthralgia/ arthritis teratogenic effect
1-6 days before swelling and up to 9 days after swelling	school age	bed rest until swelling subsides analgesics for pain encourage fluids and soft foods hot or cold compresses antipyretics	live mumps attenuated	sc	none
1-5 days before eruption until vesicles are crusts (crusts are not contagious)	2-8 years of age (no passive protection)	antihistamines to prevent itching daily bath and linen change fingernails kept cut short mittens on hands if child scratches vesicles	none available for general use	—	—
1 week before onset and as long as fever persists	all ages	complete bed rest general nursing care moist hot packs range-of-motion exercises	trivalent live oral polio vaccine	oral	rare

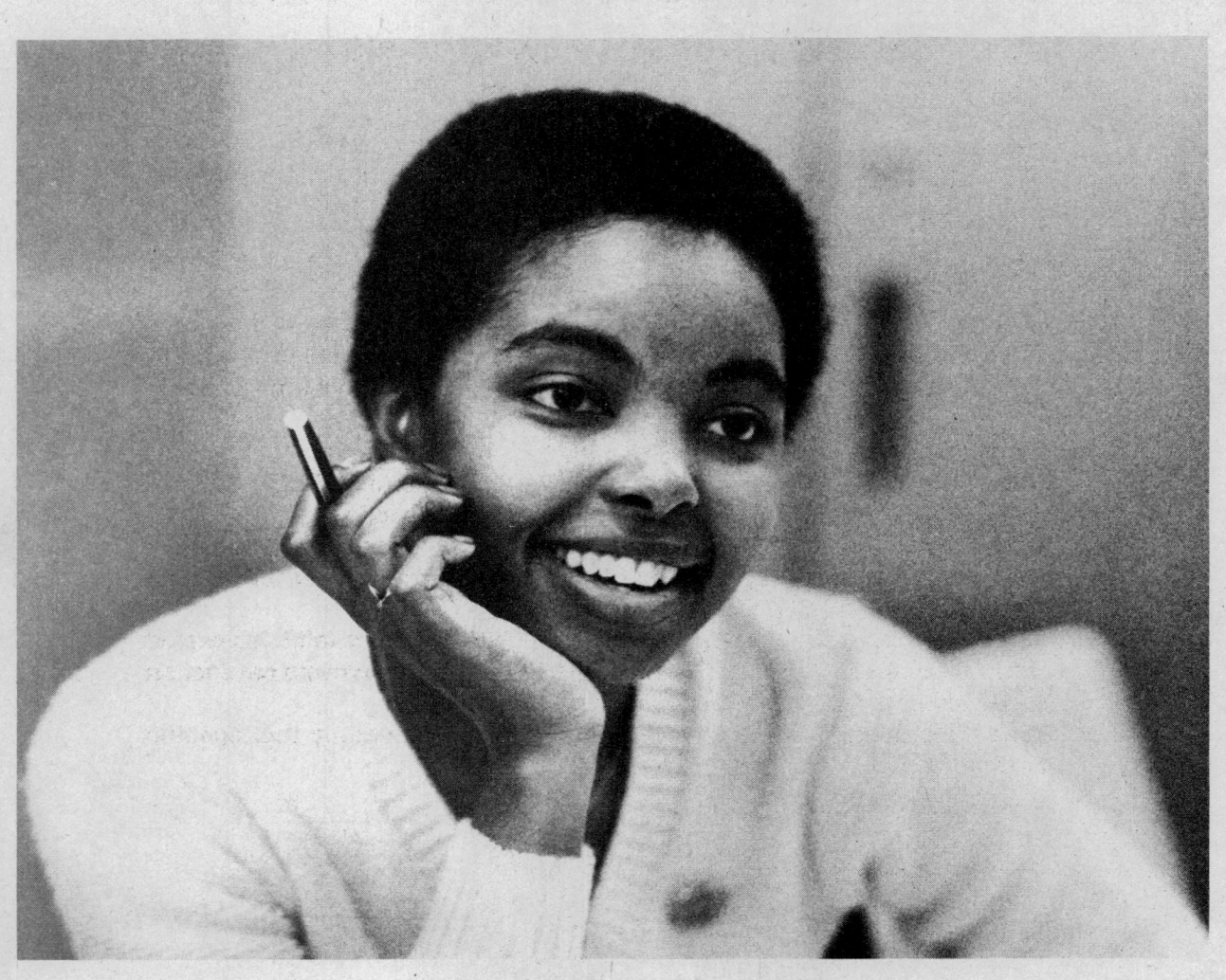

Section 6
Questions and Answers

The questions and answers in this section have been organized in such a way as to simulate the NCLEX-RN exam.

The 375 questions have been divided into four sections of 93 or 94 questions each. Each section tests your nursing knowledge in regard to care of the adult, the child, the childbearing family, and the client with psychosocial problems.

Instructions for Taking the Test
1. Review the information in Section One: Preparing for the NCLEX.
2. Time yourself, allowing one and one-half hours per section.
3. Read each question carefully and select *one* best answer to each question.
4. Don't leave questions blank, since you will not be penalized for random answers on the NCLEX.
5. Score your exam using the answer key. Count any questions left unanswered as incorrect. A score of 75% (70 questions) or more right answers per section is roughly equivalent to a passing grade.
6. Review the questions you answered incorrectly and restudy that specific material.

Section 6: Questions and Answers

BOOK ONE QUESTIONS 651
BOOK ONE ANSWERS 662
BOOK TWO QUESTIONS 667
BOOK TWO ANSWERS 677
BOOK THREE QUESTIONS 682
BOOK THREE ANSWERS 693
BOOK FOUR QUESTIONS 698
BOOK FOUR ANSWERS 710

Sample Test Questions: Book One

You are a community health nurse making a home visit to the Stephens family. Mona Stephens is a single mother with a 2½-year-old daughter, Vanessa, and a three-week-old son, Burton. The family lives on public assistance and receives food stamps. Burton's formula is supplied by the WIC program.

1. After Miss Stephens welcomes you and you sit down with her to begin the visit, which of the following is most appropriate to say?
   1. "You look tired. Are you getting enough sleep?"
   2. "Vanessa seems to like her new brother."
   3. "Tell me what a typical day is like for the three of you."
   4. "Are you having any trouble meeting your expenses?"

2. Miss Stephens tells you she is concerned about Burton's "throwing up. He does it every time he eats." What would be your best first response to further clarify this potential problem?
   1. "About how much does he throw up each time, and what does it look like?"
   2. "Are you burping him after every ounce?"
   3. "Perhaps you aren't diluting his formula correctly. Let's check."
   4. "Is he taking formula with iron?"

3. After you ascertain that Burton is experiencing normal newborn regurgitation, you reassure his mother that newborns often experience this because
   1. The newborn's stomach capacity is so small.
   2. It takes some time for the newborn to adjust to the formula's richness.
   3. The lining of the newborn's stomach is easily irritated.
   4. The cardiac sphincter between the esophagus and stomach is not fully matured.

4. Miss Stephens tells you that Vanessa has been wetting her bed again, "even though I had her completely trained when she was just two." Your best reply would be
   1. "Vanessa may have been trained a little too early and is just having some accidents."
   2. "This may be a sign of a urinary tract infection. I'll take a urine sample with me to have it checked."
   3. "Sometimes toddlers feel uncertain when a new baby comes into the family, and they go back to old habits."
   4. "Make sure you don't give her too much to drink before she goes to bed, and it will probably stop soon."

5. You make a follow-up visit in three months. Which of the following would you be most concerned about?
   1. Burton is taking 28 oz of formula daily along with 2 tbsp of cereal and pureed fruit twice daily.
   2. Vanessa continues to wet the bed two or three times a week.
   3. Miss Stephens tells you she is "always exhausted."
   4. The only toys in the home are makeshift ones, such as shoe boxes, tissue paper, and pots and pans.

6. You assess Burton's development at this visit. He should be exhibiting which one of the following behaviors?
   1. Bears some weight on his legs.
   2. Imitates speech sounds.
   3. Sits with minimal support.
   4. Uses a thumb-finger grasp.

Margaret Dunneden is a 40-year-old business woman who was admitted to the psychiatric unit two days ago for severe depression. You have been assigned to be her primary nurse therapist.

7. Mrs. Dunneden says to the nurse, "I'm terrible. I don't deserve to live." Which of the following responses by the nurse would be most appropriate?
   1. "Yes, it has occurred to us that you have that opinion of yourself."
   2. "If you continue to talk this way, I can't listen to you any more."
   3. "What has led you to think that you don't deserve to live?"
   4. "I don't think you're terrible. Don't you think you're liked here?"

8. When you tell Miss Dunneden that you will be meeting with her for regular interviews, she says, "Why would you want to do that?" What would be the most therapeutic response?
   1. "I think you're worth the time and effort."
   2. "I have been assigned as your therapist."
   3. "You need to talk about your feelings."
   4. "You can't get better without help."

9. In your first interview with Miss Dunneden, she fails to call you by name and appears anxious. What is the most likely explanation of this behavior?
   1. It is part of her depressed state.
   2. You have not made your expectations clear to her.
   3. She is probably hallucinating.
   4. This is typical of initial interviews.

10. Miss Dunneden tells you she has just received a promotion and is in line for another significant advance in her company if she does as well in the new position as she did in the last. How is this information most likely related to her depression?
    1. Success can sometimes result in a depression.
    2. Depression includes grandiose delusions.
    3. This will help validate that she is not worthless.
    4. The promotion will give her a goal.

11. One day, you notice Miss Dunneden is sitting alone in the television lounge; and although the TV is on, she is not watching it. You go to sit beside her. Which of the following would be the most therapeutic way to open a conversation with her?
    1. "What are you feeling?"
    2. "Do you like TV?"
    3. "Tell me how you're doing today."
    4. "You're not watching TV."

12. Instead of responding verbally, Miss Dunneden gets up and walks away from you. Which of the following is the most therapeutic thing for you to do?
    1. Let her go.
    2. Follow her and encourage her to talk.
    3. Follow her and confront her avoidance behavior.
    4. Send another staff person to check on her.

13. One of the staff members reports that Miss Dunneden has been eating very little at meals. Which of the following is the most likely explanation of this behavior?
    1. It is a common side effect of antidepressants.
    2. The hospital food is probably unfamiliar to her.
    3. She is trying to get attention from the staff.
    4. It is part of her psychiatric problems.

14. Miss Dunneden begins to respond to her antidepressant trazodone HCl (Desyrel), and will continue to take it after she is discharged. Which of the following is the correct information to give her about her medication?
    1. It may be addicting and should be stopped as soon as she can tolerate being without it.
    2. Dizziness can be minimized by not taking the drug on an empty stomach.
    3. The drug may cause hypertension, and she should monitor her blood pressure.
    4. She should avoid foods such as aged cheeses and yogurt and products made with yeast, beer, and wine.

15. Suicide is a primary concern when planning nursing care for depressed clients. Personnel must be particularly alert for suicidal attempts during which of the following periods?
    1. During the depth of the client's depression, and when the client is stuporous
    2. When the client begins to voice somatic complaints
    3. When the feeling of depression begins to lift
    4. The periods before and after visiting hours

16. Which of the following is accurate?
    1. Suicide is the leading cause of death in this country among all age groups and among adolescents.
    2. Depressed persons attempt suicide as an expression of anger.
    3. Hospitalized persons rarely attempt suicide.
    4. A person who talks about suicide will not attempt it.

17. When would you best begin preparing for the termination of your relationship with Miss Dunneden?
    1. At your first meeting
    2. During the working phase
    3. After rapport has been established
    4. When her discharge date is set

18. A few days before Miss Dunneden's scheduled discharge, you find her crying alone in her room. She says, "I just don't know if I'll be able to make it." What is the most therapeutic response?
    1. "You're worried that you'll get depressed again."
    2. "You won't be able to 'make' what?"
    3. "You wouldn't be leaving if you couldn't make it."
    4. "Everyone feels that way sometimes."

19. What is the most likely explanation for Miss Dunneden's behavior?
    1. She is not ready for discharge.
    2. She has become overly dependent on the hospital.
    3. She is having a common reaction to discharge.
    4. She needs to know you still care about her.

Alda Clark is a 75-year-old widow, who maintains her own residence. While cleaning the snow off her walk, she slipped and fell.

20. You notice Mrs. Clark is unable to move her left leg. Your first priority is to
    1. Extend her leg into a normal position.
    2. Try and reduce the fracture.
    3. Elevate the extremity.
    4. Treat her as if a fracture has occurred.

21. You suspect that Mrs. Clark fractured her left hip because of which of the following manifestations?
    1. Edema around the site
    2. Internal rotation of the left hip
    3. Abduction of the left hip
    4. Shortened right leg

22. Preparation of Mrs. Clark's skin before applying Buck's extension traction should include which of the following?
    1. Surgical preparation of the area where pins will be inserted
    2. Close shaving of the leg with a safety razor
    3. Washing and drying of the skin
    4. Application of talc to area

23. The diagnosis of extracapsular fracture of the left hip requiring internal fixation is made. Your plan of care in the postoperative course includes which of the following?
    1. Sedation to reduce Mrs. Clark's pain
    2. Early ambulation with weight bearing on the left leg to prevent muscle atrophy
    3. Provisions for "log-rolling" Mrs. Clark
    4. Maintaining adduction of the left hip to prevent dislocation of the prosthesis

24. Mrs. Clark has had osteoarthritis for years. She takes aspirin 600 mg q4h to relieve the pain. Side effects of aspirin are indicated by which of the following signs?
    1. Urinary retention
    2. Bradycardia
    3. Tinnitus
    4. Diplopia

25. Mrs. Clark expresses concern over her impending discharge. At the unit discharge conference, you present Mrs. Clark's case. What would be the most effective intervention for Mrs. Clark?
    1. Realize this is a normal reaction.
    2. Discuss the reality of placing her in a nursing home.
    3. Teach her about hazards in her environment.
    4. Have the social worker make a visit to Mrs. Clark's home.

Phillip Witten is employed as the manager of a real estate business. Subsequent to increasing pressures at work, hurried and irregular meals, an unhappy home and family environment, Mr. Witten developed a duodenal ulcer.

26. The nurse knows that all of the following may be manifestations of a duodenal ulcer *except* which one?
    1. Pain relieved by food
    2. Pain in the middle of the night
    3. Bloating or fullness after eating
    4. Hematemesis

27. Mr. Witten was placed on a bland diet regimen. Substances permitted on this diet include which one of the following?
    1. Creamed soup, pureed squash
    2. Potato chips, whole wheat bread
    3. Sponge cake, fried chicken
    4. Bran muffins, unsalted butter

28. Anticholinergic drugs are useful in the management of gastrointestinal problems such as Mr. Witten's duodenal ulcer. Which is their major action?
    1. Increase gastric motility
    2. Reduce production of gastric secretions
    3. Neutralize hydrochloric acid in the stomach
    4. Absorb excess gastric secretions

29. Mr. Witten has an order for antacids q2h. You are the night nurse, and at 2:00 A.M. when you go to his room to give him the antacid, he is asleep. What action is most appropriate?
    1. Wake him and give the medication.
    2. Let him sleep but wake him at 4:00 A.M. and give a double dose of medicine.
    3. Let him sleep until he wakes up and then resume the antacid q2h.
    4. Wake him but give him a double dose of medicine so you do not have to wake him at 4:00 A.M.

30. Mr. Witten requires surgical intervention and has a gastric resection. Postoperative nursing interventions include connecting his Salem sump tube to an Emerson pump. If he starts to regurgitate, which action should the nurse take?
    1. Irrigate the tube with normal saline.
    2. Notify the physician.
    3. Switch the suction to low Gomco.
    4. Reposition the tube.

31. After his abdominal surgery, the nurse must be particularly conscientious in encouraging Mr. Witten to cough and deep breathe hourly for which of the following reasons?
    1. Marked changes in intrathoracic pressure will stimulate gastric drainage.
    2. The high, abdominal incision will lead to shallow breathing to avoid pain.
    3. The phrenic nerve has been permanently damaged during the surgical procedure.
    4. Deep breathing will prevent postoperative vomiting and intestinal distention.

32. The nurse should be aware of potential complications after a total gastrectomy. For example, two months postoperatively, Mr. Witten sought help for complaints of dizziness, sweating, and tachycardia, which occurred immediately after he ate. He also had lost 10 lb. Symptoms were probably due to which of the following?
    1. Pernicious anemia
    2. Dumping syndrome
    3. Recurrence of the ulcer at the incision
    4. Pyloric stenosis

Mark Stevens, three years old, has trisomy 21. During a routine clinic visit, Mrs. Stevens relates to you that her husband is being transferred to another city. She is very concerned about the effect this move will have on Mark.

33. Which of the following suggestions would receive the highest priority when discussing the move with Mrs. Stevens?
    1. Adhere to Mark's daily routine as much as possible during and after the move.
    2. Include Mark in all the family discussions concerning the move.
    3. Have Mark stay with relatives until the move is complete.
    4. Enroll Mark in a specialized day-care program as soon as possible.

34. Mrs. Stevens is also concerned about Mark's weight. She states that "at three he should weigh approximately 30 lb. Mark is well below that." Your response is most appropriately based on which of the following statements?
    1. Mrs. Stevens needs to increase Mark's daily fluid and caloric intake.
    2. The height and weight of children with trisomy 21 is usually below chronologic norms.
    3. Mark is not a normal three-year-old.
    4. Three-year-olds are very fussy eaters, and Mark's weight will improve in time.

35. Identify which of the following childhood problems poses the most serious threat to Mark.
    1. Conjuctivitis
    2. Fracture
    3. Club foot
    4. Bronchitis

36. When Mark was an infant, a stimulation program was developed for him based on his abilities. What was the best rationale for this action?
    1. To prevent hypotonicity of his muscles
    2. To promote an optimal developmental level
    3. To involve the family in his care
    4. As a precursor for vocational training

37. Which of the following actions is likely to have had the most impact on Mark's learning during the infant-stimulation program?
    1. Giving Mark's parents written instructions explaining the exercises
    2. Observing Mark's parents performing the exercises to validate parental understanding
    3. Verbally explaining the exercises to Mark while they are being performed to increase his understanding
    4. Praising Mark for his accomplishments and cooperation with the exercises

38. In which of the following child-rearing areas will Mark's parents likely have the most trouble?
    1. Discipline
    2. Feeding
    3. Toileting
    4. Socialization

39. Assuming Mark's immunizations are up to date, which immunization will he receive next?
    1. PPD, MMR
    2. DPT, TOPV
    3. TOPV, MMR
    4. DPT, PPD

40. Which of these statements concerning learning disabilities is correct?
    1. They are the result of an emotional disturbance.
    2. The definition includes children who are blind or deaf.
    3. They involve problems with math or reading skills.
    4. They are usually treated with stimulants or tricyclic antidepressants.

Ann Cooper, aged 28, was referred to the infertility clinic after six years of unsuccessful attempts to conceive. She and her husband, Tim, wish to exhaust all possibilities before applying to a community adoption agency.

41. After taking a complete health history from both partners, you prepare them for further assessments. Which of the following fertility tests are generally suggested at the time of the initial visit?
    1. Testicular biopsy and culdoscopy
    2. Laparoscopy and hormonal studies
    3. Huhner test and thyroid screening
    4. Semen analysis and basal body temperature

42. After several months of consultation, the cause of infertility still has not been established. Mr. Cooper expresses his frustration that so little specific information has been given. Which of the following statements by the nurse is most appropriate?
    1. "I know that you want a family, but these tests take time."
    2. "Your doctor is a very competent infertility specialist."
    3. "It is hard when you don't know who is to blame."
    4. "Those feelings of frustration are understandable."

43. The physician completes all tests and finds no physical reason for the inability of Mrs. Cooper to conceive. He prescribes the drug clomiphene citrate (Clomid) and will continue with hormonal studies. You understand that a side effect of this therapy may be
    1. Uterine fibroids.
    2. Multiple gestation.
    3. Hypertension.
    4. Transitory depression.

44. Several months after initiating Clomid therapy, the couple visit the clinic for confirmation of pregnancy. The physician estimates that Mrs. Cooper is approximately eight weeks pregnant. The couple is delighted with the news. In setting a goal for antepartal care, which of the following is a priority?
    1. To promote regular clinic visits
    2. To encourage active exercise
    3. To include the father in classes
    4. To reduce the woman's work schedule

45. In the 10th week of pregnancy, Mrs. Cooper experiences scant vaginal bleeding for several days. Urine HCG levels remain elevated, and the physician believes that there is no imminent risk of abortion. As the couple prepare to return home, which of the following must be included in teaching?
    1. "Please call if you experience abdominal pain or cramping."
    2. "Notify the doctor if you are nauseated or if you vomit."
    3. "If you feel very fatigued, please let us know."
    4. "Report any signs of urinary frequency."

46. An ultrasound examination is scheduled at the next visit, in the 12th week of pregnancy. What is your understanding of the chief purpose of such a test at that time?
    1. Biparietal diameters are determined.
    2. Potential problems are identified.
    3. Fetal viability is confirmed.
    4. Placental function is assessed.

47. The pregnancy advances without complications, and Mrs. Cooper keeps all clinic appointments faithfully. After an examination in the 32nd week, you discuss her concerns and discomforts. Mrs. Cooper reports occasional nightmares about labor and delivery. You listen to her and understand that this experience
    1. May be related to the history of infertility.
    2. Is very common for the primigravida.
    3. May indicate deeper psychologic problems.
    4. Is quite usual throughout pregnancy.

48. The Coopers plan on a birthing-room delivery. Their Lamaze classes include an orientation to the unit and a tour of the nursery in addition to the usual content and practice sessions. Which of the following charted statements by the birthing-room nurse following delivery indicates that the prepared-childbirth classes met the couple's needs?
    1. Breathing and relaxation techniques were applied effectively.
    2. Early mother-father-infant bonding was initiated.
    3. No analgesics were needed during the first stage of labor.
    4. Father remained supportive throughout the delivery.

49. A 7 lb daughter initiated breast-feeding within an hour of birth. You understand that a major benefit of early nursing is to
    1. Enhance closeness to the newborn.
    2. Promote uterine contraction.
    3. Meet the nutritional needs of the infant.
    4. Stimulate meconium passage.

50. On the infant's admission to the newborn nursery, a gestational assessment is performed. Which of the following indicates that the newborn is probably full term?
    1. Apgars of 9 and 10 at one and five minutes
    2. Good reflexes
    3. Many sole creases present
    4. Birth weight at 50th percentile

51. While observing the Cooper infant, you note that she sneezes frequently and appears to be a nose breather. Which of the following assessments is appropriate?
    1. There may be a respiratory problem.
    2. Further assessment is indicated.
    3. The environment may be cold.
    4. These are normal responses.

52. You notice that the infant looks directly at her mother while breast-feeding and seems to react to voices of both the parents. Mr. Cooper asks you if their daughter can see and hear. Which of the following responses is most accurate?
    1. "We think that the newborn can see light and hear loud sounds."
    2. "Research has shown that close-up vision and hearing are present."
    3. "The newborn only appears to respond to sensory stimuli."
    4. "It is impossible to determine this in the first days of life."

53. During the first two days of rooming-in, you teach Mrs. Cooper many aspects of newborn care. On the day of discharge, you observe her feed and handle the baby. Which of the following actions indicates that Mrs. Cooper has learned safe handling of her daughter?
    1. The infant is placed on her right side after the feeding.
    2. Breast-feeding is managed comfortably and effectively.
    3. The diaper area is cleansed after passage of a stool.
    4. The mother handles the baby gently while dressing her.

54. The father asks you about laboratory charges for a PKU test. What is your understanding of the major purpose for this test?
    1. It identifies newborns with any chromosomal abnormality.
    2. State law dictates several routine screening tests.
    3. A rare metabolic disorder can be detected by such testing.
    4. Autoimmune adaptation of the newborn is measured.

Judy Rogers is a 25-year-old, Type I insulin-dependent diabetic. She works as a bookkeeper and has a young son. She has maintained fairly good diabetic control until recently and is now being admitted for reevaluation. Her insulin routine has been 22 units of NPH plus 5 units of regular insulin daily. She takes her insulin each morning before leaving the house.

55. Which piece of subjective data obtained on your admission assessment indicates a potentially serious problem with Mrs. Rogers's self-care management?
    1. "I'm not getting as much sleep as I used to. Tommy seems to wake up at least once every night."
    2. "I've been promoted at work, but the new job has more responsibility."
    3. "I can't seem to find the time for morning urine tests anymore."
    4. "I'm careful about never skipping meals, but I frequently have to eat breakfast at our morning coffee break."

56. Since Mrs. Rogers takes NPH insulin you reinforce her knowledge of a proper diet by testing her understanding of the importance of snacks at which time of day?
    1. Midmorning
    2. Midafternoon
    3. Early evening
    4. Bedtime

57. Mrs. Rogers administers her insulin in two injections. What is the most accurate evaluation of this routine?
    1. This is the only safe method because NPH should never be mixed with any other form of insulin.
    2. This is the preferred method because it prevents mistakes in measurement.
    3. There are no real advantages or disadvantages to administering the insulin in one or two injections.
    4. It is preferable to accurately mix the two insulins in one injection to decrease lipodystrophy.

58. Mrs. Rogers's pattern of site rotation can be evaluated as effective if she
    1. Uses other sites besides her thighs for injections.
    2. Uses both hands equally well to give her injections.
    3. Uses no single injection site more frequently than once a month.
    4. Can name four acceptable injection sites besides the upper arm.

Thomas O'Connor, two days old, was to be circumcised before going home from the newborn nursery, when hypospadias was noted. The physician told Mrs. O'Connor that he would not circumcise Tommy until a later date, because of the abnormal opening in the penis. He was called away and left the room without any further explanation.

59. When the nurse came into the room, Mrs. O'Connor seemed distraught. She was holding Tommy and said, "I don't see anything abnormal about Tommy's penis." The nurse should show the penis to Mrs. O'Connor and explain that the congenital anomaly is located
    1. On the dorsal surface.
    2. On the ventral surface.
    3. On the ventral curvature.
    4. On the dorsal curvature.

60. Mrs. O'Connor asks why the doctor did not do the circumsion. She says, "My baby is healthy, even though he has this problem." The nurse would best respond
    1. "Your baby can urinate without a circumcision."
    2. "When the doctor does surgery to correct the anomaly, he will circumcise Tommy then."
    3. "The skin over the end of the penis may be needed to correct the anomaly."
    4. "Your baby really doesn't need a circumcision."

61. Mrs. O'Connor asks at what age is the corrective surgery usually done. The nurse would best respond
    1. "In a month or so when Tommy is eating well and will be stronger."
    2. "Whenever you ask the doctor to do it."
    3. "When Tommy starts school, about four or five years of age."
    4. "About two years before Tommy starts school, that is, when he is about three years old."

62. When Tommy is hospitalized for his surgery, which of the following will be most traumatic for him?
    1. Separation from his family
    2. Placement in unfamiliar surroundings
    3. Association with strangers
    4. Being unable to run and play as he chooses

63. When Tommy has his corrective surgery, he will be in the cognitive-development period known as
    1. Preoperational thought.
    2. Sensorimotor development.
    3. Concrete operations.
    4. Intuitive reflex development.

Oscar Brown, aged 37, has had a cough and fatigue for several weeks. A sputum culture is positive for Mycobacterium tuberculosis.

64. Which of the following best prevents the transfer of the tuberculosis organism?
    1. Instructing all family members in effective hand washing
    2. Having all who contact Mr. Brown wear a mask
    3. Having Mr. Brown cover his mouth when talking to you
    4. Having Mr. Brown's dishes disinfected after use

65. Mr. Brown and his family ask many questions when first told about his diagnosis of active tuberculosis, e.g., "How did this happen? What can we do? What will happen?" Your best response might be which of the following?
    1. "Mr. Brown probably contracted tuberculosis from another person with tuberculosis."
    2. "Mr. Brown will be given medication and be treated at home."
    3. "You need not be concerned; tuberculosis is curable."
    4. "You seem very worried about the tuberculosis. Are you?"

66. The definitive test for the diagnosis of tuberculosis is
    1. A positive PPD skin test.
    2. A positive sputum culture.
    3. Abnormal findings on chest x-ray.
    4. Abnormal results of a pulmonary function test.

67. Screening a population for tuberculosis with tuberculin skin testing is an example of
    1. Primary health promotion.
    2. Secondary health promotion.
    3. Tertiary health promotion.
    4. Primary prevention.

Harry Collins, a 39-year-old draftsman for a small engineering firm, came to the mental health center at the insistence of his wife. In his leisure time, Mr. Collins designs household gadgets. Mr. Collins has the persistent belief that someone is attempting to steal his designs. His attempts to prevent this are interfering with his marital relationship and with other social relationships. He has installed an elaborate alarm system in their home and spends hours finding places to hide his designs. He refuses to attend social functions because "someone will steal his ideas." Other than self-imposed isolation from his co-workers, he has no difficulties at work. He completes his work on time and is respected by colleagues as a hard worker.

68. Mr. Collins's symptoms are delusions of
    1. Grandeur.
    2. Persecution.
    3. Reference.
    4. Religiosity.

69. The nurse who takes Mr. Collins's admission history understands that his delusion is related to
    1. A desire for attention.
    2. Anger at his employer.
    3. Fear of losing control.
    4. Low self-esteem.

70. Mr. Collins is given a diagnosis of chronic paranoia. Based on this, the nurse would expect Mr. Collins to have
    1. Hallucinations.
    2. Hostility.
    3. Impaired intellectual functioning.
    4. Poor reality testing in all areas.

71. Which of the following nursing diagnoses would be most appropriate for Mr. Collins?
    1. Attention-getting behavior related to mistrust of others
    2. Decreased intellectual functioning
    3. Impaired marital relationship owing to suspiciousness
    4. Paranoia

72. Initial plans for Mr. Collins would best include
    1. Allowing Mr. Collins to initiate relationships and activities.
    2. A one-to-one relationship initiated by the nurse.
    3. Participation in a competitive sport.
    4. Participation in an occupational-therapy group.

73. Mr. Collins attends his first group-therapy session the second day of hospitalization. He leaves in the middle of the session and tells his nurse, "They don't know what they're doing in there. They're all crazy. I won't go to those meetings." The nurse's most appropriate action would be to
    1. Develop a one-to-one relationship with Mr. Collins before he begins group therapy again.
    2. Explain the benefits of group therapy in helping Mr. Collins overcome his delusions.
    3. Insist that Mr. Collins return to the group session immediately.
    4. Tell Mr. Collins that he is excused today but must return to group therapy tomorrow.

74. All of the following nursing actions will be important in developing a one-to-one relationship with Mr. Collins *except*
    1. Accurate and honest communications.
    2. Clearly stated mutual expectations.
    3. Confrontation regarding delusions.
    4. Consistency in keeping appointments.

75. Mr. Collins has been hospitalized for a week. He still talks at length about the measures he can take to protect his designs. The nurse's most appropriate action is to
    1. Involve Mr. Collins in an activity on the unit.
    2. Listen attentively and encourage further discussion.
    3. Tell Mr. Collins his plans are unnecessary.
    4. Tell Mr. Collins she is aware of his actions.

76. Which of the following is the best indicator that Mr. Collins is improving?
    1. He attends occupational therapy.
    2. He attends to his personal hygiene and grooming.
    3. He freely discusses his attempt to protect his designs.
    4. He discusses feelings of anxiety with the nurse.

Sixteen-month-old Mi Lin and her family moved to the US from Southeast Asia one month ago. Mi Lin and her parents visit the pediatric clinic for the first time.

77. Which of the following is *least* important for you to consider as you initiate your interaction with Mi Lin?
    1. Developmental level
    2. Racial heritage
    3. Cultural experiences
    4. Inability to comprehend English

78. To gain Mi Lin's trust and cooperation, you should first
    1. Offer Mi Lin a toy to play with.
    2. Extend your arms to Mi Lin to encourage her to come to you.
    3. Use a puppet to "talk" to Mi Lin.
    4. Establish a positive interaction with Mi Lin's parents.

79. You measure Mi Lin's length and weight and find she is below the 5th percentile for both. A nutritional history reveals Mi Lin's caloric and nutrient intake is consistent with recommended guidelines. Which of the following interpretations is likely to be most valid?
    1. Growth norms are based on American children, who tend to be larger on the average.
    2. Mi Lin's parents may not have been truthful concerning her intake.
    3. A hormone deficiency may be causing a growth lag.
    4. Mi Lin may not be getting adequate activity and exercise.

80. When assessing Mi Lin's development, you would be most concerned about which one of the following findings?
    1. Exaggerated lumbar curve
    2. Has only 10 teeth
    3. Unable to point to her body parts
    4. Knows only one two-syllable word

81. Prior to coming to the US, Mi Lin had not received any childhood immunizations. Upon arrival, she received her first diphtheria, pertussis, tetanus vaccines (DPT) and oral polio vaccine (TOPV). Mi Lin would receive which immunizations today?
    1. DPT and TOPV vaccines
    2. Tuberculin test
    3. Measles, mumps, rubella (MMR) vaccine
    4. Tetanus and diphtheria (Td) vaccines

82. When preparing to administer Mi Lin's immunization, you
    1. Allow Mi Lin to play with a syringe for a few minutes.
    2. Talk in a soothing tone to Mi Lin while her mother holds her firmly in her lap, and proceed quickly.
    3. Explain to Mi Lin that you must give her "a shot so she won't get sick."
    4. Secure the assistance of at least one other nurse to help restrain Mi Lin.

Kathy Smith, six years old, has a condition diagnosed as noncommunicating hydrocephalus secondary to a space-occupying lesion. A ventricular bypass shunt is being considered to relieve the intracranial pressure.

83. What was probably the earliest manifestation of increased intracranial pressure that Kathy exhibited?
    1. Early morning headache
    2. Motor dysfunction
    3. Change in vital signs
    4. Papilledema

84. Following insertion of a ventriculoperitoneal shunt, how would Kathy best be positioned?
    1. Semi-Fowler's on the operative side.
    2. Semi-Fowler's on the unoperative side.
    3. Flat on the operative side.
    4. Flat on the unoperative side.

85. Monitoring for signs of increased intracranial pressure is an essential part of Kathy's care. What would be the most valuable indicator of changing intracranial pressure?
    1. Change in sensorium
    2. Tachycardia
    3. Nausea and vomiting
    4. Pulmonary rales

86. Compared to her pre-op vital signs, Kathy's vital signs 18 hours post-op reveal decreasing pulse and respiratory rates and an increasing blood pressure with an increase in pulse pressure. What is your best assessment of the situation?
    1. These are early signs of meningitis.
    2. Her intracranial pressure is increasing.
    3. This is caused by anxiety secondary to post-op stress.
    4. Her central nervous system is immature.

87. Which of the following is the most frequently seen complication of ventricular shunting?
    1. Ascites
    2. Hydrocele
    3. Ileus
    4. Infection

Julio Cortez, aged 47, is admitted with severe substernal chest pain. A diagnosis of acute myocardial infarction is made. He is in severe pain and is cold, clammy, and dyspneic.

88. All of the following interventions are important. Which should be done first?
    1. Administer oxygen.
    2. Check vital signs.
    3. Institute complete bed rest.
    4. Administer morphine.

89. Mr. Cortez is started on heparin therapy. You tell Mr. Cortez he is receiving heparin to
    1. Thin his blood.
    2. Slow the clotting of his blood.
    3. Stop his blood from clotting.
    4. Dissolve the clot in his heart.

90. Mr. Cortez begins to have blood in his stool and has episodes of epistaxis. In view of this development, which drug would you have available?
    1. Vitamin C (ascorbic acid)
    2. Vitamin K (AquaMEPHYTON)
    3. Protamine sulfate
    4. Calcium chloride

91. Mr. Cortez suffers congestive heart failure and is given digitalis. Which of the following indicates a toxic effect of digitalis?
    1. Hypokalemia
    2. Bradycardia
    3. Nausea and vomiting
    4. Gynecomastia

92. With left-sided congestive heart failure, which of the following symptoms is most expected?
    1. Nocturnal dyspnea
    2. Sacral edema
    3. Oliguria
    4. Anorexia

93. Mr. Cortez is advised to eliminate foods high in cholesterol from his diet. This means he should avoid eggs and
    1. Liver.
    2. Yogurt.
    3. Chicken.
    4. Corn oil.

Correct Answers and Rationales: Book One

1. **#3.** This opening statement allows the nurse to gain an overall perspective of family functioning, yet is specific enough to focus the response (as opposed to, "Tell me how you are doing"). The other choices focus narrowly on one aspect, which might be appropriate as the visit proceeds, but are haphazard initial questions. Also, two of them (#1 and #4) require only a "yes" or "no" response and thus do not encourage disclosure by the client.

2. **#1.** Your first response should help to clarify the problem by seeking additional information. #2 might be asked as you proceed to narrow the scope of the cause. #3 is likely to make the parent feel defensive, and #4 is irrelevant, since research does not implicate iron as a cause of regurgitation or vomiting.

3. **#4.** The young infant's cardiac sphincter is not yet fully matured and as a result often relaxes, allowing regurgitation of stomach contents.

4. **#3.** The arrival of a new family member is especially distressing to the two- to three-year-old child and may precipitate jealousy and regression to earlier dependent behaviors, such as bed-wetting, thumb sucking, or clinging.

5. **#3.** Although tiredness is a common complaint of mothers of small children, Miss Stephens's feeling "exhausted" may indicate anemia or poor coping. This needs to be further investigated. Although Burton does not need solids at this age, the caloric intake is within recommended ranges. Bed-wetting is not considered unusual in children of Vanessa's age, and she may still be adjusting to her new brother. These homemade toys provide appropriate developmental stimulation for Miss Stephens's children.

6. **#1.** Burton should be bearing some weight on his legs when held upright. Inability to do so may indicate a neuromotor delay.

7. **#3.** This is the only response that recognizes and acknowledges the client's perception of her situation and that encourages her to explore it with the nurse. This response is therapeutic and conveys respect for the client's point of view and a desire to help her learn to cope with her problems. It promotes a relationship of trust.

8. **#3.** Focus on the client's needs without risking an argument about feelings of worthlessness.

9. **#4.** Early interviews are characterized by anxiety. The client is too focused on herself to recognize the nurse as a unique individual.

10. **#1.** Success can cause depression in some persons because they fear failure, which will lead to a loss of self-esteem.

11. **#3.** Encourage the client to talk by using general, open-ended questions.

12. **#2.** Stay with her to show you care about her. Encourage her to talk but do not push or confront her.

13. **#4.** Anorexia is a common occurrence in depressed clients. It is rarely a side effect of antidepressants.

14. **#2.** The most common side effect of Desyrel is dizziness. Antidepressants are not addicting. #3 and #4 are common for MAO inhibitors.

15. **#3.** Suicide attempts occur most frequently when the feelings of depression begin to lift. The person's energy level is so low at the depth of depression that she may not have energy to carry out suicidal thoughts and wishes. In addition, having just been relieved of the extreme suffering of a deep depression, she may find the thought of a possible recurrence intolerable.

16. **#2.** Suicide is an act of self-punishment, of anger directed toward the self. The suicidal person is a depressed person who feels guilty, condemns herself, and directs her anger inward.

17. **#1.** Preparing for termination begins with the inception of the therapeutic relationship.

18. **#1.** Reflection encourages her to talk about her fears without minimizing them as #3 and #4 do.

19. **#3.** Clients often become anxious near discharge and reexperience symptoms they may not have shown for some time.

20. **#4.** The diagnosis has not been confirmed; you only suspect a fractured hip. Never attempt to reduce a fracture, or extend or elevate the extremity. You may cause more damage.

21. **#3.** Fractured hips present with abduction of the affected extremity and movement away from the main axis of the body. There is also external rotation of the hip and the leg is shortened. It is difficult to assess edema at this point.

22. **#3.** Washing and drying of the skin minimizes the risk of nicking or cutting the skin, which could result in infection. It also aids in securing the traction.

23. **#3.** When the client is moved, she needs to be "log-rolled" with abductor splint or pillows between her legs. Sedation may not be indicated in view of her age. Early ambulation is advocated, however no weight bearing is allowed on the operated side.

24. **#3.** Doses of aspirin sufficient to relieve pain may cause tinnitus. The other side effects listed are not characteristic of aspirin.

25. **#1.** Depression and worry following hip fracture are normal for this age group. Since she is independent, she may be able to care for herself at home. She needs to know about the hazards in her environment but not until after she handles her psychosocial concerns. This is a nursing concern, not a problem for a social worker to handle.

26. **#4.** Hematemesis occurs with gastric ulcers. All the other symptoms listed are indicative of duodenal ulcers.

27. **#1.** All fried foods and whole grains are prohibited.

28. **#2.** Anticholinergic drugs block the effect of acetylcholine at receptor sites thereby reducing the production of gastric secretions.

29. **#1.** Antacids are given to coat the ulcer to protect it from irritation.

30. **#2.** The Salem tube has a double-lumen feature that allows for escape of air bubbles. Irrigation is contraindicated after gastric surgery, unless ordered, to avoid trauma to the surgical site. Gomco suction is contraindicated because it is intermittent suction; to be effective, the Salem tube requires continuous suction.

31. **#2.** After abdominal surgery, the client is at greatest risk of pulmonary complications.

32. **#2.** Foods enter the duodenum too rapidly following gastrectomy.

33. **#1.** Maintaining consistency in Mark's environment is the single most effective way to promote a sense of security and continuity during the move.

34. **#2.** Children with trisomy 21 tend to be shorter than average with weight measurements below chronologic norms. Their caloric needs are based on height and weight, not age.

35. **#4.** Respiratory infections are common in children with trisomy 21 and account for high morbidity. The hypotonicity of the chest and abdominal muscles is a major predisposing factor to respiratory infections.

36. **#2.** The goal for caring for a child with trisomy 21 (as well as any form of retardation) is to promote optimal development. Children with trisomy 21 have hypotonic muscles. While including the family in Mark's care is important, it is not the primary reason.

37. **#4.** While all the options are necessary in an infant-stimulation program, motivating the child to want to learn is a critical factor. This is best accomplished through praising the child's accomplishments. This option is also helpful in promoting self-esteem.

38. **#1.** While problems may occur in all of these areas, discipline presents the greatest challenge, because parents of these children typically eliminate it completely from their child-rearing practices.

39. **#2.** Mark would receive DPT and TOPV at four to six years of age. The PPD is usually administered at 12 months of age and before the MMR. The MMR is given at 15 months of age.

40. **#3.** Learning disabilities refer to difficulties with understanding and using language; they can include problems with math, reading, listening, and talking. They do not refer to sensory deficits; nor are they the result of emotional disturbances. Medications are not routinely administered unless the child has attention-deficit problems as well.

41. **#4.** While the other tests may be performed later, they are involved or invasive. Semen analysis is a simple assessment. Basal body temperature charting is performed at home by monitoring temperature daily for one or two cycles.

42. **#4.** This response indicates understanding of common feelings about infertility. None of the other responses can be considered therapeutic communication.

43. **#2.** Clomid increases the risk of ovarian cysts and multiple births. None of the other choices are correct.

44. **#1.** A priority goal for any pregnant client is to promote good and regular prenatal care. #2 is partially correct, but the term "active" is not appropriate. At this point in early pregnancy, fathers are not usually encouraged to attend classes; nor are the mothers. Few women need to reduce work schedules at this point.

45. **#1.** If the client experiences contractions, cramping, or more bleeding, she may be experiencing a miscarriage. All other signs are normal in early pregnancy.

46. **#3.** At this time in pregnancy, when the client has a history of bleeding, the test is performed to confirm fetal viability. Biparietal diameters are a useful assessment between 18 and 24 weeks gestation. Neither #2 nor #4 is accurate.

47. **#2.** These fears and dreams are common, especially in the last trimester. There is no correlation with infertility history.

48. **#1.** The focus of Lamaze classes is the practice of breathing, relaxation, and conditioned responses for use during labor. While it is positive that bonding and support were noted, these are not criteria for evaluation of class learning. Use of analgesia during labor is not a criterion for successful outcome of Lamaze classes.

49. **#1.** While uterine contractions increase during breast-feeding, the major reason for initiating nursing immediately after delivery is to promote closeness. Nutritional needs are minimal at this time. Meconium is passed within the first 24 hours.

50. **#3.** This is the only assessment that refers to gestational-age factors. Apgar scores measure immediate adaptations to extrauterine life; birth weight is not necessarily related to length of gestation; reflexes may be good in some infants who were born before term.

51. **#4.** These are normal responses.

52. **#2.** Studies indicate that sensory development at birth is quite good.

53. **#1.** A newborn should be positioned on the abdomen or right side after feeding to prevent aspiration of milk or mucus. The other behaviors are appropriate, but do not measure *safe* care.

54. **#3.** While state laws do require these tests, the most appropriate response gives the major purpose of the test, beyond compliance with law. The other choices are inaccurate.

55. **#4.** She takes regular insulin but has long delay between insulin administration and the first meal of day.

56. **#2.** Peak action for NPH is 8-12 hours after administration.

57. **#4.** NPH and regular insulin may be safely mixed if it is accurately and consistently done. There is no need for two shots.

58. **#3.** Other choices are important, but the final goal is to prevent overuse of sites.

59. **#2.** In hypospadias, the urethal opening is abnormally located behind the glans or anywhere along the ventral surface of the penile shaft.

60. **#3.** Circumcision is avoided, since the foreskin may be needed for reconstructive surgery.

61. #4. Surgery is usually performed when the child is about three years of age. The phallus is of sufficient size and the child has not yet developed any mutilation anxiety and is not yet in school.

62. #1. Toddlers have difficulty accepting being separated from parents.

63. #1. Piaget calls the period from two years to seven years the period of preoperational thought. Now that the child has language, the child learns on a conceptual level.

64. #3. Tuberculosis is primarily transmitted by droplets from the nose and mouth. All of the interventions may be used, but #3 controls the transmissions of droplets best.

65. #4. The multiple questions suggest anxiety and fear. #4 best reflects this anxiety back and encourages Mr. Brown and his family to express their feelings. The other responses, while factually correct, will probably not allay anxiety.

66. #2. A positive sputum culture is the only test specific for active tuberculosis. The other tests are nonspecific or only indicate exposure (#1).

67. #2. The goal of tuberculin skin testing is the early diagnosis and treatment of tuberculosis, i.e., secondary health promotion.

68. #2. Delusions of persecution are defined as false beliefs that oneself has been singled out for harassment.

69. #4. Content of the delusion serves to build up the person's self-esteem. Insufficient data are given to support the other choices.

70. #2. Persons with paranoid ideation have underlying hostility. There is no evidence of hallucinations. Intellectual functioning appears intact. Reality testing remains intact except for the area related to the delusion.

71. #3. Mr. Collins has marital problems because of his behavior. There is no evidence that his behavior is attention seeking. Intellectual functioning is not disturbed. Paranoia is a medical diagnosis.

72. #2. Interventions would begin with one-to-one activities. Socialization is gradually increased. The client will need assistance to develop a relationship. Activities should be nonthreatening.

73. #1. Involve the suspicious client in group activity and relationships gradually. Begin by developing a one-to-one relationship; involve others slowly. #2, #3, and #4 do not allow for this gradual involvement.

74. #3. Do not argue with the client about his delusions. Consistency and clarity will enhance development of trust and are crucial in developing a relationship.

75. #1. Maintain a focus on reality without demeaning the client or becoming involved in arguments.

76. #4. The goal for a suspicious client is for him to recognize the anxiety that causes the delusion and to express that anxiety. No disruption of work or self-care abilities has been indicated. Discussion of delusions indicates no change.

77. #2. Although Mi Lin's racial heritage is an important factor to consider when assessing growth and physical health status, it has little bearing on how the nurse would approach Mi Lin in a clinical situation.

78. #4. At this age, it is best to allow the child to make the first move. Establishing your interaction with Mi Lin's parents first gives Mi Lin time to size you up and see that her parents demonstrate trust in you.

79. #1. Asian children are shorter and weigh less, on the average, than white children, on whom growth norms are often based. Even though the graphs have been recently revised to be more representative of children from varying backgrounds, the nurse should always consider the child's family heritage when evaluating variances from normal.

80. #4. By this age, the majority of children know at least 3 other words in addition to "mama" or "dada." Although this finding may be within normal ranges, it bears further investigation to identify a possible delay in language development. The other findings are all characteristic of toddlers at this age.

81. #3. The recommended schedule for children who have not been immunized according to the usual recommended schedule for infancy indicates that measles, mumps, and rubella vaccines should be given in a combined injection one month after the first DPT and TOPV vaccines have been given.

82. **#2.** It is best to have a parent assist with holding the child during a briefly painful procedure, such as an immunization, if possible. Proceeding quickly is the desirable approach with a child this age for a procedure that will be over quickly. Prolonged explanations only increase the child's anxiety and, in Mi Lin's case, would not be understood because she does not speak English. She may be given the needleless syringe to play with *following* the injection.

83. **#1.** Early morning headaches are frequently the earliest sign of increased intracranial pressure. The other manifestations are usually seen later.

84. **#4.** Positioning the patient flat on the unoperative side will prevent pressure on the shunt valve and allow for gradual drainage of the spinal fluid. The other positions would place additional pressure on the shunt.

85. **#1.** The primary indicator of changing intracranial pressure is changes in sensorium or level of consciousness.

86. **#2.** A decrease in pulse and respiration with an increase in blood pressure and pulse pressure are signs of increased intracranial pressure.

87. **#4.** Complications such as ascites, ileus, and hydrocele have been reported following ventricular shunts; however, infection and blockage of the shunt are the most common problems.

88. **#4.** Relief of pain is the priority goal for a client with a myocardial infarction.

89. **#2.** Anticoagulant therapy is used to prolong, not prevent clotting. Anticoagulants have no thrombolytic (clot dissolving) action. "Blood thinner" is a term commonly used by lay persons for anticoagulants, but actually anticoagulants have no effect on hemoconcentration.

90. **#3.** Protamine sulfate is the antidote for heparin. Vitamin K is the antidote for *oral* anticoagulants.

91. **#3.** Digitalis toxicity is manifested by gastrointestinal upset. Bradycardia is a side effect that may or may not indicate toxicity. Hypokalemia potentiates digitalis effects, but is not a toxic effect.

92. **#1.** *Left*-sided congestive heart failure causes pulmonary congestion and associated symptoms. Oliguria, while present in both right-sided and left-sided congestive heart failure, is primarily a symptom of right-sided failure.

93. **#1.** Organ meats are high in cholesterol.

Sample Test Questions: Book Two

Josephine Harrod has been admitted to the hospital with hepatitis Type A.

1. Mrs. Harrod's care should include which of the following precautions?
   1. Stool and needle isolation
   2. Special care of linens and food
   3. Use of a gown and gloves during client contact
   4. All of the above

2. Several months following her hospitalization for hepatitis, Mrs. Harrod reentered the hospital with complaints indicative of cholecystitis and cholelithiasis. Because she has an existing jaundice, which of the following tests should be performed prior to surgery?
   1. Lee-White Clotting time
   2. Bleeding time
   3. Prothrombin time
   4. Circulation time

3. In caring for Mrs. Harrod, the nurse would best consider which to be a major complication after gallbladder surgery?
   1. Atelectasis
   2. Pneumonia
   3. Hemorrhage
   4. Thrombophlebitis

4. Following surgery, Mrs. Harrod has a nasogastric tube in place with an order to irrigate it prn. What is the rationale for irrigating a post-op client's nasogastric tube?
   1. To remove secretions from the stomach
   2. To decrease abdominal distention
   3. To minimize bleeding
   4. To maintain patency of the tube

Barbara Tilson developed juvenile diabetes at age 11. She is now 21, insulin-dependent, but well controlled during her first pregnancy. A healthy 10 lb girl is delivered at 38 weeks gestation.

5. When caring for Baby Girl Tilson in the delivery room, what is the nurse's first priority?
   1. Ensuring proper identification
   2. Establishing a warm environment
   3. Maintaining a patent airway
   4. Facilitating parental bonding

6. Which of the following is a priority when caring for Baby Girl Tilson in the nursery?
   1. Maintaining hydration
   2. Assessing gestational age
   3. Initiating early feeding
   4. Monitoring blood sugar level

7. In preparing Mrs. Tilson for discharge you include infant-care teaching. Which of the following is most important for this mother to know?
   1. Although the baby has a problem she is normal and should be treated like any infant.
   2. Give the child 24 calorie/oz formula to counteract hypoglycemia.
   3. See the pediatrician regularly throughout infancy and childhood.
   4. Feed the child skim milk to maintain weight in infancy.

8. The nurse knows that Mrs. Tilson may develop manifestations of hypoglycemia. These include which one of the following?
   1. Acetone odor to breath, nausea, and vomiting
   2. Increased temperature, pulse, and respiration rate
   3. Increased voiding, thirst, and abdominal pain
   4. Increased hunger, trembling, and dizziness

9. The discharge teaching plan includes emphasis on proper foot care. Which of the following practices indicates that Mrs. Tilson has learned such care?
   1. Nails, corns, and calluses are trimmed weekly.
   2. She walks barefoot as much as possible.
   3. Her feet are bathed and inspected daily.
   4. Salicylate creams are applied to red areas.
10. The nurse notes lipodystrophies on Mrs. Tilson's thighs. She states that she gives all her insulin injections into her thighs. In teaching Mrs. Tilson how to prevent lipodystrophies, which response is accurate?
    1. All of her injections should be given at a 45° angle.
    2. This is an unavoidable complication of insulin administration.
    3. A change in type of insulin will eliminate the problem.
    4. Rotation of sites to include the abdomen and forearm will help alleviate the problem.
11. When assessing Mrs. Tilson's condition, which manifestations might indicate ketoacidosis?
    1. Pale, moist, cool skin; confusion
    2. Flushed skin, air hunger
    3. Extreme nervousness, shallow respirations
    4. Hunger, diplopia
12. If Mrs. Tilson develops diabetic acidosis, what will the intervention be?
    1. Regular insulin given IV
    2. NPH insulin given subcutaneously
    3. Glucagon given IV
    4. Orange juice and glucose given orally

Allen Spinet, 23 years old, was injured in an automobile accident.

13. Of the following sequences, which would be the most appropriate in the immediate posttrauma minutes?
    1. Control the hemorrhage; establish an open airway; stabilize the fractured vertebrae; splint the fractured leg.
    2. Establish an open airway; control the hemorrhage; stabilize the fractured vertebrae; splint the fractured leg.
    3. Establish an open airway; stabilize the fractured vertebrae; control the hemorrhage; splint the fractured leg.
    4. Establish an open airway; control the hemorrhage; splint the fractured leg; stabilize the fractured vertebrae.

14. Which is the most important intervention in treating hemorrhage?
    1. Allay apprehension.
    2. Give oral fluids.
    3. Prevent chilling, but don't overheat.
    4. Restore blood volume.
15. Shock causes which of the following?
    1. A Po_2 greater than 80 mm Hg
    2. A pH less than 7.34
    3. A Pco_2 less than 42 mm Hg
    4. A decrease in capillary permeability
16. If cardiopulmonary resuscitation were performed on Mr. Spinet by two persons, which of the following ratios of pulmonary inflations to cardiac compressions would be used?
    1. 1:1
    2. 1:5
    3. 2:15
    4. 2:20
17. Effective cardiopulmonary resuscitation would be best indicated by which sign?
    1. Palpable carotid pulse
    2. Dilated pupils
    3. Easily blanched nail beds
    4. Normal skin color
18. Mr. Spinet is conscious and is bleeding from a compound fracture of the right leg. The adequacy of his general tissue perfusion can be determined by assessing all of the following *except* which one?
    1. Urinary output
    2. Blood pressure
    3. Level of consciousness
    4. Skin color
19. Mr. Spinet has been admitted to the ICU. He has a mean blood pressure of 90. He is on nitroprusside drip and an epinephrine drip to be titrated to keep blood pressure at a mean of 80. What is the most appropriate action?
    1. Decrease nitroprusside.
    2. Increase nitroprusside.
    3. Decrease epinephrine.
    4. Increase epinephrine.
20. What is the primary objective of therapy for Mr. Spinet's shock?
    1. Maintain the blood pressure.
    2. Improve tissue perfusion.
    3. Maintain adequate vascular tone.
    4. Improve kidney function.

21. Mr. Spinet's injuries include a skull fracture. One of the goals of care for him is to observe for increasing intracranial pressure. Increased intracranial pressure would be indicated by which signs?
    1. Increased pulse rate and increased blood pressure
    2. Increased pulse rate and decreased blood pressure
    3. Decreased pulse rate and increased blood pressure
    4. Decreased pulse rate and decreased blood pressure

22. In addition, which of the following would best indicate increased intracranial pressure?
    1. BP change from 110/80 mm Hg to 140/50 mm Hg
    2. Pulse change from 78/minute to 92/minute
    3. Respirations change from 16/minute to 26/minute
    4. Change in level of consciousness from stupor to drowsy and restless

Mr. "X" was admitted to the psychiatric unit without an awareness of who he was or where he lived. He has no evidence of a head injury or psychosis.

23. Mr. X is diagnosed as suffering a dissociative reaction. He probably has this as a reaction to which of the following?
    1. A life-threatening situation
    2. An unresolved conflict
    3. A frustrating experience
    4. Taking the NCLEX examination

24. Mr. X is using which of the following defense mechanisms?
    1. Regression
    2. Denial
    3. Rationalization
    4. Repression

25. Mr. X is hospitalized on a psychiatric unit. The theraputic milieu will focus on which of the following?
    1. Encouraging him to remember what happened to him
    2. Keeping him from other clients until staff is more certain of who he is
    3. Expecting him to be involved in daily activities on the unit as he is able
    4. Administering electroconvulsive therapy (ECT) to help him became aware of the conflict and deal with it

As an involved nurse in the community you are teaching a sex education class for high school students.

26. One of the students asks you about the reliability of pregnancy-test kits. Which is the best response?
    1. "Discuss this with your physician."
    2. "These tests can give inaccurate results."
    3. "They confirm pregnancy 10 days after conception."
    4. "Used according to directions, they are 95% reliable."

27. You have just shown a film on female sexuality to the high school class, and several of the girls have asked you what causes cramps. What would be the most accurate response?
    1. The uterus in young girls is immature, and this creates pain during your period.
    2. If you worry about having cramps or are upset about something, you will get cramps.
    3. Your hormones are in a state of change, and this causes periodic episodes of cramps.
    4. Cramps are due to the contraction of the muscles of your uterus.

28. Several boys in the class are concerned about physical changes ocurring with puberty. The most accurate response to this concern is that all of the following are physical characteristics of male puberty *except* which one?
    1. Increased available energy
    2. Increased size of genitals
    3. Swelling of breasts
    4. Nocturnal emissions

29. Two students in the class are concerned because they are not yet menstruating. From your knowledge of the average age of menarche for the typical North American girl, you may give the following information:
    1. It is about nine years, but family tendencies vary.
    2. It is about 10½ years, so you may wish to speak with your physician.
    3. It is about 12½ years, but some variation in this pattern is normal.
    4. It is about 14 years, so you have plenty of time yet before being concerned.

Janice Carter is in the 37th week of pregnancy. She calls the physician to report that she awakened in the middle of the night and found herself lying in a pool of bright red blood.

30. Which condition is characterized by third-trimester, painless bleeding?
    1. Abruptio placentae
    2. Placenta previa
    3. Incomplete abortion
    4. Ectopic pregnancy

31. Mrs. Carter is admitted to the labor room. Which of the following is contraindicated during the admission assessment?
    1. Vaginal examination
    2. X-ray pelvimetry
    3. Type and crossmatch
    4. Perineal prep

32. Mrs. Carter is worried about her condition, and about her two-year-old twins at home. Bob Carter asks you if he should remain with Mrs. Carter or return home to check on the children and their teenaged sitter. Which response indicates an understanding of their feelings at this time?
    1. "You would feel more secure if you checked on your family."
    2. "Your wife is well cared for here. You may go home for a while."
    3. "You really belong here, now. Call home and check on the children."
    4. "Why not ask your wife what would be best for her?"

33. An ultrasound confirms that the placenta totally covers the cervical os. Mrs. Carter is prepared for a cesarean birth. Physical preparation for this surgery includes which of the following?
    1. Type and crossmatch
    2. Insertion of Foley catheter
    3. Skin prep and shave
    4. All of the above

34. Mrs. Carter will receive a spinal anesthetic. As she prepares to sign the consent forms, she asks about the possiblity of postanesthetic headaches. Your response is based on the knowledge of which of the following?
    1. They rarely occur, and are usually mild.
    2. Medication is available to counteract headaches, and is given prn.
    3. Headaches may occur if there is any allergy to the agent used.
    4. This problem may be prevented by restrictions on position changes.

35. Baby Carter, 6 lb 4 oz, is delivered by cesarean section, and appears to be in stable condition. Mrs. Carter's blood loss during delivery was 1,200 ml. She receives 2 units of blood replacement. While she is in the recovery room, you notice several changes in her condition. Which change would you report to the physician immediately?
    1. Pulse changes from 88 to 120, she appears restless.
    2. Blood pressure is stable at 100/80; she appears pale.
    3. Temperature rises to 100.2°F; her mouth is dry.
    4. Lochia rubra noted; she appears to be in pain.

36. An IV of 1,000 ml of 5% dextrose in saline with 10 units of pitocin is ordered. The solution is to infuse in 6 hours. Drop factor is 10. At what rate should the IV infuse?
    1. 27 drops per minute
    2. 2.7 drops per minute
    3. 37 drops per minute
    4. 3.7 drops per minute

37. While the intravenous pitocin is infusing, you continue to assess Mrs. Carter's condition. Which of the following assessments is most important at this time?
    1. Monitoring uterine contractions
    2. Measuring urinary output
    3. Checking IV site
    4. Monitoring respirations

Loretta Neter, a 22-year-old woman, is admitted to an inpatient psychiatric unit. Paralysis developed in her right arm, for which no physical cause can be found. The admitting diagnosis is conversion reaction.

38. The source of apparent paralysis, caused by a conversion disorder such as Miss Neter's, is which of the following?
    1. Conscious
    2. Unconscious
    3. Partially conscious
    4. Undeterminable

39. Miss Neter's physical symptoms are primarily a way for her to accomplish which of the following?
    1. Express anger at someone, probably a parent
    2. Avoid problems at work
    3. Avoid an unconscious conflict and the anxiety it produces
    4. None of the above

40. The nurse notices that Miss Neter does not appear frightened about her paralysis. In fact, she seems somewhat comfortable with it. Why is this symptom significant?
    1. It demonstrates Miss Neter's flexibility and adaptability to difficult situations.
    2. It shows that Miss Neter consciously knows that she's not physically damaged.
    3. It is a common client response to a conversion and stems from the unconscious conflict.
    4. None of the above

41. Miss Neter is using which of the following defense mechanisms?
    1. Repression
    2. Suppression
    3. Displacement
    4. Repression and displacement

42. Miss Neter tends to focus on her paralysis in her interactions with others by asking for help, even for things she can do herself, and by talking about how she feels about having a paralyzed arm. Which of the following interventions would be most appropriate when dealing with this dynamic?
    1. Allow the client to discuss her symptoms to help relieve her anxiety.
    2. Encourage the client to get involved in activities on the unit and to discuss other topics.
    3. Insist that the client not discuss her paralysis or receive help from others to force her to learn new ways of handling anxiety.
    4. Insist she discuss her physical symptoms with the nurses and the physician only, not with friends and family.

43. One day Miss Neter says to the nurse, "I suppose you think I'm faking my paralysis." Which of the following would be the best nursing response?
    1. "Yes, I think you could move your arm if you chose to do so."
    2. "I think you know that there is no physical cause for your paralysis."
    3. "I believe you are presently unable to move your arm, regardless of the cause."
    4. "I believe your paralysis is physical and that you may have been misdiagnosed."

44. Miss Neter's comment is most likely due to which of the following explanations?
    1. She is having auditory hallucinations.
    2. She is having paranoid delusions.
    3. She is seeking reassurance.
    4. She is lonely.

Jerry Smith, aged 10, is admitted to the intensive care unit with second- and third-degree burns of the face, neck, chest, and upper extremities.

45. After establishment of a patent airway, which of the following actions takes priority?
    1. Cleaning and debriding the burns
    2. Administering pain medication
    3. Establishing a good IV line
    4. Getting a history of the nature of the burns

46. During the first 24 hours postburn, most burn deaths are the result of which of the following?
    1. Hypovolemic shock
    2. Gram negative infection
    3. Respiratory complications
    4. Renal failure

47. The doctor orders the "burn budget" for Jerry. The nurse knows that means which of the following?
    1. The IV rate will remain constant for 48 hours.
    2. The "budget" includes only colloids.
    3. Vital signs and urinary output may indicate a need for the "budget" to be changed.
    4. Maintaining the prescribed IV rate will prevent further fluid loss.

48. Jerry should be observed for signs and symptoms of oxygen deprivation because of the burns on his face and chest. What is the most consistent early symptom of oxygen deprivation?
    1. Headache
    2. Tachycardia
    3. Diaphoresis
    4. Restlessness

49. Jerry is having severe pain. Meperidine (Demerol) with hydroxyzine (Vistaril) IV is ordered. Why is the IV route the most appropriate?
    1. There are decreased skin surfaces for IM sites.
    2. More rapid action will prevent agitation.
    3. Decreased peripheral circulation may prevent drug absorption.
    4. Less medication will be necessary to relieve the pain.

50. When Jerry's bowel sounds return, he is started on hyperalimentation via NG tube. A good nursing intervention when administering NG feedings is to check residual stomach contents routinely. What should you do if you note a large residual prior to a feeding?
    1. Discard it and withhold the feeding for 1 hour.
    2. Replace it and hold the feedings until the residual is decreased.
    3. Call the physician for further orders.
    4. Proceed with the feedings; it is of no concern if it does not recur.

51. As soon as Jerry's condition is stabilized, range-of-motion exercises are begun. What is the primary reason for this?
    1. To promote circulation thus aiding wound debridement
    2. To decrease further tissue breakdown from immobility
    3. To decrease pain by diverting his attention
    4. To utilize nutrients thus increasing energy production

52. Hand splints are applied in the immediate postburn period for which of the following reasons?
    1. Immobilizing the hands decreases pain.
    2. Tendon rupture and hand deformities can be prevented.
    3. Keeping the fingers extended will aid circulation.
    4. They act as restraints to prevent the client's touching the burned areas.

53. Jerry is scheduled for a skin graft to the upper part of his chest. What is the most important nursing priority during the first 48 hours postgraft?
    1. Keeping the grafted area immobilized
    2. Encouraging frequent vigorous coughing
    3. Providing nutritional supplements
    4. Turning the client q2h

54. The Smith family is presented at a nursing conference. One of the nurses states, "Jerry's parents are in crisis. I think they need crisis intervention." Which of the following assessments would provide the *least* helpful information in determining their need for crisis intervention?
    1. How they have dealt with stress in the past?
    2. What family/friend supports do they have?
    3. How do they perceive Jerry's current situation?
    4. How has Jerry's rehabilitation progressed thus far?

Olivia Carnelli, aged 76, is scheduled for a right modified mastectomy tomorrow.

55. Preoperatively, you would discuss postoperative
    1. Skin grafting.
    2. *Peau d'orange* skin changes.
    3. Treatment of intraductal edema.
    4. Use of a HemoVac.

56. Which of the following would you expect to be her biggest concern?
    1. Body-image alterations
    2. Fears her illness will not allow her to attain life's goals
    3. Loss of functional ability
    4. Concerns about the effect her surgery will have on her sexual relationship with her spouse

57. When Mrs. Carnelli returns from surgery, you monitor her for signs and symptoms of hemorrhage. In addition to assessing her vital signs, you would best
    1. Ask her if her back feels wet.
    2. Have her cough and deep breathe.
    3. Observe the amount of drainage in the HemoVac.
    4. Visually check under her back for drainage.

58. Which of the following plans would be most likely to meet Mrs. Carnelli's learning needs?
    1. Provide written materials for her to read during the day.
    2. Offer brief, frequent one-to-one sessions.
    3. Teach her during a single session taking a sufficient amount of time to provide complete factual material.
    4. Have her join a group session with peers; use charts, several speakers, and handouts.

59. You've discussed ways of minimizing lymphedema with Mrs. Carnelli. Which of the following statements indicates a need for more teaching?
    1. "I'll decrease my salt and water intake."
    2. "I'll avoid biting my nails."
    3. "I'll sleep with my arm elevated on pillows."
    4. "I'll keep my right arm elevated as much as possible during the day."

60. Before Mrs. Carnelli is discharged you would expect her to
    1. Be able to explain incision care.
    2. Have adapted to her altered body image.
    3. Have completed the grieving process.
    4. Have received an order for a Jobst pressure machine.

Mrs. Keller brings her son, Jermaine, who just turned five, to the pediatrician's office for a complete health appraisal prior to his entering kindergarten next month.

61. You would focus part of your assessment on Jermaine's achievement of psychosocial tasks. At this age, Jermaine should be trying to accomplish a sense of
    1. Autonomy.
    2. Inquisitiveness.
    3. Self-identity.
    4. Initiative.

62. You obtain a nursing history from Mrs. Keller and Jermaine. Mrs. Keller reports the following behaviors. Which one is it most important to investigate further?
    1. Jermaine has occasional nightmares and won't go to sleep without a light on.
    2. Jermaine wets the bed at night two or three times a month.
    3. Jermaine has an imaginary friend named Rudy.
    4. Jermaine cries and protests when a sitter comes to stay with him.

63. Mrs. Keller asks you to suggest some appropriate toys and activities for Jermaine. Which of the following would be *least* appropriate?
    1. Scissors, paper, and crayons
    2. A two-wheel bicycle
    3. Dolls
    4. A 50-piece jigsaw puzzle

64. You are evaluating Jermaine's readiness to attend kindergarten. He should be able to do all the following *except* which one?
    1. Recognize colors
    2. Count to 20
    3. Tell time on a clock
    4. Recite the alphabet

65. Part of your assessment of Jermaine includes vision screening using the Snellen E chart to test for visual acuity. Jermaine's results are 20/30 vision in both eyes. Which of the following would be the best action to take?
    1. Rescreen Jermaine immediately.
    2. Rescreen Jermaine in two weeks.
    3. Refer Jermaine to an ophthalmologist for a complete eye exam.
    4. Explain to Jermaine and his mother that his vision is normal.

66. While you are conducting vision screening, it is also important to screen Jermaine for
    1. Strabismus.
    2. Diplopia.
    3. Papilledema.
    4. Pupil reactivity.

67. Jermaine's height is at the 50th percentile. His weight is at the 90th percentile. A nutritional history reveals that Jermaine's diet is very high in carbohydrates and fats. You help Jermaine's mother develop a plan to ensure Jermaine gets the nutrients he needs without overeating. This diet would provide Jermaine with approximately how many calories per day?
    1. 1,200
    2. 1,700
    3. 2,400
    4. 2,800

68. Treatment of Jermaine's overweight would best include
    1. A planned program of activity and exercise.
    2. A daily appetite suppressant.
    3. Large doses of supplemental vitamins.
    4. Withholding all sweets.

69. Part of Jermaine's physical examination is an otoscopic exam. To best prepare Jermaine for this, you would
    1. Allow Jermaine to hold the otoscope and "practice" on a doll.
    2. Show Jermaine a picture of a child being examined with an otoscope.
    3. Tell Jermaine, "This won't hurt. It just helps us to look at your eardrum."
    4. Say, "Just lie down here, Jermaine, and we will be finished in a minute."

70. Jermaine returns for a follow-up visit in six months. Which of the following best indicates Jermaine is progressing satisfactorily with his nutritional plan?
    1. Jermaine has lost 5 lb.
    2. Jermaine's daily intake has been 300 calories less than recommended.
    3. Jermaine's weight is now in the 75th percentile.
    4. Jermaine has stopped craving junk food.

Kim Dombrowski is a two-year-old who has been admitted to your unit to rule out the diagnosis of cystic fibrosis.

71. Which of the following may be considered a normal variant in the toddler?
    1. Five colds in the past year
    2. Steatorrhea
    3. Voracious appetite
    4. Dyspnea on exertion

72. What test would probably be performed to confirm the diagnosis of cystic fibrosis in Kim?
    1. Chromosomal analysis
    2. Chest x-ray
    3. Sweat chloride determination
    4. Stool fat assay

73. Kim's condition has been diagnosed as cystic fibrosis, and she is ready to be discharged. When doing parental teaching, the nurse should instruct them to do which action?
    1. Use caution when Kim is actively playing outdoors on hot, sunny days.
    2. Restrict all visitors so Kim won't catch cold.
    3. Continue to tell Kim that she will soon be well.
    4. Limit caloric intake since Kim does not have sufficient enzymes to digest unrestricted intake.

Gloria Rock, gravida 5, para 4, has just delivered her fifth son vaginally following a two-hour labor. The baby weighs 9 lb 10 oz. The following questions refer to Mrs. Rock's postpartal care.

74. Mrs. Rock is especially at risk for
    1. Difficult maternal-infant bonding.
    2. Postpartal hemorrhage.
    3. Puerperal infection.
    4. Urinary retention.

75. One day postpartum, Mrs. Rock complains of night sweats that keep her awake. The most probable cause of these sweats is
    1. IV fluids administered during labor.
    2. Excessive oral intake during the day.
    3. Elimination of fluid that was retained during pregnancy.
    4. Oxytocin given IV following placental expulsion.

76. Mrs. Rock frequently comments, "I hope this is our last baby because we can't afford any more." The nurse's best response would be which of the following?
    1. "Discuss this with your physician at your six-week check-up."
    2. "You need not worry until you quit breast-feeding."
    3. "Would you like information about birth-control methods?"
    4. "Things usually work out for the best."

77. Mrs. Rock goes home from the hospital and returns to the clinic for insertion of an intrauterine device (IUD). The nurse explains to Mrs. Rock that this type of contraception is effective only if the device remains in place. The nurse's teaching has been effective if Mrs. Rock reports checking for the IUD string after
    1. Sexual intercourse.
    2. Ovulation.
    3. Menstrual periods.
    4. Physical activity.

Otis O'Shea, aged 28, is admitted to the hospital after becoming embroiled in an argument with the police during a routine traffic check. His admitting diagnosis is paranoid schizophrenia.

78. As the nurse is orienting Mr. O'Shea to the unit, he states, "They can't arrest me, I'm J. Paul Getty, and I don't have to fool with inconsequential people like the police." Which of the following would be the best initial response?
    1. "Can't arrest you?"
    2. "What made you so angry, Mr. O'Shea?"
    3. "This is your room, Mr. O'Shea."
    4. "Your record indicates your name is Otis O'Shea."

79. The defense mechanism being used by Mr. O'Shea is which of the following?
    1. Denial
    2. Fantasy
    3. Introjection
    4. Projection

80. The physician leaves orders for Mr. O'Shea to have haloperidol (Haldol) 75 mg qid. Which of the following would be the most appropriate action for the nurse to take?
    1. Call the physician; the dose is too low.
    2. Call the physician; the dose is too high.
    3. Call the physician; Haldol is not effective for paranoid schizophrenia.
    4. Administer the drug; the medication and dose are appropriate.

81. Shortly after admission, Mr. O'Shea is seen ordering the other clients around. What action should the nurse best take?
    1. Confront him with his behavior on a one-to-one basis.
    2. Encourage other clients to confront him in a group meeting.
    3. Seclude him.
    4. Spend more time with him on a one-to-one basis.

82. Shortly after breakfast one morning the nurse hears Mr. O'Shea talking loudly and notes that he is beginning to pace in the hall. What would be the best initial action for the nurse to take?
    1. Tell him, "Let's have a cup of coffee and talk about what's making you angry."
    2. Offer him a prn medication for agitation.
    3. Suggest that he use the punching bag.
    4. Isolate him before he hurts someone on the unit.

83. Mr. O'Shea has not had a bowel movement for six days. This is most likely related to which of the following?
    1. His decreased activity level
    2. Lack of fiber in his diet
    3. A side effect of Haldol
    4. Constriction of the bowel as a result of tension

84. Mr. O'Shea has a great deal of difficulty making decisions. This is most likely the result of which of the following?
    1. Autism
    2. Mixed feelings
    3. Ambivalence
    4. Apathy

85. When Mr. O'Shea's behavior becomes more appropriate the nurse decides to include him in the preparations for the next unit party. Which of the following would be the most appropriate activity for him?
    1. Assign him to the entertainment committee.
    2. Ask him to take charge of making the coffee and seeing that the pot is kept filled.
    3. Put him in charge of the clean-up committee.
    4. Ask him to arrange for the pizza to be delivered.

86. Mr. O'Shea has an erratic employment history and is at present unemployed. He is planning to secure a job before discharge. What nursing action would be the most useful?
    1. Help him read the want ads.
    2. Role play the job interview with him.
    3. Refer him for vocational testing.
    4. Encourage him to write a resume.

Mona Spires comes to the clinic because she thinks she has "an infection."

87. She tells you that she has a thick, white, cottage-cheeselike vaginal discharge. Which of the following would you also expect to find on physical examination?
    1. Erythematous and edematous vulva
    2. A painless, red, eroded lesion with an indurated border on the vulva
    3. Papillary, flesh-colored growths on the genitalia
    4. Vesicular genital lesions

88. Which of the following statements best indicates that Miss Spires understands the disease process and its treatment?
    1. "I can resume sexual activity now, because I'm being treated."
    2. "I'll apply the lotion every 12 hours."
    3. "I'll continue to take the antibiotics for 14 days."
    4. "I won't abstain from intercourse while I'm being treated, but I'll have my partner use a condom."

Jeff Tate, 34 years old, presents to the health clinic complaining of urinary burning, frequency, and urgency; hematuria; fever and chills. Lab tests on a clean catch urine reveal RBC and WBC: too many to count; numerous hyaline casts; and bacteria: more than 100,000/ml. A physical exam reveals extreme tenderness in his back at the costovertebral angle (CVA). Mr. Tate's condition is diagnosed as pyelonephritis, and he is admitted to the hospital.

89. The most important blood test of kidney filtration to be done on Mr. Tate would be
    1. Glucose.
    2. Electrolytes.
    3. Creatinine.
    4. BUN.

90. An intravenous pyelogram (IVP) is ordered for Mr. Tate. Which of the following nursing interventions would be the most important for the nurse to do the night prior to the IVP?
    1. Give a cathartic and enemas to cleanse the bowel.
    2. Instruct the client to be NPO after midnight.
    3. Identify by history any client allergies to medicines or foods.
    4. Teach the client that x-rays will be taken at multiple intervals.

91. Mr. Tate is placed on a regimen of a sulfonamide antibiotic (Bactrim). As a nurse, you know which of the following to be true concerning this drug?
    1. It is metabolized by the liver and excreted through the bile.
    2. It produces a false-negative glucose on urine tests.
    3. It will cause the urine to become acidic in pH.
    4. It can crystallize in the urine if fluid intake is insufficient.

92. Upon Mr. Tate's discharge, the physician wants him to maintain his urine in a more acidic state by eating an acid-ash diet. Which of the following foods would you teach the client can be unrestricted in his diet?
    1. Milk
    2. Carrots
    3. Grape-Nuts
    4. Dried apricots

93. Which of the following interventions would be a priority in discharge teaching for Mr. Tate?
    1. Drink at least 3-4 liters of fluid/day.
    2. Take sitz baths 3-4 times/day for urethral burning.
    3. Void immediately after sexual intercourse.
    4. Avoid exposure to persons with upper respiratory infections.

94. After three weeks, Mr. Tate returns to the ER of the hospital with severe, sharp, deep lumbar pain radiating to his right side. A repeat IVP reveals a kidney stone in the right ureter at the bifurcation of the iliac vessel. Upon his admission to the hospital, which of the following goals would take initial priority in this client's nursing care?
    1. Client will decrease risk of future kidney stones.
    2. Client will be prepared for possible urinary tract surgery.
    3. Client will be free from discomfort of kidney stones.
    4. Client will have fluid intake of 3-5 liters/day.

Correct Answers and Rationales: Book Two

1. **#4.** Hepatitis type A is virus spread via contact with oral and respiratory secretions, feces, and serum from an infected person.

2. **#3.** Prothrombin and other clotting factors are synthesized by the normal liver. The rate of prothrombin synthesis is influenced by absorption of vitamin K, which may be impaired because of obstruction of the bile duct. The prolonged prothrombin time may lead to hemorrhage.

3. **#1.** Because of the high incision and upper abdominal pain, the postoperative client resists coughing and deep breathing and is likely to develop atelectasis.

4. **#4.** Irrigation maintains the patency of the tube, which will also accomplish #1 and #2.

5. **#3.** Although all are correct, the priority is establishing and maintaining a patent airway.

6. **#4.** Excess insulin may lead to hypoglycemia. Brain damage will result if not corrected. Feeding is begun after assessment of glucose level.

7. **#3.** This infant has the usual risk related to heredity for diabetes. She should be seen regularly during childhood. No changes in feeding are indicated.

8. **#4.** The release of epinephrine in response to an abnormal drop in blood-sugar level results in dizziness and trembling. Hunger is characteristic of hypoglycemia. The other symptoms are manifestations of diabetic acidosis.

9. **#3.** Daily washing, lubricating, and drying of the feet prevents dryness and skin breakdown. The other actions listed may lead to tissue trauma or irritation.

10. **#4.** The client should use a diagram and schedule to rotate injection sites, so that injections are given in the same site no more than once a month. Injections are given subcutaneously at a 90° angle with a ½-inch needle to ensure deep subcutaneous injection.

11. **#2.** Dry, hot, flushed skin and air hunger (Kussmaul's respirations) are caused by the lungs attempting to compensate for carbonic acid buildup by blowing off CO_2. These are signs of ketoacidosis. The others are characteristics of hypoglycemia.

12. **#1.** Insulin must be given intravenously because of the dehydration and poor perfusion that occur with diabetic acidosis. Regular insulin is the only insulin which can be given intravenously.

13. **#2.** The client's airway is the first priority following trauma. Control of hemorrhage is second. Stabilization of the fractured vertebrae takes precedence over splinting of the leg.

14. **#4.** Primary intervention with hemorrhage is to stop the bleeding and restore blood volume in order to prevent irreversible shock. The other interventions are appropriate but of secondary importance.

15. **#2.** Shock causes metabolic acidosis (decreased pH). Tissue metabolism continues so that large amounts of acid are emptied and accumulate in the stagnant blood. With progressive tissue hypoxia, anaerobic metabolism produces nonvolatile lactic acid that further increases the acidosis.

16. **#2.** One lung inflation after every five cardiac compressions is the ratio currently recommended by the American Heart Association.

17. **#1.** A palpable carotid pulse would indicate adequate sternal compression.

18. **#4.** Alterations in skin color may result from changes in vasomotor tone yet give little indication of perfusion of the vital organs.

19. **#3.** Doing either #2 or #3 would bring the BP down; but since vasoconstriction causes other problems, you would want to keep epinephrine dose as low as possible. #1 and #4 would cause BP to rise further.

20. **#2.** All are goals of treatment, but tissue perfusion must be improved to prevent irreversible damage and death of tissues. If tissue perfusion improves, other goals will be accomplished secondarily.

21. **#3.** As cerebral pressure rises as a result of tissue injury, edema, and hypoxia, the BP increases in response to the hypoxic stimulation of the vasomotor center. The pulse rate slows as the blood pressure increases.

22. **#1.** A widening pulse pressure is the most characteristic symptom of increasing intracranial pressure.

23. **#2.** Dissociative reactions are hysterical reactions characterized by bizarre behavior in which the client splits off one portion of his conscious mind from the whole when that represents some major, otherwise unresolvable, conflict for him. This is a neurotic rather than psychotic reaction.

24. **#4.** Repression is the unconscious involuntary forgetting of unacceptable or painful thoughts, impulses, feelings, or acts. A dissociative reaction is the unconscious use of repression to forget events that may cause persons to recall painful material.

25. **#3.** Mr. X will best be helped by decreased anxiety and active involvement. The focus is on reality-based milieu activities. The staff relates to him within the reality of the situation (i.e., relationships and day-to-day activities of the milieu). ECT would not help because it is believed that ECT helps seal off unconscious conflicts. Therefore it would not help a client become more aware of a conflict.

26. **#4.** Detection of HCG in urine can be 95% reliable 10 days after a missed period, if the kit is used according to directions.

27. **#4.** This is the only accurate statement. Cramps are not caused by emotions or hormones.

28. **#1.** Increased size of genitals, swelling of breasts, and nocturnal emissions result from hormonal changes of puberty. Rapid growth and increased energy demands decrease available energy.

29. **#3.** Although 12½ years is the average, the age at onset of menstruation varies.

30. **#2.** Low implantation of the placenta causes painless bleeding in the third trimester.

31. **#1.** A vaginal examination is contraindicated for this client, because it might stimulate contractions and increase the risk of delivery of the placenta.

32. **#4.** This is a decision both must make.

33. **#4.** All of these are important in preparation for the cesarian birth.

34. **#4.** The bed will be kept flat for 8-12 hours after use of spinal anesthetic to avoid headaches.

35. **#1.** Rapid pulse and apprehension are signs of shock.

36. **#1.** With a drop factor of 10 drops/ml; the desired rate is 27 drops/ml.

37. **#2.** Pitocin has an antidiuretic effect; thus urinary output must be carefully monitored.

38. **#2.** Conversion disorders are unconsciously motivated.

39. **#3.** Miss Neter's symptoms are an expression of an unconscious conflict. Often this conflict has anger as a component, but the paralysis often inhibits expression of the anger rather than encourages it. If the symptom was acquired consciously, Miss Neter would be described as malingering.

40. **#3.** The symptom serves the purpose of relieving the need to directly deal with the unconscious conflict; therefore the person feels some sense of relief. The symptom is called *la belle indifférence*.

41. **#4.** She is repressing conflicting feelings that she unconsciously believes she cannot handle and displaces the resulting anxiety into the physical symptom of paralysis. In this way, her focus is on the paralysis. As a result, she is relieved of the need to deal with the original conflict. Suppression is a conscious mechanism; and if she were using suppression, she would consciously know that her paralysis was an emotional response and it would be within her conscious control.

42. **#2.** It is important to encourage her to give up the symptom by not focusing on it. However, since the symptom is a method she uses to relieve anxiety, staff members need to help her find new ways of relieving anxiety before she will give up her present method of relieving it.

43. **#3.** This is the response that demonstrates the nurse's understanding of the pain the symptom is causing Miss Neter and its reality to her.

44. **#3.** The client is seeking reassurance about the origin of her symptoms.

45. **#3.** An IV needs to be started quickly, so that fluids can be restored and pain medication given.

46. **#1.** Following fluid losses from the burned areas and fluid shift from the intravascular and intracellular compartments, hypovolemic shock can occur.

47. **#3.** The burn fluids include colloids, electrolytes, water to replace insensible losses. The amount budgeted varies with age of client and area of burn. It is simply an estimate. Changes in vital signs and urinary output would necessitate making changes.

48. **#4.** While tachycardia will occur with lack of oxygen, restlessness can be noted first.

49. **#3.** With the fluid shifts occurring during the first hours postburn, the peripheral circulation is impaired, and there may be inadequate pain relief from an IM injection. Also, after a few days when the peripheral circulation has been restored, an overdose might occur from the unabsorbed medication.

50. **#3.** Gastric dilation and gram-negative infections can result in poor gastric emptying and need to be reported immediately. Discarding the residual may deplete needed electrolytes.

51. **#2.** Jerry is already in a state of negative nitrogen balance; immobility increases catabolism.

52. **#2.** Skin surfaces on the hand are very thin, and the tendons lie very close to the skin. Immobilizing the hands prevents injury to these structures.

53. **#1.** During the immediate postgraft period, preventing any movement of the grafted surfaces takes precedence over any other activity. Deep breathing can be encouraged, but coughing is contraindicated.

54. **#4.** Assessing the progress of Jerry's rehabilitation will not provide significant information about how emotionally prepared his parents are to deal with his current problems. How they have handled stress in the past is a good indicator of how they will deal with this current stress.

55. **#4.** Postoperatively, Mrs. Carnelli will probably have a HemoVac in place. Skin grafting is rarely done. It is not needed as it is with the more extensive, Halsted radical mastectomy. *Peau d'orange* change in skin is a preoperative assessment parameter.

56. **#3.** A major concern for this age group is maintaining independence. #1 and #4 are more common for a young adult. #2 is probably not a factor at her age.

57. **#4.** Drainage is drawn to the back of the dressing by gravity. If you do not look under her back for drainage, Mrs. Carnelli may hemorrhage significantly without its being detected.

58. **#2.** This best allows the RN to assess understanding of material and provides an opportunity to adapt to the patient's concentration span. #1 is not best with this age group since they may have trouble with written content or may not be motivated to read. #3 and #4 may overtax Mrs. Carnelli and do not allow feelings about the surgery and diagnosis to be expressed.

59. **#2.** This intervention relates more to preventing infections in the arm on the side of the surgery.

60. **#1.** Prior to discharge, Mrs. Carnelli should be able to explain incision care. Adapting to an altered body image takes weeks or months, as does the grieving process. The latter may even be delayed two or three months. A Jobst pressure machine is used only if other methods for preventing lymphedema are ineffective.

61. **#4.** The psychosocial task at this age is accomplishment of a sense of initiative.

62. **#4.** By age five, children should separate from their parents with relative ease, especially when left in familiar surroundings, such as home, with a sitter.

63. **#2.** The average child does not learn to ride a two-wheel bicycle until six or seven years of age.

64. **#3.** The average five-year-old can recognize most colors, count to 20, and recite the alphabet. It is not until about age seven that children can tell clock time.

65. **#4.** These results are normal; 20/20 or 20/30 vision is considered within normal limits at this age, because visual acuity may not be fully developed.

66. **#1.** Strabismus is a common health problem that must be detected early to prevent amblyopia. The other options are used to assess neurologic status.

67. **#2.** Recommended caloric intake at this age is approximately 1,700 calories/day.

68. **#1.** A carefully planned program of diet and exercise that meets the child's continued needs for growth is essential. Focus should be on slowing weight gain to allow height to catch up over a period of several months, rather than trying to have the child lose weight. Appetite suppressants are without merit in the treatment of childhood overweight and obesity. Large doses of vitamins are unnecessary, if the child is eating a well-balanced diet, and may actually be harmful to the child. Withholding all sweets is unrealistic and may lead to cheating. The child should be helped to change his eating habits with the recognition that an occasional sweet treat is acceptable.

69. **#1.** Children at this age need to actually experience an event firsthand to know it and what it feels like. Practicing the feel of the otoscope on a doll will help lessen Jermaine's anxiety and increase his cooperation.

70. **#3.** Because of slowing of Jermaine's weight gain, his weight is now only one standard deviation from his height. Weight loss and caloric restriction are not desired outcomes. Jermaine may not be craving junk food, but this option doesn't give you enough information to evaluate his progress (e.g., he may not be eating junk food, but his caloric intake may be as high as previously if he is substituting other foods).

71. **#1.** Because of their developing immune systems and increasing chances of exposure to infectious agents, toddlers may normally have 8-10 colds per year.

72. **#3.** The normal chloride content of sweat is less than 40 mEq/liter. A concentration of greater than 60 mEq/liter is diagnostic of cystic fibrosis.

73. **#1.** Massive salt loss may occur with sweating, leading to dehydration and hypoelectrolytemia. If the fluid deficit is large, cardiovascular collapse may occur.

74. **#2.** The uterine muscle may be too exhausted to contract owing to overdistention from a large baby and the number of pregnancies. Rapid labor also overworks the uterus.

75. **#3.** Fluid shifts during the postpartal period cause a normal diaphoresis and diuresis.

76. **#3.** This is the best answer, because nurses can give this information. Breast-feeding is not a reliable contraceptive; and if she waits six weeks, she may get pregnant again.

77. **#3.** The cervix is slightly open during menses, and the menstrual flow may facilitate expulsion of the IUD.

78. **#3.** This response keeps the interaction reality oriented. #1 and #2 probe into the client's delusion. #4 may provoke an argument.

79. **#4.** Projection is unconsciously attributing one's own unacceptable qualities and emotions onto others. He is saying, "I'm not inconsequential. They are."

80. **#2.** The maximum therapeutic dose range for Haldol is 100 mg daily.

81. **#4.** The suspicious, hostile, or aggressive client should be worked with initially, and probably for an extended time, on a one-to-one basis. This will allow a trusting relationship to develop. #1 and #2 will provoke anger and hostility and will reinforce defenses. #3 isolates the client and may also reinforce defenses and perpetuate the delusional system.

82. **#1.** Intervene while the client is still able to talk about feelings. #2 will not allow the client the opportunity to learn to deal with negative feelings. #3 also will not allow client to learn verbal methods of dealing with anger. #4 is not justified by his behavior at this time.

83. **#3.** Constipation is a side effect of Haldol. The other choices can cause constipation, but no data have been given to support them.

84. **#3.** Ambivalence is the coexistence of two opposing feelings toward another person, object, or idea. The term "mixed feelings" is sometimes used, but ambivalence is the proper term.

85. **#2.** Put the suspicious, hostile, aggressive client in charge of things not people. #2 is the only response that meets that criterion.

86. **#2.** This allows the client to practice verbally what he is going to say before he is in the actual situation (one that is likely to be stressful). #3 may also be useful; but with Mr. O'Shea's employment history, vocational counseling is less likely to be useful than his learning to deal with stressful situations.

87. **#1.** This is another symptom of candidiasis. A painless, red, eroded lesion describes a chancre of syphilis; while papillary flesh-colored growths are genital warts. Vesicular genital lesions are consistent with a diagnosis of herpes.

88. **#4.** Unless the partner is going to use a condom, Miss Spires should abstain from sexual intercourse until the symptoms of the infection disappear. Candidiasis is treated with antifungals such as miconazole cream or nystatin suppositories, not antibiotics.

89. **#3.** After creatinine is removed by glomerular filtration, it is only minimally reabsorbed or it is excreted by the tubule cells. BUN, glucose, and electrolyte values are affected by many factors other than renal function, therefore, are not as specific.

90. **#3.** The dye used for an IVP is iodine based and can cause a severe allergic reaction (anaphylaxis) in sensitive individuals. Food allergies to shellfish can indicate an iodine allergy, because shellfish are high in iodine content. The other choices should be done; but because of the possible danger to the client, the allergy history takes priority.

91. **#4.** Sulfonamides dissolve well in urine and are excreted unchanged in the urine; therefore they are excellent for treating urinary tract infections. However, if fluid intake is not sufficient, the drug can crystallize, resulting in renal toxicity. While on the drug regimen, intake should be sufficient to maintain a urine output of at least 1 liter/day.

92. **#3.** Whole grains are unrestricted in an acid-ash diet. The other three foods listed would be part of an alkaline-ash diet and are either not allowed or are allowed in restricted amounts.

93. **#1.** A high urine output helps flush out bacteria from the urinary tract and maintain a low urine osmolarity. Encourage clients to void every two to three hours during the day and one to two times during the night. Sitz baths are helpful during an acute episode but are not a priority of discharge planning. Voiding after intercourse is recommended for women who have repeated urinary tract infections. Avoidance of exposure to respiratory infections would be highly desirable if the client was showing signs and symptoms of renal failure. At this point, Mr. Tate is not in this category.

94. **#3.** All of these goals are worthwhile and will need to be met prior to discharge; however, because of the severity of the renal colic, #3 must be the first priority. Only then can the client respond to teaching and begin taking increased fluids. Morphine may have to be given for the pain, depending upon the severity. IV fluids may have to be started to promote elevated intake initially.

Sample Test Questions: Book Three

Carol Perez, 21 years old, is in acute renal failure following a large loss of blood from injuries she received in a car accident. Her 24-hour urine output is 275 ml. Her serum BUN is 90 mg/100 ml and her serum creatinine is 7.2 mg/100 ml.

1. During the oliguric phase of acute renal failure, which of the following would be an appropriate nursing intervention?
   1. Increase dietary sodium and potassium.
   2. Place on fluid restriction of 1,500 ml daily.
   3. Weigh client three times weekly.
   4. Provide a low protein, high carbohydrate diet.

2. Mrs. Perez fails to respond to therapy to correct her acute renal failure. She goes into chronic renal failure with the prospect of having to start dialysis or have a kidney transplant. Which of the following indicators would you expect to see in Mrs. Perez as the renal failure becomes more severe?
   1. Anemia
   2. Hypokalemia
   3. Diaphoresis
   4. Hypotension

3. In planning Mrs. Perez's diet, which of the following food sources would be the best source of high biologic-value protein?
   1. Bananas
   2. Asparagus
   3. Chipped beef
   4. Mushrooms

4. While waiting for a suitable transplant kidney to be identified, Mrs. Perez has to begin dialysis. An arteriovenous (AV) fistula is created for hemodialysis. As a nurse, you understand that one major complication you must observe for following an AV fistula is
   1. Rejection of the silastic cannula connecting the artery and vein.
   2. Accidental dislodgement of the cannula with hemorrhage.
   3. Thrombosis of the artery and vein site.
   4. Cardiac irritation caused by the cannula's insertion.

5. Nursing assessment of the access site to the AV fistula would best include
   1. Taking blood pressures in the affected arm to monitor the presence of good circulation.
   2. Auscultation of a bruit over the fistula to rule out thrombosis.
   3. Checking skin temperatures and pulses proximal to the fistula to assess circulation.
   4. Palpating the access site for a thrill to assess circulation.

6. While waiting for the AV-fistula site to mature for hemodialysis, Mrs. Perez is maintained using peritoneal dialysis. During peritoneal dialysis, the nurse notes a retention of 600 ml of dialysate fluid after draining the peritoneal cavity. The initial response of the nurse would best be to
   1. Infuse an additional 1,400 ml of fresh dialysate and continue with dialysis.
   2. Have the client turn from side to side to help localize fluid to promote drainage.
   3. Check vital signs to assess whether a fluid overload is occurring.
   4. Notify the physician of the fluid retention.

7. Today Mrs. Perez will undergo hemodialysis for the first time. Which of the following interventions, if implemented, would be most likely to help her avoid disequilibrium syndrome?
   1. Withhold her antihypertensive medications.
   2. Dialyze her for a short period of time.
   3. Dialyze her in a sitting position.
   4. Withhold protein from her diet.

8. While waiting for a compatible kidney for transplant, Mrs. Perez will be discharged home. Because of the distance of the hemodialysis center from her home, the physician decides to maintain her with continuous ambulatory peritoneal dialysis (CAPD). When educating Mrs. Perez about CAPD, the top priority is to teach her
   1. Sterile technique to help prevent peritonitis.
   2. To maintain a more liberal protein diet.
   3. To maintain a daily written record of blood pressure and weight.
   4. To continue regular medical and nursing follow-up.

9. Mrs. Perez returns to the hospital for a kidney transplant. Which of the following interventions would do the most to help prevent transplant rejection?
   1. Transfusion of four units of typed and cross-matched blood.
   2. Psychologic and emotional preparation of the client.
   3. Hemodialysis until the transplant begins to function.
   4. Administration of immunosuppressive drugs.

Chris and Jack O'Neal delayed childbearing for several years. They now find conception difficult and consult a fertility specialist for evaluation.

10. Which of the following assessments of fertility is most easily performed?
    1. Laporoscopy
    2. Semen analysis
    3. Salpingogram
    4. Culdoscopy

11. The O'Neals are successful in conceiving. During her pregnancy, Mrs. O'Neal is carefully monitored because of a history of cardiac surgery as a child. Careful assessments are essential from weeks 28-32. Which of the following conditions is Mrs. O'Neal at greatest risk of?
    1. Premature delivery
    2. Cardiac decompression
    3. Fluid retention
    4. Infection

12. At a regular clinic visit in her eighth month, you observe that Mrs. O'Neal has gained 4 lb in two weeks and seems to have an excessive amount of amniotic fluid. You understand that this condition may be asssociated with which condition?
    1. Congenital abnormalities
    2. Diabetes
    3. Placenta previa
    4. Fibrin defects

13. Mrs. O'Neal develops severe hypertension and is hospitalized. She is given IV magnesium sulfate to prevent convulsions. Nursing assessments during administration of this drug focus on which of the following expected actions?
    1. Respiratory stimulation
    2. Analgesic effects
    3. Urinary suppression
    4. Central nervous system depression

14. Prior to delivery, Mrs. O'Neal's obstetrician administers a pudendal block. Which of the following assessments would you use to evaluate the effectiveness of the infiltration?
    1. Blocked sensation in the perineal area
    2. Reduced perception of uterine contractions
    3. Decreased response to painful stimuli
    4. Depressed central nervous system

15. Mrs. O'Neal is delivered of an 8 lb son. The infant has an initial axillary temperature of 96°F. If the infant is not warmed immediately, the nurse would observe which of the following?
    1. Shivering
    2. Cyanosis
    3. Respiratory rate increase
    4. Irritability

16. Baby Boy O'Neal appears pink and active, but you observe a slight grunting on expiration. What additional observations are important at this time?
    1. Respiratory rate
    2. Nasal flaring
    3. Chest movements
    4. All of the above

17. While performing a physical assessment of Baby Boy O'Neal, you observe a swelling on the side of the infant's head. This swelling is soft, does not pulsate or bulge when the infant cries, and does not cross suture lines. What have you observed?
    1. Intracranial hemorrhage
    2. Cephalohematoma
    3. Caput succedaneum
    4. Hydrocephalus

18. You observe Mrs. O'Neal interacting with her baby on the first day of rooming-in. Which of the following behaviors could indicate potential problems with early attachment?
    1. Mrs. O'Neal complains of episiotomy pain while sitting with her infant.
    2. She appears discouraged with early breast-feeding attempts.
    3. There is little attempt to touch or speak to the alert newborn.
    4. When the infant is quiet, Mrs. O'Neal often naps.

19. On her third postpartum day, Mrs. O'Neal is found crying and expressing inadequacy in meeting her baby's needs. Of what is this behavior characteristic?
    1. Postpartum blues
    2. Normal taking-in behavior
    3. Abnormal bonding
    4. Early psychotic depression

20. Two weeks have elapsed since Mrs. O'Neal had a normal vaginal delivery with episiotomy. She is breast-feeding Baby Boy O'Neal. What is a goal of care at this time?
    1. Avoid nipple damage to prevent puerperal mastitis.
    2. Initiate supplemental bottle feedings to provide adequate nutrition.
    3. Encourage resumption of sexual relations to promote marital harmony.
    4. Reduce caloric intake to facilitate return to prepregnant weight.

Roger Caine, a 30-year-old insurance salesman, was awarded an expense-paid Caribbean cruise for his outstanding sales record. While on his trip, he became restless and overactive. He insisted on eating every meal at the captain's table. He danced until the wee hours and was up early, ready to go. He talked fast and behaved grandiosely. Upon arrival in New York, he spent money excessively. He demanded a luxurious hotel suite and loudly berated the hotel manager because no luxurious hotel suite was available. Shortly thereafter, he was admitted to a hospital with a diagnosis of manic-depression. At the hospital, history taking revealed he had been hospitalized two years earlier for depression.

21. Care of Mr. Caine will be based on the theory that the manic phase is viewed as all of the following *except* one. Which one is incorrect?
    1. A way of coping with depression
    2. Flight into activity
    3. Displacement against depressed feelings
    4. Escape from reality

22. Which of the following actions must be *avoided* to ensure effective intervention with Mr. Caine's manipulative and/or demanding behavior?
    1. Give a short, clear definition of limits that will be set.
    2. Consistently enforce the limits that were set.
    3. Allow some leeway when limits are violated.
    4. Hold frequent staff conferences to ensure cohesiveness and consistency in carrying out the plan of care.

23. All of the following should be considered in planning Mr. Caine's physical care *except* which one?
    1. He may disregard injury.
    2. He does not take time out to eat or drink.
    3. He may ignore constipation, bladder distention, etc.
    4. He will be overly concerned about cleanliness.

24. Mr. Caine is to be maintained on a regimen of lithium carbonate. What is the therapeutic blood level for lithium?
    1. 0.8–2.6 mEq/l
    2. 0.8–1.5 mEq/l
    3. 1.6–2.4 mEq/l
    4. 2.9–3.2 mEq/l

25. Mr. Caine should be observed for side effects of lithium. Which of the following is *not* an expected side effect?
    1. Nausea and sluggish feeling
    2. Muscle weakness
    3. Thirst and polyuria
    4. Diffuse rash

26. Mr. Caine has difficulty sleeping. He rarely sleeps more than three hours at a time. All of the following might alleviate his insomnia except one. Which one?
    1. Provide an evening of quiet activity.
    2. Give him a warm drink at bedtime.
    3. Administer a sedative for sleep.
    4. Encourage him to take a cool shower before retiring.

Antoinette Davis, a newborn, has meningomyelocele. She is being transferred directly from the delivery room to a special care unit.

27. What would be the safest position for Antoinette?
    1. Semi-Fowler's
    2. Supine
    3. Modified Sims's
    4. Prone

28. Mr. and Mrs. Davis have decided to have the defect surgically repaired. Prior to surgery, what is the most appropriate way to care for the meningomyelocele?
    1. Apply dry sterile dressings.
    2. Leave it open to the air.
    3. Apply sterile saline soaks.
    4. Apply gauze impregnated with Vaseline Petroleum Jelly.

29. While you are caring for Antoinette both pre- and postoperatively, which of the following nursing actions would receive the highest priority?
    1. Maintain her legs in abduction.
    2. Measure her head circumference daily.
    3. Provide tactile stimulation.
    4. Prevent skin breakdown.

30. Twenty-four hours before surgery, Antoinette develops a fever. She is fussy, irritable, and refuses her formula. Which of the following nursing measures would be most appropriate?
    1. Check the meningomyelocele sac.
    2. Contact Antoinette's physician.
    3. Institute isolation precautions.
    4. Ask Mrs. Davis to feed Antoinette.

31. Which of the following types of problems presents the most serious threat to the longterm management of children with meningomyelocele?
    1. Orthopedic
    2. Respiratory
    3. Integumentary
    4. Renal

Henry Duboff, a 50-year-old white man, awakes in the middle of the night with severe dyspnea, bilateral basilar rales, and expectoration of frothy, blood-tinged sputum. He is brought to the hospital by the paramedics in congestive heart failure complicated by pulmonary edema.

32. Dyspnea is a characteristic sign of congestive heart failure. This is primarily the result of which mechanism?
    1. Accumulation of serous fluid in alveolar spaces
    2. Obstruction of bronchi by mucoid secretions
    3. Compression of lung tissue by a dilated heart
    4. Restriction of respiratory movement by ascites

33. Edema caused by cardiac failure tends to be which of the following?
    1. Painful
    2. Dependent
    3. Periorbital
    4. Nonpitting

34. What is the optimal bed position for the client with congestive heart failure?
    1. Position of comfort, to relax the client
    2. Semirecumbent, to ease dyspnea and metabolic demands on the heart
    3. Upright, to decrease danger of pulmonary edema
    4. Flat, to decrease edema formation in the extremities

35. Respirations of the client with congestive heart failure are usually of which kind?
    1. Rapid and shallow
    2. Deep and stertorous
    3. Rapid and wheezing
    4. Cheyne-Stokes

36. How do rotating tourniquets relieve the symptoms of acute pulmonary edema?
    1. Cause vasoconstriction
    2. Cause vasodilation
    3. Decrease the amount of circulating blood
    4. Increase the amount of circulating blood

37. When tourniquets are applied to extremities to relieve the symptoms of pulmonary edema, one tourniquet should be rotated, in order, on a regular basis. How often are they rotated?
    1. q5min
    2. q10min
    3. q15min
    4. q20min

38. Best positioning of the client who has acute pulmonary edema is
    1. Semi-Fowler's with legs slightly elevated.
    2. Dorsal recumbent with head slightly lower than the body.
    3. Prone.
    4. High-Fowler's.

39. When Mr. Duboff is admitted to CCU, his ECG shows changes indicative of an anterior myocardial infarction. Which criteria should the nurse monitor to assess his cardiac status?
    1. ECG changes, serum enzymes, and leg cramps
    2. Chest pain, ECG changes, and serum enzymes
    3. Chest pain, ECG changes, and serum creatinine
    4. ECG changes, serum electrolytes, and blood urea nitrogen

40. Mr. Duboff continues to have ventricular dysrhythmias even though he is being treated with lidocaine (Xylocaine). His second hospital day, he goes into cardiac arrest. Which of these responses by the nurse would be appropriate initially?
    1. Open his airway.
    2. Start chest compressions.
    3. Check his carotid pulse.
    4. Put him on a hard surface.

41. Mr. Duboff has been resuscitated with success and is transferred to the medical floor four days postarrest. At this time, he is scheduled for a cardiac catheterization. The nurse will emphasize to Mr. Jones that during the procedure he will be as follows:
    1. Heavily sedated and will not be able to move
    2. Under a general anesthetic and unconscious
    3. Awake, not sedated, and asked to remain still
    4. Awake, mildly sedated, and asked to change his position

42. The information gathered from the left cardiac catheterization will include all *but* one of the following:
    1. The patency of the coronary arteries
    2. The status of collateral circulation
    3. Pulmonary artery patency
    4. The condition of the myocardium

43. Postcardiac catheterization, in what position will Mr. Duboff be?
    1. Supine with affected leg extended
    2. Supine with affected leg flexed
    3. Side lying with both legs flexed
    4. Able to assume any position he desires

Jo Ellen Baxter, a 50-year-old with a diagnosis of chronic, undifferentiated schizophrenia, is hospitalized on a surgical unit for an appendectomy.

44. The day after surgery, Mrs. Baxter tells the nurse that she feels creatures eating away at her abdomen. What is the first thing the nurse needs to do?
    1. Request an increase in her phenothiozines to control the psychosis.
    2. Talk with her more often to help control her stress level.
    3. Assess for possible abdominal pains.
    4. Request an order for benztropine (Cogentin) to control her extrapyramidal symptoms.

45. The care needs of a chronic schizophrenic client such as Mrs. Baxter are best reflected in which of the following statements?
    1. Have a different staff member care for her each day to avoid intimacy.
    2. Have one staff member care for her as much as possible to increase trust.
    3. Have one staff member care for her and remain with her the entire shift to increase intimacy and closeness.
    4. There is no need to be concerned about the assignment, since Mrs. Baxter will not know the difference.

46. Oral antibiotics are started. Mrs. Baxter has been taking her phenothiozines at home reliably for years. Which of the following is the most appropriate nursing intervention?
    1. Set up a plan to describe to Mrs. Baxter the cause of her problem, the effects on her body, and physiologic changes caused by her disease.
    2. Tell her how often to take the medication and have her do it a few times while in the hospital.
    3. Insist she not be discharged until the course of the medication has been given.
    4. Request a home health nurse come into her home and give her the medication.

47. While you are talking with Mrs. Baxter one day, she tells you that the "creatures from Odum have just left my room." The creatures from Odum are probably which of the following?
    1. The result of an extrapyramidal reaction
    2. A response to a phobic fear of being alone
    3. A symbol from her autistic world
    4. An example of flight-of-ideas

48. Which of the following is the most appropriate nursing response to Mrs. Baxter's statement about the creatures from Odum?
    1. Acknowledge that the creatures have special meaning for Mrs. Baxter.
    2. Suggest a variety of interpretations of the creatures for Mrs. Baxter.
    3. Tell Mrs. Baxter to call you the next time she sees them.
    4. Tell her you don't like to talk about creatures.

Judy Jankowski brings her 9-week-old son, John, to the well-baby clinic for a visit. John weighed 6 lb 5 oz and was 19 inches long at birth.

49. When assessing John, you should be concerned about which one of the following findings?
    1. John weighs 10 lb 14 oz today.
    2. John's apical pulse rate is 124/minute.
    3. John still wakes up for a feeding at 4-5 A.M.
    4. John's posterior fontanel is closed.

50. John's mother tells you he is taking 6 oz of iron-fortified commercial formula six times a day, plus an ounce of rice cereal in the morning and at bedtime. Based on these data you concluded that
    1. John is receiving too many calories.
    2. John's diet is too high in iron.
    3. John's diet is deficient in vitamins.
    4. John's intake is appropriate for his age and weight.

51. Mrs. Jankowski asks you when she can start feeding John pureed fruits and vegetables. Which of the following is the most appropriate response?
    1. "Are you getting a lot of pressure from your family and friends to give John a greater variety of foods to eat?"
    2. "Let's take a look at John's daily intake and how he compares with current guidelines for a baby's nutrition."
    3. "Would you feel better if John was eating more 'real' food?"
    4. "We don't usually recommend adding fruits and vegetables until infants are five or six months old."

52. When discussing developmental stimulation with Mrs. Jankowski, you would best recommend which of the following toys for John?
    1. A stuffed rabbit or teddy bear
    2. A windup musical toy
    3. An activity box for the crib
    4. A teething toy

53. Mrs. Jankowski expresses concern about John's erratic sleeping patterns. She tells you that John still wakes up at least once each night. When you inquire about John's sleep environment, she tells you that John sometimes sleeps in bed with her and her husband, but most of the time he sleeps in a playpen in their bedroom. Which of the following would best guide your response to Mrs. Jankowski?
    1. Infants should get a minimum of 16 hours of sleep each day.
    2. Most infants sleep consistently through the night by the time they are six months old.
    3. Infants tend to sleep longer at night if they are given a tablespoon of cereal with their bedtime feeding.
    4. It is dangerous for infants to sleep in their parents' bed.

54. John is scheduled to receive his first immunizations today. When administering his DPT injection, you should use which site?
    1. Deltoid muscle
    2. Subcutaneous tissue of the thigh
    3. Gluteus medius muscle
    4. Vastus lateralis muscle

55. John is scheduled to return to the clinic at four months of age. At this time, which of the following areas of accident prevention is *least* important to address when counseling John's mother?
    1. Suffocation and aspiration
    2. Injuries from hot water burns
    3. Poisonous ingestions
    4. Falls

56. Anticipatory guidance concerning developmental stimulation should be based on your knowledge that John can be expected to learn which of the following before his next clinic visit?
    1. Reach for objects within visual range
    2. Sit without support
    3. Imitate speech sounds
    4. Transfer a toy from one hand to the other

57. Which of the following goals is most important when planning John's care?
    1. John will receive optimal nutrition.
    2. John will receive appropriate developmental stimulation.
    3. John will be free from accidental injury.
    4. John will be immunized against communicable diseases.

Leslie Ames is a new postpartum client. This is her second pregnancy, and she has expressed concern about breast infections. With her first pregnancy, Leslie had two episodes of mastitis that were treated with antibiotics.

58. Which of the following statements regarding breast inflammations is *incorrect*?
    1. Acute mastitis involves the overgrowth of fibrous tissue around ducts.
    2. Acute mastitis usually occurs at the beginning or end of lactation.
    3. Chronic cystic mastitis manifests itself in small, "buckshot" nodules that are palpable.
    4. Clinical manifestations of a mammary abscess include purulent discharge from the nipple, dusky red coloring of the breast, and marked sensitivity.

59. Postpartum teaching for Mrs. Ames about prevention of mastitis should include all *but* which of the following?
    1. Alternate nursing positions of infant on the breast.
    2. Clean breasts before and after nursing with clear warm water.
    3. Discontinue nursing if engorgement occurs.
    4. Apply warm, wet compresses just before feeding.

60. Each of the following observations was noted on Mrs. Ames's chart. Which one has implications for potential infection?
    1. Temperature on the first postpartum day is 100.2°F.
    2. Right nipple appears slightly cracked. No swelling noted.
    3. Urinated 2,500 ml on first postpartum day.
    4. Episiotomy slightly swollen; sutures clean; no discharge.

John Coates was admitted to a psychiatric unit two days ago. He goes to occupational therapy and becomes angry during the group activity.

61. Mr. Coates tells you that the occupational therapists don't like him. This tells you that he is probably experiencing one of the following. Which one?
    1. Trying to avoid OT because he is shy
    2. Feeling threatened by the group activity
    3. Feeling angry with someone in the group
    4. Being mistreated by the occupational therapists

62. What is a more appropriate new plan for Mr. Coates?
    1. Have him go to OT anyway so he can learn to adjust.
    2. Tell him he cannot go to OT until he learns to act properly.
    3. Put him in group therapy instead.
    4. Have him go to OT alone for awhile.

Eight-year-old Chad Fredricks is brought to the emergency room by his mother. He has multiple bruises over his entire body and a fractured right arm. His mother states he was playing with his wagon and fell on his right arm. The mother describes him as a "troublemaker" and a bad kid. He is not crying and refuses to speak to the nurse or his mother. The nurse thinks that Chad may be a victim of child abuse.

63. All *but* one of the following reasons make the nurses suspicious. Which is the one exception?
    1. The multiple bruises do not fit the description of the accident.
    2. The mother identifies him as a bad child.
    3. Chad does not turn to his mother for solace.
    4. Chad, by playing with a wagon, shows regression or retarded development for an eight-year-old.

64. Mrs. Fredricks is advised that Chad will need to have his arm set and placed in a cast; then he will be hospitalized for further assessment and treatment. She is questioned about her methods of disciplining Chad. She responds angrily by saying, "Of course, I spank him. He's such a troublemaker; he does things purposely to upset me. He's so ungrateful. Sometimes I feel overwhelmed by it all, but I do not abuse him. I'm not overly violent. I hit him only when he asks for it." The nurse knows that Mrs. Fredricks is probably which of the following?
    1. Lying to the hospital personnel to protect herself; she knows she's abusive.
    2. Is probably telling the truth and it is someone else who hits the child
    3. Isn't aware of the fact that her behavior is abusive
    4. Disciplining the child appropriately, since he seems to have a behavior problem

65. The nurse realizes that the hospital has certain legal responsibilities in Chad's case. All of the following should be done *except* which one?
    1. Document all bruises and cuts; include their placement and size.
    2. Chart interaction patterns between Chad and his mother.
    3. Document staff perceptions of the relationship between Chad and his mother.
    4. Report to the state child-welfare agency.

66. The unit to which Chad is admitted has primary care; the head nurse needs to assign a primary nurse who has which of the following skills?
    1. Can identify with Chad's problem
    2. Is able to set limits on the mother's behavior with Chad
    3. Recognizes the needs of both the mother and Chad
    4. Can discuss adoption procedures with the mother

67. The nurse needs to understand that parents who abuse their children
    1. Frequently do not know or are unable to ask for help until after they have felt overwhelmed by problems.
    2. Plan ahead as to when and how to abuse their children.
    3. Rarely were abused themselves; so they do not recognize the problem until it's too late.
    4. Usually are not concerned about their abusive actions.

68. After providing for physical care of the hospitalized child, the nurse needs to give priority to play activities that encourage the child to
    1. Describe details of the traumatic events.
    2. Maintain control over his feelings, e.g., games that are quiet or include many rules.
    3. Be distracted from unpleasant experiences.
    4. Share feelings of joy, anger, fear, or loneliness.

69. The nurse assigned to Chad recognizes her own negative feelings towards Mrs. Fredricks. The nurse's best action would be to
    1. Continue to care for Chad and relate to the mother during visiting hours and not share feelings with other staff, since they might be influenced by negativism.
    2. Be open with the mother about feelings, e.g., saying, "I can help you more if I am honest with you."
    3. Ask other nurses to discuss the case over lunch to reduce guilt feelings about disliking the mother.
    4. Discuss feelings with the head nurse, along with details of the care plan, asking for evaluation of the nursing care for the client and her mother, and discussing implications of reassignment to another case.

70. Interventions to assist Mrs. Fredricks best include which of the following?
    1. Techniques to handle angry behavior before it goes out of control
    2. Encouragement that the problems of parents lessen as a child grows older
    3. Opportunities to discuss how child abuse started in the family
    4. Discussions on how parents can make children follow rules

71. The nurse will know Mrs. Fredricks is responding to treatment when Mrs. Fredricks takes which of the following steps?
    1. Decides to place Chad for adoption
    2. Begins to talk more realistically about Chad's mistakes
    3. Talks about her own frustrations and anxieties
    4. Realizes that her needs are secondary to Chad's

72. Another good indicator of progress for both the child and the mother is which of the following?
    1. Both sleep and eat well and carry out daily activities with no thoughts about past abusive behavior.
    2. They rarely encounter frustrating conflicts.
    3. When frustrated by Chad, Mrs. Fredricks uses one or two of the alternatives to physical punishment she has learned.
    4. The mother has planned many separate activities for herself and Chad so they have much less time together.

Lan Yang, aged 60, undergoes a total laryngectomy for cancer of the larynx. He returns from surgery with a laryngectomy tube and an NG tube.

73. In the immediate postoperative period, Mr. Yang requires both nasopharyngeal suctioning and suctioning through the laryngectomy tube. When doing these two procedures at the same time, the nurse should do all of the following *except* which one?
    1. Use a sterile suction setup.
    2. Suction the nose first, then the laryngectomy tube.
    3. Suction the laryngectomy tube first, then the nose.
    4. Lubricate the catheter with saline.

74. The nasogastric tube is used to provide Mr. Yang with fluids and nutrients for approximately 10 days, for which of the following reasons?
    1. To prevent pain while swallowing
    2. To prevent contamination of the suture line
    3. To decrease need for swallowing
    4. To prevent need for holding head up to eat

75. When should Mr. Yang best start speech rehabilitation?
    1. When he leaves the hospital
    2. When esophageal suture line is healed
    3. Three months after surgery
    4. When he regains all his strength

An 18-year-old neighbor, Lucia Ortega, is in the second month of pregnancy and feels very well. She talks to you about her job in a small animal hospital, where she is an experienced helper to the veterinarian. She plans to continue working during the pregnancy.

76. Which of the following tasks would you suggest Mrs. Ortega assign to a high school student who helps part-time?
    1. Operating a computer to prepare weekly statements
    2. Preparing the surgical suite for minor procedures
    3. Handling rabies and distemper vaccines and syringes
    4. Administering antibiotic ear drops to small animals

77. Mrs. Ortega takes home a small abandoned kitten who appears to be in good condition. What teaching is most appropriate at this time?
    1. "Realize that the kitten may be jealous of your infant."
    2. "Ask your husband if he will care for the litter box."
    3. "Check to see if you and your husband have any allergies."
    4. "Be sure to keep the animal indoors at all times."

78. Several weeks later, Mrs. Ortega develops vague flulike symptoms. Which of the following statements by the client indicates she has learned what was taught at the early antepartal visits?
    1. "I know I shouldn't take any over-the-counter remedies now."
    2. "I feel so tired all the time; so I must need the rest."
    3. "I urinate frequently; so I probably am drinking too many fluids."
    4. "Between the morning sickness and the flu, I'll be happy to lose weight."

79. It is established that her symptoms are caused by toxoplasmosis. As the pregnancy advances, the physician is concerned that fetal growth is not appropriate for gestation. Which of the following tests would best provide information about the development of the fetus?
    1. Urine estriol
    2. Amniocentesis
    3. Ultrasound
    4. Nonstress test

80. Suspicions are confirmed, and the couple is told that it appears the fetus suffers from intrauterine growth retardation. The physician spends much time with them, drawing sketches of the placenta and the fetus. As you talk with them afterward, Mrs. Ortega begins to cry. "I don't think I can cope with a retarded baby." Which response is most appropriate?
    1. "Perhaps you were not listening to the doctor's explanation."
    2. "Are there other retarded children in either family?"
    3. "There are many resources available to help you."
    4. "Let's talk about what the doctor said to us all."

81. A 5 lb infant is delivered vaginally at 39 weeks. Apgars are 9 and 10 at one and five minutes. The newborn appears active, wide-eyed, and alert. There was slight meconium staining of the placenta and cord. What would you most suspect about this child's condition?
    1. The baby may have suffered chronic hypoxia.
    2. It appears that the baby's condition is normal.
    3. Assessments indicate good adaptation.
    4. This child may have been somewhat premature.

82. Although the Ortega infant appears to behave normally, you observe that the child occasionally cries, then appears to quiet himself and fall asleep. What is your best understanding of this behavior?
    1. Perhaps the baby's needs have not been met.
    2. This is normal, expected behavior.
    3. The central nervous system may be immature.
    4. The neonate is not able to deal with frustration.

83. Which of the following is most important in the discharge teaching plan for the Ortega infant?
    1. Be sure to keep the visits to the pediatric clinic.
    2. Feed the baby every two to three hours, so he will gain weight.
    3. Report any diarrhea or vomiting to the physician.
    4. Take the baby's temperature daily and keep a record.

The admission of Sam Levitt to a young-adult psychiatric unit was precipitated by his attempts to beat up his father. A history of episodic agitation and aggressive behavior for many months preceded this event.

84. The admitting nurse would best give priority attention to which one of the following areas?
    1. The client's thoughts about being harmed by others
    2. His thoughts of harming other persons at a future time
    3. Thought patterns that are disconnected and unrelated
    4. Thoughts that describe false, fixed beliefs

85. The affective pattern that Mr. Levitt is most likely to display in the next few days is
    1. Elation, silliness, and humor.
    2. Passiveness, flatness, and detachment.
    3. Tension, anger, and irritability.
    4. Remorsefulness, sadness, and gloom.

86. When the unit becomes especially active and noisy with visitors and newly admitted persons, Mr. Levitt is most likely to
    1. Insist in a loud voice that a staff member escort him to the canteen immediately.
    2. Retreat to his room for an extra nap.
    3. Initiate a pool game with another client and play to win.
    4. Engage a staff person in a heated discussion about patient-government activities.

87. A priority nursing goal for Mr. Levitt on admission is to assist him to
    1. Discuss childhood situations in which he lashed out at persons in order to increase his self-understanding.
    2. Participate in a variety of physical activities in order to dissipate his destructive feelings.
    3. Talk at length about his deep-seated anger in order to reduce the chance he will strike out again.
    4. Make plans to reapply for admission to the community college he had attended.

88. Mr. Levitt was found pacing, striking his fists in the air, and cursing another client named Mrs. Sanders. The nurse would best say
    1. "Mr. Levitt, stop cursing at Mrs. Sanders. I will stay and help you control yourself."
    2. "You must feel very angry. Maybe you should calm down."
    3. "Mr. Levitt, Mrs. Sanders did nothing to upset you; so please stop threatening her."
    4. "Mr. Levitt, calm down. You can get rid of all this energy in the gym this afternoon. Come and eat breakfast now."

89. When Mr. Levitt's father escorts his son to the unit following the son's first weekend pass from the inpatient setting, the nurse speaks to them together. The nurse's most important focus is
    1. How both the father and son felt about the weekend.
    2. What activities they did that were satisfying to both.
    3. How frequently, if at all, Mr. Levitt lost control.
    4. What events occurred that indicated progress in Mr. Levitt's ability to refrain from threatening behavior.

90. A long-term indicator of Mr. Levitt's progress will be his
    1. Ability to move from verbal to physical activities when he senses increased anger.
    2. Deliberate actions to engage in several community activities separate from his family.
    3. Assuming responsibility to be punctual for all therapy sessions.
    4. Willingness to admit that he has a bad temper and that he must do something about it.

When Edward Barden, a 37-year-old construction worker, is admitted to the nursing unit, he tells you that he has pain radiating down his right leg.

91. You would include all the following in your assessment *except* which one?
    1. Activities that occur prior to the pain
    2. What relieves the pain
    3. How he carries out activities of daily living
    4. How he got to the hospital

92. Mr. Barden is scheduled for a myelogram. Which of the following nursing care considerations is best included in the postprocedure care?
    1. Keep the client in bed for 6–8 hours.
    2. Allow the client to go to the bathroom as soon as he gets back to his room in order to excrete the dye.
    3. Limit fluids.
    4. Provide heavy sedation for his spinal headache.

93. The myelogram indicates that Mr. Barden has a ruptured intervertebral disc at L4–5. Preoperative teaching includes all the following *except* which?
    1. Postoperative "log-rolling"
    2. Getting out of bed the first post-op day
    3. Activities to be avoided after discharge
    4. Need to wear shoes when first ambulating

94. In the immediate postoperative period, Mr. Barden complains of a severe headache. Effective nursing intervention best includes telling him
    1. This is to be expected.
    2. To sit up 45° in bed.
    3. He needs to "log-roll" every 1-2 hours in bed.
    4. He needs to force fluids.

Correct Answers and Rationales: Book Three

1. **#4.** Nitrogenous waste products from protein metabolism result in an elevation of BUN; therefore, a low protein diet is needed. The protein given should be of high biologic value (i.e., contain all essential amino acids). A high carbohydrate diet will help reverse gluconeogenesis. The client should be weighed daily. Intake is calculated on urine output plus 500–1,000 ml of insensible water loss every 24 hours. Her potassium is already elevated; therefore, the diet should be restrictive of potassium and may even require the administration of ion-exchange resins such as Kayexalate.

2. **#1.** One contributing cause to the anemia seen in chronic renal disease is that renal erythropoietin production is decreased and the bone marrow is depressed by the increasing uremia. Because of the decreased ability of the kidneys to excrete waste products and maintain normal fluid and electrolyte balance, the body will develop hyperkalemia and hypertension. The stimulation of the renin-angiotension mechanism also contributes to the hypertension. The skin becomes very dry because of atrophy of the sweat glands.

3. **#3.** Milk, meats, fish, and eggs are considered the best sources of high biologic-value protein. Some vegetables have all of the essential amino acids but are not consistently the best sources. In contrast, fruits are poor sources for high biologic-value protein.

4. **#3.** An AV fistula is an *internal* access created by a side-to-side or end-to-end anastomosis of an adjacent vein and artery. This results in an enlarged vein, which is caused by the high pressure in the artery. The resulting vessel provides an easy access for venipuncture. Thrombosis at this site can be a major complication. Rejection does not occur, because no foreign material is involved. Dislodgment is not a problem, because the fistula is internal. (An AV *shunt* is external.) Cardiac irritation is a problem with subclavian catheters used for temporary access for hemodialysis.

5. **#4.** The presence of a bruit and a thrill indicates good circulation. Skin temperatures and pulses should be assessed *distal* to the fistula. Blood pressure and venipunctures should never be done in the affected limb in order to help promote the longevity of the fistula.

6. **#2.** Any fluid retention greater than 300 ml needs to be assessed prior to continuing with dialysis. Turning the client from side to side may help drain the remaining dialysate thereby eliminating the need for contacting the physician. Vital signs must be monitored at frequent intervals throughout the dialysis.

7. **#2.** Disequilibrium syndrome is believed by some to be caused by too rapid or excess fluid removal from the circulatory system. Dialysis for a short time (two to four hours) and at a reduced rate of blood flow is effective in decreasing its occurrence and severity.

8. **#1.** The most common recurring problem with peritoneal dialysis is peritonitis; therefore, education on proper techniques to help decrease its occurrence should take priority. All the other listed interventions are also important and should be included in the teaching.

9. **#4.** The main defense against transplant rejection is immunosuppresive drugs (e.g., azathioprine [Imuran], prednisone). This therapy is begun prior to surgery and continues following surgery. It is important for the client not to discontinue this drug therapy unless instructed to do so by a physician, and then the reduction is done slowly over an extended period of time.

10. **#2.** All are invasive tests except for the examination of semen for sperm motility.

11. **#2.** This is a period of maximum cardiac output, and as a result, cardiac decompensation may occur.

12. **#1.** Many anomalies are associated with excessive amniotic fluid.

13. **#4.** Magnesium sulfate may depress central nervous function, including respiratory rate.

14. **#1.** This is the desired response. There is no CNS effect or change in pain of contractions.

15. **#3.** Cold stress increases metabolic efforts; respiratory distress can result.

16. **#1.** All are important assessments of respiratory function.

17. **#2.** Cephalohematoma is an effusion of blood between the bone and the periosteum.

18. **#3.** Talking to the infant in the first 24 hours is part of early bonding.

19. **#1.** Fatigue and hormone changes cause this behavior.

20. **#1.** Mastitis can occur two to three weeks after delivery as organisms enter through the nipple.

21. **#3.** Behavior in the manic phase of manic-depressive psychosis has been termed mirror-image depression. Close observation of the client during a manic phase will periodically reveal fleeting comments, facial expressions, or mannerisms that are depressive. The client's behavior indicates an attempt to cope with his feelings of depression.

22. **#3.** Manipulative and/or demanding behavior of the manic client is most effectively controlled by limit setting that is clearly spelled out to him, is fair, and is consistently enforced. Since his behavior often provokes staff anger, staff-client arguments and rejection of the client are common. This reaffirms the client's feelings of rejection. Only frequent staff conferences and staff planning can provide a therapeutic plan of care and the support for staff, which is essential if they are to give the needed care.

23. **#4.** The manic client's hyperactivity permits him no time or thought for his physical needs. Nursing responsibilities include careful observation of his physical state and the nursing measures necessary to ensure his physical well-being.

24. **#2.** Lithium toxicity is closely related to serum-lithium levels and can occur at doses close to therapeutic levels. Adverse reactions are seldom encountered at levels below maximum therapeutic levels, except in clients sensitive to lithium.

25. **#4.** #1 through #3 are clinical signs of toxicity that must be detected and reported to the physician immediately.

26. **#4.** Activities that decrease stimuli may help counteract insomnia. Rest and sleep are vital for the manic client, because hyperactivity may lead to dangerous exhaustion.

27. **#4.** Antoinette must be kept in the prone position to reduce tension on and prevent trauma to the sac. The supine and semi-Fowler's position would place tension on the sac. The Sims's position is difficult to maintain in a newborn.

28. **#3.** Before surgical closure of the sac, it is important to prevent drying of the sac. Sterile saline soaks help to prevent drying. Dry sterile dressings or leaving the sac open to the air is advocated only if surgery is to be delayed.

29. **#2.** While all these nursing actions would be appropriate, measuring head circumference daily is essential. Hydrocephalus is a possible complication of meningomyelocele, and a major sign of hydrocephalus in infants is head enlargement. Any change in the size of the infant's head can be assessed with daily measurements.

30. **#1.** An elevated temperature accompanied by behavioral changes may be an early sign of infection. Any leak, abrasion, or tear of the meningomyelocele sac would further support the possibility of infection (e.g., meningitis). Assess the sac before notifying the physician. Isolation precautions should be instituted to protect the other babies and would be appropriate once the sac has been assessed. While Mrs. Davis might help calm Antoinette, it is not appropriate until the nursing assessment is complete.

31. **#4.** Renal problems present a major threat to the life of the child with spina bifida as well as to her self-image and willingness to become involved with activities and individuals outside the home. The other areas may become problematic but are generally not life threatening.

32. **#1.** Congestive heart failure causes pulmonary circulatory congestion and the characteristic symptom is dyspnea.

33. **#2.** Because of gravity, dependent edema occurs in cardiac failure.

34. **#2.** The client with congestive heart failure can breathe with more ease in a Fowler's or semi-Fowler's position since gravity promotes drainage of secretions from the pulmonary bed. Also maximal lung expansion is permitted, because there is less pressure from the abdominal organs.

35. **#1.** Respirations in congestive heart failure are rapid and shallow, because of the pulmonary circulatory congestion.

36. **#3.** Rotating tourniquets are used in pulmonary edema to decrease venous return to the right side of the heart.

37. **#3.** This ensures that the venous return of a single extremity is compressed for no more than 45 minutes.

38. **#4.** This position aids in drainage of secretions from the lungs. Also it is more comfortable than a lying-down position. It helps to decrease the pooling of blood in the lungs.

39. **#2.** Chest pain, ECG changes, and serum enzymes best assess a post-myocardial infarction client. All will show definite changes as the infarction process evolves.

40. **#1.** The first step in a cardiac arrest is to ensure the client has an open airway.

41. **#4.** During a cardiac catheterization, the client must be alert in order to follow the requests of the health team. The client will be asked to make verbal responses, change his position, and cough and deep breathe.

42. **#3.** The left-sided cardiac catheterization will not demonstrate any pathologic condition in the pulmonary artery or the right side of the heart.

43. **#1.** During the left-sided cardiac catheterization, the catheter is introduced into the femoral artery of the leg and retrograde into the left side of the heart. Postcatheterization, the client is cautioned to keep the affected leg extended to avoid any increase in pressure to the puncture site.

44. **#3.** Chronic schizophrenics will sometimes incorporate pain into their delusional system.

45. **#2.** Sameness will increase trust in Mrs. Baxter, but intimacy will frighten her and cause her to withdraw more into herself.

46. **#2.** Lengthy explanations will be too confusing. Rather tell her how to take the drugs and show her, and she will probably be as reliable with them as she has been with her phenothiazines.

47. **#3.** The creatures are part of her hallucinatory world into which she withdraws at times.

48. **#1.** This statement acknowledges the importance of the hallucination for Mrs. Baxter without undermining her need for the symptom; it also does not indicate that the nurse regards the hallucination content as real.

49. **#1.** John should not double his birth weight until he is at least five months old. At the current rate, he will do so at a much younger age. He is gaining weight too rapidly. The other findings are all within normal limits.

50. **#1.** John should be receiving 53 calories/lb/day, or about 560 calories daily (at his current weight). He is currently taking 780 calories in formula alone, plus the cereal.

51. **#2.** This response lessens the parent's defensiveness and increases the likelihood of parent compliance with recommendations. It involves the parent in the decision-making process.

52. **#2.** Hearing is well-developed by this age. John cannot yet reach for the stuffed animal and doesn't have the motor skills to manipulate the activity box. Teething does not begin in the average infant until at least four months of age.

53. **#2.** The majority of infants sleep through the night by six months of age. There is no set recommended minimum amount of sleep an infant should get; the infant's growth and activity patterns are better indicators of adequate sleep than number of hours slept. Research does not support the idea that solids lengthen nighttime sleep. Sleep arrangements vary with cultural patterns; many infants sleep in their parents' bed.

54. **#4.** The vastus lateralis is the safest site for administering injections to infants, because it is free of major nerves and blood vessels.

55. **#3.** Because John is not yet old enough to be mobile in his environment, he is at minimal risk for poisonous ingestions.

56. **#1.** The average infant learns to reach for objects by four months of age. The other milestones are characteristic of infants over six months of age.

57. **#3.** Accident prevention is the priority goal because it is concerned with safety.

58. **#1.** Acute mastitis involves a localized infection of a breast gland and/or duct, usually requiring treatment with antibiotics.

59. **#3.** Continued nursing is essential to promote drainage and decrease milk tension.

60. **#2.** A cracked nipple provides an entryway for bacteria. Continued breast-feeding will increase the risk of infection.

61. **#2.** He is using projection and indicating that he is uncomfortable in a group setting.

62. **#4.** He will have the benefit of OT without feeling threatened by the group.

63. **#4.** While a symptom of child abuse is that the child exhibits behavior not appropriate to age, playing with a wagon is appropriate for an eight-year-old.

64. **#3.** Some abusive parents do not see their behavior as inappropriate. They may have been abused as children and so raise their children as they were raised.

65. **#3.** The nurse documents behaviors and factual information, which may become evidence. Ideas about what might have happened are not the hospital staff's responsibility to report.

66. **#3.** The mother has strong unmet needs and, as a result, has difficulty controlling her anger. Similiarly, Chad too has unmet needs. The nurse needs to address the problems of both mother and child in order to be most effective.

67. **#1.** Complex, lifelong dynamics of being abused or unable to handle frustration leave the parent overwhelmed by problems. The parent loses control and the ability to change the behavior.

68. **#4.** Recovery for the abused child can be facilitated by the freedom to express emotion in a caring, safe environment. Although sharing details and gaining emotional control are important to the healing process, the expression of emotion is a priority if therapeutic interventions are to be successful.

69. **#4.** Negative feelings toward abusing parents are not uncommon, and the nurse can handle them professionally by discussing them with the head nurse.

70. **#1.** Effective control of anger is important in order to reduce abuse. Problems of child raising tend to increase with the child's age. The complexity of child abuse does not allow for finding a starting point. Focusing on making children follow rules usually reflects negative feelings rather than fostering a positive environment.

71. **#3.** In discussing her own feelings, Mrs. Fredericks can learn how to control stress more effectively.

72. **#3.** Frustrations are a real part of parenting. Handling, not avoiding them, is most important.

73. **#2.** The laryngectomy tube enters directly into the trachea and is considered sterile; it should be suctioned first. The nose can then be suctioned using the same suction catheter.

74. **#2.** The NG tube prevents food and fluid from contaminating the pharyngeal and esophageal suture line.

75. **#2.** Speech rehabilitation can be started as soon as the esophageal suture line has healed.

76. **#3.** This is a task that poses potential danger to a pregnant woman in the first trimester. There would appear to be no risks with the other tasks.

77. **#2.** There is danger in handling cat litter; so this is an essential aspect of teaching.

78. **#1.** This response indicates she has learned *essential* content of antepartal teaching. #2 has some validity and #3, urinating often, is not a sign of good health during pregnancy. Both #3 and #4 would indicate poor health habits during pregnancy.

79. **#3.** An ultrasound examination would provide information on the fetal development. Estriol and nonstress tests indicate placental-fetal well-being, while the amniocentesis may provide a variety of information from genetic information to extent of lung development.

80. **#4.** This best meets the couple's needs. Apparently they have misunderstood the physician's explanation.

81. **#1.** The signs indicate hypoxia. While the Apgar score is normal, the deprivation of nutrients and oxygen in utero causes an infant's intrauterine growth to be retarded.

82. **#2.**

83. **#1.** Since the baby was exposed to infection and deprived of nutrients and oxygen during pregnancy, it is essential to monitor health and growth throughout infancy and childhood. Diarrhea and vomiting should always be reported, but are not unique to this situation. Feeding the infant more frequently may or may not be indicated. Temperature monitoring is not necessary if the infant appears well.

84. **#2.** The nurse would give priority to collecting data relevant to the known past history. The safety of others takes precedence over thought disorders.

85. **#3.** A common dynamic of threat to others is the affective theme of anger.

86. **#1.** The high-activity milieu may precipitate a sense of losing control in angry clients. Likewise, they rarely can give to others, or sustain interaction. Seeking self-centered attention from staff might be viewed as a plea for help. It is the most likely action of this client under the circumstances.

87. **#2.** Only after anger is constructively released can the client focus on specific feelings and self-understanding. Future plans, although important, cannot be realistically developed until anger is reduced.

88. **#1.** To disrupt angry outbursts, get the client's attention by using his name. Give firm, simple directions. Stay with client in order to help him gain internal control. Weakly stated interventions do not provide structure.

89. **#4.** Although feelings are important, it is still more important to learn about situations that the potentially violent person has handled well. This information can disclose strengths and give the nurse a chance to give positive reinforcement and assess the effects of hospitalization.

90. **#2.** The ability to extend relationships beyond the family indicates developing security and independence. It also dilutes the intense family situations that often precipitate violence.

91. **#4.** The mode of transportation to the hospital is not significant as part of your initial assessment.

92. **#1.** Bed rest is necessary for six to eight hours to prevent a spinal headache. Although the client may need to void, he cannot get out of bed. Fluids are to be encouraged. Only mild sedation is required for a spinal headache.

93. **#3.** This would be included in discharge instructions. All the other answers need to be included in the preoperative teaching.

94. **#4.** All the other interventions would increase the severity of the headache.

Sample Test Questions: Book Four

A new client, John Small, has been admitted to a 20-bed unit of a university hospital. He was brought in by the police after getting in a fight and tearing up a bar. He is 6 ft 3 in tall and weighs 275 lb. At the present time, he is pacing in the unit recreation room, mumbling. His jaws are tight and his hands are clenched. Other clients are afraid of him and are trying to avoid him by going to their rooms.

1. Which of the following would the nurse best use initially in an attempt to prevent a crisis on the unit?
   1. Keep the other clients away and observe Mr. Small's behavior until he calms down.
   2. Place Mr. Small in seclusion immediately and then help him to verbally express his anger.
   3. Approach Mr. Small on a one-to-one basis and offer him a prn medication immediately.
   4. Approach Mr. Small on a one-to-one basis, help him identify his anger, and offer him alternatives.
2. The milieu (environment) is a very important tool in working with an angry client. The environment may be therapeutic or nontherapeutic. Which of the following descriptions suggests an environment that would be most helpful in preventing a crisis for Mr. Small?
   1. Body bags, large outside grounds, art activities, and a variety of places for Mr. Small to be alone
   2. Many programmed activities that encourage him to become involved in his own goals and treatment
   3. Setting firm, clear rules and limits
   4. A milieu in which the clients determine the privileges for each other
3. Mr. Small continues to exhibit increasing signs of anxiety. He is shouting at and threatening the other clients. The nurse would need to do all *but* one of the following. Which one?
   1. Offer Mr. Small a chance to dice the carrots for the salad being served at dinner.
   2. Call a crisis team that could, if necessary, quickly subdue Mr. Small.
   3. Prepare Mr. Small a prn medication and a seclusion room with restraints.
   4. Keep the other clients away from Mr. Small.
4. Mr. Small continues to become more agitated, and he attempts to hit another client. The nurse decides that he needs to be placed in seclusion with full, leather restraints. Which one of the following interventions would *not* be utilized when restraining a client?
   1. Have an established team that can move as quickly as possible.
   2. Remove the glasses and jewelry of staff and the client to prevent Mr. Small from destroying anything.
   3. Identify for Mr. Small the positive behaviors the staff expects from him.
   4. Utilize more staff and security guards whenever possible as members of the team.

5. Mr. Small has been out of seclusion for several hours. He is expressing that his rights have been violated and he demands to leave the hospital. The law includes several important provisions that apply to seclusion, restraints, and medication. Which one of the following statements would *not* apply in this situation?
   1. Mr. Small can refuse to be placed in seclusion and restraints.
   2. He can refuse to take his medication.
   3. He can be retained in the hospital against his will if he is admitted by the state under an emergency or involuntary admission.
   4. Mr. Small is entitled to legal counsel to discuss his future plans and concerns.

6. Mr. Small expresses concern about others knowing all about his "private life and behavior." Provisions have been made in the law to speak to his concerns. Which one of the following would *not* pertain to his concern?
   1. Clients should have access to phones where others cannot hear conversations.
   2. Information in clinical records should not be a part of the public record.
   3. Information cannot be released without the client's consent.
   4. Staff must include specific information in a separate document that is not part of the hospital record.

7. An interdisciplinary conference is held. Various points of view are expressed in attempting to arrive at a plan of care for Mr. Small. The various members of the team represent a number of beliefs about the frame of reference or models that could be used to assist him. The nurse is able to identify each model by its major characteristics. Which of the following would *not* be a point of view supportive of the medical-biologic model?
   1. Mr. Small is suffering from an illness or defect.
   2. The source of his illness can be located in his body.
   3. His illness has a course that has a positive prognosis.
   4. Mr. Small's illness can be treated properly only by physicians.

8. One team member believes the psychoanalytic model would be most helpful. Which of the following ideas is most supportive of this model?
   1. The diagnosis includes identifying the client's strengths.
   2. The clarification of the psychologic meanings of Mr. Small's experiences, feelings, and behavior will lead to insight.
   3. People can control others, whether or not they want to be controlled.
   4. Illness symptoms acquire a meaning only within the context of the client's social system.

9. Which of the following would *not* be expressed by a staff member who favors the behaviorist model?
   1. Behavior is unconsciously stimulated and determined by a mental mechanism.
   2. The self is a sum of all past conditioning.
   3. Behavior can be observed, described, and recorded.
   4. People are products of both what they do and what they are reinforced for doing by conditions in their environment.

10. Several staff members wish to utilize the social-interpersonal model with Mr. Small. The major ideas from this model that might be applicable include all *but* which one of the following?
    1. Mr. Small's anger should be viewed as a knowledge deficit regarding what to do with his impulses.
    2. Interventions should focus on improving interactions between Mr. Small and others.
    3. Interventions should focus on helping Mr. Small gain a perspective on his life-style and environment.
    4. Interventions should focus on including and involving all the significant systems that have an impact on Mr. Small's life.

11. The timing of interventions for angry, aggressive behavior is best when the intervention occurs
    1. Before the initial anxiety is converted to aggressive behavior.
    2. After the aggressive act has occurred.
    3. During the aggressive act.
    4. After the initial anxiety.

Michael Hampton, two years old, is admitted to the pediatric unit for evaluation of seizure activity.

12. Mrs. Hampton begins to describe Michael's seizures. She states, "He gets real stiff and then starts to shake all over. After a couple of minutes it stops, and he falls asleep." What has most likely happened?
    1. Grand mal seizure
    2. Petit mal seizure
    3. Jacksonian seizure
    4. Psychomotor seizure

13. Which of the following lab tests would be most helpful in determing the cause of Michael's seizures?
    1. Hemoglobin electrophoresis
    2. Lead and protoporphyrin levels
    3. Serum amylase
    4. Sedimentation rate

14. Michael is placed on a regimen of phenytoin elixir (Dilantin) PO. Which of the following of Michael's needs would receive particular emphasis when discussing this drug with Mrs. Hampton?
    1. Frequent naps
    2. Oral hygiene
    3. Prophylactic antibiotics
    4. Isometric exercises

15. Which of the following immunizations should Michael *not* receive?
    1. Tetanus
    2. Diphtheria
    3. Pertussis
    4. Polio

You are monitoring the induction of labor for a primigravida, Mary Albert.

16. In evaluating the action of the medication oxytocin (Pitocin) which of the following evaluations would indicate an adverse effect?
    1. A contraction lasting over 120 seconds
    2. An decrease in blood pressure
    3. Urinary output of 100 ml per hour
    4. Increasing intensity of contractions

17. Mrs. Albert, now in active labor, expresses concern about her ability to continue to behave as she would wish during the remainder of labor. Which of these nursing interventions would be most supportive of her?
    1. Tell the client that her responses are influenced by her culture.
    2. Inform her that medication is available if she needs it.
    3. Instruct the client in relaxation and breathing exercises.
    4. Reassure Mrs. Albert that she will be accepted regardless of her behavior.

18. An external monitor has been applied to Mrs. Albert. The following assessment is made: a fetal heart deceleration of uniform shape, beginning just as the contraction is under way and returning to the baseline at the end of the contraction. Which of the following nursing interventions is appropriate?
    1. Administer O_2.
    2. Turn the mother on her left side.
    3. Notify the physician.
    4. Continue observations of labor.

19. One-half hour after her delivery, you make the following assessment of Mrs. Albert: fundus firm, 1 inch below the umbilicus; lochia rubra; complains of thirst; slight tremors of lower extremities. Analysis of these data is suggestive of which condition?
    1. Impending shock
    2. Circulatory overload
    3. Sub-involution
    4. Normal postpartum adaptation

20. Mrs. Albert, two hours postdelivery, complains of severe perineal pain. Which nursing action would take priority?
    1. Administer prescribed pain medication.
    2. Initiate sitz baths.
    3. Inspect the perineum.
    4. Teach perineal muscle exercises.

21. Which of the following nursing assessments could indicate bladder distention six hours after Mrs. Albert's normal vaginal delivery?
    1. Poor abdominal muscle tone
    2. Increased lochia rubra with clots
    3. Uterus contracted below umbilicus
    4. Uterus soft to the right of midline

You are summoned to the home of your neighbor, a multigravida, during a severe snowstorm. She appears to be in active labor. Both she and her husband are very apprehensive.

22. What is the most appropriate initial action?
    1. Call for an ambulance.
    2. Calm both parents.
    3. Prepare a clean delivery field.
    4. Assess the mother's status.

23. Your assessment reveals the infant in a vertex presentation, crowning. As you assist in the delivery of the head, which would be appropriate instructions to the mother?
    1. Push during the contraction to aid in delivery.
    2. Pant during contractions to avoid forceful expulsion.
    3. Bear down continuously to assist the abdominal muscles.
    4. Breathe slowly and deeply to ensure proper oxygenation of the fetus.

Juanita Sanchez, aged 78, has been living with her daughter since her husband's death five years ago. She has become increasingly forgetful and unable to care for herself. She wanders away from home frequently and is argumentative, because of organic brain syndrome. The family has decided to place Mrs. Sanchez in a nursing home.

24. Based on the diagnosis of organic brain syndrome, nursing assessment of Mrs. Sanchez would most likely reveal which of the following intellectual changes?
    1. Decreased ability to handle anxiety
    2. Disorientation to time and place
    3. Emotional lability
    4. Paranoid ideation

25. Mrs. Sanchez becomes more confused after she has been admitted to the nursing home. Which of the following actions would be most helpful to decrease her confusion?
    1. Assist Mrs. Sanchez with all activities of daily living.
    2. Find out from the family what her usual daily routine is and follow it as closely as possible.
    3. Restrict visitors during the first two weeks so she can adjust to the nursing home.
    4. Wait for the confusion to decrease as Mrs. Sanchez adjusts to her new environment.

26. Mrs. Sanchez's increased confusion is probably caused by
    1. Anger at her daughter.
    2. Decreased personal space.
    3. Increased brain deterioration.
    4. Unfamiliar surroundings.

27. Mrs. Sanchez frequently wanders from her room into other clients' rooms or out to the street. The most effective nursing intervention would be to
    1. Accompany Mrs. Sanchez when she wanders and guide her to her room or the dayroom.
    2. Ask Mrs. Sanchez to explain why she cannot remain in her room or public areas.
    3. Confine Mrs. Sanchez to her room, because she gets lost too frequently.
    4. Restrain Mrs. Sanchez in her chair so she will not disturb others or become lost.

28. Mrs. Sanchez repeatedly attempts to leave the nursing home stating, "My husband is waiting at home for me. I have to leave work now." The nurse's most appropriate response is
    1. "He knows you're staying here tonight; come back in now."
    2. "Mrs. Sanchez, you know you retired 13 years ago and your husband is dead."
    3. "You can't leave now; you have to stay here."
    4. "Your husband died five years ago, and you're in the nursing home now."

29. Mrs. Sanchez's daughter states that Mrs. Sanchez had lost 11 lb in the past three months. Which of the following would be the most appropriate nursing intervention to ensure adequate nutrition?
    1. Feed Mrs. Sanchez when she doesn't finish her meal.
    2. Give Mrs. Sanchez six small feedings during the day.
    3. Tell Mrs. Sanchez that she will be tube-fed if she doesn't eat.
    4. Observe Mrs. Sanchez's eating and weigh her before developing a plan.

30. Which of the following will be most effective in assisting Mrs. Sanchez to maintain a reality orientation?
    1. Call Mrs. Sanchez by name and identify yourself each time you enter her room.
    2. Encourage Mrs. Sanchez to spend her time watching television in her room.
    3. Plan a different schedule of activities every day to prevent boredom.
    4. Rotate staff assignments; so she will know each staff member.

31. Mrs. Sanchez is most likely to demonstrate which of the following?
    1. Decreased attention span and ability to learn new things
    2. Equal recall of both recent and past events
    3. Increased ability to adapt to change in her environment
    4. Increased interest in hygiene and grooming

32. The nurse notes that Mrs. Sanchez frequently confabulates when asked about her everyday activities. She does this in order to
    1. Fill in memory gaps.
    2. Get attention from the nurse.
    3. Increase her attention span.
    4. Prevent regression.

33. The night nurse reports that Mrs. Sanchez is very confused, is in and out of bed, and makes multiple requests for assistance throughout the night. Which of the following nursing actions would most effectively lessen her confusion?
    1. Alter her bedtime routine to increase physical activity.
    2. Give her a detailed explanation of her need for adequate rest.
    3. Turn on night-lights in her bedroom and bathroom.
    4. Give her a sedative to help her sleep.

34. Mrs. Sanchez has difficulty deciding what to wear in the morning. The most effective nursing intervention would be to
    1. Give her as much time as she needs to make her own decision.
    2. Help her select an outfit and get dressed.
    3. Lay out her clothes each morning before she awakens.
    4. Tell her she must hurry or she will miss breakfast.

35. Mrs. Sanchez tells her daughter she might as well not visit since she doesn't care enough to let her own mother stay at home. The daughter tells the nurse, "I don't know what to do. Mother's so angry she doesn't want to see me. But I had to do something. We couldn't take care of her anymore." The nurse's most appropriate initial response would be
    1. "Wait a few days and she'll get over this."
    2. "She'll be OK once she gets settled here; don't worry."
    3. "You feel guilty about leaving your mother here."
    4. "This is a very difficult time for you and your mother."

36. The daughter asks if she should come back the next day to visit. The nurse's most appropriate response would be
    1. "Come back tomorrow; your interest is important for your mother."
    2. "Is there anyone else who could visit your mother?"
    3. "Wait until your mother calls you to say she wants to see you."
    4. "Your mother will be busy with the staff and clients. She won't miss you if you don't come."

37. An hour after her daughter leaves, Mrs. Sanchez tells the nurse, "I haven't seen my daughter in days. Something must be wrong." The nurse's most appropriate response would be,
    1. "Are you afraid she won't come back to visit you?"
    2. "I'm sure you'll hear from her again soon."
    3. "You're confused; she was here earlier tonight."
    4. "Your daughter was here before dinner this evening."

38. Which of the following would be most helpful in providing ongoing care for Mrs. Sanchez?
    1. Follow her usual routine as much as possible.
    2. Involve her in all unit activities to decrease her loneliness.
    3. Provide one-to-one teaching sessions to help her understand her limitations.
    4. Adhere strictly to the unit's routine.

Eleven-year-old Gail is hospitalized with rheumatic fever with carditis and polyarthritis. She also has Sydenham's Chorea.

39. Which of the following is true concerning this disease?
    1. It is usually associated with glomerulo-nephritis.
    2. Symptoms disappear shortly after the fever abates and the temperature returns to normal.
    3. The child should resume normal activities as soon as she feels well.
    4. It usually follows a strep infection.

40. In planning your nursing care, you note that Gail is on bed rest. What is the rationale for this?
    1. To help the pain of the arthritis
    2. To minimize the effects of the carditis
    3. So other children will not see Gail's choreiform movements
    4. To help alleviate the febrile effects of the disease

41. Which of the following is likely to be the major psychologic stressor of Gail's illness and hospitalization?
    1. Fear of bodily damage
    2. Separation from friends
    3. Loss of control
    4. Threat to identity and self-esteem

42. Which of the following children should the nurse select as Gail's roommate?
    1. Seven-year-old Susan who also has rheumatic fever
    2. Ten-year-old Amy with insulin-dependent diabetes
    3. Thirteen-year-old Sharon with sickle cell vaso-occlusive crisis
    4. Twelve-year-old Evelyn with fever of unknown origin

43. Which of the following activities is most appropriate for Gail?
    1. Listening to records and the radio
    2. Watching television
    3. Playing ping pong in the game room
    4. Crocheting a small afghan

44. Gail is taking prescribed salicylates. These medications are used to achieve all of the following actions in treating polyarthritis associated with rheumatic fever *except* which one?
    1. Reduce inflammation
    2. Reduce leukocytosis
    3. Relieve pain
    4. Reduce fever

45. Gail's blood tests show the following results. Which is the most indicative of an improvement in her condition?
    1. Positive C-reactive protein
    2. White blood cell count of 11,000
    3. Decreased erythrocyte sedimentation rate (ESR)
    4. Elevated antistreptolysin O titer

46. Gail is readmitted to the hospital two months later for a cardiac catheterization. When preparing Gail for the procedure, the nurse should take into account which of the following?
    1. Concrete explanations and experiences will be most meaningful.
    2. Gail is likely to misinterpret the procedure as punishment for previous misbehavior.
    3. Gail should be given a full verbal explanation of the procedure using correct medical terminology.
    4. Gail should be allowed to make all decisions concerning her care.

Elizabeth Johnson, 21, delivered her first child this morning.

47. She is in the "taking-in" phase of the postpartum period, as identified by Rubin. Which of these behaviors is common during this time of restoration?
    1. Requesting "no visitors" so she can rest
    2. Asking if "rooming in" could begin immediately
    3. Talking constantly about the labor and delivery
    4. Experiencing mild transient feelings of depression

48. Which of the following assessments on the day after delivery indicates normal reproductive adaptation?
    1. Fundus firm, 1 cm below the umbilicus
    2. Scant lochia serosa
    3. Moderate breast engorgement
    4. Perineal sutures healed

49. On the third day after delivery Mrs. Johnson complains of breast engorgement. Her 6 lb infant seems quite sleepy when put to breast. An appropriate nursing intervention would be which of the following?
    1. Teach her breast massage/manual expression of milk.
    2. Suggest she use ice packs to breasts immediately prior to nursing.
    3. Teach her to use the electric breast pump when the baby is sleepy.
    4. Advise her to increase her protein and fluid intake.

50. Mrs. Johnson asks you if breast-feeding will change the shape of her breast. Which of the following would be the most appropriate response?
    1. "Yes, the shape of your breast may be affected if the baby is allowed to nurse too vigorously."
    2. "Breast-feeding does not affect the shape of the breast. However, wearing a proper breast support is important."
    3. "If you breast-feed for more than six months, the shape of the breast will change."
    4. "Breast-feeding may change the shape of the breast, however, this shouldn't be the most important consideration."

51. Mrs. Johnson seems very discouraged about breast-feeding. She says, "Neither baby Tim nor I seem to be successful at this breast-feeding. Maybe it's because I am so small." Your response to the mother is based on the understanding of which of the following?
    1. Hormone levels may vary in individual women.
    2. Desire to breast-feed affects milk production.
    3. Primigravidas are usually apprehensive about feeding.
    4. Breast size is not a factor in volume of milk produced.

52. Prior to discharge, both Mr. and Mrs. Johnson attend several classes on infant care. Which statement by the new father indicates he has a realistic understanding of newborn behavior?
    1. "I hope we can get him on a schedule of two naps and a full night's sleep."
    2. "I don't want him to be spoiled, so he'll learn quickly not to cry for attention."
    3. "If we can get him on a schedule for feedings, he'll nurse better."
    4. "It looks like the next weeks will be mostly feeding, changing, and caring for baby."

Twenty-two-month-old Katie is admitted to the pediatric unit with acute, spasmodic laryngitis (croup). Katie shares a bedroom at home with her brother, who has a history of several attacks of croup.

53. When a nursing history is taken, Katie's mother tells the nurse that Katie is toilet trained. Which additional information is the most important for the nurse to ascertain?
    1. The age at which Katie began toilet training
    2. Katie's toileting habits and routine at home
    3. Katie's mother's understanding of the possibility of regression in Katie's toileting habits while she is hospitalized
    4. Katie's willingness to accept help from the nursing staff with her toileting needs

54. Developmentally, Katie should exhibit which of the following behaviors?
    1. Dress and undress herself without help
    2. Share her toys with other children
    3. Speak in five to six word sentences
    4. Feed herself well with a spoon

55. When assessing Katie's respiratory status, the nurse will likely note which of the following symptoms?
    1. Bradypnea
    2. Rales and rhonchi
    3. Inspiratory stridor
    4. High fever

56. Katie is in a croup tent with compressed air. Nursing care of Katie should include all the following measures *except* which one?
    1. Frequent monitoring of vital signs
    2. Restricting fluid intake
    3. Administering a mild sedative as prescribed
    4. Changing wet bed linens frequently

57. Katie is hospitalized for four days. Katie's parents visit every evening but are unable to stay with her overnight. Which behavior is Katie most likely to demonstrate when separating from her parents?
    1. Readily seeks comfort from the nurse
    2. Sucks her thumb, whines, and curls up in a corner of her crib
    3. Cries loudly and tries to cling to her parents
    4. Waves and blows them a kiss

58. Which toy would be most appropriate for Katie when her parents are not with her?
    1. A large ball
    2. A push-pull toy
    3. Wooden blocks
    4. A pegboard and hammer

59. When Katie is discharged, the nurse should provide her parents with the following guidance *except* which one?
    1. Katie may show some regression in her behavior for a few weeks.
    2. Katie should not be separated from her parents for lengthy periods of time until she feels secure again.
    3. Katie should be allowed to sleep with her parents for a few nights until she readjusts to being home.
    4. Katie's parents should reinstitute limits that were in effect prior to her hospitalization.

Stanley Brown, a 50-year-old man who has been a heavy smoker for the past 20 years, is admitted to the hospital with a diagnosis of emphysema with right lower lobe pneumonia. Upon his arrival at the medical floor, the nurse carries out her assessment, which is as follows: extremely dyspneic, ashen in color, perspiring profusely, very agitated, and coughing up large amounts of tenacious white sputum. Mr. Brown's orders include stat blood gases; O_2 at 2 liters; aminophylline IV drip; sputum for C&S; start ampicillin (Polycillin) 1 gm after sputum is obtained.

60. All of the following information is provided by Mr. Brown. What probably precipitated his emphysema flare-up?
    1. He wore a new cotton suit 2 days ago.
    2. He smoked more cigarettes than usual three days ago.
    3. He went bowling last week.
    4. He has had a cold for the past week.

61. What is the expected action of aminophylline?
    1. Increase the production of sputum
    2. Relax the bronchial muscle
    3. Promote sleep and relieve anxiety
    4. Liquefy tenacious sputum

62. To detect a common side effect of aminophylline, the nurse should assess Mr. Brown for the possible development of which symptom?
    1. Generalized dermatitis
    2. Hematuria
    3. Urinary retention
    4. Tachycardia

63. Mr. Brown's blood-gas results demonstrate a pH of 7.37, Po_2 of 65 mm Hg, and a Pco_2 of 50 mm Hg. On the basis of this information, which statement is most justified?
    1. Mr. Brown has acute respiratory insufficiency and needs to have his O_2 turned up to 8 liters.
    2. Mr. Brown has acute pulmonary failure and needs to be placed on a ventilator.
    3. Mr. Brown has adapted to his high level of arterial CO_2 and is in chronic respiratory acidosis.
    4. Mr. Brown demonstrates chronic respiratory acidosis and will soon display neurologic changes.

64. Mr. Brown produces sputum, which is sent to the lab for culture and sensitivity. Then, IV ampicillin (Polycillin) is started. You know that this drug belongs to the penicillin family of antibiotics and that the pencillins, among all the antimicrobials, are most often responsible for which of the following?
    1. Anaphylaxis
    2. Urinary retention
    3. Nausea and vomiting
    4. Gastric perforation

65. Mr. Brown does not improve. On the third day post-hospital admission, his temperature is 103.4° F (39.7° C), he has right-sided chest pain, and decreased right-sided chest excursion. A portable chest x-ray reveals further extension of his pneumonia with a spontaneous pneumothorax. Mr. Brown is informed that a chest tube must be inserted immediately. To assist Mr. Brown to comply with this procedure, which of the following pieces of information does the nurse need to have in order to be of most help in answering his questions?
    1. The pneumothorax is caused by disruption in the integrity of the pleura.
    2. A rib has fractured and is causing changes in thoracic pressures.
    3. Air has collected in the mediastinal space.
    4. The pneumothorax is caused by the accumulation of pus in the lung tissue.

66. Mr. Brown asks the nurse how the chest tube will help him to breathe with greater ease. Which of the following responses by the nurse would be *inappropriate*?
    1. The chest tube will allow for the drainage of fluid and air from the pleural space.
    2. The chest tube will aid in reestablishing positive pressure in the pleural space.
    3. The chest tube will aid in reexpansion of the lung.
    4. The chest tube will aid in reestablishing negative pressure in the pleural space.

67. After the chest tube is inserted and connected to the Pleur-evac, Mr. Brown wants to know why there are water "bubbles" in the water-seal container. Which of these responses by the nurse would be best?
    1. "You should ask your doctor for more information."
    2. "It indicates that the system is working correctly."
    3. "Oh! don't worry about it. I am taking good care of you."
    4. "It indicates that your lung has not fully expanded."

68. Mr. Brown progresses well. One week post-op, his chest tube is removed. Mr. Brown tells the nurse he realizes proper nutrition is very important for his future health, but he just doesn't have much of an appetite. Which of these responses by the nurse would be most helpful for him?
    1. Eat three large meals a day that are high in carbohydrate.
    2. Eat three large meals a day that are high in protein.
    3. Eat six small meals a day that are high in carbohydrate.
    4. Eat six small meals a day that are high in protein.

69. When Mr. Brown is discharged, he and his wife are referred to the Visiting Nurse Association. Mr. Brown and his wife will more readily accept aid from this organization if which of the following is noted?
    1. The need that they think they have for such help
    2. The enthusiasm of the nurse who plans their care
    3. The availability of the help
    4. The willingness of Mrs. Brown to accept the help

Michael Lamaroux, a 34-year-old construction worker, is admitted to a medical-surgical unit following an auto accident for treatment of fractured femurs and his right hip. He had been drinking and hit another car. Although Mr. Lamaroux's blood-alcohol level is high, he insists that he only had one beer. He is to have surgery for reduction of his fractured hip.

70. He tells his nurse that he is especially sensitive to pain and has used Percodan for headaches in the past. What is the best initial statement the nurse can make?
    1. "Do you have any medications with you that were not prescribed by a physician?"
    2. "Be sure not to take any medications except what we give you for pain."
    3. "Have you ever felt like you needed medication to help you get through the day?"
    4. "I need you to make a verbal contract with me right now that you will not take any medication except what is ordered for you at this time. Other drugs may interfere with your anesthesia tomorrow."

71. In order for withdrawal symptoms to occur in a person with a substance use disorder, which of the following is *unnecessary*?
    1. Physiologic dependence
    2. Marked tolerance
    3. Diminished intake
    4. Cessation of intake

72. Which of the following ego-defense mechanisms is a top and continuing priority in dealing with alcoholic clients?
    1. Dependency
    2. Denial
    3. Paranoia
    4. Projection

73. Of all the following approaches to the treatment of alcoholism, which has been found to be the most effective to date?
    1. Membership in Alcoholics Anonymous
    2. Family-systems approach
    3. Treating the alcoholism as a chronic disease
    4. Individual psychotherapy

74. Following inpatient treatment for his fractures and for his substance abuse, Mr. Lamaroux agrees to involve himself in therapy. Which of the following would have the *least* influence on the structure of family-therapy sessions?
    1. Genetic factors and chronic disease effects of alcoholism
    2. History of alcoholism in other family members and the previous generation
    3. Over- and underfunctioning within the family
    4. How closeness and distance are dealt with in the family

75. Following weeks of treatment for his fractures and detoxification for his alcoholism, Mr. Lamaroux tells his visiting best friend that he had someone bring him a dose of phencyclidine (PCP). If this is true and if he ingests it, his anticipated behavior may resemble which of the following?
    1. Major depression
    2. Antisocial personality disorder
    3. Acute schizophrenia
    4. Morphine overdose

76. All *but* which of the following statements are correct about PCP?
    1. May produce acute panic and anxiety states
    2. May produce habituation
    3. May produce physical dependence
    4. Is also referred to as angel dust

77. In revising the goals, the nurse writes, "Client will decrease drug-seeking, manipulative, and acting-out behavior." Which of the following nursing orders is *not* appropriate for the updated care plan in light of Mr. Lamaroux's drug and alcohol problems?
    1. Set firm and consistent limits.
    2. Clearly define acceptable and unacceptable behavior.
    3. Hold a care conference to assure that entire staff adopt a consistent approach to client's behavior.
    4. Provide a high level of sympathy and empathy for his difficulties.

Sylvia Marlin, a 28-year-old newlywed, is admitted to the hospital with an enlarged thyroid gland.

78. In taking a nursing history, which of the following is considered a risk factor in the development of cancer of the thyroid?
    1. A diet low in iodine
    2. A diet high in iodine
    3. A history of streptococcal sore throat
    4. A history of irradiation of the head or neck

79. In carrying out an initial and daily assessment of a client with thyroid enlargement, the nurse will carefully observe for which of the following?
    1. Difficulty in swallowing or breathing
    2. Cough and sputum production
    3. Muscle twitching
    4. Diminished hearing

80. In addition to having an enlarged thyroid gland, Mrs. Marlin has been experiencing symptoms suggestive of hyperthyroidism. What might these symptoms include?
    1. Fatigue, weight gain, dry skin, cold intolerance
    2. Decreased pulse rate, slurred speech, constipation, cold intolerance
    3. Nervousness, weight loss, tachycardia, heat intolerance
    4. Abdominal pain, diarrhea, fatty food intolerance, heat intolerance

81. Mrs. Marlin's laboratory workup will probably indicate which of the following?
    1. Deficiency of serum T_3 and/or T_4
    2. Increased levels of serum T_3 and/or T_4
    3. Deficiency of serum TSH
    4. Increased levels of serum ACTH

82. A serious form of hyperthyroidism results in a condition known as what?
    1. Myxedema
    2. Cretinism
    3. Graves' disease
    4. Addison's disease

83. Mrs. Marlin's hyperfunctioning thyroid results in exophthalmos. Nursing interventions specific for this problem should include which of the following?
    1. Frequent mouth care using a soft toothbrush and normal saline mouthwash
    2. A private room with decreased environmental stimulation and light
    3. Lubricating eye drops and instructions to blink at regular intervals
    4. Frequent monitoring of vital signs and body temperature

84. Mrs. Marlin's diagnostic workup includes a radioactive iodine (RAI) uptake. In preparing the patient for this procedure, what should the nurse do?
    1. Take a history of all recent medications and x-ray examinations.
    2. Place the client on a low sodium diet for 3 days prior to the test.
    3. Prepare the client for isolation using radiation precautions.
    4. Instruct the client in 24-hour urine collection techniques.

85. To inhibit thyroid hormone synthesis, Mrs. Marlin is given propylthiouracil (PTU). In reviewing this medication with her prior to discharge, the nurse would include all of the following *except* which one?
    1. Report weight loss and increased pulse rate.
    2. Report fever, sore throat, rash.
    3. Take the drug once daily at the same time each day.
    4. Expect some weight gain.

86. Antithyroid drug therapy has proved to be ineffective. Mrs. Marlin is readmitted to the hospital for thyroidectomy. Prior to thyroidectomy, an iodine solution has been administered for several weeks in order to decrease the vascularity and size of the thyroid gland. When giving an iodine solution, the nurse should do which of the following?
    1. Give the drug on an empty stomach to speed its rate of absorption.
    2. Dilute the drug in fruit juice, milk, or water.
    3. Not give the drug with milk or antacids
    4. Not give the drug at bedtime

87. Prior to her surgery, Mrs. Marlin acquires coryza, stomatitis, and swollen salivary glands. What should the nurse do?
    1. Request a consult from an ear, nose, and throat specialist.
    2. Isolate the client from other preoperative clients.
    3. Evaluate the client's diet for excessive iodine intake.
    4. Hold the iodine solution and report the client's symptoms.

88. Postoperative care of the client following thyroidectomy includes which of the following?
    1. Keep the head of the bed flat to prevent neck flexion.
    2. Avoid coughing and deep breathing to prevent injury to the suture line.
    3. Restrict ambulation until the suture line is healed.
    4. Check the back of the neck and upper part of the back when assessing the dressing.

89. Following thyroidectomy, the nurse frequently assesses the client's voice and ability to speak. What is the nurse trying to evaluate?
    1. Changes in level of consciousness
    2. Recovery from anesthesia
    3. Injury to the parathyroid gland
    4. Spasm or edema of vocal cords

90. Mrs. Marlin begins to experience respiratory distress. A check of the surgical dressing reveals it to be tight about her neck with a small amount of bloody drainage. What should the nurse do?
    1. Perform a tracheostomy.
    2. Reinforce the dressing and notify the doctor.
    3. Loosen the dressing and notify the doctor.
    4. Place the patient in high-Fowler's position and notify the doctor.

91. The nurse will instruct Mrs. Marlin to avoid which of the following activities for several weeks following a thyroidectomy?
    1. Turning the head
    2. Sitting in a chair
    3. Brushing the teeth
    4. Side-lying position

92. The nurse observes Mrs. Marlin for injury to the parathyroid gland as a result of her surgery. Which of the following is *not* a sign or symptom of parathyroid damage?
    1. Painful muscle spasms
    2. Numbness and tingling
    3. Increased serum calcium
    4. Increased serum phosphorus

93. Treatment of parathyroid hormone deficiency can be expected to include which of the following?
    1. Thyroid preparations
    2. Digitalis
    3. Calcium gluconate
    4. High phosporus diet

94. Following a total thyroidectomy, what should the nurse teach the client?
    1. Take thyroid medication daily for the rest of life.
    2. Thyroid medication will be prescribed for 1-2 years.
    3. Restrict sea food, iodized salt, and green vegetable intake.
    4. Take iodine solution daily for the rest of life.

Correct Answers and Rationales: Book Four

1. **#1.** Many clients interpret the nurse's entering "their space" as a threat, and Mr. Small is exhibiting signs of increased anxiety. His history indicates that he has utilized violent, aggressive behavior in response to increased anxiety. The nurse and the client do not have an established nurse-client relationship, and the nurse has not assessed his behavior and responses to others. Therefore, the nurse should reduce the environmental stimuli and assess his response to the decrease.

2. **#3.** Mr. Small is having difficulty maintaining self-control. Clear, firm limits will reduce his anxiety by providing a sense of control. Rules provide a sense of security until the client can provide his own controls.

3. **#1.** The client is showing signs of escalating anxiety. He has a history of doing harm to others. The nurse needs to offer simple, limited, alternative behaviors without providing the client access to any weapons that could be used to do harm to himself or others.

4. **#3.** When a client is placed in seclusion, communication should be kept simple and aimed at helping the client understand that the staff are assuming control until he can control his own behavior. When the staff are placing the client in restraints his anxiety level will be raised and hearing will become more selective. Expectations should be communicated at a time when the client's anxiety is lower.

5. **#1.** Client's rights are addressed in state laws. State laws have statutes to include the conditions under which restraints can be used. Mr. Small's aggressive, violent behavior supports the need to protect others.

6. **#4.** The law does deal with confidentiality concerns of clients. Limiting the documentation of staff is in violation of the portion of most state laws that indicates the record must contain specific data.

7. **#3.** The medical model, while describing a characteristic course, does not guarantee a positive resolution.

8. **#2.** All other choices are characteristic of the medical-biologic, behavioral, or sociologic models.

9. **#1.** The concept of unconscious motivation is a characteristic of the psychoanalytic model.

10. **#1.** The social-interpersonal model focuses on society and groups. The behaviorist model focuses on learning theory.

11. **#1.** Anger is cyclic. Once the client works out his anger and frustration in an aggressive act, he feels guilty and needs to justify and explain his behavior. While his anxiety is temporarily decreased, he experiences a decrease in self-esteem, which further increases the anxiety and can result in more acting-out behavior. The best intervention is to stop the anger cycle before it begins.

12. **#1.** A grand mal seizure is characterized by a tonic phase (stiffening) and a clonic phase (rhythmic shaking of the trunk and extremities). During a petit mal seizure, the child appears to be daydreaming or gazing off into space. Jacksonian seizures (not usually seen in children) are focal seizures in which twitching and jerking occur usually at the distal end of an extremity. The child is usually awake during the seizure and frequently the twitching may involve the entire side of the body. A psychomotor seizure usually begins with the child staring into space. Behaviors or automatisms such as chewing and smacking the lips also occur.

13. **#2.** Lead intoxication causes increased intracranial pressure and the sequelae of convulsions, retardation, and sensory deficits. Incidence of lead poisoning peaks between two and three years of age. The most frequently used lab tests for lead screening are lead levels and the erythrocyte-protoporphyrin levels. Hemoglobin electrophoresis identifies hemoglobin disorders; serum amylase identifies pancreatic and liver disorders; the sedimentation rate is usually elevated in the presence of inflammatory problems and is useful in determining the progress of inflammatory diseases.

14. **#2.** Hypertrophy of gum tissue is frequently seen in children who receive phenytoin over long periods of time. Oral hygiene and frequent dental checks can be very effective in preventing the occurrence of this problem.

15. **#3.** Pertussis immunization is contraindicated in all children who have neurologic disorders.

16. **#1.** If contractions exceed 90 seconds in duration, there is a danger of the uterus rupturing. Increasing intensity of contractions is desirable.

17. **#4.** Acceptance is needed in time of stress.

18. **#4.** This is a normal occurrence. Continue to observe fetal heart rate and contractions.

19. **#4.** These are normal adaptations.

20. **#3.** Such pain may be associated with the development of a hematoma. Assessment should precede intervention.

21. **#4.** A full bladder displaces the uterus and prevents contraction.

22. **#4.** Before taking any other action, assessment is a priority.

23. **#2.** A precipitous delivery may result in a perineal tear.

24. **#2.** This is the only symptom listed that is indicative of a problem with intellectual function. #1, #3, and #4 indicate changes in emotional functioning.

25. **#2.** A familiar, established routine decreases confusion and the demands on the client's coping mechanisms. Efforts should be made to follow previous patterns. #1 would increase dependence, #3 would lead to increased feelings of isolation. Waiting will not lessen the confusion.

26. **#4.** Admission to a care facility often exacerbates symptoms because of the new environment.

27. **#1.** Confinement and restraints increase feelings of hopelessness and inadequacy, which may lead to increased confusion. These clients will not be able to explain their behavior, and requests for such explanations may increase argumentativeness.

28. **#4.** This provides reality orientation without degrading or arguing with the client.

29. **#2.** Provide smaller meals that require less attention to complete. The other choices would decrease independence, threaten the client, or allow the problem to continue.

30. **#1.** Identify yourself to avoid misidentification and call the client by name to reinforce her sense of identity. #2 would decrease her interaction with others, possibly increasing confusion. #3 and #4 provide an inappropriate degree of stimulation.

31. **#1.** Decreased ability to learn because of decreased attention span are characteristics of organic brain syndrome. Recent and remote memory changes are variable. As memory changes occur, the person will have more difficulty adapting to change and attending to usual activities of daily living.

32. **#1.** Confabulation involves using old memories or inventing information to fill in memory gaps about present experiences.

33. **#3.** Avoiding shadows and darkness will help decrease her disorientation. Maintain the usual bedtime routine. These clients will not understand or remember explanations. Sedatives often increase activity and confusion in the elderly.

34. **#2.** Provide assistance and direction with activities of daily living as needed. Giving her time will not increase her decisiveness or lessen confusion. Laying out her clothes makes the decision for her and decreases independence. Rushing her will increase confusion.

35. **#4.** Assist family members to explore their feelings. Maintaining family contact is necessary for orientation and self-identity. Reassurance will not help family members deal with feelings or the situation. There is insufficient evidence to justify an inference of guilt.

36. **#1.** Assist with feelings and client situations so family members will not withdraw from the client. Encourage regular visits.

37. **#4.** Provide concrete information that reinforces reality without emphasizing the client's deficits. Probing for feelings increases confusion and argumentativeness in these clients.

38. **#1.** Decreasing the number of adjustments needed in a new environment lessens confusion. Do not overstimulate or confront clients with deficits. Provide for individualization of care.

39. **#4.** Two possible sequelae of a strep infection are rheumatic fever and glomerulonephritis, but the two do not necessarily occur in conjunction with each other.

40. **#2.** The major sequela of rheumatic fever is heart damage, particularly scarring of the mitral valve. Bed rest is recommended for the client with carditis to minimize metabolic needs and ease the workload of the heart.

41. **#2.** All are potential stressors, but the school age child is especially vulnerable to separation from friends.

42. **#2.** Seven-year-old Susan is somewhat young to be the best choice, even though she has the same health problem. Because Gail has carditis, she should not be placed with Sharon; Gail had a recent strep infection and Sharon's condition may be aggravated by exposure to a potential source of infection. On the other hand, Evelyn has a fever, which may indicate a concurrent infection to which Gail should not be exposed. Amy is the best choice, because she is close enough in age, has no infectious condition, and, like Gail, has a chronic illness.

43. **#4.** Gail is on bed rest with bathroom privileges and cannot go to the playroom. Listening to records and watching television are passive activities. Crocheting requires minimal exertion, promotes joint mobility, and also fosters Gail's feelings of accomplishment.

44. **#2.** Salicylates have no effect on white blood cell production or destruction.

45. **#3.** A decreasing ESR indicates a decrease in the body's inflammatory response.

46. **#3.** Gail is able to cognitively understand full explanations using correct terminology. Such explanations also consider her emotional needs and foster feelings of control. However, while she should be included in making decisions that affect her, she is not legally able to give consent for or refuse necessary care.

47. **#3.** There is a need during this phase to integrate the experience of delivery into reality.

48. **#1.** This indicates normal uterine involution. At this stage lochia should be rubra.

49. **#1.** Complete emptying of the breasts is important for the comfort of the mother. Engorgement is a normal physiologic process.

50. **#2.** The shape of the breast will not be changed by breast-feeding. The bra will prevent breakdown of breast musculature and provide comfort.

51. **#4.** Breast size is not a factor in volume of milk produced.

52. **#4.** The neonate sleeps more than 20 hours daily, nurses every two to three hours, urinates, and has frequent stools.

53. **#2.** Although all these pieces of information may be important and may be ascertained at some point during Katie's hospital stay, the nurse must know Katie's usual patterns in order to develop an appropriate care plan to meet Katie's toileting needs.

54. **#4.** Dressing without supervision, sharing with other children, and using complete sentences are characteristics of preschoolers, not toddlers. Katie should have learned to use a spoon well by 18-20 months of age.

55. **#3.** Croup is characterized by inspiratory stridor and a metalliclike cough. The respiratory rate will be increased (tachypnea). Because this form of croup is usually viral, Katie is not likely to have a high fever. The disease is an upper-airway inflammation; so rales and rhonchi will be absent.

56. **#2.** A liberal fluid intake helps liquefy secretions so that Katie can expectorate them. Vital signs should be monitored frequently, especially respiratory status, to detect further airway obstruction. Bed linens should be changed frequently to prevent chilling and promote comfort. Mild sedatives are often used to decrease the child's anxiety and, therefore, facilitate breathing.

57. **#3.** Protest behavior most characterizes the toddler's separation from parents. Despair or detachment behavior is unlikely to appear when hospitalization is short, especially when parents visit daily.

58. **#4.** A pegboard and hammer allow Katie to release her anger about separation and her frustration over her loss of control in a socially acceptable way.

59. **#3.** Allowing Katie to sleep with her parents may increase Katie's insecurity, since this was not part of her routine prior to hospitalization.

60. **#4.** Respiratory infections such as a flu, colds, etc. are the most frequent cause of exacerbations in clients with emphysema (COPD).

61. **#2.** Aminophylline has a beta-adrenergic effect that results in the relaxation of bronchial muscle.

62. **#4.** A common, untoward effect of aminophylline is tachycardia, because it stimulates the cardiac muscle.

63. **#3.** A normal pH with elevated CO_2 indicates chronic respiratory acidosis. The client has adjusted to the high level of arterial CO_2, and signs of neurologic involvement are usually not present.

64. **#1.** Among the antimicrobial drugs, penicillins are most often responsible for anaphylaxis because of their allergic properties.

65. **#1.** Disruption in the integrity of the pleura allows air from the lung to enter the pleural space.

66. **#2.** The primary purpose of a chest tube is to reestablish subatmospheric pressure in the pleural space.

67. **#4.** Correct information allays anxiety.

68. **#4.** Clients with emphysema may not be able to tolerate eating large meals; they must eat frequent small meals. Also they may have an intolerance to foods high in carbohydrates, but they need proteins for tissue repair.

69. **#1.** The willingness to accept professional help depends upon the need as the client sees it.

70. **#3.** This response encourages the client to discuss his feelings and can provide important clues to what is troubling him or what has been difficult for him.

71. **#4.** Even diminished intake can lead to withdrawal. Cessation is not a prerequisite to the occurrence of withdrawal symptoms.

72. **#2.** The alcoholic client knows something is wrong, but cannot connect it with alcohol use.

73. **#1.** Regardless of what other approaches are used, membership in Alcoholics Anonymous is crucial.

74. **#1.** Although genetic factors and chronic disease effects are important; #2 through #4 are important areas to explore and focus upon in the family therapy sessions.

75. **#3.** A PCP reaction may present with florid psychosis, severe hallucinations, and may very much resemble schizophrenia.

76. **#3.** Hallucinogens such as LSD and PCP do not produce a physical dependence.

77. **#4.** Too much sympathy and empathy reinforce the client's view of himself as a victim of alcohol, drugs, or other people. The client will not accept responsibility for himself, nor will he be able to break through his denial if a high level of sympathy and empathy is given. The client would then manipulate his nurse and avoid dealing with his problems. #1 through #3 are critical to setting the stage for the client to work on his problems. The client needs to internalize limits.

78. **#4.** While a dietary deficiency of iodine may cause goiter and hypothyroidism, dietary iodine is not now regarded as implicated in the development of thyroid cancer. However, a history of irradiation of head, neck, or chest—for acne, enlarged thymus or tonsils, Hodgkin's disease, etc.—is now strongly associated with the development of thyroid cancer.

79. **#1.** An enlarged thyroid may encroach on organs in close proximity. Swallowing and breathing are usually the first functions to be affected. Muscle twitching would be the result of parathyroid involvement.

80. **#3.** #1 and #2 suggest hypofunction of the thyroid gland. The symptoms listed in #4 are not, as a group, specific for thyroid dysfunction.

81. **#2.** Primary thyroid hyperactivity is characterized by elevations in serum triiodothyronine (T_3) and/or thyroxine (T_4). Secondary hyperthyroidism, caused by malfunction of the pituitary gland, is characterized by an overproduction of thyroid-stimulating hormone (TSH). Serum ACTH levels remain unaffected unless hyperpituitarism in involved.

82. **#3.** Graves' disease is hyperthyroidism accompanied by goiter and/or exophthalmos. It is thought to be autoimmune in nature because of the presence of long-acting thyroid stimulators (LATS) in the blood of many, but not all, affected persons. Myxedema is caused by hypofunction of the thyroid; cretinism is caused by congenital hypothyroidism. Addison's disease is caused by adrenocortical hypofunction.

83. **#3.** Exophthalmos is characterized by bulging eyes. To prevent drying of the overly exposed eyeballs, lubricating eye drops, such as methylcellulose drops, are frequently prescribed. In addition, self-lubrication and protection through regular blinking are encouraged. While not specific to exophthalmos, placement of clients in areas of low environmental stimuli in order to decrease adrenergic activity and frequent monitoring of vital signs for changes are considered important aspects of the nursing care plan.

84. **#1.** Results of the test are affected by the client's intake of iodides (in medications or x-ray contrast media) and thyroid hormones. Proper interpretation of results requires this information be noted on laboratory slips.

85. **#3.** Propylthiouracil should be taken every 8 hours to ensure adequate levels over a 24-hour period. Too low a dosage will be evidenced by a return of weight loss and rapid pulse rate. A serious side effect of this drug is agranulocytosis, evidenced by indications of infection (fever, sore throat, or rash). In returning to a euthyroid state, the client can be expected to regain previously lost weight.

86. **#2.** To disguise the salty taste and to decrease gastric irritation, iodine solutions should be well diluted in a full glass of fruit juice, milk, or water and administered after meals and at bedtime.

87. **#4.** These symptoms are indicative of iodine poisoning (iodism). The nurse's first action should be to discontinue iodine therapy and report the client's signs and symptoms to the physician. A secondary consideration is any additional sources of iodine in the diet (iodized salt, seafood, vegetables grown near the seaside, etc.). Isolation of the client is not required, and symptoms will subside with adjustment of iodine intake.

88. **#4.** Hemorrhage is a serious complication following thyroidectomy. Because of gravity, drainage may not be visible along the suture line on the anterior neck dressing, but rather at the back of the neck and upper part of the back. The preferred position for the postthyroidectomy client is semi-Fowler's with good neck support. Turning, coughing, and deep breathing as well as early ambulation can be accomplished while the head and neck are supported in a neutral position.

89. **#4.** Increasing hoarseness postthyroidectomy may indicate injury to the recurrent laryngeal nerve or swelling in the area of the glottis. Parathyroid injury will be evidenced by muscular tingling or twitching.

90. **#3.** Respiratory distress and a tightening neck dressing may indicate hemorrhage into tissues or increasing edema in the neck area. Loosening the dressing to prevent further tracheal compression should be the nurse's first action. Reinforcement of the dressing would only increase tracheal compression. High-Fowler's position alone will not decrease swelling; the dressing must also be loosened.

91. **#1.** Sitting in a chair, brushing the teeth, and lying on one's side may all be accomplished without the flexion, extension, or rotation of the neck that should be avoided in the early postoperative period because of the strain they place on the suture line. The client must be instructed to turn the whole body, not just the head during this time.

92. **#3.** Injury to the parathyroid gland would be accompanied by decreased levels of calcium.

93. **#3.** The treatment of choice, both on an emergency and long-term basis, is the administration of calcium gluconate. Thyroid preparations have no influence on parathyroid functioning. Digitalis is a cardiotonic and requires normal levels of calcium to produce desired effects. Since phosphate levels increase in hypoparathyroid conditions, dietary phosphorus would be contraindicated.

94. **#1.** Following total removal of the thyroid gland, the client must take thyroid medication daily for the rest of life to supply the hormones essential for maintenance of body metabolism. Since the thyroid hormones themselves are taken, dietary iodine is no longer needed to support their synthesis within the body. Dietary iodine need not be advised or restricted.

Appendix
Approved Nursing Diagnoses from the North American Nursing Diagnosis Association, April, 1984

Activity intolerance*
Activity intolerance, potential*
Airway clearance, ineffective
Anxiety*
Bowel elimination, alteration in: constipation
Bowel elimination, alteration in: diarrhea
Bowel elimination, alteration in: incontinence
Breathing pattern, ineffective
Cardiac output, alteration in: decreased
Comfort, alteration in: pain
Communication, impaired: verbal
Coping, family: potential for growth
Coping, ineffective family: compromised
Coping, ineffective family: disabling
Coping, ineffective individual
Diversional activity, deficit
Family process, alteration in*† (formerly Family dynamics)
Fear
Fluid volume, alteration in: excess*†
Fluid volume deficit, actual
Fluid volume deficit, potential
Gas exchange, impaired
Grieving, anticipatory
Grieving, dysfunctional
Health maintenance, alteration in*
Home maintenance management, impaired
Injury, potential for: (poisoning, potential for; suffocation, potential for; trauma, potential for)
Knowledge deficit (specify)
Mobility, impaired physical

Nutrition, alteration in: less than body requirements
Nutrition, alteration in: more than body requirements
Nutrition, alteration in: potential for more than body requirements
Oral mucous membrane, alteration in*
Parenting, alteration in: actual
Parenting, alteration in: potential
Powerlessness*
Rape trauma syndrome
Self-care deficit: feeding, bathing/hygiene, dressing/grooming, toileting
Self-concept, disturbance in: body image, self-esteem, role performance, personal identity
Sensory-perceptual alteration: visual, auditory, kinesthetic, gustatory, tactile, olfactory
Sexual dysfunction
Skin integrity, impairment of: actual
Skin integrity, impairment of: potential
Sleep pattern disturbance
Social isolation*†
Spiritual distress (distress of the human spirit)
Thought processes, alteration in
Tissue perfusion, alteration in: cerebral, cardiopulmonary, renal, gastrointestinal, peripheral
Urinary elimination, alteration in patterns
Violence, potential for: self-directed or directed at others

*Addition from 1982 Conference
†Moved from to-be-developed list

Index

Abdomen
  physical examination of, 211
Abduction, 313
Abortion, 394
  spontaneous, 394
Abruptio placentae, 398, 398f
Absorption
  in digestion, 209
Abuse, victims of, 61
Abused adults, assessment of, 62
Abused children, assessment of, 62
Abusers, assessment of, 62
Accident prevention
  adolescent, 522
  infant, 516
  preschooler, 520
  school-age child, 521
  toddler, 519
Acetaminophen (Tylenol)
  poisoning, 586t
Acid-base balance
  regulation of by kidneys, 252
Acidosis
  child, 555
  metabolic, 588
Acting out behavior, 60, 67, 83t
Activities
  age appropriate in hospital,
    703 [41-43]
Addiction, 90, 98
Addison's disease, 241
Adduction, 313
Adenoidectomy, 579
Adenosine diphosphate (ADP), 210
Adenosine triphosphate (ATP), 210
Admission to mental hospital, 34
Adolescent pregnancy, 407
Adolescent, 521
  age-related needs and fears, 528
  developmental responses to
    hospitalization, 527
Adrenal crisis, 242
Adrenal glands, 233
  hyperfunction of, 240
  hyposecretion of, 241
Adrenergic blockers, 181t
Adrenergic drugs, 195t
Adrenergic stimulation, 179
Adroyd, 558
Affect, 77, 98
Affective Disorders
  See Elated-Depressive Behavior
After-birth pains, 432
Aggression, 83t, 691 [84-901], 698 [1-5]
Aggressive behavior, 64
Airway obstruction, 533, 535

Alcohol abuse, 91, 706 [70-77]
Alcohol, in pregnancy, 387, 390
Alcoholics Anonymous, 93
Alcoholism, 91
  treatment of, 93
  stages of, 94
Aldosterone, 252
Alkalosis
  child, 555
  metabolic, 588
  respiratory, 588
Alphafetoprotein, 574
Alzheimer's disease, 48
Ambivalence, 79, 98, 675 [84]
Amenorrhea, 378
Aminophylline, 705 [61-62]
Amnesia, 41
Amnesics, use of during labor, 414
Amniocentesis, 392
Amniotic fluid analysis, 391t, 393
Amniotic fluid embolism, 430
Amniotic fluid, 385
Amphetamines, abuse of, 96
Amputation, 318
Anabolism, 210
Anal fissure, 282
Analgesics, 168t
  aspirin, 653 [24]
  use of in labor, 414
Anaphylactic shock, 178
Android pelvis, 375
Anemia in pregnancy, 404
Anemia, iron deficiency
  child, 547
Anesthesia
  general, 166t
  regional, 166t
  stages, 166t
  use of in labor, 414
Anger, 83t
  in organic brain syndrome, 702 [35]
Angina pain
  distribution of, 180f
Angina pectoris, 179
Angiography, 175
  renal, 255
Animism, 517
Anorexia nervosa, 42
Antacids, 219, 654 [29]
Antepartal care, 381, 655 [44,47]
Anthropoid pelvis, 375
Anticholinergic drugs, 219
Anticholinesterase medications, 305
Anticoagulant antagonists, 184t
Anticoagulants, 184t
  heparin, 660 [89]

Anticonvulsants, 303t, 400
Antidepressants, 51t, 652 [14]
Antihypertensive drugs, 191t, 192, 400
Antilactation agents, 419
Antiparkinsonian drugs, 300t
Antisocial behavior, 72
Antispasmodic drugs, 225
Anuria, 252
Anxiety, 36, 98
  discharge, 653 [18,19]
  diagnosis of, 37
  four levels of, 37
  manifestations of, 37t
Anxious behavior
  See Anxiety; Phobias
Anxiousness, 83t
Apgar score, 453
Apgar scoring chart, 453t
Aphasia
  client with, 292
  motor (expressive), 288
  sensory (receptive), 288
Aphasia, expressive
Apical pulse, 174
Apnea, 460
Appendicitis, 225
Arterial blood gases, 176
  infants and children, 538
Arteriography, renal, 255
Arteriosclerosis obliterans, 193
Arteriovenous fistula, 267, 682 [4,5]
Arteriovenous shunt, 266
Arthritis, 319
Arthroplasty, 320
Ascites, 231
Aspirin (salicylate poisoning), 586t
Assaultive behavior, 64
Assessment
  activity and rest problems, 314
  normal neonate, 452
Associative looseness, 79, 83t
Asthma, bronchial, 196
Astrocytoma, 609
Athetosis
  See Dyskinesis
Atrial fibrillation, 186

KEY: f following the page number
         refers to a figure
      t following the page number
         refers to a table
   [10] numbers in brackets refer
         to individual question
         numbers.

720 INDEX

Atrial flutter, 186
Atrial septal defect, 540, 541f
Attachment deprivation syndrome
    See Failure-to-thrive (FTT) syndrome
Audiogram, 291
Audiometry, pure tone, 523
Autism, 78, 83t, 98
Autonomic nervous system, 286
Autosomal recessive disorder, 558
Babinski's reflex, 448
Backache, 388
Ballottement, 384
Barium enema, 213, 274
Bartholin's glands, 376
Basal body temperature, 378f
Bath, neonate, 455-6
Behavior
    acting out, 60
    aggressive, 64
    antisocial, 72
    assaultive, 64
    controlling, 83t
    hostile, 64
    hyperactive, 58
    interventions for, 83t
    passive-aggressive, 64
    socially maladaptive, 60
    suspicious, 75
    withdrawn, 77
Behavioral Model, 20t
Benign prostatic hypertrophy, 271
Billroth I
    See Gastrectomy, subtotal
Billroth II
    See Gastrectomy, subtotal
Binocularity tests (for strabismus), 523
Biopsy
    colon, 275
    renal, 255
Birth control methods, 674 [77]
Birth injuries, 464
Birthmarks, 445
Bishop's Scale, 426t
Bladder cancer, 259, 332
    radiation therapy, 260
    surgery, 260
Bladder, 250
    cancer of, 259
    postpartum, 433
Blindness, 293
Blood levels, normal, 547t
Bone scan, 314
Bone-marrow aspiration, 604
Bowel
    child, 562
    postpartum, 433
Bowel, large
    See Large bowel
Bradypnea, 460
Brain scan, 290
Brain tumors, 609
Brain, 285
Brainstem glioma, 610
Braxton Hick's contractions, 381, 384, 388, 410
Brazelton, 444
Breasts, 376
    cancer, 333
    changes, postpartum period, 433
    engorgement, relief of, 435
    tenderness in pregnancy, 388
Breast-feeding, 456, 656 [49], 684 [20], 704 [50-51]
Breath holding, 576

Brecht feeder, 557
Breech presentation, 408, 420
Bronchial asthma, 196
    child, 536
Bronchiolitis, 536
Bronchitis, chronic, 196
Bronchodilators, 197t, 537t
Bronchoscopy, 174
Brudzinski's sign, 578
Brushfield spots, 571
Buerger's disease, 193
Burn budget, 671 [47]
Burn surface area, estimation of, 590f
Burns, 589, 671 [45-54]
    systemic responses, 589t
Bursa, 313
Calcium gluconate, 400
Calculus (calculi), urinary, 258
Cancer, 326
    assessment, 327
    bladder, 259, 332
    breast, 333
    cervix, 332
    chemotherapy, 328
    childhood, 602
    classification, 327
    colon, 282, 332
    diagnostic tests for, 327
    early detection of, 330
    larynx, 310, 332
    lung, 205, 302
    medical treatment of, 327
    physiology/pathophysiology, 326
    prognosis, 327
    prostate, 273, 332
    radiation therapy, 328
    risk factors, 326
    surgery, 327
Candidiasis, 675 [87,88]
Caput succedaneum, 446
Carcinoma, 326
Cardiac catheterization, 175, 686 [42,43], 703 [46]
    infants and children, 538, 593t
Cardiac compensation, 188
Cardiac disorders
    in pregnancy, 402
    congenital, 540
Cardiac glycosides, 179, 189t
Cardiac output, 170
Cardiogenic shock, 178
Cardiopulmonary arrest, 176, 686 [40]
Cardiopulmonary resuscitation, 177, 668 [16,17]
Cardiovascular system, 170
    child, 532
    in pregnancy, 382
Carditis, 545
Cartilage, 313
CAT scan
    See Computerized axial tomogram, 290
Catabolism, 210
Cataracts, 306
Catatonic schizophrenia, 86
Caudal block, 416
CBC, 176
Cellular aberration, 326, 602
Central nervous system, 285
Central venous pressure, 171
Cephalic presentation, 408
Cephalohematoma, 446, 464, 684 [17]
Cephalopelvic disproportion, 420
Cerebral arteriogram, 291

Cerebral palsy, 572
Cerebrovascular accident, 295
Cervical cancer, 332
Cervix, 376
Cesarean birth, 428, 670 [35]
Cesarian incisions, 429f
Chadwick's sign, 381, 384
Chemotherapeutic drugs, 329-330t, 603-604t
Chemotherapy, 328
Chest drainage, closed, 544
Chest surgery, 203
Chest tubes, 203, 706 [66-67]
Chickenpox, 581
Child abuse, 61, 688 [63-72]
    legal responsibilities, 689 [65]
Child, 513
    feeding assessment, 651 [2,3]
    ill and hospitalized, 525
    immunologic differences, 568
    integumentary differences, 568
    neurologic differences, 568
    normal growth and development, 651 [1]
    nutrients, 687 [50,51]
    toilet training, 651 [4]
Childbearing
    normal, 381, 408, 432
    high risk, 389
Childbirth
    classes, 656 [48]
    education, 389
Childhood cancer, 602
Childhood schizophrenia, 87
Chloasma, 381
Cholangiogram, 213
Cholecystectomy, 226
Cholecystitis, 225, 667 [2]
Cholecystogram, 213
Cholecystostomy, 225, 667 [3]
Choledocholithotomy, 226
Cholelithiasis, 225
Cholesterol, 186t
Cholinergics, 304t
Chordee, 563
Chorea (Saint Vitus' dance or Sydenham's chorea), 545
Chronic obstructive lung disease (COLD), 196
Chronic obstructive pulmonary disease (COPD), 196
Chronic organic brain syndrome, 48
Chvostek's sign, 240
Cirrhosis, 229
Cleft lip, 556
Cleft palate, 556
Clomid, 655 [43]
Clubfoot, congenital, 599
Coarctation of the aorta, 540, 542f
Cocaine, abuse of, 96
Cognitive development
    adolescent, 521
    infant, 513
    preschooler, 519
    school-age child, 520
    toddler, 517
Colectomy, 280
Colitis, ulcerative, 277, 278t
Collagen disease, 322
Colon
    cancer, 282, 332
    obstruction of, 281
Colonoscopy, 275
Colostrum, 433

INDEX

Commitment procedure, 98
Communicable diseases, 524, 580
Communication skills, 24t
Community Mental Health Model, 20t
Compensation,
   as defense mechanism, 23
Competency, legal aspect of, 34
Computerized axial tomogram, 290
Concussion, 293
Conduction, cardiac, 170, 187
Conduction tests (hearing testing), 523
Condylomata in pregnancy, 406
Confabulation, definition of, 98
Conflict, definition of, 98
Confused behavior, nursing process, 48
Confusion, 48
   organic brain syndrome, 701 [24-38]
   chronic, 48
Congenital anomalies, 465, 683 [12]
Congestive heart failure, 188, 188t, 661 [92], 685 [32,38]
Conjoint therapy, 98
Conjunctivitis, chemical, 446
Constipation, 276, 675 [83]
   in pregnancy, 388
Controlling behavior, 83t
Contusion of the head, 293
Conversion disorders, 45, 670 [38-44]
Conversion, as defense mechanism, 23
Convulsions in pregnancy, 400
Coomb's test, 419
Coping mechanisms, parental, 527
Coronary arteries, 182f
Coronary artery disease, 179
Corrosives (lye, bleach, ammonia), poisoning, 587t
Corticosteroids, 537t
Countertransference, definition of, 99
Covert, definition of, 99
CPR
   See Cardiopulmonary resuscitation
Craniectomy, 294
Craniopharyngioma, 610
Cranioplasty, 294
Craniotomy, 294
Creatinine clearance, 254
Credé's method, 575
Cretinism, 238
Crib death
   See Sudden infant death syndrome
Crisis intervention, 26, 99, 672 [54]
Crohn's disease, 277, 278t
Croup tent, 535
Croup, spasmodic
   See Laryngitis, acute spasmodic
Cultural variables, 18
Curling's ulcer, 592
Cushing's syndrome, 240
Cutaneous ureterostomy, 260
Cystectomy, 260
Cystic fibrosis, 558, 674 [71-73]
Cystitis, 257
   postpartum, 441
Cystography, 255
Cystoscopy, 255
Cytomegalovirus, in pregnancy, 405
Daily fetal movement count, 391
Deafness
   conductive, 289
   sensorineural, 289
Death and dying, 28
   nursing process, 30
Death, child's understanding of, 29
Decerebrate posture, 289, 290f

Decorticate posture, 289, 290f
Defense mechanisms, 21, 669 [24], 671 [41], 675 [79]
Dehydration, 592
   signs of, 552
Delirium tremens, definition of, 99
Delusion, definition of, 99
Delusions, 78, 83t, 658 [68,69]
Denial, 21
Denis-Browne splint, 599
Dental care, 523
   toddler, 518
   school-age child, 521
Denver Developmental Screening Test, 570
Dependence, 83t
Depersonalization, 41, 79, 99
Depression, 52, 652 [7-19]
   types, 53-54
   See also Bipolar depression, 54
Descent during labor, 410
Desquamation, 445
Developmental disabilities, 568
Developmental responses to hospitalization, 525
Developmental screening tools, 523
Developmental stimulation, infant, 687 [52-57]
Diabetes mellitus, 243, 657 [55-58]
   care of skin and feet, 246
   diet, 245t, 245
   foot care, 668 [9]
   insulin administration, 246
   medical treatment of, 244
   pregnancy, 401, 667 [5-12]
   types, 243
   urine testing, 246
Dialysis, 264
   psychologic adjustment to, 269
Diaper rash, 456
Diarrhea, 276, 554
Diets, 185, 186, 192, 221-223, 245, 264, 265, 279, 389, 450, 515
   acid-ash, 676 [92]
   bland, 654 [27]
   diabetic, 657 [55]
   low cholesterol, 661 [93]
Differentiation, 326
Digestion, 208
Digestive system
   anatomy, 208
   assessment of, 210
   child, 552
   in pregnancy, 383
   process, 208
   secretions, 208
Digitalis, 660 [91]
Digoxin, 544
Dilantin, 700 [14]
   See also Anticonvulsants
Disabled infant,
   parental reaction to, 466
Discharge teaching,
   child and family, 528
Discipline, toddler, 518
Displacement, as defense mechanism, 23, 41, 43
Dissociation, 21
Dissociative reactions, 41, 669 [23,25]
Diuretics, 232, 544,
Diverticulitis, 224
Diverticulosis, 224
Dizygotic twins, 406
Double bind, definition of, 99

Down's Syndrome, 570
Drug abuse, 96
Drug addiciton in pregnancy, 390
Drugs
   adrenergic, 195t
   adrenergic blockers, 181t
   analgesics, 168t
   anticholinergic, 654 [28]
   anticoagulant antagonists, 184t
   anticoagulants, 184t
   anticonvulsants, 303t, 576
   antidepressants, 51t
   antihelminthics, 584
   antihypertensive, 191t
   bronchial asthma, 537t
   bronchodilators, 197t
   cardiac glycosides, 189t
   disulfiram (Antabuse), 95
   emergency, 177t
   expectorants, 198t
   glucocorticoids, 242
   lithium carbonate, 51t, 684 [24,25]
   magnesium sulfate, 424
   MAO inhibitors, 51t
   mineralocorticoids, 242
   oxytocic agents, 419
   phenothiazines, 80t, 100
   potassium iodine, saturated solution of (SSKI), 237
   propranolol (Inderal), 238
   ritodrine, 424
   salicylates, 703 [44]
   terbutaline, 424
   thioxanthenes, 80t
   tokolytic agents, 424
   tranquilizers, major, 80t
   tranquilizers, minor, 39t
   vasodilators, 181t
   vesicants, 331
DSM III, 13
Dumping syndrome, 224, 654 [32]
Duncan mechanism, 418
Duodenal ulcer, 654 [26-32]
Dyad, definition of, 99
Dying child, nursing process, 32
Dysarthria, 288
Dyskinesis (athetosis), 572
Dysmenorrhea, 378
Dysrhythmias, 185
   atrial, 185
Dystocia, 420
Ear
   external, 287
   inner, 288
   middle, 288
ECG, 175
Echocardiography, 175
Eclampsia, classification of, 399, 399t
Ectoderm, 384
Ectopic pregnancy, 395, 395f
Edema in pregnancy, 388
EEG, 291
Ego, definition of, 99
Elated-Depressive Behavior, 50
Elation, 58
Elderly (over 65), physiologic characteristics, 161
Electrocardiogram, 175
Electroconvulsive therapy, 50
Electroencephalogram, 291
Electrolyte imbalance, 592
Electrolytes, 176
Electromyogram, 314

722 INDEX

Elimination, 250, 562
   toddler, 518
Emergency birth, 425
Emergency drugs, 177t
Emerson pump, 654 [30]
Emphysema, 196, 705 [60-61]
Encephalitis, signs of, 582
Endocarditis, 539
Endocardium, 170
Endocrine system, 233
   assessment of, 235
   child, 552
Endoscopy, 213
Engagement
   fetus, 408
   in labor, 410
Engorgement, 433
Entoderm, 384
Ependynoma, 610
Epicardium, 170
Epidural block, 416
Epiglottitis, acute, 534
Epilepsy, 302
Episiotomy, 426, 427f
Epistaxis, 309
Epstein's pearls, 447
Erikson, Eric, 20t, 22t, 513, 517, 519, 521
   stages of development, 19, 514t
Erythema marginatum rheumaticum, 545
Erythema toxicum, 445
Erythroblastosis fetalis, 458
Erythromycin, 545
Erythropoietin, 252
Esophageal varices, 231
Estrogen, 377, 382
Examination, neurologic, 288
Exanthema subitum
   See Roseola
Exercises
   range-of-motion, 313, 672 [51]
   isometric, 314
Exophthalmos, 707 [83]
Expectorants, 198t, 537t
Extension, 313
Extracapsular fracture, 653 [20-25]
Extrapyramidal reaction,
   definition of, 99
Eye
   exterior, 286
   interior, 286
Failure-to-thrive syndrome, 553
Faintness in pregnancy, 388
Fallopian tubes, 376
False labor, 410
Family therapy, 27, 99
Family, violence in, 61
Fantasy, 23
Fascia, 313
Fat soluble vitamins, 558
Ferrous sulfate (Fer-In-Sol), 547
Fertility assessment, 379t, 655 [41], 683 [10]
Fertilization, 377
Fetal alcohol syndrome, 463
Fetal blood sampling, 393
Fetal circulation, 385
Fetal development, 384
Fetal heart rate, 411f, 416
   acceleration, 413f
   baseline, 411t
   decelerations, 412f, 413t
   during labor, 411
Fetal hypoxia, chronic, 691 [81]

Fetal monitoring, 411
Fetal positions with cephalic presentation, 409f
Fetal weight, 387
Fetal well-being,
   laboratory studies of, 391t
Fissurectomy, 283
Fixation, 23
Flexion during labor, 410
Flexion, 313
Flight of ideas, definition of, 99
Fluid and electrolyte balance, 250
Fluid overload, 592
Follicle-stimulating hormone (FSH), 376
Fontanels, 446
Food allergies, infant, 516
Footling breech, 420
Forceps, 427
Formula preparation, neonate 456
Fractured hip, 317
Fractures
   medical treatment, 315
   types of, 315
Fredet-Ramstedt procedure, 556
Freud, Sigmund, 20t, 22t
   stages of development, 19
Friedman curve, 421, 422f
Fugue, psychogenic, 41
Fundal height, 386
   fourth stage of labor, 419
   postpartum, 432
Fundus, 376
Gastrectomy, subtotal, 219, 654 [32]
Gastric analysis, 216
Gastritis, 217
Genetic transmission, 549f
Genitalia
   female external, 376f
   male, 271f
Gestational age variations, 450, 656 [50]
GI tract obstruction, lower, 566
Glands
   See name of individual gland
Glaucoma, 308
Glomerulonephritis, acute, 565
Gonorrhea in pregnancy, 405
Goodell's sign, 381, 384
Gout, 320
Grasp, neonate, 448
Graves' disease, 237
Gravida, 386
Grief and Mourning Process, 28
   stages of, 466
Group therapy, 26, 99
Guthrie test, 455
Gynecoid pelvis, 375
Habituation, 90
Hallucinations, 78, 83t, 99, 687 [47]
Hallucinogenics, 97
Hand splints, 672 [52]
Head injury, 293
Health, characteristics of, 159
Health care, infant, 516
Health promotion, levels of, 159, 658 [67]
Healthy adult, physiologic characteristics, 159
Hearing, 287
   screening, 523
Heart, abnormal, 541f
Heart defects
   acyanotic, 540
   cyanotic, 540
Heart, normal, 171f

Heart sounds, normal, 174
Heart valves, 173f
Heartburn in pregnancy, 388
Heat loss in neonate, 449
Heberden's nodes, 320
Hegar's sign, 381, 384
Helplessness, 83t
Hemarthrosis, 550
Hematologic problems, 546
Hematologic system, child, 532
Hematoma, postpartum, 438
Hemiparesis, 295
Hemiplegia, 295
Hemodialysis, 266, 683 [7]
Hemophilia, 550
Hemorrhage, 591, 668 [13-15], 672 [57]
   epidural, 293
   extradural, 293
   postpartum, 437
   subconjunctival, 446
   subdural, 293
Hemorrhoidectomy, 283
Hemorrhoids, 282
   in pregnancy, 388
Hepatic encephalopathy, 232
Hepatitis
   type A, 227, 667 [1]
   type B, 228
Hernia, hiatus, 217
Herniated nucleus pulposus, 323
Herpes, in pregnancy, 405
Hiatus hernia
   See Hernia, hiatus
Hip
   dislocation, 599
   fractured, 317
   congenital dysplasia, 599
Hirschsprung's disease, 567
Hodgkin's disease, 608, 608t
Homan's sign, 435
Home care, 534
   child, 545
Hopelessness, 83t
Hormones, 208t, 234t
   See also Glands
Hormones, female, 376-377
Hospitalization, preparation for, 527
Hostile behavior, 64
Hostility, 83t
Human chorionic gonadotropin, 382
Human chorionic
   somatomammotropin, 382
Hyaline membrane disease
   See Respiratory distress syndrome
Hydaditiform mole, 396, 396f
Hydramnios, 466
Hydrocarbon poisoning, 587t
Hydrocephalus, 421, 660 [83-87]
   congenital, 573
Hymen, 376
Hyperactive behavior, 58
Hyperbilirubinemia
   See Jaundice, neonatal
Hypercapnia, 196
Hyperemesis gravidarum, 396
Hyperglycemia
   See Ketoacidosis
Hyperparathyroidism, 239
Hyperpituitarism, 236
Hypertension, 191
   portal, 229
   pregnancy, 399, 683 [13]
Hyperthyroidism, 707 [78-94]
   See also Grave's disease

Hypertonic uterine dysfunction, 420
Hypoglycemia, 247t, 248, 461, 561, 667 [8]
  neonatal, 450
Hypokalemia, 588
Hypoparathyroidism, 240
Hypopituitarism, 236
Hypospadias, 563, 657 [59-61]
Hypothermia, 457
  neonatal, 450
Hypothyroidism, 238
Hypotonic uterine dysfunction, 420
Hypovolemic shock 178, 671 [46]
Hypoxemia, 196
Id, definition of, 99
Idealization, 21
Ideas of reference, as defense mechanism, 23
Identification, as defense mechanism, 21
Identified client, definition of, 99
Ileal conduit, 260
Ileostomy, 280
Illusion, definition of, 99
Immobility, 525
  infant, 525
  preschooler, 526
  school-age child, 527
  toddler, 526
Immobilization, complications of, 316
Immunity, 581
Immunization, 524, 655 [39], 660 [81,82], 687 [54]
  contraindications to, 516, 517t
  infant, 516
  recommended schedule, 517t
Immunology, neonatal, 449
Impetigo contagiosa, 585t
Implantation, 378
Incompetent cervical os, 395
Indigestion in pregnancy, 388
Induction of labor, 425
Infant (1 month to 1 year), 513
  age-related needs and fears, 527
  developmental responses to hospitalization, 525
  feeding, 656 [53]
  safety, 656 [53]
  stimulation, 655 [36]
Infantile spasms, 576
Infection
  neonatal, 462
  postpartum, 439
  pregnancy, 404
  systemic, 592
  wound, 592
Infertility, 379t, 655 [41-43]
Inflammatory bowel disease, 277
Injury, 525
  preschooler, 526
  toddler, 525
Insanity, legal aspects of, 35
Insight, definition of, 99
Insomnia, 685 [26]
Insulin-dependent diabetes mellitus, 560, 560t
Insulin, 657 [56]
  administration, 246
  See also Drugs, hypoglycemic
Internal organs, female, 377f
Internal rotation during labor, 410
Interpersonal, definition of, 99
Interstitial-cell stimulating hormone, 377
Intervertebral disk, ruptured, 691 [91-94]
Intracranial hemorrhage, neonate, 464

Intracranial pressure increased, 291, 660 [83,85,86], 669 [21,22]
  in infants and older children, 574t
Intracranial surgery
  See Surgery, intracranial
Intradural blocks, 416
Intrapartal care, 408
Intrapsychic, definition of, 100
Intrauterine growth retardation, 691 [80]
Intravenous pyelogram, 676 [90]
Introjection, as defense mechanism, 23
Intussusception, 567
Iodine, radioactive, 237
Ipecac, 534
Iron dextran (Imferon), 547
Isolation, as defense mechanism, 21
IV rates, 167t
Jaundice, neonatal, 445, 457
Joints, 313
Kernicterus in neonate, 458
Kernig's sign, 578
Ketoacidosis, 247, 248, 561, 668 [11,12]
Kidneys, 250, 251t
  assessment of, 252
  diagnostic tests, 252
  fluid and electrolyte balance, 250
  stones, 676 [94]
  transplantation, 270, 683 [9]
Koplik's spots, 581
Korsakoff's syndrome, 48
Kubler-Ross, Elizabeth, 28
La belle indifférence, 45
Labia majora, 376
Labia minora, 376
Labor
  abnormal fetal position or presentation, 423
  abnormal position, 420
  analgesics, used during, 414
  bloody show, 410
  breathing techniques, 417
  emergency at home, 701 [22-23]
  essential factors in, 408
  excessive size of fetus, 421
  faulty presentation, 420
  fetal heart deceleration, 700 [18]
  fetal positional response to, 410
  first stage, 416
  fourth stage, 419
  lie of the fetus, 408
  monitor, 700 [18]
  onset theories, 410
  passageway, 408, 420
  passenger, 408, 420
  person, 421
  physiologic alterations during, 410
  position, 409
  powers, 420
  premature, 423
  presentation, 408
  second stage, 418
  signs of, 410
  stages and phases of, 415t
  station, 409
  third stage, 418
  uterine contractions, 408
Laceration of the head, 293
Lactation, 433
Laminectomy, 323
Lanugo, 445
Large bowel
  assessment, 274
  diagnostic tests, 274

Large-for-gestational age infant, 451t, 452
Laryngeal cancer, 310, 332
Laryngectomy, 690 [73-75]
Laryngitis
  acute spasmodic, 534, 704 [53-57]
Laryngotracheobronchitis, 535
Latent, definition of, 100
LaVeen shunt, 231
Laxatives, bulk, 225, 276t
Lead, chronic poisoning, 587t
Learning disabilities, 655 [40]
Leg cramps in pregnancy, 388
Legal implications
  psychiatry, 699 [5,6]
  record keeping, 699 [6]
  seclusion, 699 [5]
Leopold's maneuver, 421
Lethality, 90
Leukemia, 606
Level of consciousness, 288
Lice (pediculosis), 585t
Life cycle stages, 22t
Ligaments, 313
Lightening, 410
Limit setting, definition of, 100
  toddler, 518
Linea nigra, 381
Lipodystrophies, 657 [57,58], 668 [10]
Liver biopsy, percutaneous, 216
Liver disease, complications of, 231
Lochia, 419, 432t
Logan bar, 557
Longitudinal lie of the fetus, 408
Loss of control, 525
  infant, 525
  preschooler, 525
  school-age child, 526
  toddler, 525
Loss, 28
  nursing process, 29
Lumbar puncture, 289
Lung cancer, 205, 302
Lung scan, 174
Luteinizing hormone (LH), 377
Lymphedema, 673 [59]
Lysozyme, 435
Mafenide acetate (Sulfamylon), 591
Magnesium sulfate, 401, 401t
Malformed infant, parental reaction to, 466
Mania, 58
Manic-depression, 54, 684 [21-26]
Manipulation, 83t, 100
Mastectomy
  Halstead radical, 333
  modified radical, 333, 672 [55-60]
Mastitis, 440, 688 [58-60]
Maternal psychologic adaptation, 434t
Maternal-infant bonding, 434
  after cesarean, 430
McBurney's point, 225
McDonald procedure, 395
McDonald's rule, 386-387, 386t
Mean arterial pressure, 170
Measles, 581
Meconium ileus, 559
Meconium stool, 449
Meconium-aspiration syndrome, 460
Medical-biologic model, 20t
Medication administration, young children, 530t
Medication guide, children, 529t
Medulloblastoma, 609

Megacolon
  See Hirschsprung's disease
Meningitis
  bacterial 577
  neonate, 462
Meningocele, 574
Meningomyelocele, 574, 685 [27-31]
Menopause, 377
Menses, postpartum, 437
Menstrual cycle, 376-377, 669 [29]
Mental retardation, 570, 571t
Mesoderm, 384
Metabolism
  child, 552
  definition of, 210
  See also Nutrition and metabolism
Metastasis, 326
Milia, 445
Milieu, definition of, 100
Milieu therapy, 26, 81, 698 [2]
Milk, nutritional comparison of human and cow's, 450t
Models, theoretical
  Behavioral, 20t
  Community Mental Health, 20t
  Medical-Biologic, 20t
  Psychoanalytic, 20t
  Social-interpersonal, 20t
Molding, 445
Mongolian spots, 445
Mongolism
  See Down's Syndrome
Monozygotic twins, 406
Morning sickness, 388
Moro's reflex, 448
Motility, in digestion, 209
Mourning, definition of, 28
Mucolytics, 198t
Multiple gestation, 406
Multiple personalities, 41
Multiple sclerosis, 300
Mumps, 581
Musculoskeletal system, 313
  in pregnancy, 382
Myasthenia gravis, 304
Myelogram, 314, 691 [92]
Myocardial infarction, 181, 660 [88-93], 686 [39-43]
  blood tests for, 182f, 183t
Myocardial scan, 175
Myocardium, 170
Myringotomy, 578
Myxedema, 238
Naegele's Rule, 385t, 386
Narcissism, definition of, 100
Narcosis, 198
Narcotic drug addiction, neonatal, 463
Narcotics
  for pancreatitis, 227
  use of during labor, 414
Nasal problems, 309
Nasogastric tube, 667 [4]
Necrotizing enterocolitis, neonatal, 465
Neologism, definition of, 100
Neonate, 444
  high-risk, 451t, 457
  jaundice, 449
  maturity rating and classification, 454f
  reflexes, 448
Neoplasm, 326
Nephrectomy, 258
Nephritis, 564
  poststreptococcal, 565
  compared to nephrosis, 565t

Nephroblastoma
  See Wilms' tumor
Nephrolithotomy, 258
Nephron, 250, 251
Nephrosis, 564
Nephrosis, compared to nephritis, 565t
Nephrotomogram, 254
Nephrotoxic agents, 252
Nervous system, functions of, 285
Neuroblastoma, 611
Neurogenic shock, 178
Neurologic problems, child, 570
Neurosis, definition of, 100
Nevi in newborn, 445
Nitroglycerin, 180
Nongonococcal urethritis in pregnancy, 406
Nonstress testing, 391
Normal development, 513
  Asian child, 659 [77-82]
  infant, 687 [49-57]
  psychosocial tasks, 673 [61]
  toddler, 704 [53-59]
Nose, 288
Nurse-client relationship, phases of, 23
Nutrition and metabolism, 208
Nutrition, 523
  adolescent, 522
  child, 552
  during pregnancy, 388, 390t
  infant, 515, 515t
  neonatal, 449
  preschooler, 519
  school-age child, 521
  toddler, 518
Nystagmus, 301
Obsessive-compulsive disorders, 41
Oil embolism, 609
Oligohydramnios, 466
Oliguria, 252
Opiates, abuse of, 96
Organic brain syndrome, 701 [24-38]
  anger, 702 [35]
  confabulation, 702 [32]
  reality orientation, 701 [30]
  See also Confusion
Ortolani's sign, 600
Osmotic diuretics, 291
Osteoarthritis, 320
Osteodystrophy, renal, 263
Osteomyelitis, 601
Osteotomy, 320
Otitis media, 557, 578
Ovaries, 376
Overt, definition of, 100
Overweight child, 673 [67-70]
Ovulation, 377
Oxygen deprivation, 671 [48]
Oxygenation, 170
  assessment of, 172
  child, 532
Oxytocin, 427t
  challenge test, 392
  during labor, 421
Pacemaker, 187
Pain, 525
  angina pectoris, 180
  child, 529
  child's responses to, 527, 529
  infant, 525
  preschooler, 526
  school-age child, 527
  toddler, 526
Palliation, 326

Pancreas, 235
  disorders of, 243
Pancreatic enzymes, 558
Pancreatitis, 226
Papanicolaou (Pap) smear, 379
Paracervical block, 416
Paradoxical communications, definition of, 100
Paranoia, 75, 100, 658 [68-76]
Paranoid schizophrenia, 86, 675 [78-86]
Parathormone, 252
Parathyroid, 233
  damage, 708 [92]
  disorders of, 239
  hormone deficiency, 709 [93]
Parent-infant bonding, 419
  See also Maternal-infant bonding
Paresthesias, 301
Parity, 386
Parkinson's disease (parkinsonism), 299
Parotitis
  See Mumps
Paroxysmal atrial tachycardia, 186
Passive-aggressive behavior, 64
Patent ductus arteriosus, 540, 541f
Paternal reactions to pregnancy, 383
Pavlov, 20t
Pelvic measurements, 375
Pelvis, female, 375, 375f
Penicillin, 545, 705 [64]
Peplau, H., 20t
Peptic ulcer disease, 218
Pericardium, 170
Peridural block, 416
Perineum, 376
  healing, 433
  lacerations, 428
Peripheral nervous system, 286
Peripheral vascular disease, 193
  manifestations, 194f
Peritoneal dialysis, 682 [6]
Peritonitis, 267
Personality disorders, 72
Personality, definition of, 100
Phencyclidine (PCP), 707 [75-76]
Phenobarbital, 534
Phenothiazines, 100
Phenylketonuria (PKU), 455, 657 [54]
Pheochromocytoma, 240
Phlebothrombosis, 193
Phobias, 40, 100
Phototherapy, neonate, 459
Physical growth
  adolescence, 521
  infant, 513
  preschooler, 519
  school-age child, 520
  toddler, 517
Piaget, Jean, 513, 517, 519, 520
Pilocarpine electrophoresis
  See Sweat chloride test
Pinworms (Helminths), 584
Piperazine citrate, 584
Pitocin
  See Oxytocin
Pituitary, 233, 236
Placenta previa, 397, 397f, 670 [30-37]
Placenta, 382
  delivery of, 418
Platypelloid pelvis, 375
Play
  preschooler, 519
  school-age child, 520-1

toddler, 518
  infant, 514
Pneumoencephalogram, 291
Pneumonia, 199, 705 [64-65]
Pneumonitis, 539
Pneumothorax, tension, 203
  spontaneous, 705 [65]
Poisonous ingestions, 584, 586t
Polycythemia, 459, 544
Polydrug abuse, 89
Polymyositis, 322
Polyuria, 252
Portacaval shunt, 231
Postmature infant, 451
Postpartal care, 432, 674 [74-77]
Postpartum
  adaptation, 700 [19], 703 [48]
  bladder distention, 700 [21]
  blues, 434, 684 [19]
  breast engorgement, 703 [49]
  exercise, 436
  pericare, 435
  maternal psychologic adaptation, 433
  perineal pain, 700 [20]
  physiologic status, 433
  taking-in phase, 703 [47]
Post-traumatic stress disorder, 46
Posture
  decerebrate, 289, 290f
  decorticate, 289, 290f
Potassium
  food content, 192t
Potentiation, 90
PPD (purified protein derivative), 202
Prednisone, 564
Preeclampsia, 399
Pregnancy-induced hypertension, 399
Pregnancy
  adolescent, 407
  antepartal teaching, 690 [76-77]
  diagnostic tests, 391, 669, [26]
  discomforts of, 387-388
  maternal adaptations to, 383
  paternal reactions to, 383
  psychologic tasks of, 383
  psychosocial changes, 383
  schedule of visits, 385
  signs and symptoms of, 384, 384t
Premature atrial contraction, 186
Premature infant, 450
Premature ventricular contraction, 186
Preoperational thought, 658 [63]
Preschooler, 519
  age-related needs and fears, 528
  developmental responses to
    hospitalization, 526
Pressure transducer, 413
Prevention
  primary, 20t
  secondary, 20t, 658 [67]
  tertiary, 20t
Proctoscopy, 275
Progesterone, 377, 382
Projection, 23, 675 [79]
Prolapsed cord, 423
Propylthiouracil, 708 [85]
Prostaglandins, 377
Prostate cancer, 273, 332
Prothrombin time, 667 [2]
Psychiatric nursing
  description of, 13
  legal aspects of, 34
  roles, 14
Psychoanalysis, definition of, 100

Psychoanalytic model, 20t
Psychodrama, definition of, 100
Psychodynamics, definition of, 100
Psychogenic, definition of, 100
Psychologic maladaptations,
  postpartum, 443
Psychosis, definition of, 100
Psychosocial characteristics
  of the healthy client
    elderly, 16
    middle adult years, 16
    young adult years, 15
Psychosocial development
  adolescent, 521
  infant, 513
  preschooler, 519
  school-age child, 520
  toddler, 517
Psychosomatic disorders, 43
Psychotherapy, definition of, 26, 100
Psychotic disorders, miscellaneous, 87
Puberty, 521, 669 [28]
Pudendal block, 416, 683 [14]
Puerperium, 432
Pulmonary edema, 190, 685 [32-38]
Pulmonary embolus
  postpartum, 443
Pulmonary function tests, 174
Pulmonary volumes, 175f
Pulse deficit, 174
Pyelogram, 254
Pyelolithotomy, 258
Pyelonephritis, 257, 676 [89-94]
Pyloric stenosis, 556
Pyloroplasty, 219
Pylorotomy, 556
Pyrvinium pamoate (Povan), 584
Queckenstadt's test, 289
Quickening, 384
Radiation therapy
  external, 328
  internal, 328
Radioactive iodine uptake, 708 [84]
Rales, 174
Rape, 68
  child victim, 69
  the emergency room, 68
Rationalization, 21
Raynaud's disease, 193
Reaction formation, 23
Reality-oriented therapy,
  definition of, 101
Reality, definition of, 100
Recommended Dietary Allowances,
  females aged 11-50, 389t
Reed-Sternberg cell, 609
Regression, 23, 78
Renal colic, 259
Renal failure
  acute, 260, 682 [1-9]
  chronic, 262, 682 [2,3]
Renal system in pregnancy, 383
Renin, 252
Repression, 21, 41, 43
Reproductive anatomy and physiology
  (female) 375
Reproductive system, 381
Respiratory distress syndrome, 450, 459
Respiratory distress, 535, 592
  neonate, 459
Respiratory system
  adult, 170
  child, 532
  in pregnancy, 383

Rest, 313, 523
Restraints
  pediatric 526t
  physical, 66, 698 [4]
Retinal detachment, 307
Rh sensitization, 458f
Rheumatic fever, 545, 703 [39-46]
Rheumatic heart disease, 545
Rheumatoid arthritis, 319
RhoGam, 435
Rhonchi, 174
Ringworm (tinea), 585t
Ritodrine hydrochloride, 424t
Ritualistic behaviors, 83t
Rooting, 448
Roseola, 581
Rubella in pregnancy, 405
Rubin, Reva, 383, 433, 434t
Ruptured uterus, 430
Saddle block, 416
Safety, child, 523, 568
Salem sump, 654 [30]
Sarcoma, 326
Scarlet fever, 581
Schilling's test, 216
Schizophrenia
  catatonic, 86
  childhood, 87
  paranoid, 86
  undifferentiated, 87, 686 [44-48]
Schizophrenogenic, definition of, 101
School-age child, 520
  age-related needs and fears, 528
  developmental responses to
    hospitalization, 566
Schultze mechanism, 418
Scoliosis, 600
Seclusion, legal implications, 699 [5]
Secondary gain, 83t
Sedatives, 400
  abuse of, 96
  use of during labor, 414
Seizures
  akinetic, 576
  febrile, 576
  Jacksonian, 576
  focal motor, 302
  grand mal, 302, 576, 700 [12-15]
  petit mal, 302, 576
  psychomotor, 302, 576
Self-esteem, 83t
Self-help groups, 27
Self, therapeutic use of, 19
Sengstaken-Blakemore tube, 231
Sensory development, 656 [51,52]
Sensory problems, child, 570
Separation anxiety, 658 [62]
  toddler, 525, 527
Separation
  infant, 525
  preschooler, 526
  school-age child, 526
  toddler, 525
Septic shock, 178
  neonate, 462
Serum estriol, 391t
  determination in pregnancy, 393
Sex education, 669 [26-29]
Sexual acting out, 68
Sexual intercourse
  postpartum, 437
Sexuality, 524
  preschooler, 520
  healthy client, 17

Sexually transmitted diseases, 582, 583t
Shirodkar procedure, 395
Shock, 178, 668 [15], 670 [35]
Shortness of breath, 388
Sibling reactions to pregnancy, 383
Sick infant, parental reaction to, 466
Sickle cell anemia, 548
Sigmoidoscopy, 275
Significant others, definition of, 101
Silver nitrate, 591
Silver sulfadiazine (Silvadene), 591
Silverman-Andersen scale, 460, 460t
Sinus arrest, 186
Sinus bradycardia, 185
Sinus tachycardia, 185
Skeletal deformity, 595
Skene's ducts, 376
Skin grafts, 672 [53]
Skin infections, 584, 585t
Skin infestations, 584, 585t
Skinner, B.F., 20t
Skull, neonate 446f
Sleep, 524
 infant, 516
 neonate, 456
 preschooler, 519
Small-for-gestational age infant, 451t
Smoking during pregnancy, 387, 391
Snellen test, 291
Social determinants of mental health and illness, 21t
Social-interpersonal model, 20t
Socialization
 adolescent, 522
 infant, 514
 preschooler, 519
 school-age child, 520
 toddler, 518
Socially maladaptive behavior, 60
Socioeconomic-cultural status in pregnancy, 390
Sodium, food content, 185t
Somatic behaviors, 83t
Spasticity, 572
Speech rehabilitation, 690 [75]
Spina bifida, 574
Spinal anesthetic 670 [34]
Spinal block, 416
Spinal cord, 285
 injuries of, 296
Spinal fusion, 323, 600
Sprain, 313
Status asthmaticus, 536
Status epilepticus, 302
Steroids, 295
Stool examination, 274
Stools, neonatal, 449
Strabismus, 673 [66]
Strain, 313
Stranger anxiety, infant, 525, 527
Streptococcal infection
 in pregnancy, 405
Striae gravidarum, 381
Stroke
 See Cerebrovascular accident
Subaortic stenosis, 542f
Sublimation, 23
Subluxation, 599
Substance abuse, 89
Substitution, as defense mechanism, 23
Suctioning, 690 [73]
Sudden infant death syndrome (SIDS), 533

Suicide, 653 [15,16]
 methods of, 55t
 potential for, 55
Sullivan, H.S., 20t, 22t
Sunset eyes, 573
Superego, definition of, 101
Superiority, 83t
Suppression, 21
Surgery
 adult client, 164
 child, 528
 complications, 164
 discharge, 167
 for cancer, 327
 intracranial, 294
 intraoperative period, 165
 perioperative procedures, 164
 postopertive period, 167
Suspicious behavior, 75
Sweat chloride test, 558
Symbiosis, definition of, 101
Symbolization, 21
Synovectomy, 320
Synovium, 313
Syphilis in pregnancy, 405
Systemic lupus erythematosis, 322
T-tubes, 226
Tachypnea, 460
Taking-hold, 434t
Taking-in, 434t
Temperature guide, children 529t
Tendons, 313
Tensilon test, 305
Tetany, 238
Tetralogy of Fallot, 542f, 543
Therapeutic communication, 23, 655 [42]
Therapeutic relationships, 14
Therapist, definition of, 101
Therapy
 conjoint, 98
 crisis intervention, 99
 family, 27, 99
 group, 26, 99
 milieu, 81
 reality-oriented, 101
Thought disorder, 83t
Throat, 288
Thrombophlebitis, 193
Thyroid storm, 238
Thyroid
 diagnostic tests for, 233
 disorders of, 237
Thyroidectomy, 708 [86-94]
Tidal volume, 174
Toddler, 517
 age-related needs and fears, 527
 developmental responses to hospitalization, 525
Tokodynamometer, 413
Tolerance, 90
Tonic neck reflex, 448
Tonsillectomy, 579
Tonsillitis, 579
TORCH complex, 405
Tourniquets, rotating, 190, 685 [36,37]
Toxemia, 399
Toxoplasmosis in pregnancy, 405, 690 [78-79]
Traction, Buck's, 317, 653 [22]
Traction, types of, 596t, 597f
Tranquilizers
 use of during labor, 414
 major, 80t

 minor, 39t
 side effects of, 81t
Transference, definition of, 101
Transplant, kidney, 270
Transposition of the great vessels, 542f, 543
Transverse lie of the fetus, 408
Trauma, 668 [13-22]
Trendelenburg's sign, 600
Triad, definition of, 101
Trisomy 21, 571, 654 [33-40]
Trousseau's sign, 240
True labor, 410
Tube feedings, 672 [50]
Tuberculosis, 201, 658 [64-67]
 in pregnancy, 405
Tympanometry, 578
Ulcer
 duodenal, 219
 gastric, 219
 peptic, 218
Ulcerative colitis, 277, 278t
Ultrasonic transducer, 413
Ultrasonography, 392
Ultrasound, abdominal, 215
Umbilical cord, 382, 447
 care, 456
Unconscious client, 292
Unconscious, definition of, 101
Undifferentiated schizophrenia, 87
Undoing, 23, 41
Upper GI series, 211
Uremic fetor, 263
Ureteral colic, 259
Ureteral reimplantation, 564
Ureterolithotomy, 258
Ureters, 250
Urethra, 250
Urethroplasty, 563
Urinalysis, 252
Urinary antiseptics, 564
Urinary elimination, child, 562
Urinary estriol, 391t
 determination in pregnancy, 393
Urinary frequency in pregnancy, 388
Urinary meatus, 376
Urinary tract infection, 564
 in pregnancy, 405
Urine output, child, 562
Uterine contractions, 388, 413, 416
 assessment of, 414f
Uterine dysfunction in labor, 420t
Uterine fibroids, 442
Uterine prolapse, 441
Uterus, 376
 ruptured, 430
Vacuum extraction, 428
Vagina, 376
Vaginal bleeding, in pregnancy, 656 [45]
Vagotomy, 219
Valsalva maneuver, 182
Varicella zoster
 See Chickenpox
Varicose ulcers, 193
Varicose veins, 193
 in pregnancy, 388
Vascular pressures, 172f
Vaso-occlusive crisis, 548
Vasoconstrictors, 309
 epinephrine, 668 [19]
 nitroprusside, 668 [19]
Vasodilators, 179
 coronary, 181f

Vasopressors, 179
Ventricular
    contraction, premature, 186
    dysrhythmias, 186
    fibrillation, 186
    septal defect, 540, 541f
    tachycardia, 186
Ventriculogram, 291
Ventriculoperitoneal shunt, 660 [84,87]
Vernix caseosa, 445
Violence, 61
Vision screening, 673 [65]
    healthy child, 523
Vision, 286

Visual acuity tests, 523
Vital capacity, 174
Vital sign ranges, children, 515t
Vitamin D, 252
Vitamin K in neonate, 449
Vocalization
    infant, 514
    preschooler, 519
    school-age child, 520
    toddler, 518
Vomiting, child, 554
Water requirements, child 552
Water-seal drainage, 706 [67]

Weight gain
    during pregnancy, 386
    infant, 513
    neonate, 456
    school-age child, 520
Wharton's jelly, 447
Wheezing, 174
White's classification, 401
Wilms' tumor, 611
Withdrawal, 23, 90
    from alcohol, 92
Withdrawn behavior, 77
Wolpe, 20t
Word salad, definition of, 101

Notes

Notes

Notes

Notes